Psoriasis

BASIC AND CLINICAL DERMATOLOGY

Series Editors

ALAN R. SHALITA, M.D.

Professor and Chairman
Department of Dermatology
State University of New York
Health Science Center at Brooklyn
Brooklyn, New York

DAVID A. NORRIS, M.D.

Director of Research
Professor of Dermatology
The University of Colorado
Health Sciences Center
Denver, Colorado

1. Cutaneous Investigation in Health and Disease: Noninvasive Methods and Instrumentation, *edited by Jean-Luc Lévêque*
2. Irritant Contact Dermatitis, *edited by Edward M. Jackson and Ronald Goldner*
3. Fundamentals of Dermatology: A Study Guide, *Franklin S. Glickman and Alan R. Shalita*
4. Aging Skin: Properties and Functional Changes, *edited by Jean-Luc Lévêque and Pierre G. Agache*
5. Retinoids: Progress in Research and Clinical Applications, *edited by Maria A. Livrea and Lester Packer*
6. Clinical Photomedicine, *edited by Henry W. Lim and Nicholas A. Soter*
7. Cutaneous Antifungal Agents: Selected Compounds in Clinical Practice and Development, *edited by John W. Rippon and Robert A. Fromtling*
8. Oxidative Stress in Dermatology, *edited by Jürgen Fuchs and Lester Packer*
9. Connective Tissue Diseases of the Skin, *edited by Charles M. Lapière and Thomas Krieg*
10. Epidermal Growth Factors and Cytokines, *edited by Thomas A. Luger and Thomas Schwarz*
11. Skin Changes and Diseases in Pregnancy, *edited by Marwali Harahap and Robert C. Wallach*
12. Fungal Disease: Biology, Immunology, and Diagnosis, *edited by Paul H. Jacobs and Lexie Nall*
13. Immunomodulatory and Cytotoxic Agents in Dermatology, *edited by Charles J. McDonald*
14. Cutaneous Infection and Therapy, *edited by Raza Aly, Karl R. Beutner, and Howard I. Maibach*
15. Tissue Augmentation in Clinical Practice: Procedures and Techniques, *edited by Arnold William Klein*
16. Psoriasis: Third Edition, Revised and Expanded, *edited by Henry H. Roenigk, Jr., and Howard I. Maibach*

ADDITIONAL VOLUMES IN PREPARATION

Psoriasis

Third Edition, Revised and Expanded

edited by

Henry H. Roenigk, Jr.
Northwestern University Medical School
Chicago, Illinois

Howard I. Maibach
University of California School of Medicine
San Francisco, California

MARCEL DEKKER, INC. NEW YORK • BASEL

ISBN: 0-8247-0108-9

This book is printed on acid-free paper.

Headquarters
Marcel Dekker, Inc.
270 Madison Avenue, New York, NY 10016
tel: 212-696-9000; fax: 212-685-4540

Eastern Hemisphere Distribution
Marcel Dekker AG
Hutgasse 4, Postfach 812, CH-4001 Basel, Switzerland
tel: 44-61-261-8482; fax: 44-61-261-8896

World Wide Web
http://www.dekker.com

The publisher offers discounts on this book when ordered in bulk quantities. For more information, write to Special Sales/Professional Marketing at the headquarters address above.

Current printing (last digit):
10 9 8 7 6 5 4 3 2

PRINTED IN THE UNITED STATES OF AMERICA

Series Introduction

During the past decade there has been a vast explosion in new information relating to the art and science of dermatology as well as fundamental cutaneous biology. Furthermore, this information is no longer of interest only to the small but growing specialty of dermatology. Scientists from a wide variety of disciplines have come to recognize both the importance of skin in fundamental biological processes and the broad implications of understanding the pathogenesis of skin disease. As a result, there is now a multidisciplinary and worldwide interest in the progress of dermatology.

With these factors in mind, we have undertaken a series of books specifically oriented to dermatology. The series has been purposely broad in focus and has ranged from pure basic science to practical, applied clinical dermatology. Thus, while there is something for everyone, all editions in the series should ultimately prove to be valuable additions to the dermatologist's library.

It is an honor and privilege to add the third edition of Henry H. Roenigk, Jr., and Howard I. Maibach's *Psoriasis* to our series. This outstanding text involves well-known authors throughout the world and addresses both basic science as well as clinical aspects of this troublesome disease. It has become the reference standard for authoritative discussion of psoriasis and should prove to be a valuable addition to the libraries of clinicians and researchers.

Alan R. Shalita
SUNY Health Science Center
Brooklyn, New York

Preface

The third edition of *Psoriasis* has been significantly expanded and contains much new and innovative information. The first edition, published in 1985, contained 56 chapters. The third edition, which now contains 73 chapters, has a more condensed and compact clinical section and a broader view of the therapeutic options for psoriasis.

A great deal of new information from the field of molecular biology has begun to assist our understanding of the mechanisms that produce and flare psoriasis. One area that has undergone dramatic development since the second edition is genetics. This new field explores the epidemiology of psoriasis. There are several conflicting conclusions in this area, and we have tried to present all views. It is hoped that genetics will result in the final "cure" for psoriasis.

We have extensively updated the chapters on former therapies. For example, there are now new guidelines on methotrexate, with less need for liver biopsies. There are newer systemic retinoids with shorter half-lives. Cyclosporin is used more, and a new preparation with better absorption is available. Topical vitamin D therapy has also found a significant place in the therapy of psoriasis. While PUVA therapy is still being used to treat psoriasis, the recent finding of increased incidence of malignant melanoma from the 16-center PUVA follow-up study has caused some concern.

Section VIII, New Treatments and Innovations, contains information on new therapies that are still in the developmental stages. Many of these therapies have not yet been approved. Newer topical retinoids have just been approved and seem helpful in stable plaque disease. New systemic cyclosporin and vitamin D products have also proven effective in large trials. New topical immunosuppressive agents will be safe and effective. The work with DAB-389 has given insight into the pathogenesis of psoriasis, as well as providing different forms of therapy. And the pharmaceutical industry is continually generating new ideas for psoriasis therapy.

Finally, the physician, as well as organizations such as the National Psoriasis Foundation, is key in giving the emotional support necessary for the patient to deal with this disfiguring disease. Physicians need to spend more time dealing with quality of life issues that face the patient. This is sometimes difficult in an era of managed care.

This book is intended for the practicing physician, whether internist, rheumatologist, family physician, pediatrician, dermatologist, or resident. Each chapter attempts to convey all new information in a way that enables the reader to develop a solid understanding of how to properly treat and advise patients about psoriasis. *Psoriasis* should prove to be a key reference book for anyone treating patients with this disease.

We would like to express our deep appreciation to our extensive collection of international contributors, who have lent their expertise in the development of this text. Coordinating text and meeting deadlines is not always an easy task. We aspire to update this volume every 5 years, so as to keep this publication current and beneficial to the reader. We will be back in 2003.

Henry H. Roenigk, Jr.
Howard I. Maibach

Contents

IX. Patient Involvement in Psoriasis

Contributors

Setsuya Aiba, M.D., Ph.D. Department of Dermatology, Tohoku University School of Medicine, Sendai, Japan

Smita Amin, M.D., F.R.C.P.(C) Department of Medicine, The Toronto Hospital, Western Division, University of Toronto, Toronto, Ontario, Canada

Ole Baadsgaard, M.D. Department of Dermatology, University of Copenhagen, Gentofte Hospital, Copenhagen, Denmark

Joanna Badger, M.D. Department of Dermatology, University of California Medical Center, San Francisco, California

Shanta Bantia, Ph.D. University of Alabama, Birmingham, Alabama

Ronald Barr University of California, Irvine, California

Alfred A. Bartolucci, Ph.D. BioCryst Pharmaceuticals, Inc., Birmingham, Alabama

Saqib J. Bashir University of California School of Medicine, San Francisco, California

Enzo Berardesca, M.D. Department of Dermatology, University of Pavia, Pavia, Italy

Timothy G. Berger, M.D. Department of Dermatology, University of California Medical Center, San Francisco, California

Bruno Berretti, M.D. Department of Dermatology, Polyclinique d'Aubervilliers, Aubervilliers, France

Jayant Bhalerao, Ph.D. Department of Pediatrics, University of Texas Southwestern Medical Center, Dallas, Texas

Joseph B. Bikowski, Jr., M.D. Department of Dermatology, University of Pittsburgh School of Medicine, Pittsburgh, Pennsylvania

Jan D. Bos, M.D., Ph.D., F.R.C.P. Department of Dermatology, Academic Medical Center, University of Amsterdam, Amsterdam, The Netherlands

Anne M. Bowcock, Ph.D. Department of Pediatrics, University of Texas Southwestern Medical Center, Dallas, Texas

Irwin M. Braverman, M.D. Yale University School of Medicine, New Haven, Connecticut

Roshantha A.S. Chandraratna, Ph.D. Retinoid Research, Allergan, Inc., Irvine, California

R.C. Chou Clinical Pharmacology, F. Hoffmann-La Roche, Ltd., Basel, Switzerland

Enno Christophers, M.D. Department of Dermatology, University of Kiel, Kiel, Germany

William J. Cook, M.D., Ph.D. BioCryst Pharmaceuticals, Inc., Birmingham, Alabama

Roger C. Cornell, M.D. Department of Dermatology, Scripps Clinic and Research Foundation, La Jolla, California

Mark D.P. Davis, M.D. Mayo Graduate School of Medicine, Rochester, Minnesota

Elke M.G.J. de Jong University Hospital Nijmegen, Nijmegen, The Netherlands

F. Distante, M.D. Department of Dermatology, University of Pavia, Pavia, Italy

Louis Dubertret Dermatologie, Hôpital Saint Louis, Paris, France

Madeleine Duvic, M.D. Department of Dermatology, M.D. Anderson Cancer Center, Houston, Texas

Alan Elias University of California, Irvine, California

Charles N. Ellis, M.D. Department of Dermatology, University of Michigan, Ann Arbor, Michigan

Ernst Epstein University of California School of Medicine, San Francisco, California

Eugene M. Farber, M.D. Psoriasis Research Institute, Palo Alto, California

Torkel Fischer, M.D. National Institute for Working Life, Solna, Sweden

David A. Fisher Department of Dermatology, University of California, San Francisco, California

Thomas J. Franz, M.D. BioCryst Pharmaceuticals, Inc., Birmingham, Alabama

Elaine Fuchs University of Chicago Medical Center, Chicago, Illinois

Charles Gambla, M.D. Department of Dermatology, University of California Medical Center, San Francisco, California

Christoph C. Geilen Free University, Berlin, Germany

Brian Gemzik Research Division, Abbott Laboratories, Chicago, Illinois

Lawrence E. Gibson, M.D. Department of Dermatology, Mayo Clinic and Mayo Medical School, Rochester, Minnesota

Richard G. Glogau Department of Dermatology, University of California, San Francisco, California

Michael H. Gold, M.D.* Northwestern University Medical School, Chicago, Illinois

Michael T. Goldfarb, M.D. Department of Dermatology, University of Michigan, Ann Arbor, Michigan

Ernesto Gonzalez, M.D. Newtonville, Massachusetts

Alice Bendix Gottlieb, M.D., Ph.D. Clinical Research Center and Division of Clinical Pharmacology, University of Medicine and Dentistry of New Jersey—Robert Wood Johnson Medical School, New Brunswick, New Jersey

Maximilian Grassberger Novartis Research Institute, Vienna, Austria

Christopher E.M. Griffiths, M.D., F.R.C.P. Department of Dermatology, University of Manchester, Manchester, England

Charles Grupper Department of Dermatology, Polyclinique d'Aubervilliers, Aubervilliers, France

Marek Haftek, M.D., Ph.D. INSERM Unit 346/CNRS, Edouard Herriot Hospital, Lyon, France

David J. Hecker, M.D. Department of Dermatology, Mount Sinai School of Medicine, New York, New York

Tilo Henseler, M.D., Ph.D. Laboratory for Epidemiology and Genetics, Department of Dermatology, University of Kiel, Kiel, Germany

Michael F. Holick, M.D., Ph.D. Department of Medicine, Boston University Medical Center, Boston, Massachusetts

Herbert Hönigsmann, M.D. Department of Dermatology, University of Vienna Medical School, Vienna, Austria

A. Inerot Göteborg University, Sahlgrenska University Hospital, Göteborg, Sweden

Ross S. Kaplan University of California School of Medicine, Irvine, California

Lloyd E. King, Jr., M.D., Ph.D. Department of Medicine, Vanderbilt University School of Medicine, and Department of Dermatology, Department of Veterans Affairs Medical Center, Nashville, Tennessee

John Y.M. Koo, M.D. Psoriasis Treatment Center, Department of Dermatology, University of California Medical Center, San Francisco, California

Stefan Kraft Department of Dermatology, Ludwig Maximilians University, Munich, Germany

**Current affiliation*: Gold Skin Care Center, Nashville, Tennessee.

Knud Kragballe, M.D., Ph.D. Marselisborg Hospital, Aarhus, Denmark

Sven Krengel Free University, Berlin, Germany

James G. Krueger, M.D., Ph.D. Laboratory for Investigative Dermatology, The Rockefeller University, New York, New York

Arto Lahti University of Oulu, Oulu, Finland

Antti I. Lauerma, M.D., Ph.D. Department of Dermatology, University of Helsinki, Helsinki, Finland

Mark Lebwohl, M.D. Department of Dermatology, Mount Sinai School of Medicine, New York, New York

Jaeho Lee Department of Dermatology, University of California Medical Center, San Francisco, California

Noreen Lemak, M.D. Department of Dermatology, University of Texas Medical School, Houston, Texas

Yung-Hian Leow University of California School of Medicine, San Francisco, California

Ruth S. Lewis School of the Art Institute of Chicago, Chicago, Illinois

Elissa J. Liebman Harvard Medical School and Massachusetts General Hospital, Boston, Massachusetts

Nicholas J. Lowe, M.D. Southern California Dermatology and Psoriasis Center, Santa Monica, and UCLA School of Medicine, Los Angeles, California

Pamela S. Lowe, RPT Southern California Dermatology and Psoriasis Center, Santa Monica, California

Howard I. Maibach, M.D. University of California School of Medicine, San Francisco, California

Jonathan Mansbridge, Ph.D. Advanced Tissue Sciences, La Jolla, California

T. Martinsson Göteborg University, Sahlgrenska University Hospital, Göteborg, Sweden

Janice Matsunaga, M.D. Associate Clinical Professor, Section of Dermatology, John A. Burns School of Medicine, Honolulu, Hawaii

Jerry L. McCullough, M.D. Department of Dermatology, University of California School of Medicine, Irvine, California

Marian T. McEvoy, M.D., M.R.C.P., F.A.C.P. Department of Dermatology, Mayo Clinic and Mayo Foundation, Rochester, Minnesota

Josef G. Meingassner Novartis Research Institute, Vienna, Austria

M. Alan Menter, M.D. Psoriasis Center, Baylor University Medical Center, Dallas, Texas

John A. Montgomery, Ph.D. BioCryst Pharmaceuticals, Inc., Birmingham, Alabama

Vera B. Morhenn, M.D. Department of Dermatology, University of California, San Diego, California

Lexie Nall, M.D. Epidemiology Laboratory, Stanford University School of Medicine, Stanford, California

Lillian B. Nanney, Ph.D. Department of Plastic Surgery & Cell Biology, Vanderbilt University School of Medicine, Nashville, Tennessee

Patricia W. Noah, Ph.D. Department of Medicine, University of Tennessee, Memphis, Tennessee

George A. Omura, M.D. BioCryst Pharmaceuticals, Inc., Birmingham, Alabama

Constantin E. Orfanos, M.D. Department of Dermatology and Venerology, Free University, Berlin, Germany

Bernhard Ortel, M.D. Department of Dermatology, Harvard Medical School and Massachusetts General Hospital, Boston, Massachusetts

Carle Paul Hôpital Saint Louis, Paris, France

Harold O. Perry, M.D. Mayo Clinic and Mayo Medical School, Rochester, Minnesota

Carlo Pincelli, M.D. Department of Dermatology, University of Modena, Modena, Italy

Mark R. Pittelkow, M.D. Departments of Dermatology, and Biochemistry and Molecular Biology, Mayo Clinic and Mayo Medical School, Rochester, Minnesota

Klemens Rappersberger Department of Dermatology, Vienna General Hospital, Vienna, Austria

Siba Prasad Raychaudhuri, M.D. Psoriasis Research Institute, Palo Alto, California

Narra Reddy, Ph.D. BioCryst Pharmaceuticals, Inc., Birmingham, Alabama

Henry H. Roenigk, Jr., M.D. Department of Dermatology, Northwestern University Medical School, Chicago, Illinois

Anne-Marie Ros, M.D., Ph.D. Department of Dermatology, Karolinska Hospital, Stockholm, Sweden

E. William Rosenberg, M.D. Department of Medicine, University of Tennessee, Memphis, Tennessee

W. Mitchell Sams, Jr., M.D. University of Alabama, Birmingham, Alabama

Gundula M. Schaumburg-Lever, M.D. Department of Dermatology, Eberhard Karls University, Tübingen, Germany

Richard K. Scher, M.D., F.A.C.P. Professor, Department of Dermatology, College of Physicians and Surgeons, Columbia University, New York, New York

Jens-Michael Schröder, Ph.D. Department of Dermatology, University of Kiel, Kiel, Germany

Jørgen Serup, M.D., Ph.D. Director, Department of Pharmaceutical Research, Leo Pharmaceutical Products, Copenhagen, Denmark

Joan L. Shelk Leone Dermatology Center, Arlington Heights, Illinois

Braham Shroot, Ph.D. Centre International de Recherches Dermatologiques, Sophia-Antipolis, France

John Siebenlist, M.D. Department of Dermatology, University of Texas, San Antonio, Texas

Alan K. Silverman, M.D. Professional Practice, Dallas, Texas

Robert B. Skinner, Jr., M.D. Department of Medicine, University of Tennessee, Memphis, Tennessee

Richard B. Stoughton, M.D.† Department of Dermatology, University of California School of Medicine, San Diego, California

Anton Stütz Novartis Research Institute, Vienna, Austria

John Paul Sundberg, D.V.M., Ph.D. The Jackson Laboratory, Bar Harbor, Maine

Gunnar Swanbeck, M.D., Ph.D. Department of Dermatology, Göteborg University, Sahlgrenska University Hospital, Göteborg, Sweden

Hachiro Tagami, M.D., Ph.D. Department of Dermatology, Tohoku University School of Medicine, Sendai, Japan

Charles R. Taylor, M.D. Department of Dermatology, Harvard Medical School and Massachusetts General Hospital, Boston, Massachusetts

Peter C.M. van de Kerkhof, M.D., Ph.D. Department of Dermatology, University of Nijmegen Hospital, Nijmegen, The Netherlands

Tacey X. Viegas, Ph.D. BioCryst Pharmaceuticals, Inc., Birmingham, Alabama

J. Wahlström Göteborg University, Sahlgrenska University Hospital, Göteborg, Sweden

Gerald M. Walsh, Ph.D. BioCryst Pharmaceuticals, Inc., Birmingham, Alabama

Louis Weinrauch, M.D. Bell Dermatology Associates, Jerusalem, Israel

Gerald D. Weinstein, M.D. Department of Dermatology, University of California School of Medicine, Irvine, California

Göran Wennersten, M.D., Ph.D. Associate Professor, Department of Dermatology, Karolinska Hospital, Stockholm, Sweden

Ulf W. Wiegand Clinical Pharmacology, F. Hoffmann-La Roche, Ltd., Basel, Switzerland

Klaus Wolff, M.D. Department of Dermatology, Vienna General Hospital, Vienna, Austria

---

†Deceased.

Stephen Wright, M.D. Research Division, Abbott Laboratories, Chicago, Illinois

Eva Zachariae, M.D. Department of Rheumatology, Aarhus University Hospital, Aarhus, Denmark

Hugh Zachariae, M.D. Department of Dermatology, Aarhus University Hospital, Aarhus, Denmark

Herschel S. Zackheim, M.D. Department of Dermatology, University of California, San Francisco, California

Gail M. Zimmerman National Psoriasis Foundation, Portland, Oregon

Part I

CLINICAL FEATURES

1

Skin Manifestations of Psoriasis and Eczematous Psoriasis: Maturation

Henry H. Roenigk, Jr.
Northwestern University Medical School, Chicago, Illinois

Ernst Epstein and Howard I. Maibach
University of California School of Medicine, San Diego, California

PSORIASIS

Psoriasis, a common, chronic, intractable skin disease, affects 1–3% of the American population. The true incidence may be even higher, because individuals with minor clinical manifestations may not seek medical attention, but elect to treat the condition themselves. Men and women are equally affected; women have an earlier onset of disease.

The skin lesions of psoriasis usually first appear between the ages of 20 and 50 (mean age at onset is 28 years), but the initial lesions may appear as early as age 1 or as late as age 80. Regardless of the time of onset of the disease, the patient faces a lifelong struggle to eradicate the erythematous scaling plaques that are a source of anxiety and embarrassment.

In ancient times, people considered psoriasis a form of leprosy. The biblical term "lepra" included what is now called psoriasis (as well as several other diseases). Undoubtedly, many psoriatic patients suffered the same physical and mental abuses as lepers of the era. Confusion between leprosy and psoriasis lasted for almost 19 centuries. Not until 1841 was the word "lepra" eliminated in the consideration of psoriasis. The pathogenesis of the disease remains unexplained.

Psoriasis is classified as a papulosquamous disease. Other papulosquamous diseases which can be confused with psoriasis include:

- Pityriasis rosea
- Seborrheic dermatitis
- Pityriasis rubra pilaris
- Secondary syphilis
- Lichen planus
- Parapsoriasis guttate
- Parapsoriasis en plaque
- Lupus erythematosus
- Tinea infections of skin and nails

The primary lesion is an erythematous papule, topped by a silvery scale. Gradually or explosively these papules coalesce to form plaques of varying shapes and patterns. The plaques may be coin-shaped (guttate), geographic, annular or circinate (ringlike), figurative, gyrate, or serpiginous. The individual lesions distribute themselves in a pattern. Areas of the skin most commonly affected include the elbows, knees, scalp, groin, and nails.

Psoriasis may have eczematous features. Termed eczematous psoriasis, this is usually the result of superimposed irritation or contact dermatitis, i.e., secondary eczematous psoriasis. However, sometimes psoriasis resembles eczema without apparent exogenous cause; we call this primary eczematous psoriasis. Consequently, psoriasis may be morphologically indistinguishable from:

Nummular eczema
Contact dermatitis, irritant and/or allergic
Atopic dermatitis
Other chronic endogenous dermatoses

There are many varieties of lesions; the different sizes and shapes often mislead the physician. Clinical recognition by referral to a dermatologist and occasionally the examination of a skin biopsy specimen may help confirm the diagnosis. Most commonly, the characteristic cutaneous lesions of psoriasis are round, erythematous, dry patches of various sizes covered by abundant grayish-white imbricated scales. The Auspitz sign is a pinpoint of bleeding that occurs when scales are picked off plaques of psoriasis. The plaques of psoriasis are generally symmetrically located on both elbows and knees. There may be a burning sensation and pruritus in acute flares of psoriasis, but more frequently the lesions are asymptomatic except for the cosmetic embarrassment. The lesions can be so extensive as to cover the entire body with an erythroderma.

Clinical Forms of Psoriatic Skin Lesions

Classic Plaque

These well-defined erythematous plaques are shown in Figure 1 (Color Plate 1). The borders are sharp and usually a silvery gray scaling on the surface is easily removed. Plaques tend to be symmetrical in distribution with knees [Fig. 2 (Color Plate 2)] and elbows being the most common locations. Active psoriatic plaques have a rapid peripheral extension which may form a ring with central clearing. Physical trauma in the active phase results in linear patterns of psoriasis (the Koebner phenomenon) in the areas of injury to epidermal tissue [Fig. 3 (Color Plate 1)]. Hat band pressure, hair brushing, vaccination, sunburn, or simply rubbing or scratching may provide sufficient trauma to induce the formation of lesions. This may also be seen on the hands of factory workers and golf or tennis players. Intertriginous areas (groin, axilla) produce erythematous plaques which are moist and lack the characteristic scale and elevation (inverse psoriasis) [Fig. 4 (Color Plate 2)].

Hands and Feet

The plaques of psoriasis are less erythematous here but are well demarcated and have white scales. There may be sterile pustules in the plaques [Fig. 5 (Color Plate 1)]. Hyperkeratosis and fissures can lead to severe disabilities [Fig. 6 (Color Plate 1)].

Scalp

Scalp lesions of psoriasis [Fig. 7 (Color Plate 2); Fig. 8 (Color Plate 1)] present with erythema, scaling, and pruritus similar to seborrheic dermatitis. The plaques are usually well demarcated. While hair loss is common in scalp psoriasis, it is usually temporary. There may be plaques along the forehead extending from the scalp.

Figure 1 Classic plaque of psoriasis with well-defined borders and silvery gray scaling.

Figure 3 Koebner phenomenon: new psoriatic lesions in areas of previous epidermal trauma.

Figure 5 Psoriasis of plantar surface of foot with fissuring and pustulation.

Figure 6 Psoriasis of the palms with hyperkeratotic plaquelike lesions.

Figure 8 Psoriasis of scalp.

Figure 11 Annular type of pustular psoriasis.

Figure 14 Psoriatic nails.

Figure 15 Psoriatic arthritis of distal interphalangeal joints with extensive skin and nail changes.

Intertriginous Psoriasis

Psoriasis has an affinity for skinfold areas with the gluteal cleft, retroauricular folds as well as inguinal, axillary, and inframammary areas being favored sites. The red, often glazed, and well-dermarcated plaques may closely resemble seborrheic dermatitis, candidiasis, or a dermatophyte infection. The typical silver scale is generally absent in this form.

Guttate

Small erythematous papules with a fine scale, frequently generalized, may follow upper respiratory infections, streptococcal pharyngitis, and viral flu. This form tends to occur in younger persons and frequently is the initial episode of psoriasis. The disease consists of an explosive eruption of teardrop-shaped lesions, primarily on the trunk [Fig. 9 (Color Plate 2)].

Pustular

Pustular psoriasis of adults is divided into two groups: disease that evolves from preexisting psoriasis and the pustular form of disease that develops de novo. Patients with preexisting psoriasis tend to develop either localized pustular reactions around preexisting psoriatic plaques, or a generalized systemic erythema covered by waves of sheeted pustulation and scarlatiniform peeling [Fig. 10 (Color Plate 2)]. These patients are severely ill with fever to 104°F, leukocytosis, and lymphopenia. Up to one-third of the described cases are believed to be due to the withdrawal of systemic corticosteroids, but other associations include pregnancy, infection, stress, sunlight, and the use of salicylates, sulfonamides, phenothiazines, and lithium.

The second type of pustular psoriasis in adults evolves in patients without preexisting psoriasis and is rare. These patients are older, generally over 40 years of age. Their disease may present as an annular form, characterized by a low-grade, subacute infection, gyrate form, and annular pustular lesions; each with minimal systemic effects [Fig. 11 (Color Plate 1)]. A less common presentation is that of a short-lived, exanthematous dermatosis associated with systemic infections and drug exposure.

Typical plaques of psoriasis may develop pustules, usually after topical treatment with irritants. Cultures of the pustular contents usually do not show bacteria. The pustules are usually confined to psoriatic lesions, but short-lived generalized eruptions may occur. Systemic symptoms are usually absent, and with topical treatment the pustules usually subside.

Pustular psoriasis in infants, like infantile psoriasis, is uncommon. Most of these children have seborrheic dermatitis initially, and more than 50% develop psoriasis as adults.

Pustular psoriasis of the palms and soles may occur concurrently with psoriasis elsewhere on the body. The lesions are distributed symmetrically on the hands and feet, and patients are subject to periodic painful exacerbations.

Eczematous Psoriasis

Psoriasis may present as nondescript patches of chronic dermatitis lacking the morphology of plaque type psoriasis. At times eczematous features are so prominent that a diagnosis of nummular eczema or contact dermatitis is made.

Erythroderma

Rarely psoriasis will present as diffuse generalized erythroderma with no typical plaque or guttate lesions.

Figure 2 Symmetrical distribution of psoriatic plaques.

Figure 4 Inverse psoriasis in moist area of intertriginous skin.

Figure 7 Psoriasis of the scalp after hair has been shaved off.

Figure 9 Guttate psoriasis.

Figure 10 Acute generalized pustular psoriasis of von Zumbusch.

Figure 12 Erythrodermic psoriasis.

Figure 13 Infantile psoriasis presenting as diaper dermatitis.

The differentiation from pityriasis rubra pilaris or mycosis fungoides (Sézary syndrome) may require examination of a skin biopsy specimen.

Exfoliative erythroderma is an acute condition resulting from a progressive worsening of the psoriasis in either an acute or chronic fashion. The skin becomes diffusely red, warm, and profoundly scaling [Fig. 12 (Color Plate 2)] to the point of generalized desquamation. Cutaneous blood flow may increase to more than two-thirds normal, and can result in high-output congestive heart failure. Venous pressure is increased, hypervolemia ensues, temperature control is erratic, and the patient becomes systemically ill. There may be protein loss and electrolyte imbalance. This condition has been described following the withdrawal of systemic steroid therapy, following antimalarial therapy, and following nonspecific harsh therapies for psoriasis.

Diaper Psoriasis

Infantile psoriasis presenting as diaper dermatitis [Fig. 13 (Color Plate 2)] has increased in frequency in the past decade, and is related to the increased use of topical steroids and the effects of their withdrawal on these common dermatoses. Seventeen percent of babies with psoriasiform diaper dermatitis develop classic psoriasis. It is probable that repeated trauma to the diaper area in infancy produces an isomorphic response in those infants genetically predisposed to psoriasis.

Nails

Nail changes are common in psoriasis and may occur on several or all fingernails. There may be stippling or pitting of the nail plate. There is yellowing or altered transparency followed by heaping up of scale resulting in distortion of the nail plate. Secondary bacterial or fungal infection can result in the nail plate being colored black or green. Frequently there is swelling, redness, and scaling of the paronychial margins, and often there is associated arthritis of the terminal phalangeal joint [Fig. 14 (Color Plate 1)].

Arthritis

Five distinct forms of arthritis are associated with psoriasis. The most common type is a monarticular, nonsymmetrical type affecting mainly the hand joints. In rheumatoid-type arthritis (RA factor negative), severe mutilating types are seen. HLA-B27 histocompatibility antigen is strongly associated with psoriatic arthritis, ankylosing spondylitis, and Reiter's disease [Fig. 15 (Color Plate 1)].

Differential Diagnosis of Psoriasis

While the diagnosis of psoriasis is often obvious at a glance, it can be a challenge and is easily overlooked. This is especially true of localized forms. A patient may be treated for otitis externa by his otolaryngologist, while receiving treatment for "pruritus ani" from the proctologist and applying a fungicide to a foot rash presumed to be "athlete's foot" when the correct—and unifying—diagnosis is psoriasis. Psoriasis localized to the hands is often labeled "contact dermatitis"—a label that is sometimes partially correct as irritants or allergens may cause a superimposed contact dermatitis. The diagnosis of psoriasis may be made only because typical psoriatic lesions were found on asymptomatic and supposedly uninvolved skin areas such as the feet and gluteal cleft. When in doubt, examine the entire skin. Morphological criteria for psoriasis vary in significance; they are summarized in Table 1.

Psoriasis can mimic many diseases. The most common confounders, and some diagnostic hints, are listed below.

Seborrheic Dermatitis

The scalp scaling is more diffuse and there are no individual plaques. Face and chest lesions are erythematous with fine scales but no plaques.

Lichen Planus

Plaques are small, similar to guttate psoriasis, but occur more on flexor than extensor surfaces; the latter is more common in psoriasis. There is less scaling but fine striae on papules of lichen planus.

Pityriasis Rosea

These small plaques have a fine scale at the periphery. They are distributed over the trunk in a "Christmas tree" pattern.

Secondary Syphilis

The guttate or small plaques resemble pityriasis rosea more than psoriasis. The lesions often extend to the palms and soles.

Table 1 Criteria for Diagnosing Psoriasis

Major signs
Erythematous, usually sharply marginated plaques that often have silvery scales in hairy areas
Severe dandruff, often with marginated plaques
Nail changes
Multiple pitting
Dystrophic nails and nail separation without evidence of fungus
Seronegative arthritis
Intermediate signs
Hyperkeratoses, localized, with or without scaling on elbows (extending on the forearms), knees, ankles, soles, palms, and knuckles
Pruritus ani or other intertrigo with sharp margination of erythema
Corticoid-responsive penile macules, especially on the glans
Recalcitrant, scaly otitis externa
Persistent, localized patches of nummular eczema
Sterile paronychia, often multiple
Minor signs
Eczematous plaques of palms, soles, or both
Acute onset of keratolysis like lesions of the palms or soles
Recurrent eczematous discoid eruptions of trunk and extremities
Koebner's phenomenon: new lesions appearing at sites of trauma

Source: Adapted from Ref. 5

Mycosis Fungoides

Plaques of mycosis fungoides may look identical to psoriasis and only a skin biopsy specimen will help to differentiate them. The erythrodermic forms of mycosis fungoides and psoriasis are similar.

Tinea and Onychomycosis

Fungal infections are generally localized on the feet, groin, and hands, although trunk lesions may be similar to plaque psoriasis. Generally, the scale is at the periphery with central clearing. The nails infected with fungus are thick and dystrophic, but usually there is no pitting. Potassium hydroxide exams will identify the hyphae of fungi and fungal cultures will confirm the diagnosis.

Eczematous Disorders

Nummular eczema, hand eczema, and other chronic eczematous disorders are disguises sometimes assumed by psoriasis. Prolonged observation may be required before the correct diagnosis is evident. Chronicity and resistance to therapy should arouse the clinician's suspicion of possible psoriasis. Examine the entire skin since typical psoriasis in another location clinches the diagnosis.

Palmo-Plantar Keratoderma

Sharply dermarcated hyperkeratotic lesions of the palms and soles are often found in patients with typical psoriasis. However, there is a population with chronic palmar and/or plantar hyperkeratotic dermatitis without evidence of psoriasis elsewhere. Various labels have been applied to these patients (keratoderma climactericum, hyperkeratotic dermatitis of the palms, tylotic eczema); they probably reflect a reaction pattern rather than nosological or etiological entities.

Pustulosis Palmaris et Plantaris

Pustular lesions on the palms and soles are a well-recognized part of the psoriatic diathesis. Recurrent crops of palmar and/or plantar pustules may occur without psoriatic lesions elsewhere. Named pustulosis palmaris et plantaris, this poorly understood syndrome appears to have multiple causes. Some, but not all, patients with palmo-plantar pustulosis eventually develop psoriasis.

ECZEMATOUS PSORIASIS: WHAT IS IT?

Classic teaching suggests that psoriasis is a distinctive papulosquamous eruption readily diagnosable on morphologic grounds. In evaluating patients in private practice and a psoriasis clinic, we have recognized a significant overlap between psoriasis and the eczematous dermatoses. We encountered patients diagnosed by ourselves and our colleagues for years as having nummular eczema, or chronic hand dermatitis, whose disease had evolved into typical psoriasis. Furthermore, in patients with psoriasis, it is common to find areas with frank eczematous features that—if examined alone—would not permit a diagnosis of psoriasis. We coined the phrase "eczematous psoriasis" to describe this overlap phenomenon.

The analogous situation of psoriasis and seborrheic dermatitis is accepted by clinicians and discussed in most texts. The term "sebopsoriasis" describes disease with features of psoriasis and seborrheic dermatitis. Who has not treated a patient with typical seborrheic dermatitis of the scalp which, over the years, became increasingly stubborn until finally it became classic scalp psoriasis?

Clinical Overview

Our interest in the eczematous aspect of psoriasis developed from clinical experience, especially in two situations. The first pattern consisted of disseminated chronic dermatoses, usually labeled nummular eczema, which either failed to respond to antieczematous remedies or would promptly relapse once treatment was discontinued. Often there was a suspicion of contact dermatitis: commonly results of several patch tests were positive and patients were labeled as having "chronic allergic contact dermatitis." On retesting these patients in the patch test clinic, we were frequently unable to duplicate the previous positive results, and believed that they represented false-positive tests: the phenomenon known as the "angry back" or "excited skin" (3). In other patients we confirmed the existence of true contact allergy by patch testing. However, in most cases the allergens were not relevant to the *presenting dermatitis*.

On what evidence did we diagnose psoriasis in these patients? Careful examination of the *entire* skin often showed unequivocal localized areas of psoriasis, for example: (1) a patch of typical scalp psoriasis or retroauricular dermatitis, (2) the sharply demarcated erythematous scaling of the ear canals so characteristic of psoriasis, (3) fingernail dystrophy or pitting in the presence of normal nail folds, or (4) the frequent finding of typical perianal psoriasis with sharply demarcated erythema and fissuring extending up the gluteal cleft. Chronic, sharply marginated skin thickening over the elbows and knees, frequently extending down the forearm or leg, is easily missed, as are similar lesions over the malleoli. Peculiar, and often evanescent, "peeling" of the palms or soles, reminiscent of keratolysis exfoliativa, is often not appreciated unless specifically sought. Many of these patients had never had their *entire* skin examined.

We emphasize that many lesions were eczematous, and not morphologically suggestive of psoriasis. Others were psoriasiform in that they were sharply marginated, but instead of being scaly, plaques were eczematous.

Adapted from *Seminars in Dermatology* 2:45–50, 1983.

Patients with chronic "contact dermatitis" of the hands and/or the feet referred for patch testing formed the second category which led to our awareness of eczematous psoriasis. In many the morphology suggested psoriasis: sharply demarcated plaques of the palms stopping at the wrists; grouped, deep-set tiny blisters of the palms and volar aspects of the fingers; sharp demarcation of the eruption at the sides of the digits. Dorsal involvement was frequently absent, or if present was often limited to plaques located over the joints. Fingernail dystrophy, such as onycholysis and pitting, with normal nail folds pointed to an endogenous process. The foot lesions were often considered a consequence of irritation or allergy to footwear.

Many of these patients had been diagnosed as having industrial contact dermatitis and had impressive positive patch test results. However, analysis of most of these cases established the industrial nature to be simply irritation from friction or chemicals at work superimposed on psoriasis of the hands. In a few, confirmed positive patch test results did correlate with previous exposure to these materials. Unfortunately, the patients' conditions failed to clear once exposure to the allergen was stopped. In retrospect it was clear these patients had an allergic contact dermatitis superimposed on psoriasis.

Primary and Secondary Eczematous Psoriasis

It is useful to differentiate between primary eczematous psoriasis and secondary eczematous psoriasis. Primary eczematous psoriasis represents a wholly endogenous process. The eczematous features are simply part of the spectrum of psoriatic skin changes (see Cases 1 and 3, below). By contrast, secondary eczematous psoriasis represents an exogenous factor superimposed on psoriasis. The exogenous factors are most commonly irritants (Case 4), but may be allergens (Case 2). The exogenous factors in eczematous psoriasis pose formidable problems to clinicians. It is easy to fall into the trap of attributing the entire skin disorder to contact allergy, especially when a relevant allergen is demonstrated on patch testing. The failure of the rash to clear when the allergen is withdrawn frustrates patient and physician. The dilemma does not end here; when confronted with eczematous psoriasis, how far should one pursue the search for exogenous factors? Particularly vexing is the matter of irritants; we know these aggravate psoriasis, yet we lack diagnostic tests for them. To complicate the situation further—requiring an ever alert diagnostician—occult contact urticaria may also occur. Recognizing contact urticaria on normal skin is difficult; identifying it on dermatitic skin is not possible on *morphological* grounds. Only by frequently inquiring if topical exposure causes burning, stinging, or itching, and following these leads with appropriate *immediate* testing, will this factor be identified (4).

Dermatopathology

Our experience is that the histological findings conform to the gross morphology. Biopsied eczematous lesions in psoriatic patients reveal just that; nonspecific eczematous histological results. Such reports, while misleading to the inexperienced, no longer confuse us. We are not microscopists; our experience is based on reports by consulting dermatopathologists. Since, at present, histological examination is not helpful in differentiating eczematous dermatoses from psoriasis with eczematous overtones, we usually spare our patients the discomfort of this procedure.

Diagnosis

The diagnosis of eczematous psoriasis rests on inclusion and exclusion. Essential to this diagnosis is the presence of stigmata of psoriasis. Eczematous psoriasis is not a wastebasket term for chronic dermatitis; the patient must have morphological evidence of psoriasis. We have characterized the major and minor stigmata of psoriasis (Table 1).

Exclude specific causes of skin disorders such as contact dermatitis, a fungus infection, drug eruption, and the mycosis fungoides syndrome. However, these may coexist with psoriasis; this is particularly true of irritant dermatitis and, to a lesser extent, allergic contact dermatitis. Often the diagnosis of psoriasis is made only after prolonged observation and study. We emphasize the importance of suspecting eczematous psoriasis when evaluating a patient with chronic dermatitis.

Why Diagnosis Is Important

The diagnosis of eczematous psoriasis has profound prognostic and therapeutic significance. Patients must be informed that they have a chronic skin disorder for which we have no instant cure but which may eventually resolve. While exogenous factors may aggravate the rash, it is not the result of industrial contactants, other contactants, food allergy, or a host of other possible environmental factors. This is *not* something patients like to hear; temper it by explaining that psoriasis often improves spontaneously, and we do have measures for controlling it. Patients must understand that the search for a *cause* is over: they have psoriasis. The emotional and physical benefit to patients is often remarkable. Their lengthy search—from dermatologist to dermatologist—for a cause and instant cure is ended.

Treatment

Therapeutically these patients should be managed as psoriatic patients with eczematous symptoms. Systemic corticosteroids are to be avoided. Irritating vehicles, especially those containing high concentrations of propylene glycol, may not be tolerated. Frequently topical corticoids will only be effective under occlusion; often high concentrations and high-potency formulations are required. Judicious use of coal tar may clear the previously recalcitrant process. At times ultraviolet (UV) therapy, either in conjunction with coal tar or the newer psoralen and UVA (PUVA) approach may be indicated. Appropriate topical therapy often brings sufficient control so that patients can function normally. In the most recalcitrant examples, carefully monitored methotrexate therapy may be required.

Diagnosing eczematous psoriasis is only an important step in patient management. We must be continually on our guard that the eczematous features are not a consequence of some industrial or other environmental contact, or irritations, or allergy to a topical medicament. The following cases illustrate some of the ways eczematous psoriasis has presented in our practices.

Case 1

A 52-year-old woman presented with extensive patches of oozing dermatitis on her trunk and armpits [Figs. 16A, B (Color Plate 3)]. She had been diagnosed as having "neurodermatitis" and "eczema" and treated by two dermatologists with topical corticoids and repeated courses of systemic corticoids and tranquilizers. Scalp and elbow involvement suggested eczematous psoriasis. Two months of topical corticoids under occlusion and coal tar caused the dermatitis of the trunk to subside. At this point, the dermatitis of the scalp [Fig. 16C (Color Plate 3)] and elbow [Fig. 16D (Color Plate 3)] had lost its eczematous features and was morphologically psoriasis. In the following 4 years, the patient had several flare-ups of her psoriasis, each time with marked eczematous features. Potent topical corticoids used under occlusion controlled the glabrous skin lesions; anthralin controlled the scalp psoriasis.

Case 2

A 10-year-old girl was seen for an eczematous dermatitis of her feet [Fig. 17A (Color Plate 3)] which had been treated unsuccessfully for 6 months with many topicals. Family history was relevant: her mother had chronic hand dermatitis, a sibling had dermatitis, and an uncle and an aunt had psoriasis. While the dorsa of the feet showed a possible eczematous eruption, perhaps shoe allergy, the vesicles of the soles [Fig. 17B (Color Plate 3)] and the sharply demarcated rash of the heels [Fig. 17C (Color Plate 3)] pointed to psoriasis. A perianal dermatitis [Fig. 17D (Color Plate 3)] typical of psoriasis led to an initial diagnosis of eczematous psoriasis. However, repeated flare-ups raised the question of shoe allergy; patch testing showed her to be highly allergic to her sneakers, the rubber additive mercaptobenzothiazole, and coal tar [Fig. 17E (Color Plate 3)]. The diagnosis was revised to psoriasis with shoe contact dermatitis. The patient readily controlled her psoriasis with topical corticoids when she wore only leather sandals. However, over the next 6 years she had several flare-ups of foot dermatitis after wearing rubber-containing shoes. In this patient, the eczematous features of psoriasis were clearly related to superimposed contact dermatitis.

Case 3

A 25-year-old man presented with a 3-year history of hand dermatitis that had been treated by several physicians with topical corticoids. Examination revealed a dermatitis affecting digits 3, 4, and 5 of both hands with scaling, erythema, and fissuring limited to the dorsa and sides [Fig. 18A (Color Plate 4)]. The thumbs and forefingers were clear. All 10 fingernails showed pitting, including fingers free of dermatitis. Based on morphology, persistence, and the fingernail pitting, he was diagnosed as having "hand dermatitis, probably on the basis of psoriasis." The entire skin was carefully examined and was clear except for the hands. The patient's hand dermatitis improved with betamethasone valerate cream used under occlusion.

The patient returned 7 months later with nondescript patches of dermatitis on his upper extremities, and fairly well demarcated scaling plaques on the penis [Fig. 18B (Color Plate 4)]. He was told he had psoriasis. The patient returned the next year having developed classic psoriatic patches on his trunk [Fig. 18C (Color Plate 4)]. Since then his psoriasis has been treated intermittently at a regional university medical center.

Case 4

A 53-year-old male bartender presented with a dermatitis of his right hand [Fig. 19A (Color Plate 4)] that had been present for several weeks and which the patient believed was caused by his work. He was unaware of any family history of eczema or psoriasis and denied other skin problems. Examination revealed dermatitis of the dorsa and sides of digits 2–5 of the right hand with prominent involvement of the interdigital webs. Many fingernails showed pitting, including several fingers on the *uninvolved* left hand [Fig. 19B (Color Plate 4)]. The remainder of the skin was unremarkable except for perianal dermatitis extending up the gluteal cleft. *After* being examined, the patient changed his history and admitted to having had perianal irritation for the past 3 weeks.

The diagnosis was hand dermatitis, probably due to psoriasis with aggravation from contactants. Since the patient strongly suspected an industrial cause, he was patch tested with a routine screening series as well as materials from work. Results of all tests were negative except for a few obvious irritants. The hand dermatitis cleared with topical corticoids used under occlusion and routine hand protection. The patient was able to return to work and had no further problems over the next 15 months.

This patient has mild psoriasis which remained latent until apparently irritated by factors at work. The

Figure 16 (A) Eczematous psoriasis in a 52-year-old woman. (B) Eczematous morphology in axilla. (C) After 2 months of treatment the scalp dermatitis was typical psoriasis. (D) The elbows now show psoriasis.

Figure 17 (A) Foot dermatitis in a 10-year-old girl. (B) Vesicles on soles suggest an endogenous process. (C) Sharply demarcated rash at heel suggests psoriasis. (D) Perianal fissuring dermatitis typical of psoriasis. (E) Positive results of patch test to shoes and rubber additives. Patient has *both* psoriasis and shoe contact dermatitis.

Plate 1

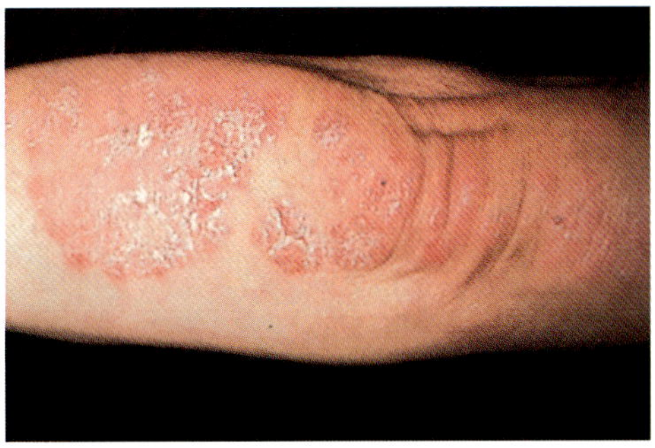

Figure 1

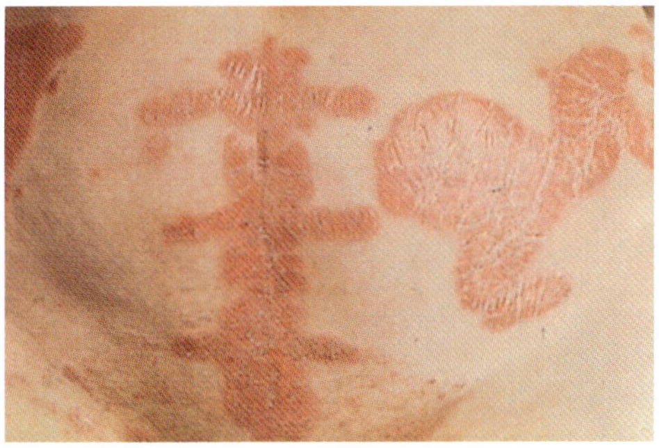

Figure 3

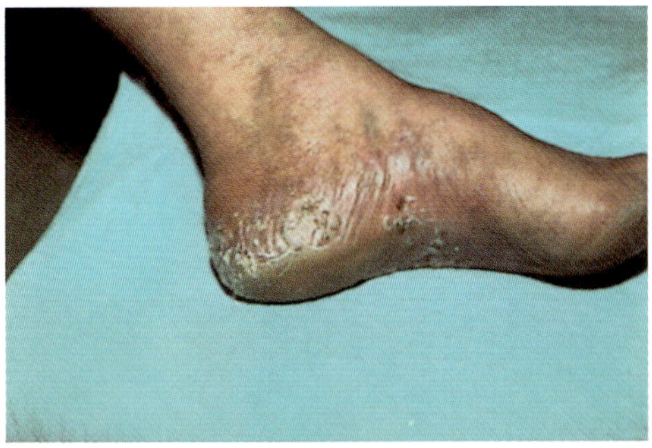

Figure 5

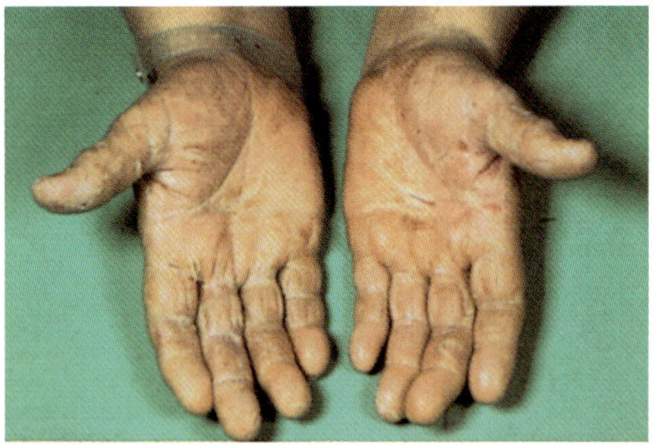

Figure 6

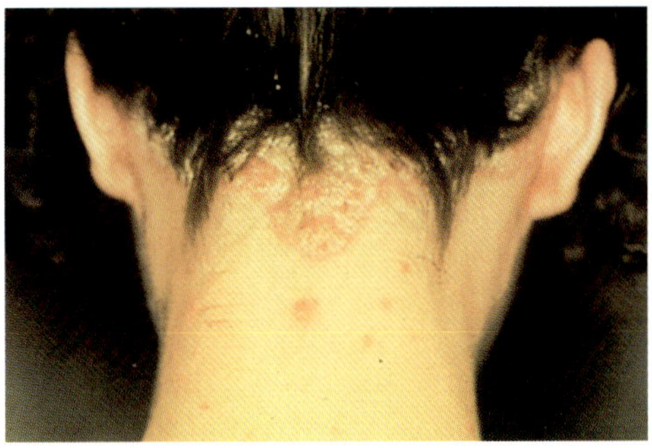

Figure 8

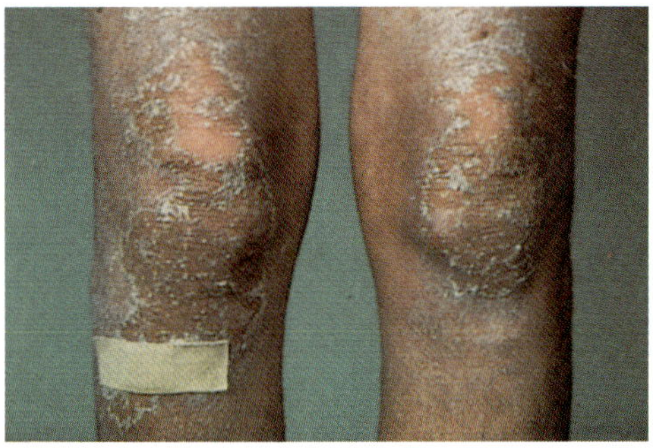

Figure 11

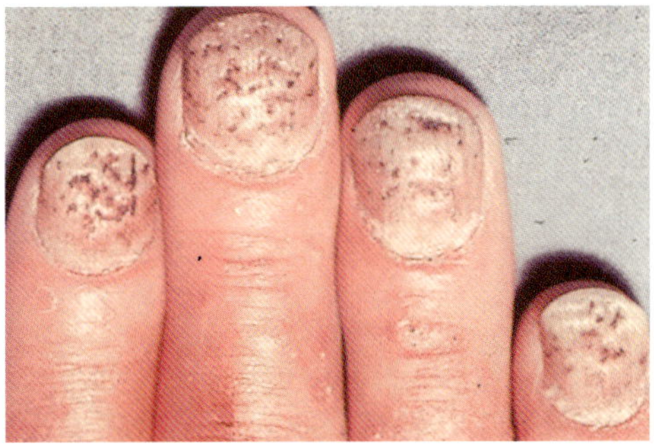

Figure 14

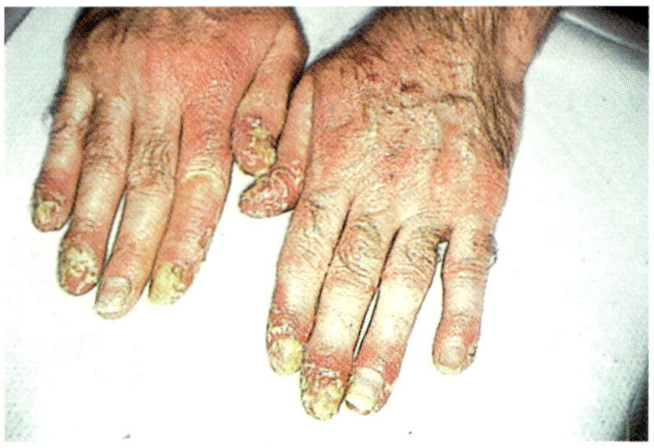

Figure 15

Plate 2

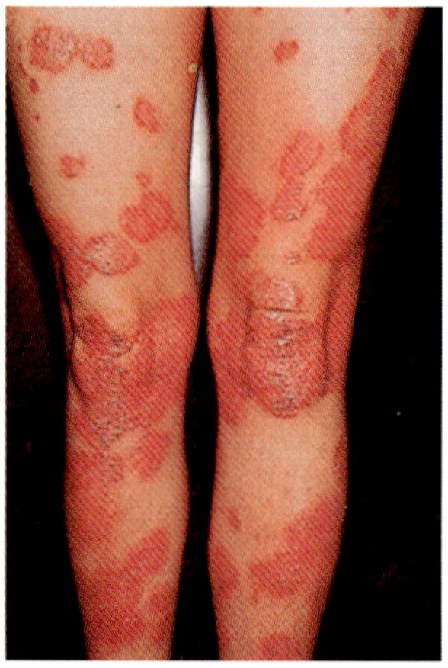

Figure 2

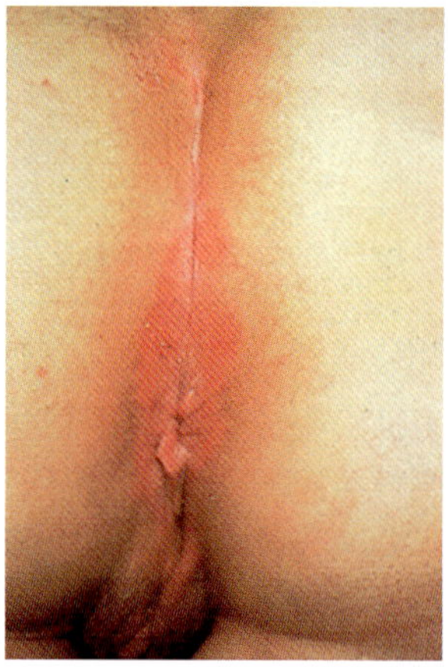

Figure 4

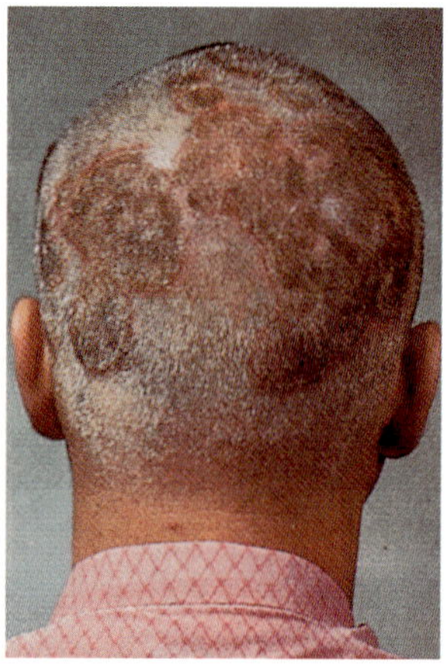

Figure 7

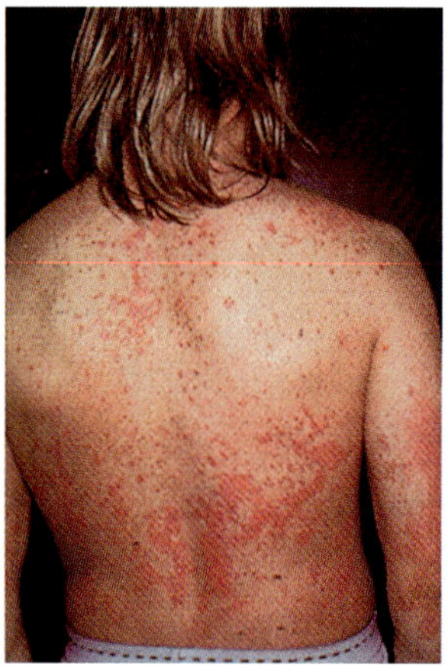

Figure 9

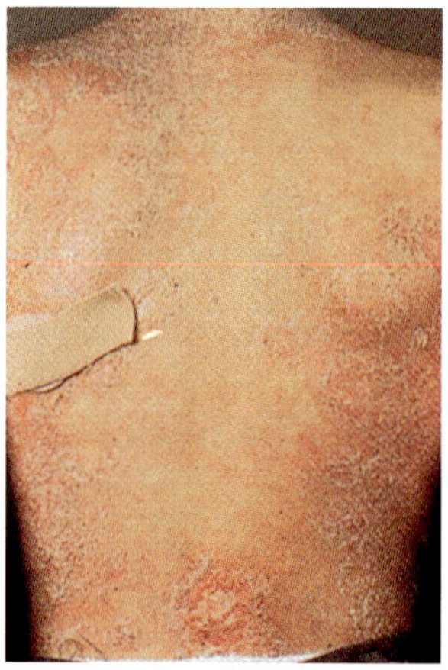

Figure 10

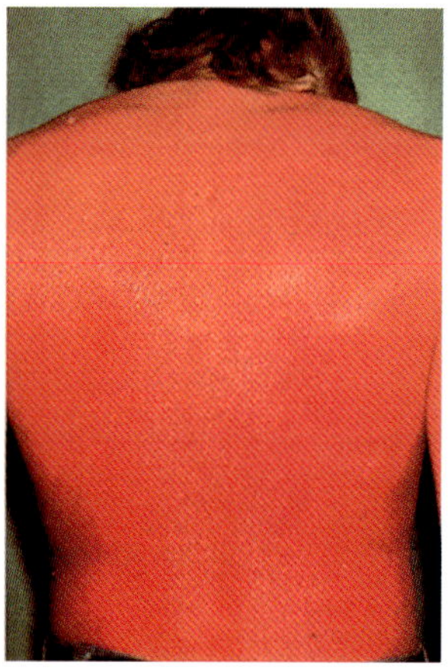

Figure 12

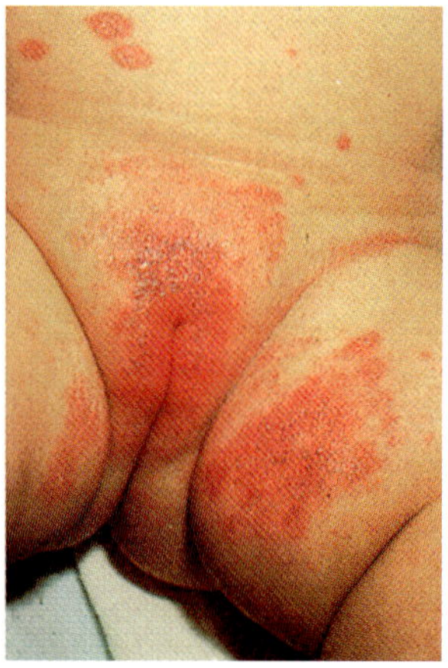

Figure 13

Plate 3

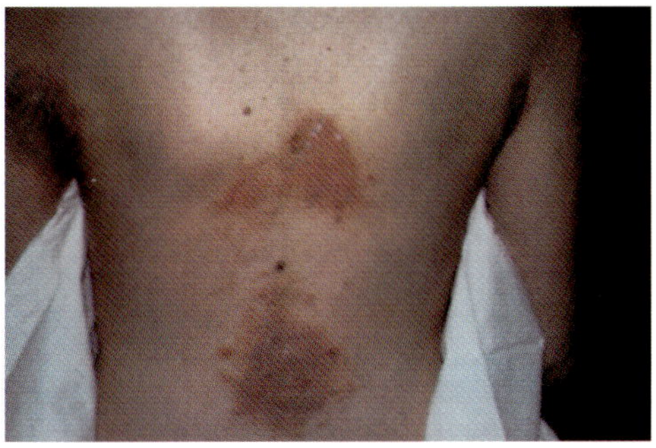

Figure 16A

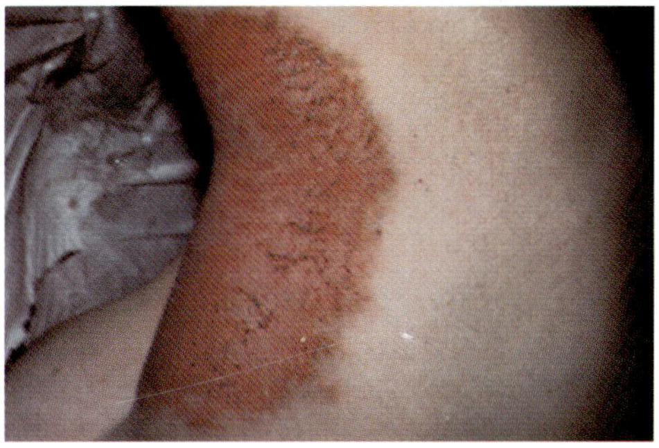

Figure 16B

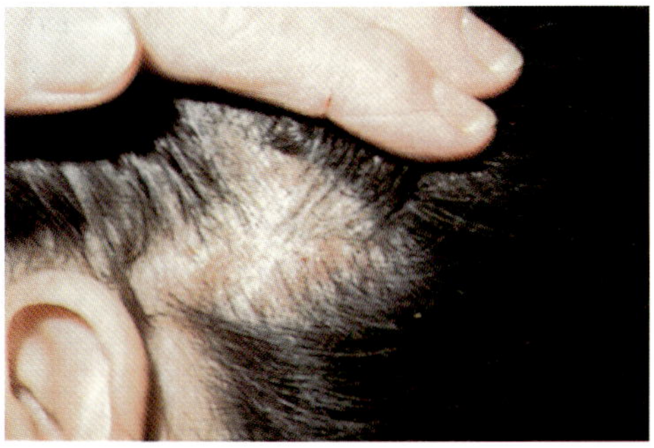

Figure 16C

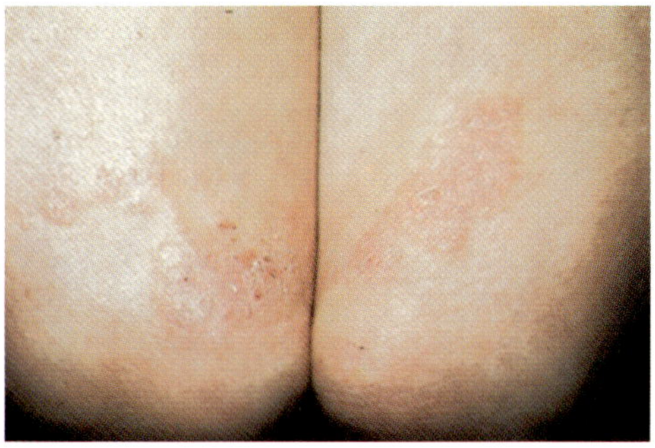

Figure 16D

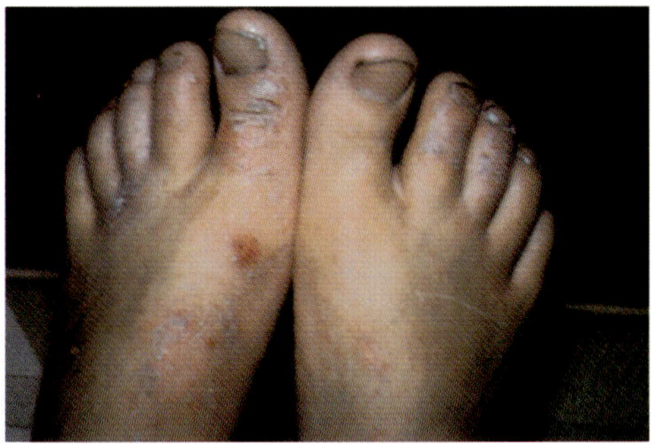

Figure 17A

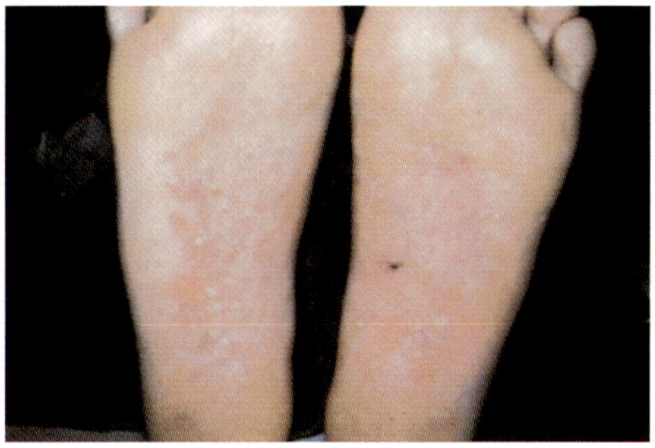

Figure 17B

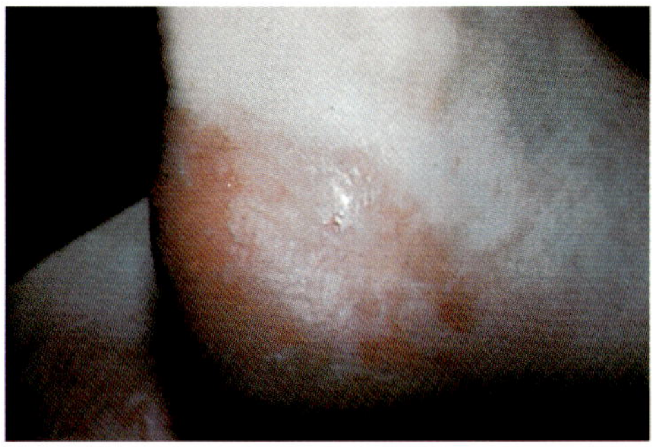

Figure 17C

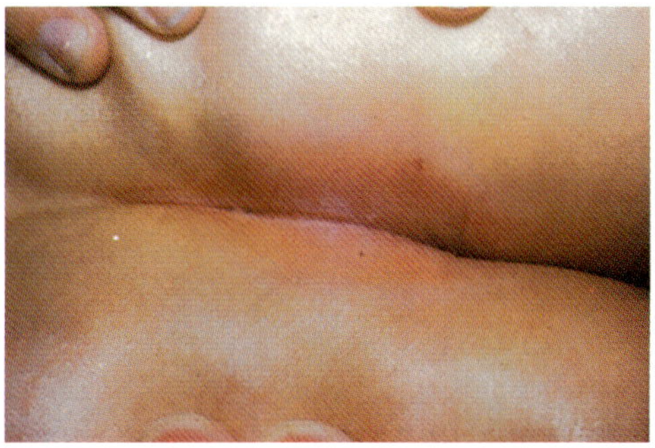

Figure 17D

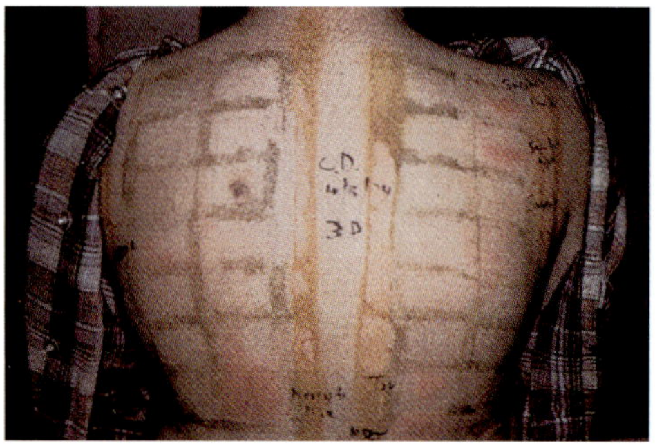

Figure 17

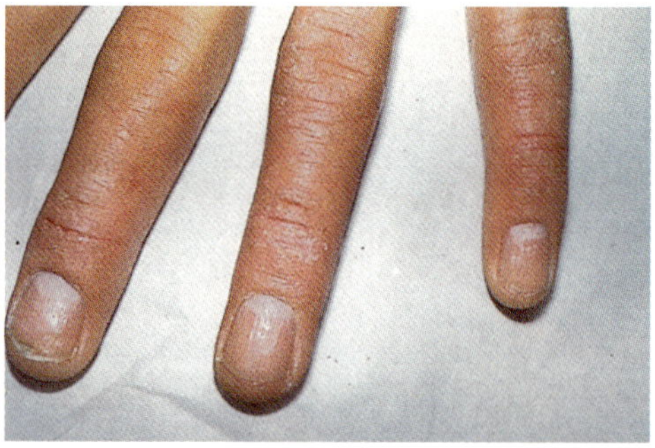

Figure 18A

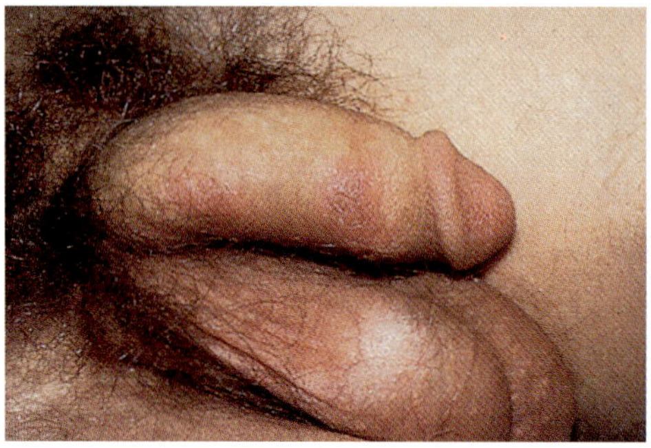

Figure 18B

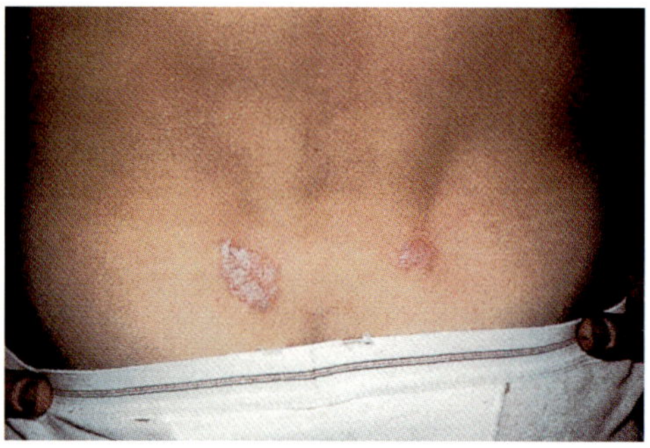

Figure 18C

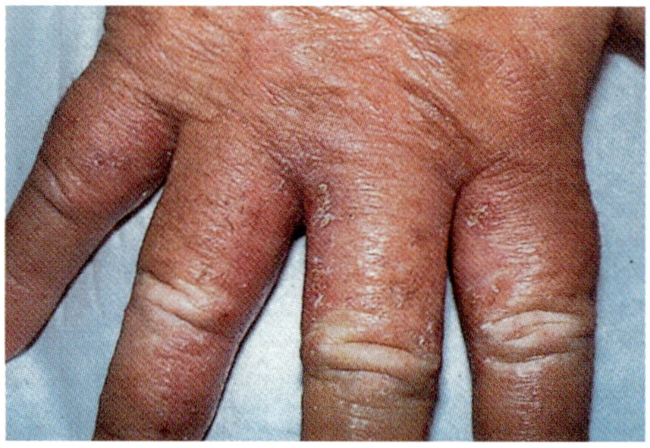

Figure 19A

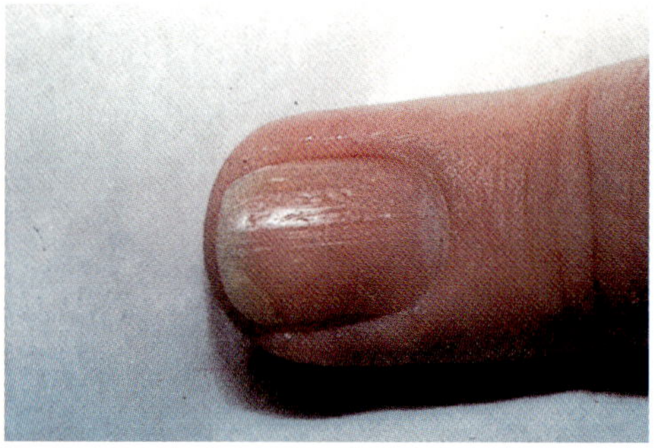

Figure 19B

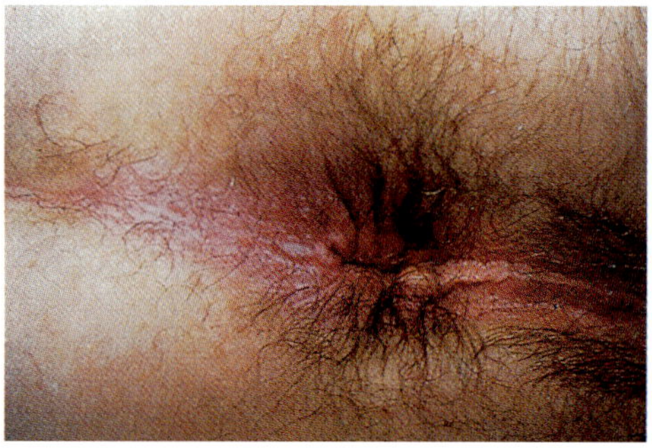

Figure 19C

Figure 18 (A) Dermatitis of digits 3, 4, and 5 in a 25-year-old man. (B) Seven months later patient returns with psoriasiform plaque of penis. (C) Two years later; classic psoriasis of trunk.

Figure 19 (A) A 54-year-old male bartender with "industrial" hand dermatitis limited to right hand. (B) Pitting of fingernail of uninvolved *left* hand. (C) Perianal dermatitis extending up gluteal cleft; a major marker for psoriasis—and a reason for examining the entire skin.

fingernail pitting involving normal fingers and the perianal dermatitis were the clues to his psoriatic state.

Conclusion

The concept of eczematous psoriasis is presented as an approach to handling a special subset of chronic, difficult-to-manage eczema cases. Determining its exact locus in the spectrum of the psoriatic rainbow awaits biochemical definition of the psoriatic genotype and phenotype. While we await this definition, knowledge of the existence of this population aids both patient and physician by simplifying diagnostic methods and improving therapeutic results. The dermatologist in the primary care setting will more frequently encounter patients with localized disease (cases 2, 3, 4). In a tertiary care center, the more atypical and extensive forms will predominate. In either instance, recognition makes for improved management.

REFERENCES

1. deBerker, D.A.R., Baran, R., and Dawber, R.P.R. (1995). *Handbook of Diseases of the Nails and Their Management.* Blackwell Scientific, Oxford, 1995.
2. Zaias N. (1990). *The Nail in Health and Disease,* Appleton & Lange, Norwalk, CT. 2nd ed.
3. Mitchell, J.C., and Rook, A.J. (1982). Diagnosis of contact dermatitis from plants. *Semin. Dermatol.* 1:25–32.
4. von Krogh, C., and Maibach, H. (1982). The contact urticaria syndrome—1982. *Semin. Dermatol.* 1:59–66.
5. Drake, T., and Maibach, H. (1975). Taking the heartbreak out of psoriasis. *Modern Med.* 43:90–96.

2

Pustular Psoriasis: Generalized and Localized*

Smita Amin
The Toronto Hospital, Western Division, and University of Toronto, Toronto, Ontario, Canada

Howard I. Maibach
University of California School of Medicine, San Francisco, California

GENERALIZED PUSTULAR PSORIASIS

Definition

Generalized pustular psoriasis (GPP) is an uncommon form of psoriasis in which a widespread acute, subacute, or, rarely, chronic eruption of sterile pustules occurs.

Classification

1. Acute generalized pustular psoriasis
2. Generalized pustular psoriasis of pregnancy
3. Circinate and annular pustular psoriasis
4. Juvenile and infantile pustular psoriasis
5. Localized forms (not acral or palmoplantar)

Relationship to Psoriasis Vulgaris

Unlike palmoplantar psoriasis, GPP is clearly part of the psoriatic spectrum. Four main strands of evidence support this contention. First, patients may have phases of psoriasis vulgaris before, during, or after the pustular episodes (1). Second, family data concerning psoriasis are similar to those found in ordinary psoriasis (1,2). Abnormalities of neutrophil chemotaxis found in psoriasis vulgaris are similar to those found in GPP (3,4). Finally, several therapeutic agents of proven efficacy in psoriasis vulgaris, such as methotrexate, psoralen and ultraviolet A (PUVA), and etretinate, are also efficacious in GPP.

Provocative Factors

Provocative factors are most clearly recognized in acute GPP of the von Zumbusch type. The disease in von Zumbusch's original patient (5) was provoked by pyrogallol. Strongly irritating topical therapy, for example, with coal tar, can certainly be provocative (6). Occasionally, injudicious continuation of anthralin therapy of psoriasis vulgaris may be a triggering factor (1,7). Generalized pustular psoriasis is a rare but well-documented complication of pregnancy (see below). Sunlight has been implicated occasionally (8). A recent case report documents recurrent flares of GPP associated with well-documented episodes of cholestatic jaundice (9). Hypocalcemia following accidental parathyroidectomy has precipitated GPP (12). A number of drugs have precipitated acute GPP, including salicylates (13), iodine (14), lithium (15), phenylbutazone (16), oxyphenbutazone (16), trazodone (17), and penicillin (18a). More recently, topical calcipo-

*This is an updated version of Chapters 3 and 4 by Stephen Wright and Harvey Baker from previous edition of this book.

triol was reported to precipitate GPP (18b). Recombinant interferon-beta has caused a pustular form of preexisting psoriasis (18c). Table 1 contains a more complete list of the drugs reported to have provoked attacks of GPP.

The role of corticosteroid therapy in causing or aggravating GPP has been controversial. Nevertheless, there is substantial evidence that withdrawal of systemic steroid therapy can precipitate the disease (1,8,26). In a study of 103 patients with GPP in the United Kingdom, 37 patients had received oral steroids before the onset of the first pustular phase. In 21 of these patients, the GPP closely followed steroid dosage reduction or complete withdrawal (1). Similarly, the use of potent topical corticosteroids under occlusion for widespread psoriasis has certainly precipitated GPP (1,27,28). Chronic previously stable acral pustulosis has been converted to GPP by high-dosage prednisolone therapy followed by sudden withdrawal (29). In our opinion, there can be no doubt that intensive corticosteroid therapy, whether topical or systemic, can provoke GPP in previously nonpustular psoriasis (30a).

Annular pustular psoriasis (APP) differs from GPP by its more subacute and limited course of activity and lack of toxicity (1). APP has been reported to be induced by UV radiation after tanning salon use (30b). Other interesting documentations have been the occurrence of APP in association with affective psychosis (30c) and with systemic lupus erythematosus (30d).

Table 1 Drugs Reported to Provoke Pustular Psoriasis

Drug	Ref.
Amiodarone	19a
Atenolol	19b
Calcipotriol	18b
Hydroxychloroquine	22a, 22b
Interferon-β	18c
Lithium carbonate	15
Morphine	23
Oxyphenbutazone	16
Penicillin	18
Phenylbutazone	16
Potassium iodine	14
Procaine	20
Propranolol	21
Salicylates	13
Sulphanamides	24
Sulphapyridine	13
Trazodone	17

HLA Antigens

Generalized pustular psoriasis is positively associated with HLA B27 (2,31). This is not surprising in view of the strong clinical association of GPP with polyarthritis (1,2,31). In a Finnish series, 9 of 16 patients carried the B27 antigen and all had arthritis (2). The effect of B13, B17, B37, CW6, and DR7, all of which are positively associated with psoriasis vulgaris (32), is unclear at present owing to lack of adequate data.

Histopathology

In acute GPP, intense inflammation characterizes the histopathological features (33–36). There is acanthosis with elongation of rete ridges (31). The earliest cellular infiltration is lymphocytic (35). Intense edema of the epidermis follows with marked intercellular and intracellular swelling. Neutrophils pour into the epidermis, producing spongiform pustules of Kogoj, microabscesses, and very quickly macroabscesses. Initially, the overlying stratum corneum may be orthokeratotic, but later it is parakeratotic. The pustule is subcorneal. As it dries it is shed and a parakeratotic stratum corneum grows below it.

It has been claimed that the initial events are at the acrosyringium, causing sweat duct obstruction and pustule formation (36), but this has not been substantiated.

In the subacute and chronic form of GPP, the histopathological features are less dramatic. Parakeratosis may be slight and the epidermal neutrophil invasion less intense.

Pathogenesis

The accumulation of polymorphonuclear leukocytes (PMNLs) which characterizes generalized pustular psoriasis has been attributed to abnormalities of PMNL chemotaxis, either due to an intrinsic PMNL defect (37), or to the elaboration of chemoattractant substances by psoriatic epidermis (38). A number of studies of PMNL chemotaxis have produced varying results (39–44), partly perhaps due to variations in experimental technique. Furthermore, groups of patients with GPP have generally been too small to allow meaningful statistical interpretation of results, and as yet, no clear correlation has emerged between PMNL chemotactic abnormalities and the clinical severity of GPP.

Chemoattractant factors elaborated by psoriatic epidermis include leukotriene B_4 (45), C5a (46), and interleukin 1 (47), but other unidentified peptides are certainly present in the psoriatic "leukotactic factor" which can be derived from affected epidermis (48). Again, there is no clear relationship between the severity of the psoriasis and the quantity of chemoattractant present in the skin, perhaps because interactions between several chemotactic substances may alter the biological responses to each one.

Acute Form (von Zumbusch)

Clinical Features

At the onset of an attack of acute GPP of the von Zumbusch type, the skin becomes very red and tender. The patient may complain of anorexia, nausea, apprehension, or fever. As the temperature rises, malaise may be severe. Preexisting psoriasis vulgaris becomes bright red and new areas of erythema and edema develop, and are sometimes very widespread. Within hours, myriad pinhead-sized pustules appear, studding the erythematous background (Fig. 1). The flexures may be involved as well as the genitalia, fingers (Fig. 2), toes, and nail beds. Annular, circinate, and other patterned lesions may be seen, or the inflammation may be universal. Sometimes it supervenes on a preexisting psoriatic erythroderma.

Within a day, many of the pustules have enlarged and may have become confluent, producing lakes of pus (Fig. 3), which dry out and peel off with accompanying corneal sheets (Fig. 4), leaving a glazed smooth erythematous surface on which a fresh crop of pustules may soon appear. The buccal mucosa and tongue can be involved with frank pustules, or, more commonly, an acute "geographic tongue" (1,8,49,50) (Fig. 5).

The disease may undergo remission after one or two waves of pustulation, or it may recur every day or two for weeks, progressively exhausting the patient. Two main groups of patients can be discerned (1,26). In the first, a preexisting banal psoriasis vulgaris may have lasted for years and a provocative GPP-inducing factor may be evident. In the second group, the onset of psoriasis tends to be later in life and the disease is atypical from the outset. Such atypical patterns may be flexural (51) (sometimes initially misdiagnosed as seborrheic dermatitis or candidosis), or acral and indistinguishable from acropustulosis (acrodermatitis continua of Hallopeau). A fairly rapid and apparently spontaneous progression to GPP follows within weeks or months.

In addition to these two groups of patients, a third pattern has been called exanthematic GPP (1). In the absence of any form of previous psoriasis, the patient develops an acute GPP which tends to resolve over a few weeks and which may not recur (1). Rarely, the eruption begins as an acute palmoplantar pustulosis which spreads after an upper respiratory infection but clears rapidly (52). Possibly some of these cases represent an acute leukocytoclastic vasculitis which can mimic this clinical picture (53,54). Immune complex deposition has been identified in such cases (54).

In due course remission of the episode may leave the patient in an erythrodermic state, or discoid lesions of psoriasis vulgaris may become apparent as the wave of inflammation retreats. The nails may have been shed and, if so, will usually regrow.

Differential Diagnosis

Acute generalized exanthematous pustular dermatitis may mimic GPP closely with a clinical picture which comprises generalized erythema, sterile pustules, fever, and spontaneous healing (55,56). Histologically there are subcorneal and spongiform eosinophilic pustules and a leukocytoclastic vasculitis (57). It may be precipitated by a viral infection (57), and is probably the same entity as the generalized eruptive pustular drug rash described consequent to various antibiotic therapy, including cephalosporins (58,59), amoxicillin (60), and chloramphenicol (61) as well as to other drugs such as phenytoin (62), piperazine, and furosemide (61). The distinction is important in order that the relatively aggressive therapy often used for pustular psoriasis may be avoided. The term toxic pustuloderma has been proposed as an alternative name for this entity (63).

Acute pemphigus foliaceus can mimic GPP but the evolution of lesions is slower. Subcorneal pustular dermatosis of Sneddon and Wilkinson remains a controversial entity (64). Necrolytic migratory erythema associated with glucagonoma must be remembered, but the wasting, anemia, glossitis, and ulcerative mouth involvement, with a histological picture showing prominent epidermal necrosis, should allow differentiation.

Banal staphyloderma, rampant candidiasis, and pustular eruptions due to iodine or bromide may oc-

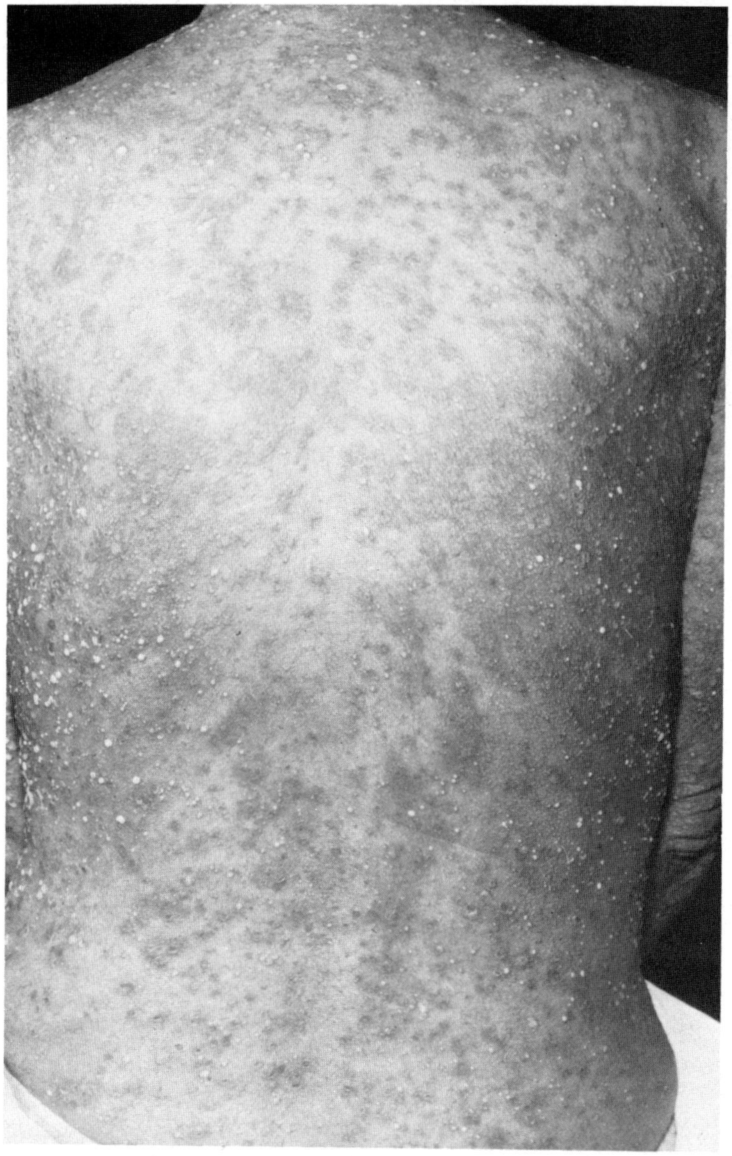

Figure 1 Acute generalized pustular psoriasis; early stage with numerous pinhead pustules.

casionally pose difficulty. Gram-negative or other septicemias, particularly those occurring in immunosuppressed patients, may be complicated by a generalized pustular eruption and should be considered.

Complications

In the absence of effective treatment, death can occur in the acute stage of GPP, cardiorespiratory failure being the most common cause of death. Hypoalbuminemia may be profound, perhaps because of a sudden loss of plasma protein into the tissues (65).

In one patient, albumin half-life was shortened to 4 days (normal 11–12 days) (65). Hypocalcemia may be a consequence of the hypoalbuminemia (1,66). The consequent oligemia may cause acute and fatal renal tubular necrosis (67). There may be evidence of liver damage or even jaundice, owing to a combination of oligemia, general toxicity, and perhaps drugs (11,67,68). Deep vein thrombosis in a leg may cause fatal pulmonary embolism. Staphylococcal infection may complicate GPP, usually because of hospital cross infection. *Staphylococcus aureus* may be grown

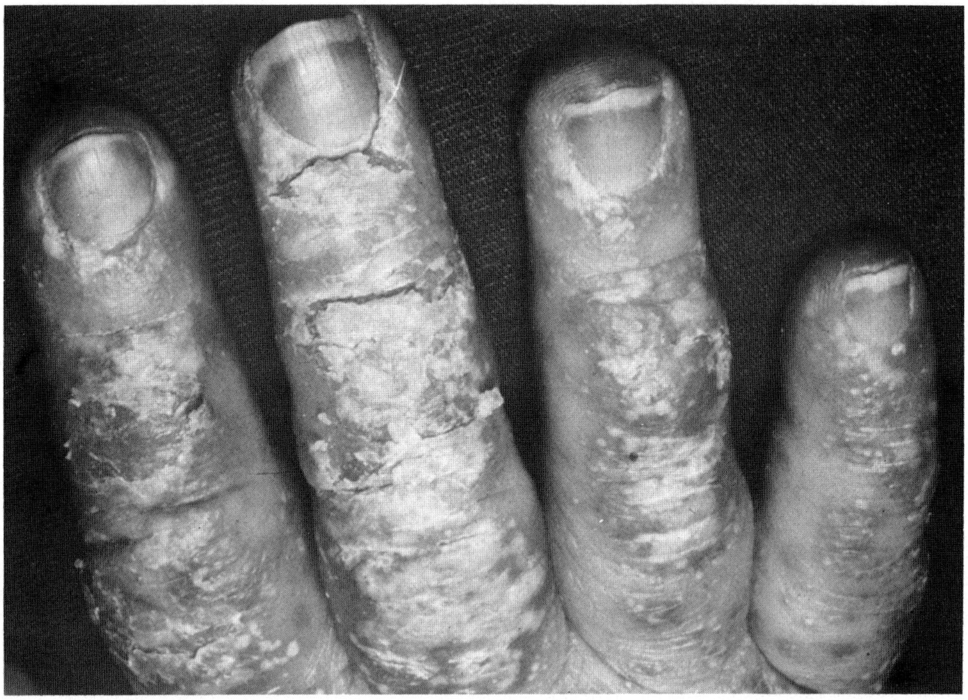

Figure 2 Acute generalized pustular psoriasis; later stage involving the fingers.

from pustules and rarely from blood cultures. However, claims that most GPP is due to staphylococcal bacteremia (69) have not been substantiated (70a).

Inflammatory polyarthritis is common. In one large series, one-third of the patients were eventually affected (1). In another series, 9 of 16 patients had polyarthritis (2). Ophthalmologic complications of GPP include sterile purulent conjunctivitis, iridocyclitis, corneal ulceration, and exfoliation of the cornea (1). Uveitis has been reported (70b). Malabsorption may be a feature of the acute episode (66,71) and may further contribute to hypocalcemia (66). The absorption of therapeutic drugs may be impaired. Amyloidosis is a rare complication (72,73). The obstetrical complications of GPP in pregnancy are discussed below.

If GPP lasts more than a few days, gross hair loss from all areas of the body may follow. This may be immediate and a consequence of any erythrodermic state. Occasionally, a telogen effluvium follows 2–3 months after the worst of the illness.

Laboratory Features

Absolute lymphopenia at the outset of episodes of GPP has been documented in several patients (74), coinciding with a rapidly climbing polymorphonuclear leukocytosis. The latter may be extreme. Levels of 40,000 or more have been seen occasionally in this leukemoid reaction (1,74). The lymphopenia was attributed to increased sequestration of these cells (74).

Hypoalbuminemia and hypocalcemia have already been mentioned. The plasma globulins may be raised. A raised erythrocyte sedimentation rate (ESR) is usual. If oligemia is marked, plasma creatinine and urea will rise. The appearance of albumin and casts in the urine is a warning of impending renal tubular necrosis if the patient is not rapidly rehydrated. Previous reports of an abnormally low plasma zinc level in GPP (75) have been confirmed, and occur in parallel with low zinc levels in suction blister fluid (76). Zinc levels in the skin, however, appear to be increased in GPP (76). The significance of these findings and their relationship to neutrophil chemotaxis is obscure. Hyperlactatemia is likely to be secondary to the hyperproliferation and leukocytosis (77).

GPP of Pregnancy

Generalized pustular psoriasis of pregnancy (first described by Hebra in 1872) (78), sometimes called impetigo herpetiformis (71), sometimes occurs also in

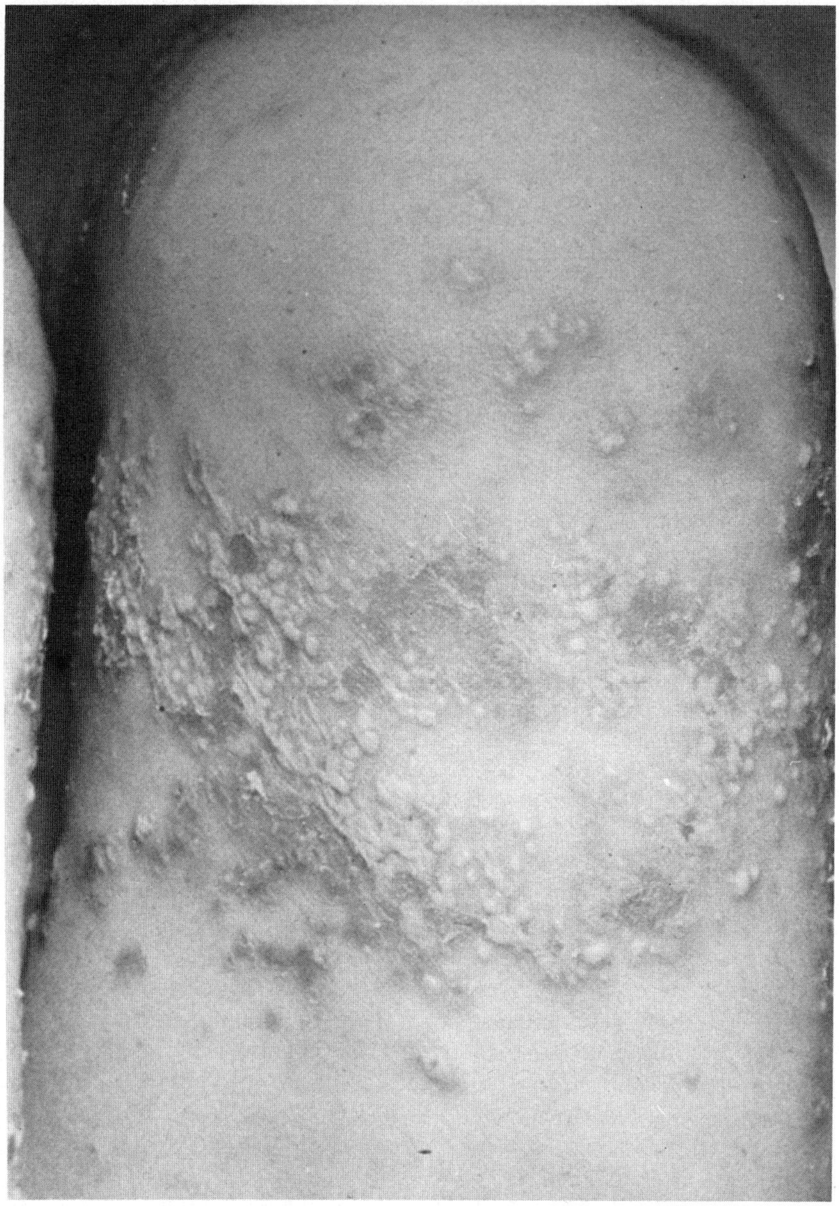

Figure 3 Acute generalized pustular psoriasis; pustules becoming flaccid and confluent.

the puerperium It is rare and only about 100 cases have been documented in the literature (71), although this certainly understates its incidence. Essentially, the clinical features are of an acute or subacute GPP of the von Zumbusch type. Onset is unusual before the sixth month, but the disease may last until the child is born and for several weeks afterward.

Constitutional disturbance may be severe and death may occur, attributable to heart failure, disturbance of thermoregulation, or renal failure. The more severe and long-standing the disease, the greater the risks of placental insufficiency, leading to stillbirth, neonatal death, or fetal abnormalities (79,80).

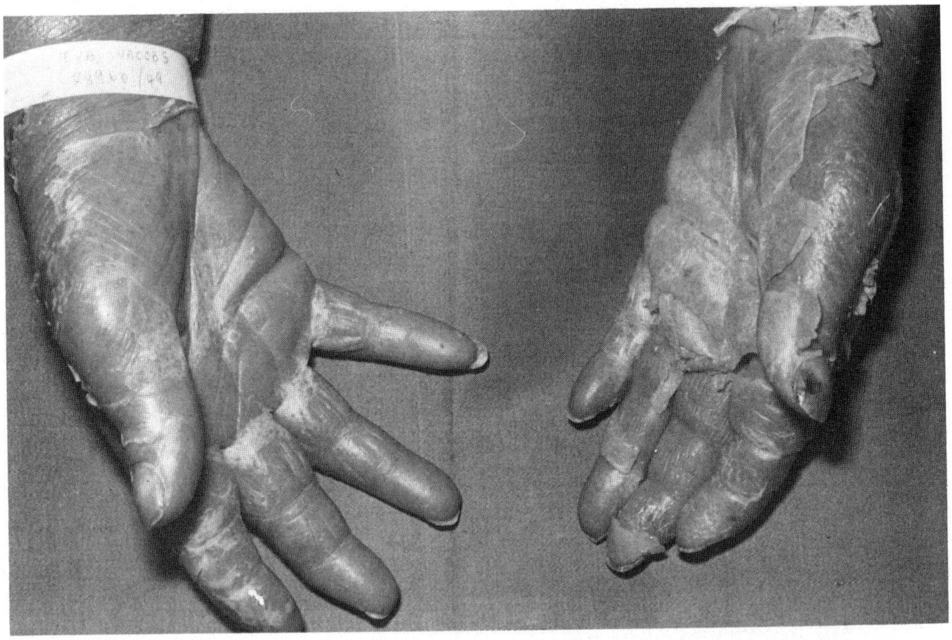

Figure 4 Exfoliation of corneal sheets as the wave of generalized pustulation subsides.

Characteristically, the disease recurs in subsequent pregnancies (71). Recurrence has been described in up to nine pregnancies (71,80).

The laboratory features are similar to those in any form of acute GPP (see above). Lowered levels of vitamin D have been reported (71), probably attributable to impaired intestinal absorption.

It has become generally accepted that "impetigo herpetiformis" is not a separate entity, but is GPP in pregnancy, although there is some disagreement on this (81). The frequent relationship with psoriasis vulgaris in the patient or her family strengthens this belief. In one patient, a brother had had GPP (80). Large mononuclear cells have been described in the dermis and epidermis in some cases, and it has been postulated that these define true impetigo herpetiformis as opposed to pustular psoriasis occurring in pregnancy (81). This observation awaits confirmation.

Circinate and Annular Pustular Psoriasis

Annular and other patterned lesions may be seen in acute GPP, but are more characteristic of the subacute or chronic forms of widespread pustular psoriasis (1,82,83). Lesions begin as discrete areas of erythema which become raised and edematous. Slow centrifugal spread may mimic erythema annulare centrifugum (84) (Fig. 6). Pustules appear peripherally on the crest of the advancing edge, become desiccated, and leave a trailing fringe of scale as the lesion slowly advances (Fig. 7). Most of the detail descriptions of these patterns have been in the French literature (82,83,85).

Some authors (86) have separated a related pattern, well-described by Lapiere (87), as recurrent circinate erythematous psoriasis (85). It was originally described in 1907 as recurrent circinate erythema. It may occur alone (in the complete absence at any stage of recognizable psoriasis), or as a phase in what is clearly generalized pustular psoriasis.

Juvenile and Infantile Pustular Psoriasis

All forms of pustular psoriasis are rare in childhood. Five cases were seen in one series of 479 psoriatic patients (88); two cases in 590 psoriatic patients in another (89). In a series of 104 cases of GPP, there were only five children (1).

Although GPP can begin at any age in childhood, in more than 25% of the reported series, onset has been in the first year (90,91). The disease may begin in the first few weeks of life and two cases of congenital GPP have been described (91). Other pustular conditions of infancy and childhood which should be

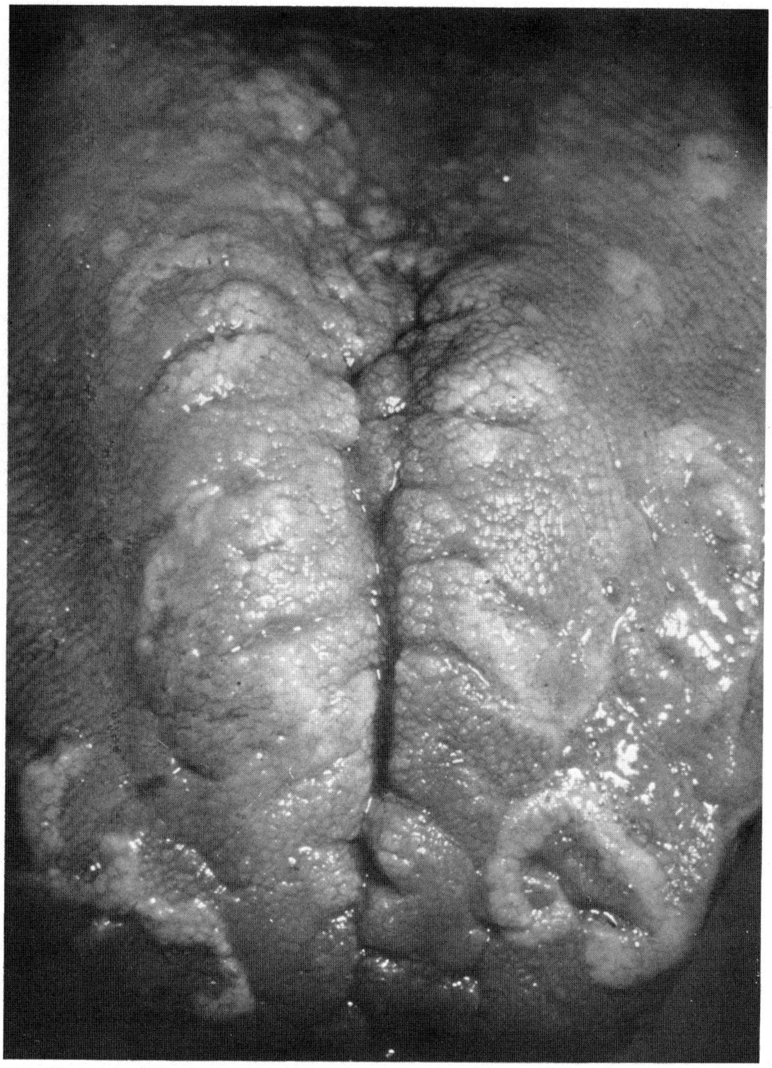

Figure 5 Geographic tongue (annulus migrans) in generalized pustular psoriasis.

considered in the differential diagnosis are shown in Tables 2 and 3, respectively.

In contrast to psoriasis vulgaris in childhood (92) and GPP in adults (1), a male preponderance is seen in GPP of childhood (about 3:2 male/female ratio) (90,91).

Also, unlike the adult forms, childhood GPP tends to have a more benign course (91). Infantile cases are also often benign; circinate and annular forms are common (Fig. 8). Systemic symptoms are often absent and spontaneous remissions occur (93). In at least one-third of infantile cases, a history of an eruption diagnosed as seborrheic dermatitis, diaper dermatitis, or diaper psoriasis is obtained (90,94). More severe forms with fever and toxicity do occur, necessitating active treatment (Fig. 9). Rarely, pustulosis has supervened on a congenital erythroderma (95,96a).

The majority of children are aged 2–10 years at onset. The disease may be of a von Zumbusch pattern, but annular and circinate forms and mixed patterns are seen as well (91,96b). Onset of the von Zumbusch type may be abrupt with fever and toxicity, and an erythrodermic background can rapidly become generalized flares of sterile pustules. Attacks settle within 2 to 4 days but repeated waves of inflammation may follow (93). These patients tend to develop psoriasis vulgaris (91).

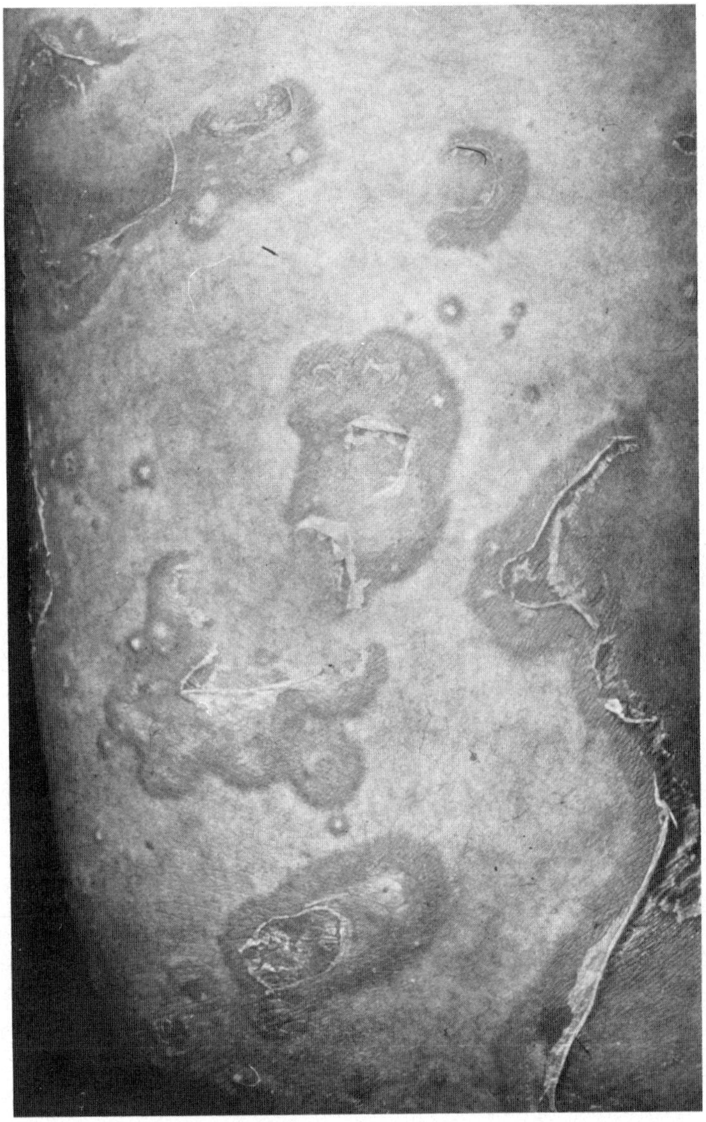

Figure 6 Subacute annular and circinate pustular psoriasis; annular erythematous and urticate plaques with sparse pustules.

In older children, the disease resembles that in the adult and may be of any of the recognized patterns. Transient solitary episodes of exanthematic GPP occur rarely in childhood.

A rare case of juvenile GPP was reported in a pair of monozygotic twins (96c). They presented with strikingly similar clinical courses and interestingly they also shared the same HLA types.

Chronic recurrent multifocal osteomyelitis (CRMO) is usually a rare association with palmoplantar pustulosis. However, it has been described in a child with GPP (96d). Sterile lytic bone lesions, possibly early CRMO, has also been reported in an infant with GPP (96e).

Localized Forms of Generalized Pustular Psoriasis

Localized forms of GPP (1) must be distinguished from palmoplantar pustulosis or acropustulosis. The term psoriasis with pustules is perhaps more appropriate. Diaper psoriasis may be so complicated especially if Candida growth is encouraged. One or more plaques of psoriasis vulgaris may develop pustules

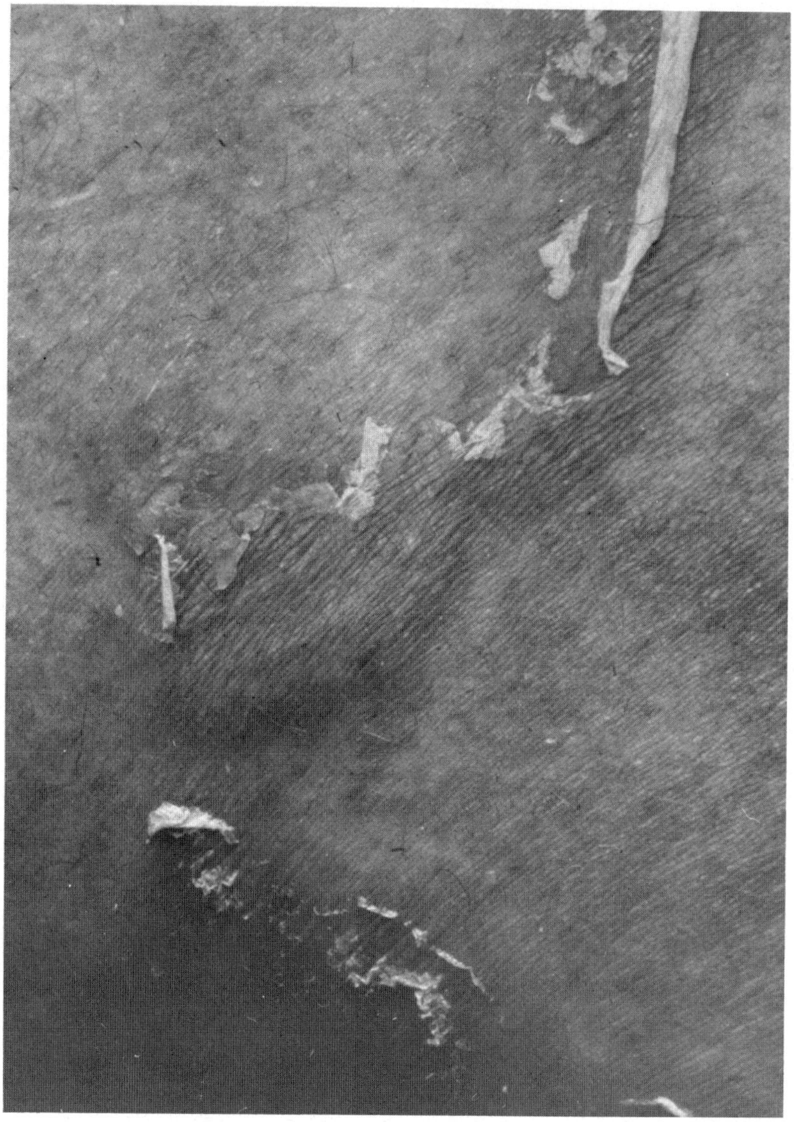

Figure 7 Subacute annular and circinate pustular psoriasis; spreading edge leaves a fringe of scaling.

Table 2 Differential Diagnosis of Infantile Pustular Psoriasis

Impetigo
Acropustulosis of infancy
Toxic erythema of the newborn
Miliaria
Candidosis
Congenital syphilis
Hand, foot, and mouth disease
Primary herpes simplex infections
Histiocytosis

following prolonged irritant topical therapy. Overenthusiastic use of anthralin on the anterior legs below the knees may produce flat glazed plaques in which pustules appear (1). Resolution is usually prompt with bland topical treatment.

Management

The care and treatment of acute GPP may confront dermatologists with the most difficult and complex problems they are likely to encounter in practice. Management requires attention to possible provocative

Table 3 Differential Diagnosis of Childhood GPP

Staphylococcal scalded skin syndrome
Pityriasis rubra pilaris
Toxic epidermal necrolysis
Erythrodermic psoriasis
Generalized atopic or seborrheic dermatitis
Reiter's disease
Generalized candidiasis

Source: Ref. 96b.

factors, general support measures, nursing of the skin, and the use of specific drugs.

Possible Provocative Factors

If a provocative drug, such as lithium, aspirin, or other drugs recognized to precipitate GPP (see Table 1) can be implicated, then it should be withdrawn. Similarly, inappropriate topical therapy with irritating tar or anthralin preparations or massive use of potent corticosteroids under occlusion must be withdrawn. Tar or

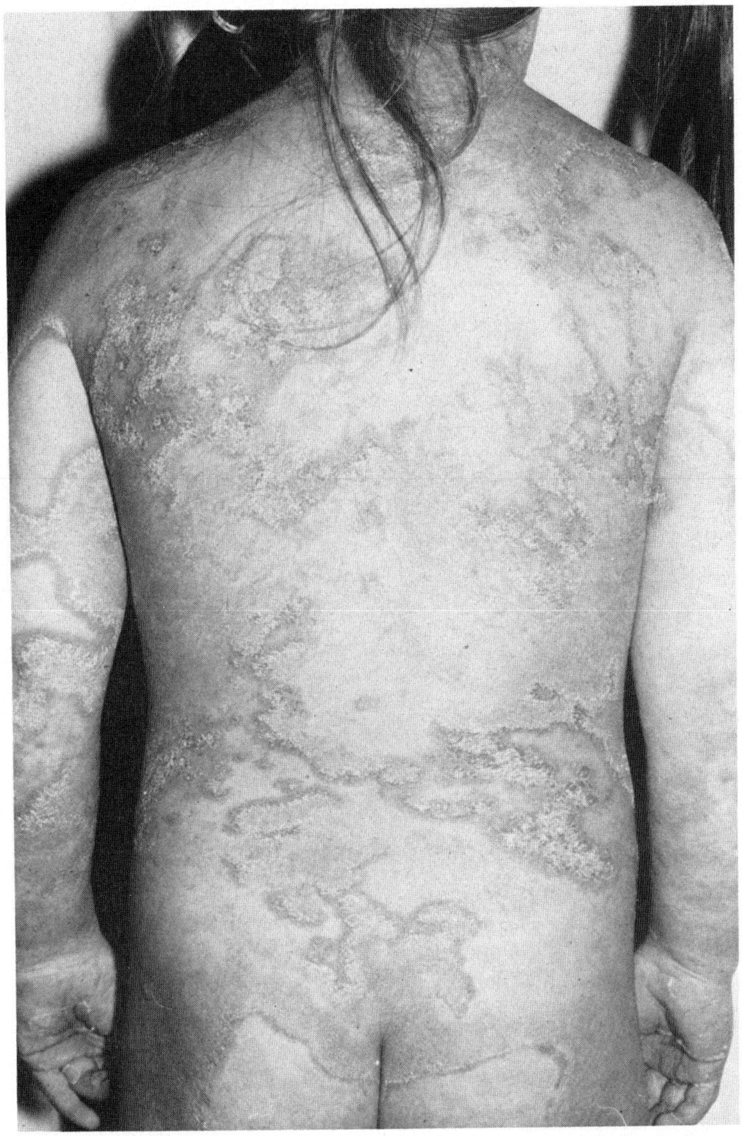

Figure 8 Subacute annular and circinate phase of generalized pustular psoriasis in a child.

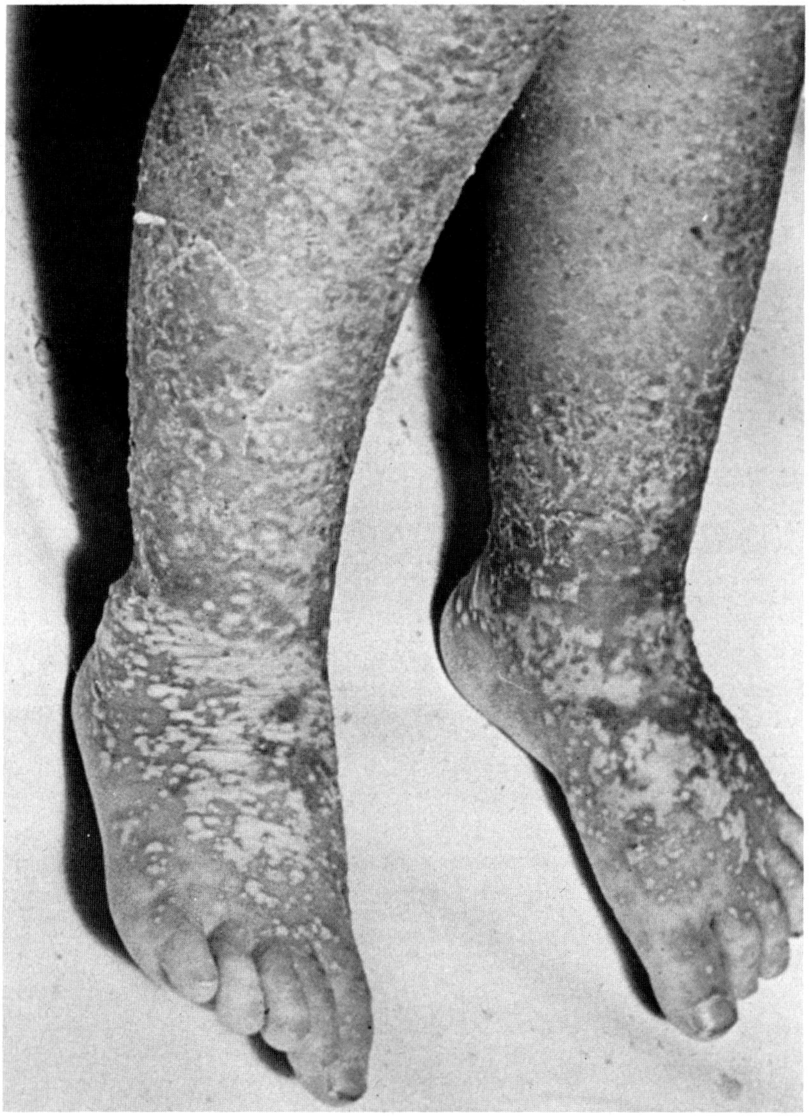

Figure 9 Acute generalized pustular psoriasis (von Zumbusch) in a child.

anthralin can be replaced abruptly by completely bland local applications, but potent corticosteroids may have to be withdrawn slowly to minimize the risk of pituitary-adrenal failure and, separately, exacerbation of the skin condition. Serial dilution of the corticosteroid in mineral oil (soft white paraffin) slowly over several days may be the safest course. Where infection has clearly played a part in precipitating GPP, it should be treated vigorously with the appropriate (usually anticoccal) antibiotic. Cloxacillin and erythromycin are generally the antibiotics of choice. Rarely, when GPP in pregnancy is threatening the patient's life, termination or early delivery may be needed.

General Measures

When life is not immediately threatened nor the patient in gross distress, initial management should be conservative. This is particularly important in infants and children (97). Bed rest in the hospital, mild sedation, bland local therapy, maintenance of adequate hydration, and avoidance of excessive heat loss may allow spontaneous remission (1,94,97). This course is particularly appropriate if there is a previous history of ordinary psoriasis and evidence of a provocative factor, such as recent steroid therapy (1,26). However, in acute GPP of the von Zumbusch type, repeated waves of pustulosis may exhaust the patient, especially if elderly, and the risks of hypostatic chest infection or deep vein thrombosis in the legs (with the consequent hazard of pulmonary embolism) are ever present. In such circumstances, the clinician must resort to drugs in an attempt to terminate the episode and maintain subsequent suppression. In subacute and chronic forms of GPP, the decisions can be less hurried. At all times, the physician has to weigh the hazards of the disease against the different hazards of active therapy.

If the skin background is erythrodermic, percutaneous heat losses will be considerable and are increased if the patient is nursed close to an open window on a bright but cool day. The patient may feel hot and throw aside bedding or bedclothing, which exacerbates heat losses. A low-reading thermometer should always be available to the nursing staff. Water loss through the skin may be increased 10-fold or more so that more than 1 liter of water is so lost. Fortunately, electrolyte loss is not a problem. A fluid intake of at least 3 liters a day is usually needed, and the nursing staff may need determination to achieve this. Careful monitoring of fluid balance is mandatory.

Drug Therapy

Methotrexate. This is the drug of choice providing renal function is adequate, marrow function is normal, and liver disease is absent (68). A creatinine clearance test may be necessary to assess glomerular function. In very acute GPP, small intravenous doses (5–10 mg), repeated every 5–7 days, *never* more frequently, may be safest and the most effective. The intramuscular route may be used, but in either case, each dose should only rarely exceed 0.3 mg/kg. In acute GPP, fever, toxicity, and pustulation may respond to methotrexate within 24–48 hr, but erythema or erythroderma is slower to respond. Sometimes, pustular relapse is seen after 5 or 6 days as the effect of the drug diminishes; dose frequency must be determined accordingly.

Oral therapy is less predictable and absorption of the drug may be variable in these circumstances. If the oral route is used, 0.2–0.4 mg/kg will be needed, repeated every 6–10 days (usually weekly) according to response. In the context of acute GPP, the cutaneous effects of methotrexate toxicity due to overdosage can be catastrophic, with widespread erosion and ulceration in an already ill patient; overdosage must be avoided. Plasma creatinine and albumin levels may have to be monitored daily for a short period. As control is established, weekly oral doses usually suffice, and later even doses every 14 days may be effective. Occasionally, better control is achieved with the Weinstein-Frost regimen in which the weekly dosage is divided into three parts given at 12-hr intervals. Methotrexate has been used in combination with other cytotoxic drugs.

Hydroxyurea. There is only one report of successful use of hydroxyurea in GPP (102), and follow-up was short. It is a disappointing agent when used alone; in GPP the activity of hydroxyurea compared with methotrexate parallels that in psoriasis vulgaris. It is occasionally of value in combination with PUVA therapy or etretinate.

Dapsone. This sulfone and its use in dermatology have been usefully reviewed by Lang (103). Its successful use in pustular dermatoses was first described in 1956 by Hellier (104) in GPP, and by Sneddon and Wilkinson in subcorneal pustular dermatosis (105). Dapsone proved effective for long periods in GPP evolving from acrodermatitis continua, a form of the disease with a particularly bad prognosis (97). Isolated confirmatory reports have followed, suggesting that dapsone is particularly valuable in atypical variants of GPP (106). The drug was apparently of no value in the treatment of one infant case (95), but much higher dosages were beneficial in another infant (107). A further case report documents a good response to 50 mg daily in a 9-year-old child (108).

Sulfapyridine. This early sulfonamide was used successfully in various localized forms of pustular psoriasis, and its effective prescription in GPP has been occasionally documented (104,105,109).

Corticosteroids. The role of oral or parenteral corticosteroids is controversial (30,68,110). The immediate beneficial effects of large dosages of prednisolone or a fluorinated derivative are beyond doubt, but it is well documented that as the dosage is reduced serious pustular relapses tend to occur (1,68,111,112). There is substantial evidence that corticosteroids in large dosages destabilize psoriasis (1,30,68), making management more difficult in the medium and long terms. However, corticosteroids may be needed occasionally as a life-saving measure when metabolic (particularly cardiovascular) complications threaten to overwhelm the patient and when methotrexate has failed or is contraindicated. Furthermore, even when successful, although methotrexate can suppress pustulation, fever, and toxicity within 48 hr, intense generalized erythema may remain for much longer, so that the cardiovascular load is not dramatically diminished by this antimetabolite. In such dire circumstances, prednisolone, 40 mg daily, will generally have markedly beneficial effects within 24 hr, lessening inflammation, and reducing cutaneous blood flow. After a few days, the dosage can be progressively reduced, but another potent form of therapy is likely to be needed to allow the patient to be subsequently weaned off the corticosteroid. If methotrexate is chosen, its introduction is best delayed until the dosage of prednisolone has been reduced, if possible, to 20 mg daily or less to lessen the risk of additive hazards such as immunosuppression and consequent risk of infection. There may be a particular risk from disseminated herpes zoster or measles in young children (1).

Etretinate. This synthetic derivative of vitamin A has undoubted antipsoriatic efficacy in a dosage of 0.5–1.0 mg/kg body weight daily by mouth, but even in full dosage it is not always sufficient alone in GPP. Nevertheless, GPP may improve quite quickly on 1 mg/kg used alone and complete clearance within 3 weeks has been reported (113–115a). However, if GPP occurs against a background of universal erythroderma, full dosages of etretinate may be irritating, producing exacerbation of the disease and worsening the erythema (113). In this situation, lower dosages (0.3–0.5 mg/kg) are more appropriate and treatment may have to be continued for many weeks, so that in fulminating life-threatening disease, etretinate monotherapy is not sufficient. The use of etretinate in children with GPP has been reported (115b,c). The results were excellent without skeletal complications. However, until more data are available, etretinate should be used with caution in children. Combination with PUVA therapy (see below) may be valuable. There is very little data concerning the use of acitretin, the deethylated metabolite of etretinate, in pustular psoriasis (116). It is probably slightly less effective than etretinate, but has a much shorter half-life and may therefore be of therapeutic value in certain circumstances. Further studies are awaited.

Photochemotherapy (PUVA). In psoriasis vulgaris, PUVA ranks with methotrexate in antipsoriatic efficacy (117). Far fewer data are available for GPP, but successful treatment has been reported in 32 patients (118). In this series, the cumulative UVA dosage to clearance was 52 ± 43 J cm^2, with a mean of 14.5 ± 6.8 treatments given over 3.5 ± 1.9 weeks. In general, at clearance, individual dosages of UVA of about 5 J cm^2 were being used.

Severely ill patients may have to be treated in the horizontal position. Adequate follow-up data and information on the role of maintenance PUVA therapy are still lacking.

Retinoid-PUVA Combined Therapy. The rationale for combined therapy is to achieve results not attainable with either form of treatment alone to accelerate response which is particularly important in acute GPP, and to reduce the dosage and, therefore, the potential toxicity of each component. These aims can be achieved (119,120).

Experience has shown that in GPP, especially with an erythrodermic background, the etretinate should be started in a modest dosage of 0.25–0.5 mg/kg daily. After 7–10 days PUVA is added given on 3 or 4 days weekly. At the point of clearance, the etretinate can be withdrawn and maintenance PUVA continued for about 2 months only. Emollients and very weak topical steroids may be needed at the same time (119,120).

Essential Fatty Acids. Essential fatty acids of the n-3 series, derived from alpha-linolenic acid, have been used in plaque psoriasis, and a single case report documents a good response in GPP (121a). This observation remains to be confirmed.

Clofazimine. The beneficial effect of clofazimine in GPP has been reported in the literature (121b,c).

Cyclosporin A. Since the initial report of good therapeutic results in psoriasis with cyclosporin A (122) further studies have confirmed its efficacy (123,124). Several case reports now document a good response in GPP to treatment with cyclosporin A (124, 125) and in acrodermatitis continua (126a,b), but controlled clinical trials remain to be published.

Pristinamycin. A single case report documents the response of GPP in pregnancy to pristinamycin, a macrolide-related antibiotic which is safe in pregnancy (127a).

Topical Calcipotriol. Response of acute GPP to topical calcipotriol was recently reported in 3 patients (127b).

Choice of Therapy

Therapeutic options may be limited by the availability of certain forms of therapy in individual countries or hospitals. In our opinion, therapy should always be conservative and expectant in the hope of spontaneous remission of the GPP, where the clinical circumstances allow. In this phase, topical therapy is invaluable, but it must be nonirritant and overexposure to steroids must be avoided. If systemic treatment cannot be avoided, methotrexate and retinoid-PUVA combined therapy are the most effective modalities and choice will depend on the overall clinical situation and the availability of the drugs or apparatus needed. The emergence of more information on retinoid-PUVA combinations and of the therapeutic possibilities of cyclosporin A in particular make more effective treatment of resistant pustular psoriasis a realistic target. Furthermore, the relative freedom from teratogenicity of cyclosporin A compared to retinoids or retinoid-PUVA combinations may be of value in the treatment of GPP during pregnancy. More concentrated forms of fish oil, or combinations of essential fatty acids may provide a nontoxic alternative to other systemic therapy.

Prognosis

There are few data on the long-term prognosis of GPP. Von Zumbusch's patient (5) survived many acute episodes over a number of years and perhaps was lucky to live before potent (and dangerous) remedies were available. Ryan and Baker (97) reported on the prognosis in 155 patients with all types of GPP. Thirty-four of 106 patients who were followed up had died; 26 of these deaths were attributable to the disease or its treatment. Generalized pustular psoriasis developing from acropustulosis (acrodermatitis continua) had the worst prognosis; 7 of 11 patients died and another remained severely disabled. To some extent this particularly poor outlook reflected the age at onset of these patients, who were predominantly elderly. However, death was a direct result of GPP in all of these cases, owing to cardiac failure or respiratory infection during uncontrolled pustular psoriasis.

In general, patients with preceding ordinary psoriasis had a better prognosis than those with atypical prepustular psoriasis (1,97).

The better prognosis of GPP of pregnancy reflects the abrupt removal of the main provocative factor by childbirth or, in extremis, termination of the pregnancy (71,80). Generalized pustular psoriasis of childhood also carries a more benign prognosis (90,91), providing the use of oral corticosteroids and methotrexate can be avoided (94). Khan and his colleagues (1,94) stressed the hazard of fatal viral infections in corticosteroid-treated children, and advocated bland topical therapy, if necessary in a hospital, for up to 3 months in anticipation of spontaneous remission. In their patients, where the use of oral corticosteroids was avoided, growth and development progressed unimpaired despite GPP.

LOCALIZED PUSTULAR PSORIASIS

The accumulation of polymorphonuclear leukocytes (PMNLs) in the epidermis to form microabscesses is one of the salient histological features of psoriasis. Histologically, all psoriasis is "pustular" but, by convention, the term is reserved for those forms of psoriasis in which the PMNL collections become macroscopic so that pustules appear visible to the naked eye. It is convenient and rational to separate the localized forms, which are generally acral and chronic, from the generalized forms which may be subacute or acute. Generalized pustular psoriasis has been discussed earlier in this chapter.

Classification

Any classification of localized pustular psoriasis must be arbitrary, and it should be remembered that it is not known whether or not psoriasis is a single entity. The two major divisions are (1) palmoplantar pustulosis (including pustular bacterid), and (2) acropustulosis (acrodermatitis continua). These patterns are not mutually exclusive; combinations may be seen at the same time, or at different times in the same patient.

Palmoplantar Pustulosis

Nomenclature

Crocker first used the term dermatitis reopens for a recurring pustular eruption of the hands and feet over 100 years ago (128). A mild form limited to the palms and soles was described by Audry (1901) as relapsing phylctenular dermatitis of the extremities (129), and by Dore (1928) as acrodermatitis Dore (130). A relationship between this eruption and psoriasis was proposed by Barber, and by Ingram, in 1930 (131,132), when the name psoriasis pustulosa was suggested.

Andrews was of the opinion that the rash was a response to a distant septic focus and named it pustular bacterid (133,134) (see below). Sachs et al. showed that most patients had no apparent forms of infection, nor were psoriatic, and called it acrodermatitis pustulosa perstans (135), but the descriptive term pustulosa palmoplantaris had been used by Bonnevie in 1939 (136), and endorsed by Lever (137). These authors believed palmoplantar pustulosis to be the most acceptable term (138), and we will use it throughout this chapter.

Definition

Palmoplantar pustulosis (PPP) is a common condition in which erythematous and scaly plaques studded with sterile pustules develop on the palms and soles. It is characteristically indolent and resistant to treatment.

Precipitating Factors

Septic foci have been blamed for PPP (133,134,139), but their removal may not cure the eruption (140,141), and PPP certainly occurs in the absence of any demonstrable focus of sepsis. A 50% clearance rate of PPP following tonsillectomy has been reported (142), renewing interest in the role of distant sepsis.

British studies have proposed a link between cigarette smoking and PPP (143,144), a finding confirmed in a Swedish study (157), although discontinuation of smoking had no effect on the eruption. The condition has occurred after 6 months treatment with lithium carbonate (145). Remission of PPP following ileojejunal bypass for obesity in three patients is an intriguing finding which awaits confirmation and explanation (146).

Histopathology

The primary histopathological event in PPP is a vesicle in the lower layers of the epidermis containing mononuclear cells. As the vesicle migrates upward it is invaded by polymorphonuclear leukocytes to form a pustule (147,148). Spongiosis may be evident (149). It may not be possible to differentiate PPP and psoriasis vulgaris histologically (147).

Pathogenesis

Not all authorities accept that PPP is part of the psoriatic entity. It can be confidently accepted as psoriatic if typical psoriasis is found elsewhere on the body, or if an unequivocal history of previous ordinary psoriasis is obtained. In the absence of such evidence, the presence of psoriasis in one or more first-degree relatives is circumstantial support. However, typical PPP often occurs in the absence of any such findings; at present it is not possible to confirm or refute the association with psoriasis. HLA data do *not* support such an association. The characteristic psoriatic associations with HLAs B13 and B17, CW6, and DR7 are not seen in PPP (150–152). These findings have been confirmed in Denmark (142), Finland (143), the United Kingdom (135), and France (150). A study combining all previous European studies confirms this lack of a definite HLA association in PPP (153). In Japan, where the B locus associations are different, B37 was associated with psoriasis vulgaris, but not with PPP (139). Neutrophil chemotaxis is enhanced in patients with PPP (154,155), but no definite relationship between the degree of abnormality or neutrophil chemotaxis and the clinical severity of PPP has yet been defined.

It remains unclear whether differences in neutrophil chemotaxis exist between patients with PPP and GPP (155), or whether they are secondary to the disease itself. Differences in epidermal phospholipase A_2 activity between PPP and psoriasis vulgaris have been advanced as further evidence that the two conditions are separate (156).

Clinical Picture

Palmoplantar psoriasis, a disease of adults, is rare in children. It is uncommon in early adult life; most patients develop the disease in the fifth or sixth decade. A population study in Sweden showed a prevalence of 0.05% (13), and PPP was found in 0.66% of patients visiting a Swedish dermatology outpatient clinic in 1986 (157). A modest female preponderance is seen in most series (158,159).

Typically, the patient with PPP presents with one or more well-defined plaques. On the hands, these are seen on the thenar and hypothenar eminences. Less frequently, the center of the palm or the distal palm is involved. On the feet, favorite sites are the insteps (Fig. 10), the medial or lateral side of the foot (Fig. 11) at the level of the insteps, the sides or back of the heel (Fig. 12), often spreading onto the plantar aspect of the heel. Less frequently, the distal sole is involved. Digital involvement is uncommon. The first lesion may remain solitary for months or longer, but other lesions may follow in the characteristic sites. Sometimes a striking symmetry of lesions is apparent, especially on the feet (Fig. 13). The affected skin is dark red and may be scaly. Removal of scale, such as by treatment, may leave a glazed dull red surface. Rubbing of the surface may reveal the silvery scale of psoriasis.

Set in this plaque are multiple superficial pustules varying from 2–8 mm in size. The pustules are yellow

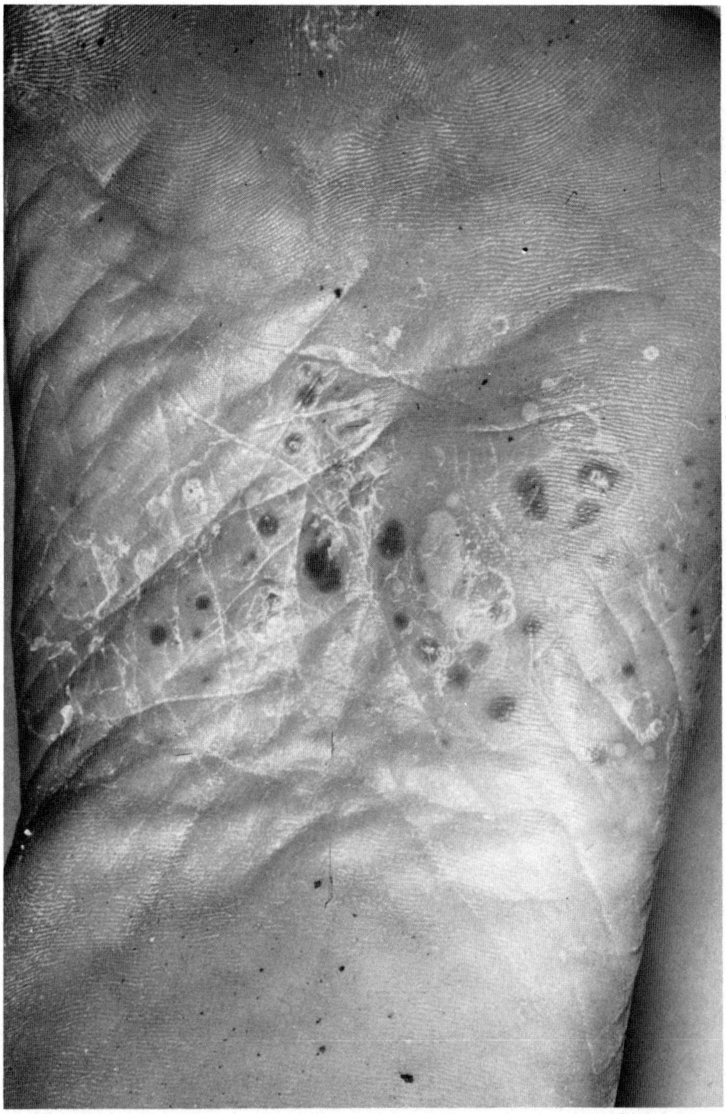

Figure 10 Pustular psoriasis of the instep showing pustules at different stages of evolution.

when fresh, but later become yellow-brown and even dark brown as the contents are desiccated. Eventually the dried pustule scales off. Typically, pustules at all stages of evolution are apparent.

A very uncommon variant of this clinical picture is an eruption of much smaller lesions, or even spattered individual pustules, more diffusely on the palms or soles (Fig. 14).

Differential Diagnosis

Tinea and eczema are the important alternatives to PPP. Tinea often affects the toe clefts, which are spared in PPP. The nails may be affected.

Vesicular eczema may pose difficulties in diagnosis. Translucent vesicles are rarely seen in PPP, but transitional forms may cause difficulty. It is not rare for experienced clinicians to modify their diagnosis during prolonged observation of the patient. Secondary infection of eczema may cause difficulty, but is more painful than PPP, and bacteriological cultures of the contents of a pustule is helpful. The term pustular bacterid describes what is essentially an acute leukocytoclastic vasculitis which can mimic PPP (160). It has been reported after streptococcal upper respiratory infections (160), and immune complex deposition has been detected (161).

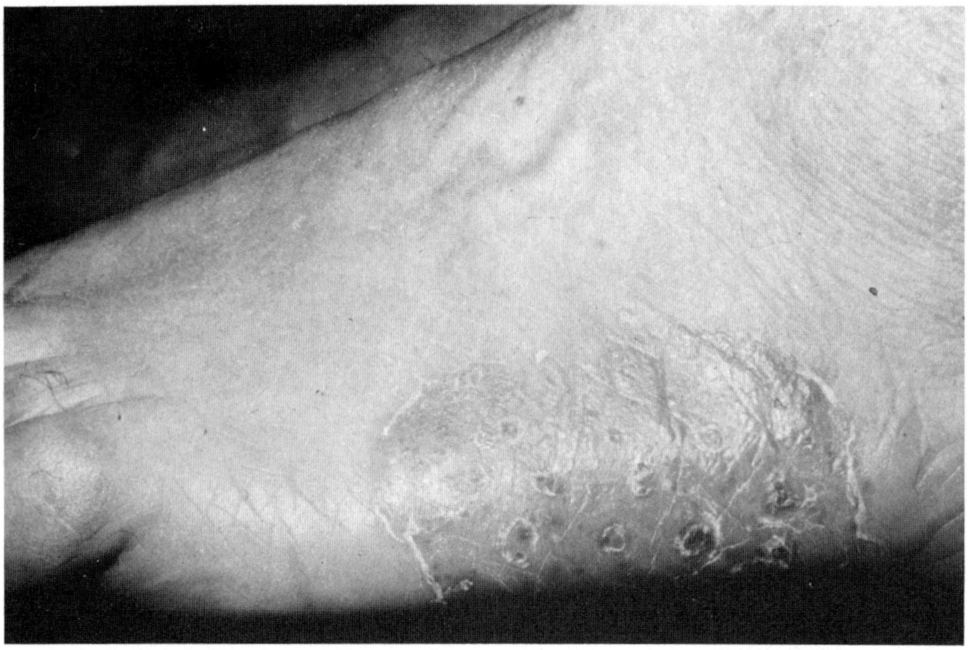

Figure 11 Pustular psoriasis on lateral border of the foot.

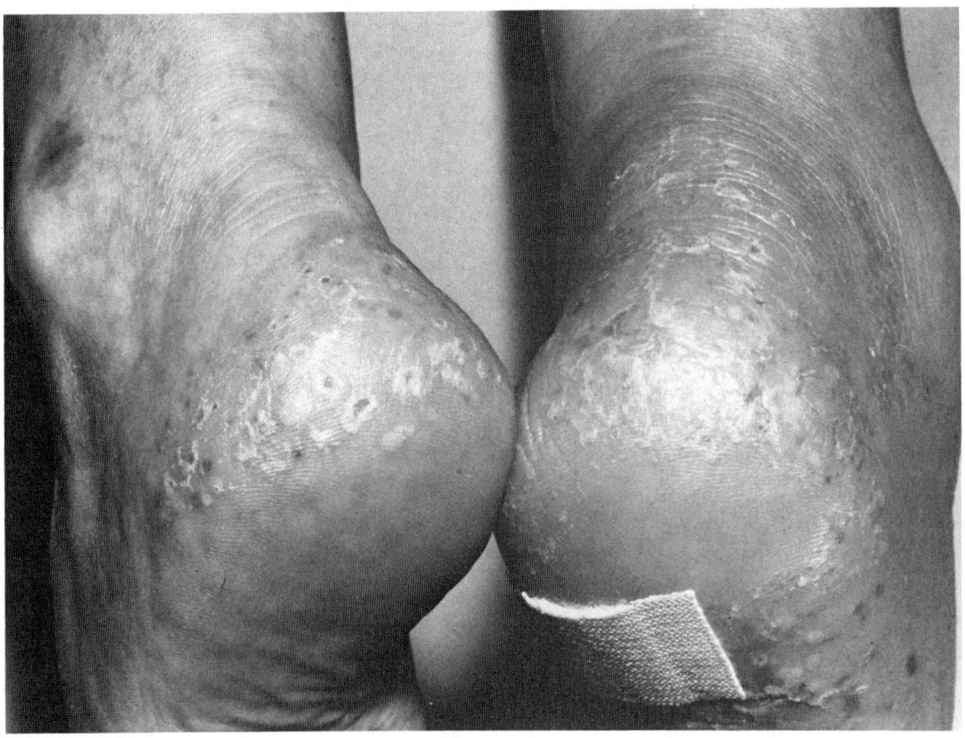

Figure 12 Pustular psoriasis of heels.

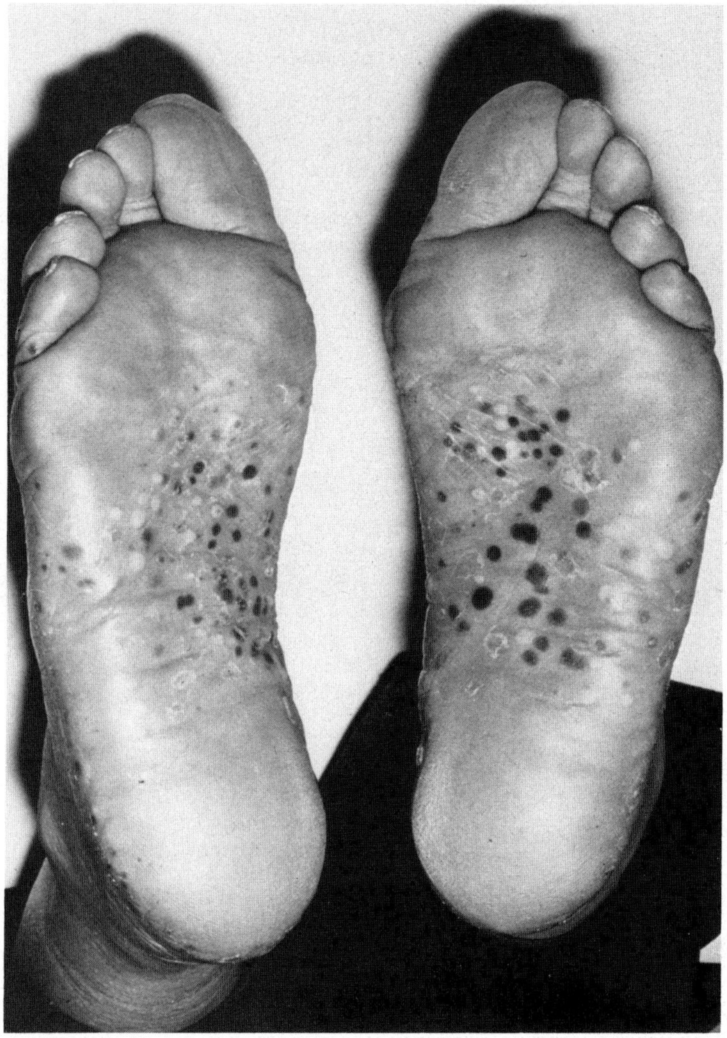

Figure 13 Pustular psoriasis of feet, demonstrating characteristic symmetry.

Prognosis

Untreated PPP may disappear spontaneously. The more usual course is prolonged, lasting years, sometimes with slow spread or extension. Five years after diagnosis, 75% of patients still have active disease (140), and 10 years after diagnosis, only 30% are clear of skin lesions (162).

Disease Associations

Pustulotic Arthro-Osteitis

Anterior chest wall joint symptoms were described in association with PPP by Ishibashi in 1977 (163). Since then, involvement of the manubriosternal joint has been described in 6% and of the sternoclavicular joints in 10% of patients (164). Japanese reports document an incidence of sternocostoclavicular arthritis of 9.4–10.6% (165,166). Scintigraphic evidence of sternocostoclavicular joint involvement was present in 22% of 73 Swedish patients (167). While Japanese experience has been of a severe arthritis, often requiring surgery, European experience is that the joint involvement is invariably mild, but may signal more significant joint involvement elsewhere.

Autoimmune Thyroid Disease

In a study of 50 patients with PPP, the incidence of clinically evident thyroid disease and thyroid autoan-

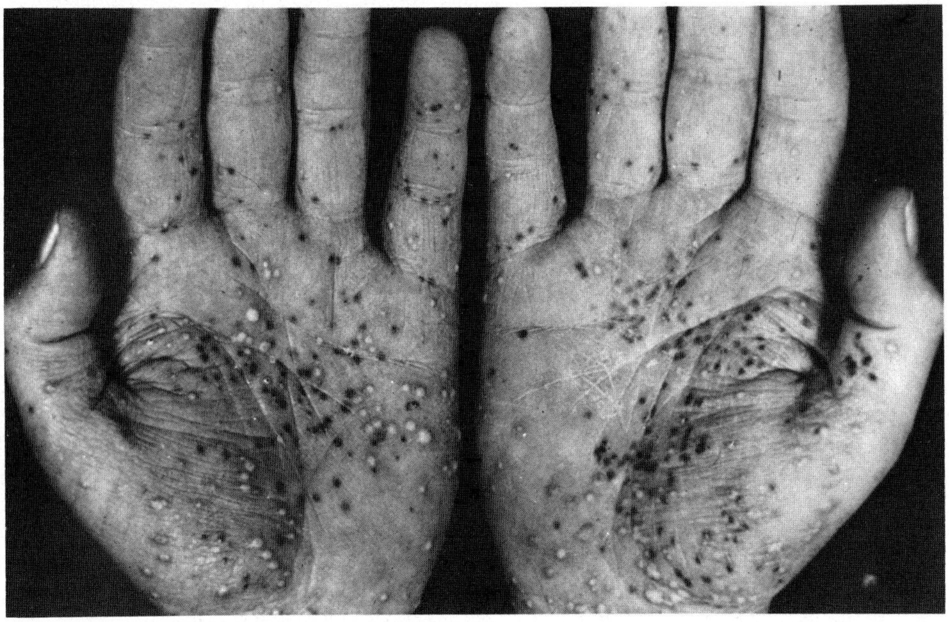

Figure 14 Diffuse pattern of pustular psoriasis on palms.

tibodies was significantly higher than in a matched control group (157). It is suggested that patients with PPP should be screened for thyroid disease.

Pustular Bacterid

The term pustular bacterid (PB) was introduced by Andrews (133,134) to describe a rare acute monomorphic sterile pustular eruption of the hands and feet. It begins abruptly, so that within a few days many large (4–8 mm) pustules are spread evenly on the palms and palmar aspects of the fingers. The plantar aspects of the feet may be similarly involved. In some patients, pustules are also seen on the dorsal aspects of the hands. The term pustular bacterid implies that the eruption is provoked by a remote form of bacterial infection (133,139). Probably this is occasionally so, but in most cases PB simply represents an acute exanthematic variant of PPP or a totally unrelated leukocytoclastic vasculitis (160,161) with immune complex deposition (161) provoked by infection.

Acropustulosis

Acrodermatitis Continua

Synonyms for this condition of acropustulosis (AP), or acrodermatitis continua (AC), have included pustular acrodermatitis, acrodermatitis perstans continua (168), and dermatitis repens (169).

Definition

Acrodermatitis continua is a chronic localized sterile pustular and scaly inflammation beginning acrally on a finger or toe and tending to remain localized to one or more digits for months or years.

Clinical Picture

Whereas PP is predominantly a disease of middle age, the age spread of AC is much wider. The disease may occur in children. It is rare in young adults but, unlike PPP, it not infrequently begins in old age. It is more common in females.

Typically, the patient relates the onset to minor trauma or infection at or near the tip of a single digit, more often a finger than a toe. A small area of inflammation persists and becomes scaly. One or more small pustules develop and desiccate into psoriasiform scaling. Frequently, the initial lesion is at the tip of the digit, but soon the nail folds may be involved and the nail plate becomes dystrophic (Fig. 15). The nail bed skin may be inflamed and pustules may appear under the nail plate (Fig. 15). Slowly the inflammation extends proximally, the advancing edge often having a fringe of epidermis just before or beyond which are tiny pustules. At times, scaling may be less evident and the whole affected area has a smooth, red, glazed appearance and is sore and tender. The secondary nail

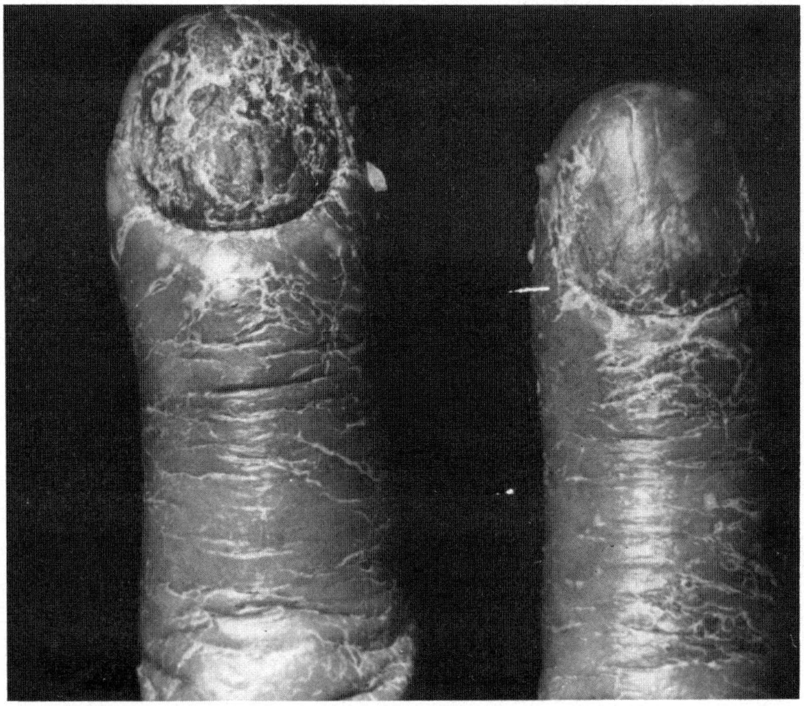

Figure 15

changes include separation of the plate, ridging, crumbling and destruction of the nail, and, occasionally, gross subungual keratosis.

Complications

If AC persists for months and years as is usual, the nail plate may be completely destroyed. Bony changes can occur (131,170) with osteolysis of the tufts of the distal phalanx (170). Occasionally, frank synovitis is seen in terminal or even proximal interphalangeal joints. The free end of the digit may become tapered with loss of pulp and changes mimicking those of scleroderma. In such digits, the circulation may be secondarily affected, so that discomfort is greatest in cold weather. Acropustulosis (AP) may evolve into generalized pustular psoriasis, especially in the elderly (171). The tongue may become involved, showing fissuring or the geographic pattern of pustular psoriasis (172,173).

Differential Diagnosis

In the earliest stage of AC, staphylococcal impetigo, pulp infection, or herpetic whitlow may be suspected. Later, infective eczematoid dermatitis and tinea must be excluded. Candidiasis is likely to be a problem only in the immunodeficient patient. The dubious entity of parakeratosis pustulosa (174) should be considered in children. Subungual malignant melanoma should be considered when only a single nail is involved.

Prognosis

Acrodermatitis continua in young people tends to persist for years. After months or years, a second digit may be involved and, occasionally, multiple fingers or toes are involved. Slow proximal extension along the digit is usual. Painful secondary fissuring may lead to a permanent flexion deformity of the digit. In the elderly, evolution of the disease into generalized pustular psoriasis is a definite hazard.

Histopathology

In the early lesion of AC, epidermal edema and spongiosis are present (148). Soon neutrophilic invasion of the epidermis is evident with the formation of neutrophilic abscesses. The fully formed pustule stretches the epidermis. The dermis contains a mixed inflammatory infiltrate (139). Parakeratosis and loss of granular layer may be striking or absent according to the lesion's stage of evolution.

Management

We do not have effective therapy for localized pustular psoriasis; its management is often as frustrating for the physician as for the patient. Treatment is discussed here in the usual approach to the problem, using simple treatments first.

Topical Therapy

In both PPP and AC, topical therapy is the usual starting point. Coal tar preparations are more likely to be helpful in AC than PPP, but the patient may need to be encouraged to persevere for several weeks. Occlusive tar ointments or tar-impregnated bandages are appropriate for AC, but creams, gels, or lotions may be more acceptable in PPP. Dithranol (anthralin) has been disappointing and has very little place in the treatment of AC. Occasionally, weak preparations can be tried. Higher strengths may aggravate AC. Almost always topical corticosteroids will be used early and are of limited value. In AC, scaling may be reduced, but pustulation is usually little affected. In PPP, corticosteroid creams or ointments (the latter sometimes combined with coal tar) seem to bring about partial remission in perhaps a third of patients, but continued treatment may not maintain the improvement. Often it is only feasible to treat the hands or feet at night. The effect of corticosteroids is enhanced by polythene occlusion. Hydrocolloid dressings applied every third day on a medium strength corticosteroid is highly effective against PPP (175). On the hands, the hazard of secondary coccal infection is minimal, but atrophy of the skin of the dorsa of the hands can appear quickly. The benefits of such treatment, if any, are usually only temporary (176).

Methotrexate has been used topically, but is not of established value. An aqueous solution containing 1 mg/ml can be applied as a wet compress under polythene occlusion overnight. It is more likely to be helpful in AC than PPP.

Oral Therapy

Tetracycline

The use of tetracycline is time honored in PPP. It seemed to help 40% of patients in one double-blind crossover trial (158,177). The therapy is without risk as well as without rationale and is worth trying for a few weeks. Tetracycline, 250 mg three times daily, is appropriate dosage.

Colchicine

Because colchicine is known to influence neutrophil function, it has been tried in psoriasis vulgaris topically (178) and orally (179) and success has been claimed (180). Its use in PPP was first reported in 1976 (179). Good results have been claimed in a larger series (36). Takigawa and colleagues (18) claimed that in 13 of 32 patients there was complete clearing of pustulation with some improvement in most of the others. These results were achieved with doses of 1–2 mg daily, later reduced to 0.5–1.0 mg daily. These observations were uncontrolled and treatment was begun during periods of disease exacerbation, so spontaneous fluctuation and improvement would be expected in a proportion over the following 4 weeks. Nausea and diarrhea can be troublesome problems for patients receiving higher dosages. Wright and Baker have not had the same success in a small number of patients with PPP: Mann's report documents failure in PPP (182).

Clofazimine

There is evidence that clofazimine can enhance neutrophil phagocytosis, and success in PPP has been reported (183). No larger studies have followed.

Sulfapyridine and Sulfones

There is anecdotal evidence that sulfapyridine and sulfones have sometimes been of value (184,185), but there is no well-documented or controlled evidence of their efficacy in PPP or AC.

Methotrexate

Oral methotrexate is the most effective systemic treatment of psoriasis, but it has long been recognized that PPP and AC are relatively resistant. Nevertheless, some patients can be controlled with conventional dosage of 0.2–0.4 mg/kg once weekly (186). A methotrexate effect on PMNL chemotaxis can be demonstrated (187).

Hydroxyurea

The cytotoxic agent hydroxyurea is less effective than methotrexate in most patterns of psoriasis and this is also true of PPP. Nevertheless, modest success has been reported in PPP (60). There are no reports of its use in AC. Hydroxyurea is known to inhibit neutrophil chemotaxis (187).

Corticosteroids

Oral steroids should be used with caution in pustular psoriasis. Very high dosages of prednisolone followed by abrupt withdrawal in the treatment of chronic AC have precipitated generalized pustular psoriasis (189). There is evidence that small dosages of triamcinolone, not exceeding 8 mg daily with maintenance dosage of 2–4 mg daily, may be effective and safe in PPP (190); this is also our experience. Pulse treatment with adrenocorticotropin (ACTH) or injected steroid should be avoided.

Etretinate

The retinoid etretinate has provided an important new weapon in the management of various patterns of psoriasis. The drug is of value in PPP in a substantial proportion of patients in a dosage of 0.5–1.0 mg/kg daily (191–195). Therapy is not without problems. Apart from the usual well-known effects of synthetic retinoids on the skin, lips, hair, and elsewhere, the strong antiproliferative effect on the epidermis of the palms and soles may abolish scaling and reduce pustulation, leaving a sore, painful bright red glazed skin surface which the patient is unable to tolerate. This problem is not always solved by reducing the dosage.

PUVA Therapy

The introduction of PUVA (psoralen and ultraviolet A) therapy was a real advance in the management of PPP, although it is far from dramatic in its effects. After initial reports of success using oral or topical 8-methoxypsoralen (8-MOP) (196–199), controlled studies have confirmed the value of oral therapy (200). In the latter study 14 to 22 treatments were needed to achieve clearance with mean final UVA dosages between 12 and 17 J/cm^2 (200). The efficacy of topical PUVA has also been demonstrated in a controlled study (201) confirming other reports (202,203). However, response tends to be slower and less complete than with psoriasis vulgaris; up to 40 treatments are sometimes needed to achieve good control (202).

Retinoid-PUVA Therapy

The first open study of retinoid-photochemotherapy combination treatment showed complete clearance of all lesions in 12 patients (204). Controlled studies have confirmed the superiority of Re-PUVA over PUVA alone (205,206). All these studies are marked by the rapid and high relapse rate which follows cessation of therapy.

Cyclosporin A

There have, as yet, been no controlled studies of cyclosporin A (CyA) in localized pustular psoriasis. One case report documents a good response to high-dose CyA (14 mg/kg/day) in a single patient with acrodermatitis continua (207).

REFERENCES

1. Baker, H., and Ryan, T.J., (1968). *Br. J. Dermatol.* 80:771.
2. Karvonen, J., Tillikainen, A., and Lassus, A. (1977). In *Psoriasis: Proceedings of the 2nd International Symposium.* E.M. Farber et al. (Eds.). Yorke Medical Books, New York, p. 405.
3. Michaelson, G. (1980). *Br. J. Dermatol.* 103:351.
4. Ternowitz, T. (1986). *J. Am. Acad. Dermatol.* 15: 1191.
5. Von Zumbusch, L.R. (1910). *Arch. Dermatol. Syphilol. Berlin.* 99:335.
6. Ogawa, M., Baughman, R.D, and Glendenning, W.E. (1969). *Arch. Dermatol.* 99:671.
7. Maguire, A. (1966). *Br. J. Dermatol.* 78:360.
8. Schuppener, H.J. (1958). *Dermatol. Wochenschr.* 138: 841.
9. Aronsson, A, and Nilsson, A. (1986). *Acta Derm. Venereol. (Stockh.)* 66:164.
10. Risum, G. (1973). *Br. J. Dermatol.* 89:309.
11. Craig, J.A. (1974). *Br. Med. J.* 3:43.
12. Feiwel, M., and Ferriman, D. (1957). *Proc. R. Soc. Med.* 50:392.
13. Shelley, W.B. (1964). *JAMA* 189:985.
14. Shelley, W.B. (1967). *JAMA* 201:133.
15. Lowe, N.J., and Ridgeway, H.B. (1978). *Arch. Dermatol.* 114:1788.
16. Reshad, H., Hargreaves, G.K., and Vickers, C.F.H. (1983). *Br. J. Dermatol.* 109:111.
17. Barth, J.H., and Baker, H. (1986). *Br. J. Dermatol.* 115:629.

18a. Katz, M., Seidenbaum, M., and Weinrauch, L. (1987). *J. Am. Acad. Dermatol.* 17:918.

18b. Georgala, S., Rigopoulous, D., Aroni, K., and Stratigos, J.T. (1994). *Int. J. Dermatol.* 33:515–516.

18c. Webster, G.F., Knobler, R.L., Lublin, F.D., Kramer, E.M., and Hochman, L.R. (1996). *J. Am. Acad. Dermatol.* 34:365–367.

19a. Muri, A.D. (1982). *N. Z. Med. J.* 95:711.

19b. Wakefield, P.E., Berger, T.G., and James, W.D. (1990). *Arch. Dermatol.* 126:968–969.

20. Hadida, E., Sayag, J., Tramier, G., and Valette, P. (1969). *Bull. Soc. Fr. Dermatol. Syphiligr.* 76:1095.
21. Hu, C.H., Miller, C.M., Peppercorn, R., and Farber, E.M. (1985). *Arch. Dermatol.* 121:1326.
22a. Hays, S.B., Camisa, L., and Luzar, M.J. (1984). *J. Am. Acad. Dermatol.* 10:619.
22b. Friedman, S.J. (1987). *J. Am. Acad. Dermatol.* 16: 1257.
23. Lindgren, S., and Groth, O. (1976). *Acta Derm. Venereol. (Stockh.)* 56:139.
24. Ryan, T.J., and Baker, H. (1971). *Br. J. Dermatol.* 85: 407.
25. Nicholas, J.F., Mauduit, G., Haoud, J., Chouvet, B., and Thivolet, J. (1988). *Ann. Dermatol. Venereol.* 115:289.
26. Agache, P., Barale, T., and Bonjean, J.M. (1970). *Arch. Belg. Dermatol. Syphilol.* 26:115.
27. Boxley, J.D., Dawber, R.P.R., and Summerly, R. (1975). *Br. Med. J.* 2:255.
28. Carruthers, J.A., August, P.J., and Staughton, R.C.D. (1975). *Br. Med. J.* 4:203.
29. Miyachi, Y., Danno, K.,Yanase, K., and Imamura, S. (1980). *Acta Derm. Venereol. (Stockh.)* 60:66.
30a. Baker, H. (1976). *Br. J. Dermatol.* 94(Suppl. 12):83.
30b. Rosen, R.M. (1991). *J. Am. Acad. Dermatol.* 25: 336–337.
30c. Shimamoto, Y., and Shimamoto, H. (1990). *Cutis* 45: 439–442.
30d. Rongioletti, F., Casciaro, S., Boccaccio, P., and Rebora, A. (1990). *Int. J. Dermatol.* 29:290–292.
31. Zachariae, H. (1977). In *Psoriasis: Proceedings of the 2nd International Symposium.* E.M. Farber et al. (Eds.). Yorke Medical Books, New York, p. 163.
32. Zachariae, H., Petersea, H.O., Nielsen, F.K., and Lamm, L. (1977). *Dermatologica* 154:73.
33. Civatte, A. (1957). *Atlas d'Histologie.* Masson, Paris.
34. Pinkus, H., and Mehregan, A.H. (1969). *A Guide to Dermatohistopathology.* Butterworth, London.
35. Ueharam, M., and Ofuji, S. (1974). *Arch. Dermatol.* 109:518.
36. Neumann, E., and Hard, S. (1974). *Acta Derm. Venereol. (Stockh.)* 54:141.
37. Cotterill, J.A., Roberts, M.M., Freeman, R., King, B., and Moystoufi, K. (1974). *Proc. Ry. Soc. Med.* 67: 874.
38. Tagami, H., and Ofuji, S. (1976). *Br. J. Dermatol.* 95: 1–8.
39. Michaelsson, G. (1980). *Br. J. Dermatol.* 103:351.
40. Preissner, W.C., Schroder, J.M., and Christophers, E. (1983). *Br. J. Dermatol.* 109:1.
41. Langer, A., Chorzelski, T.P., Fraczykowska, M., Jablonska, S., and Szymancyzk, J. (1983). *Arch. Dermatol. Res.* 275:226.
42. Krueger, G.G., Hill, H.R., and Jederberg, W.W. (1978). *J. Invest. Dermatol.* 71:189.
43. Tigonalowska, M., Glinski, W., and Jablonska, S. (1983). *J. Invest. Dermatol.* 81:6.
44. Ternowitz, T. (1986). *J. Am. Acad. Dermatol.* 15: 1191.
45. Brain, S.D., Camp, R., Cunningham, F.M., et al. (1984). *Br. J. Pharmacol.* 83:313.
46. Schroder, J.M., and Christophers, E. (1985). *J. Invest. Dermatol.* 84:444.
47. Takematsu, H., Terui, T., Ohkohchi, K., Tagami, H., Suzuki, R., and Kumagai, K. (1986). *Acta Derm. Venereol. (Stockh.)* 66:93.
48. Luger, T.A., Chavon, J., Colot. M., and Oppenheim, J. (1983). *J. Immunol.* 131:818–820.
49. O'Keefe, E., Braverman, I.M., and Cohen, I. (1973). *Arch. Dermatol.* 107:240.
50. Dawson, T.A.J. (1974). *Br. J. Dermatol.* 91:419.
51. Ridley, C.M. (1981). *Br. J. Dermatol.* 105(Suppl. 19): 39.
52. Hellgren, L., and Mobacken, H. (1971). *Arch. Derm. Venereol. (Stockh.)* 51:284.
53. Tan, R.S.H. (1974). *Br. J. Dermatol.* 91:209.
54. Miyachi, Y., Danno, K., Yanase, K., and Imamura, S. (1980). *Arch. Dermatol. Venereol. (Stockh.)* 60:66.
55. Beylot, C., Bioulae, P., and Doutre, M.S. (1980). *Ann. Dermatol. Venereol.* 107:37.
56. Janier, M., Jayle, D., Laloux, S., and Valensi, F. (1985). *Ann. Dermatol. Venereol.* 112:719.
57. Rouchouse, B., Bonnefoy, M., Pullot, B., Jacquelin, L., Dimoux-Dime, G., and Clandy, A.L. (1986). *Dermatologica* 173:180.
58. Kalb, R., and Grossman, M.E. (1986). *Cutis* 38:58.
59. Jackson, H., Vion, B., and Levy, P.M. (1988). *Dermatologica* 177:292.
60. Binet, O., Beltzer-Garelly, E., and Rougeot, M.A. (1987). *Journ. Dermatol. de Paris,* March.
61. MacMillan, A.L. (1973). *Dermatologica* 146:285.
62. Stanley, J., and Fallou Pellicci, V. (1978). *Arch. Dermatol.* 114:1350.
63. Staughton, R.C.D., Rowland Payne, C.M.E., Harper, J.I., and McMichen, H. (1984). *J.R. Soc. Med.* 77(Suppl. 4):6.
64. Chimenti, S., and Ackerman, B. (1980). *Am. J. Dermatopathol.* 3:363.
65. Braverman, I.M., Cohen, I., and O'Keefe, E. (1972). *Arch. Dermatol.* 105:189.
66. Copeman, P.W.M., and Bold, A.M. (1965). *Proc. R. Soc. Med.* 58:425.
67. Warren, D.J., Winney, R.J., and Beveridge, G.W. (1974). *Br. Med. J.* 2:406.
68. Ryan, T.J., and Baker, H. (1969). *Br. J. Dermatol.* 81: 134.
69. McFadyen, T., and Lyell, A. (1971). *Br. J. Dermatol.* 85:274.
70a. Matta, M. (1974). *Br. J. Dermatol.* 90:309.
70b. Yamamoto, T., Yokozeki, H., Katayama, I., and Nushioka, K. (1995). *Br. J. Dermatol.* 132:1023–1024.

71. Ott, F., Krakowski, A., Tur, E., Lipitz, R., Weisman, Y., and Brenner, S. (1982). *Dermatol.* 4:458.
72. Berger, P.A. (1969). *Br. Med. J.* 2:351.
73. Mackie, R.M., and Burton, J. (1974). *Br. J. Dermatol.* 90:567.
74. Sauder, D.N., Steek, W.D., Bailin, P.B., and Krakauer, R.S. (1981). *J. Am. Acad. Dermatol.* 4:458.
75. Thune, P. (1980). *Dermatologica* 161:179.
76. Dreno, B., Vandermeeren, M.A., Boiteau, H.L., Stalder, J.F., Barriere, H. (1986). *Dermatologica* 173: 209.
77. Yung, C.W., Stephen, R., Soltani, K., and Lorinez, A.L. (1982). *Arch. Dermatol.* 118:432.
78. Von Hebra, F. (1872). *Wien Med. Wochenschr.* 22: 1197.
79. Beveridge, G.W., Harkness, R.A., and Livingstone, J.R.B. (1966). *Br. J. Dermatol.* 78:106.
80. Oumeish, O.Y., Farraj, S.E., and Bataineh, A.S. (1982). *Arch. Dermatol.* 118:103.
81. Pierard, G.E., Pierard-Franchimont, C., and de la Brassine, M. (1983). *Am. J. Dermatopathol.* 5:215.
82. Degos, R., Civatte, J., and Arroy, M. (1966). *Bull. Soc. Franc. Dermatol. Syphilol.* 73:356.
83. Milian, G., and Katchoura, V. (1953). *Bull. Soc. Franc. Dermatol. Syphilol.* 40:851.
84. Rajka, G., and Thune, P.O. (1979). *Acta Derm. Venereol. (Stockh.)* 59(Suppl. 89):143.
85. Bazex, A. (1967). *Bull. Soc. Franc. Dermatol. Syphilol.* 74:689.
86. Baker, H. (1986). Psoriasis. In *Textbook of Dermatology,* 4th edition. A. Rook, D.S. Wilkinson, and J. Ebling (Eds.). Blackwell Scientific Publications, Oxford, p. 1528.
87. Lapiere, S. (1959). *Arch. Belg. Dermatol.* 15:7.
88. Maril, F.G., and Vodov, I. (1974). *Bull. Soc. Franc. Dermatol. Syphilol.* 81:590.
89. Beylot, C., Grupper, C., and Desmons, F. (1973). *Ann. Dermatol. Syphilol.* 100:121.
90. Beylot, C., Bioulac, P., Grupper, C., Desmons, F., Larregue, M., and Maleville, J. (1977). In *Psoriasis: Proceedings of the 2nd International Symposium.* E.M. Farber et al. (Eds.). Yorke Medical Books, New York.
91. Beylot, C., Puissant, A., Bioulac, P., Saurat, J.H., Pringuet, R., and Doutre, M.S. (1979). *Acta Derm. Venereol. (Stockh.)* 59(Suppl. 87):95.
92. Nyfors, A. (1981). *Acta Derm. Venereol. (Stockh.)* 61(Suppl. 95):47.
93. Hubler, W.R. (1984). *Arch. Dermatol.* 120:1174.
94. Khan, S.A., Grant Peterkin, G.A., and Mitchell, P. (1972). *Arch. Dermatol.* 105:67.
95. McGibbon, D.H. (1979). *Clin. Exp. Dermatol.* 4:115.

96a. Henrikson, L., and Zachariae, H. (1972). *Dermatologica* 144:12.

96b. Zelickson, B.D., and Muller, S.A. (1991). *J. Am. Acad. Dermatol.* 24:186–194.

96c. Takematsu, H., Masakazu, R., Takahashi, K., and Tagami, H. (1992). *Arch. Dermatol. Venereol. (Stockh.)* 72:443–444.

96d. Prose, N.S., Fahrner, L.J., Miller, C.R., and Layfield, L. (1994). *J. Am. Acad. Dermatol.* 31:376–379.

96e. Ivker, R.A., Grin-Jorgensen, C.M., Vega, V.K., Hoss, D.M., and Grant-Kels, J.M. *Pediatr. Dermatol.* 10: 277–282.

97. Ryan, T.J., and Baker, H. (1971). *Br. J. Dermatol.* 85: 407.
98. Piamphongsant, T., Nimsuwan, P., Gritiyarangsan, P. (1985). *Clin. Exp. Dermatol.* 10:552.
99. Tuyp, E., Mackie, R.M. (1986). *J. Am. Acad. Dermatol.* 14:70.
100. Shoji, A., Kitajima, J., Hamada, T. (1987). *J. Dermatol. (Tokyo)* 14:274.
101. Zachariae, H. (1988). *Lancet* 1:422.
102. Stein, K.M., Shelley, W.B., and Weinberg, R.A. (1971). *Br. J. Dermatol.* 85:81.
103. Lang, P.G. (1979). *J. Am. Acad. Dermatol.* 68:395.
104. Hellier, F.F. (1956). *Br. J. Dermatol.* 68:395.
105. Sneddon, I.B., and Wilkinson, D.S. (1956). *Br. J. Dermatol.* 68:385.
106. Peachey, R.D.G. (1977). *Br. J. Dermatol.* 97(Suppl. 15):64.
107. Staughton, R. (1977). *Proc. R. Soc. Med.* 70:286.
108. Judge, M., and Black, M.M. (1988). Case presented at The Royal Society of Medicine, London, October 1988.
109. Hall, A.F. (1944). *Arch. Dermatol.* 50:107.
110. Telfer, N.R., and Dawber, R.P.R. (1987). *J. Am. Acad. Dermatol.* 16:144.
111. MacMillan, A.L., and Champion, R.H. (1973). *Br. J. Dermatol.* 88:183.
112. Olsen, E.A., and Cornell, R.C. (1986). 16, 144.
113. Orfanos, C.E. (1982). In *Psoriasis: Proceedings of the 3rd International Symposium* E.M. Farber and A.J. Cox (Eds.). Grune & Stratton, New York, p. 197.
114. Lorand, T., Pierard-Franchimont, J., and de la Brassine, M. (1983). *Dermatologica* 167:159.

115a. Wolska, H., Jablonska, S., Langner, A., and Fraczkowska, M. (1985). *Dermatologica* 171:297.

115b. Rosińska, D., Wolska, H., Jablonska, S., and Konca, I. (1988). *Pediatr. Dermatol.* 5:266–272.

115c. Shelntiz, L.S., Esterly, N.B., and Honig, P.J. (1987). *Arch. Dermatol.* 123:230–233.

116. Gollnick, H., Bauer, R., Brindley, C., Orfanos, C.E., Plewig, G., Wokalek, H., Hoting, E., et al. (1988). *J. Am. Acad. Dermatol.* 19:458.
117. Fitzpatrick, T.B., Stern, R.S., and Parrish, J.A. (1982). In *Psoriasis: Proceedings of the 3rd International Symposium.* E.M. Farber and A.J. Cox (Eds.). Grune & Stratton, New York, p. 149.
118. Henseler, T., Wolff, K., Honigsmann, H., and Christophers, E. (1981). *Lancet* 1:853.

119. Wolff, K., and Fritsch, P.O. (1982). In *Psoriasis: Proceedings of the 3rd International Symposium.* E.M. Farber and A.J. Cox (Eds.). Grune & Stratton, New York.
120. Orfanos, C.E. (1984). *Acta Derm. Venereol. (Stockh.)* (Suppl. 112):37.
121a. Kettler, A.H., Baughn, R.E., Orengo, I.F., Black, H., and Wolf, J.E. (1988). *J. Am. Acad. Dermatol.* 18: 1267.
121b. CHuprapaislip, T., and Piamphongsant, T. (1978). *Br. J. Dermatol.* 99:303–305.
121c. Nair, L.V. and Shercef, P.H. (1991). *Int. J. Dermatol.* 30:151.
122. Mudler, W., and Hermann, B. (1979). *N. Engl. J. Med.* 301:555.
123. Harper, J.I., Keat, A.C.S., Staughton, R.D.D. (1984). *Lancet* 2:981.
124. Wentzeu, J.M., Baughman, R.D., O'Connor, G.T., and Bernier, G.M. (1987). *Arch. Dermatol.* 123: 163–165.
125. Meinardi, M.M.H.M., Westerhof, W., and Bos, J.D. (1987). *Br. J. Dermatol.* 116:269–270.
126a. Zachariae, H., and Thesdup-Pederson, K. (1987). *Dermatologica* 175:29–32.
126b. Peter, R.U., Ruzicka, T., Donhauser, G., and Braun-Falco, O. (1990). *J. Am. Acad. Dermatol.* 23: 515–516.
127a. Aubin, F., Blanc, D., Quencez, E., Zultak, M., and Agache, P. (1988). *Dermatologica* 177:247–248.
127b. Berth-Jones, J., Bourke, J., Bailey, K., Graham-Brown, R.A.C., and Hutchinson, P.E. (1992). *Br. Med. J.* 305:868–869.
128. Crocker, H.R. (1888). *Diseases of the Skin.* H.K. Lewis, London, p. 128.
129. Audry, C.H. (1901). *Ann. Dermatol. Syphilol. Paris.* 12:913.
130. Dore, S.E. (1928). *Br. J. Dermatol.* 40:12.
131. Barber, H.W. (1930). *Br. J. Dermatol.* 42:500.
132. Ingram, J.T. (1930). *Br. J. Dermatol.* 42:489.
133. Andrews, G.C. (1934). *Arch. Dermatol. Syphilol.* 29: 548.
134. Andrews, G.C., and Machacek, G.F. (1935). *Arch. Dermatol. Syphilol.* 32:766.
135. Sachs, W., Mackee, G.M., and Rothstein, M.J. (1947). *Arch Dermatol. Syphilol.* 56:766.
136. Bonnevie, P. (1939). *Aetiologie und Pathogenese der Ekzemkrankheiten.* Copenhagen, p. 28.
137. Lever, W.F. (1967). *Histopathology of the Skin.* J.B. Lippincott, Philadelphia, p. 149.
138. Baker, H. (1984). *Dermatol. Clin. North. Am.* 2:455.
139. Ashurst, P.J.C. (1964). *Br. J. Dermatol.* 76:169.
140. Hellgren, L., and Mobacken, H. (1971). *Acta Derm. Venereol. (Stockh.)* 51:284.
141. Everall, J. (1957). *Br. J. Dermatol.* 69:269.
142. Ono, T., Jono, M., Kito, M., Tomoda, T., Kageshita, T., Eguwa, K., and Kuriya, N. (1983). *Acta Otolaryngol.* 401(Suppl.):12.
143. O'Doherty, C.J., and MacIntyre, C. (1985). *Br. Med. J.* 291:864.
144. Cox, N.H., and Ray, S. (1987). *Int. J. Dermatol.* 26: 445.
145. White, S.W. (1982). *J. Am. Acad. Dermatol.* 7:660.
146. Hallberg, D., and Molin, L. (1974). *Acta Derm. Venereol. (Stockh.).* 54:155.
147. Lever, W.F., and Shaumberg-Lever, G. (1983). *Histopathology of the Skin.* J.B. Lippincott, Philadelphia, p. 146.
148. Uehara, M., and Ofuji, S. (1974). *Arch. Dermatol.* 109:518.
149. Pierard, J., and Kint, A. (1978). *Ann. Dermatol. Venereol. (Paris)* 105:681.
150. Ward, J.M., and Barnes, R.M.R. (1978). *Br. J. Dermatol.* 99:477.
151. de la Brassine et al. (1982). In *Psoriasis: Proceedings of the 3rd International Symposium.* E.M. Farber et al. (Eds.). Grune & Stratton, New York, p. 285.
152. Okhaido, M., Ozawa, A., Nakagawa, M., Tsuji, K. (1982). In *Psoriasis: Proceedings of the 3rd International Symposium.* E.M. Farber et al. (Eds.). Grune & Stratton, New York, p. 287.
153. Rosen, K., Lindholm, A., Mobacken, H., and Sandberg, L. (1982). *Dermatol. Monatsschr.* 168:182.
154. Ternowitz, T. (1986). *J. Am. Acad. Dermatol.* 15: 1191.
155. Jurik, A.G., Ternowitz, T., and Grundal, H. (1988). *Dermatologica* 176:161.
156. Cartwright, P.H., Ilderton, E., Sowdon, J.M., and Yardley, H.J. (1988). Paper presented at the British Society for Investigative Dermatology, Manchester, England, September 1988.
157. Rosen, K. (1988). *Acta Derm. Venereol. (Stockh.)* 68(Suppl. 121):1.
158. Thomsen, K., and Osterbye, P. (1973). *Br. J. Dermatol.* 89:293.
159. Zone, J. (1986). In *Clinical Dermatology.* D.J. Dermis, R.G. Crowise, R.L. Dobson, and J.S. McGuire (Eds.). Harper & Row, Philadelphia, 1 Unit 1–4:1.
160. Tan, R.S.H. (1974). *Br. J. Dermatol.* 91:209.
161. Miyachi, Y., Danno, K., Yanase, K., and Imamura, S. (1980). *Acta Derm. Venereol. (Stockh.)* 60:66.
162. Enfors, W., and Molin, L. (1971). *Acta Derm. Venereol. (Stockh.)* 51:289.
163. Ishibashi, A., Nishiyama, Y., Endo, M., Kawaji, W., and Kato, T. (1977). *J. Dermatol. (Tokyo)* 4:53.
164. Bergdahl, K., Bjorksten, B., Gustavson, K.H., and Liden, S. (1979). *Dermatologica* 159:37.
165. Sonozaki, H., Kawashima, M., Hongo, O. et al. (1981). *Ann. Rheum. Dis.* 40:547.
166. Sonozaki, H., Mitsui, H., Miyanaga, Y. et al. (1981). *Ann. Rheum. Dis.* 40:554.

167. Hradil, E., Gentz, C.F., Matilainen, T., Moller, H., Sanzen, L., and Uden, A. (1988). *Acta Derm. Venereol. (Stockh.)* 68:65.
168. Hallopeau, H. (1897). *Ann. Dermatol. Syphilol. Paris.* 8:473.
169. Crocker, H.R. (1903). *Diseases of the Skin,* 3rd edition. H.K. Lewis, London, p. 196.
170. Mahowald, M.L., and Parrish, R.M. (1982). *Arch. Dermatol.* 118:434.
171. Baker, H., Ryan, T.J. (1968). *Br. J. Dermatol.* 80:771.
172. Moulin, G. (1974). *Bull. Soc. Franc. Dermatol. Syphilol.* Paris 8:473.
173. O'Keefe, E., Braverman, I.M., and Cohen, I. (1973). *Arch. Dermatol.* 107:240.
174. Hjorth, N., and Thomsen, K. (1967). *Br. J. Dermatol.* 79:527.
175. Kragballe, K., and Larsen, F.G. (1991). *Acta. Derm. Venereol. (Stockh.)* 71:540.
176. Allenby, C.F. (1966). *Br. J. Dermatol.* 78:154.
177. Ward, J.M., Corbett, M.F., and Hanna, M.J. (1976). *Br. J. Dermatol.* 95:317.
178. Kaidbey, K.H., Petrozzi, J.W., and Kligman, A.M. (1975). *Arch. Dermatol.* 60:515.
179. Mori, S., Hino, K., and Izumi, H. (1976). *Jpn. J. Dermatol.* 86:671.
180. Wahba, A., and Cohen, H. (1980). *Acta Derm. Venereol. (Stockh.)* 60:515.
181. Takigawa, M., Miyachi, Y., Uchara, M., and Tagami, H. (1982). *Arch. Dermatol.* 118:458.
182. Mann, R.J. (1982). *Br. J. Dermatol.* 106:373.
183. Molin, L. (1975). *Acta Derm. Venereol. (Stockh.)* 55:151.
184. Ridley, M. (1981). *Br. J. Dermatol.* 105(Suppl. 19):39.
185. Lang, P.G. (1979). *J. Am. Acad. Dermatol.* 1:479.
186. Thomsen, K. (1971). *Acta Derm. Venereol. (Stockh.)* 51:397.
187. Cream, J.J., and Pole, D.D. (1980). *Br. J. Dermatol.* 102:557.
188. Hattel, T., and Sondergaard, J. (1974). *Acta Derm. Venereol. (Stockh.)* 54:152.
189. Calkins, E., Reznick, L., and Bauer, W. (1957). *N. Engl. J. Med.* 256:245.
190. Robinson, T.W.E. (1966). *Br. J. Dermatol.* 78:158.
191. Thune, P. (1982). *Dermatologica* 164:67.
192. Reymann, F. (1982) *Dermatologica* 164:209.
193. Jansen, C. et al. (1979). *Acta Derm. Venereol. (Stockh.)* 59:271.
194a. White, S.I., Puttick, L., and Marks, J.M. (1986). *Br. J. Dermatol.* 115:577.
195. White, S.I., Marks, J.M., and Shuster, S. (1985). *Br. J. Dermatol.* 113:581.
196. Menne, J. (1976). *Ugeskr. Laeger.* 138:3119.
197. Weber, G. (1974). *Br. J. Dermatol.* 90:317.
198. Lakshmipathi, T., Gould, P.W., Mackenzie, L.A., Johnson, B.E., and Frain-Bell, W. (1977). *Br. J. Dermatol.* 96:587.
199. Mizuno, N., Uematsu, S., and Ohno, M. (1976). *Arch. Dermatol.* 112:883.
200. Morison, W.L., Parrish, J.A., and Fitzpatrick, T.B. (1978). *Br. J. Dermatol.* 99:297.
201. Murray, D., and Warin, A.P. (1979). *Br. J. Dermatol.* 101(Suppl. 17):13.
202. Abel, E.A., Goldberg, L.H., and Farber, E.M. (1980). *Arch. Dermatol.* 116:1257.
203. Wilkinson, J.D., Ralfs, I.G., Harper, J.I., and Black, M.M. (1979). *Acta Derm. Venereol. (Stockh.)* 59(Suppl. 89):193.
204. Fritsch, P.O., Honigsmann, H., Jasche, E. et al. (1978). *J. Invest. Dermatol.* 70:178.
205. Lawrence, C.M., Marks, J.M., Parker, S. et al. (1984). *Br. J. Dermatol.* 110:221.
206. Rosen, K., Mobacken, H., and Swanbeck, G. (1987). *Arch. Dermatol.* 123:885.
207. Zachariae, H., and Thesdrup-Pedersen, K. (1987). *Dermatologica* 175:29.

3

The Nails

Richard K. Scher
College of Physicians and Surgeons, Columbia University, New York, New York

CLINICAL FEATURES

The clinical features of psoriasis of the nails depend upon which foci of the nail unit are involved (1). A thorough understanding of the anatomy is essential to comprehend the features seen in the nail unit grossly (2).

The components of the nail consist of the following parts: the proximal and lateral nail folds, the nail matrix, the nail bed, and the hyponychium (3) (Fig. 1). Some regard the distal phalanx to be part of the nail unit (4). Since the distal phalanx is the location of the psoriatic arthritis [Fig. 2 (Color Plate 1)] with its concomitant nail changes in more than 90% of cases, it is best included here as a nail unit component. The proximal nail fold is a skin fold that lies over the proximal portion of the matrix and the proximal portion of the plate (the nail root). The lateral nail folds encompass the nail plate on both sides. Psoriatic involvement of these structures produces the typical clinical appearance of psoriasis of the skin [Fig. 3 (Color Plate 1)].

Lying beneath the proximal fold is the matrix, which is responsible for the manufacture and development of the plate (5). The plate represents the horny end product of the matrix. Structurally the matrix may be divided into three parts: a proximal portion, producing the superficial portion of the plate; an intermediate, producing the central part of the plate; and a distal, the lunula, producing the under surface of the plate. The lunula is visible in certain digits as the half moon (6).

When psoriasis involves the proximal portion of the nail matrix, the nail plate reveals pitting [Fig. 4 (Color Plate 1)]. The pathogenesis involves abnormal keratinization with parakeratosis in the proximal nail matrix which produces retained nuclei on the surface of the nail plate (7). As the nail plate grows beyond the proximal nail fold, these retained nuclei are cast off and give rise to pitting. Pitting in psoriasis tends to occur in a random, disorderly fashion; the pits generally tend to be large and deep. This is in contradistinction to the pitting in other conditions such as alopecia areata in which the indentations tend to be in rows and are more superficial. When the intermediate portion of the matrix is involved and the proximal nail matrix is normal, the clinical appearance is generally seen as a focus of leukonychia. The abnormal keratinization is within the plate, appearing as a white spot. Distal nail matrix or lunula involvement may be more difficult to detect because its clinical manifestation may be either as a focus of onycholysis or a somewhat thinned nail plate [Fig. 5 (Color Plate 1)]. Other changes noted in the plate secondary to nail matrix disease would be longitudinal grooves and ridges when the psoriatic involvement is arranged in a longitudinal fashion throughout the nail matrix. Conversely, transverse depressions (Beau's lines) may ap-

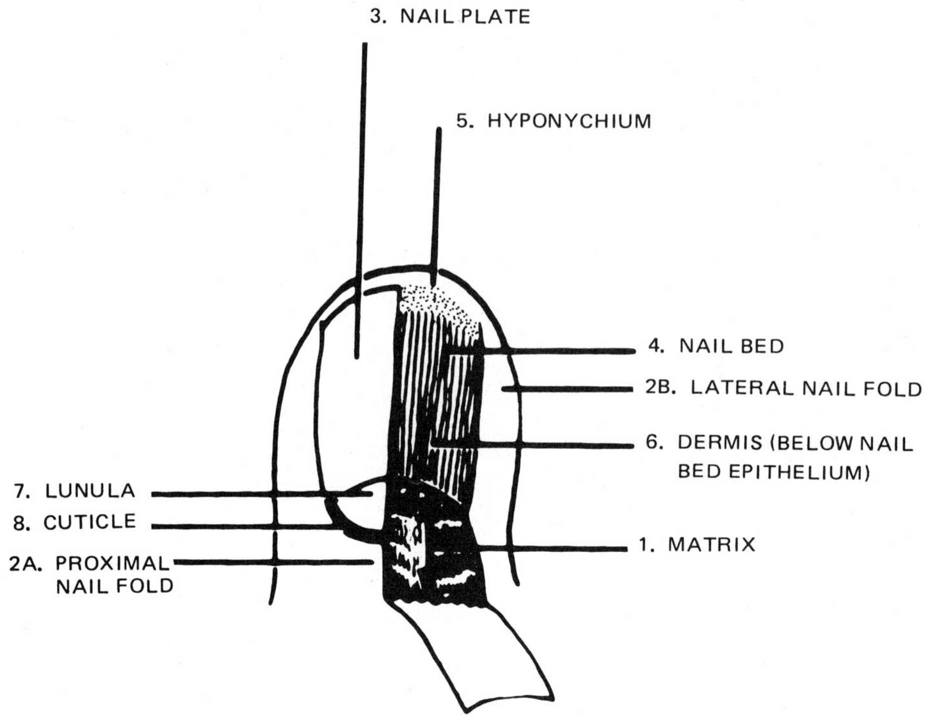

Figure 1 Anatomy of the nail unit. (From Ref. 1.)

pear if the psoriatic process has that configuration. Erythema of the lunula may also occasionally be evident. Nail bed psoriasis may present clinically as a reddish brownish discoloration of the nail bed and appear as an "oil drop" [Fig. 6 (Color Plate 1)] change beneath the plate (8). Other changes seen clinically are simple erythema and hyperkeratosis of the epithelium of the nail bed, resulting in prominent subungual hyperkeratosis [Fig. 7 (Color Plate 1)]. When the subungual hyperkeratosis is extensive, it causes crumbling of the plate [Fig. 8 (Color Plate 1)] with actual secondary destruction of this portion of the nail unit. Splinter hemorrhages are common [Fig. 9 (Color Plate 1)]. Hyponychial psoriasis can present as a combination of distal onycholysis, "oil drop" change, and subungual hyperkeratosis.

Figure 2 Distal interphalangeal joint psoriatic arthritis associated with psoriatic onychodystrophy.

Figure 3 Psoriasis of the proximal and lateral nail folds associated with psoriatic onychodystrophy.

Figure 4 Psoriatic stippling of the nail plate; randomly arranged, deep-seated pits.

Figure 5 Onychatrophy: thinning of the nail plate due to focal psoriasis mainly in the distal matrix.

Figure 6 "Oil drop" sign of the nail bed: discoloration secondary to psoriasis at this site.

Figure 7 Subungual hyperkeratosis secondary to hypertropy of the cornified cells of the nail bed and hyponychium.

Figure 8 Crumbling of the nail plate secondary to extensive subungual hyperkeratosis.

Figure 9 Splinter hemorrhages of the nail bed: a consequence of focal bleeding points analogous to Auspitz' sign in the skin.

Plate 1

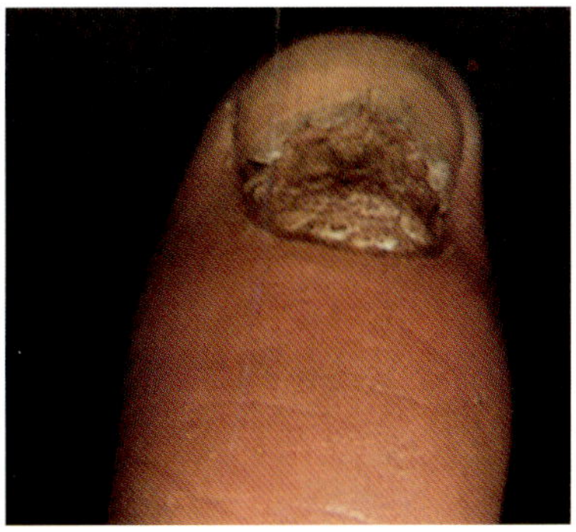

Figure 2

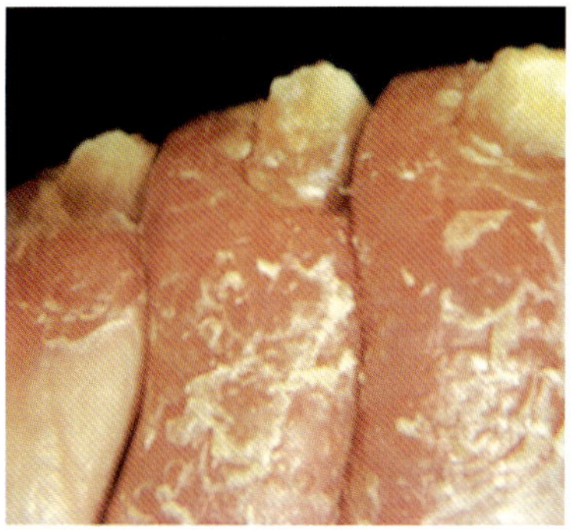

Figure 3

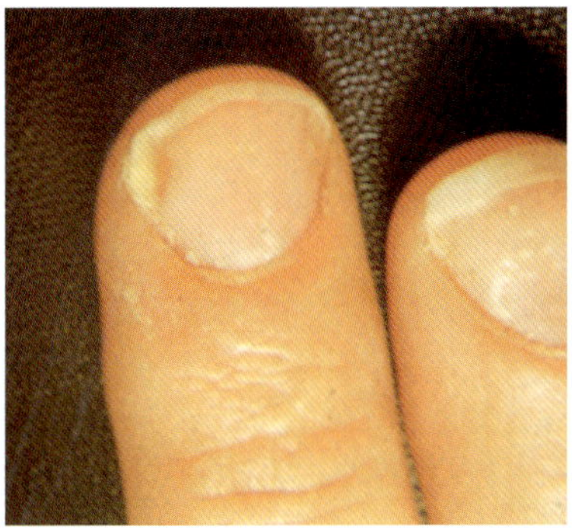

Figure 4

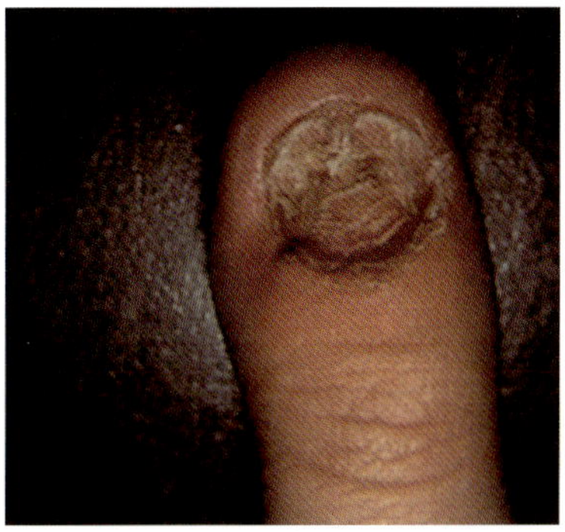

Figure 5

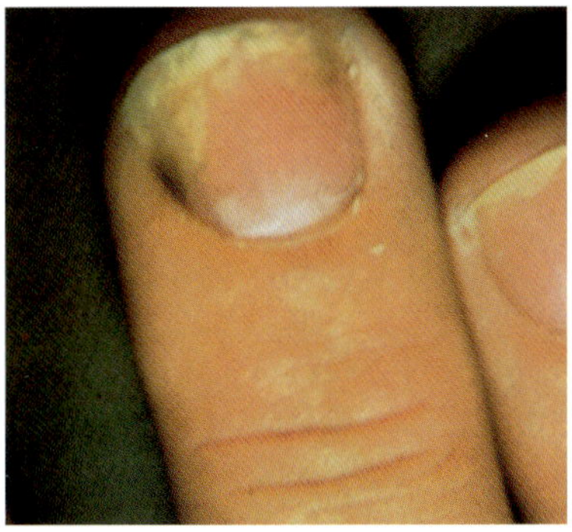

Figure 6

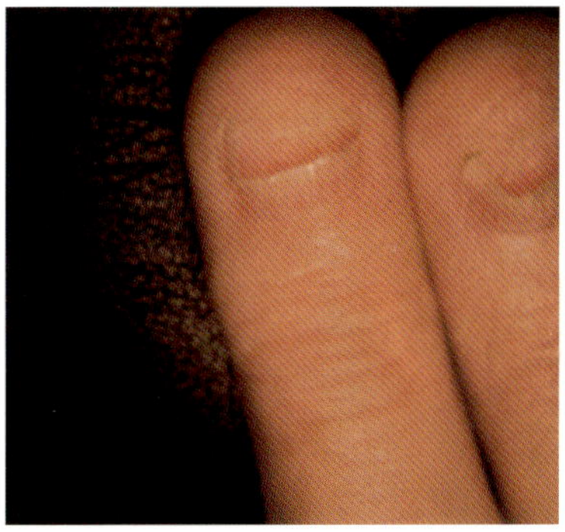

Figure 7

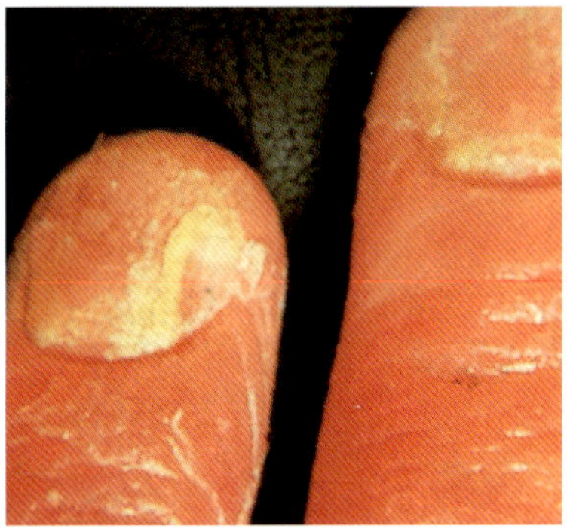

Figure 8

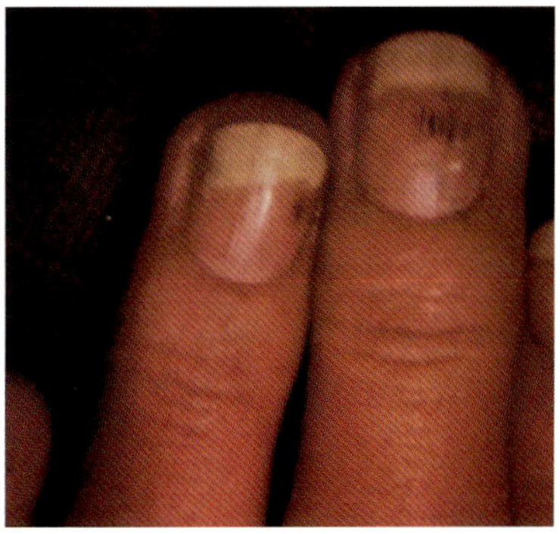

Figure 9

In summary, the clinical manifestations of psoriasis of the nail unit may range from minimal, in the form of simple pitting, to extensive changes involving virtually the entire nail apparatus with extensive destruction and changes sufficient to interfere with normal function.

THERAPY

The mainstay treatment of psoriatic nails consists of intralesional corticosteroids. This involves the use of triamcinolone acetonide in a concentration of 2.5 mg/ml injected into the proximal nail fold every 3–4 weeks for a total of four to six injections (9). The need for subsequent injections depends upon frequency and extent of recurrences. The corticoid may be diluted with normal saline or a 1% plain local anesthetic such as lidocaine. A 30-gauge needle should always be used and a freezing spray applied first to minimize pain. This modality is most effective for pitting, longitudinal ridging, and leukonychia because matrix psoriasis is responsible. Since the proximal nail fold overlies the matrix, the steroid is being instilled at the ideal site.

When the clinical manifestation is subungual hyperkeratosis, the "oil drop" sign, or distal onycholysis, this treatment is less effective. Logically, the intralesional injection in these instances should be placed in the nail bed—the site of the pathology. Since this would be too painful, it is not feasible unless prior anesthesia is administered. However, injecting the lateral nail folds close to the bed will often overcome this disadvantage. Another alternative is to use high-potency topical steroids under occlusion (10) after cutting back all of the onycholytic nail and gently curetting the foci of the hyperkeratosis. This approach unfortunately affords less than optimal results. In any case, it is not recommended for children under 12 years of age or for more than two weeks at a time. Atrophy and telangiectasia of the skin may occur as well as damage to the underlying distal phalanx. One percent 5-fluorouracil solution may be effective (11). Its use should be limited to those patients who have either matrix disease (i.e., pitting) or marked subungual hyperkeratosis due to nail bed disease. For distal onycholysis, this regimen is not indicated, as it often aggravates the condition.

In severe cases of psoriasis of the nails, methotrexate has been used similarly to its use in incapacitating cutaneous psoriasis. However, the use of this approach for nail disease alone seems highly questionable.

UVA—with oral or topical psoralens—is effective (12), as has been oral etretinate (13) and acitretin.

Recently, calcipotriol has been successful for cutaneous psoriasis. Its efficiency in psoriatic nails has not yet been proved.

REFERENCES

1. Basuk, P.J., Scher, R.K., Ricci, A.R. (1997). Dermatologic diseases of the nail unit. In *Nails: Therapy, Surgery, Diagnosis.* R.K. Scher and C.R. Daniel, III (Eds.). W.B. Saunders Co., Philadelphia, pp. 172–200.
2. Scher, R.K. (1989). The nail. In *Dermatologic Surgery,* Principles and Practice. R.K. Roenigk and H.H. Roenigk, Jr. (Eds.). Marcel Dekker, New York, p. 509.
3. Scher, R.K. (1979). Nail surgery. In *Techniques in Skin Surgery.* E. Epstein and E. Epstein, Jr. (Eds.). Lea & Febiger, Philadelphia, pp. 164–166.
4. Baran, R., and Dawber, R.P.R. (Eds.). (1994). *Diseases of the Nails and Their Management.* Blackwell Scientific Publications, Oxford, p. 2.
5. Zaias, N. (1990). *The Nail in Health and Disease.* S.P. Medical and Scientific Books—Spectrum Publications, Inc., New York, pp. 2–3.
6. Samman, P.D., and Fenton, D.A. (1986). *The Nails in Disease,* 4th ed. William Heinemann Medical Books Ltd., London, pp. 6–7.
7. Zaias, N. (1966). Psoriasis of the nail. *Arch. Dermatol.* 99:567–579.
8. Kouskoukis, C.E., Scher, R.K., and Ackerman, A.B. (1983). Biopsies of nails: the "oil drop" sign of psoriatic nails—a clinical finding specific for psoriasis. *Am. J. Dermatopathol.* 5:259–260.
9. Scher, R.K. (1981). Nail diseases. In *Office Dermatology.* H.H. Roenigk, Jr. (Ed.). Williams & Wilkins, Baltimore, p. 144.
10. Scher, R.K. Psoriasis of the nail. In Daniel, III, C.R., (Ed.). Symposium on the Nail. *Dermatol. Clinics.* 3: 387–394, 1985. W.B. Saunders Co., Philadelphia.
11. Fredriksson, T. (1974). Topically applied fluorouracil in treatment of psoriatic nails. *Arch. Dermatol.* 110: 735–736.
12. Marx, J.L., and Scher, R.K. (1980). Response of psoriatic nails to oral photochemotherapy. *Arch. Dermatol.* 116:1023–1024.
13. Rabinovitz, H.S., Scher, R.K., and Shupack, J.T. (1983). Response of psoriatic nails to the aromatic retinoid etretinate. *Arch. Dermatol.* 119:627–628.

4

Scalp and Hair, Palms and Soles

Janice Matsunaga
John A. Burns School of Medicine, Honolulu, Hawaii

Howard I. Maibach and Ernst Epstein
University of California School of Medicine, San Francisco, California

SCALP AND HAIR

Psoriasis is a dermatological disorder that affects not only the cutaneous surface but also other ectodermal structures such as nails, hair, and rarely, mucous membranes. Psoriatic alopecia was described by Schuster (1); the hairs in plaques of psoriasis were noted to be clinically less dense, with many dystrophic or telogen bulbs [Fig. 1 (Color Plate 1)]. Several of his patients also showed some thinning of the hair in unaffected areas of their scalp. In still others, he noted a "scarring" alopecia, showing perifollicular inflammation and fibrosis histologically. Recently, Wright and Messenger (1a) described three patients with scalp psoriasis that had never been pustular or erythrodermic. They developed true scarring alopecia. Histologically these cases showed "chronic inflammatory cells around the infundibular region of the hair follicle." Sebaceous glands were also noted to be absent, along with partial to complete destruction of the follicular epithelium. Even though the histologic picture was not specific for psoriasis, the authors suggest an association between the inflammatory changes of the scalp psoriasis resulting in a scarring alopecia. It is already well known that the erythrodermic and pustular forms of psoriasis can and often do involve extensive hair loss.

Proper epidemiological and complete biological description does not exist. With the exception of antimetabolite treatment-induced anagen alopecia, the mechanisms of hair loss remain obscure. In the former, mitotic inhibition is assumed to be the mechanism. Fortunately, most psoriatic patients' plaques respond to dosages of methotrexate and thioguanine sufficiently low to make this kind of alopecia uncommon. When present, regrowth occurs with lowered dosages of medication. The pathognomonic broken, tapered hair shaft allows differentiation of this drug etiology from the more obscure idiopathic hair loss of psoriasis (2).

In the "idiopathic" form, loss ranges from minimal or slowly developing telogen effluvium to rapid acute shedding of clumps of hair, leading to almost total alopecia. Possibly because of observer bias (i.e., our inpatient unit), the most striking examples occur in patients with the greatest extent and severity of scalp plaques. Although hair loss is more obvious in women, we do not know if a true sex difference exists. Loss may occur in areas with minimal or no obvious plaque involvement; possibly in response to a systemic factor, reminiscent of the typical acute telogen effluvium.

On scanning electron microscopy hair shafts may be significantly thinner in psoriatic plaques than in unaffected skin or in normal persons. Dystrophy of the hair is also seen more frequently in psoriatic patients (3). This may facilitate breakage of the hair from traumatic rubbing while medications are applied and scales removed.

It is interesting that despite increased epidermal turnover in psoriatic plaques all compartments of the hair follicle except for the upper external root sheath show normal epidermopoiesis (4). Hair growth rate is similar in normal controls and lesional as well as nonlesional skin in psoriatic patients (5), implicating a dermal rather than epidermal regulator in this condition.

Treatment Failures: Role of Debridement

In countries where patients have free choice of physicians, many go from dermatologist to dermatologist seeking a panacea for their troublesome, itching, scaling scalp. There are very few more dramatic causes of needless dissatisfaction with dermatological counsel.

Failures relate largely to three factors. First, for reasons not documented, most topical treatments fail to resolve scalp lesions until thick, hyperkeratotic scales have been removed [Figs. 2 and 3 (Color Plate 1)]. The conventional theory is that scales minimize drug flux. Although this may be the case for the scalp, it is not so for plaques on glabrous skin where the penetration of hydrocortisone quantitatively resembles that on normal skin (6).

Scales can be nontraumatically removed after softening. This can be done with commercial oil solutions such as Baker's P & S solution, but we have found liberal amounts of inexpensive mineral oil to be quite adequate. Some minutes later, gentle debridement with a fine-toothed baby's comb removes the scales easily. With extensive involvement this is best done by a nurse, parent, spouse, or someone else in the home. Commercial shampoo machines such as those used in beauty salons are useful for psoriasis day care centers or for inpatients. After one or two such debridements (which may require repetition from time to time), recalcitrant lesions suddenly respond. A bland shampoo after the oil and comb debridement helps make the procedure tolerable. Keratolytics such as Kerilyte gel or Epilyte lotion may also effectively aid in the softening of the scales.

The second cause of failure is a lack of recognition that picking and scratching in themselves will perpetuate the process via the isomorphic Koebner response. Like many habits, this may be difficult to break. Nevertheless with appropriate topical therapy and careful explanation of the mechanism to the patient, most cases of difficult scalp psoriasis will respond.

The third and last cause is occult irritation or allergic contact dermatitis. Neither demonstrate typical morphology on the scalp and are only diagnosed with a high index of suspicion and appropriate patch testing.

Therapy

Corticosteroid Lotions

Application of corticosteroid lotions (e.g., triamcinolone acetonide 0.025% or 0.1% in propylene glycol, clobetasol propionate scalp solution, fluocinonide solution, hydrocortisone butyrate solution) to the scalp results in clinical improvement in psoriasis. The major effects of topically applied corticosteroids include vasoconstriction, reduction in inflammation, and a decrease in epidermal mitotic activity (7,8). Absorption through the skin is doubled by skin stripping and enhanced up to 10 times by occlusion (9). This can be accomplished with a plastic shower cap or plastic wrap under a bathing cap. The scalp is many times more permeable to hydrocortisone (and some other chemicals) than the forearm (10). Keratolytics (salicylic acid) may also be used in conjunction with topical steroids to facilitate penetration. Occasionally, corticoid lotions may cause irritation, especially on broken or damaged skin. Often the vehicle (e.g., propylene glycol) may produce severe subjective irritation, burning, and stinging. With respect to the current potent and superpotent topical corticosteroids, prolonged use can result in development of atrophy, striae, telangiectasias, and tachyphylaxis. Caution is

Figure 1 Psoriatic alopecia of the scalp.

Figure 2 Abundant micaceous psoriatic scaling of scalp.

Figure 3 Thick hyperkeratotic psoriatic scale.

Plate 1

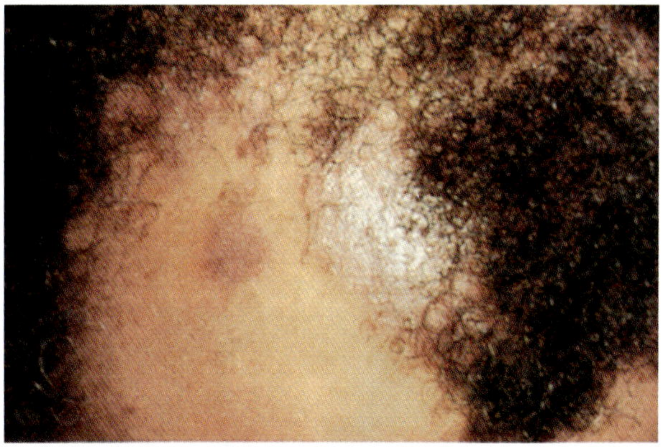

Figure 1

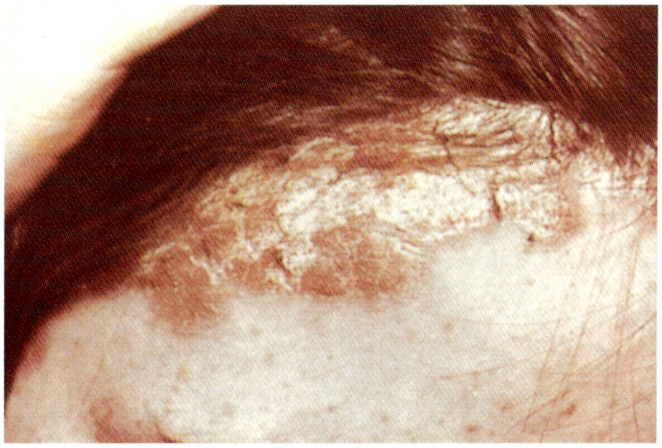

Figure 2

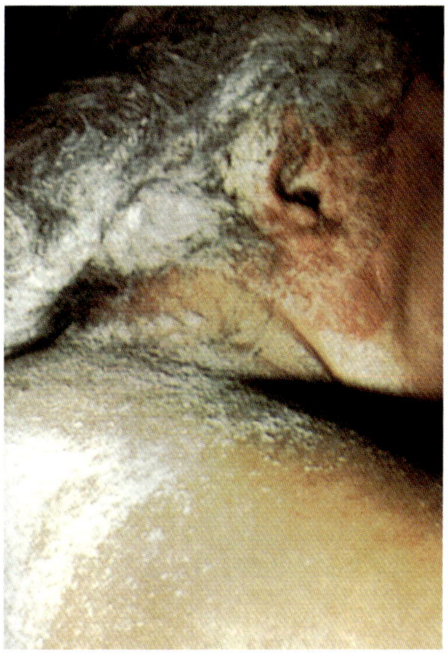

Figure 3

Table 1 Tar Shampoos

Formulation	Percentage active substance
DHS Tar Shampoo	0.5 Coal tar
Denorex Shampoo, gel	9 Coal tar solution
Neutrogena T/Gel Therapeutic Shampoo	2 Solubilized coal tar extract
P & S Plus	8 Coal tar solution (1.6 crude coal tar), 2 salicylic acid
Pentrax Tar Shampoo	4.3 Crude coal tar
Tegrin Medicated Shampoo	5 Alcohol extract of coal tar
Sebutone	0.5 Coal tar, 2 sulfur, 2 salicylic acid
X-seb T	10 Coal tar solution, 4 salicylic acid
Zetar	1 Whole coal tar

needed to avoid these potential side effects from occurring by limiting the amount and duration of treatment and refraining from use of occlusion.

The side effects of topical corticoids chronically applied to the scalp have not been specifically examined. One would expect more adrenal suppression potential per unit area of scalp than most other sites because of enhanced penetration. Corticoids are potent antimitotic agents in human skin (11). We have produced marked suppression of hair growth on the forearm in experimental studies with high-potency topical corticoids. We still do not have a well-documented dose-response curve for these preparations, however.

Intralesional Steroids

In certain cases of psoriasis of the scalp, a few localized, discrete plaques are present. These may respond to topical corticosteroids as described above, or medicated shampoos. Another alternative is injection of the corticosteroid directly into the psoriatic plaques. This obviates the need to have the steroid penetrate the stratum corneum into the epidermis. This method is particularly useful for the smaller, thick, resistant plaques.

Tar Preparations

Crude coal tar contains a mixture of many hydrocarbons. Its presumed primary mode of action is suppression of epidermal cell deoxyribonucleic acid (DNA) synthesis, as shown in the hairless mouse model (12). There is also evidence that the epidermis becomes atrophic with prolonged use after a transient hyperplasia in human skin (13). Coal tar shampoos (Table 1) containing between 2.00 and 8.75% coal tar extract have been proven to be effective and safe in the treatment of psoriasis and other scaling dermatoses of the hair and scalp (14). Use of these shampoos suppresses DNA synthesis substantially better than vehicle alone (15). The shampoo is generally applied to the hair, lathered, then left on for 5–10 min before being rinsed thoroughly.

Patients' acceptance of tar shampoos varies. Some are unable to tolerate the strong odor and others will note staining of their light hair after prolonged use. On damaged or broken scalp, tar can irritate. When it is used as the sole treatment of areas with thick plaques, it is often insufficient to eradicate the problem.

Liquor carbonis detergens (LCD) in concentrations of 5–20% can be applied to the scalp as a lotion overnight to treat particularly thick plaques. Keratolytics may be added to enhance sloughing of the scale. A shower cap is required to protect bed linens, however. Shampooing in the morning will remove the residue.

Zinc Pyrithione

One and 2% zinc pyrithione (Table 2) in a shampoo base has been shown to be safe and effective for scalp psoriasis (16,17). Presumably it decreases the cell

Table 2 Zinc Pyrithione Shampoos

Formulation	Percentage zinc pyrithione
Danex Protein-Enriched Dandruff Shampoo	1
DHS Zinc	2
Head and Shoulders	2
Zincon Dandruff Shampoo	1

turnover rate in hyperproliferative dermatoses such as psoriasis. It is not easily absorbed through intact epidermis or mucous membranes, but is soluble in sebum and penetrates into hair follicles, thereby resisting removal by rinsing (18). Irritation and hypersensitivity are generally low. Between shampoos, a 0.1–0.25% zinc pyrithione hair tonic can be used.

Anthralin

Anthralin was extensively used by Ingram in treating psoriasis, and he found it to be highly effective (19). Since that time, interest in anthralin has been sporadic because of the major side effects of irritation and staining of normal skin and the rapid oxidation of the compound. Lowe and Breeding tested various strengths of anthralin and found that at a concentration between 0.1 and 0.4% anthralin in Eucerin there was a significant suppression in DNA synthesis in the hairless mouse model (20). Baxter and Stoughton observed a decreased epidermal mitotic index with anthralin and even with simple occlusion, though to a much lesser extent in the latter (21). Anthralin can be separated by column chromatography into its pure form, an anthralin dimer and 1,8-dihydroxyanthroquinone (22). Only the pure form was found to be active, however. A scalp pomade of 0.4% anthralin in petrolatum has also been shown to be effective in psoriasis when applied with warm mineral oil under occlusion for 2 hr and then washed off with a tar shampoo (23). Commercial preparations of anthralin in various dosages can also be applied to the scalp for 15–60 min daily before shampooing completely. A major limiting factor with anthralin scalp pomades is the possibility of inadvertent transfer to the eyes with resultant potentially severe irritation.

"20:10:5" Ointment

Oil of Cade, 20%, 10% precipitated sulfur, and 5% salicylic acid in petrolatum are used together for resistant cases of psoriasis of the scalp. The salicylic acid softens the stratum corneum which is subsequently shed. Sulfur also causes injury to the epidermis and contributes to exfoliation. The use of this time-honored remedy is mainly limited to the inpatient or day care center because of the odor and inconvenience.

Chloroxine (Capitrol)

Chloroxine (5,7-dichloro-8-hydroxyquinoline) is a synthetic antibacterial and cytostatic compound which can be formulated with a shampoo base and used in the treatment of scalp psoriasis. Irritation of the scalp has been reported as has allergic contact dermatitis to some of the ingredient compounds. As with other shampoos, blond, gray, or bleached hair can become discolored. Excessive drying and pruritus of the scalp have also been noted in some patients.

Selenium Sulfide

Other shampoos effective in decreasing the epidermal turnover rate in psoriasis are those containing selenium sulfide 1.0–2.5% (e.g., Exsel, Selsun) (24). When used on undamaged skin this compound appears to be just as effective or slightly superior to 2.0% zinc pyrithione, 2.0% sulfur with 2% salicylic acid, or 0.5% selenium sulfide. Among the drawbacks with this preparation are; (1) discoloration of hair, especially red tones, if the shampoo is poorly rinsed off; (2) rebound "oiliness" of the hair and scalp once the shampoo is stopped; (3) stinging of the eyes with conjunctival contact; and (4) excessive dryness of the hair necessitating the use of a conditioner. If it is used for prolonged periods of time on open or damaged skin, it can cause tremors, hyperhidrosis, lower abdominal pain, weakness, lethargy, decreased appetite, and emesis (25).

Sulfur-Salicylic Acid

Another shampoo formulation containing precipitated sulfur and salicylic acid has been found safe and effective for use in the treatment of psoriasis of the scalp (e.g., Fostex, Sebulex). One main drawback is the strong odor.

Ketoconazole and Imidazoles

Recently, the role of topical and systemic ketoconazole in the treatment of recalcitrant scalp psoriasis has been discussed, but controlled studies have yet to be done to prove its efficacy. Some believe that Candida or Pityrosporum may be partially involved in psoriasis. Treatment with oral or topical ketoconazole or imidazoles have, in some instances, reversed some of the psoriatic lesions. Combinations of tar shampoos, topical corticosteroids, and ketoconazole appear to be superior to ketoconazole alone (26). Because of the usual necessity for a prolonged course of ketoconazole to improve the scalp, the risk of hepatic toxicity must constantly be borne in mind.

Calcipotriene/Calcipotriol

The vitamin D_3 analog, calcipotriene has recently been released for use in psoriasis. Its benefits have been documented in studies. Its effectiveness does not seem to be as dramatic as with the superpotent topical corticosteroids or with betamethasone 17-valerate solution, but the long-term side effects of corticosteroids are not seen and tachyphylaxis does not seem to be a risk factor. Its main side effect is local irritation and pruritus especially if it is inadvertently applied to the face. It was once thought that hypercalcemia might present a problem with this medication, but if less than 100 g/week is applied, this problem rarely occurs.

At present, the ointment solution and cream are available in the United States. Some patients object to applying the greasy ointment preparation to their scalp. One technique that can be utilized is to mix equal amounts of calcipotriene ointment and a hair conditioner together and then apply it directly to the affected areas in the scalp. Future studies of calcipotriene combinations with other topical as well as systemic psoriasis therapies may further define its role in the armamentarium of treatment modalities.

Antimicrobials

Although considered somewhat controversial at the present time, various antimicrobial agents may be helpful in addition to the traditional therapies for psoriasis. It has long been known that group A or B beta-hemolytic *Streptococcus* can produce a guttate flare of psoriasis. In the process of working up a particularly difficult patient, a history, physical examination, and laboratory assessment can sometimes shed some light on possible microbial factors that may be present.

For instance, psoriasis which affects the seborrheic distribution may be due to *Malassezia.* A patient who is immunosuppressed or has diabetes may have colonization with *Candida.* Involvement of the hands and feet may signal a dermatophyte secondary infection. Stains, culture, KOH preparations, streptococcal titers, and other laboratory examinations may further clarify a significant source for treatment. Appropriate antimicrobial therapy can then be initiated.

Fluorouracil

Although infrequently used today, topical 5% fluorouracil under occlusion, particularly on relatively sparse hair-bearing areas of the scalp, has been used successfully in the past. If it is applied daily, it can cause painful erosions to occur. A pulse regimen when used 2–3 days/week produces less side effects. Erythema is another possible side effect. In studies conducted using this medication on psoriatic plaques, there were no systemic toxicities.

Comments

Scaling of the scalp is often unsightly and symptomatic. Fortunately, although none of our therapies is curative, the compounds described above, when appropriately utilized, control the process in most. Nevertheless, much work remains to be done. Most agents have a far from dramatic effect when judged objectively. They decrease scale and reduce itching but only partially. They are more effective at reducing loose scale than adherent scale. More potent agents or ones with improved pharmacokinetics are needed. Furthermore, we need controlled information on drug tolerance. Most dermatologists and patients empirically change from one drug to another as a result of a lack of satisfaction and knowledge of the likelihood of drug tolerance. Measures to prevent and control psoriasis of the scalp can help to limit the extent of the disease. Avoidance of trauma to the scalp, such as vigorous massaging, combing, brushing, permanents, hair dyes, and scratching away the scale, should be taught to our patients.

PALMS AND SOLES

Psoriasis of the palms and soles may occur by itself with no evidence of psoriasis elsewhere, or be part of typical psoriasis. When severe, the fissuring and hyperkeratosis of palmar and plantar psoriasis often interferes with the patient's daily life, especially working and walking. While mild palmoplantar psoriasis requires little more than lubricants, severe palmoplantar psoriasis responds poorly to treatment and is a major challenge for the dermatologist.

Diagnosis

When there is psoriasis elsewhere, the diagnosis of palmoplantar psoriasis can usually be made confidently on clinical grounds except on the feet where dermatophytosis not uncommonly coexists with psoriasis. When the diagnosis of psoriasis is not obvious, i.e., when there is no clear-cut psoriasis elsewhere, the patient must be questioned closely as to personal and family history of endogenous dermatitis and psoriasis. Sometimes only persistent questioning—almost an interrogation—yields the vital information of a parent or sibling with psoriasis. Persons who have had episodes of localized psoriasis in the past often need their memory jogged to recall an episode of elbow scaling or gluteal cleft fissuring and perianal itching. In the absence of obvious psoriasis elsewhere, it is mandatory to examine the entire skin of the patient. This includes the perianal area, the penis, the soles, and the ears. Those who undress patients often find clear-cut psoriasis perianally or a patch of dermatitis on a sole or ankle in patients who repeatedly denied skin problems other than on their hands.

The morphology of palmar psoriasis is often typical with sharply demarcated, red scaling plaques stopping on the palm-wrist juncture. Involvement of the digits generally stops at the sides of the fingers. Frequently, there is hyperkeratosis over the knuckles. Pitting of the fingernails in the presence of normal-appearing paronychial skin is practically pathognomonic of psoriasis. Palmoplantar psoriasis is almost always bilateral; when only one palm or sole is involved, repeated searches for dermatophyte infection by microscopic examination of scales cleared with potassium hydroxide (KOH) is mandatory.

Tiny deep-set vesicles appearing in clusters are a common feature of palmoplantar psoriasis. When deep-set blisters predominate, and only the palms and soles are involved, the differential diagnosis between psoriasis limited to the palms and soles versus pustulosis palmaris et plantaris is impossible. There is evidence, based on HLA studies (31,32), that palmoplantar pustulosis is a different entity from palmoplantar psoriasis. Nevertheless, some patients with the clinical picture of pustulosis palmaris et plantaris will, after a course of years, develop psoriasis elsewhere.

Table 3 Differential Diagnosis of Palmoplantar Psoriasis

1. Dermatophytosis
2. Contact dermatitis: mainly feet
3. Other chronic lichenified palmoplantar dermatoses; i.e., keratoderma climactericum
4. Pompholyx (dyshidrosis)
5. Pustulosis palmaris et plantaris
6. Keratosis palmaris et plantaris and related genodermatoses
7. Unusual presentations of lichen planus, discoid lupus erythematosus, bullous pemphigoid, and other endogenous skin disorders
8. Bowen's disease, amelanotic melanoma, and other skin neoplasms

Differential Diagnosis (Table 3)

Dermatophytosis

Dermatophytosis heads the differential diagnostic list because we are dealing with a disorder much more treatable than palmoplantar psoriasis. Tinea manum can perfectly mimic palmar psoriasis. Tinea pedis not only mimics plantar psoriasis, but on the feet psoriasis and a dermatophyte infection may coexist. It is sometimes difficult to demonstrate fungi in tinea manum and tinea pedis; repeated microscopic examination of KOH-cleared scales should be done when a dermatophyte infection is suspected.

Contact Dermatitis

While bilateral palmar dermatoses are practically never solely caused by contact allergy, contact allergy to topical medicaments may significantly aggravate them. More commonly, irritation from topical medicaments is a frequent aggravating factor in palmar psoriasis. Unilateral palmar psoriasiform rashes should trigger some searching questions by the dermatologist, since there are cases where contact allergy to a wooden knife handle or other grasped object has produced a lichenified contact dermatitis morphologically simulating psoriasis. Allergy to shoe insoles may produce contact dermatitis of the feet clinically indistinguishable from psoriasis. Shoe contact dermatitis coexisting with psoriasis is fortunately uncommon, but the possibility should be kept in mind.

Other Chronic Lichenified Palmoplantar Dermatoses

There are significant numbers of patients with chronic lichenified palmar and/or plantar dermatoses which defy accurate classification (33). Physicians label these according to their training or current fashion. Chronic eczema, keratoderma, and hyperkeratotic eczema are such "waste basket" terms. Chronic hyperkeratotic dermatitis appearing in women at menopause has been termed keratoderma climactericum; there is doubt whether this is an entity. All these disorders are endogenous, that is, the result of an unknown skin dysfunction, and share a similar response to treatment.

Pompholyx

Pompholyx is the preferred term for a condition characterized by recurring groups and crops of small- to medium-sized blisters on the palms, soles, and often affecting the sides of the digits. Although the term dyshidrosis is frequently used to describe this disorder, we dislike this term as it implies malfunction of the sweat glands, which is not the case.

Pustulosis Palmaris et Plantaris

As mentioned earlier, pustulosis palmaris et plantaris may be indistinguishable from psoriasis.

Keratosis Palmaris et Plantaris

Keratosis palmaris et plantaris is usually morphologically distinct, differing from psoriasis by its uniformity of involvement and lack of inflammation. Almost always inherited as a dominant trait, a positive family history can usually be obtained. Occasional cases will present diagnostic difficulty, as may keratosis palmaris et plantaris punctata.

Other Skin Disorders

On rare occasion, lichen planus, discoid lupus erythematosus, bullous pemphigoid, granuloma annulare, and other skin disorders may present on the palmar or plantar surfaces with little or no involvement elsewhere (34). Usually, the morphology provides diagnostic clues; at times a biopsy is required for diagnosis.

Neoplasms

Bowen's disease, amelanotic melanoma, and other neoplasms may mimic a patch of chronic dermatitis. When confronted with a solitary patch of palmar or plantar dermatitis which fails to clear with therapy, perform a biopsy.

Biopsy

Biopsies of classic palmar and plantar psoriasis rarely show the features diagnostic of psoriasis. This is basically a clinical diagnosis, biopsy confirmation is rarely obtained and, in our experience, is not needed. Biopsies are indicated when another disorder, such as lichen planus or discoid lupus erythematosus, is suspected.

Treatment

Treating palmoplantar psoriasis often tests the skill of the dermatologist and the endurance of the patient. Patients need the stimulation of a positive and directed therapeutic approach while being gently led to an understanding of the chronic nature of their disorder. Guarded optimism is justified, for in many patients palmoplantar psoriasis, once controlled, retains its improved state with simple lubrication and protective measures. Treatment depends on severity. Table 4 outlines the therapeutic sequence we favor.

Protective Measures

Protective measures must be combined with topical or systemic agents. This is mainly a problem for the hands. Psoriasis damages the skin's barrier function. Consequently, water, detergents, fruit juices, etc., which are innocuous to normal palmar skin, will significantly aggravate dermatitic skin. Not only do soaps, solvents, and repeated wetting and drying aggravate palmar psoriasis, so does friction. Repetitive friction is poorly tolerated; glove protection is critical. Gloves should be worn for gardening, hammering, and other similar tasks to avoid friction. When the patient's hands are performing wet work or are exposed to paints and irritating solvents, waterproof or other impermeable gloves should be worn.

A systematic program for hand protection is essential. A printed instruction sheet (Table 5) provides details. The patient should not be simply handed the hand protection sheet; significant points should be emphasized by the physician and the patient instructed to read this daily for 1 week. On follow-up visits, question patients in detail as to their implementation of protective gloves and avoidance of irritants. The irritant effect of dry and cold air is often overlooked; leather gloves should be worn to protect the hands from the desiccating effects of dry and cold air.

A common source of irritants are topical medicaments. Many over-the-counter lubricants, creams, lotions, and healing ointments are mild but definite irritants. Frequently, patients severely aggravate their palmoplantar psoriasis by treatment with highly irritating antifungal preparations. The printed treatment instructions—which we urge you to use—emphasize that the patient is not to apply anything to the rash except what you prescribe. It is important to stress this repeatedly verbally as well.

Unfortunately, physicians may fall into the trap of prescribing an irritant in the form of a corticoid-containing gel or solution or a strong urea preparation. Most corticoid gels and solutions contain solvents which have a significant irritant potential. While they are useful on the scalp, do not routinely use them on palms or soles.

Table 4 Treatment of Palmoplantar Psoriasis

A. MINIMAL PSORIASIS. Hydrocortisone-containing lubricant (HCL*) plus protective measures (PM†)
B. MILD PSORIASIS. HCL* plus mid-strength corticoid ointment applied bedtime without occlusion plus PM†
C. MODERATE PSORIASIS. 1% or 2.5% hydrocortisone ointment (petrolatum base) used overnight with plastic occlusion‡ plus daytime HcCL* plus PM†
D. SEVERE PSORIASIS OR MODERATE PSORIASIS NOT RESPONDING TO ABOVE MEASURES. A stepwise approach is useful, beginning with the simplest measures. In addition to the procedures outlined, all patients should use HCL* and PM†.
   1. A mid-strength topical corticoid, e.g., 0.1% triamcinolone acetonide ointment, used under occlusion.‡ Caution: skin thinning.
   2. Localized psoriasis responds to intralesional injections of repository corticoids; we recommend triamcinolone acetonide suspension 10 mg/ml.
   3. Acute cases may benefit from a 2–4 week course of oral prednisone, preferably in an every other day schedule.
   4. PUVA therapy. If performed with topically applied 8-methoxypsoralen, eye precautions are not needed.
   5. Cytotoxic drugs, e.g., methotrexate
   6. Retinoids, e.g., etretinate, acitretin
   7. Topicals: tar, anthralin, 5 FU.
   8. Cyclosporine
   9. Other radiation modalities: high-dose UVB, grenz ray, superficial x-ray.

*HCL = hydrocortisone-containing lubricant. A useful formulation is 2.5% hydrocortisone ointment (petrolatum base) 20 g, 1% hydrocortisone cream q.s. 120 g. See discussion in text.
†PM = protective measures. Described in Figure 2.
‡For hands use *pliable* disposable plastic gloves. They can usually be reused for 2–3 days. For foot occlusion, cover with a plastic kitchen storage or sandwich bag cut off at the ankle and held in place with socks.

Lubrication

Lubricating palmoplantar skin is an important part of treatment, for it helps to prevent the painful fissuring as well as the scaling. White petrolatum (Vaseline) is an ideal lubricant; however, most patients find it messy to use. If used thinly—applying it microscopically thinly and then wiping off the excess with a paper tissue—some patients will use white petrolatum successfully as a lubricant.

There are many commercial hand and other skin lubricants available. These are usually oil and water emulsions and in general have only a mild lubricating effect. They are simply not greasy enough. Some are irritating because of the surfactants and preservatives used in their systems. White petrolatum can be mixed into a water-washable cream base to provide additional lubrication. We have found that as long as the percentage of white petrolatum is kept below approximately 20%, most patients find the lubricant cosmetically acceptable.

One of us employs 1% hydrocortisone in such a petrolatum-water washable cream mixture to lubricate and control mild dermatitis. A practical way to provide such a hydrocortisone-containing lubricant is to have the pharmacist mix 20 g of hydrocortisone ointment 2.5% (petrolatum base, i.e., Hytone ointment, etc.) with 1% hydrocortisone cream to a total of 120 g. This provides a white petrolatum concentration of about 17% and a hydrocortisone concentration slightly over 1%. It is useful to have the pharmacist dispense this in two jars of 60 g each. One jar is to be kept in the kitchen, the other in the bathroom. Instruct the patients not to screw the lid down after each use so that after each hand washing it is just a matter of seconds to lift the cap off, scoop up a small amount of the lubricant with a finger, and then massage it thinly into the entire skin of both hands. It is also helpful to provide the patient with an empty 15-g jar which they are to fill from the larger jars and take with them to work or when traveling. In those patients fortunate enough to have clearing of their psoriasis, we encourage continuing systematic long-term use of lubricants.

Topical Agents

Corticosteroids are the mainstays of topically applied medicaments. While we use tar and anthralin with enthusiasm on psoriasis elsewhere, on the palms and soles our experience with them has been disappointing. Topical and intralesional 5-fluorouracil have recently been described as being effective in plaque psoriasis (35). To our knowledge, there are no studies on

Table 5 Instruction Sheet Detailing Protective Measures To Be Followed By All Patients with Hand Dermatitis

Hand Protection for Hand Dermatitis
Hand dermatitis (hand eczema is another name for the same thing) is common. Hand rashes usually result from a combination of (1) sensitive skin; and (2) irritation or allergy from materials touched. Everyone's hands routinely touch irritating soaps and detergents several times a day. Add the raw foods, solvents, paints, oils, greases, acids, glues, and so on that most of us touch at work or in the home, and you can see that the skin of your hands takes a beating.
Not everyone gets hand dermatitis. Many lucky persons have "tough" skin, but, unfortunately, some persons have skin that's easily damaged. The result is dermatitis. Persons with hand dermatitis often have dermatitis elsewhere, and frequently blood relatives have hand dermatitis. We can't toughen your skin, but we have effective treatment to heal your dermatitis.
Skin protection is an important part of treatment. This instruction sheet gives you detailed directions on how to protect your hands. Please read it carefully every day for a week to fix these instructions in your mind.
1. Protect your hands from direct contact with soaps, detergents, scouring powders, and similar irritating chemicals by wearing waterproof, heavy-duty vinyl gloves. Heavy-duty vinyl gloves (such as Allerderm brand) are better than rubber gloves, since you may become allergic to rubber. Heavy-duty vinyl gloves are usually available at paint and hardware stores. Buy four or five pairs so they can be conveniently located in kitchen, bathroom, and laundry areas. If a glove develops a hole, *discard it immediately*! Wearing a glove with a hole is worse than wearing no gloves at all.
2. The waterproof, heavy-duty vinyl gloves may be lined or unlined. You should have enough waterproof gloves so that the insides of the gloves can dry between wearings.
3. Wear waterproof gloves while peeling and squeezing lemons, oranges, or grapefruit, peeling potatoes, and handling tomatoes.
4. Wear leather or heavy-duty fabric gloves when doing dry work and gardening. Dirty your gloves—not your hands. If you keep house for your family, scatter a dozen pairs of cheap cotton gloves about your home and use them while doing dry housework. When they get dirty, put them in the washing machine. Wash your gloves—not your hands.
5. If you have an automatic dishwasher, use it as much as possible. If you don't, let a member of your family do the dishes. Do your laundry by machine, not by hand.
6. Avoid direct contact with turpentine, paint thinner, paints, and floor, furniture, metal, and shoe polishes. They contain irritating solvents. When using them, wear heavy-duty waterproof gloves.
7. When washing your hands, use lukewarm water and very little mild soap. Rinse the soap off carefully and dry gently. All soaps are irritating. No soap is "gentle to your skin" except in the minds of advertising writers—so don't waste your money on special soaps or "soap-free" cleansers.
8. Rings often worsen dermatitis by trapping irritating materials beneath them. Remove your rings when doing housework and before washing your hands.
9. When outdoors in cold or windy weather, wear unlined leather gloves to protect your hands from drying and chapping.
10. Use only the prescribed medicines and lubricants. Do not use other lotions, creams, or medications—they may irritate your skin.
11. Protect your hands for at least four months *after* your dermatitis has healed. It takes a long time for skin to recover, and unless you're careful the dermatitis may recur.
There is no fast, "magic" treament for hand dermatitis. Your skin must be given a rest from irritation. Follow these instructions carefully.

palmoplantar psoriasis with this agent. While the future holds promise of other topical agents, such as the vitamin D analogues, at present we are forced to rely on topical corticoids.

For minimal psoriasis, a lubricant, preferably containing about 1% hydrocortisone, is often all that is needed to control scaling and dryness. When there is mild psoriasis, it is useful to augment this daytime hand lubrication regimen with bedtime use of a midstrength corticoid ointment applied without occlusion. Triamcinolone acetonide ointment, 0.1%, in petrolatum is an inexpensive and practical choice. If there is a poor response, one is tempted to increase the bedtime corticoid and go to a high-strength corticoid or even one of the superhigh-strength (class I) corticoids. Unfortunately, superpotent corticoids, such as clobetasol propionate (Temovate in the United States; Dermovate in Britain), can cause skin thinning even when used only once daily. We generally prefer a trial of hydrocortisone in petrolatum under occlusion rather than increasing the strength of the bedtime corticoid.

For moderate psoriasis, or mild psoriasis that does not respond to a midstrength corticoid at bedtime without occlusion, use of 1.0 or 2.5% hydrocortisone in petrolatum applied at bedtime and occluded with plastic gloves overnight is often very effective. Long-term occlusion increases the penetration of a corticoid approximately 10-fold, but this is not its only beneficial effect. It has been shown that occlusion by itself may heal plaque-type psoriasis (36). By using a hydrocortisone ointment overnight with occlusion, one gets the benefit of a corticoid which does not cause significant skin thinning along with the beneficial effects of occlusion. For patients to properly use overnight occlusive treatment on the hands, detailed instructions are helpful. They are provided in Table 6. Once the psoriasis is controlled, the patient is gradually weaned off the occlusion, and this approach is described in another patient instruction sheet (Table 7). When using occlusive treatment, it is best to use a corticoid in petrolatum to avoid the irritant or allergenic effects of the surfactants and preservatives present in all cream-type bases.

For severe psoriasis, or moderate psoriasis not responding to the measures described above, a mid-strength topical corticoid ointment used under occlusion is often effective. Skin thinning is a troublesome complication, especially on the fingertips. Often, the skin thinning effect with its fissuring, tenderness, and easy bleeding is misdiagnosed as part of the psoriasis and ever increasingly stronger topical corticoids are employed. The palms and soles are more resistant to this skin-thinning effect. In fact, in severe hyperkeratotic psoriasis of the soles, it is sometimes desirable to use superpotent corticoids under occlusion for their skin-thinning effect. This should be carefully monitored by the physician to ensure the patient uses this only on the greatly thickened areas, and the treatment is modified as soon as the excessive hyperkeratosis is controlled.

Psoriasis Not Responding to Topical Corticoids

Unfortunately, many psoriatics do not respond well to topical corticoids. Even with skillfully employed occlusion, the psoriasis continues to blister, fissure, and

Table 6 Hand Dermatitis Instructions: Initiation of Occlusive Treatment

1. Covering skin overnight with plastic increases the penetration and effectiveness of cortisone medicines. For hand dermatitis, you should wear plastic gloves overnight after applying a cortisone to your rash. You will receive a special cortisone to be used only at bedtime. Please follow these directions carefully.
2. At bedtime, apply ______________________ (a cortisone) thinly to the rash areas only, do *not* apply it to normal skin. Then put on the plastic gloves, taking them off in the morning. The plastic gloves should be soft and pliable. Our office uses B-D Disposable Vinyl Examining Gloves and they can be re-used until they develop holes. They are made in four sizes, your proper size is: Small Medium Large Extra-large. If your druggist does not stock them, our receptionist can tell you where to buy them.
3. At first, wearing the plastic gloves may be uncomfortable. It usually takes a few days to get used to them.
4. The cortisone ointment–plastic glove treatment can make your skin become thin. You should use it exactly as directed on this sheet. It is important to apply the cortisone medicine *only to the rash* when using plastic gloves. Do *not* apply the cortisone medicine to normal skin. If your fingertips are normal, cut the fingertips off your gloves, as the plastic covering softens skin. If your rash is on only one or two fingers, cut fingers from the plastic glove and hold them in place with a nonirritating paper tape such as Micropore tape.
5. Housewives can benefit from plastic covering by applying the cortisone medicine to the *rash areas only* before putting on their heavy-duty plastic (or rubber) gloves for dishwashing and other wet work.
6. During the day, apply the prescribed medicated hand lubricant thinly to the *entire* skin of both hands. The daytime lubricant can be used as often as desired, and should be used after each hand washing. Apply the hand lubricant at least 10 times a day! If the daytime hand lubricant is not greasy enough, you may apply white petrolatum (Vaseline) very thinly *after* applying the daytime hand lubricant.
7. DO NOT USE ANY CREAMS, LOTIONS, OR OINTMENTS EXCEPT AS INSTRUCTED.
8. Pamper your hands by following the hand-protection instructions.
9. When washing your hands, use lukewarm water and very little mild soap. Rinse the soap off well and dry gently. Then apply a little medicated hand lubricant and massage in well.
10. CAUTION: Strong cortisones covered with plastic may cause your skin to thin and crack easily. The strong cortisone-plastic covering combined treatment should be used only under close medical supervision. As soon as your rash is better, we will provide directions for long-term control of your hand dermatitis.

Table 7 Hand Dermatitis Instructions: Continuation of Occlusive Treatment

1. When your hand dermatitis is better, the overnight plastic treatment will be used less often. It is important to gradually decrease the treatment and not suddenly stop it.
2. When your skin has nearly healed, start using the cortisone medicine and plastic covering every *other* night. If your hand dermatitis improves as expected, you should start this about ____________________. On the nights you are not wearing plastic gloves use ____________________ at bedtime.
3. If you do well wearing gloves only every other night, after about 2 weeks, wear them only every third night. If your hands remain clear while using the plastic covering every third night, after 3–4 weeks you may try stopping the plastic glove treatment.
4. These directions are rough guides; the exact timing depends on the condition of your skin. If your rash gets worse when you switch to plastic every *other* night, return to the every night treatment. Later when the rash gets better, again try starting the every other night plastic covering.
5. While you are gradually using less and less of the nighttime plastic glove treatment, keep up frequent applications of the daytime hand lubricant. It is also important that you continue to protect your hands carefully, as described in the hand-protection instructions.
6. Some patients find that as soon as they completely stop wearing plastic gloves, the hand rash returns. If this happens, use the cortisone medicine overnight plastic glove treatment one or two times a week as needed to keep the rash under control.
7. IMPORTANT CAUTION. Strong cortisones covered with plastic may cause skin thinning, which results in skin cracking easily. To prevent skin thinning, be sure to use the strong cortisone–plastic glove treatment less often as soon as the rash is better.
8. When your hand rash has cleared, see if regular use of the medicated hand lubricant and careful hand protection will keep your skin free of rash. Continue the medicated hand lubricant and the hand protection routines for at least 4 months after healing. It takes a long time for skin to recover.
9. Cortisone medicines keep for years at room temperature. As long as the prescriptions are refillable, if you need more medicine, take the *original container* to your pharmacist for your refill. If you have used up all the authorized refills, please make an appointment for a check-up visit.
10. Patients with hand dermatitis often have recurrences. Should your hand dermatitis recur, begin with every night plastic covering until you are better, then use it less and less. If your rash does not get better after 1 week of every night treatment, stop it and return to this office so your treatment can be changed.

otherwise incapacitate the patient. Our approach is a stepwise one, proceeding from the simpler to the more complex and more toxic methods.

Repository Corticoid Injection

If there are only a few areas of psoriasis, intralesional injection of a repository corticoid is usually dramatically effective in providing a remission of 3–6 months. We prefer triamcinolone acetonide, 10 mg/ml, injected with a tuberculin-type syringe and 30-gauge needle. The procedure is painful; refrigeration analgesia using ethyl chloride or a similar spray makes it more tolerable.

Prednisone

Patients with acute swelling and blistering may benefit from a 2–4 week course of prednisone. The aim is to prepare the skin for topical corticoid therapy. Every other day prednisone is preferable to a daily dose. The risk is that of corticoid addiction with the patient flaring severely whenever the corticoid is stopped.

Psoralen and Ultraviolet A Therapy

In a significant number of psoriatic patients who fail to respond to topical corticoids (37,38), PUVA will clear and control the lesions. The treatment is slow and can be tricky, especially when topical 8-methoxypsoralen is used because of the small margin between an effective dose and burning. However, topically applied 8-methoxypsoralen has the advantage that eye protection is not needed. The treatment can be adapted to home maintenance use with commercially available black light bulbs (39).

Cytotoxic Drugs

Patients with life-ruining palmoplantar psoriasis who fail to respond to simpler measures may be controlled with oral methotrexate. The toxicity of this drug, especially on the liver when used over a long time, means that it should be an agent of last resort.

Retinoids

Etretinate (40) and acitretin may be dramatically effective in clearing psoriasis. As with cytotoxic agents, their significant toxicity limits long-term use.

Cyclosporine

Cyclosporine, a potent, albeit toxic, suppressor of psoriasis is covered in another chapter. Low-dose cyclosporine has been found effective in the closely related palmoplantar pustulosis (41).

Radiation Therapy

Conventional superficial x-ray therapy is effective in temporarily suppressing palmoplantar psoriasis. Most dermatologists feel that radiation therapy has no place in a benign, chronic disorder. The less toxic grenz ray therapy is of little benefit on the thick palmoplantar skin.

Summary of Treatment

The majority of patients with palmoplantar psoriasis can be controlled with careful use of lubricants, avoidance of irritants, and application of topical corticoids. Occlusion is of great benefit, both in increasing penetration of corticoids and because of its beneficial effect on psoriasis. Skin thinning with resultant fissuring and skin fragility remains a common side effect of potent topical corticoids, which is often unrecognized by physicians. There remain a significant number of patients who do not respond to these measures; therapy for them is difficult and frustrating.

REFERENCES

1. Schuster, S. (1972). Psoriatic alopecia. *Br. J. Dermatol.* 87:73–77. 1a. Wright, A.L., and Messenger, A.G. (1990). Scarring alopecia in psoriasis. *Acta Derm. Venereol. (Stockh).* 70:156–159.
2. Maguire, H., and Maibach, H. (1964). Acute hair loss from drug-induced abortion. *N. Engl. J. Med.* 270: 1112–113.
3. Wyatt, E., Bottoms, E., and Comaish, S. (1972). Abnormal hair shafts in psoriasis on scanning electron microscopy. *Br. J. Dermatol.* 87:368–373.
4. Shahrad, P., and Marks, R. (1976). Hair follicle kinetics in psoriasis. *Br. J. Dermatol.* 94:7–12.
5. Comaish, S. (1969). Autoradiographic studies of hair growth in various dermatoses: investigation of a possible circadian rhythm in human hair growth. *Br. J. Dermatol.* 81:283–288.
6. Wester, R.C., Bucks, D.A.W., and Maibach, H.I. (1983). In vivo percutaneous absorption of hydrocortisone in psoriatic patients and normal volunteers. *J. Am. Acad. Dermatol.* 8:645–647.
7. Maibach, H., and Stoughton, R. (1973). Topical corticosteroids. *Med. Clin. North Am.* 57(5):1253–1264.
8. Engel, D.J.C., Marx, A.F., Rekker, R.F., and van Wijk, L. (1974). Topically active corticosteroids. *Arch. Dermatol.* 109:863–865.
9. Feldmann, R.J., and Maibach, H. I. (1965). Penetration of ^{14}C hydrocortisone through normal skin, the effect of stripping and occlusion. *Arch. Dermatol.* 91: 661–666.
10. Robertson, D., and Maibach, H. (1983). Topical corticoids. *Semin. Dermatol.* 2(4):238–249.
11. Fisher, L., and Maibach, H. (1973). Topical antipsoriatic agents and epidermal mitosis in man. *Arch. Dermatol.* 108:374–377.
12. Walter, J.F., Stoughton, R.B., and DeQuoy, P.R. (1978). Suppression of epidermal DNA synthesis by ultraviolet light, coal tar and anthralin. *Br. J. Dermatol.* 99:89–96.
13. Lavker, R.M., Grove, G.L., and Kligman, A.M. (1981). The atrophogenic effect of crude coal tar on human epidermis. *Br. J. Dermatol.* 105:77–82.
14. Olansky, S. (1980). Whole coal tar shampoo: a therapeutic hair repair system. *Cutis* 25:99–104.
15. Lowe, N.J., Breeding, J.H., and Wortzman, M.S. (1982). New coal tar extract and coal tar shampoos. *Arch. Dermatol.* 118:487–489.
16. Snyder, F.H., Buehler, E.V., and Winek, C.L. (1965). Safety evaluation of zinc 2-pyridine-thiol 1-oxide in a shampoo formulation. *Toxicol. Appl. Pharmacol.* 7: 425–437.
17. Orentreich, N. (1972). A clinical evaluation of two shampoos in the treatment of seborrheic dermatitis. *J. Soc. Cosmet. Chem.* 23:189–194.
18. Rutherford, T., and Black, J.G. (1969). The use of autoradiography to study the localization of germicides in skin. *Br. J. Dermatol.* 4:75–86.
19. Ingram, J.T. (1953). The approach to psoriasis. *Br. Med. J.* 2:591–594.
20. Lowe, N.J., and Breeding, J. (1981). Anthralin: different concentration effects on epidermal cell DNA synthesis rates in mice and clinical responses in human psoriasis. *Arch. Dermatol.* 117:698–700.
21. Baxter, D.L., and Stoughton, R.B. (1970). Mitotic index of psoriatic lesions treated with anthralin, glucocorticosteroid and occlusion only. *J. Invest. Dermatol.* 54(5):410–412.

22. Fisher, L.B., and Maibach, H.I. (1975). The effect of anthralin and its derivatives on epidermal cell kinetics. *J. Invest. Dermatol.* 64(5):338–341.
23. Farber, E.M., Abel, E.A., and Charuworn, A. (1983). Recent advances in the treatment of psoriasis. *J. Am. Acad. Dermatol.* 8(3):311–321. 23a. Murdoch, D., and Cussold, S.P. (1992). Calcipotriol: a review of its pharmacological properties and therapeutic use in psoriasis vulgaris. *Drugs* 43:415–429. 23b. Ramsay, C.A. (1992). Calcipotriol and psoriasis. *Int. J. Dermatol.* 31: 549–550. 23c. Klaber, M.R., Hutchinson, P.E., Pedvis-Leftick, A., et al. (1994). Comparative effect of calcipotriol solution (50 micrograms/ml) and betamethasone 17-valerate solution (1 mg/ml) in the treatment of scalp psoriasis. *Br. J. Dermatol.* 131(5): 678–683. 23d. Russell, S., and Young, M.J. (1994). Hypercalcemia during treatment of psoriasis with calcipotriol. *Br. J. Dermatol.* 130:795–796.
24. Plewig, G., and Kligman, A.M. (1969). The effect of selenium sulfide on epidermal turnover of normal and dandruff scalps. *J. Soc. Cosmet. Chem.* 20:767–775.
25. Ransome, J.W., Scott, N.M., and Knoblock, E.C. (1961). Selenium sulfide intoxication. *N. Engl. J. Med.* 264:384–385.
26. Cutaneous Fungal Infections and Ketoconazole Therapy in *Mycology Observer* 2/16/89. A discussion with Drs. Odom, Hazen, and Faergeman.
27. Skinner, R.B., Jr., Rosenberg, E.W., and Noah, P.W. (1995). Antimicrobial treatment of psoriasis. *Dermatol. Clin.* 13(4):909–913.
28. Ljunggren, B., and Moller, H. (1972). Topical use of fluorouracil in the treatment of psoriasis. *Arch. Dermatol.* 106:263.
29. Tsuiji, T., and Sugai, T. (1972). Topically administered fluorouracil in psoriasis. *Arch. Dermatol.* 105: 208–212.
30. Pearlman, D., Youngberg, B., et al. (1986). Weekly pulse dosing schedule of fluorouracil: a new topical therapy for psoriasis. *J. Am. Acad. Dermatol.* 15: 1247–1252.
31. Ward, J.M., and Barnes, R.M.R. (1978). HLA antigens in persistent palmoplantar pustulosis and its relationship to psoriasis. *Br. J. Dermatol.* 99:477–483.
32. Rosen, K., Lindholm, A., Mobacken, H., and Sandberg, L. (1982). HLA antigens associated with pustulosis palmoplantaris. *Dermatol. Monatsschr.* 168: 182–185.
33. Hersle, K., and Mobacken, H. (1982). Hyperkeratotic dermatitis of the palms. *Br. J. Dermatol.* 107:195–202.
34. Barth, J.H., Venning, V.A., and Wojnarowska, F. (1988). Palmoplantar involvement in autoimmune blistering disorders—pemphigoid, linear IgA disease and herpes gestationis. *Clin. Exp. Dermatol.* 13:85–86.
35. Pearlman, D.L., Youngberg, B., and Engelhard, C. (1987). Weekly psoriasis therapy using intralesional fluorouracil. *J. Am. Acad. Dermatol.* 17:78–82.
36. Friedman, S.J. (1987). Management of psoriasis vulgaris with a hydrocolloid occlusive dressing. *Arch. Dermatol.* 123:1046–1052.
37. Morison, W.L., Parrish, J.A., and Fitzpatrick, T.B. (1978). Oral methoxsalen photochemotherapy of recalcitrant dermatoses of the palms and soles. *Br. J. Dermatol.* 99:297–302.
38. Abel, E.A., Goldberg, L.H., and Farber, E.M. (1980). Treatment of palmoplantar psoriasis with topical methoxsalen plus long-wave ultraviolet light. *Arch. Dermatol.* 116:1257–1261.
39. Epstein, E. (1989). Home PUVA treatment for chronic hand and foot dermatoses. *Cutis* 44:423–427.
40. White, S.I., Marks, J.M., and Shuster, S. (1985). Etretinate in pustular psoriasis of palms and soles. *Br. J. Dermatol.* 113:581–585.
41. Reitamo, S., Erkko, P., Remitz, A., Lauerma, A.I., Montonen, O., Harjula, K. (1993). Cyclosporine in the treatment of palmoplantar pustulosis. *Arch. Dermatol.* 129:1273–1279.

5

Photosensitive Psoriasis

Anne-Marie Ros and Göran Wennersten
Karolinska Hospital, Stockholm, Sweden

TERMINOLOGY AND DEFINITION

Patients with psoriasis usually benefit from ultraviolet light exposure, but some deteriorate and their lesions are worsened by sunlight. Only psoriatics with no obvious reason for their light sensitivity, e.g., other skin disease with photoaggravation, concomitant photodermatosis, or drug reaction, should be considered to have the diagnosis of *photosensitive psoriasis.* Thus, photosensitive psoriasis is here defined as psoriasis where the *psoriasis lesions* deteriorate after sun exposure or new psoriasis lesions appear.

Psoriatic patients may believe that their psoriasis is photosensitive for several reasons (Table 1). Absence of expected improvement after sun exposure is sometimes interpreted as if sunlight had worsened their psoriasis. Increased susceptibility to severe sunburn in patients with fair complexions, skin type I or II, may lead to confusion with actual worsening of psoriasis lesions. Concomitant photodermatoses such as polymorphous light eruption (PMLE), chronic actinic dermatitis, solar urticaria, and porphyria *with no relation to psoriasis* must be excluded in differential diagnosis, as must other skin diseases with photoaggravation, e.g., seborrheic dermatitis, lupus erythematosus (1–4), hypocomplementemia (5), and vitiligo (6,7). Photoallergic and phototoxic contact reactions induced by chemicals should also be considered, as should reactions elicited by photosensitizing drugs.

Table 1 Differential Diagnostic Aspects to Be Considered in Photosensitive Psoriatics

Fair complexion with *skin type I or II* but *no* other sign of specific psoriasis lesions provoked by sunlight
Absence of expected improvement in psoriasis lesions after sun exposure
Concomitant photodermatosis *unrelated* to psoriasis such as PMLE, chronic actinic dermatitis, solar urticaria, porphyria
Preexisting dermatosis with photoaggravation but *no relation* to psoriasis, e.g., seborrheic dermatitis, lupus erythematosus
Photosensitizing drugs
Phototoxic or photoallergic contact reactions induced by chemicals

HEREDITY

The heredity for photosensitive psoriasis has not been detailed earlier. In a recent questionnaire study, 2000 psoriatics were asked about the occurrence of photosensitivity among their relatives (8). Twenty-eight percent of the photosensitive psoriatics reported some kind of photosensitivity, 14% had relatives with PMLE, and 7% had relatives with photosensitive psoriasis. The corresponding figures among nonphotosensitive psoriatics were that 11% had a positive heredity for light sensitivity of any kind, 9% had relatives with PMLE, and 1% had relatives with photosensitive psoriasis. The heredity for psoriasis was the same in both groups, i.e., 32% (8).

EPIDEMIOLOGY

The reported prevalence of photosensitive psoriasis varies considerably between different studies. Lane et al. found in 1937 (9) a prevalence of 14.3% photosensitivity among 231 psoriatics. Lomholt studied different aspects of psoriasis in the Faroe Islands in 1963 (10), and found a prevalence of 14% photosensitivity in men and 24% in women. In Farber and co-workers' large questionnaire study among 2144 psoriatics in 1968 (11) and 5600 psoriatics in 1974 (12), photosensitivity was observed in 15 and 20%, respectively. In Braun-Falco and co-workers' questionnaire study in 1972 (13), the prevalence was estimated at 14%. However, the existence of photosensitivity was one question among many in these studies, and was not analyzed in detail. The figures reported seem fairly high and most probably are cases with other concomitant diseases with light sensitivity included; consequently, photosensitive psoriasis as defined above would therefore be less frequent.

In our questionnaire study of 2000 psoriatics (8), the issue of photosensitive psoriasis was investigated in more detail. The written questionnaire answers were confirmed and supplemented with telephone interviews, and the prevalence of photosensitive psoriasis, as defined above, was estimated to be only 5.5%.

CLINICAL FINDINGS IN PHOTOSENSITIVE PSORIASIS

Publications with descriptions of clinical findings in photosensitive psoriasis are sparse and documented mainly as case reports. As early as 1933, Matras reported a 13-year-old female with psoriasis which flared after sun exposure (14).

In 1964, Bielicky and Kvicalova (15) investigated 14 photosensitive psoriasis patients who had been exposed to intensive sun before flaring of their psoriasis. Most of their patients had fair skin and half were blonde. All but one had a lowered erythema threshold for UVB. The finding of a fair complexion and a tendency to sunburn in patients with photosensitive psoriasis was also emphasized by Frain-Bell (16).

Thus, a light complexion and skin type I is one important factor for susceptibility to photosensitive psoriasis. This was confirmed in our recent questionnaire study (8) of 2000 psoriatics, where 20% of photosensitive psoriatics had skin type I compared to 4% in our nonphotosensitive patients. In that study, however, most patients developed psoriasis first and the photosensitivity occurred years later in many. This would not be the case if skin type alone explained the appearance of photosensitivity. Further, as many as 54% of the photosensitive psoriatics had skin type III or IV, which supports the theory that causes other than a fair complexion contribute to their light sensitivity.

Increased photosensitivity has been found in patients with an unstable, eruptive form of psoriasis (17), but this was not confirmed in our study (18).

Exacerbation of photoinduced psoriasis lesions is for obvious reasons usually observed in early spring (8). In 34% of our photosensitive psoriatics, debut symptoms of light sensitivity appeared suddenly, and 26% had been sunbathing intensively at the onset (8). Twenty percent stated that their psoriasis was previously improved by exposure to sunlight (8).

Exacerbation of psoriasis from sun exposure was observed mostly on the arms (74%), legs (63%), or the back of the hands (49%), followed in frequency by the back (33%), breast (31%), feet (30%), and face (21%). Skin type I, psoriasis affecting the hands, heredity for photosensitivity and increased age were all significantly ($p \leq 0.001$) more common in the photosensitivity group than in the nonphotosensitive psoriatics. With advanced age, the chance to develop photosensitive psoriasis increases, corresponding to a long duration of psoriasis (8). Other variables such as joint symptoms, pruritus, or psoriasis worsened by stress or infection did not differ significantly between the photosensitive and nonphotosensitive psoriatics (8).

Further, we found that about half of our photosensitive psoriatics had a *history of PMLE with psoriasis appearing as a sequela in their PMLE lesions.* The other half, slowly developed psoriasis after sun exposure, but with no preceding PMLE reaction (18). The mechanisms behind the latter direct reaction are unknown. The importance of a Koebner reaction in this context has been advocated and will be discussed later.

LIGHT SENSITIVITY AND ELICITING WAVELENGTHS

Light Testing

UVB Erythema Threshold

A lowered erythema threshold for UVB irradiation in photosensitive psoriatics has been reported earlier (15,16), but was not confirmed in our recent study, where only 7 of 35 of the photosensitive psoriatics investigated had a lowered erythema threshold for UVB (18).

UVA Erythema Threshold

A lowered erythema threshold for UVA irradiation has not been reported, but data are lacking except for our own report (18), where only 1 of 35 of the photosensitive psoriatics investigated had a lowered threshold for UVA.

UVB Provocation Studies

Provocation with high doses of artificial UVB irradiation (3 and 5 MED) may provoke new psoriatic lesions in some, but not all photosensitive psoriatics, in our experience (18). Positive provocation occurred in 12 of 35 patients tested (18). New psoriasis lesions appeared 11–48 days after the test procedure. The lesions came gradually and were histologically confirmed. In some of these patients, PMLE lesions first provoked by UVB were seen within 3–6 days, developing into psoriasis lesions after about 17–24 days (18). Even suberythematous UVB doses has been described to elicit a psoriatic response 3 weeks after light testing in a patient with an otherwise normal MED within the UVB range (18a).

UVA Provocation Studies

Very high doses of UVA irradiation may also provoke psoriasis lesions in some photosensitive psoriatics. In our study, 17 of 35 patients tested reacted pathologically after UVA provocation with doses of 25–75 J/cm^2 (18). Even here it was found that some patients (12 of 17) first developed a PMLE reaction, which in 6 of 17 patients was followed by psoriasis lesions in the test areas, 17–59 days after testing. However, in 29% (5 of 17) of our patients, the UVA provocation induced specific photosensitive psoriatic lesions without any preceding PMLE lesions. These specific lesions occurred gradually 17–48 days after testing and were documented histologically.

PMLE followed by psoriasis was provoked more easily with UVA than was photosensitive psoriasis with no preceding PMLE, which was easier to provoke with UVB.

RELATION TO POLYMORPHOUS LIGHT ERUPTION

About 50% of our light sensitive psoriasis patients investigated with light testing had a history of PMLE with psoriasis developing in the previous PMLE lesions. It may be of interest to compare some clinical data of this group with the other 50% who on phototesting experienced no sign of any preceding PMLE lesion, but who exhibited new psoriatic lesions successively after ultraviolet irradiation (Table 2).

An abrupt appearance of the light sensitivity, often after overexposure to sunlight, was most common in the PMLE group. The hands, arms, and legs were often involved in both groups, but in the PMLE group the chest and back were more often also involved. In the photosensitive psoriasis group, the hands were involved in 82% compared to 61% in the PMLE group. Improvement by hardening was more frequent in the PMLE group (39%) than in the photosensitive psoriasis group (24%). The duration of psoriasis and the light sensitivity was about the same in both groups (18).

PMLE is a common disease, more recent epidemiological studies showing prevalence figures of 11% (19) and 17% (20). It is therefore not surprising that many patients with psoriasis could also be susceptible to PMLE causing their psoriasis to flare as a secondary phenomenon, which may be part of a Koebner reaction. However, our experience shows that *in many psoriasis patients the PMLE reaction never develops into psoriasis lesions.* The reason for this discrepancy is unknown.

RELATION TO THE KOEBNER PHENOMENON

Earlier analysis of photosensitivity in psoriatics has focused on skin type and has often attributed the light sensitivity to a Koebner phenomenon in patients with a fair complexion and a tendency to sunburn easily (16,21,22). This may be true for some patients but not all. In our study a *history* of a Koebner reaction to trauma was found in 61% of those with PMLE followed by psoriasis, and in 65% of the photosensitive psoriatics (18). However, when these patients were light tested there seemed to be no difference in the likelihood of developing PMLE with psoriasis, or psoriasis with no preceding PMLE reaction, as regards an actual positive or negative history of Koebner reactions. The frequency of Koebner reactions in psoriatics is not fully known, but it has been estimated at 33% in a population with ordinary psoriasis (23). Much higher frequencies have been reported in other studies. The topic has recently been meritoriously reviewed in an article in which the huge amount of ex-

Table 2 Clinical Data for 35 Investigated Paients with Photosensitive Psoriasis

	PMLE followed by psoriasis	Photosensitive psoriasis
Abrupt appearance of light sensitivity	61%	12%
Overexposure prior to debut	33%	12%
Psoriasis previously improved by sunlight	39%	24%
Improvement by hardening	39%	24%
History of Koebner phenomenon	61%	65%
Mean duration of psoriasis, years	22.7 (5–45)	25.4 (6–50)
Mean duration of light sensitivity, years	9.7 (2–30)	11.5 (2–40)

Source: Ref. 18.

isting documentation is analyzed and summarized (24). In our investigated patients (18), a history of Koebner reactions seemed to be common, but there was no correlation concerning psoriatics with positive or negative phototests on provocation. The importance of the Koebner phenomenon in photosensitive psoriatics remains to be investigated further.

IMMUNOLOGICAL INVESTIGATIONS

Immunological investigations of photosensitive psoriasis are sparse. We investigated the cellular infiltrate in our light-sensitive psoriasis patients with monoclonal antibodies after light provocation with UVA and UVB (25). We thought it of special interest to investigate whether there was any difference between the group with PMLE followed by psoriasis and those with psoriasis occurring with no preceding PMLE reaction after light provocation.

The dermal infiltrate after UV irradiation consisted mainly of T lymphocytes with a dominance of cells of T helper/inducer phenotype and less staining of T suppressor/cytotoxic phenotype cells except in a few cases where the latter were more abundant. This pattern was seen in both groups investigated, but also in a group of nonpsoriatic PMLE patients (25). Exocytosis with mainly T suppressor/cytotoxic phenotype cells in the epidermis was seen in most patients in both groups after psoriasis had developed, a common finding also in nonphotosensitive psoriasis (26). CD15 positive cells in the dermis (monocytes, granulocytes) were also sparse, but increased in most patients after psoriasis had developed. Langerhans cells in the dermis were mostly sparse and did not seem to be affected by the development of lesions into psoriasis. These findings do not permit any substantial conclusions as to the role of T lymphocytes in photosensitive psoriasis.

PROGNOSIS

In the detailed examination of 35 patients with PMLE followed by psoriasis (18 of 35) and with photosensitive psoriasis not preceded by a PMLE reaction (17 of 35), a hardening phenomenon was reported in 39 and 24%, respectively. The light sensitivity had remained unchanged in 21 of 35 patients, worsened in 13 of 35, and improved in only 1 of 35. Mean duration of the light sensitivity for the two groups was 9.7 (2–30) and 11.5 (2–40) years, respectively (18).

TREATMENT

Adequate clothing protection from sun exposure and the regular use of an efficient sunscreen to UVB and UVA irradiation are the simplest and most important basic means of protecting light-sensitive psoriatics, and should always be emphasized. Beta-carotene orally in fairly high daily doses (100–200 mg) may be tried in some cases, but there are not enough studies to substantiate the clinical effect in photosensitive psoriasis.

The best therapy seems to be photochemotherapy with PUVA, which may be given either as a prophylactic before expected flaring of psoriasis in the spring or summertime, or as a treatment if extensive psoriasis has already appeared. PUVA administered with oral trimethylpsoralen was found by us in a recent study, and confirmed by light test procedures (27), to have a good-to-excellent effect as a prophylactic to prevent solar exacerbation of psoriatic lesions. However, if extensive psoriasis lesions preexist, trimethylpsoralen cannot be recommended as an effective treatment measure (28). However, 8-methoxypsoralen could be tried with careful increase and monitoring of the light doses to prevent any initial flaring of psoriasis during treatment.

CONCLUSIONS

Photosensitive psoriasis, i.e., psoriasis worsened after sun exposure, is rare, the prevalence in a recent survey among 2000 psoriasis patients being estimated at 5.5% (Table 3). The reaction pattern of photosensitivity divided into two groups, where about 50% first had PMLE reactions which further developed into classic psoriatic lesions, and the other 50% slowly developed psoriatic skin changes with no preceding PMLE reaction. Photosensitive psoriatics have a significantly ($p \leq 0.001$) higher frequency of skin type I, heredity for photosensitivity, advanced age, and psoriasis affecting the hands than do nonphotosensitive psoriatics. Light testing revealed normal erythema thresholds to UVB and UVA in most patients. Ultraviolet A provoked most easily PMLE with subsequent psoriasis, and psoriasis with no preceding PMLE most easily with UVB. The prognosis is unfavorable. Besides basic measures with adequate clothing and use of efficient broad-spectrum sunscreens, PUVA therapy is advocated. Trimethylpsoralen may be given as a prophylactic therapy before the spring and summertime. If widespread psoriasis already preexists, 8-methoxypsoralen should be used with a very careful monitoring of UVA dosimetry.

Table 3 Characteristics of Photosensitive Psoriasis Found in a Recent Survey of 2000 Psoriasis Patients

Prevalence about 5.5%
Skin type I overrepresented
Psoriasis affecting hands common
Reaction pattern of photosensitivity in two groups: about 50% had first PMLE reactions which further developed into classic psoriatic lesoins, and the other 50% slowly developed psoriatic skin lesions with no preceding PMLE reaction
Erythemal thresholds to UVB and UVA mostly normal
Photosensitive psoriasis lesions appear slowly from 11–17 days after light testing up to 48–59 days
PMLE followed by psoriasis most easily provoked with UVA
Photosensitive psoriasis with no preceding PMLE most easily provoked with UVB
The disease is protracted and the prognosis unfavorable

Source: Refs. 8 and 18.

REFERENCES

1. O'Leary, P.A. (1927). Chronic lupus erythematosus disseminatus and psoriasis vulgaris. *Arch. Dermatol. Syphilol.* 15:92.
2. Millns, J.L., McDuffie, F.C., Muller, S.A., and Jordan, R.E. (1978). Development of photosensitivity and an SLE-like syndrome in a patient with psoriasis. *Arch. Dermatol.* 114:1177–1181.
3. Millns, J.L., and Muller, S.A. (1980). The coexistence of psoriasis and lupus erythematosus. An analysis of 27 cases. *Arch. Dermatol.* 116:658–664.
4. Kulick, K.B., Mogavero, H., Provost, T.T., and Reichlin, M. (1983). Serologic studies in patients with lupus erythematosus and psoriasis. *J. Am. Acad. Dermatol.* 8:631–634.
5. Doyle, J.A. (1984). Photosensitive psoriasis. *Aust. J. Dermatol.* 25:54–58.
6. Koransky, J.S., Roenigk, H.H., Jr. (1982). Vitiligo and psoriasis. *J. Am. Acad. Dermatol.* 7:183–189.
7. Powell, F.C., Dicken, C.H. (1983). Psoriasis and vitiligo. *Acta Derm. Venereol.* (Stockh.) 64:246–249.
8. Ros, A.-M., and Eklund, G. (1987). Photosensitive psoriasis—an epidemiologic study. *J. Am. Acad. Dermatol.* 17:752–758.
9. Lane, C.G., and Craford, G.M. (1937). Psoriasis. A statistical study of 231 cases. *Arch. Dermatol.* 35: 1051–1061.
10. Lomholt, G. (1963). Infuence of sun- and sea-bathing. In *Psoriasis. Prevalence, Spontaneous Course and Genetics. A Census Study on the Prevalence of Skin Diseases on the Faroe Islands.* G.E.C. GAD, Copenhagen, pp. 113–114.
11. Farber, E.M., Bright, R.D., and Nall, M.L. (1968). Psoriasis. A questionnaire survey of 2144 patients. *Arch. Dermatol.* 98:249–259.
12. Farber, E.M., and Nall, M.L. (1974). The natural history of psoriasis in 5600 patients. *Dermatologica* 148: 1–18.
13. Braun-Falco, O., Burg, G., and Farber, E.M. (1972). Psoriasis. Eine Fragebogenstudie bei 536 Patienten. *Munch. Med. Wschr.* 114:1105–1110.
14. Matras, A. (1933). Psoriasis vulgaris—Eruption nach Sonnenbestrahlung. *Zentralbl. Haut. Geschl. Kr.* 46: 413.
15. Bielicky, T., and Kvicalova, E. (1964). Photosensitive psoriasis. *Dermatologica* 129:339–348.
16. Frain-Bell, W. (1979). What is that thing called light? *Clin. Exp. Dermatol.* 4:1–29.

17. Szabo, E., and Horkay, I. (1965). Untersuchungen über die Lichtreaktionen bei Psoriasis-patienten. *Zeitschrift Haut. Geschl. Kr.* 39:425–429.
18. Ros, A.-M., and Wennersten, G. (1986). Photosensitive psoriasis—clinical findings and phototest results. *Photodermatology* 3:317–326.
18a. Kudoh, K., Obata, M., Torinuki, W., and Tagami, H. (1988). Photosensitive psoriasis provoked by a suberythematous dose of ultraviolet-B light. *Dermatologica* 176:138–142.
19. Morison, W.L., and Stern, R.S. (1982). Polymorphous light eruption: a common reaction uncommonly recognized. *Acta Derm. Venereol.* (Stockh.) 62:237–240.
20. Ros, A.-M., and Wennersten, G. (1986). Current aspects of polymorphous light eruption in Sweden. *Photodermatology* 3:298–302.
21. Pillsbury, D.M., and Lofgren, R. (1941). Psoriasis with Koebner phenomenon following ultraviolet irradiation. *Arch. Dermatol.* 44:123–124.
22. Gross, P. (1956). The Koebner phenomenon in its relationship to photosensitivity. *Arch. Dermatol.* 74: 43–45.
23. Melski, J.W., Bernhard, J.D., and Stern, R.S. (1983). The Koebner (isomorphic) response in psoriasis. *Arch. Dermatol.* 119:655–659.
24. Eyre, R.W., and Krueger, G.G. (1985). The Koebner response in psoriasis. In *Psoriasis.* H.H. Roenigk, Jr., and H.I. Maibach (Eds.). Marcel Dekker, New York, pp. 105–116.
25. Ros, A.-M., and Wennersten, G. (1987). Photosensitive psoriasis—an immunohistochemical study after light provocation with UVA and UVB. *Photodermatology* 4: 79–87.
26. Hammar, H., Gu, S.-Q., Johannesson, A., Sundqvist, K.-G., and Biberfeld, P. (1984). Subpopulations of mononuclear cells in microscopic lesions of psoriatic patients. Selective accumulation of suppressor/cytotoxic T cells in epidermis during the evolution of the lesion. *J. Invest. Dermatol.* 83:416–420.
27. Ros, A.-M., and Wennersten, G. (1987). PUVA therapy for photosensitive psoriasis. *Acta Derm. Venereol.* (Stockh.) 67:501–505.
28. Seghal, V.N., Rege, V.I., Kharangate, V.N., and Reys, M. (1975). Photochemotherapy of psoriasis with 4,5′,8 trimethylpsoralen. *Dermatologica* 150:316–319.

6

Human Immunodeficiency Virus and Psoriasis

Joanna Badger, Timothy G. Berger, Charles Gambla, and John Y.M. Koo
University of California Medical Center, San Francisco, California

Infection with the human immunodeficiency virus (HIV) may be complicated by psoriasis and/or an inflammatory arthritis. The clinical features of the arthritis are variable and may resemble psoriatic arthritis or Reiter's syndrome (1,2).

The fact that both psoriasis and Reiter's syndrome may present for the first time or be exacerbated by HIV infection suggests that HIV infection enhances or triggers the expression of these diseases in a susceptible individual (1,3). These diseases show significant etiological, clinical, and histological overlap and are considered to be part of the same disease spectrum (2).

EPIDEMIOLOGY

In one of the most definitive studies to date, Garbe and colleagues (4) followed a cohort of 456 HIV-infected individuals from 1982 to 1992. During this 10-year period, psoriasis occurred in 6.4%. This figure is much higher than the prevalence of 2% found in the general population. A study undertaken by Berman et al. reported a similar figure of 5% (5).

Researchers at the San Francisco General Hospital (3) found that one-third of HIV-infected patients with psoriasis develop psoriasis prior to HIV infection, while two-thirds note the onset of psoriatic symptoms following seroconversion. The prevalence of 6.4% correlates well with this data. If one-third develop psoriasis before HIV infection, then the prevalence figure for this subgroup will reflect that of the general population, i.e., 2%. If two-thirds develop psoriasis after seroconversion, then the prevalence for this subgroup will be double that associated with the general population, i.e., 4%. When combining the prevalence figures for both subgroups, the overall prevalence for HIV-associated psoriasis would be expected to be approximately 6%. Others (6,7) have, however, reported prevalences of 1.3–2%, similar to the general population.

The prevalence figures for psoriatic arthritis in HIV-infected individuals also vary. Berman et al. (5) and Solinger and Hess (8) report prevalences of 2% and 1.2%, respectively. Psoriatic arthritis occurs in 5–10% of non-HIV-infected individuals with psoriasis and 0.05–0.14% of the general population. These two studies suggest that the prevalence of psoriatic arthritis is higher in the HIV-infected population.

No study has demonstrated a correlation between the severity of the psoriatic skin lesions and the prevalence of arthritis in HIV-infected persons (1).

Controversy also exists over the prevalence of Reiter's syndrome in the HIV-infected population, particularly as the prevalence in the general population has not yet been firmly established. Reported prevalences have ranged from a high of 5–10% (5,9) to a low of 0.3–0.5% (10,11). This figure is similar to the prevalence in non-HIV-infected homosexual men, but much higher than the reported prevalence in the general population of 0.0035–0.004% (12,13). These differences may relate to different rates of exposure to infectious agents known to trigger Reiter's syndrome.

Twenty percent of persons with HIV-associated psoriasis have their presentation with a CD4+ count >400 (3,4). Approximately half of cases present before clinical findings of immunodeficiency (except for low CD4+ count) (3,4). Therefore, both psoriasis and Reiter's syndrome may be the initial clinical manifestation of HIV infection.

ETIOLOGY

Although etiology of psoriasis remains unclear, a multifactorial pattern has emerged with certain etiological factors having a strong association with both psoriasis and Reiter's syndrome. In particular, both diseases have a strong genetic component and may be precipitated by infectious agents and certain drugs. These etiological factors remain true regardless of the HIV status of the individual, and the bulk of the evidence so far strongly suggests that psoriasis is the same disease in both groups.

Association with class 1 HLA antigens is well recognized. Although the frequency of HLA antigens in HIV-associated Reiter's syndrome is well established, little is known about the frequency of HLA antigens in HIV-associated psoriasis or psoriatic arthritis.

Reiter's syndrome is associated with HLA B27 in 80% of HIV-negative individuals and a similar value of 70–80% has been found in HIV-infected individuals (2,5,14). This marked association strongly suggests a genetic predisposition.

Reveille and colleagues examined the HLA antigen frequencies in HIV-infected male patients with psoriasis and psoriatic arthritis compared with noninfected controls (2). HLA B27 was found in 45% of all patients with psoriasis, including those with arthritis, compared with only 6% in the control group. Those with psoriatic arthritis were found to have HLA B27 in 78% of cases whereas only 23% of patients with psoriasis alone were found to have this particular antigen. Twenty-three percent of the patients with psoriasis alone expressed HLA B17, a figure that is 3 times higher than the 6% found in the control group, and 61% were found to have one or more B7 "CREG" antigens. Although these figures suggest a marked increase in HLA frequency, particularly HLA B27 and B17, the results did not attain statistical significance due to insufficient sample size (2).

Another important etiological aspect of Reiter's syndrome and psoriasis is the role played by infectious agents. The fact that Reiter's syndrome may be precipitated by a gastrointestinal or genitourinary-urinary infection has been well established. The definition of reactive arthritis is based on the temporal relationship between an infection distant to the joint and the subsequent development of arthritis. HIV-infected individuals are at increased risk of acquiring a range of bacterial, viral, and fungal infections including recognized arithrogenic organisms such as: (1) *Shigella*, (2) *Salmonella*, (3) *Campylobacter*, and (4) *Chlamydia trachomatis*. Certain studies have identified a pathogen in 30% of HIV-positive Reiter's patients (9). A higher-than-expected frequency of *Yersinia*-induced Reiter's syndrome in HIV-positive individuals has been reported in the United Kingdom (15). Low *Chlamydia* antibody titers in 60% and high *Chlamydia* antibody titers in 33% of HIV-positive subjects compared with 8% and 1.7%, respectively, in HIV-negative healthy subjects have also been reported (16).

Bacterial, fungal, and viral agents have all been implicated as trigger factors in the onset or exacerbation of psoriasis. Guttate psoriasis is frequently precipitated by streptococcal infection perhaps triggered by a streptococcal "superantigen" (17). Patients with this form of psoriasis improve following treatment with systemic antibiotic therapy. HIV-associated guttate psoriasis may also show a dramatic response to antibiotic therapy. Some *Staphylococcus aureus* toxins can also act as "superantigens" (18) and staphylococcal sepsis has been linked with psoriatic flares in HIV-infected individuals (19). However, whether the infection triggers the psoriatic flare or whether septicemia follows the secondary infection of psoriatic plaques remains unclear (19). Regardless of the specific initiating event, the resolution of psoriasis following intravenous antibiotic therapy is well documented (19). A psoriatic flare in an HIV-infected individual should always raise the possibility of an occult staphylococcal infection even if the patient does not appear to be particularly unwell.

Drugs are also known to trigger or exacerbate psoriasis in both HIV-negative and HIV-positive individuals. Drugs identified in HIV-infected psoriatics as having a triggering effect include lithium, beta blockers, and systemic corticosteroids. Corticosteroid withdrawal following treatment of *Pneumocystis carinii* pneumonia or as a part of chemotherapy premedication for treatment of Kaposi's sarcoma have caused flares of psoriasis in patients followed by the authors. Removal of the corticosteroid component of chemotherapy resulted in improvement of the psoriasis.

PATHOGENESIS

The advent of HIV infection and its recognized association with psoriasis and Reiter's syndrome has shed some light on the pathogenesis of these two closely related diseases.

Does HIV infection have a unique role or does it facilitate the pathogenic mechanisms that occur in non-HIV-infected individuals? The bulk of the evidence to date strongly supports the latter interpretation. The histological findings and etiological factors associated with psoriasis remain consistent regardless of the HIV status of the individual. Psoriasis is therefore considered to be the same disease in both HIV-negative and HIV-positive individuals and the same pathogenic model for psoriasis can be applied to both groups.

Why is psoriasis more prevalent in HIV-positive individuals and why does it tend to follow a more aggressive course? The CD4+ lymphocyte targeting by HIV results in the progressive depletion of CD4+ cells. The removal of such down-regulating agents probably facilitates a variety of pathogenic mechanisms that are no longer held in check. Many unrelated conditions, for example, seborrheic dermatitis and pruritic folliculitis, are known to occur more frequently in HIV-infected individuals. No unifying process has been linked with this diverse list of diseases other than a reduced CD4+ count and a relative increase in CD8+ cells.

Attention has therefore been focused on the pathogenic effects of the progressive CD4+/CD8+ imbalance and the possible direct effects of HIV itself. However, the possibility that CD4+ cells may have an active role cannot be discounted as several patients with end-stage AIDS and extremely low CD4+ counts have been noted to have a spontaneous remission (20).

A Primary Immune Mechanism

The immunohistochemical characteristics of psoriatic lesions include the preferential localization of CD4+ lymphocytes in the dermis and CD8+ lymphocytes in the epidermis (21). It has also been shown that the onset and exacerbation of psoriatic lesions is linked to the accumulation of CD8+ lymphocytes in affected areas whereas remission following treatment is associated with a decrease in CD8+ lymphocytes (22,23). An expansion of CD8+ cells could be induced by interleukin-2 (IL-2), released by HIV-infected lymphocytes. The activated CD8+ lymphocytes may then infiltrate the epidermis with subsequent keratinocyte activation and proliferation. HIV infection may set the stage for this postulated CD8+-mediated process through the HIV-associated reduction in CD4+ count and relative increase in CD8+ count.

HIV and Arthritogenic Organisms

This theory is based on the increased incidence of opportunistic infections associated with HIV infection that may act as arthritogenic pathogens. In addition, a reduced immune reaction and response to infecting organisms was seen in HLA B27 and B7 positive individuals who developed a reactive arthritis following a *Salmonella* epidemic (24). The HIV-associated immunodeficiency may compound such an immune defect as well as facilitating the emergence of opportunistic and potentially arthritogenic pathogens.

A Direct Role for HIV Involving Epidermal Langerhans Cells and Dermal Dendrocytes

In HIV infection and in psoriasis, epidermal Langerhans cells (ELC) are reduced (25). In HIV-infected persons with psoriasis this reduction is more marked (25). It is unknown if this reduction of ELC in HIV-infected patients is due to infection of ELC by HIV. What pathogenic role this reduction of ELC may play in psoriasis and whether the enhanced reduction of ELC associated with HIV disease is related to the increased severity of psoriasis in some HIV infected patients is unknown.

Psoriatic lesions are associated with increased numbers of dermal dendrocytes (26). Dermal dendrocytes are potential targets for HIV infection because they express CD4+ receptors and can function as phagocytes. Using in situ hybridization with confocal laser scanning microscopy, HIV transcripts have been demonstrated within the dermal dendrocytes of psoriatic lesions of HIV-positive individuals but not in normal skin from HIV-positive patients or from the skin biopsies of seronegative psoriatic patients (27). The finding of HIV-1 RNA sequences in the psoriatic lesions and not in the normal skin suggests that HIV may play a local role in triggering psoriatic lesions. The exact mechanism by which this may occur is unknown, but HIV itself directly triggering keratinocyte proliferation or HIV-infected dermal dendrocytes stimulating keratinocyte proliferation indirectly through cytokine production has been proposed (27). However, the role of dermal dendrocytes in HIV-associated psoriasis is not clear-cut. Although the density of dermal dendrocytes is increased in the psoriatic lesions of both HIV+ and HIV− individuals, there is no significant difference in density between the two groups (26). Therefore, the sudden onset or worsening of psoriatic lesions associated with HIV infection cannot be attributed to HIV-induced dermal dendrocyte proliferation. However, the results do not exclude a qualitative or functional abnormality.

HIV May Have a Direct Effect on Keratinocytes

Evidence for a direct role for HIV is produced by transgenic mice studies. In one study, the entire HIV proviral genome was inserted into mouse embryos. Forty-five percent of the offspring of one of these mice developed a syndrome with skin lesions that resembled psoriasis, suggesting that the HIV genome may drive epithelial proliferation (28). It has been noted that some psoriatic HIV-positive patients receiving zidovudine (AZT) show marked and dramatic remission of their skin lesions (29). More recently, AZT has been found to have a beneficial effect on the psoriatic skin lesions of HIV-negative individuals although the benefit appears to be less dramatic than in HIV-positive individuals (30). AZT is a thymidine analog that inhibits viral reverse transcriptase. It also inhibits host DNA synthesis so its effect on psoriasis may be explained by direct inhibition of keratinocyte proliferation by the drug itself (20), a possibility supported by its therapeutic effect in HIV-negative psoriatic patients.

Bacterial Agents Acting as Triggers

S. aureus toxins have been shown to function as superantigens that interact with T cells (18). Once activated, the T cells may induce a generalized psoriatic flare (19), as observed in HIV-infected patients with *S. aureus* septicemia. In immunocompetent individuals psoriatic lesions, although colonized, uncommonly become infected. By comparison, more than 50% of HIV-positive psoriatic patients have been found to have staphylococcal skin infections, in particular, folliculitis and intertriginous impetigo (6). In addition, *Candida albicans* infections are increased in HIV-infected patients, and there are reports of non-HIV-infected patients with chronic plaque psoriasis whose symptoms were exacerbated by cutaneous infections with superantigen secreting *C. albicans* (31).

In summary, while it appears that HIV-associated psoriasis may occur due to the imbalance of CD4+/CD8+ cells caused by HIV infection, increased infections with arthrogenic pathogens, infection of cutaneous antigen presenting cells (dermal dendrocytes and perhaps epidermal Langerhans cells) by HIV, a direct effect of HIV on epidermal proliferation, and increased rates of infection with agents that produce "superantigens" may all play a role. Most likely, during the course of HIV disease, some or all of these factors may exert an effect on the psoriasis of the HIV-infected persons.

CLINICAL FEATURES

The spectrum of psoriasis, psoriatic arthropathy, and Reiter's syndrome is broad with substantial clinical overlap, and the distinction between them on clinical grounds is often difficult. For instance, typical lesions of keratoderma blenorrhagica can occur in a patient with otherwise typical psoriasis in the absence of arthritis. Although the clinical manifestations of HIV-associated psoriasis are similar to those of non-HIV-infected individuals, there are some variations. Researchers at UCSF found that HIV-associated psoriasis falls into two main clinical groups (3).

Group 1 (Psoriasis Begins Before HIV Seroconversion)

The onset of symptoms precedes seroconversion and characteristically occurs in the second decade with a mean age of onset of 19 years (range 10–30 years). There is often a positive family history of psoriasis. While any pattern of psoriasis can occur in this group, the clinical features correspond to the classical psoriatic patterns seen in non-HIV-infected individuals and are most commonly one of three patterns.

1. Typical psoriasis vulgaris
2. Guttate psoriasis—A common pattern even in the absence of a preceding streptococcal infection.
3. Erythrodermic psoriasis

Group 2 (Psoriasis Begins After HIV Seroconversion)

The onset of psoriasis follows HIV seroconversion usually by about 5 years. This group is older, with a mean age of psoriasis onset of 36 years (range 23–58 years). A family history of psoriasis is generally absent. The clinical features tend to differ from those associated with classic psoriasis. In particular, inverse psoriasis and involvement of the palms and soles are more common and may be indistinguishable from Reiter's syndrome. The patterns of psoriasis observed in the group include:

1. Psoriasis vulgaris
2. Acral psoriasis with palmoplantar keratoderma (keratotic papules and pustules); keratoderma blenorrhagicum (Fig. 1)
3. Inverse psoriasis with prominent plaques in the scalp, axillae, and groin (Fig. 2)
4. Pustular psoriasis
5. Erythrodermic psoriasis (may occur as frequently in this group as in group 1)

Multiple types of psoriatic lesions may occur simultaneously in the same patient (3,6). The prevalence of psoriatic arthritis varies between the two groups, occurring with greater frequency in group 2 (3).

Psoriasis may appear at any clinical stage of HIV disease and the features may be mild, moderate, or severe (3). Some researchers report that the severity of psoriasis tends to reflect the stage of HIV disease

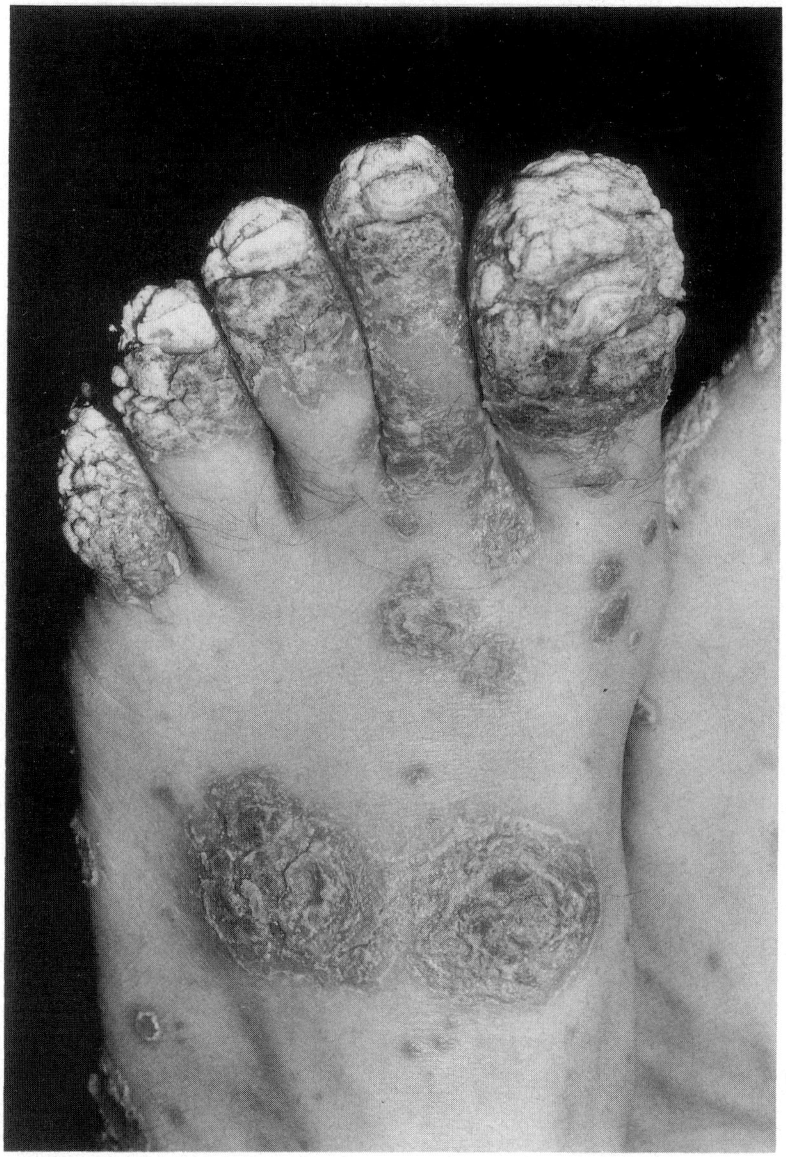

Figure 1 Markedly hyperkeratotic plaques of the foot. These lesions resolved with low-dose etretinate (37.5 mg daily) and aggressive local measures (tar soaks, topical tar ointments, and quartz light treatments).

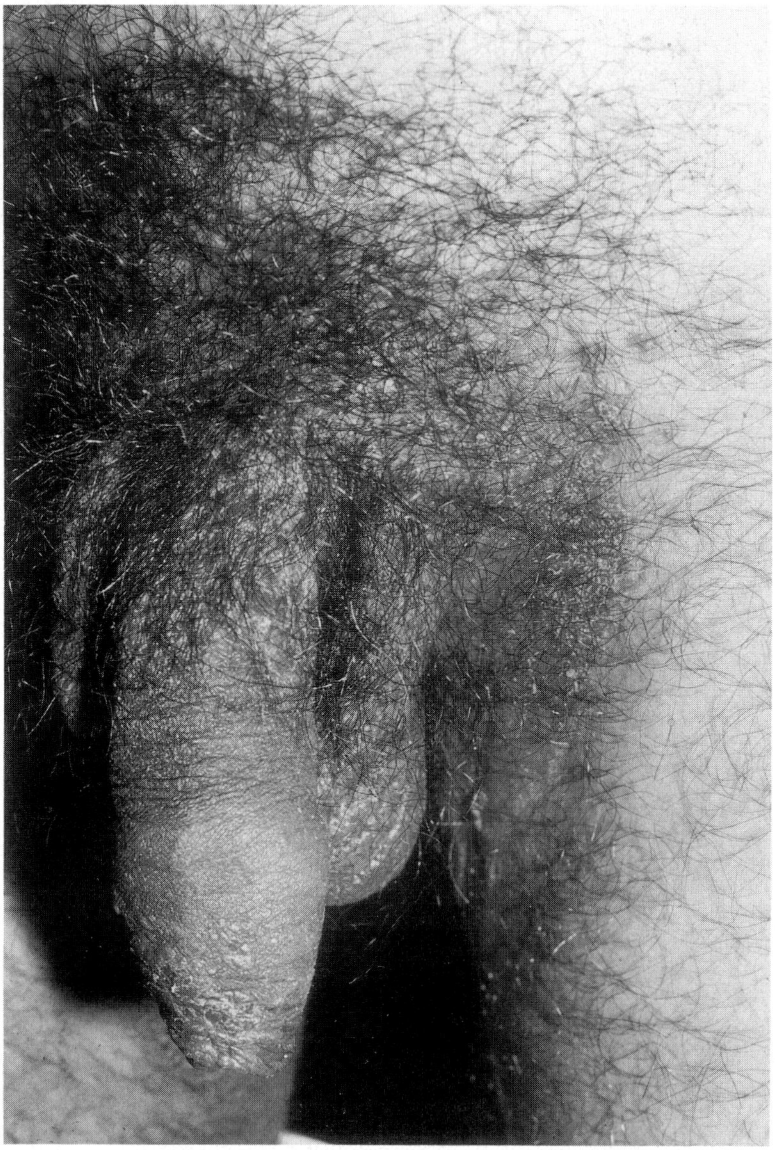

Figure 2 Fixed, red, scaling plaque of the groin extending onto the scrotum and penis in a patient with Reiter's syndrome and AIDS.

and often worsens as HIV disease progresses (1). Not all studies have detected such a direct correlation. Researchers in San Francisco found all grades of psoriasis in patients with a range of HIV disease (3). However, either extreme of the HIV disease spectrum is often associated with a corresponding degree of skin involvement. Patients with asymptomatic HIV infection tend to have mild psoriasis and patients with low CD4+ counts generally have severe psoriasis (3).

Factors known to exacerbate psoriasis in HIV-negative psoriatic patients may also worsen the skin lesions of HIV-infected individuals. These include infectious agents and certain drugs. The sudden flare of HIV-associated psoriasis may reflect an underlying staphylococcal infection even if the patient does not appear to be severely ill, and an occult infection must always be excluded (19).

Subtle histological features distinguish HIV-associated psoriasis from psoriasis in the seronegative. These include the presence of individually necrotic keratinocytes in the epidermis and plasma cells in the dermal infiltrate. These features are also seen in other

HIV-associated skin conditions and are more reflective of the pattern of HIV-associated skin diseases than HIV-associated psoriasis in particular. As in psoriasis in the uninfected patient, if the clinical lesions are atypical, the histology is atypical. Clinically typical HIV-associated psoriasis usually has typical histological features. We have found biopsies most useful at the onset of psoriasis, when small papules and plaques are not clinically typical, but usually histologically have sufficient features to allow us to diagnose psoriasis.

Psoriasis does not appear to adversely affect the survival of HIV-positive patients (3). However, studies so far have not been large enough to detect a significant difference.

The joint and tendon involvement in HIV-associated psoriasis and Reiter's syndrome tends to be more severe than in the general population and less responsive to anti-inflammatory drugs (1). In addition, the numbers of joints affected tends to increase with time.

Psoriatic arthropathy in HIV disease is clinically identical to the joint involvement in immunocompetent psoriatics. It primarily affects the foot and ankle and is often accompanied by intense enthesopathy and dactylitis especially in the feet, which may be the major source of disability. The pattern of arthritis in both HIV-associated psoriatic arthritis and Reiter's syndrome is as follows (1):

1. Predominantly lower limb oligoarthritis
2. Dactylitis
3. Heel and foot enthesis
4. Distal interphalangeal joint involvement
5. ± polyarthritis

The radiological appearance of hands and feet in psoriatic arthritis often reveals classic psoriatic arthritis features with "pencil and cup" deformities and osteolysis (32).

In summary, the clinical features of HIV-associated psoriasis and Reiter's syndrome are often modified by HIV infection resulting in a shift in the presentation and natural history of these conditions.

TREATMENT

In treating an HIV-infected psoriatic, several simple management tips are often useful. First, look for secondary infection. Flares of HIV-associated psoriasis are not infrequently associated with skin infections. Often a course of antistaphylococcal antibiotics will improve HIV-infected psoriatics. Chronic antibiotic treatment and the control of nasal carriage may lead to improvement or stabilization of HIV-associated psoriasis. Even erythrodermic psoriasis may be the result of subclinical staphylococcal sepsis, as noted above (19). Blood cultures are in order in the HIV-infected patient with sudden development of psoriatic erythroderma.

Zidovudine can be added to the anti-HIV regimen of the patient. When the drug is used as sole treatment, AZT toxicity is often limiting; AZT in lower doses added to other antivirals is often well tolerated and may have some benefit on the patient's psoriasis (7,29,33).

The treatment of psoriasis in a HIV-infected individual can be difficult because many of the therapeutic modalities involve some degree of immunosuppression. The reduced range of options can pose a significant therapeutic challenge. The three-tiered treatment approach for standard psoriasis also applies to HIV-associated psoriasis with some modification.

The first level of treatment involves the application of topical agents, which are most effective in mild or localized disease. Topical steroids and calcipotriol can be prescribed as in any psoriatic patient (34). Other alternatives in this group include anthralin (including short-contact therapy) and tar preparations. The use of high-concentration tar products may be associated with folliculitis. Topical therapy requires high compliance for benefit. Unfortunately, in patients with advanced HIV infection, associated fatigue, depression, dementia, or the presence of multiple other medical requirements often prevents the regular application of topical medications. In the very ill patient, simple occlusion of lesions with semipermeable dressings is an effective alternative. Duoderm or similar dressings are applied to the affected areas and left on for a week at a time. Lesions tend to begin to fade in about 3 weeks with no other management. Where occlusion is not an option, we are more likely to move to retinoid or phototherapy in the HIV-infected patient, recognizing the severe limitations of topical treatment in this setting. This is especially true if the psoriasis is gradually worsening.

The intermediate treatment level covers the various forms of phototherapy. The indications include extensive involvement or severe localized psoriasis as in keratoderma blenorrhagicum. There is some debate as to whether phototherapy is immunosuppressive and whether it may cause viral activation (35). While serum HIV titers may be transiently elevated by light therapy, the clinical importance of this finding is unclear. When looked at as a group, HIV-infected psoriatics treated with phototherapy do not seem to clinically suffer acceleration of their HIV disease (35,36). Kaposi's sarcoma, however, does seem to be exacerbated by phototherapy and is therefore a relative contraindication to phototherapy.

In addition, HIV-infected individuals (more commonly those with dermatitis or folliculitis rather than psoriasis) are often more photosensitive. This may be related to HIV disease itself or the photosensitizing medications HIV-infected patients frequently require, for example trimethoprim/sulfamethoxazole and the nonsteroidal anti-inflammatory agents. For these reasons, our phototherapy unit has modified phototherapy in HIV-infected patients in the following ways. First, phototherapy is initiated and increased with caution. Initial dosing is begun at the level for one skin type less than the HIV patient's actual skin type—i.e., the HIV-infected patient with type IV skin is begun as if his skin was type III. Patients are carefully observed for erythema, and frequent dose modifications may be required. Second, because of the concern about immunosuppression, patients receive phototherapy to only the areas required. We attempt local treatment, such as quartz light, more aggressively in HIV-infected patients. When the patients are treated in a light box, they expose only the targeted area. Patients may be treated on only half the body, for instance, if the psoriasis involves predominantly that area. The head and face are frequently shielded.

For the reasons outlined above, standard outpatient phototherapy is more difficult in the HIV-infected patient. We have found, however, that retinoid therapy is well tolerated in general, and many patients are therefore begun on retinoids in low doses in anticipation of using phototherapy in the future. With low-dose etretinate treatment (25 mg daily), psoriasis may improve or stabilize. The combination of retinoids plus phototherapy allows less light to be used and results in more rapid clearing of the psoriasis. Most patients with HIV-associated psoriasis in our center who get phototherapy receive RE-UVB. We have avoided PUVA, because of theoretical concerns of immunosuppression. This is not based on actual data, but the fact that PUVA delivers light deeper into the skin, reaching the dermis where HIV-infected dermal dendrocytes have been demonstrated. Other centers have used PUVA without complications. Should PUVA be required, we would still recommend prior initiation of retinoids and the use of RE-PUVA for the reasons mentioned above. We have made regular use of topical PUVA for hand and foot psoriasis, in combination with oral retinoids, with success.

When outpatient phototherapy, as outlined above, is ineffective, in the uninfected patient we might proceed to methotrexate or cyclosporin A (37,38). In the setting of HIV, because of our concern in the use of these immunosuppressives, we have favored the "Day Treatment" approach. Patients are admitted to the Day Treatment Center and given very intense Goeckerman or Ingram therapy. Patients with even the most recalcitrant disease tend to respond well to either regimen. With 3–4 weeks of intensive treatment, very severe patients can be improved. In Day Treatment maximal use can be made of local therapies to target problem areas, usually the hands and feet. These patients are put into a remission that is maintained with oral retinoids and intermittent phototherapy, avoiding immunosuppressive agents. The disadvantage of this approach is its higher cost, but we feel that is warranted to avoid the use of potentially life-threatening immunosuppressives in an already immunocompromised host.

The third level of treatment includes the oral agents. As mentioned above, we begin retinoid therapy early and use it aggressively in the HIV-infected patient with psoriasis. It has been of tremendous benefit, and toxicity has been minimal. This is because it seems to work at reasonably low doses in some HIV-infected patients. Many of our patients have hepatitis B and C virus infection, but liver function test abnormalities have only occasionally required us to discontinue retinoid therapy.

Cyclosporin and methotrexate are last-line agents, and we consider them relatively contraindicated on the basis that they theoretically could accelerate immunosuppression. However, there are case reports describing the beneficial use of both agents in HIV-associated psoriasis without significant worsening of HIV disease, and we have used methotrexate when required in the photosensitive psoriatic intolerant or failing retinoid therapy (37,38). In fact, an HIV-positive renal transplant patient has been described as receiving cyclosporin for 8 years without experiencing adverse effects (39). There is insufficient survival data to comment on the outcome of such treatment.

It appears that MTX and CSA are better tolerated early in HIV disease and are of greater risk in patients with advanced disease, when additional immunosuppression can lead to life-threatening opportunistic infections. If MTX or CSA is to be considered in an HIV-infected patient, adequate prophylaxis for *Pneumocystis* pneumonia, mucosal candidiasis, cryptococcosis, *M. avium*-complex, herpes simplex, and perhaps cytomegalovirus and toxoplasmosis in the person seropositive for these latent agents, should be considered. A high level of vigilance must be maintained for the development of one of these infections. These agents should be used as required, and once the psoriasis has improved, the dose reduced, and attempts made to change to safer treatment. For instance, treat with MTX and then switch to retinoid or RE-UVB for maintenance.

REFERENCES

1. Arnett, F.C., Reveille, J.D., and Duvic, M. (1991). Psoriasis and psoriatic arthritis associated with human immunodeficiency virus infection. *Rheum. Dis. Clin. North Am.* 17:59–78.
2. Reveille, J.D., Conant, M.A., and Duvic, M. (1990). Human immunodeficiency virus-associated psoriasis, psoriatic arthritis and Reiter's syndrome: a disease continuum? *Arthritis Rheum.* 33:1574–1578.
3. Obuch, M.L., Maurer, T.A., Becker, B., and Berger, T.G. (1992). Psoriasis and human immunodeficiency virus infection. *J. Am. Acad. Dermatol.* 27:667–673.
4. Garbe, C., Husak, R., and Orfanos, C.E. (1994). HIV associated dermatoses and their prevalence in 456 HIV infected individuals. Relation to immunological status and diagnostic significance. *Hautartz* 45:623–629.
5. Berman, A., Espinoza, L.R., Diaz, J.D., Aguiler, J.L., Rolando, T., Vasey, F.B., Germain, B.F., and Lockey, R.F. (1988). Rheumatic manifestations of human immunodeficiency virus infection. *Am. J. Med.* 85:59–64, 1988.
6. Duvic, M., Johnson, T.M., Rapini, R.P., Freese, T., Brewton, G., and Rios, A. (1987). Acquired immunodeficiency syndrome-associated psoriasis and Reiter's syndrome. *Arch. Dermatol.* 123:1622–1632.
7. Kaplin, M.H., Sadick, N.S., Wieder, J., Farber, B.F., and Neidt, G.W. (1989). Antipsoriatic effects of zidovudine in human immunodeficiency virus associated psoriasis. *J. Am. Acad. Dermatol.* 20:76–82.
8. Solinger, A.M., and Hess, E.V. (1990). HIV and arthritis. *Arthritis Rheum.* 17:562 (letter).
9. Winchester, R., Brancato, L., Itescu, S., Skovron, M.L., and Soloman, G. (1988). Implications from the occurrence of Reiter's syndrome and related disorders in association with advanced HIV infection. *Scand. J. Rheumatol.* 74(Suppl):89–93.
10. Clark, M., Kinsolving, M., and Chernoff, D. (1989). The prevalence of arthritis in two HIV infected cohorts. *Arthritis Rheum.* 32(Suppl):S85.
11. Hochberg, M.C., Fox, R., Nelson, K.R., and Saah, A. (1990). HIV infection is not a risk factor for Reiter's syndrome (abstract). *Clin. Res.* 37:318A.
12. Michet, C.J., Machado, E.B.V., Ballard, D.J., and McKenna, C.H. (1988). Epidemiology of Reiter's syndrome in Rochester Minnesota 1950–1980. *Arthritis Rheum.* 31:428–431.
13. Noer, H.R. (1966). An 'experimental' epidemic of Reiter's syndrome. *JAMA* 198:693–698.
14. Winchester, R., Bernstein, D.H., Fischer, H.D., Enlow, R., and Solomon, G. (1987). The co-occurrence of Reiter's syndrome and acquired immunodeficiency. *Ann. Intern. Med.* 106:19–26.
15. Hughes, R.A., and Keat, A.C.S. (1990). *Yersinia* reactive arthritis and human immunodeficiency virus infection. *Arthritis Rheum.* 33:758–759 (letter).
16. Silveiro, L.H., Gutierrez, F., Scopelitis, E., Cuellar, M.L., Citera, G., and Espinosa, L.R. (1993). *Chlamydia*-induced reactive arthritis. *Rheum. Dis. Clin. North Am.* 19:351–362.
17. Leung, D.Y.M., Travers, J.B., Giorno, R., Norris, D.A., Skinner, R., Aelion, J., Kazemi, L.V., Kim, M.H., Trumble, A.E., Kotb, M., and Schlievert, P.M. (1995). Evidence for a streptococcal superantigen driven process in acute guttate psoriasis. *J. Clin. Invest.* 96: 2106–2112.
18. Choi, Y., Kotzin, B., Herron, L., Callahan, J., Marrack, P., and Kappler, J. (1989). Interaction of staphylococcal aureus 'superantigens' with human T cells. *Proc. Natl. Acad. Sci. USA.* 86:8941–8945.
19. Jaffe, D., May, L.P., Sanchez, M., and Moy, J. (1991). Staphylococcal sepsis in HIV antibody seropositive psoriasis patients. *J. Am. Acad. Dermatol.* 24: 970–972.
20. Duvic, M. (1990). Immunology of AIDS related to psoriasis. *J. Invest. Dermatol.* 95(Suppl):38S–40S.
21. Gottlieb, S.L., Gilleaudeau, P., Johnson, R., Estes, L., Woodworth, T.G., Gottlieb, A.B., and Krueger, J.G. (1995). Response of psoriasis to a lymphocyte selective toxin (DAB 389 IL-2) suggests a primary immune, but not keratinocyte pathogenic basis. *Nature Med.* 1: 442–447.
22. Baker, B.S., Griffths, C.E.M., Lambert, S., Powles, A.V., Leonard, J.N., Valdimarsson, H., and Fry, L. (1987). The effects of cyclosporin A on T lymphocyte and dendritic cell sub-populations in psoriasis. *Br. J. Dermatol.* 116:503–510.
23. Gottlieb, A.B., Grossman, R.M., Khandke, L., Carter, D.M., Sehgal, P.B., Fu, S.M., Granelli-Piperno, A., Rivas, M., Barazani, L., and Krueger, J.G. (1992). Studies of effect of cyclosporin in psoriasis in vivo: combined effects on activated T lymphocytes and epidermal regenerative maturation. *J. Invest. Dermatol.* 98:302–309.
24. Inman, R.D., Chiu, B., Johnson, M.E.A., Vas, S., and Falk, J. (1989). HLA class 1-related impairment in IL-2 production and lymphocyte response to microbial antigens in reactive arthritis. *J. Immunol.* 142: 4256–4260.

25. Zemelman, V., Van Neer, F., Roberts, N., Patel, P., Langtry, J., and Straughton, R.C.D. (1994). Epidermal Langerhan's cell, HIV-1 infection and psoriasis. *Br. J. Dermatol.* 130:307–311.
26. Van Neer, F., Zemelman, V., Cerio, R., Langtry, J., and Straughton, R.C.D. (1993). The role of factor XIIIa-positive dermal dendrocytes in HIV-positive psoriatics. *Br. J. Dermatol.* 128:29–33.
27. Mahoney, S.E., Duvic, M., Nickoloff, B.J., Minshall, M., Smith, L.C., Griffiths, C.E.M., Paddock, S.W., and Lewis, D.E. (1991). Human immunodeficiency virus transcripts identified in HIV-related psoriasis and Kaposi's sarcoma lesions. *J. Clin. Invest.* 88:174–185.
28. Leonard, J.M., Abramczuk, J.W., Pezen, D.S., Rutledge, R., Belcher, J.H., Hakim, F., Shearer, G., Lamperth, L., Travis, W., Fredrickson, T., Notkins, A.L., and Martin, M.A. (1988). Development of disease and virus recovery in transgenic mice containing proviral DNA. *Science* 242:1665–1670.
29. Duvic, M. (1987). Remission of AIDS associated psoriasis with zidovudine therapy. *Lancet* 2:627(letter).
30. Townsend, B.L., Cohen, P.R., and Duvic, M. (1995). Zidovudine for the treatment of HIV negative patients with psoriasis: a pilot study. *J. Am. Acad. Dermatol.* 32:994–999.
31. Leung, D.Y.M., Walsh, P., Giorno, R., and Norris, D.A. (1993). A potential role for superantigens in the pathogenesis of psoriasis. *J. Invest. Dermatol.* 100: 225–228.
32. Lane, N. (1994). Psoriasis and psoriatic like arthritis. IN: Cohen, P.T., Sande, M.A., and Volberding, P.A., eds: *The AIDS Knowledge Base*, 2nd ed. Little Brown, Boston, pp 5.37-1–5.37-3.
33. Ruzicka, T., Froschl, M., Hohenleutner, U., Holzman, H., and Braun-Falco, O. (1987). Treatment of HIV induced retinoid resistant psoriasis with zidovudine. *Lancet* 2:1469–1470 (letter).
34. Gray, J.D., Bottomley, W., Layton, A.M., Cotterill, J.A., and Monteiro, E. (1992). The use of calcipotriol in HIV related psoriasis. *Clin. Exp. Dermatol.* 17: 342–343.
35. Meola, T., Soter, N.A., Ostreicher, R., Sanchez, M., and Moy, J.A. (1993). The safety of UVB phototherapy in patients with HIV infection. *J. Am. Acad. Dermatol.* 29:216–220.
36. Fotiades, J., Lim, H.W., Jiang, S.B., Soter, N.A., Sanchez, M., and Moy, J. (1995). Efficacy of ultraviolet B phototherapy for psoriasis in patients infected with human immunodeficiency virus. *Photoimmunol. Photomed.* 11:107–111.
37. Maurer, T.A., Zackheim, H.S., Taffanelli, L., and Berger, T.G. (1994). The use of methotrexate for the treatment of psoriasis in patients with HIV infection. *J. Am. Acad. Dermatol.* 31:372–375.
38. Allen, B.R. (1992). Use of cyclosporin for psoriasis in HIV positive patient. *Lancet* 339:686 (letter).
39. Jacobson, S.K., Calne, R.Y., and Wreghitt, T.G. (1991). Outcome of HIV infection in transplant patient on cyclosporin. *Lancet* 337:794 (letter).

7

Psoriatic Arthritis

Eva Zachariae and Hugh Zachariae
Aarhus University Hospital, Aarhus, Denmark

Although Jean Louis Alibert described an association between psoriasis and arthritis as early as 1818 (1), the recognition of psoriatic arthritis (PA) as a separate entity has been questioned up to the last decades (2). However, the increasing radiological, serological, clinical, and genetic evidence enables us to place PA as a specific disease in the group of seronegative spondyloarthropathies.

DEFINITION

In 1964, PA was listed as a clinical entity by the American Rheumatism Association (3). Diagnostic clinical criteria, however, have not been agreed upon (3a) and several definitions have been suggested stressing separate features of this multifaceted disease. The high incidence of distal joint involvement compared to rheumatoid arthritis (RA) as well as arthritis mutilans, also seen in RA, have received special attention (4,5). The great variety of clinical manifestations can be framed in the definition suggested by Moll and Wright in 1973 (6): Inflammatory arthritis associated with psoriasis, usually with a negative serological test for rheumatoid arthritis. Other, more detailed sets of criteria have been suggested (7,8). The term psoriatic arthritis is suggested by the American Rheumatism Association (3) and is widely used.

EPIDEMIOLOGY

Extensive studies have reported on the prevalence of psoriasis (9). There is, however, no agreement in the reports on the frequency of arthritis in psoriatics. The criteria for evaluating the arthritis differ widely, the variety reflecting the differences of the patient populations examined (10–19). Inpatients in a dermatology department treating severe cutaneous disease will show a higher incidence than those of an outpatient clinic diagnosing and treating less severe skin complaints, or patients interviewed in a general population survey. In the arthritis clinic, the rheumatologist may overlook slight skin lesions that have been ignored by the patient, but would be clinically and histologically confirmed by the dermatologist. A family history of skin complaints may reveal a genetic disposition which together with a thorough investigation of the skin will change the diagnosis from seronegative rheumatoid arthritis to psoriatic arthritis. Also, the rare patients with HLA B27 negative ankylosing spondylitis on close examination may reveal a psoriasis (20) or a spondylitis characteristic of that disease. On the other hand, the dermatologist may have difficulties in distinguishing osteoarthritis, arthralgia, or soft tissue rheumatism from inflammatory arthritis. The fact that the symptoms of psoriasis as well as psoriatic arthritis can be very slight, causing little inconvenience to the patient so that the condition is never diagnosed, contributes to the conception of PA as a not uncommon disease, with a prevalence around 20 in psoriatic patients (17).

GENETICS

Early epidemiological surveys confirmed the importance of heredity in the etiology of psoriasis (9,10,13). A familial occurrence of PA was thoroughly investigated by Moll and Wright in 1973 (21), and at the same time the first reports on HLA antigens in PA made clear that genetic factors also play an important part in this disease (22,23). No clear Mendelian pattern could be established from these investigations, and it was concluded that as in psoriasis, the genetic transmission is a multifactorial inheritance with environmental factors playing a part in triggering arthritis in the genetically predisposed.

Since then numerous studies have contributed to our knowledge of PA and enabled us to divide it into clinical subgroups (24–32). The first recognized and most conspicuous association was that of HLA B27 and spondyloarthropathies (30). HLA B27, moderately raised in the PA group as a whole, as would be expected was found significantly increased in the spondylitic group, though not as high as in akylosing spondylitis (AS), whereas B27 was normal or only slightly raised in patients with peripheral arthritis alone (24,26–28,31,32). The antigens HLA A26 and B17 are also found significantly raised in PA by most investigators (25–27,32). HLA B17, if present, seems to be linked to severe arthritis, but as is well known it is also found to be high in psoriasis without arthritis (28,32). HLA B38 is found by some authors to be a marker of severe peripheral arthritis (25–28,31). Spondylitis in one study was present in all B39-positive patients (33).

HLA DR typing has shown as association between PA and DR3, DR4, and DR7 (26–28,31). DR4 is recognized as linked to severe seropositive RA, but several authors have found the prevalence of this antigen normal in seronegative arthritis, while others have found no difference from RA (28,34).

The significantly raised frequency of Cw6 in psoriasis is well recognized (35). This probably is reflected in the significant increase also found in PA (27,28,31). Armstrong suggests a primary association of Cw6 with psoriasis with DR4 as an additional marker for psoriatic arthritis (28). HLA DR7 is increased in PA at a higher frequency than in psoriasis without arthritis, and seems to be connected with severe disease of long duration (28). Of interest is the recent report by Sakkas, who detected a particular DNA pattern in 60% of patients with PA, but only in 12% of patients with psoriasis alone (36).

LABORATORY FINDINGS

The abnormalities in laboratory findings to some extent can be explained as a result of joint inflammation and vary with the severity of the joint disease, whereas none are diagnostic for this special arthritis entity.

Of greatest significance is the negative *SCA test* used in the definition of the disease (6). A positive SCA test is, however, found in 5% of normal individuals (37) and would therefore also be expected in the true PA population. A high titer, however, should alert us to look for other symptoms of RA, i.e., nodules, the absence of which are characteristic for PA. Considering the incidence of RA in the general population a coincidence of PA and RA should be expected in a small percentage of patients.

Antinuclear antibodies, which are often present in RA, are not found in PA in most reports (17,38).

A number of nonspecific markers for joint inflammation are used to assess disease activity. Among these, the *erythrocyte sedimentation rate* (ESR) is most widely used to evaluate the effect of drug treatment. *Hemoglobin* (Hb), *white blood cell* (WBC) *count*, *platelet count*, and *C-reactive protein* (CRP) are other such markers. Recently, new parameters have been investigated. *Plasma viscosity* and *serum histidine* may prove useful in assessing disease severity (39). Rubins found a decrease in *T helper/T suppressor cells*, corresponding to a more severe clinical course of the disease (40). *Circulating immune complexes* have also been found as markers of disease activity and tissue damage, the incidence decreasing after improvement of the disease following treatment (41).

Serum uric acid is often found elevated in psoriatics and has been found raised in PA patients in a number of studies (15,42). This is explained as a result of increased purine metabolism owing to high cell turnover. The slightly elevated levels usually do not give rise to attacks of gout. Lambert and Wright (42) found a high prevalence of values above normal, but a mean value inside the normal range. This would be influenced by the intake of nonsteroidal anti-inflammatory drugs (NSAIDs) blocking the renal secretion of uric acid.

Examination of serum complement levels have shown normal values (43). *Amino-terminal procolla-*

gen III peptide has been found significantly raised in patients with active RA (44); this is also the case in PA (44a). Danielsen (45) found elevated levels of *immunoglobulin A* (IgA) in PA. Tapanes (46) measured IgG, IgA, and IgM in serum and found normal ranges in PA as compared to elevated levels in RA. However, IgA has also been found elevated in other spondyloarthropathies, and has lead to glomerulonephritis as described by several authors (47,48).

PATHOGENESIS

Psoriasis is a unique example of excess cellular proliferation and inflammation. Psoriasis and PA share several features. As already mentioned, the patterns of inheritance are multifactorial and polygenic in both and some HLA antigens are shared by both. Both the arthritis and psoriasis may be induced or exacerbated by infection, and the histology of the skin in psoriasis and the joints in PA have great similarities. Both the skin (23) and joint disease (50), however, are also pleomorphic with several subtypes. The striking clinical similarity of PA and Reiter's disease suggest that we may be dealing with the same type of process in both entities; this is especially true for associations with pustular psoriasis.

Though PA has not definitely been proved to be caused by immunological disturbances, there is proof that immunological factors are important in the etiology. The importance of the T-cell (50a) is demonstrated by the early influx of these cells. This influx comes prior to the neutrophil infiltration. The IL-2 receptor is a relative specific marker of early T-cell activation and is associated with T-cell proliferation. T-cell activation is as in the psoriatic plaques followed by neutrophil activation and vasodilatation. Endothelial swelling and thickening of the vessel wall follow (8,51). Involved cytokines are, among others, IL-1, IL-2, IL-6, IL-8, and IFN-γ. Tumor necrosis factor (TNF) has also been implicated in the formation of the articular lesions. Released from immunocompetent cells, it activates the inflammatory process and may cause bone reabsorption. The conception of PA as a clinical entity not identical with RA is also confirmed by pathological findings. The synovitic processes have been considered nearly indistinguishable in RA and PA (50). Newer investigators, however, found some differences (50b). Espinoza in light and electron microscopy studies found vascular changes the most prominent feature in PA. They included endothelial cell swelling, inflammatory cell infiltration, and thickening of the vessel wall (8,51). In chronic disease, marked deposition of newly formed collagen in the subsynovial tissue, the changes differing qualitatively from what is found in RA, was in agreement with the clinical findings of severe capsular fibrosis (52). In vitro studies of skin and synovium fibroblasts supported the concept of the importance of this cell in the pathogenesis of PA (52a,52b).

The pathology of psoriatic synovitis appears to depend upon the joint involved and the duration of the disease (52). With advanced synovitis, the difference between PA and RA become discernible pathologically, especially in the distal interphalangeal (DIP) joints. The hyperplasia of the synovial lining cells is found less pronounced than in RA, also in weight-bearing joints. Capsular fibrosis is prominent with thickening of small- and medium-sized arteries. Nail fold capillary changes distinguish PA from RA and probably account for the involvement of DIP joints (53,58).

Types I and II synoviocytes found in chronic PA confirm that immunological mechanisms are maintaining the tissue injury (54). Neuropeptides have been studied in synovium and synovial membrane and seem to have a role in the development of arthritis (54a). Fibrinogen and fibrin-related antigens have been demonstrated in synovium (55). C_3 levels are found normal (56).

The radiological periosteal changes so characteristic of the seronegative spondyloarthropathies have been shown to be due to elevation of periosteum by proliferation of periosteal cells without inflammatory infiltrate, large quantities of osteoblasts being overlaid by fibroblasts. This induces the destruction and remodeling so typical of PA (57).

Focal inflammatory lesions, known as enthesopathies, of the attachment of ligaments and tendons have been seen in patients with PA, but not much knowledge of this exists. The histopathology of the flexor tendon synovitis with "ray" involvement of digits is not clear and can hardly be explained as a kind of Koebner phenomenon otherwise seen in the selection of arthritic joints. That trauma can influence the onset of PA has been described and discussed by several authors (6,60,63). This phenomenon is found related to the T4/T8 ratio and number of dendritic cells in skin (59), but has not been investigated in arthritic lesions.

A marked increase in the frequency of PA in psoriatics with HLA DR^+ keratinocytes was demonstrated recently by Gottlieb (61), her patients having severe psoriasis not responding to outpatient management.

Synovial fluid findings have not been found much different from what is seen in RA. In acute synovitis, the WBC count is usually high, consisting mainly of polymorphonuclear neutrophils (PMNs). In chronic synovitis, low cell counts are usual with an increase in mononuclear cells.

The wide spectrum of symptoms accompanying acquired immunodeficiency syndrome implies dysfunction of the musculoskeletal system. The increased incidence of psoriasis and PA in HIV-positive patients may help to elucidate the pathogenesis of these conditions. It indicates that CD4+ T-helper cells are not necessary for their development.

CLASSIFICATION

The varied picture of PA has made it necessary to distinguish between subgroups. The classification by Moll and Wright (6) covers most purposes:

1. Oligoarticular asymmetrical arthritis (70%). This is by far the most often seen. We find the typical "sausage digit" (Fig. 1) here and the monoarthritis belongs to this group.
2. Symmetrical involvement often clinically difficult to distinguish from RA (15%). Metacarpophalangeal (MCP) joint involvement is more common than in the oligoarticular form. For diagnosis, a thorough search for nodules, repeated SCA tests, and a careful screening of the x-rays is helpful. Patients with severe disease are often found in this group.
3. Arthritis involving mainly or exclusively the DIP joints (5%). This group, although conspicuous, is rare and the condition is not always disabling, depending on the physical demands on the patient. Severe nail psoriasis in these patients may be the major problem.
4. Arthritis mutilans (5%), in which there is typical telescoping of fingers and toes caused by extensive bone resorption, is also seen in RA. It is not always accompanied by severe general disease. Wright, in a later classification, has included the type dominated by peripheral ankylosis in this group (60).

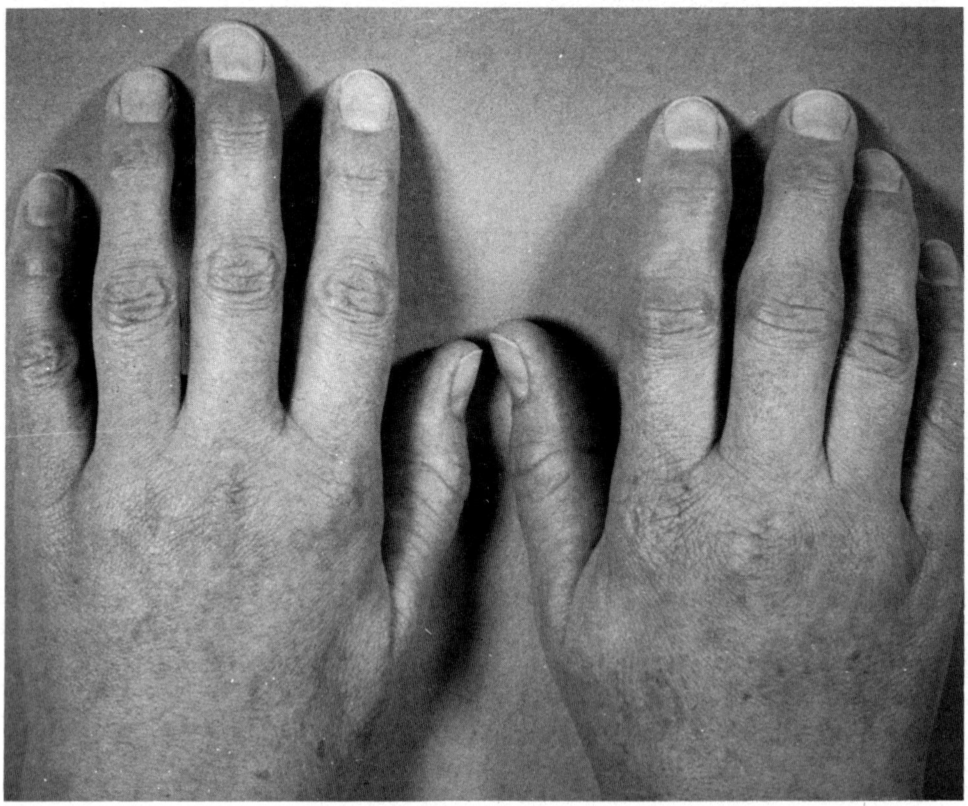

Figure 1 Psoriatic arthritis. Asymmetric swelling of DIP joints and "sausage digit" of right third finger.

5. The spinal form (5%) resembles but is not necessarily identical with ankylosing spondylitis. This interesting group appears in different forms. Patients with anterior chest wall symptoms and arthritis mainly affecting the axial joints could be placed in this group. This will be discussed in the following.

The significant overlap between these groups presents problems, and several suggestions for a reclassification have been published (60a,60b). Convenient for clinical use is Veale's suggestion of three groups (60c):

1. An asymmetric arthritis usually, but not invariably, involving a small number of joints with few erosions, infrequent deformity, and good preservation of function.
2. A symmetric polyarthritis, frequently erosive, deforming, and functionally disabling, but distinguishable from RA by association with DIP joint arthritis, spondylitis, and negative RF (titer < 80).
3. Predominant spondylitis, similar to AS, which may accompany a peripheral arthritis but behaves independently of it.

SPONDYLOARTHROPATHY

Attention has been called to the relationship to other inflammatory joint diseases affecting the spinal joints by Wright and Reed, who described the link between Reiter's disease and PA (62). After discovery of the HLA B27 antigen, this link has been more closely defined (64,65). In the group of seronegative spondyloarthropathies the association of PA to Reiter's syndrome seems closest, the skin manifestations being histologically identical and also affecting the mucous membranes. The frequency of psoriasis in inflammatory bowel disease has been found increased (66,66a). In this condition, the presence of sacroiliitis is connected with HLA B27 (67). The radiological picture of psoriatic spondylitis may be indistinguishable from ankylosing spondylitis, although in many patients there are obvious differences. Often the pain and restriction of spinal mobility seem less pronounced in PA (68,69). Sixty percent of HLA B27–negative patients with ankylosing spondylitis have been found to have psoriasis (10). Many patients have less severe cervical complaints, although there seems to be special groups of cervical involvement (32,74).

In psoriasis vulgaris, there is no increase of HLA B27, whereas the relationship between generalized pustular psoriasis and this antigen has been established (64,65). Though histologically indistinguishable, the localized type of pustular psoriasis and pustulosis palmoplantaris (persistent palmoplantar pustulosis), appear less closely connected to this antigen, and the type of axial involvement seems to differ.

THE SAPHO SYNDROME

During the last decades increasing attention has been paid to the appearance of arthritis in the anterior chest wall accompanied by sclerotic bone lesions and sacroiliitis, usually unilateral in patients with palmoplantar pustulosis or acne (70–72). The acronym SAPHO syndrome (synovitis, acne, pustulosis hyperostosis, osteitis) (72a) has been widely accepted for this condition. The axial involvement including sacroiliitis, the moderately increased incidence of HLA B27 as well as the significant association to inflammatory bowel disease, and the similarities between the pustulotic and psoriatic lesions have established the relationship to the spondyloarthropathies. Lately, reports of arthritis in the temporomandibular joints, another axial site, have drawn attention to the problems of this localization.

Eye inflammation in the form of conjunctivitis and iritis occurs mainly in the HLA B27–positive patients.

RADIOLOGICAL FINDINGS

In 1961, Wright described the characteristic x-ray picture in PA compared to RA (75), the recognition of which can be conclusive in the differential diagnosis. A number of special features distinguish these radiographic findings.

The simultaneous appearance of destruction and bony proliferation is among the most typical radiographic findings. The destruction, especially in DIP and PIP joints, can be severe, concentrating on the "bare areas" (76) of the joints and spreading to the subchrondal bone, creating the typical pencil shape of the distal end of the phalanx. Adjacent to the erosions, new bone formation is seen, which starts as fluffy masses (Figs. 2 and 3), and later develops into well demarcated bone. This is seen in the joint area as well as along the shafts of the bones, and typically at insertions of tendons and ligaments (Fig. 4). Cortical erosions in the tufts of the distal phalanges are regularly seen (77), resulting in whittling of bone in both fingers and toes (Fig. 5). Typically this is found in relation to nail involvement (75). Relative sparing of

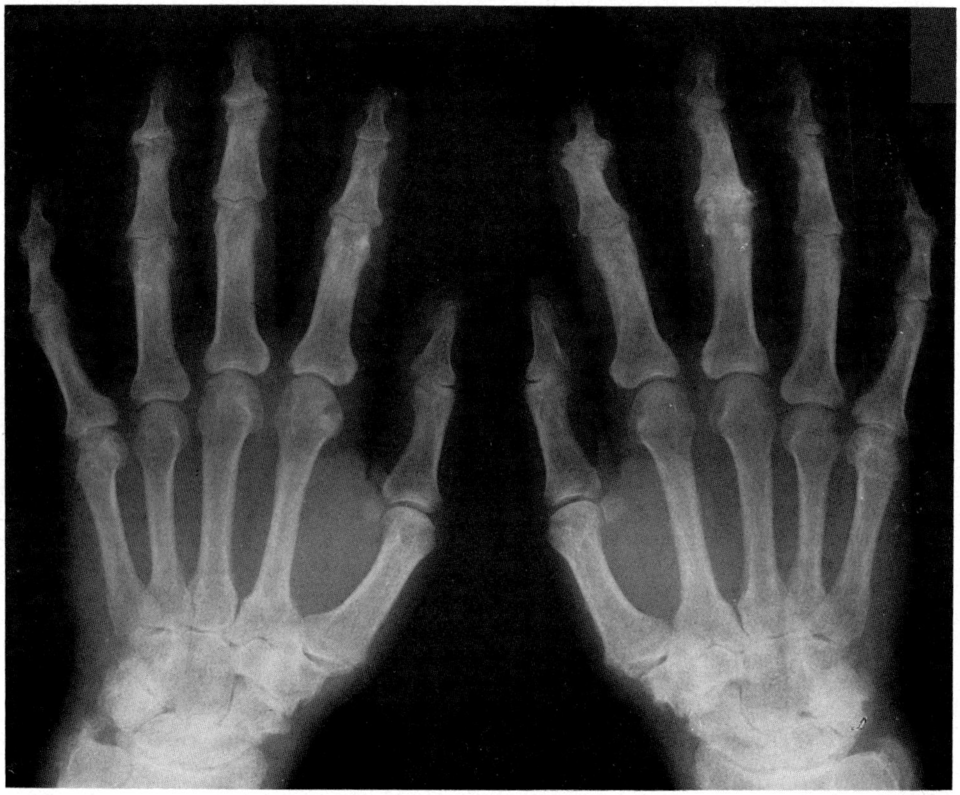

Figure 2 Classic radiographic changes of psoriatic arthritis of the hands. Asymmetrical erosions with bony proliferation and fluffy periosteal changes especially at ulnar styloid, relative sparing of MCPs, bony ankylosis of both fifth DIPs, and normal mineralization.

the metacarpophalangeal (MCP) joints with affection of DIP and proximal interphalangeal (PIP) joints is common (78). Sausage digit involvement of a single ray showing soft tissue swelling due to flexor tendon sheath inflammation accompanied by arthritis of the joints of the finger or toe is another characteristic feature. In the feet, severe destruction of the toes may be encountered even in patients who had had no complaints at this site (75).

The osteoporosis seen in psoriatic arthritis remains controversial. A low-grade osteoporosis compared to RA is accepted by most investigators (75,79), especially in the hands and feet. The distal forearm bone mineral content of patients with severe polyarticular disease, however, was found to be similar to that of a comparable group of RA patients (80). Ankylosis of the joints occurs more often and earlier in PA than in RA.

The radiographic differential diagnosis between erosive osteoarthritis and PA may present problems in patients with slight symptoms. The difference between the "mouse ear" appearance caused by the marginal erosions of PA and the "seagull" picture in the joint destruction of erosive osteoarthritis has been described by Martel (76).

In the axial skeleton, the changes are asymmetrical (Fig. 6) compared to what is seen in ankylosing spondylitis, and are similar to those of Reiter's disease (81), whereas the findings of ankylosing spondylitis and inflammatory bowel disease have more in common. The reports on the incidence of sacroiliitis varies from 10 to 50% (75,78,82). On x-ray screening of patients who have never had low back complaints, sacroiliitis is often found. On the other hand, psoriatics may show spinal involvement without sacroiliitis. The arthritis of the sacroiliac joint is often unilateral or asymmetrical, as are the characteristic nonmarginal syndesmophytes and paravertebral ossifications in the thoracolumbar spine with often large nonmarginal parasyndesmophytes bridging the vertebrae at irregu-

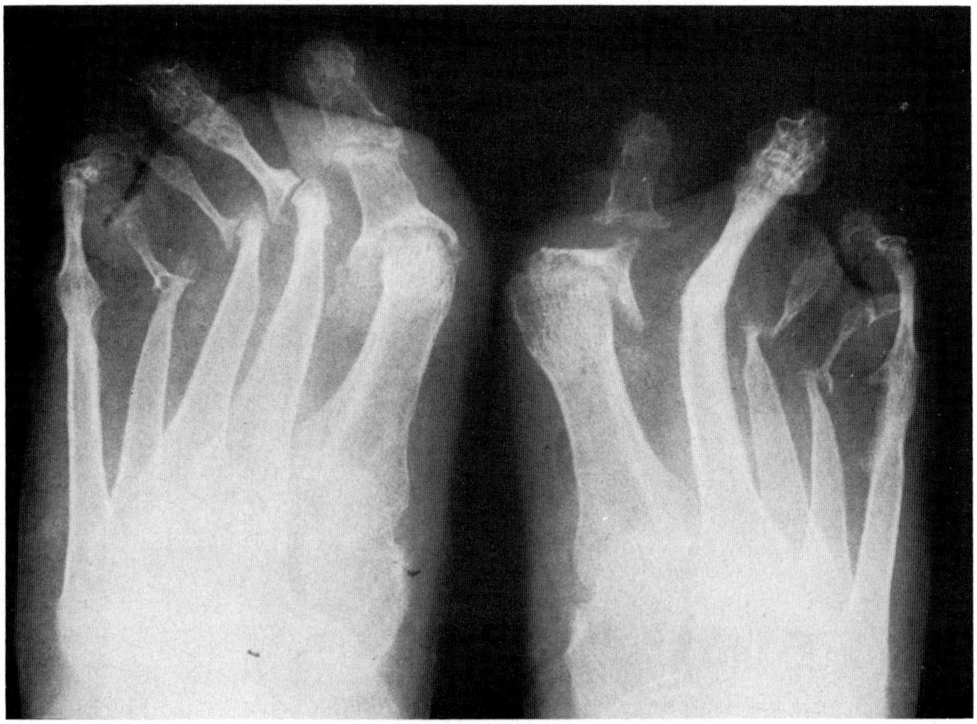

Figure 3 Arthritis mutilans of the feet. Note "pencil and cup" deformity in the right fourth toe and the bony ankylosis of the right second and both fifth rays.

lar sites, distinguishing the lesions from those of ankylosing spondylitis (81,83,84). A spinal form indistinguishable from ankylosing spondylitis is also seen, particularly in HLA B27–positive patients.

Inflammation at the site of tendon insertions characterizes the seronegative spondyloarthropathies (83), producing fluffy bone formations commonly seen around shoulders, knees, or pelvic bones, occasionally resulting in calcification of ligaments and tendons around the pelvis. Inflammation of the Achilles tendon and the plantar fascia at the insertion at the heel bone, resulting in erosion and spur formation, is also seen as in Reiter's disease (see Fig. 4).

The radiological findings are an important tool in the diagnosis of PA. For screening purposes of patients suspected of PA, x-rays of the hands and wrists, the feet (including lateral view), and the sacroiliac joints are usually sufficient. If this fails, more sophisticated examinations of special areas related to the complaints may be employed (Fig. 8).

Bone scintigraphy (Fig. 9) has been useful in detecting arthritis in the early stages. Increased periarticular uptake in psoriatics was found by one investigator (85). This could not be reproduced in another study (86).

Computed tomography (CT) has proved valuable especially in joints that are difficult to evaluate clinically. Magnetic resonance imaging (MRI) of inflamed joints seems highly promising as it gives information of nonosseous intra-articular tissue (86a).

CLINICAL PICTURE

The variety of the clinical course ranges from severe disabling arthritis to slight symptoms not demanding any therapy. In general, the disease is less severe than RA, allowing most patients to lead an almost normal life. A considerable number, however, develop erosive arthritis that may lead to functional impairment and requires active systemic treatment.

The *age at onset* shows a peak at about 40 years, although the symptoms in patients developing a severe disease usually start earlier (87).

Distribution between sexes is equal. The male/female ratio for the group as a whole is 1.00–1.04 (6),

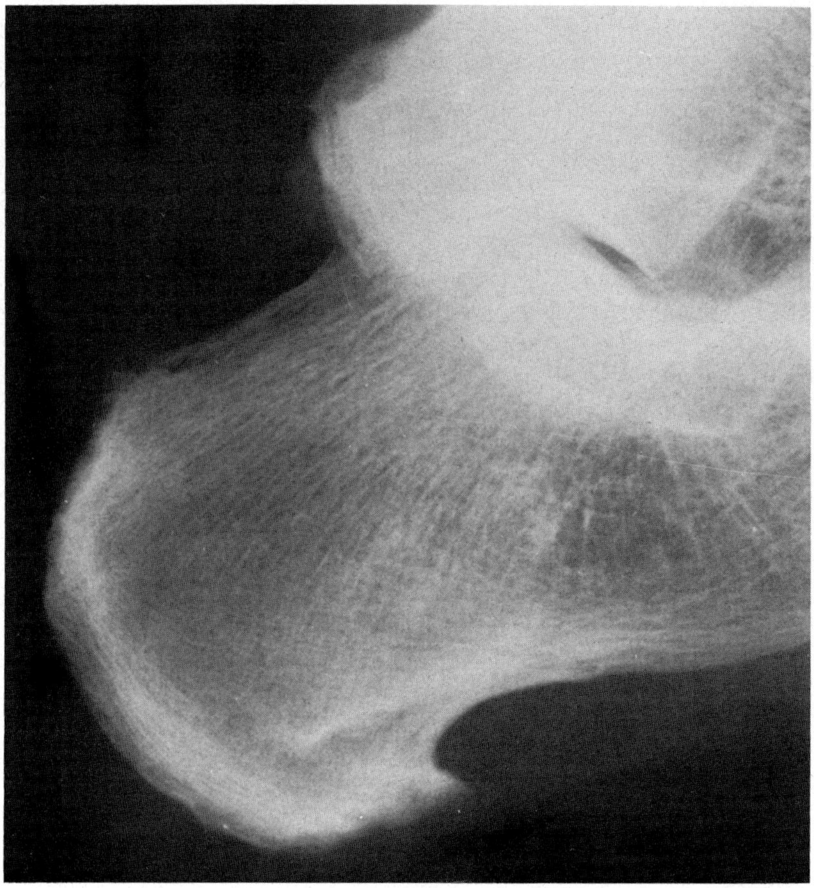

Figure 4 Heel of a patient with psoriatic arthritis. Note erosions and bony proliferation at attachment of Achilles tendon and plantar aponeurosis, cloudy bone formation at talus.

but this varies in the subgroups. The difference in the patient selection responsible for the varied figures reported (13,88). The distal joint group is more common in men. The same is the case in the group resembling ankylosing spondylitis. Females more often have an RA-like picture.

In about half the cases, the onset is acute (87), often without any triggering factors. The initial symptoms may be mistaken for gout, particularly when located to the first toe and accompanied by a raised serum uric acid. Urate crystals are not found, however, and the course of the disease will prove the right diagnosis. This mistake is common, and PA should be ruled out through thorough investigation of the x-ray findings and family history. In a patient with psoriasis, a deep Koebner phenomenon (6,60) must be suspected if there is a complaint of a sprained ankle, a suspected meniscal tear, or a traumatized finger or toe showing persistent swelling and tenderness. Fever and malaise accompanying the initial arthritis may be the sign of progressive polyarticular disease.

The most common clinical type is asymmetrical oligo- or monarticular and slowly progressing. This type, however, though still characterized by mild arthritis, can develop into polyarticular disease. Usually the joints of the fingers and toes are the first involved, starting with synovitis in the sheath of the flexor tendon where quantities of fluid can accumulate. At the same time, the joints of the digit are involved, creating the picture of the typical sausage digit (see Fig. 1). This localization in single rays of the hands and feet is a classic manifestation of PA. Effusions of extensor tendon sheaths are rarely seen (60). Widespread involvement of the toe joints, often causing little trouble to the patient, is not unusual (Fig. 7).

The clinical picture, however, can also be almost indistinguishable from RA, involving larger weight-

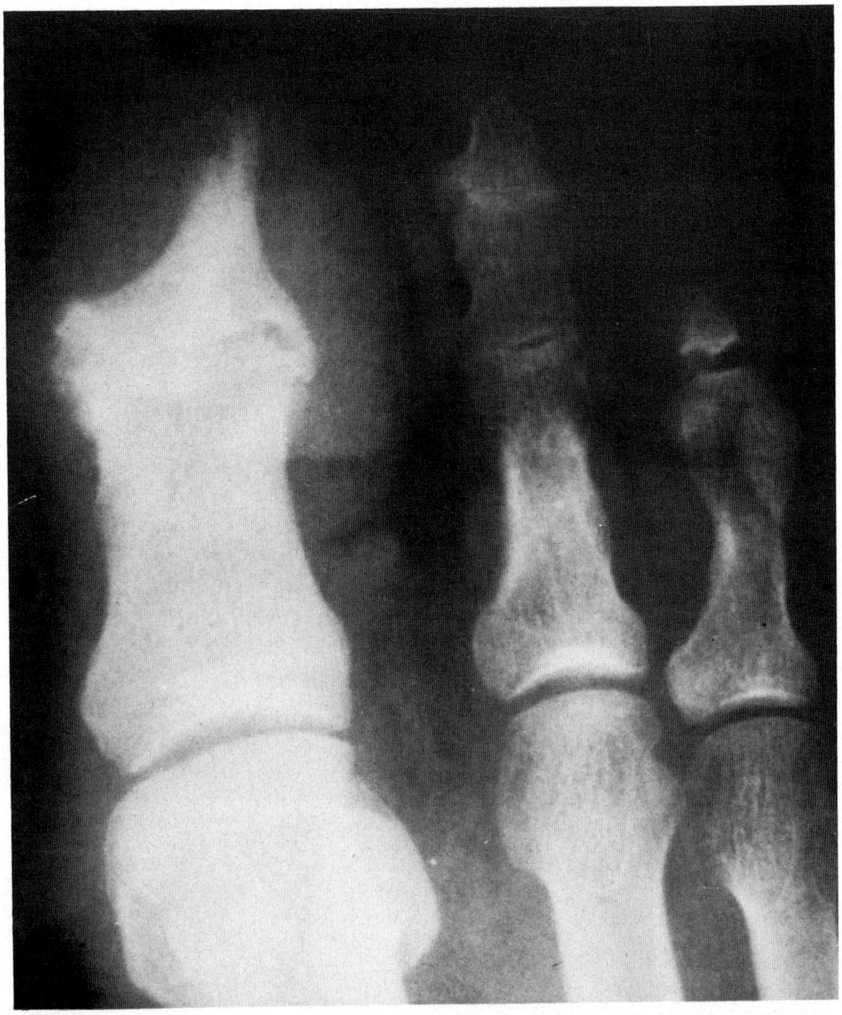

Figure 5 Psoriatic arthritis. Acro-osteolysis of distal phalanx of first toe.

bearing joints as well as the wrists and MCPs in a symmetrical fashion (78).

Several patterns of spinal involvement can be identified (84). Some cases appear indistinguishable from AS, displaying symmetrical involvement of the spine, including the sacroiliac joint. These patients are often HLA B27 positive and complain of pain and stiffness of the back. In another group, the spine involvement is typically asymmetrical and not always accompanied by sacroiliitis, which when present may be confined to one joint. In this type, the pain and restriction of movement can be less severe (89). Some patients may show isolated involvement in the cervical spine (74,84). The incidence of sacroiliitis varies in different reports (79). On x-ray screening of patients with peripheral arthritis, a high incidence of asymptomatic cases will be found. This type of sacroiliitis is not closely linked to the HLA B27 antigen (90).

Concomitant sacroiliitis is usual in the conspicuous, but rare, arthritis mutilans dominated by severe osteolysis. Another rare but severely mutilating type dominated by ankylosis may be included into this group (60,84).

Little attention has been paid to the probably large group suffering from severe disabling pain with few clinical findings (91). Vilanova has eminently described this "algic" form, the incidence of which he estimates as being 20% (12). It may be caused by enthesopathies, but the absence of histological evidence has made assessment difficult. Vilanova may be right in considering it "a simply evolutionary phase of arthropathic psoriasis" (Fig. 8).

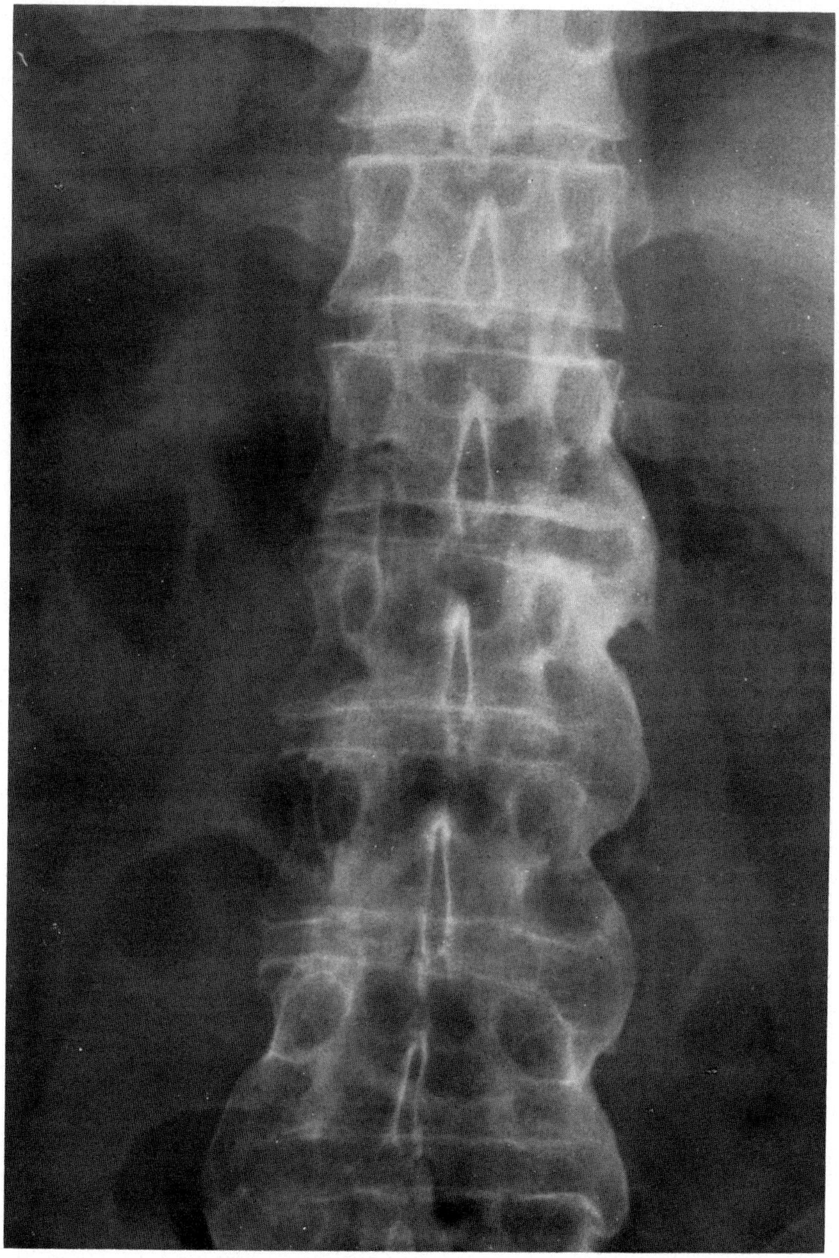

Figure 6 Psoriatic arthritis. Lumbar spine with asymmetric syndesmophytes.

Enthesitis (92) is well known in PA, and may appear on radiographs as ossification of tendon insertions.

In 74% of cases, the skin lesions precede the arthritis. Simultaneous onset occurs in only 10%, and it is not the characteristic feature as postulated in some early reports. In the remaining 16%, the arthritis comes first (87), causing difficulties in diagnosis. In patients with a typical clinical picture, i.e., classic radiographic findings and a negative SCA test and a family history of psoriasis, one must justify classifying the patient as having "psoriatic arthritis sine psoriasis," despite the absence of skin lesions. Psoriatic arthritis can be seen in all types and severities of skin involvement. The skin lesion in the patient with severe arthritis may be barely detectable. On the other hand,

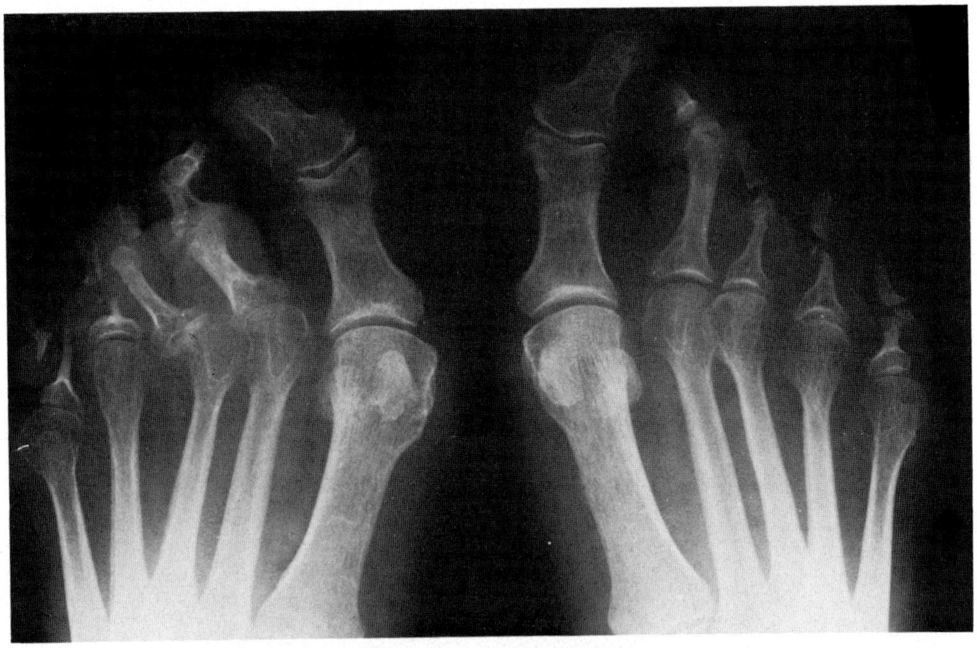

Figure 7 Arthritis mutilans of the toes. Note the relative sparing of the MTP joints. The patient had few complaints concerning the toes. Also, she had only two small erosions in her fingers and an asymptomatic sacroiliitis.

there is increased frequency and severity of arthritis in patients with widespread and serious skin involvement (14).

Pustular psoriasis is accompanied by arthritis in 30% (93) of cases. Here the arthritis may be severe. This type of skin lesion shows a linkage disequilibrium with HLA B27, present in 56% (90), and is in general connected with the spinal arthritis form. In pustulosis palmoplantaris, there is no increase of HLA B27. One type of localized pustular psoriasis is acrodermatitis continua, in which the skin lesion starts at the fingertip. This condition is often HLA B27 positive (23) and may be accompanied by severe peripheral arthritis (Fig. 10). It has much in common with Reiter's disease, as the mucous membranes and the spine may also be involved.

Nail involvement is present in a higher incidence in PA than in uncomplicated psoriasis, being found in 85% of arthritis compared to 31% in psoriasis (60). In the distal joint type, onycholysis is common.

Extra-articular manifestations are not the rule. Aortic insufficiency (8) and mitral valve prolapse (94) have been described, but one must bear in mind that chest pain can be caused by arthritis of the sternal joints. Eye inflammation as in Reiter's disease is reported to be common (95). Rheumatic nodules are not seen in PA, their presence, which is often accompanied by a significantly positive SCA test, would place the patient in the group of coincidental PA and RA. The effect of pregnancy has been studied by Østensen (96), who found that it had a beneficial effect on PA.

PSORIATIC ARTHRITIS IN CHILDHOOD

Juvenile psoriatic arthritis is rare. The incidence of this subset of juvenile chronic arthritis is about 4–9 percent. The publications on this subject are scarce (97–101). Lambert (97) reported 43, Southwood (97a) 35, Sills (100) 24, and Shore (101) 60 children with arthritis before the age of 16 and psoriasis at onset of arthritis or occurring within the subsequent 15 years. The incidence was about twice as high in girls as in boys, and the age at onset was found higher than in juvenile chronic arthritis; about 10–12 years. When the onset was early the course was severe and progressing in some cases. There was an even distribution of oligo- and polyarticular onset. In one-half of the children, the skin disease occurred first; few had simultaneous onset. In the half in whom arthritis occurred first, the diagnosis was difficult. However, the pattern of arthritis resembled what is seen in adults, including sausage digits, asymmetry, and DIP and sacroiliac involvement. All in all, the course was mild,

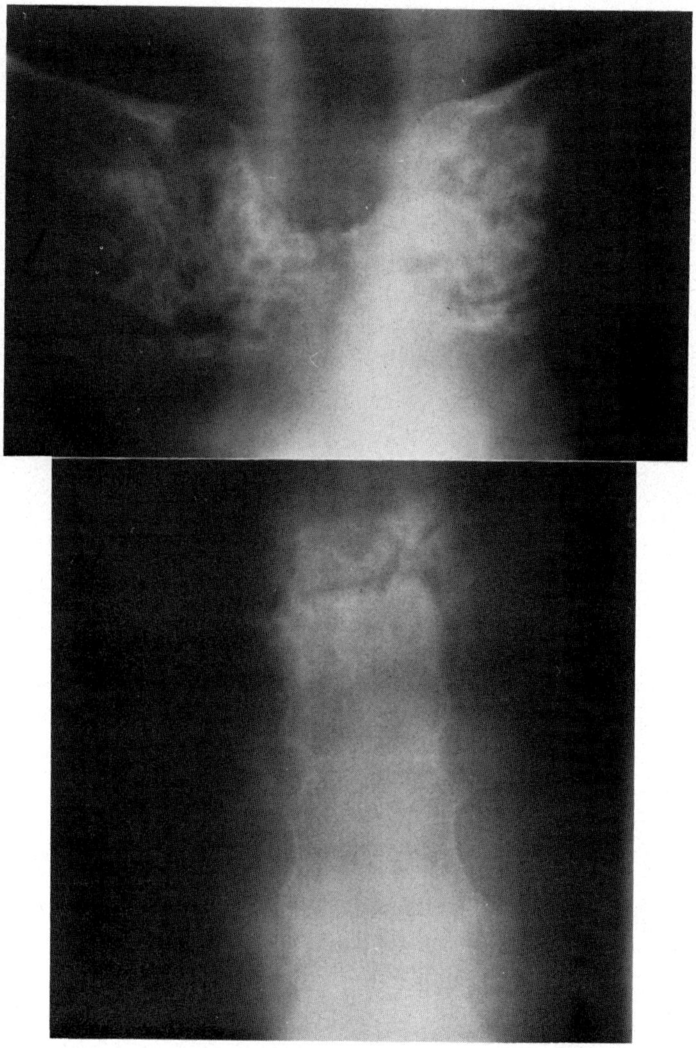

Figure 8 Zonograph of sternal joints in psoriatic arthritis. Radiographs of sternal joints can be difficult to evaluate because of overlapping with other thoracic structures. Zonography often reveals lesions otherwise overlooked.

but more serious than is seen in oligoarticular juvenile chronic arthritis, the arthritis spreading to polyarticular disease in most cases. In 10%, the course was severe and disabling. It is obvious that several subsets exist, probably with different genetic patterns (101a,101b,101c). The recognition of the progressive and erosive cases is important, as early disease-modifying medical intervention is indicated.

TREATMENT

In a number of patients, the arthritis is mild and needs little therapy. Many manage well with an occasional aspirin. Others may require treatment with nonsteroidal anti-inflammatory drugs for shorter or longer periods. Several drugs have been evaluated, none of which seem to be more effective or less toxic than others. Indomethacine has been reported to induce exacerbation of psoriasis when used topically (102) or orally (103). If this is significant for PA, it has not been established.

In oligo- or monarticular disease, intra-articular steroid injections are extremely useful. Also, injections at extra-articular sites are extensively used, helping to keep the patient physically active with little discomfort. No controlled studies of the injection of

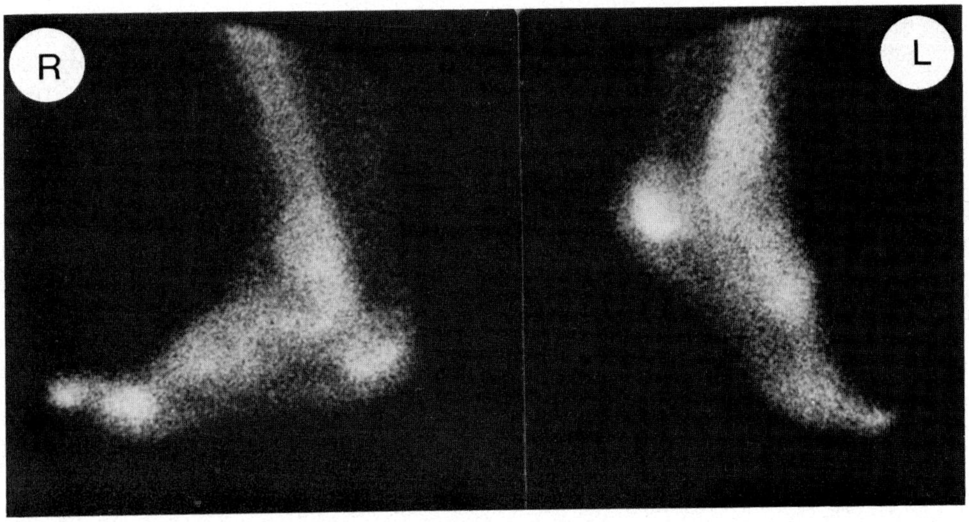

Figure 9 Scintigraphic findings in a psoriatic, who had complained of severe pain in the right first toe and left heel for 10 years. Two years later, periosteal proliferation and erosions were found at these sites.

joints or tendons of this special disease are reported. The pronounced clinical effect on the inflammation is well known. The risk of infection when injecting through affected skin is insignificant when highly scaly plaques are avoided, the skin lesion being of noninfectious origin. Intra-articular methotrexate has not been widely used (104). It does not seem more effective than saline irrigation of the joint. This cor-

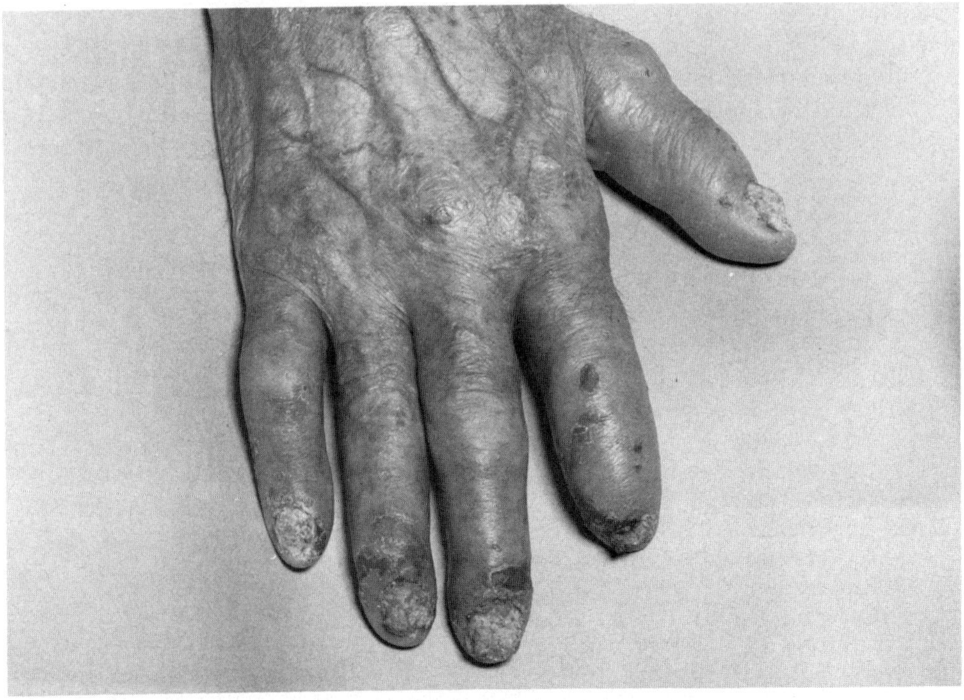

Figure 10 Acrodermatitis continua with arthritis of DIP and PIP joints.

responds to the lack of effect of topical methotrexate on psoriatic skin lesions.

In more severe disease that cannot be controlled by these measures, we have a wide spectrum of effective disease-modifying antirheumatic drugs at our disposal.

The use of systemic corticosteroids is controversial. It has been tempting because of the good short-term effect on skin lesions and arthritis. The rebound phenomenon at withdrawal with deterioration of skin symptoms, however, prevents its long-term use.

Methotrexate

Methotrexate for years has been one of the most valuable agents in controlling severe psoriasis. Dermatologists have been aware of its effect on arthritis; therefore, in many clinics it has been the drug of first choice in cases of disabling psoriasis with arthritic complaints. Lately, rheumatologists have overcome the fear provoked by the report by Black (105), who in a placebo-controlled study administered methotrexate in high dosage, inducing severe side effects. The dosages now used are much lower. Usually 15 mg in weekly dosages is sufficient. The effect on the arthritis is significant (106), with improvement of arthritis activity after 1–3 months (Table 1). After discontinuation, the arthritis usually flares up. It is often possible, however, to reduce the dose. Long-term treatment should be continued at the lowest dosage that can control the complaints from joints and skin. It is obvious that this treatment demands maximum compliance and regular control of liver and bone marrow parameters. The Toronto group in a 24-month study found that methotrexate did not significantly prevent radiological damage (106a). Some of their patients, however, had failed to respond to other DMARDS. It is likely that methotrexate is most effective when given early after disease onset (106b).

It is mandatory that both physician and patient are aware of drug interactions. Salicylates and sulfonamides should be avoided (107). NSAIDs may be given, but not on methotrexate treatment days. Methotrexate has now proved valuable also in RA.

In general, rheumatologists abstain from using liver biopsies in their control of RA patients treated with methotrexate. We recommend that the guidelines for methotrexate in psoriasis (106c) be followed in PA. Even with low-dose methotrexate (7.5 mg weekly) we have experienced a cirrhosis proceeding to a fatal outcome with normal routine liver tests (106d). PIIINP was not available at that time. PIIINP has been proposed to be used to limit the number of liver biopsies necessary for the control of liver toxicity in psoriasis (44a). Although PIIINP in a number of patients with PA may be increased due to arthritis alone and not to liver toxicity, as long as the test remains normal no significant fibrogenesis in the liver is taking place. An elevated PIIINP indicates that a liver biopsy should be performed according to the guidelines (106c).

Sulfasalazine

Sulfasalazine in controlled studies has proved to induce remission in PA (107a). Like methotrexate its effect appears after 3 months of treatment, and it

Table 1 ESR and Clinical Evaluation (7) in 28 Patients with Psoriatic Arthritis Treated with MTX, Before and After 3 Months and 6 or 12 Months After Start of Treatment

Evaluation ± SE	Before	3 months[a]	6 or 12 months[a]
1. ESR	43 ± 6	17 ± 3	17 ± 4
2. No. of swollen joints	8.5 ± 0.7	2.9 ± 0.7	2.3 ± 0.6
3. Joint tenderness score	11.5 ± 1.3	3.5 ± 0.6	2.0 ± 0.5
4. Morning stiffness	12.5 ± 2.4	3.4 ± 1.2	2.4 ± 0.9
5. Grip strength	10.8 ± 1.6	6.0 ± 1.6	6.8 ± 1.6
6. Analgesic consumption	9.6 ± 1.5	4.1 ± 1.4	3.6 ± 1.4
7. Pain assessment	3.8 ± 0.3	1.6 ± 0.3	1.3 ± 0.3
8. General condition	3.2 ± 0.2	2.3 ± 0.2	1.4 ± 0.2

[a]All parameters were significantly improved after 3 and 6 or 12 months. Statistical significance was assessed using Wilcoxon's test for two samples. A p-value below 0.05 was considered significant.

Source: Ref. 106.

is well tolerated. It seems to have some effect on the skin symptoms. Like methotrexate it is a good first-choice drug in active progressive arthritis, especially where the skin symptoms are not dominant. In therapy-resistant cases combination therapy with these two drugs may be tried.

Azathioprine

Azathioprine has been proved to induce remission in arthritis with less effect on the skin. One study compared its effect to that of methotrexate (108).

Antimalarials

Antimalarials have had the reputation of causing severe exfoliative dermatitis. New studies suggest that the exacerbation of the skin disease is rare (43), but it can be severe (109).

Gold Salts

Gold salts have been avoided because of the fear of flare-up of psoriasis. In small groups of patients, gold has had a beneficial effect on the arthritis without causing severe rash (110,111). In another report, two patients with psoriasis developed a severe pustular psoriasis after the first injection of gold (112). The oral gold compound auranofin has been found safe, although not quite as effective as intramuscular gold (113). Further studies are needed to reveal in which patients these remission-inducing drugs can be safely used.

Penicillamine

Penicillamine does not seem to have been used much in PA, and no significant reports on this drug have appeared.

Colchicine

Colchicine appeared to have a significant beneficial effect in a placebo-controlled study; the side effects were few (114). This drug has been proved to influence the chemotaxis of PMN leukocytes.

Etretinate and Acitretine

Etretinate in open studies seems to have a beneficial effect on arthritis (115,116). Others, however, could not confirm this (115). Today acitretine has substituted etretinate in a number of countries. In both cases fertile female patients need to be on safe birth control procedures during therapy and up to 2 years after discontinuation of the drug.

Photochemotherapy

Photochemotherapy with PUVA (psoralen and ultraviolet A) in one study proved effective in patients without spondylitic involvement, whereas in spondylitis skin clearing was not associated with improvement of arthritis (118).

Cyclosporin

Cyclosporin has been used in PA with significant effect on psoriasis, whereas the improvement of arthritis was moderate (119). Low to medium doses of cyclosporin (2–5 mg/kg) have been found less potent than methotrexate, 15 mg weekly (120). Other workers, however, have used cyclosporin with great success as a disease-moderating agent (120a). The guidelines for using cyclosporin should be followed (120b). Dosages should in general not exceed 5 mg/kg/day. The renal toxicity is clearly the limiting factor for long-term therapy (120c). Some patients with PA may need to continue to be on NSAID. However, NSAID therapy should be discontinued when possible, because these drugs have a synergistic nephrotoxic effect with cyclosporin (120d). If cyclosporin therapy for PA is to be given for more than 2 years, we advise a kidney biopsy due to the structural renal changes that invariably appear after this length of treatment (120c,120e,120f).

Reconstructive Surgery

Reconstructive surgery can be helpful and necessary in patients with joint deformities. The tendency to fibrosis and spontaneous fusion contribute to maintaining the stability of the joints in a functional position; on the other hand, mobilization after surgery may prove difficult (60). Fear of increased tendency to infection has led to restraint from surgery. Belsky found a significant increase of infection in hand surgery compared to that in RA (121). This can be accidental, as it occurred only in two implant arthroplasties out of 81 (121). Others have found no increase (60). The fact that PA is rarely treated with systemic steroids would contribute to this. Methotrexate and azathioprine may be discontinued preoperatively (122) for a short period.

Overall Management

While much attention has been paid to medical treatment, the importance of overall management has received little comment, but must not be underestimated. Collaboration between the dermatologist and rheumatologist is mandatory for the success of the treatment. While dermatologists treat the severe skin conditions, the joint status has to be looked after to prevent loss of function, and, if possible, to improve the functional capacity of the patient.

The different needs of patients in different disease categories should be taken into consideration. Only the relatively small group of patients with symmetrical erosive nonproliferative disease indistinguishable from RA is in need of the joint protective measures so necessary in RA, as only this group develops palmar subluxation of wrists and MCP joints (121). The increased risk of fibrosis and ankylosis indicate that the main effort should be concentrated on maintaining the joints in a functional position.

There are no reports on the effects of joint-mobilizing exercises in this special group. In a study of spondylitic cases (68), little deterioration of spinal mobility was found during a long term follow-up. It is well known that exercise improves the spinal mobility in ankylosing spondylitis (123) to some degree. It would be expected that an effort to improve or at least preserve mobility by exercise would be worthwhile. The fact that arthritis can be provoked by trauma and excessive strain implies that an effort to avoid such strains would be purposeful.

PROGNOSIS

Psoriatic arthritis has been considered a mild disease with a better prognosis than RA (6,87,124). The majority of patients are only slightly incapacitated and able to work, and hospital admissions are few (87). However, in a group of patients, the percentage varying in different reports (6,17,18,78,87,124,125) the course is progressive and involves joint destruction and disability. Several factors influence the outcome. Early onset under the age of 20 (87) inaugurates a malignant course. Also, early childhood onset is a sign of more severe progressive and erosive disease (99). The general impression of an association between the severity of skin disease and arthritis has been confirmed (14,17,117). Hereditary factors also play a part (6). HLA DR3 predisposes to erosions (28), and DR4 to a progressive RA-like course (28,34). DR7 seems to have an association with long duration and early onset (28), and B27 is a marker of spinal disease.

There is a female preponderance in the severe group in most reports (18,78).

Pustular psoriasis, not least the generalized type, can be associated with treatment-resistant progressive disease. Other subgroups have a mild course; this includes the oligoarticular group and the type mainly affecting the distal joints. Even with widespread spinal disease, the prognosis of pain and restriction of movement seems good in most of these patients.

All the aforementioned will have to be taken into consideration when trying to predict the course of disease in the individual patient. In most cases, one can assure the patient that the prognosis is good and the risk of disablement slight (87,124,125). But the physician must select the patients with more progressive disease and be prepared to treat them early and aggressively (127). All approaches to differential diagnosis have to be taken into account to place the patient in the right prognostic group. In therapy, close cooperation of the dermatologist and rheumatologist and, if necessary, the physiotherapist, occupational therapist, and social worker is needed to assure the best possible final outcome for the patient.

REFERENCES

1. Alibert, J.L. (1818). *Précis Theorique et Pratique sur les Maladies de la Peau.* Caille et Ravier, Paris, p. 21
2. Cats, A. (1971). Psoriasis and arthritis. In *Psoriasis. Proceedings of the 1st International Symposium,* Stanford, 1971. E.M. Farber and A. Cox (Eds.). Stanford University Press, Stanford, California.
3. Blumberg, B.S., Bunim, J.J., Calkins, E., Pirani, C.L., and Zvaifler, N. (1964). ARA nomenclature and classification of arthritis and rheumatism (tentative). *Arthritis Rheum.* 7:93–97.

3a. Gladman, D. (1995). Psoriatic arthritis. *Bailliere's Clin. Rheumatol.* 9:319–329.

4. Fawcitt, J. (1950). Bone and joint changes associated with psoriasis. *Br. J. Radiol.* 23:440–453.
5. Bauer, W., Bennett, G.A., and Zeller, S.W. (1941). Pathology of joint lesions in patients with psoriasis and arthritis. *Trans. Assoc. Am. Physicians* 56: 349–352.
6. Moll, J.M.H., and Wright, V. (1973). Psoriatic arthritis. *Semin. Arthritis Rheum.* 3:55–78.
7. Bennett, R.M. (1979). Psoriatic arthritis. In *Arthritis and Allied Conditions.* D.J. McCarty (Ed.). Lea & Febiger, Philadelphia, pp. 642–655.

8. Vasey, F.B., and Espinoza, L.R. (1984). Psoriatic arthropathy. In *Spondylarthropathies*. A. Calin (Ed.). Grune & Stratton, Orlando, Florida, pp. 151–185.
9. Lomholt, G. (1963). Psoriasis, spontaneous course and genetics, a census study on the prevalence of skin diseases on the Faroe Islands. Copenhagen, *C.E. Gad.* 163–165.
10. Hellgren, L. (1969). Association between rheumatoid arthritis and psoriasis in total populations. *Acta Rheum. Scand.* 15:316–326.
11. Leczinsky, C.G. (1948). The incidence of arthropathy in a ten year series of psoriasis cases. *Acta Derm. Venereol.* (*Stockh.*) 28:483–487.
12. Vilanova, X., and Pinòl, J. (1951). Psoriasis arthropatica. *Rheumatism* 7:197–208.
13. Baker, H. (1966). Epidemiological aspects of psoriasis and arthritis. *Br. J. Dermatol.* 78:349–261.
14. Little, H., Harvie, J.N., and Lester, R.S. (1975). Psoriatic arthritis in severe psoriasis. *Can. Med. Assoc. J.* 112:317–319.
15. Leonard, D.G., O'Duffy, J.D., and Rogers, R.S. (1978). Prospective analysis of psoriatic arthritis in patients hospitalized for psoriasis. *Mayo Clin. Proc.* 53:511–518.
16. Biondi Oriente, G., Scarpa, R., Pucino, A., Torella, M., Vignone, L., and Oriente, P. (1984). Prevalence of psoriatic arthritis in psoriatic patients. *Acta Derm. Venereol.* (*Stockh.*) 113:109–112.
17. Stern, R.S. (1985). The epidemiology of joint complaints in patients with psoriasis. *J. Rheumatol.* 12: 315–320.
18. Gladman, D.D., Schuckett, R., Russel, M.L., Thorne, J.C., and Schachter, R.K. (1987). Psoriatic arthritis (PSA), an analysis of 220 patients. *Q. J. Med.* 62: 127–141.
19. Kononen, M., Torppa, J., and Lassus, A. (1986). An epidemiologic survey of psoriasis in the greater Helsinki area. *Acta Derm. Venereol.* (*Stockh.*) 66(Suppl. 124):8.
20. Møller, P., Vinje, O., and Berg, K. (1982). HLA antigens in psoriasis and anterior uveitis in Bechterews syndrome (ankylosing spondylitis). *Clin. Genet.* 21: 215–221.
21. Moll, J.M.H., and Wright, V. (1973). Familial occurrence of psoriatic arthritis. *Ann. Rheum. Dis.* 32: 181–201.
22. Karvonen, J., Lassus, A., Sievers, V., and Tillikainen, A. (1964). HL-A-antigens in psoriatic arthritis. *Ann. Clin. Res.* 6:304–307.
23. Zachariae, H., Hjortshøj, A., Kissmeyer-Nielsen, F., Svejgaard, A., Svejgaard, E., and Zachariae, E. (1974). HL-A-antigens in psoriatic arthritis. *Acta Derm. Venereol.* (*Stockh.*) 54:443–447.
24. Lambert, J.R., Wright, V., Rajah, S.M., and Moll, J.M.H. (1976). Histocompatibility antigens in psoriatic arthritis. *Ann. Rheum. Dis.* 35:526–530.
25. Espinoza, L.R., Vasey, F.B., Oh, J.A., Wilkinson, R., and Osterland, C.K. (1978). Association between HLA-BW38 and peripheral psoriatic arthritis. *Arthritis Rheum.* 21:72–75.
26. Espinoza, L.R., Vasey, F.B., and Haylord, S.W., Dietz, C., Bergen, L., Bridgeford, P., and Germain, B.F. (1982). Histocompatibility typing in the seronegative spondylarthropathies. *Semin. Arthritis Rheum.* 11:375–381.
27. Murray, C., Mann, D.L., Gerber, L.N., Barth, W., Perlman, S., Decher, J., and Nigra, T.P. (1980). Histocompatibility alloantigens in psoriasis and psoriatic arthritis. *J. Clin. Invest.* 66:670–675.
28. Armstrong, R.D., Panayi, G.S., and Welsh, K.I. (1983). Histocompatibility antigens in psoriasis, psoriatic arthropathy and ankylosing spondylitis. *Ann. Rheum. Dis.* 42:142–146.
29. Marcusson, J., Møller, E., and Thyresson, N. (1975). HLA-antigens in psoriasis with special reference to patients with arthritic lesions. *Acta Derm. Venereol.* (*Stockh.*) 55:297–300.
30. Schlosstein, L.P., Teresaki, P., and Pearson, C.M. (1973). High association of an HLA-antigen W27 with ankylosing spondylitis. *N. Engl. J. Med.* 288: 704–706.
31. Gerber, L.M., Murray, C.L., Perlman, S. Barth, W.F., Decker, I.L., Nigra, T.A., and Mann, D.L. (1982). Human lymphocyte antigens charcterizing psoriatic arthritis and its subtypes. *J. Rheumatol.* 9:703–707.
32. McHugh, N.J., Laurent, M.R., Treadwell, B.L.J., Tweed, S.M., and Dagger, J. (1987). Psoriatic arthritis: clinical subgroups and histocompatibility antigens. *Ann. Rheum. Dis.* 46:184–188.
33. Crivellato, E., and Zacchi, T. (1987). HLA-B39 and the axial type of psoriatic arthritis. *Acta Derm. Venereol.* (*Stockh.*) 67:249–273.
34. Gran, J.T., and Husby, G. (1987). Seronegative rheumatoid arthritis and HLA-DR4: proposal for criteria. Editorial. *J. Rheumatol.* 14:1079–1082.
35. Tillikainen, A., Lassus, A., Karvonen, J., Vartainen, P., and Juhlin, L. (1980). Psoriasis and HL-A-Cw6. *Br. J. Dermatol.* 102:179–180.
36. Sakkas, L.I., Demaine, A.G., Panayi, G.S., and Welsh, K.I. (1988). Arthritis in patients with an immunoglobulin gene polymorphism. *Arthritis Rheum.* 31:276–278.
37. Waller, M., and Toone, E.C. (1968). Normal individuals with positive test for rheumatoid factor. *Arthritis Rheum.* 11:50.
38. Zachariae, H., and Zachariae, E. (1969). Antinuclear factor, the anti-human-globulin consumption test and Wasserman reaction in psoriatic arthritis. *Acta Rheum. Scand.* 16:62–67.
39. Sitton, N.G., Dixon, J.S., Bird, H.A., and Wright, V. (1987). Serum biochemistry in rheumatoid arthritis,

seronegative arthropathies, osteoarthritis, SLE and normal subjects. *Br. J. Rheumatol.* 26:131–135.
40. Rubins, A.V., and Merson, A.G. (1987). Subpopulations of T-lymphocytes and their changes during immunotherapy. *J. Am. Acad. Dermatol.* 17:972–977.
41. Espinoza, L.R., Gaylord, S.W., Bocanegra, T.S., Vasey, F.B., and Germain, B.F. (1982). Circulating immune complexes in the seronegative spondylarthropathies. *Clin. Immunol. Immunopathol.* 22:384–393.
42. Lambert, J.R., and Wright, V. (1977). Serum uric acid levels in psoriatic arthritis. *Ann. Rheum. Dis.* 36: 234–267.
43. Kammer, G.M., Soter, N.A., Gibson, O.J., and Schur, P.H. (1979). Psoriatic arthritis, a clinical immunological and HLA study of 100 patients. *Sem. Arthritis Rheum.* 9:79–97.
44. Seibel, M.J., Raimann, S., and Seglias, J. (1988). Serum hyaluronic acid and aminoterminal procollagen III peptid in inflammatory and degenerative joint disease. *Z. Rheumatol.* 47:98–106.
44a. Zachariae, H., Aslam, H., Bjerring, P., Søgaard, H., Zachariae, E., and Heickendorff, L. (1991). Serum aminoterminal propeptide of type III procollagen in psoriasis and psoriatic arthritis: relation to liver fibrosis and arthritis. *J. Am. Acad. Dermatol.* 25:50–53.
45. Danielsen, L. (1965). Immunoelectrophoretic analysis of serum proteins in psoriasis and psoriatic arthritis. *Acta Rheum. Scand.* 11:112–118.
46. Tapanes, F.J., Rawson, A.J., and Hollander, J.L. (1972). Serum antiimmunoglobulins in psoriatic arthritis as compared with rheumatoid arthritis. *Arthritis Rheum.* 15:153–156.
47. Jenette, J.C., Ferguson, A.L., Moore, M., and Freeman, D. (1982). IgA nephropathy associated with seronegative spondylarthropathies. *Arthritis Rheum.* 25: 144–149.
48. Cawling, P., Ebringer, R., and Ebringer, A. (1980). Association of inflammation with raised serum IgA in ankylosing spondylitis. *Ann. Rheum. Dis.* 39: 545–549.
49. Espinoza, L.A., Berman, A., Vasey, F.B., Cahalin, C., Nelson, R., and Germain, B.F. (1988). Psoriatic arthritis and acquired immunodeficiency syndrome. *Arthritis Rheum.* 25:144–149.
50. Wright, V., and Moll, J.M.H. (1976). In *Seronegative Polyarthritis.* North Holland Publishing Company, Amsterdam, pp. 209–210.
50a. Gottlieb, A. (1988). Immunologic mechanisms in psoriasis. *J. Am. Acad. Dermatol.* 18:1376–1380.
50b. Veale, D., Yanni, G., Rogers, S., Barnes, L., Bresnihan, B., and Fitzgerald, O. (1993). Reduced synovial membrane macrophage numbers, ELAM-1 expression, and lining layer hyperplasia in psoriatic arthritis as compared with rheumatoid arthritis. *Arthritis Rheum.* 36:893–900.
51. Espinoza, L.R., Vasey, F.G., Espinosa, C.G., Bocanegra, T.S., and Germain, B.F. (1982). Vascular changes in psoriatic synovium. A light and electromicroscopic study. *Arthritis Rheum.* 25:677–684.
52. Kahn, M.H., and Kammer, G.M. (1985). Laboratory findings and pathology of psoriatic arthritis. In *Psoriatic Arthritis.* L. Gerber and L.R. Espinosa (Eds.). Grune & Stratton, Orlando, FL, pp. 109–124.
52a. Espinoza, L., Aguilar, J., Espinoza, C., Cuellar, M., Scopelitis, E., and Silveira, L. (1994). Fibroblast function in psoriatic arthritis I. *J. Rheumatol.* 21: 1502–1506.
52b. Espinoza., L., Espinoza, C., Cuellar, M., Scopelitis, E., Silveira, L., and Grotendorst, G. (1994). Fibroblast function in psoriatic arthritis II. *J. Rheumatol.* 21:1507–1511.
53. Redisch, W., Messina, E.J., Hughes, G., and McEwen, C. (1970). Capillaroscopic observations in rheumatic disease. *Ann. Rheum. Dis.* 29:244–250.
54. Taccari, E., Fatorossi, A., Moretti, S., Rieccieri, V., Fasani, M., and Zappini, A. (1987). Phenotypic profile of major synovial cell populations of long standing psoriatic arthritis. *J. Rheumatol.* 14:525–530.
54a. Veale, D., Farrell, M., and Fitzgerald, O. (1993). Mechanism of joint sparing in a patient with unilateral psoriatic arthritis and a longstanding hemiplegia. *Br. J. Rheumatol.* 32:413–416.
55. Fyrand, O., and Melbye, O.F. (1977). Deposition of fibrinogen in skin diseases. *Acta Derm. Venereol. (Stockh.)* 157:399–402.
56. Fyrand, O., Melbye, O.J., and Natvig, J.B. (1977). Immunofluorescence studies for immunoglobulins and complement C3 in synovial membranes in psoriatic arthritis. *Clin. Exp. Immunol.* 29:422–427.
57. Fassbender, H.G. (1976). Morphologic aspects of rheumatoid arthritis and psoriatic arthritis. In *Chronic Forms of Polyarthritis.* F.J. Wagenheuser (Ed.). Hans Huber Publishers, Bern, pp. 17–26.
58. Zaric, D., Worm, A.M., Stahl, D., and Clemmensen, O.J. (1981). Capillary microscopy of the nailfold in psoriatic and rheumatoid arthritis. *Scand. J. Rheum.* 10:247–252.
59. Baker, B.S., Powles, A.V., Lambert, S., Valdimarsson, H., and Fry, L. (1988). A prospective study of the Koebner reaction and T-lymphocytes in uninvolved psoriatic skin. *Acta Derm. Venereol. (Stockh.)* 68: 430–434.
60. Wright, V. (1985). Psoriatic arthritis. In *Textbook of Rheumatology.* W.N. Kelly, E.D. Harris, S. Ruddy, C.B. Sledge (Eds.). W.B. Saunders Company, Philadelphia, pp. 1021–1031.
60a. Kammer, G., Soter, N., Gibson, D., and Schur, P. (1979). Psoriatic arthritis, a clinical, immunological and HLA study of 100 patients. *Semin. Arthritis Rheum.* 9:75–97.

60b. HelliWell, P., Marchesoni, A., Peters, M., Barker, M., and Wright, V. (1991). A reevaluation of the osteoarticular manifestations of psoriasis. *Br. J. Rheumatol.* 33:133–138.
60c. Veale, D., Rogers, S., and Fitzgerald, O. (1994). Classification of clinical subsets in psoriatic arthritis. *Br. J. Rheumatol.* 33:133–138.
61. Gottlieb, A.B., Shumman, F., Carter, D.M., and Fabino, M. (1987). Marked increase in the frequency of psoriatic arthritis in patients with HL-A-DR[1] keratinocytes. *Arthritis Rheum.* 30:901–907.
62. Wright, V., and Reed, W.B. (1965). The link between Reiter's syndrome and psoriatic arthritis. *Ann. Rheum. Dis.* 23:12–21.
63. Wright, V. (1976). In *Seronegative Polyarthritis.* North Holland Publishing Company, Amsterdam, p. 181.
64. Karvonen, J., Tillikainen, A., and Lassus, A. (1975). HLA antigens in psoriasis with persistent palmoplantar pustulosis and pustular psoriasis. *Ann. Clin. Res.* 7:112–115.
65. Zachariae, H., Petersen, H.O., Kissmeyer-Nielsen, F., and Lamm, L. (1977). HLA-antigens in pustular psoriasis. *Dermatologica* 154:73–77.
66. Yates, N.M., Watkinson, G., and Kelman, A. (1982). Further evidence for association between psoriasis, Crohn's disease, and ulcerative colitis. *Br. J. Dermatol.* 106:323–330.
66a. Schattemann, L., Mielants, H., Veys, E., Cuvelier, C., deVos, M., Gyselbrecht, L., Elewaut, D., and Goemaere, S. (1995). Gut inflammation in psoriatic arthritis: a prospective ileonoscopic study. *J. Rheumatol.* 22:680–683.
67. Morris, R.I., Metzger, A.L., Bluestone, R., and Teresaki, P.A. (1974). HLA-W27—a useful discriminator in the arthropathies of inflammatory bowel disease. *N. Engl. J. Med.* 290:1117–1119.
68. Hanly, J.G., Russel, M.L., and Gladman, D.D. (1988). Psoriatic spondyloarthropathy, a long term prospective study. *Ann. Rheum. Dis.* 47:386–393.
69. Scarpa, R., Oriente, P., Pucino, A., Vignone, E., Cosentini, E., Minerva, A., and Biondi Oriente, C. (1988). The clinical spectrum of psoriatic spondylitis. *Br. J. Rheumatol.* 27:133–137.
70. Jurik, A.G., Graudal, H., and de Carvalho, A. (1985). Monarticular involvement of the manubrio-sternal joint. *Skeletal Radiol.* 14:99–103.
71. Jurik, A.G., Helmig, O., and Graudal, H. (1988). Skeletal disease, arthro-osteitis in adult patients with pustulosis palmoplantaris. *Scand. J. Rheumatol.* 70(Suppl.):3–15.
72. Sonozaki, H., Mitsui, H., Miyanaga, F., Okitsu, K., Garashi, M., Hayashi, Y., Matsuwara, M., Azuma, A., Okai, K., and Kawashima, M. (1981). Clinical features of 53 cases with pustulotic arthro-osteitis. *Ann. Rheum. Dis.* 40:554–557.
72a. Kahn, M.F., and Khan, M.A. (1994). The SAPHO syndrome. *Bailliere's Clin. Rheumatol.* 8:333–362.
73. Kononen, M. (1986). Subjective symptoms from the stomatognatic system in patients with psoriatic arthritis. *Acta Odont. Scand.* 44:377–383.
74. Blau, R.H., and Kaufman, R. (1987). Erosive and subluxing cervical spine disease in patients with psoriatic arthritis. *J. Rheumatol.* 14:111–117.
75. Wright, V. (1961). Psoriatic arthritis. A comparative radiographic study of rheumatoid arthritis and arthritis associated with psoriasis. *Ann. Rheum. Dis.* 20: 123–132.
76. Martel, W., Stuck, K.S., Dworin, A.M., and Hyland, R.G. (1986). Erosive osteoarthritis and psoriatic arthritis: a radiologic comparison in the hand, wrist, and foot. *Am. J. Radiol.* 134:125–135.
77. Lomuto, M., Cammisa, M., and Ditano, G. (1984). On arthropathic psoriasis: x-ray peculiarities. *Dermatologica* 168:82–86.
78. Wright, V., and Mod, J. (1976). In *Seronegative Polyarthritis.* North Holland Publishing Company, Amsterdam, pp. 169–218.
79. Brower, A.C. (1985). The radiographic features of psoriatic arthritis. In *Psoriatic Arthritis.* L. Gerber and L.R. Espinosa (Eds.), Grune & Stratton, Orlando, Florida, pp. 125–146.
80. Cooper, C., Poll, V., McLaren, M., Daunt, S.O'N., and Cawley, M.I.D. (1988). Alterations in appendicular skeletal mass in patients with rheumatoid, psoriatic and osteo-arthropathy. *Ann. Rheum. Dis.* 47: 481–484.
81. McEwen, C., Ditata, D., Lingg, C., Porini, A., Good, A., and Rankin, A. (1971). Ankylosing spondylitis and spondylitis accompanying ulcerative colitis, regional enteritis, psoriasis, and Reiter's disease. *Arthritis Rheum.* 14:291–318.
82. Lambert, J.R., and Wright, V. (1977). Psoriatic spondylitis. A clinical and radiological description of the spine in psoriatic arthritis. *Q. J. Med.* 184:411–425.
83. Bywaters, E.G. (1985). Pathology of the spondylarthropathies. In *Spondyloarthropathies.* A. Calin (Ed.). Grune & Stratton, Orlando, Florida, pp. 43–68.
84. Moll, J.M.H. (1986). Psoriatic arthropathy. In *Textbook of Psoriasis.* P.D. Mier and P.C.M. van de Kerkhof (Eds.). Churchill Livingstone, Edinburgh, pp. 55–83.
85. Namey, T., and Rosenthal, L. (1976). Periarticular uptake of 99m and technetium diphosphonate in psoriatics. *Arthritis Rheum.* 19:607–612.
86. Bachmann, E., Clemmensen, O.J., Dyrbye, M., and Larsen, K. (1983). Joint involvement in psoriasis. Scintigraphic, radiologic, and clinical findings. *Dermatologica* 166:250–254.
86a. Porter, C. (1994). Plain radiology and other imaging techniques. *Bailliere's Clin. Rheumatol.* 8:465–482.

87. Roberts, M.E.T., Wright, V., Hill, A.S.G., and Mehra, A.C. (1976). Psoriatic arthritis. Follow-up study. *Ann. Rheum. Dis.* 35:206–212.
88. Wright, V. (1959). Psoriasis and arthritis. *Arch. Dermatol.* 80:27–35.
89. Jajic, I. (1968). Radiological changes in the sacroiliac joints and the spine of patients with psoriatic arthritis. *Ann. Rheum. Dis.* 27:1–6.
90. Arnett, F.C. (1985). Psoriatic arthritis, relationship to other spondyloarthropathies. In *Psoriatic Arthritis.* L. Gerber and L.R. Espinosa (Eds.). Grune & Stratton, Orlando, FL, pp. 95–108.
91. Perlman, S. (1985). Psoriatic arthritis, natural history and prognosis. In *Psoriatic Arthritis.* L. Gerber and L.R. Espinosa (Eds.). Grune & Stratton, Orlando, Florida, pp. 83–85.
92. Kahn, M.A., and Kammer, G.M. (1985). Laboratory findings and pathology of psoriatic arthritis. In *Psoriatic Arthritis.* L. Gerber and L.R. Espinosa (Eds.). Grune & Stratton, Orlando, FL, pp. 109–124.
93. Baker, H., and Ryan, T.J. (1968). Generalized pustular psoriasis. A clinical and epidemiological study of 104 cases. *Br. J. Dermatol.* 80:171–193.
94. Pines, A., Ehrenfeld, M., and Fisman, E.Z. (1986). Mitral valve prolapse in psoriatic arthritis. *Arch. Int. Med.* 146:1371–1373.
95. Lambert, J.R., and Wright, V. (1976). Eye inflammation in psoriatic arthritis. *Ann. Rheum. Dis.* 35: 354–356.
96. Oestensen, M. (1988). Pregnancy in psoriatic arthritis. *Scand. J. Rheumatol.* 17:67–70.
97. Lambert, J.R., Ansell, B.M., Stephenson, E., and Wright, V. (1976). Psoriatic arthritis in childhood. *Clin. Rheum. Dis.* 2:339–352.
97a. Southwood, T., Petty, R., Malleson, P., Delgado, E., Hunt, D., Wood, B., and Schroeder, M-L. (1989). Psoriatic arthritis in children. *Arthritis Rheum.* 32: 1007–1013.
98. Calabro, J.L. (1977). Psoriatic arthritis in children. *Arthritis Rheum.* 20(Suppl.):415–416.
99. Singsen, B.H. (1977). Psoriatic arthritis in childhood. *Arthritis Rheum.* 20(Suppl.):403–410.
100. Sills, E. (1980). Psoriatic arthritis in childhood. *Johns Hopkins Med. J.* 146:49–53
101. Shore, A., and Ansell, B.M. (1982). Juvenile psoriatic arthritis—an analysis of 60 cases. *J. Pediatr.* 100: 529–535.
101a. Ansell, B. (1994). Juvenile psoriatic arthritis. *Bailliere's Clin. Rheumatol.* 8:317–332.
101b. Ansell, B., Beeson, M., Hall, P., Bedford, P., and Woo, P. (1993). HLA and juvenile psoriatic arthritis. *Br. J. Rheumatol.* 32:836–837.
102. Ellis, C., Fallon, J., Hezen, J., and Voorhees, J. (1983). Topical indomethacine exacerbates lesions of psoriasis. *J. Invest. Dermatol.* 80:362.
103. Katayama, H., and Kawada, A. (1981). Exacerbation of psoriasis induced by indomethacine. *J. Dermatol.* 8:323–337.
104. Hall, G.A., Jones, B.H., Head, A.C., and Jones, V. (1978). Intraarticular methotrexate. *Ann. Rheum. Dis.* 37:351–356.
105. Black, R.L., O'Brien, W.M., van Scott, E.J., Auerbach, R., Eesen, A.Z., and Bunim, J.J. (1964). Methotrexate therapy in psoriatic arthritis. *J.A.M.A.* 189: 743–747.
106. Zachariae, H., and Zachariae, E. (1987). Methotrexate treatment of psoriatic arthritis. *Acta Derm. Venereol. (Stockh.)* 67:270–273.
106a. Abu-Shakra, M., Gladman, D., Thorne, J., Long, J., Gough, J., and Farewell, V. (1995). Longterm methotrexate therapy in psoriatic arthritis: clinical and radiological outcome. *J. Rheumatol.* 22:241–245.
106b. Kragballe, K., Zachariae, E., and Zachariae, H. (1982). Methotrexate in psoriatic arthritis, a retrospective study. *Acta Dermatol. Venereol. (Stockh.)* 63: 165–167.
106c. Roenigk, H., Auerbach, R., Maibach, H., and Weinstein, G. (1988). Methotrexate in psoriasis: revised guidelines. *J. Am. Acad. Dermatol.* 19:145–156.
106d. Zachariae, H., Søgaard, H., and Heickendorff, L. (1996). Methotrexate-induced liver cirrhosis: a further 10 years follow-up. *Dermatology.* 192:343–346.
107. Roenigk, H., Auerbach, R., Maibach, H., and Weinstein, G. (1988). Methotrexate in psoriasis: revised guidelines. *J. Am. Acad. Dermatol.* 19:145–156.
107a. Farr, M., Kitas, G., Waterhouse, L., Jubb, R., Felix-Davies, D., and Bacon, P. (1990). Sulfalazine in psoriatic arthritis: a double-blind placebo-controlled study. *Br. J. Rheumatol.* 29:46–49.
108. Feldges, D.H., and Barnes, C.J. (1974). Treatment of psoriatic arthropathy with either azathioprine or methotrexate. *Rheumatol. Rehab.* 13:120–124.
109. Luzar, M. (1982). Hydroxychloroquine in psoriatic arthropathy: exacerbations of psoriatic skin lesions. *J. Rheumatol.* 9:462–464.
110. Doorwart, B.B., Gall, E.P., and Schumacher, R.P., Krauser, R.F. (1978). Chrysootherapy in psoriatic arthritis. *Arthritis Rheum.* 21:513–515.
111. Richter, M.B., Kinsella, P., and Corbette, M. (1980). Gold in psoriatic arthropathy. *Ann. Rheum. Dis.* 39: 279–280.
112. Nolting, S., and Kastrup, W. (1978). Gold terapie in Psoriasis Arthropatica (German). *Hautarzt* 39: 266–269.
113. Palit, J., Carey, J., Capell, H., Hill, J., Bird, H.A., and Nold, G. (1986). Multicenter double-blind placebo controlled comparative trial of oral gold and intramuscular gold in psoriatic arthritis. *Br. J. Rheumatol.* 25:A1/51.

114. Seidemann, P., Fjellner, B., and Johannesson, A. (1987). Psoriatic arthritis treated with Colchicine. *J. Rheumatol.* 14:777–779.
115. Cheregato, G.C., and Leoni, A. (1986). Treatment of psoriatic arthropathy with etretinate, a two year follow-up. *Acta Derm. Venereol. (Stockh.)* 66:321–324.
116. Kaplan, R.P., Russel, D.H., and Loeve, N.J. (1983). Etretinate therapy for psoriasis. Clinical responses, remission time, epidermal DNA, and polyamin response. *Am. Acad. Dermatol.* 8:95–102.
117. Orfanos, C., and Goertz, G. (1978). Oral psoriasis therapie mit einem neuber aromatischen retinoid. *Dtsch. Med. Wochenschr.* 103:195–199.
118. Perlman, S.G., Gerber, L.H., Roberts, R.M., Nigra, T.P., and Barth, W.F. (1979). Photochemotherapy and psoriatic arthritis. *Ann. Intern. Med.* 91:717–722.
119. Mueller, W., and Graft, V. (1981). The use of cyclosporine, a new immunosuppressant in the treatment of psoriatic arthritis. *Schweiz. Med. Wochenschr.* 111 /12:408.
120a. Steinsson, K., and Valdimarsson, H. (1993). The case for cyclosporin in psoriatic arthritis. *Inflammopharmacology* 2:131–139.
120b. Mihatsch, M., and Wolff, K. (1990). A consensus report: cyclosporin A therapy for psoriasis. *Br. J. Dermatol.* 122(Suppl. 36):1–3.
120c. Zachariae, H. (1996). Long term use of cyclosporine in dermatology. *Arch. Dermatol.* 132:692–694.
120d. Altman, R., Perez, G., and Sfakianakis, G. (1992). Interaction of cyclosporine A and nonsteroidal anti-inflammatory drugs on renal function in patients with rheumatoid arthritis. *Am. J. Med.* 93:396–402.
120e. Zachariae, H., Hansen, H., Kragballe, K., and Olsen, S. (1992). Morphological renal changes during cyclosporin A treatment of psoriasis—studies on pre- and posttreatment kidney biopsies. *J. Am. Acad. Dermatol.* 26:415–419.
120f. Zachariae, H., Kragballe, K., Hansen, H., Marcussen, N., and Olsen, S. (1997). Renal biopsy findings in long term cyclosporin. *Br. J. Dermatol.* 136:531–535.
121. Belsky, M.R., Feldon, P., Millender, L.H., Nalebuff, E.A., and Phillips, C. (1982). Hand involvement in psoriatic arthritis. *J. Hand. Surg.* 7:203–207.
122. Gerber, L. (1985). Pharmacologic, surgical, and rehabilitative management. In *Psoriatic Arthritis.* L. Gerber and L.R. Espinosa (Eds.). Grune & Stratton, Orlando, FL, pp. 147–165.
123. Kahn, M.A. (1984). Ankylosing spondylitis. In *Spondylarthropathies.* A. Calin (Ed.). Grune & Stratton, Orlando, FL, pp. 69–117.
124. Nissilä, M., Isomäki, H., Kaarela, K., Kiviniemi, P., Martio, J., and Sarna, S. (1983). Prognosis of inflammatory joint disease. *Scand. J. Rheumatol.* 12:33–38.
125. Coulton, B.L., Thomson, K., Symmons, D.P.G., and Propert, A.J. (1988). Outcome in patients hospitalized for psoriatic arthritis. *Br. J. Rheumatol.* 27(Suppl. 2): 191, p. 106.
126. Anonymous (1988). Prognosis of psoriatic arthritis. Editorial. *Lancet* 375–376.

8

Psychological Aspects of Psoriasis

Mark D.P. Davis
Mayo Graduate School of Medicine, Rochester, Minnesota

Marian T. McEvoy
Mayo Clinic and Mayo Foundation, Rochester, Minnesota

My torture is skin deep: there is no pain, not even itching; we lepers [psoriatics] live a long time, and are ironically healthy in other respects. . . . The name of the disease . . . is Humiliation . . . I should have been smashed at birth. Strategies of concealment ramify and self-examination is endless.

—Updike, *The New Yorker*

Psoriasis is a chronic disease, the course of which is punctuated by exacerbations and remissions. It is estimated that 1–3 million Americans have psoriasis. Because there is no cure for psoriasis, the aim of therapy is to control disease and to induce remission. Thus, psoriasis is potentially a lifelong disease with which the patient must deal daily.

In biblical times, people were ostracized because of skin disease: "The one who bears the sore of leprosy shall keep his garments rent and his head bare, and shall muffle his beard; he shall cry out 'Unclean, unclean!' " (Lev. 13:45–46). Ignorance and fear of contracting a skin disease led to the isolation of people with various skin conditions in leper colonies. Although we no longer isolate people with psoriasis, fear and ignorance persist and have an impact on the daily life of these individuals. Many feel isolated by their disease and become self-conscious and withdrawn. These reactions may lead to depression and, rarely, suicide. Fortunately, most patients with psoriasis compensate well, learning to live with and control their disease.

Dermatological disease has a strong impact on a patient's psyche because of its visibility. People infrequently die of skin disease; more importantly, they must live with their disease. Sulzberger (1) stated that of all illness, skin disease most affects the psyche and can be a great handicap in work and social settings. The recognition and management of psychological factors have become part of dermatological practice because of the complex interaction between the skin and the psyche.

EFFECT OF STRESS ON PSORIASIS

Acute, stressful events are frequently related temporally to a flare of psoriasis, such as the woman who experienced a guttate flare the day after her son was arrested (2). Commonly, psoriatic flares have been attributed to life events such as divorce, death of someone close to the patient, bankruptcy, and loss of a job. However, Mazzetti et al. (3) reported that 67.6% of stressful events were objectively mild in a group of 80 inpatients with psoriasis and that it was the patient's perception of the stressor that was important. In general, skin reactivity, as measured by itching (in healthy skin, psoriatic skin, and atopic dermatitis skin), is affected by psychosocial stress, but coping styles and other cognitive factors modulate such effects (4).

Polenghi et al. (5) studied 179 psoriatic patients using the Paykel Scale for stressful events and showed that 72% of psoriatics had experienced significant stressful events about 1 month before the appearance of psoriasis. Bolgert and Soulé (6) studied 200 cases in France and attributed a primary role to emotional factors in 48% of psoriatic flares and a minor role to them in 30%. Janula and Novotný (7) reported that 24% of 2202 patients had a flare of psoriasis after emotional trauma. Al'Abadie et al. (8) found that stress was more likely to predate the onset and exacerbations of psoriasis than of other skin conditions. The most common types of life events associated with psoriasis were family upsets, such as bereavement, and work or school demands, but chronic difficulties were also common. They found no relationship between the severity of stress and time to onset or exacerbations.

In a British study, Seville (9) prospectively followed a group of 132 patients with psoriasis for 3 years. Thirty-nine percent recalled the occurrence of a stressful event within 1 month prior to a flare compared with 10% of the control group. The stresses included death, accidents, examinations, and sexual assault. Of those who noted this relationship, 53% (27 of 51) were free of disease at 3 years, whereas 17% (14 or 81) of those who did not report stress-associated flares were disease free at 3 years. In a later study from the same center (10), 74% of patients (23 of 31) in whom stress was associated with exacerbations of psoriasis were free of psoriasis at 3 years, whereas 20% of those not identifying stress as a precipitating factor were free of psoriasis. This implied a significantly better prognosis in those patients assessed as having an insight into stress. Farber et al. (11), in a retrospective survey of 2144 patients with psoriasis, studied the relationship between the appearance or worsening of psoriasis with times of worry. Forty percent of patients reported that their psoriasis appeared at a time of worry, and 37% reported on exacerbation associated with worry.

Unfortunately, these studies are subjective, largely uncontrolled, and do not exclude observer bias. Shuster (12) argued that these studies are flawed because patients learn to give the expected response. He believed that the relationship between the skin and the mind may be a consequence of the skin's role as an organ of communication and the response of society fearing the infectious nature of skin disease (13).

Attempts have been made to *quantify* stress and to identify its relationship to skin disease (11,17–24). Baughman and Sobel (23) used the Social Readjustment Rating Scale to assess stress retrospectively. In this questionnaire, 40 common life events (such as death of a spouse or job change) were assigned different scores related to the degree of associated stress, and patients were asked to complete one questionnaire for each of the preceding 5 years. These results were correlated with the severity of their psoriasis during the same period. The authors concluded that there was a modest correlation between stress and psoriasis. Seville (25) argued that, because the incubation period between stress and flare is usually 1 month or less, these studies may underestimate the association by examining life events occurring in the preceding year.

Possible *mechanisms* whereby stress leads to exacerbations of psoriasis have been discussed. There has been some speculation that stress may induce alterations in psoriatic lesions by causing an imbalance in the neuropeptide content in lesions. An increase in the neuropeptide content with a decrease in the activity of neuropeptide-degrading enzymes, especially mast cell chymase, has been reported (26). An imbalance of the neuropeptides vasoactive intestinal peptide and substance P in psoriatic lesions has also been reported (27). However, the finding of psoriasis exacerbated by psychological factors cannot be satisfactorily explained merely by alterations of neuropeptides in the skin.

Are certain individuals more prone to stress-related psoriasis? Various psychological tests have been administered to persons with psoriasis in an attempt to define specific psoriatic personality traits. The most commonly used tests are questionnaires. The individual responses are compared with those of a control population and those of patients with known psychiatric disorders. Most of these studies failed to demonstrate a characteristic psoriatic personality (21,23,28–30).

Matussek et al. (31) measured factors of aggression in a group of 38 patients with psoriasis, 113 with depression, and 32 healthy controls. They reported that those with psoriasis demonstrated marked aggression toward others and low autoaggression. Fava et al. (24) reported high anxiety, depression, and inadequacy scores on the Kellner-Sheffield Symptom Rating Test in a group of 20 patients with psoriasis. The Minnesota Multiphasic Personality Inventory was used by

Goldsmith et al. (32) to evaluate a group of 13 inpatients with psoriasis. They noted higher scores on the psychasthenia and hysteria subscales. The Brek Depression Inventory and the Leyton Obsessional Inventory were used by Hardy and Cotterill (33) to evaluate a group of patients with psoriasis. They found that the group was more obsessive and depressed than the control population. Patients with psoriasis were compared with patients having known psychosomatic disease by using the Amsterdam Biographic Questionnaire (30). The groups scored similarly on scales measuring neuroticism, extroversion, and ability to develop self-defense mechanisms.

The validity of these studies is difficult to interpret. The populations are small and often uncontrolled. None of the authors have performed sequential studies during the course of the disease. Demonstration of a particular trait does not necessarily imply cause and effect. The abnormalities reported may simply be the patients' response to a chronic, unpredictable, visible, and often disfiguring disease.

EFFECT OF PSORIASIS ON PSYCHOSOCIAL WELL-BEING

Social Implications

Psoriasis is a disease with profound social implications. With regard to employment, limitations stemmed from the anticipated or real response of others: 38% reported no employment difficulties, 15% reported limited opportunity, 44% suffered functional difficulty, and 12% experienced interpersonal difficulty related to their psoriasis (34). Finlay and Coles (35) attempted to quantify the level of handicap experienced by patients with severe psoriasis being admitted for inpatient care or starting systemic therapy. Of the 180 patients not working, 33.9% attributed not working to their psoriasis. Of the 150 patients currently working, 59.3% had lost a mean of 26 days from work during the preceding year because of their psoriasis.

Psychological Implications

Embarrassment about one's appearance has been cited as the worst feature of having psoriasis, according to patients who have been interviewed (34,36,37). This problem is compounded further by public ignorance regarding psoriasis. Finlay and Coles (35) reported that 49% of 369 patients would be prepared to spend 2 or 3 hours each day on treatment if this might result in normal skin for the rest of the day. This statistic underscores the degree of anxiety aroused by this disease.

Ginsburg and Link (38) reported that 19 of their 100 subjects experienced a total of 50 episodes of gross rejection as a result of their psoriasis, most often in the setting of a gym, pool, or hairdressing salon or with regard to employment. Jowett and Ryan (34) interviewed 38 patients with psoriasis, 32 with eczema, and 30 with acne in an attempt to quantify the handicapping effect of skin disease. In the psoriatic group, 87% reported that itching was a prominent symptom. When asked about the worst aspect of having psoriasis, most said that it was the appearance and consequent embarrassment. Most had encountered ignorance and misunderstanding about psoriasis. Feelings of shame and embarrassment were reported by 89% of those with psoriasis, and 56% expressed anxiety about the unpredictable nature of psoriasis with regard to exacerbations, remissions, associated arthritis, and possible side effects of medication. A lack of confidence was reported by 42% and depression by 24%; 25% thought that psoriasis had caused friction within the family. Most felt that their choice of clothing, with regard to color and style, was restricted by psoriasis. This complaint was most noticeable in the female group, some of whom would not wear skirts, nylons, or short-sleeved clothing.

Ramsay and O'Reagan (36) surveyed a group of 104 patients with psoriasis with regard to the social and psychological effects of their disease. They were asked specifically about seven common social activities: swimming, sunbathing, going to a hairdresser, playing sports, communal bathing or showering, dancing, and going out of one's home. Swimming and sunbathing were avoided by 72% and 60%, respectively, and 34% avoided going to a hairdresser. Many (70%) avoided four or more of these activities, and only 11.5% did not avoid any of the seven social situations. Fifty percent of the group thought that psoriasis had inhibited their sexual relationships. This perception correlated with extensive disease and genital involvement. Eleven percent of patients said that they would avoid having children because of the fear that their offspring might develop psoriasis. Emotional disturbances in individuals who have psoriasis may not be detected on psychological testing (such as the Minnesota Multiphasic Personality Inventory) (32).

Sexual problems are also reported. In another questionnaire, one-third of patients with psoriasis had problems with dating and starting sexual relationships. This was associated with low self-esteem and emotional complaints rather than the extent or distribution of the psoriasis (39).

Depression is a frequently reported sequela to psoriasis. Fried et al. (40) surveyed 64 patients undergoing outpatient treatment for psoriasis. Approximately half the patients were found to have moderate to extreme levels of anxiety, depression, and anger during their disease flares and during periods of remission. They also had moderate to extreme levels of pruritus associated with their flares. Significant levels of social embarrassment, life disruption, and social withdrawal were also found. Gupta et al. (41) observed that degree of pruritus (as measured by a self-rated 10-point scale) correlated with degree of depression (as measured by the Carroll Rating Scale for Depression) in 77 outpatients with mild-moderate psoriasis. They concluded that depression modulated pruritus perception. More alarmingly, 9.7% of 217 psoriasis patients completing the Carroll Rating Scale for Depression reported a wish to be dead, and 5.5% reported active suicidal ideation at the time of the study. The death wish and suicidal ideation were associated with higher depression scores ($p < 0.0001$) and higher patient self-ratings of psoriasis severity ($p < 0.05$). Patient self-reports of psoriasis severity correlated directly with the overall depression scores ($r = 0.39$; $p < 0.0001$).

Psychotropic drugs can exacerbate psoriasis. The use of lithium may precipitate or exacerbate psoriasis. Lithium-induced psoriasis is often resistant to conventional antipsoriatic therapy and may necessitate stopping the drug (14,15). Acute pustular psoriasis has been reported with the antidepressant trazodone (16). The phenothiazine group of drugs may cause photosensitivity with koebnerization, and theoretically they may cause problems if introduced during the course of phototherapy.

An association between alcohol abuse or alcoholism and psoriasis has been suspected on the basis of anecdotal reports (42). The high incidence of liver biopsy abnormalities in patients with psoriasis further supports the association (43). Morse et al. (42) used the Self-Administered Alcoholism Screening Test to assess the prevalence of alcoholism among a group of 99 patients hospitalized with psoriasis. A control group of patients hospitalized with other dermatological disorders was matched for age and sex. Alcoholism was diagnosed in 11 (10 males, one female) of the patients with psoriasis and three of the control patients (one male, two females). A study (44) of 55 women aged 18–50 years suggested that smoking is a risk factor for psoriasis in women and that alcohol intake worsens psoriasis. Smoking and negative life events were more common among psoriasis patients than among controls, perhaps as consequences of the disease.

Baughman et al. (45) compared the history of alcohol use with the severity of psoriasis in a population of 1200 patients. During a 3-year follow-up, no strong association was noted between the severity of psoriasis and alcohol consumption. However, they identified some patients in whom alcohol consumption clearly was related to the exacerbation of psoriasis. Delaney and Leppard (46), in a comparison of patients with psoriasis and a dermatological control group, found no difference between the groups in alcohol consumption or drinking problems based on a single questionnaire item.

Several measurements of the disability and handicap associated with psoriasis have been developed. The psoriasis area and severity index is widely used in clinical studies to assess psoriasis severity. The psoriasis disability index (PDI) is a method to give a rapid overall measure of psoriasis disability from answers to a series of 15 questions. The PDI has been shown to be sensitive to changes in the extent of lesions and to covary with the UK Sickness Impact Profile, a more general measure of the effects of disease on quality of life used to compare the disability experienced by psoriatic patients with that experienced by patients suffering from other systemic diseases. The overall score reflects the impact that the skin disease had on the patient during the previous month, a period chosen to enable the PDI to be used to reflect change in disability after therapy (47,48). The mean PDI in a study of 369 patients with severe psoriasis was 38.2% (35).

CHILDHOOD PSORIASIS

Psoriasis in childhood presents special psychological problems. The onset of psoriasis in childhood or adolescence may magnify the psychological aspects of the disease. These patients are usually girls (female: male ratio 2:1), and during a lifetime their psoriasis will be more severe (49). At this age, patients are more vulnerable and more sensitive to the opinions of others. These children often are embarrassed and fear social ostracism. They hide their psoriasis with makeup and clothing. They avoid group activities, such as swimming and sports, that might expose them to ridicule. A young person growing up with psoriasis has to come to terms with the disease with regard to self-image, self-esteem, and relationships with others.

An experience of rejection may leave the patient apprehensive about the future (38).

The relationships within the family are complex. The parent with psoriasis or a family history of psoriasis may feel guilty and overprotect the child. Alternatively, the parent may develop a pattern of denial and ignore the child's skin problems. Sibling rivalry may be a secondary problem in the setting of overprotection. Hostility may be expressed toward the parent from whom the trait has been inherited (50).

In addition to the standard therapy, the management of childhood psoriasis includes the following: (1) educating family and friends about psoriasis, emphasizing that psoriasis is not contagious; (2) encouraging a normal life-style, with the warning that trauma to the skin may cause koebnerization; and (3) listening to and encouraging the child to voice his or her concerns.

THERAPY

Various psychotherapeutic and psychopharmacological interventions have been applied in the treatment of psoriasis. If stress is implicated as a precipitating factor, it should be addressed and eliminated if possible. Stress as a consequence of the psoriasis is universal and its treatment should play a large part in the management of the psoriasis. Psychological support is essential. This can be achieved in an outpatient or an inpatient setting. Hospitalization is the simplest form of psychotherapy—removing the patient from outside stress and assuming responsibility for skin care. McHenry and Doherty (51) reported that outpatient clinic attendance improved psoriasis in 34 of 45 patients and lessened the reports of major psychosocial effects of psoriasis on life-style from 67% (30 of 45 patients) at initial visit to 40% (18 of 45 patients) at review after 3 months.

Anxiolytic drugs have been advocated when stress is a major factor (52,53). In selected cases, antidepressant therapy may be appropriate.

In recent years, psoriasis support groups have been established, often in association with psoriasis day care centers (54). Feelings of isolation are reduced; coping skills and self-efficacy are enhanced (55). Interaction among patients helps to decrease the sense of isolation. Patient education is also an important feature of such groups. A psoriasis support group may be of particular benefit for children and adolescents with psoriasis and for their parents. The National Psoriasis Foundation, through its newsletters, reaches many persons with psoriasis. It is of particular value to those living in rural areas who might not otherwise avail themselves of a support group. The newsletters serve to update patients on advances in psoriasis research and therapy, and they provide a forum for the exchange of ideas. Psoriasis research also is sponsored by this organization. Participation in a support group is a personal decision and many persons with psoriasis will elect not to join, feeling more comfortable dealing with their skin disease privately.

Polenghi et al. (5) reported a 64% decrease in the psoriasis area and severity index for severity and the extent of psoriasis and also fewer recurrences at the 1-year follow-up in patients who received biofeedback training. Price et al. (56) reported a reduction in anxiety levels and a modest trend toward physical improvement of psoriatic patients when they attended a short series of meetings conducted by a clinical psychologist to discuss problems created by their skin complaint and were taught specific relaxation techniques. Meditation was reported to lead to an improvement in four of 10 patients with scalp psoriasis (57). Frankel and Misch (58) and Waxman (59) reported success with hypnosis as an adjunct to antipsoriatic therapy.

CONCLUSIONS

Stress may precipitate psoriasis, and psoriasis very definitely may exacerbate stress. We must identify the subgroup in whom stress is a significant precipitating factor. By elimination of these precipitating factors and by minimizing the psychological effects of stress, longer remissions may be induced. The special needs of the child or adolescent with psoriasis should be recognized.

Education of patients, their families, and the community will help to decrease feelings of isolation and stigmatization. Psychological support is an integral component in the management of patients with psoriasis (54).

REFERENCES

1. Hoffmann, N.Y. (1983). Marion Sulzberger, MD: "Mr. Dermatology," *J.A.M.A.* 249:1243, 1247–1249.
2. Lomholt, G. (1945). Acute guttate psoriasis provoked by a psychic trauma. *Acta Derm. Venereol.* (*Stockh.*) 25:524–525 (abstract).
3. Mazzetti, M., Mozzetta, A., Soavi, G.C., Andreoli, E., Foglio Bonda, P.G., Puddu, P., and Decaminada, F. (1994). Psoriasis, stress and psychiatry: psychody-

namic characteristics of stressors. *Acta Derm. Venereol. (Stockh.)* 186(Suppl.):62–64.
4. Arnetz, B.B., Fjellner, B., Eneroth, P., and Kallner, A. (1991). Endocrine and dermatological concomitants of mental stress. *Acta Derm. Venereol. (Stockh.)* 156(Suppl.):9–12.
5. Polenghi, M.M., Molinari, E., Gala, C., Guzzi, R., Garutti, C., and Finzi, A.F. (1994). Experience with psoriasis in a psychosomatic dermatology clinic. *Acta Derm. Venereol. (Stockh.)* 186(Suppl.):65–66.
6. Bolgert, M., and Soulé, M. (1955). Étude clinique et psychosomatique de 200 cas de psoriasis. *Semin. Hop. Paris* 31:1251–1261.
7. Janula, J., and Novotný, F. (1965). Zur statistischen Erforschung der Psoriasis. *Hautarzt* 16:241–246.
8. Al'Abadie, M.S., Kent, G.G., and Gawkrodger, D.J. (1994). The relationship between stress and the onset and exacerbation of psoriasis and other skin conditions. *Br. J. Dermatol.* 130:199–203.
9. Seville, R.H. (1977). Psoriasis and stress. *Br. J. Dermatol.* 97:297–302.
10. Seville, R.H. (1978). Psoriasis and stress. II. *Br. J. Dermatol.* 98:151–153.
11. Farber, E.M., Bright, R.D., and Nall, M.L. (1968). Psoriasis. A questionnaire survey of 2,144 patients. *Arch. Dermatol.* 98:248–259.
12. Shuster, S. (1979). Stress and psoriasis. *Br. J. Dermatol.* 100:614–616 (letter to the editor).
13. Shuster, S. (1978). *Dermatology in Internal Medicine.* Oxford University Press, New York, pp. 77–78.
14. Selmanowitz, V.J. (1986). Lithium, leukocytes, and lesions. *Clin. Dermatol.* 4:170–175.
15. Skoven, I., and Thormann, J. (1979). Lithium compound treatment and psoriasis. *Arch. Dermatol.* 115: 1185–1187.
16. Barth, J.H., and Baker, H. (1986). Generalized pustular psoriasis precipitated by trazodone in the treatment of depression. *Br. J. Dermatol.* 115:629–630.
17. Shanon, J. (1979). Psoriasis: psychosomatic aspects. *Psychother. Psychosom.* 31:218–222.
18. Hellgren, L. (1964). Psoriasis: a statistical, clinical and laboratory investigation of 255 psoriatics and matched healthy controls. *Acta Derm. Venereol. (Stockh.)* 44: 191–207.
19. Nyfors, A., and Lemholt, K. (1975). Psoriasis in children. A short review and a survey of 245 cases. *Br. J. Dermatol.* 92:437–442.
20. Savin, J.A. (1970). Patients' beliefs about psoriasis. *Trans. St. Johns Hosp. Dermatol. Soc.* 56:139–142.
21. Suskind, W., and McGuire, R.J. (1959). The emotional factor in psoriasis. *Scott. Med. J.* 4:503–507.
22. Wittkower, E.D., and Russell, B. (Eds.) (1953). *Emotional Factors in Skin Disease.* Paul B. Hoeber, New York, pp. 109–120.
23. Baughman, R., and Sobel, R. (1971). Psoriasis, stress, and strain. *Arch. Dermatol.* 103:599–605.
24. Fava, G.A., Perini, G.I., Santonastaso, P., and Fornasa, C.V. (1980). Life events and psychological distress in dermatologic disorders: psoriasis, chronic urticaria and fungal infections. *Br. J. Med. Psychol.* 53:277–282.
25. Seville, R.H. (1989). Stress and psoriasis: the importance of insight and empathy in prognosis. *J. Am. Acad. Dermatol.* 20:97–100.
26. Harvima, I.T., Viinamaki, H., Naukkarinen, A., Paukkonen, K., Neittaanmaki, H., Harvima, R.J., and Horsmanheimo, M. (1993). Association of cutaneous mast cells and sensory nerves with psychic stress in psoriasis. *Psychother. Psychosom.* 60:168–176.
27. Pincelli, C., Fantini, F., Magnoni, C., and Giannetti, A. (1994). Psoriasis and the nervous system. *Acta Derm. Venereol. (Stockh.)* 186(Suppl.):60–61.
28. Wittkower, E. (1946). Psychological aspects of psoriasis. *Lancet* 1:566–569.
29. Gilbert, A.R., Rodgers, D.A., and Roenigk, H.H., Jr. (1973). Personality evaluation in psoriasis. *Cleve. Clin. Q.* 40:147–152.
30. van der Schaar, W.W. (1976–1977). Psychometric investigation in 48 Dutch patients suffering from psoriasis. *Psychother. Psychosom.* 27:159–162.
31. Matussek, P., Agerer, D., and Seibt, G. (1985). Aggression in depressives and psoriatics. *Psychother. Psychosom.* 43:120–125.
32. Goldsmith, L.A., Fisher, M., and Wacks, J. (1969). Psychological characteristics of psoriatics. Implications for management. *Arch. Dermatol.* 100:674–676.
33. Hardy, G.E., and Cotterill, J.A. (1982). A study of depression and obsessionality in dysmorphophobic and psoriatic patients. *Br. J. Psychiatry* 140:19–22.
34. Jowett, S., and Ryan, T. (1985). Skin disease and handicap: an analysis of the impact of skin conditions. *Soc. Sci. Med.* 20:425–429.
35. Finlay, A.Y., and Coles, E.C. (1995). The effect of severe psoriasis on the quality of life of 369 patients. *Br. J. Dermatol.* 132:236–244.
36. Ramsay, B., and O'Reagan, M. (1988). A survey of the social and psychological effects of psoriasis. *Br. J. Dermatol.* 118:195–201.
37. Jobling, R.G. (1976). Psoriasis—a preliminary questionnaire study of sufferers' subjective experience. *Clin. Exp. Dermatol.* 1:233–236.
38. Ginsburg, I.H., and Link, B.G. (1989). Feelings of stigmatization in patients with psoriasis. *J. Am. Acad. Dermtol.* 20:53–63.
39. van Dorssen, I.E., Boom, B.W., and Hengeveld, M.W. (1992). Seksualiteitsbeleving bij patienten met psoriasis en constitutioneel eczeem. *Ned. Tijdschr. Geneeskd.* 136:2175–2178.
40. Fried, R.G., Friedman, S., Paradis, C., Hatch, M., Lynfield, Y., Duncanson, C., and Shalita, A. (1995). Trivial or terrible? The psychosocial impact of psoriasis. *Int. J. Dermatol.* 34:101–105.

41. Gupta, M.A., Gupta, A.K., Schork, N.J., and Ellis, C.N. (1994). Depression modulates pruritus perception: a study of pruritus in psoriasis, atopic dermatitis, and chronic idiopathic urticaria. *Psychosom. Med.* 56: 36–40.
42. Morse, R.M., Perry, H.O., and Hurt, R.D. (1985). Alcoholism and psoriasis. *Alcohol Clin. Exp. Res.* 9: 396–399.
43. Zachariae, H., and Sogaard, H. (1973). Liver biopsy in psoriasis. A controlled study. *Dermatologica* 146: 149–155.
44. Poikolainen, K., Reunala, T., Karvonen, J. (1994). Smoking, alcohol and life events related to psoriasis among women. *Br. J. Dermatol.* 130:473–477.
45. Baughman, R.D., Landeen, R.H., Maloney, M.E., and Stern, R.S. (1982). Psoriasis and alcohol. In *Psoriasis: Proceedings of the Third International Symposium, Stanford University, 1981.* E.M. Farber, A.J. Cox, L. Nall, and P.H. Jacobs (Eds.). Grune & Stratton, New York, pp. 323–324.
46. Delaney, T.J., and Leppard, B. (1974). Alcohol intake and psoriasis. *Acta Derm. Venereol.* 54:237–238.
47. Finlay, A.Y., and Kelly, S.E. (1987). Psoriasis—an index of disability. *Clin. Exp. Dermatol.* 12:8–11.
48. Finlay, A.Y., Khan, G.K., Luscombe, D.K., and Salek, M.S. (1990). Validation of Sickness Impact Profile and Psoriasis Disability Index in Psoriasis. *Br. J. Dermatol.* 123:751–756.
49. Farber, E.M., and Carlsen, R.A. (1966). Psoriasis in childhood. *Calif. Med.* 105:415–420.
50. Loeffel, E.D. (1978). Psoriasis in adolescence. *Major Probl. Clin. Pediatr.* 19:143–162.
51. McHenry, P.M., and Doherty, V.R. (1992). Psoriasis: an audit of patients' views on the disease and its treatment. *Br. J. Dermatol.* 127:13–17.
52. Levy, S.W. (1963). A psychosomatic approach to the management of recalcitrant dermatoses. *Psychosomatics* 4:334–337.
53. Padilla, M.A. (1965). El Diazepam en el tratamiento de las neurodermatosis. *Medicina* 45:219–221.
54. Cram, D.L., and King, R.I. (1976). Psoriasis day care centers. *J.A.M.A.* 235:177–178.
55. Abel, E.A., Moore, U.S., and Glathe, J.P. (1990). Psoriasis patient support group and self-care efficacy as an adjunct to day care center treatment. *Int. J. Dermatol.* 29:640–643.
56. Price, M.L., Mottahedin, I., Mayo, P.R. (1991). Can psychotherapy help patients with psoriasis? *Clin. Exp. Dermatol.* 16:114–117.
57. Gaston, L., Crombez, J.C., Lassonde, M., Bernier-Buzzanga, J., and Hodgins, S. (1991). Psychological stress and psoriasis: experimental and prospective correlational studies. *Acta Derm. Venereol. (Stockh.)* 156(Suppl.):37–43.
58. Frankel, F.H., and Misch, R.C. (1973). Hypnosis in a case of long-standing psoriasis in a person with character problems. *Int. J. Clin. Exp. Hypn.* 21:121–130.
59. Waxman, D. (1973). Behaviour therapy of psoriasis—a hypnoanalytic and counter-conditioning technique. *Postgrad. Med. J.* 49:591–595.

Part II

INCIDENCE AND GENETICS

9

Epidemiology: Natural History and Genetics

Eugene M. Farber
Psoriasis Research Institute, Palo Alto, California

Lexie Nall
Stanford University School of Medicine, Stanford, California

PREFATORY COMMENTS

Over 5 years have passed since the second edition of this text was issued. During that time significant advances have been made in clinical, epidemiological, and experimental investigations applicable to unraveling the etiology and pathogenesis of psoriasis and developing improved therapeutic modalities. The areas that have witnessed exponential growth are in genetic epidemiology and immunogenetics. In addition, we have seen a broadening of multidisciplinary collaboration even among scientific regions that at one time were far afield from molecular biology as seen in the study of evolutionary factors that have influenced the natural selection of the immune system. Integrating and linking these fields of study is the World Wide Web and videoconferencing on the Internet—revolutionary informational resources for transmitting the most up-to-date medical developments (43,67–70, 111–113, 173, 186, 218, 224, 279, 282, 284, 288, 316, 362,374,419).

This chapter reviews and synthesizes current knowledge on the genetics and natural history of psoriasis from worldwide studies that employ traditional epidemiological and recently developed seroepidemiological methods (111–113, 127, 128, 224, 236, 282, 284,377,419). One of its primary themes is the epidemiology of wellness (99,228,266,377,406), which not only promotes positive attitudes toward health but also advocates *disability prevention* in psoriasis (80,129).

INTRODUCTION

More than three decades ago, Sulzberger (365,366) made the following remarks:

> Medicine in ancient times taught that the causes of disease were such things as the possession by evil spirits, miasmas, too much blood, too much bile, or too much rheum. At the beginning of the bacteriologic age and of modern medicine, it was believed and hoped that single microbial agents would be found as the causes of individual diseases.

In recent times, it has come to be recognized that diseases are not due to single simple causes. Today, after many decades of clinical and laboratory investigations aimed at ferreting out the pathogenesis of psoriasis, it is the consensus that indeed this specific disorder is not precipitated by any single simple etiology, but by a complex disease mechanism of interacting factors. Naldi (282) suggests that epidemiology, by imposing methodological control and a numerate approach, can provide major contributions to “capture" and understand psoriasis, and that multidisciplinary research and large study networks are needed.

Epidemiology is widely recognized as the basic science of preventive medicine and is often defined as the branch of medical science dealing with the study of the distribution and determinants of disease frequency in humans (76,171,237,403). In recent times the term *dermatoepidemiology* has been coined, which concentrates on the application of epidemiological methods in dermatoses (78,405).

Epidemiology differs from other medical disciplines in one important aspect. Patients are studied in their natural habitat, as members of a community and in reference to both their genetically determined susceptibility and the influence of ecological environment and the artificial environment mankind has created. An epidemiological model for psoriasis can be demonstrated by a Venn diagram (Fig. 1): a person with specific genetic and behavioral characteristics (uppermost circle); the environment (ecological and artificial) (circles to the right and left); and where the three circles intersect the manifestation of the disease appears (200).

Investigation of the epidemiology and sociology of skin disease has been largely neglected in the past (169); however, several recent studies (44,94,163,175,181,220,221,242) have shown that skin diseases make sizable contributions to the total morbidity at different levels of medical care and therefore deserve attention in their relationship to other diseases (44).

DATA COLLECTION

When one inspects the studies of the natural history of a disease, it is essential to assess the sampling technique employed by the investigator (282,290). Reliable epidemiological information rests upon drawing a valid sample from which accurate interpretations can be deduced. In general, four methods have been utilized in gathering statistical data on psoriasis.

First are the classic epidemiological field studies of total populations. Here one is able to determine the prevalence of the disease in the general population and to identify prevailing genetic and environmental factors (183,184,203,234,243).

Second is the analysis of hospital inpatient/outpatient records, which show the frequency of new cases of psoriasis relative to other hospital/clinic-treated dermatoses. This approach supplies valuable data for retrospective studies. However, the factors determining referral to a hospital vary greatly; thus the reliability of the data is unpredictable and may introduce bias. The more serious illnesses are treated in a hospital, whereas less severely affected cases are cared for elsewhere or not at all (34).

The third employs data collected by a physician in his or her particular private practice. This approach is fraught with problems of bias, since individual practices reflect specific socioeconomic levels within a community rather than the community as a whole (271).

Fourth is the questionnaire survey (369). In-depth field census studies are prohibitively expensive. Therefore, the questionnaire survey is a viable alternative. As part of the overall psoriasis research program at Stanford University carried out from 1960 to the mid-1980s, which continues today at the Psoriasis Research Institute, we (121,122,124) initiated an international cooperative epidemiological study. Various dermatological facilities participated in collecting data on the course of psoriasis in their specific geographic region, which provided information on the similarities and differences in the natural history of this disorder throughout the world. Although the questionnaire method has many pitfalls (285), it nonetheless is useful in collecting large amounts of information at low cost and in providing standardized data recording, which facilitates computer manipulation and analysis of findings that can then be compared among varying investigators (369).

EPIDEMIOLOGICAL METHODOLOGY

Traditional Techniques

Six traditional epidemiological techniques have been employed in gathering prevalence, natural history, and genetic information over the past few decades: (1) census studies of large populations; (2) familial aggregation; (3) twin-pair investigations; (4) pedigree; (5) conjugal; and (6) half-sibship analyses (127,246).

Seroepidemiological Techniques

With the advent of knowledge about the association of varying frequencies of the human leukocyte antigens (HLAs) to the expression of certain diseases, seroepidemiology has provided the clinician, geneticist, and epidemiologist with a new tool for medical research and the chromosome mapping of the human genome (18, 33, 39–41, 86–89, 91–93, 96, 97, 104, 161, 219, 230, 255, 257, 262, 265, 268, 277, 303, 311,

323, 336, 341, 353, 354, 373, 379, 392, 409, 410, 414, 426, 427).

Since the discovery of the ABO blood system by Landsteiner earlier in this century, serum proteins, enzymes in serum and blood cells, and components of saliva have also been utilized as genetic markers in many diseases, including psoriasis (27–29,278,285, 322,408,425).

The fact that the frequency of certain HLA specificities, such as HLA B13, B17, B37, Cw6, and DR7 as well as others, is greatly increased in some psoriasis patients (but not in all) as compared to nonpsoriatic controls has led geneticists to consider the HLA antigens in the major histocompatibility complex of chromosome 6 as potential genetic markers for this disease. Investigators suggest that more than one genetic locus is involved in the expression of psoriasis (111–113,252,404,419), for example, chromosome 17q has recently been offered as a potential location for another gene (279,385). However, the latter has been challenged by certain investigators (279).

Many hypotheses for the mechanisms for the association between HLA and disease have been developed: (1) "molecular mimicry" in which the structure of an environmental pathogen mimics that of the HLA antigen, allowing the pathogen to induce disease; (2) the HLA antigen may act as a receptor for the disease-causing agent; and (3) the antigen itself may not be important, but it may be closely linked to a yet undiscovered immune response or disease-causing gene (91,392).

NATURAL HISTORY

Prevalence and Incidence

There is often confusion in the use of the terms *incidence* and *prevalence*. *Incidence* refers specifically to the development of *new* cases of a disease in a population (32). *Prevalence* refers to a static picture or "snapshot" of a number of persons who have a disease in a population at *one* point in time (6,58, 78,154,282).

An early report has indicated that in dermatology clinics in the United States the frequency of psoriasis as compared with other dermatological diseases is between 2nd and 12th place with a 6th position as an average (407). Recent studies have revealed that 20 dermatological disorders account for about 72% of office visits to dermatologists. Of these 20, Ramsey and Fox (324) reported that psoriasis accounted for 4.8% of office visits, ranking third after acne (27.4%) and warts (6.7%). A similar finding was made by Gundawardena and his colleagues (175); they observed that psoriasis was 3rd (8.7%) of the five most common diseases seen in their Sri Lanka dermatology clinic. Rea et al. (327) determined that psoriasis ranked 11th of 13 skin diseases studied in a British community.

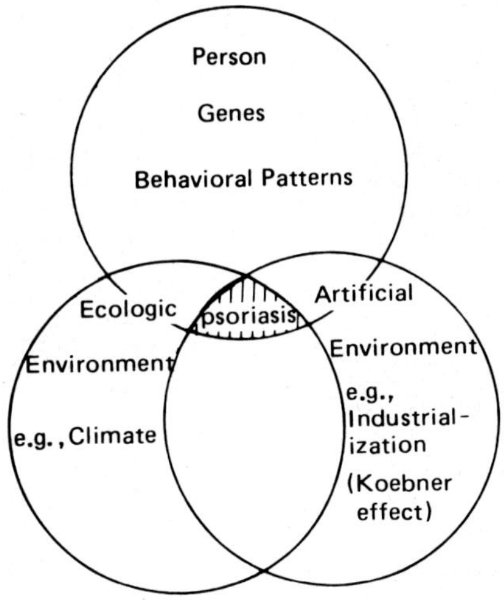

Figure 1 A Venn diagram demonstrating the interaction between genetics and environmental factors based on Ref. 200.

The prevalence of psoriasis in the general population varies from 0.1 to 2.8% in published reports (53, 121, 175, 177, 179, 183, 221, 223, 243, 305, 327, 333,395,428). Present data on different racial groups reveal much geographic variation in the occurrence of psoriasis (Figs. 2–5) (101,106,127,278). Recent geographic studies (Table 1) have shown psoriasis to occur at a rate of 1.6% in the United Kingdom (327), 1.55% in Croatia (22), 1.4% in Norway (45), 0.7% in the eastern Africa country of Rwanda (391), 0.4% in the Henan District of the People's Republic of China (184), and as high as 11.8 in Kazach'ye, located in the Arctic region of the former Soviet Union (107). Yip (425) summarized several studies stemming from Hong Kong, Japan, and the People's Republic of China and concluded that in spite of the climatic geographic differences represented in these regions, the surveys showed a constant and uniformly low prevalence of psoriasis (1%).

Through the Health and Nutrition Examination Survey (HANES 1) dermatologists in the United States examined a sample of 20,749 Americans between the ages of 1 and 74 years, who were selected without consideration for illness or complaint as they repre-

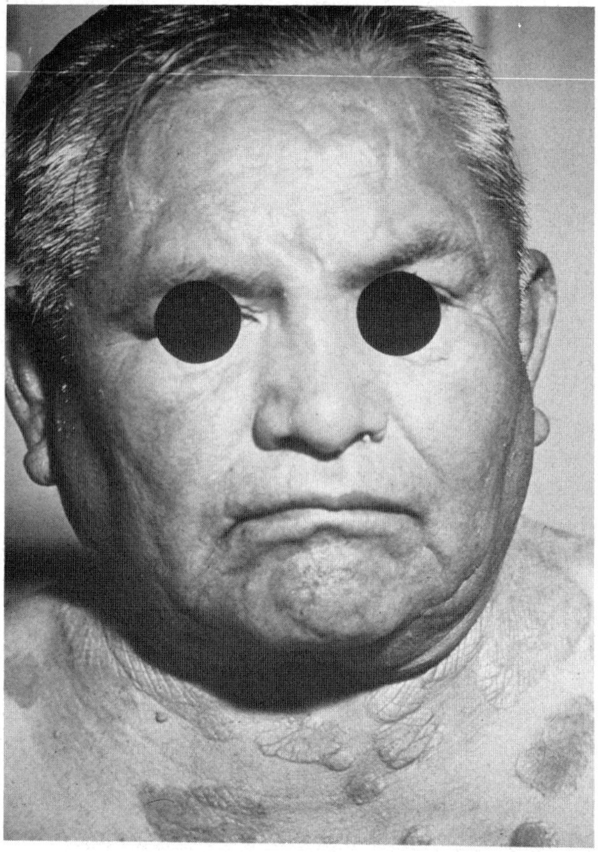

Figure 2 Psoriasis in a Native American of the southwestern United States. The occurrence of psoriasis in Native Americans of both the north and south continents is exceedingly rare, which may reflect the absence or low frequency of the HLA B13 and B17 antigens in these populations (124).

sented ethnically, socioeconomically, by age, and by sex the 194 million people in the United States at that time (203). Nearly one-third of those examined, or an estimated 60.6 million Americans, had one or more skin conditions. Excluded from these figures were those who had had dermatological ailments, but were in remission at the time of the examination, and those hospitalized for severe dermatological problems. Therefore, the estimate of the total number of individuals affected is actually understated (202,203,221). The prevalence rate for psoriasis was found to be 0.5%, which is lower than observed in other surveys.

A study group on psoriasis (221) has reported that between 150,000 and 260,000 *new* cases are seen in the United States each year. In an investigation of psoriasis patients seen in Rochester, Minnesota, from 1980 to 1983, the annual incidence rate was estimated to be 60.4/100,000 people (54.4 for men, 60.2 for women). Many authors have recommended that there is a definite need for studies of incidence rates in this and other countries, which would allow for more precise comparison of findings (282).

Pediatric Psoriasis

To determine the frequency and types of pediatric dermatological problems encountered by primary care physicians, dermatologists, and other physicians, Krowchuk and colleagues (223) examined the 1990 National Ambulatory Medical Care Survey and observed that 163.3 million physician office visits were made by patients 18 years of age or younger for all diagnoses (including psoriasis).

Dermatologists and pediatricians in the United States do not frequently consider psoriasis in the differential diagnosis of attention to the occurrence of psoriasis in young patients. Farber and Jacobs (126)

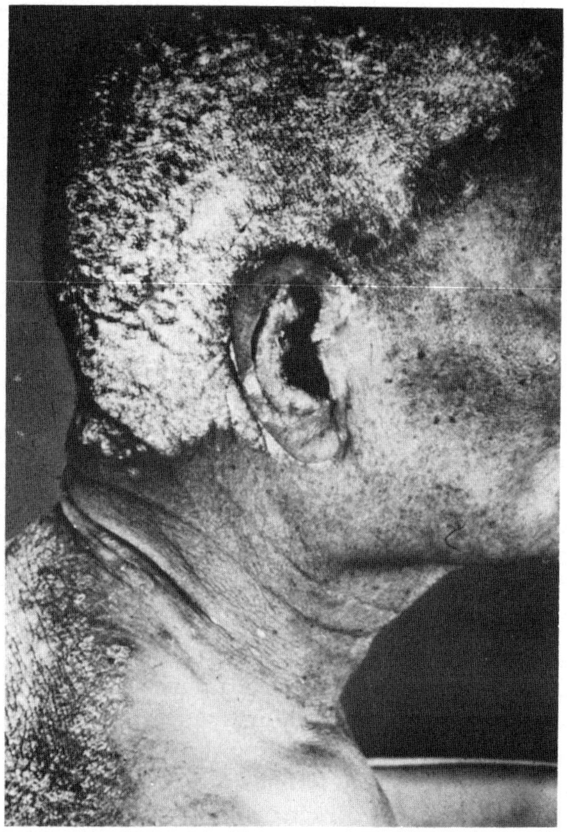

Figure 3 Psoriasis occurs in Asians, but has not been reported to be as high as in whites (124,127,144).

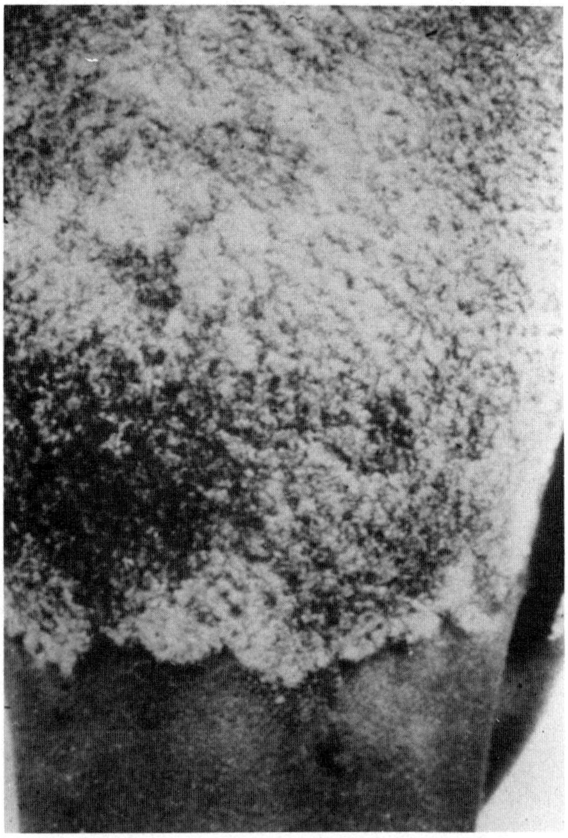

Figure 4 Prevalence of psoriasis in African blacks varies between a high rate in the eastern part of the continent and a very low rate in the western part (124,127,144).

studied 14 infants younger than 2 years of age and found that three had lesions while in the newborn nursery. Four developed lesions between 1 week and 3 months, five between 3 months and 6 months. Their investigation did not provide evidence of congenital psoriasis except in one infant in whom the obstetrician had observed nail pitting. Recently, Farber and his associates (130) performed a follow-up study on these children. In reexamination 6–13 years later, seven of nine children had recurrent psoriatic lesions, and two remained completely clear after the resolution of the initial eruption.

In infants, the diaper area is commonly observed to be the first appearance of psoriasis. The diagnosis here may be obscured by the fact that the characteristic scale is often absent. It is later when the typical psoriasis lesions appear elsewhere on the body that the diagnosis becomes clear. Psoriasis at this site in infants may be mistaken for a diaper rash, but it is actually due to fecal material and urine, which can convert minimal psoriasis to a more severe form (126,130,145).

It is common to find young children who develop psoriasis to have a family member with psoriasis. Children may present with psoriasis for the first time after scraping their knees. The scalp, face, and extremities are common sites in this age group as well as pitting of the nails. Less commonly, children may develop pustules or generalized psoriasis.

The occurrence of psoriasis varies in childhood as in other age classes. In a retrospective study in the National Skin Centre of Singapore (160), out of 75,589 new patients in 1994, 9273 (12.4%) were less than age 16. Of this pediatric group, only 100 children (1.1%) had psoriasis, whereas 2476 (3.3%) of the adult group were affected. There were significant differences in the types of disease between children and adults. For example, in children, eczema was the most common (50%), followed by viral infection (7%), bacterial infection (5%), and insect bite reactions (5%), all significantly higher than in adults.

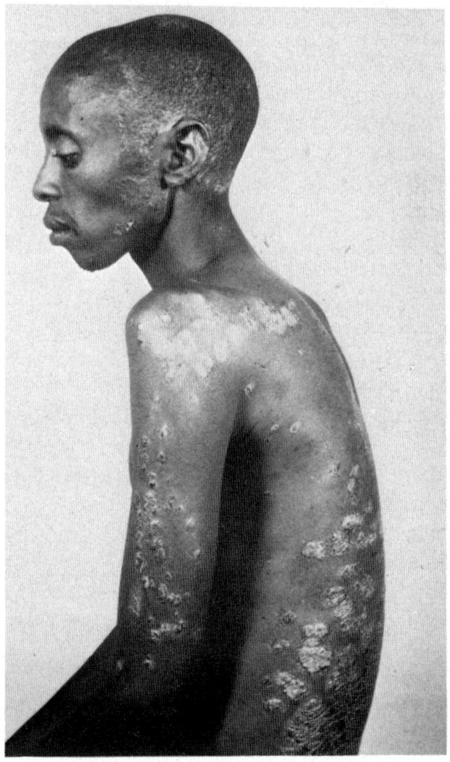

Figure 5 It has been speculated that the low occurrence of psoriasis in American blacks is due in part to their origins in the western regions of Africa (124,127,144).

Table 1 Prevalence of Psoriasis in Various Geographic Regions

Country	Frequency (%)	Sample size (number)	Source	Ref.
General populations				
Am. Samoa	0	12,569	GP	26
Czechoslovakia	1.2	NG	GP	PC 1974
Denmark	2.9	4,000	GP	48
England	1.6	2,180	GP	327
Faroe Is.	2.8	11,000	GP	243
France	2–3	NG	GP	PC 1974
Hungary	2.0	NG	GP	PC 1974
Italy	1–2	NG	GP	PC 1974
Netherlands	1.8	3,795	GP	65
Norway	1.4	10,576	GP	45
	4.8	14,482	GP	209
Lapps	0.6	2,000	GP	210
Lapps	1.4	2,508	GP	118
PR China	0.4	105,545	GP	184
	0.2	5,742,066	GP	348
	1.23	6,617,917	GP	238
So. Am. Andes	0	25,915	GP	82
Sweden	1.4	39,571	GP	183
Sweden	2.3	159,200	GP	239
United States	0.5	20,749	GP	203
USSR	2.0	NG	GP	PC 1974
Arctic-Kazach'ye	11.8	NG		107
Yugoslavia	1.6	8,416	GP	22
Specific populations (hospital, clinic, private practice)				
North America				
Am. blacks	0.7	3,860	PP	211
	1.4	2,400	PP	212
Canada	4.7	12,578	PP	271
Greenland	1.4	NG	Cl	243
United States	4.6	27,000	PP	407
	2.2	24,009,272	PP	152
Middle America, Mexico, Central America				
Mexico City	3.0	NG	PP/Cl	59
Guatemala				
Rural	0.7	3,140	Cl	115
Urban	3.0	NG	PP	59
Honduras	3.0	NG	PP	115
Jamaica	1.3	Est	FS	401
Nicaragua	0.7	3,140	Cl	115
Trinidad/Tobago	6.0	4,048	Cl	321
South America				
Bolivia	0	3,140	Cl	115
Brazil	1.3	NG	Cl	339
Colombia	0.4	3,140	Cl	115
Paraguay	4.2	3,410	Cl	115
Peru (Cuzco)	0.08	1,277	Cl	116
Venezuela (Caracas)	2.0	NG	Cl	213

Table 1 Continued

Country	Frequency (%)	Sample size (number)	Source	Ref.
Europe				
Germany	6.5	NG	Cl	PC 1974
Ireland	5.5	14,231	Cl	177
Scotland	4.8	68,400	Cl	326
Spain	3.7	4,600	Cl	332
Africa				
Central Africa				
Zambia	1.0	12,610	Cl	325
East Africa				
Ethiopia	1.3	6,580	Cl	340
Kenya	2.6	NG	Cl	294
Rwanda	0.7	1,958	Cl	390
	1.1	861	FS	390
Tanzania	3.5	230	Cl	260
	3.3	990	Cl	260
Uganda	2.8	3,371	Cl	245
West Africa				
Angola	0.3	1,459	Cl	309
Mali	0	20,000	Cl	338
Nigeria	0.5	1,156	Cl	343
	0.08	9,806	Cl	197
Senegal	0.6	45,000	Cl	363
North Africa				
Egypt	3.0	NG	Cl	110
South Africa				
Bantu	1.5	NG	Cl	346
White (Transvaal)	4.0	16,676	Cl	148
Asia				
Near East				
E. Pakistan	0.5	150,000	Cl	214
E. India (Goa)	0.7	NG	Cl	348
W. India (Calcutta)	0.5–1.5	NG	Cl	20
Malaysia				
Kuala Lumpur	1.1	5,375	Cl	2
Perak	5.5	14,544	Cl	249
No. India	0.8	20,000	Cl	31
Middle East				
Kuwait	3.1	12,225	Cl	347
Far East				
Hong Kong	1.5	52,307	Cl	425
Japan	0.29–1.18	NG	9 Series	424
	0.99–1.03	NG	4 Series	13
Australia				
Aborigines	0	NG	NG	167
White	2.6	25,296	PP	367

Cl: hospital/clinic; FS: field survey; GP: general population; NG: not given; PC: personal communication; PP: private practice.

Larsson and Liden (229) also found that psoriasis was less common in a study of 8298 schoolchildren between 12 and 16 years; 0.5% had the disease. (See also Age Onset and Pattern Distribution of Lesions and Extent of Involvement.)

Geriatric Psoriasis

Johnson (201) has alerted dermatologists to the enormity of the increase in the number of elderly who will need skin care in the future and poses the observation that this urgent problem is not being fully addressed at present (98,201,258,299).

Changes observed in the aging process both in chronological aging and in photoaging have been studied intensively in recent years. Due to many interrelated genetic, physiological, and environmental factors, people are living longer and yet no satisfactory theory to explain the longer life span has been developed (286–289).

In 1990 persons 65 years and older numbered 31.2 million, representing 12.6% of the U.S. population. This age category has increased by 22% since 1980 compared to the increase of 8% for the under-65-year-olds (286). Psoriasis can occur at any age. In their questionnaire survey of 5600 psoriasis patients, Farber and Nall (124) found the mean age onset was 27.8 ± 0.38 years. Of more than 5550 people, 273 (5%) were between the ages of 60 and 90 years (289). Hellgren (183) published a higher percentage for psoriasis in the decades 60–90; at the time of study, 105 (21%) of 502 psoriasis patients had mild to moderately severe psoriasis in their later years.

In a population-based study (32) of 132 newly diagnosed cases of psoriasis, 13% were in the age class 60–69. Swanbeck et al. (374) found a prevalence of 5% elderly in a population study of over 5000 families with psoriasis. Yap and co-workers (422) found 6.4% elderly in a study of 40,000 individuals in a Singapore skin clinic; psoriasis occurred less commonly than in the general population, whereas in another Singapore clinic study, Chua-Ty and associates (79) found 14.7% out of 2476 psoriasis patients (>60) were observed in a population of 74,589 persons. In fact, psoriasis was the most common dermatosis among the elderly (>60 years).

SEX RATIO

The occurrence of psoriasis in males and females has been nearly equal in most studies (Table 2). However, in the Scandinavian population study performed by Hellgren (183), it was found in a sample of 39,571 that 758 people were affected with psoriasis. Of these, 62% were male (473) and 38% (285) female.

In the Henan Survey (107) of the People's Republic of China, of 105,545 individuals examined, 387 had psoriasis: 57% were male, 43% female. Li (234), in analyzing the sex ratio in other Chinese series, reported nearly equal distribution between the sexes in Anhwei, but a definitely higher rate in males in a Shanghai series.

Lomholt (243), examining 10,984 inhabitants of the Faroe Islands, found that 2.8% were affected with psoriasis: 51% males, 49% females. In a mailed questionnaire survey conducted by Farber and Nall (124), among 5600 psoriasis patients, 46% were male, 54% female. The investigators did not attach any significance to the higher percentage of females to males in the sample.

AGE ONSET

General Comments

Steinberg et al. (358,359) contended that age of onset is that reported by the patient and is subject to many inaccuracies. In some cases, this is the age at which the patient recalls the presence of the first eruption. An additional source of inaccuracy is introduced by the human characteristic of vagueness about dates. While it is possible to compare the clinical results of one study with another, it is impossible to provide an accurate distribution of age onset.

Swanbeck et al. (374) underscored the problems inherent in age onset indicating, as have others, that psoriasis may go undiagnosed in the scalp, for example, until skin lesions develop in other body areas. Hence, the reported age onset may be later than the true age onset. These investigators define age onset of psoriasis as "the age at which an individual, or relative, becomes aware that that individual has the disease."

Analyzing age onset can be correct only if all the patients are seen immediately or shortly after the first eruption. If the patients are seen at a varying number of years after the onset, it must be expected that a smaller proportion of patients who acquire the disease at a more advanced age will have survived. Naldi (282) points out that only in rare situations, such as in guttate psoriasis, do onset and diagnosis virtually overlap. Beylot (36) concurs with this observation and states that in 15% of her cases, psoriasis begins before

Table 2 Sex Ratio in Selected Series of Psoriasis Patients

Reference	Year	Locale	Psoriasis patients		
			Total	% Male	% Female
190	1931	Germany	1,437	58	42
359	1951	USA	464	54	46
243	1963	Faroe Is.	312	51	49
183	1967	Sweden	758	62	38
19	1969	Russia	452	56	44
21	1971	Poland	750	51	49
424[a]	1971	Japan	2,645	64	36
335	1971	Germany	963	47	53
53	1972	Germany	536	48	52
124	1974	USA	5,600	46	54
31	1977	No. India	162	72	28
175	1978	Sri Lanka	1,366	53	47
327	1978	England	69	75	25
2	1980	Malaysia	203	67	33
319	1982	Ireland	406	37	63
12	1982	Germany	2,994	56	44
234	1982	PR China			
		Henan	387	57	43
		Anhui	280	51	49
		Shanghai			
		City	307	73	27
		Rural	23	70	30
218	1985	Sweden	1,050	45	55
281	1987	Japan	4,622	65	35
297	1990	India	112	51	49
79	1992	Singapore	2,476	62	38
95	1993	Yugoslavia	808	61	39
374	1994	Sweden	5,197	45	55

[a]Pooled data.

the age of 10 years, usually in the form of guttate psoriasis occurring soon after an upper respiratory infection.

The average age of onset is usually in the 20s, ranging from birth to the 8th or 9th decade (Figs. 7 and 8); an age onset of 108 years was reported for a black woman in the southern part of the United States (55). In their study on the natural history of psoriasis in 5600 patients, Farber and Nall (124) reported that 35% of the sample had an onset of psoriasis before the age of 20 years (10% before 10 years, 58% before the age of 30) (Fig. 9). In a review of the literature on the subject, they found that in the majority of studies, there is evidence of a greater percentage of females having an onset before the age of 30 than males (Table 3).

Using a questionnaire, Melski and Stern (267) determined that among first-degree relatives of 1209 patients with severe psoriasis, patients with onset before the age of 15 were more than three times as likely to have psoriasis as siblings of patients with onset after the age of 30.

Age onset of psoriasis varies in different geographic areas (Table 4) (148,253,274,349,428). Lomholt (243) indicated that in exploring the influence of environmental factors, the age onset of psoriasis is perhaps the most important piece of epidemiological information obtained. According to his study on the Faroe Islands, where the climatic conditions are cold and damp, the age of onset of the disease is one of the earliest reported by investigators. Of the 312 inhabitants with psoriasis, men were 33 years old, women 29 (ranging from 11 months to 90 years) at the time of examination, but the median age onset was 13 years for males, 12 years for females.

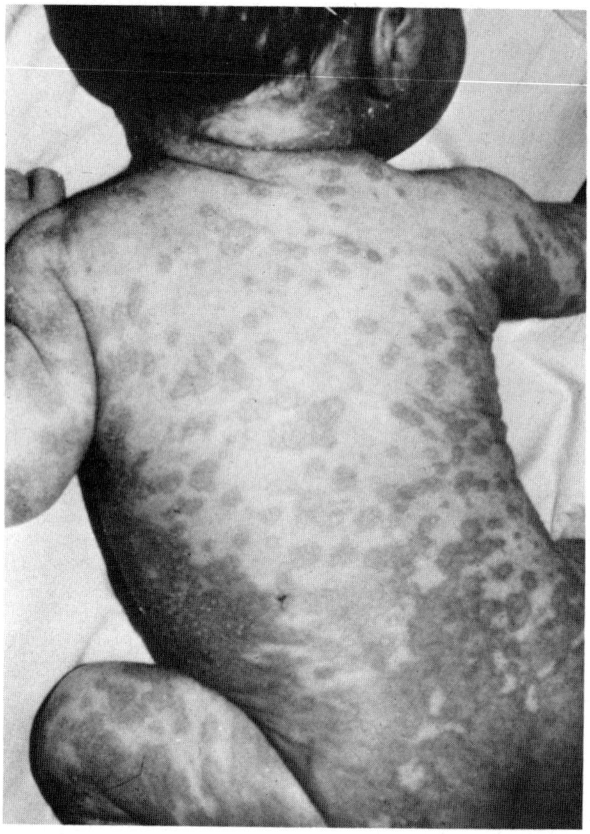

Figure 6 Infant who developed psoriasis within 3 weeks of birth.

Bimodality

In many studies, an observed frequency distribution departs from normality. One such case is skewedness, which is another term for asymmetry. Frequency distribution curves are skewed to the right or left depending on whether the right or left tails are drawn out. The age-onset graph documenting 5544 psoriasis patients (Fig. 9) in the Farber and Nall (124) study reflects an asymmetrical curve (skewed to the right) and does not agree with the bimodality curves reported by several investigators (55,108,175,195,319, 335,352), who claim two peaks in age-onset distribution in their data (Table 5).

In an analysis of the frequency distribution of age-onset in 1356 patients in a study by Ingram (195), Burch and Rowell (56,57) found evidence of bimodality in the females and males: a considerable peak during puberty and another minor peak at the climacteric. From their analysis, the investigators concluded that two genotypes predispose to psoriasis in female and at least two in males. They postulated the existence of distinct but related genetic subpopulations for both sexes, with their so-called genotype I having an "early onset" and genotype II having "late onset."

Gunawardena and his co-workers (175) observed that the frequency distribution curve for age onset was bimodal with peaks at the 2nd and 5th decade (Fig. 10). His group reported that bimodality of age onset is discernible in some of the frequency distributions presented by Hellgren (183) and Holgate (192), but noted that Farber and Nall (124) did not describe a late-onset peak in their series. Gunawardena et al. (175) stated that a late-onset peak may be overlooked because of a systematic error that nearly always arises in analyzing the age of onset (244). Ross (335), analyzing his own material and that of Lomholt (243), also supports the idea of bimodality in age onset.

Christophers and Henseler (77,185) conducted a retrospective study on a database of 2147 psoriasis patients seen in Kiel to determine age onset as well

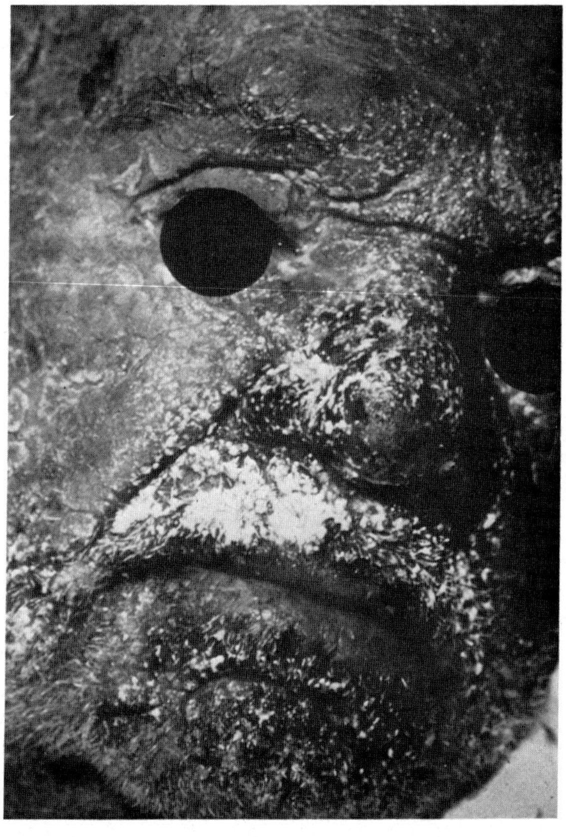

Figure 7 Psoriasis can appear in the last decades of life.

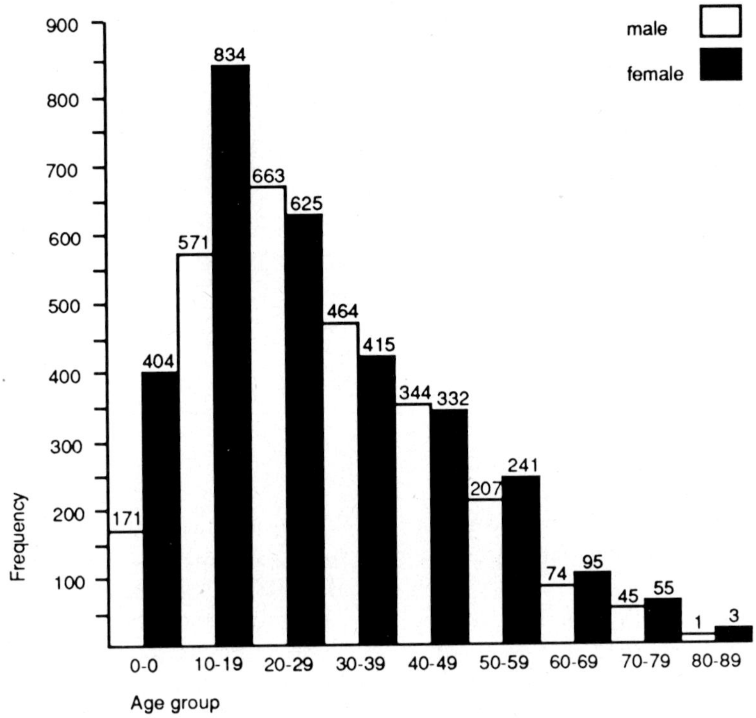

Figure 8 Age at onset of disease in 5544 psoriatic patients (124).

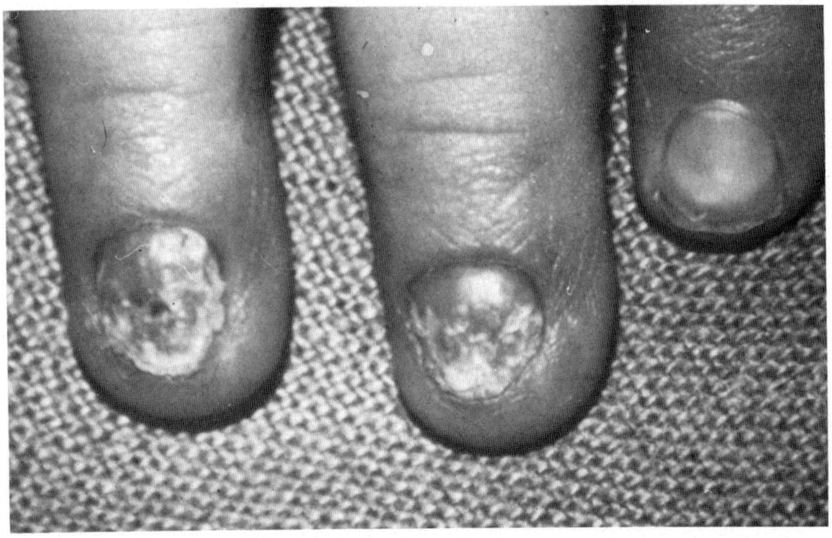

Figure 9 Nail dystrophy in a 10-month-old infant who exhibited nail pitting at birth.

Table 3 Prevalence of Onset of Psoriasis Before the Age of 30 Years in Selected Series of Patients

			Sex of patients			
Reference	Year	Locale	Male number	%	Female number	%
243	1963	Faroe Is.	103	93	143	90
329	1968	France	807	50	671	62
183	1967	Sweden	473	29	285	26
424	1971	Japan	191	50	117	48
272	1973	Sweden	127	51	173	84
124	1974	USA	2,513	56	2,991	62
31	1977	No. India	99	61	120	74
297	1990	India	57	51	55	49
79	1992	Singapore	1,537	62	939	38

as other parameters for support of their hypothesis that psoriasis vulgaris is a disease of two entities: early and late onset.

Other investigators concur with this hypothesis: Smith and co-workers (352) recorded age-onset distribution between 211 males and 245 females and found the distributional curve to be bimodal. The separation in the bimodal curve was at age 40, thus supporting the thesis that there are two genotypes for psoriasis: an early onset and late onset. Economidou et al. (108) also confirm biomodality in their study of 212 Greek psoriatic patients.

To compare a U.S. population with that of Kiel, Nall and Marder (293) selected a group of 3562 patients stemming from a nonpublished Stanford University Life Histories Survey for analysis of age onset

Table 4 Distribution of Age Onset in Selected Series of Psoriasis Patients

				Mean or modal	
Reference	No. of patients	Source	Locale	Male	Female
194	1,346	PP	England	16–20	11–15
359	464	Cl	USA	32	28
357	902	PP	Germany	16–30	16–30
243	312	GP	Faroe Is.	13[a]	12[a]
183	758	GP	Sweden	20–30	15–29
423	313	Cl	Japan	20–29	20–29
424	338	Cl	Japan	35	29
281	4,622	Cl	Japan	39	35
272	300	Cl	Sweden	23	18
124	5,600	Qu	USA	29	27
302	245	Cl/children	Denmark	9	8
31	162	Cl	No. India	28	22
175	1,366	Cl	Sri Lanka	30	20
2	203	Cl	Malaysia	21–30	21–30
267	1,209	Qu	USA	15–29	15–29
242	387	GP	PRChina	26	27
429	4,133,156	GP	PRChina	20–25	25–30
127	100	Qu	Denmark	23	
	88	PI	Hong Kong	36	
	120	PI	Kuwait	23	

[a]Median.
Cl: clinic; GP: general population; PI: physician interview; PP: private practice; Qu: questionnaire.

Table 5 Bimodality in Age Onset in Selected Series of Psoriasis Patients

			First peak (years)		Second peak (years)	
Reference	Year	No.	M	F	M	F
195	1954	1,346	16–20	11–15	NG	41–45
243	1963	312	NG	16	NG	51
335	1971	963	28	16	55	55
175	1978	1,366	18		40	
319	1982	406	15–20		>55	
185	1985	2,147	22	16	57	60
352	1993	456	>40		>40	

NG: not given.

and certain clinical course variables. Controlling the size of the population at large by weighting yielded a generalized distribution of age onset (mean = 36 years). The curve reflecting their data showed a distribution of three peaks for the total sample, with the highest peak at 22 years, next at 44 years, and a third at 53 years. Neither the shape of the age-onset distribution nor the clinical course of the patients in their study indicated that psoriasis is a two-entity disease with early and late onset, but showed that age onset can begin in infancy or at any point in the life span of an individual.

Naldi (282) reviewed the Christophers/Henseler thesis that patients with an age onset before age 40 (type I psoriasis) are more likely than patients with age onset after age 40 (type II psoriasis) to have affected first-degree relatives, and to experience severe and recurrent disease. He stated that this is an interesting concept, but that aside from study design issues, such as case definition and selection (e.g., the selection of juvenile cases may be conditioned by their family history more frequently than cases in the older age groups), a fundamental problem in their analyses arises from the fact that the numerical distribution by age of psoriasis patients is a function of the age-specific disease rate and the age distribution of the population. He commented that variations in numerator data (the number of people experiencing onset at different ages) may reflect the age distribution of the population sample. In his opinion, age-specific rates of appearance of psoriasis calculated on representative samples of the general population would be more convincing.

Swanbeck et al. (374) state that the existence of two types of psoriasis vulgaris has been proposed mainly on the basis of a peak in the age-at-onset curve at about 50 years of age. They point out that this peak can be seen only in women and coincides with menopause.

In a study by Svejgaard and his colleagues (371,372), an interesting set of findings were revealed that may provide an explanation for the bimodality in onset reported by the above-mentioned investigators. Figure 11 shows three age-onset curves for three groups of patients that had been studied not specifically for age onset. Curve (a) represents the frequency distribution of 31 patients with pustular psoriasis; curve (b) represents 79 patients with psoriasis vulgaris who were negative for the HLA B13 and B17; and curve (c) represents 77 patients with psoriasis vulgaris who were positive for these antigens. The authors point out that the frequency of the HLA B13 and/or B17 was significantly higher (59%) in patients with onset before 35 years than in those with late onset (23%). The increased frequency in the early-age-onset group was found in both antigens and in both sexes. The average age-onset for HLA B13 and/or B17 patients was 22.3 years, whereas it was 28 years for the remaining patients with psoriasis vulgaris. Furthermore, the HLA B13 and B17 group had only one mode (at about 15 years), whereas there were two modes (at 15 and 55 years) for the negative HLA B13 and/or B17 group. For the pustular psoriasis, the curve was also multimodal, with peaks at 25 and 55 years. Although the authors give no explanation for the various modes found in their curves, one might speculate that the bimodality found in the various series by Ingram and others may reflect the presence or absence of certain HLA specificities.

Sex Ratio

In 1975, Holgate (192) studied 419 patients (42% male, 58% female). The ages of onset were earlier in

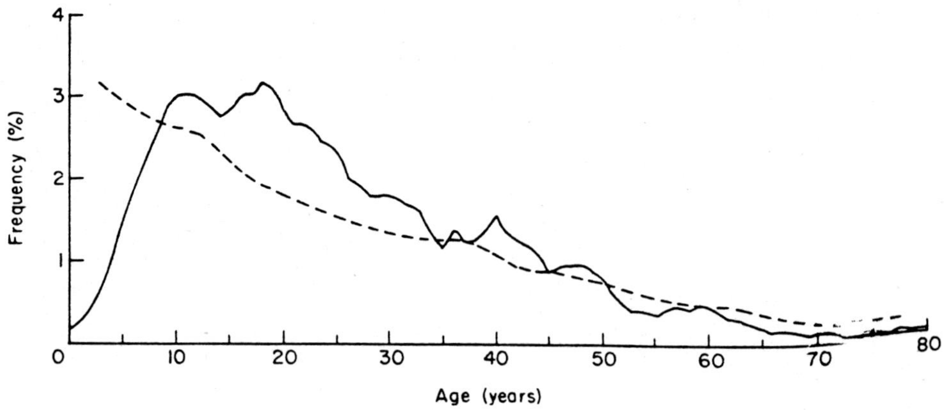

Figure 10 Gunawardena and associates (175) have reported a frequency distribution for age onset that is bimodal with peaks at the 2nd and 5th decades (straight line, psoriasis onset; perforated line, general population). (From Ref. 175.)

females than in males: between 5 and 9 years and between 15 and 19 years, respectively.

Gunawardena and associates (175) speculated that females with a family history of psoriasis and a low age onset form a natural subpopulation. Since Woodrow et al. (418) found that HLA B17 was more common in female patients and its presence was associated with early onset, Gunawardena's group concluded that there appears to be a genetic basis for the subpopulation of females with an early age of onset that may correspond to the female genotype I postulated by Burch and Rowell (56). Also, early onset and B17 were demonstrated by White et al. (410).They reported that although the male/female ratio as determined in their series of 155 psoriasis patients was relatively similar (73:82), there was a female preponderance in patients with the HLA B12, B13, and B17.

In a recent population study of 1264 psoriasis patients from the region of Karlovac, Yugoslavia, females had earlier age onset than males (94).

Family History

Age onset and family history for psoriasis are variable. In correlating age onset of psoriasis in 1942 patients with familial occurrence of the disease, Farber and Nall (124) found the highest number (33%) of probands with a family history had age onset between 10 and 19 years. One-quarter of the sample was found in the interval of 20–29 years. In all, 73% of the pso-

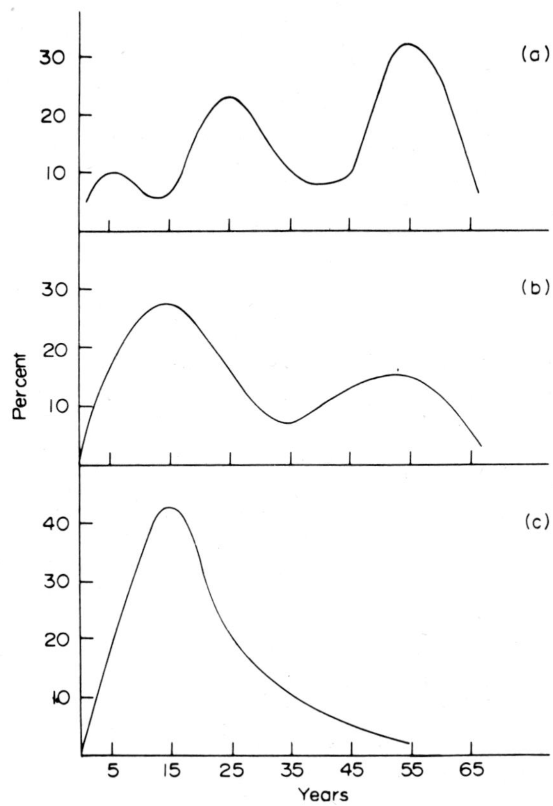

Figure 11 Svejaard and co-workers (372) found three separate curves for three HLA series: (a) 31 pustular psoriasis patients; (b) 70 psoriasis vulgaris patients negative for HLA B13 and B17, and (c) 77 psoriasis vulgaris positive for these two specificities. (From Ref. 372.)

riasis patients, indicating familial aggregation of the disease, had an age onset before 30 years.

Melski and Stern (267) found that nearly 50% of siblings of patients in their study, who had had a positive parental history of psoriasis with onset of the disease before age 15, had psoriasis by age 60 as compared with a 3% occurrence among patients' siblings in families without a positive history of psoriasis and whose disease began after age 20.

Lomholt (243) did not observe early onset in the psoriasis patients when one parent was affected, nor was there a relationship between the age of manifestation in the parent and his or her children.

In a Yugoslavian population sample of 808 psoriasis patients, del Toso-Depeder (95) found that patients with a family history of psoriasis had a 10-year earlier onset of the disease, particularly in females. By 25 years of age, 58% of the patients with positive familial psoriasis were affected; while 35% without a family history developed psoriasis.

In a study of 112 children in a province of India, 9.8% reported familial history (297); however, in an investigation of 190 children in Kuwait, 28% of the patients had a positive family history. The latter also manifested an earlier onset than those with negative history and were also more severely affected by the disorder (5). The Yugoslavian survey of 808 psoriasis patients indicated a family history in 33.3% of the cases.

Course

Late onset (after age 25) in the Faroe Island series seemed to indicate a milder future course than an early onset. An onset before the age of 10 more often resulted in a more severe course (243).

As indicated earlier, Christophers and Henseler (77,185) reported that patients with onset before age 40 (their type I early psoriasis) experienced a more severe form of the disease and had more recurrent episodes than patients with type II, late onset of psoriasis (after age 40).

Clinical Type

No evidence has been found that there is a positive correlation between age onset and clinical type. Neither Holgate (192) nor Gunawardena and his group (175) were able to establish a significant association between age onset and clinical pattern of the disease.

Severity

In examining the medical charts of 100 patients with mild psoriasis and comparing the course of their disease with 100 patients with severe psoriasis, Farber and his co-workers (123) reported that patients with a severe form had an onset of the disease earlier in life than did patients with mild disease. The latter patients appeared to have had their disease for a shorter time period.

As stated, Lomholt (243) reported that from his analysis a late onset (after the age of 25) tended to a milder course of the disease than an early onset. A considerably higher percentage of patients who had psoriasis from the age of 10 had a more severe course.

Molin (272) found a significantly more severe course of the disease with increasing age among the male patients, whereas no such finding was observed among the female patients (Table 6).

In addition to the findings by Krulig and his associates (225) in the United States, a strong association between HLA B17 and psoriasis with skin involvement of more than 50% was observed by Turowski and her colleagues (388) in Poland. However, White et al. (410) found that no particular HLA specificity was associated with a more severe form of psoriasis, but that varying degrees of severity appeared to distribute evenly among all HLA groups.

Melski and Stern (267) found no association of age onset with severity.

HLA Frequency Distribution

Age onset is apparently earlier for patients positive for HLA B13 and B17 (225,341,355,370). Patients with onset between 10 and 20 years were found by Brenner et al. (54) to show significantly higher prevalence of HLA Cw6 than patients with an onset between 35 and 45 years, as has been reported by Chris-

Table 6 Relationship of Degree of Disease Severity to Increasing Age in Psoriasis Patients

Degree of severity	Male (n = 127) (%)	Female (n = 173) (%)
Milder	24	43
Worsened	32	18
Unchanged	40	32

Source: Ref. 272.

tophers and Henseler (77,185). Such findings have been corroborated in Histocompatibility Testing Workshop reports by Hawkins et al. (182). They also observed that the HLA DR7 is increased to a higher degree in psoriasis patients. This was the case with both North American and European whites as well as Japanese patients, but in neither population was the increased frequency in HLA DR7 as large as that for HLA Cw6.

The relative risk of onset of the first symptoms of psoriasis before the age of 10 in individuals with HLA B13 and B17 was 9.63 in the work done by Turowski et al. (388). They found the reverse relationship expressed by the decrease of these specificities when the age onset was after 20 years.

Economidou et al. (108) studied the frequencies of HLA A, B, and C in a group of 212 Greek psoriasis patients and 202 control subjects. An increased frequency of B13, B16, and Cw6 antigens and a low frequency of B14 was noted in all patients. Early onset (less than 25 years of age) was associated with a high frequency of A1, B17, B37, and Cw6 antigens, whereas patients with late onset (greater than 25 years) had a significantly lower occurrence of A1, B17, and Cw6, which did not differ from that of the control subjects. In patients with familial history, no significant association with any particular HLA antigen was seen.

PATTERN DISTRIBUTION OF LESIONS AND EXTENT OF INVOLVEMENT

Biometry: Assessment of Area Involvement and Outcome

The ability to assess the severity of dermatoses and outcome in health care is important in both clinical practice and research (151,382,420). Recently, Marks and Burton (259) summarized clinical assessment techniques in 30 published studies and criticized a lack of uniformity as well as other parameters required in area measurement. They emphasized that although area measurement is probably the single most important clinical parameter of disease severity, other clinical signs may also be quantified to assist with the evaluation of psoriasis.

Nall (288) has traced the development of biometric techniques from the 1400s to the present. Patterns of distribution of psoriatic lesions were included in the early versions of the Stanford and/or Psoriasis Research Institute Life Histories Questionnaire and are still being analyzed to the present time (122,124). Anterior and posterior views of an outline figure provide the patient with the opportunity to shade in areas, of involvement. Below the figure is a listing of 18 potential areas that correspond to the involved regions in the outline figures and are coded along with the other variables in the questionnaire.

The outline configuration is called the Surface Area Model (SAM) and not only is sketched for "time of study" when the patient fills out the questionnaire, but also appears in subsequent pages as "when psoriasis was at its worst" and "at age of onset." These three sets of figures provide a rough interpretation of the course of the disease over time (124).

Since 1951, dermatologists have used Wallace's "Rule of Nines" (400) to estimate lesional involvement. Widely used since its conception, the Psoriasis Area and Severity Index (PASI) measures more precisely areas of involvement as well as assessing degree of severity. Recently a structured PASI-like form (patient PASI) (152) was developed for self-measurement of severity as a quick estimate of lesional involvement and suggested consideration for future large-scale epidemiological studies. The ultimate in assessing extent and severity of lesions is a three-dimensional approach, whereby a stereophotogram provides not only length and width of the lesion, but its depth as well (187,420).

Outcome measures refer to all the possible results that stem from exposure to causal factors. Fries et al. (158) claim that outcome in health care evaluation can be recognized as consisting of several dimensions, which can be viewed in measurable components: disability, discomfort, cost, and death. Finlay and Kelly (149) comment that in clinical research on psoriasis, more attention has been given to the dermatologists' views on treatment effects than to those of the patients. Only recently have psychological and social factors relevant to outcome been appraised (Sickness Impact Profile and Psoriasis Disability Index) (149,150).

Marks and Burton (259) suggest that since virtually every other specialty in medicine has recognized the usefulness of quantification of clinical signs, it is their belief that this would assist dermatological practice as well, and that conflicting results of clinical trials in psoriasis points out the need for objective clinical measurements.

Sites of Involvement

Pattern distribution of lesions and extent of involvement have been reviewed recently by Farber and Nall:

scalp (131), ear (119), face (120), genitalia (133), nails (132), and perianal and intergluteal regions (134). They also reviewed certain clinical variants: nonpustular palmoplantar (135), pustular (136,204), erythrodermic (137), and guttate (138).

The highest frequencies of lesions are found in the scalp and elbow, trunk, and lower extremities (53,124,183,243,423). The frequency of distribution of clinical types of psoriasis varies from series to series. Powell and his group (319) found the following morphological types in 401 patients: plaque ($n = 78$), guttate ($n = 71$), nummular ($n = 45$), annular ($n = 4$), palmar planter pustulosis ($n = 7$), and generalized pustular psoriasis ($n = 1$). Nyfors and Lemholt (302) observed, as have others (5,15,36,131,138,297), that in children guttate psoriasis follows upper respiratory infections.

In a study of childhood psoriasis in 190 Kuwaiti children (5), plaque psoriasis was the most common type found (84%), followed by guttate psoriasis (22%). Areas of involvement included extensor surfaces (63%), scalp (53%), nails (36%), and the mucosa (7%).

Another pediatric group was investigated in an Asian Indian population of 112 patients (297). Plaque psoriasis was observed in 69.6% followed by guttate (25.9%) with scalp involvement (58%) and face (46%).

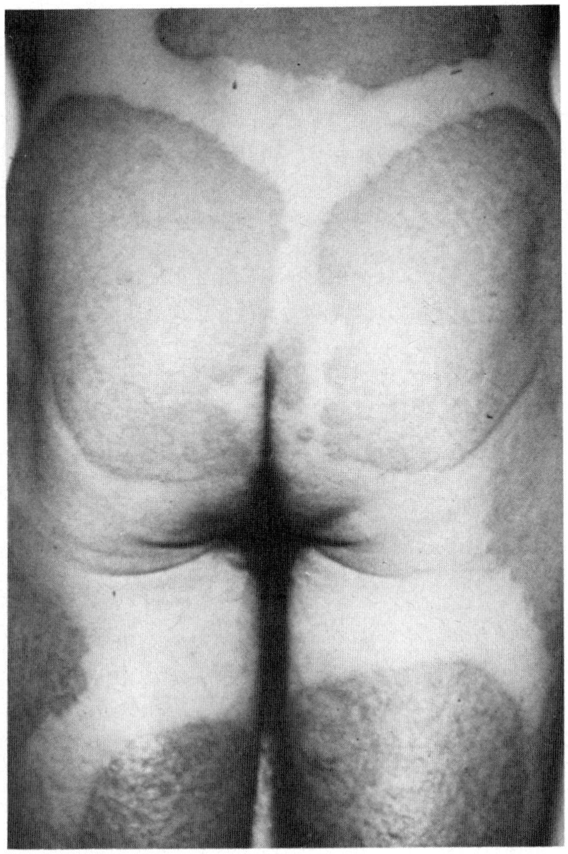

Figure 12 Symmetry in the distribution pattern of psoriasis is a characteristic factor.

Distribution Pattern of Lesions

Farber and Nall (124) have shown that psoriasis becomes more widespread over time, indicating that it is a progressive disease. They have noted that asymmetrical patterns of plaque psoriasis appear at onset and become symmetrical during the latter course of the disease (Fig. 12).

In examining 61 twin pairs for patterns of distribution of lesions, Farber and co-workers (125) observed that eight of 29 concordant monozygotic pairs had similar patterns at the onset of psoriasis, but the course of the disease varied in five of these pairs. Three pairs of the monozygotic twins had striking similarities in the pattern at onset and in the course of severity of their disorder. In these three pairs the onset occurred at the ages 4 and 4 years, 8 and 6 years, and 10 and 10 years, respectively. The striking behavior of their psoriasis might be explained on the basis of identical genetic endowment and nearly identical environmental conditions. None of the concordant dizygotic twin pairs had a similar course or degree of severity of psoriasis.

Pattern Determination

Goudie and his co-investigators (164–166) explored the possibility that vascular clones determine developmental patterns of cutaneous lesions. Their work has been with vitiligo, but the potential of their concept in defining genetic factors that influence distribution of lesions can be of significance for psoriasis research as well.

They proposed that the human skin contains a series of discrete clones of cells that occupy predetermined anatomical sites in the vascular system. These clones are thought to provide topographic information that determines that the behavior of neighboring cells is appropriate to the position they occupy in the body, for example, the varying activity of melanocytes in different regions of the skin. For this mechanism to be effective there must be systematic activation of a large set of genes whose products ensure that the vascular clones are always arranged in the same order.

Farber and Nall (145) suggest that a concept of genetic control of positioning information in patterning of lesions should not be restricted to the vascular system, but may also involve the neural system, which is being studied intensely under the rubric of psychoneuroimmunology.

DURATION

The duration of psoriasis varies with the investigation being reported (124). Farber and Nall (127) determined from a cooperative international study the following mean values for duration of psoriasis in years: Denmark, 19; United States, 17; Sri Lanka, 8; Kuwait and Hong Kong, 7.

In conducting a study in which two populations of psoriasis patients were being investigated, Nall (286,290) found that for 557 outpatients attending a Psoriasis Day Care Center the mean age at the time of the study was 47.1 years and the mean length of duration of psoriasis was 15.2 years. In the comparison group of 1114 inpatients, the mean age at time of study was 49.1 years with a mean length of duration of psoriasis of 16.5 years.

REMISSION

Remissions may occur in the course of psoriasis in varying frequencies (282). In the Stanford epidemiological study, 39% of patients stated they had experienced a remission ranging from 1 to 54 years; 29% said that their psoriasis disappeared without treatment by a physician. What causes this spontaneous remission in the course of the disease is unknown (124,282). Later these investigators examined remission rates in a comparative study of five different geographic areas (290). They determined the percentage of psoriasis patients reporting remissions and the mean length (in months) of the remissions: Denmark (55%, 35), United States (41%, 46), Hong Kong (36%, 9), Kuwait (42%, 18), and Sri Lanka (46%, 22).

Lomholt (243) stated that in his studies from the Faroe Islands 48% of patients reported periods without symptoms and 48% experienced periodic major eruptions. The corresponding values for patients with psoriasis of more than 5 years' duration are 44.9% and 42%, respectively. Yasada et al. (423,424) reported that in 197 patients, 55% indicated a remission at some time in the course of their disease. Kononen et al. (218) reported from surveying cross-sectional studies that the percentage of remissions may vary from 17% to 55%.

PREVENTION AND CONTROL

Farber and Nall (131) proposed that prevention in a broad sense refers to limiting the progress of disease at any stage of its course; control refers to reduction in frequency and/or severity of a disease in a population. Measures to prevent and control psoriasis require the education of the patient regarding environmental and genetic components that affect onset and course of the disease (129).

As soon as children can comprehend, they should be taught to take control of their life and avoid injury (e.g., contact sports), drugs, low humidity, and emotional stress. All age groups should avoid even minimal trauma. Where a disease such as psoriasis is well established, as stated earlier, a decrease in morbidity can be described as *disability prevention* (80,129).

There has been an increasing public awareness of health care issues, such as wellness programs, self-help and self-care, and the importance of taking personal responsibility for one's health (99,266,406).

TRIGGERING FACTORS

The first appearance of psoriasis often is associated with external injury (burn, cut, or scratch). The induction of lesions by such injury is known as the Koebner phenomenon, or isomorphic response. Internal factors may also precipitate or exacerbate the disease, e.g., low humidity, antecedent infection, emotional stress, or systematically administered drugs, such as lithium. A rebound flare of psoriasis may follow discontinuation of systemic corticosteroids or intensive topical corticosteroids for psoriasis (129,145, 423,424).

The triggers associated with the onset or subsequent worsening of psoriasis are the following:

Direct Injury

Traumatizing the skin by repeated picking or scratching, and injuries from cuts, burns, and bruises may be responsible for creating new lesions at the exact site of injury.

Climate

In general, patients report that cold weather has an adverse effect on their psoriasis, whereas hot weather and sunlight are beneficial. Lomholt (243) in his census study on the Faroe Islands, where the cold, foggy climate permits little chance for sunbathing, reported that in 46 psoriasis patients who went abroad and were exposed to sunlight, 80% showed improvement. Prolonged periods of low humidity have been shown to be injurious to the skin (144). Yasada et al. (424), in a study in Japan, noted that the prevalence of psoriasis is high in the cold, northeastern part of the country and low in the warmer, humid, southern regions.

In the Stanford series of 5600 psoriasis patients, Farber and Nall (124) found that 80% of the patients reported their psoriasis improved during the hot weather and when exposed to sunlight; 89% indicated that their condition worsened during cold weather. In a subsequent survey of 704 psoriasis patients, these investigators observed that more than half of the respondents said that swimming and sunbathing were beneficial; 18% stated that sea water plus sun was more effective than fresh water and sun (9%). Neither fresh nor sea water alone had any positive effect (128).

The investigators in the Henan Dermatoses Survey (184) found that onset of psoriasis as well as flare-ups occurred in the winter months.

Infections

Many bacterial, viral, or fungal infections are deleterious in psoriasis. Recently, Farber and Nall reviewed the literature on guttate psoriasis (138). They reported that investigators indicate that the most common factor provoking the onset or worsening of psoriasis is streptococcal infection associated with upper respiratory infections as well as the recently published association between guttate psoriasis and perianal streptococcal disease (15,124,126,138,302,376,415,416).

The pathogenesis of a guttate eruption is not clearly understood although it has been studied widely. One such study by Telfer et al. (376) explored 111 patients with a sudden onset or worsening of psoriasis for evidence of streptococcal infection. Of these patients, 34 had acute guttate psoriasis, 30 had a guttate flare of chronic psoriasis, 37 had chronic plaque psoriasis, and 59 had other types of psoriasis. *Streptococcus pyrogenes* was isolated from 19 (17%) of the 111 patients. Other beta-hemolytic streptococci were found with equal frequency in the study and matched control populations. The authors reported that these serotypes were similar in distribution and prevalence to those present in the local community, and that their study confirms the strong association between prior infection with *S. pyogenes* and guttate psoriasis, but suggest that the ability to trigger guttate psoriasis is not serotype specific.

Drugs

A number of medications, including antimalarials, beta-blockers, and lithium, have been implicated in provoking psoriasis (98,145). As mentioned earlier, the withdrawal of systemic corticosteroids as a treatment modality induced a flare of psoriasis. Stern (362) recommends that since the severity of psoriasis may vary spontaneously, claims that a given drug exacerbates psoriasis should be tested with appropriate protocols. Farber and Nall (145) also suggest that dermatologists prompt their patients to reveal drugs that have been prescribed for other medical purposes to avoid problems with treatment of the psoriasis.

Smoking

The potential risk factor of smoking as a trigger in causing psoriasis is debatable. Naldi et al. (283) conducted a multicenter case-control study. Interviews were performed by trained medical investigators using a structured questionnaire. A total of 215 patients, aged 16–65 years (median age 38), and 267 controls, aged 15–65 years (median age 36), were interviewed and it was found that the risk of psoriasis was higher for current smokers (15 cigarettes per day) than for those who had never smoked. In another case-control study by Mills et al. (270) the smoking habits of 108 patients with psoriasis and matched controls were investigated. The exploration revealed that the relative risk of psoriasis in those currently smoking more than 20 cigarettes per day was significantly elevated. In a large Norwegian population of 10,576 individuals, 48% indicated that they smoked cigarettes daily, while 36% were nonsmokers. Among the 149 psoriatic patients in that large sample, 58.2% reported smoking daily or occasionally as compared with 43.5% of nonpsoriatics.

Williams (415) suggests that intervention studies are needed to examine the effect of smoking on chronicity of psoriasis and response to treatment.

Alcoholism

Many countries are suffering from an epidemic of alcoholism (289). There is ample literature depicting a direct relationship between alcoholism and various social problems and a wealth of information on diagnostic techniques for screening, treatment, and evaluation of patient outcome (143,176,241,286,300,350). Genetic studies suggest a possible link between the DCD2 dopamine gene and severe alcoholism (143), but demonstrating a direct correlation between alcoholism and psoriasis is still controversial.

Only a few studies on the subject of cutaneous diseases and alcoholic intake have been reported over the past few decades (25). Some have shown a positive relationship between the manifestation of psoriasis and alcohol abuse (143,176,188,273,283), while others reject such an association (143).

In the Stanford Department of Dermatology, Nall (286,289) conducted a preliminary study on the level of alcohol consumption in 557 outpatients in the Psoriasis Day Care Center (PDCC) and 1114 inpatients (ward patients), using the Stanford University Medical Center hospital discharge summaries as a data source. A nomogram developed by Mellor furnished a uniform method for quantifying alcoholic consumption in the two groups of patients (143,241). The two populations were similar for mean age at onset: PDCC patients 32.0 years, ward patients 32.7. Whereas the age at time of study varied by 2 years—PDCC patients 47.1 years (mean length of duration of psoriasis, 15.2 years), ward patients 49.1 years (mean duration of psoriasis, 16.5 years)—the familial occurrence of psoriasis was similar for both groups, 41.7% and 41.8%, respectively.

The outstanding difference was the finding that the mean alcohol consumption (in g/day) was 41.2 for the PDCC patients and 76.1 for the inpatients; both groups reflect higher consumption rates than the national average of 27 g/day. No conclusions can be drawn to account for the increased consumption of alcohol by the PDCC and inpatients as compared with the national average other than to speculate that severe psoriasis may invoke patients to increase their ethanol consumption.

Monk and Neill (273) studied the relationship between the severity of psoriasis and alcohol consumption in 100 patients with chronic plaque psoriasis. Male patients, who were heavy drinkers, were found significantly more common in the group with severe psoriasis, and alcohol-related medical or social problems were also frequently observed. Alcohol excess and alcohol-related problems were significantly less common in women irrespective of the severity of psoriasis.

Emotional Stress

In 1993, Farber and Nall reviewed the world literature as well as their own earlier studies on the impact of stress on the onset or exacerbation of psoriasis (140) and established that emotional stress is a trigger for psoriasis. Stress may be precipitated as a consequence of a loss of or change of a job, financial worries, domestic turmoil, or loss of a loved one (145,261,423). In one study, Farber, Nall, and Charuworn (128) demonstrated that in 102 hospitalized patients with severe psoriasis, 72% reported emotional stress as contributing to the severity of their disorder. In another study, Al'Abadie and colleagues (3) investigated the role of stressful life events on the course of various skin conditions. Psoriasis patients were more likely to report that an experience of stress predated the onset and exacerbations of their disease than patients with other skin conditions (urticaria, acne, alopecia, and nontopic eczema). They concluded that their results support the notion that stress is more likely to be associated with the onset of psoriasis than other provoking factors, but also that there may be considerable individual variation in the ability to cope, suggesting psychological interventions may be helpful for certain patients.

One study exemplifies findings in a survey of triggering factors in 338 Japaneses patients (male,213, 63%; female, 125,37%). Yasada and co-workers (423) found the following triggers: climate (60.3%), stress (46.9%), sleeping disturbance (34.6%), irregular lifestyle (32.2%), and low humidity (22.5%).

Williams (415) has summed up the importance of studying triggering factors: ". . . despite the high heritability of psoriasis, manipulation of environmental risk factors, such as smoking, alcohol, exposure to streptococci, trauma, drugs, and emotional stress open up the possibility of substantial prevention of the disease in the future."

ASSOCIATED DISEASES

In addition to arthritis, a number of common diseases are associated with psoriasis (159,238,399). A defined general population of 159,200 male and female native Swedes stemming from a hospital population in Gotenberg and born in the period 1911–1940 were followed over a decade (1970–1979) with regard to inpatient hospitalization for a variety of diagnoses (238). The investigators found that psoriasis cases ($n = 372$) were significantly associated with a spectrum of diseases: male and female psoriatics seemed to show excess rates of viral infections, alcoholism, hypertension, pneumonia, liver cirrhosis, urticaria, and rheumatoid arthritis.

Henseler and Christophers (186) recently reviewed disease concomitance in psoriasis. They analyzed data from more than 40,000 patients and learned that compared with age-matched control patients *without* psoriasis, cutaneous immune disorders were underrepresented in patients *with* psoriasis. In contrast, certain systemic disorders, such as diabetes, heart disease, and obesity, occur significantly more often in psoriasis patients than in control subjects.

In Norway Braathen et al.'s (46) self-assessment health survey of 10,576 individuals demonstrated that among the 149 psoriatics, 65.8% suffered from additional disorders, while among nonpsoriatics, 54.6% experienced one or more diseases. The difference was statistically significant and indicated that in psoriatic patients there is an increased susceptibility to concurrent diseases.

Skin Cancer

In a review, Farber and Nall (142) reported that skin cancer is a worldwide disease that varies in occurrence with the intensity of solar radiation and skin type. In the United States skin cancer is reaching epidemic proportions, prompting national and local health agencies to increase their efforts to provide preventive education, including skin cancer screening facilities, to lower the morbidity of this problem.

Patients with psoriasis would be expected to have a higher-than-normal occurrence of skin cancer, since they are frequently subjected to physical and chemical agents that may be either carcinogenic or cytotoxic (196). Although some investigators have found that skin cancer occurs only rarely in psoriasis patients, Farber (personal observation) has claimed that skin cancer occurs in psoriasis patients at the same frequency as in the general population. To test this hypothesis, an analysis of the Stanford Psoriasis Life Histories Questionnaire database was undertaken. The Stanford findings supported Farber's hypothesis: The frequency of skin cancer in psoriasis patients (without previous exposure to photochemotherapy) (240) was approximately 3%, which is considered to be the occurrence in the general population (291). However, because the study was based on a self-administered questionnaire, the results might well be faulted based on the method of data collection. An empirical approach warrants investigation (389).

In a British study (37), the prevalence of skin and internal malignancies was estimated from the general practitioners' notes of 2247 psoriasis patients and 4494 age- and sex-matched controls. No significant association was found in the occurrence of skin cancer and psoriasis with the exception of a subgroup analysis, which showed an increase in skin cancers in women. There was no difference in the age of onset of skin cancers between psoriatics and controls nor any difference in the frequency of nonskin cancers in either group.

An up-to-date analysis of worldwide investigations on skin cancer has been published by Armstrong and Kricker (14).

Diabetes

There is much disagreement on the association of diabetes to psoriasis. In their sample of 5600 patients, Farber and Nall (124) found that 194 (3.5%) reported that they had diabetes. In an unpublished study (Farber and Hamlin, 1968) of 504 pedigrees of psoriatic probands (41% male, 59% female ranging in age from 2 to 94 years; mean age, 42.9 years), the prevalence of diabetes was 3.57%. Although many authors suggest that the association between psoriasis and diabetes is merely one of chance, investigators such as Binazzi and co-workers (38) and Henseler and Christophers (186) have found a significantly higher positive correlation between psoriasis and diabetes. The latter state that diabetes and obesity may well be due to dietary habits and nutritional status.

Diet

There is a dearth of information on the impact of diet on the course of psoriasis. In an assessment of the effect of diet both as a triggering factor and as a treatment for psoriasis, Stern (362) suggests that there is little systematic evidence to suggest a strong relationship between diet and psoriasis. Naldi et al. (284) have indicated from their observations that neither coffee consumption nor vitamin A levels appear to be significant in the risk of developing psoriasis. Dietary fish oil supplementation has received a great deal of attention in recent years, but clinical studies [e.g., Soyland et al. (355)] fail to find any beneficial effect of fish oil in the diets.

AIDS

Almost two decades have passed since acquired immunodeficiency syndrome (AIDS) and AIDS-related complex (ARC) became a growing international problem. The need to monitor the scope of and trends in the human immunodeficiency virus (HIV) epidemic continues (351). Such data are crucial for identifying targets for primary and secondary interventions, evaluating prevention efforts, and allocating resources for HIV-related clinical and social services, planning for the future need for HIV-related services, and educating the public (289).

Early in the understanding of AIDS, Lazar and Roenigk (233) published several cases of AIDS patients with coexisting psoriasis, along with other investigators (105,232,233). They have focused their attention on the use of antipsoriatic agents for treating psoriasis and cautioned against employing immunosuppressing agents on those AIDS patients whose immune function is already depressed.

Coopman et al. (83) have reported that frequency of psoriasis visits per year had been one or more a year and is now increased 12 times among HIV-positive persons with psoriasis more than control subjects. It might seem that since the prevalence of psoriasis ranges approximately between 1.5% to 2%, psoriasis would be expected to occur by chance in a person infected with HIV, who is genetically predisposed to psoriasis (141). Obuch and associates (306) recently published their findings on psoriasis associated with HIV-positive individuals. They conducted a cohort study of 50 HIV-positive persons with psoriasis, who were followed during a 2-year period. In one-third of the patients, psoriasis appeared before 1978 (the year when HIV seroconversion began in San Francisco) (group I). In two-thirds psoriasis developed after 1978 (group II). Group I had a lower mean age of onset (19 vs. 36 years) and more commonly had a family history of psoriasis. Severe psoriasis occurred in one-fourth of survivals in this group (19 months after diagnosis of AIDS), which is comparable to the median survival for all AIDS patients diagnosed in San Francisco between 1984 and 1990. In conclusion, the investigators stated that psoriasis in the setting of HIV disease may be mild, moderate, or severe. Survival does not seem to be adversely affected by the presence of psoriasis or its therapy.

GENETIC AND ENVIRONMENTAL FACTORS

General Comments

Opinions regarding the mode of inheritance of psoriasis vary widely (162). There are three primary theories: some have suggested that psoriasis is a monogenic or polygenic disease caused by a dominant gene(s); others have supported recessivity as a mode; and recently the mulifactorial mode of inheritance, in which both predisposing gene(s) and environmental factors play roles in the expression of the disease, has received much attention. The following sections deal with the application of various epidemiological methods for investigating heritability in psoriasis.

Three points should be considered in assessing genetic data: (1) the method employed in collecting data; (2) the geographic region involved; and (3) how the extent of the disease is defined in families and the designation of "family member." Caution must be taken in comparing one set of research findings with another. The fact that one investigator determines a low frequency of a specific variable and another investigator finds a higher occurrence of that variable may be due to the data-gathering method rather than a reflection of an actual difference in the variable figures.

It is customary to consider the environment in which an organism exists as divisible into an external and internal milieu. The external environment (milieu externe) consists of (1) an environment endowed by nature, and (2) an environment created by a particular culture. The internal environment (milieu intérieur) maintains a remarkable constancy by homeostatic mechanisms against external environmental stimuli that tend to disturb this homeostasis.

Genetic Markers

The application of molecular genetics and biochemical techniques in the studies of the HLA system and the Human Genome Project over the past several years has resulted in tremendous advances in our knowledge of genetic immunology (315). The current nomenclature for factors of the HLA system is published under the aegis of the WHO Nomenclature Committee, which considers additions and revisions to the nomenclature of specificities defined by both molecular and serological techniques (39,413).

In the human being there is an array of genes on the short arm of chromosome 6 that is initimately involved in expression of antigens on cell surfaces (227). This immunologically active genetic area of human chromosome 6 is called the *major histocompatibility complex* (MHC) or *histocompatibility locus A* (HLA) (91). There are a number of genetic loci that produce HLA antigens. These loci are designated as HLA-A, -B, -C, -D, -DR, -DQ, and -DP antigens. Each HLA locus exhibits a polymorphism of allelic genes (266,368,381,384,387,417).

The association of an HLA antigen with a given disease means that there is a higher incidence of that antigen in a group of patients with the disease than in a group of people without the disease.

Relative risk (RR) calculations are used to quantify and collate the information obtained from various studies.

$$RR = \frac{(\%\text{ of disease population with given HLA})\ (\%\text{ of controls without})}{(\%\text{ of controls with given HLA})\ (\%\text{ of patients without})}$$

The higher the relative risk, the more significant the association and the more useful HLA antigen typing would be to establish a diagnosis. Dahl (91) states that the RR calculation are destined to be used extensively in genetic counseling and preventive medicine and associates psoriasis with specific antigens with approximate relative risk (in brackets): B13 [4]; B17 [5]; B16 [4], B37 [6]; Cw6 [13]; and Dw7/DR7 [10].

Evidence for a genetic contribution in psoriasis stems from epidemiological and immunogenetic data (75,91,100,111–113,235,257,364,419). Psoriasis is one of a number of autoimmune diseases that display significant HLA associations (112). A disequilibrium exists between certain HLA antigens and psoriasis. To link psoriasis with known markers within the human genome, serological studies have been carried out with a variety of blood group and polymorphic protein antigens (91,335).

Wuepper et al. (419) in a recent review indicate a weak association has been identified in the MNS and Lewis blood group systems (relative risk, 3.5). Stronger associations with class I B-locus and class II D-locus genes (relative risk, 8–12) have also been determined by studies of the HLA system. According to these authors, the strongest association appears to be between HLA Cw6 (relative risk, 24) and various forms of psoriasis. Hammond et al. (178) reported that psoriasis seems to be the first disease more closely associated with the C locus. The previously observed associations between psoriasis and the HLA B13 and B17 may be due to linkage disequilibrium with the Cw6 antigen. This suggests that Cw6 is perhaps a genetic marker for the gene determining susceptibility to psoriasis. However, only about 10% of Cw6-positive individuals develop the disease, suggesting that other genetic and/or environmental factors must be involved. An interesting point has been put forth by Christophers and Henseler (77,185). From their clinical explorations and HLA typing, they have divided plaque psoriasis into *early onset*, which is a severe form associated with the presence of Cw6, B13, and Bw57 (B17), and a less severe form with a *late onset*, associated with Cw2 and B27.

The frequency distribution of HLA antigens has been examined in children from the ages of birth to 12 years (301). The results showed an increase of HLA B27 in minimal psoriasis, B2 in the guttate form, and B41 in inverted psoriasis. In the total sample an increase in B17, Cw6, and DR 6 was also noticed.

The reason for the association between HLA antigens and psoriasis is not known. In analogy with the findings in experimental immunology (331), it has been suggested that it is due to immune response (Ir) genes closely linked to a linkage disequilibrium (the extent to which the genetic frequencies of linked genes deviate from those expected from their allele frequencies in the population) with the genes coding the HLA antigens. Whether all genes predisposing to psoriasis are linked to the HLA region or whether the HLA system only constitutes part of a polygenic system causing psoriasis is still an open question (239,342).

The number of loci that could be used as markers for linkage analysis was limited until a decade ago when the concept of restriction fragment length polymorphism (RFLP) became available (269,310,312). The new techniques of molecular biology that have been developed over the last decade are now being routinely applied to the study of human disease. In addition to the use of restriction enzymes, the ability to clone and sequence selected segments of DNA by the proteinase chain reaction, and the creation of a high-resolution map of the human genome using RFLP detected on Southern blots, have evolved to solve many problems in genetics (269).

The application of this new technology can be seen in the work of Ozawa and colleagues (312), who analyzed the RFLP of 13 patients with psoriasis vulgaris and six healthy controls who were all positive for at least one allele of HLA Cw6. The investigators suggest that finding the RFLP in the HLA C gene indicates genetic linkage between Cw6 and psoriasis vulgaris, and that these specific fragments may well cause the onset of the disease in people predisposed to it, or may impact its course.

Genetic imprinting is a genetic mechanism that attempts to explain why the children more often have psoriasis if their fathers have psoriasis than when mothers have the disease. Support for this hypothesis is pending contingent upon further research on this matter (374,378).

Population Genetics

As indicated at the beginning of this chapter, the study of the history and geography of human genes is being integrated into new knowledge of immunogenesis and, in turn, will be added to the growing corpus of data on the relationship of molecular genetics and the onset or exacerbation of psoriasis. Cavalli-Sforza and his colleagues (40,41,43,67–70,316) have performed exhaustive analyses of human genetic data over the past 50 years, mapping the worldwide distribution of hundreds of genes. Cavalli-Sforza (67) states that genes, people, and languages have diversified in tandem through a series of migrations that apparently began in Africa and spread throughout all parts of the globe. Reconstruction of human evolution is being achieved by bringing together immunogenetic, archeological, and linguistic data. These allied disciplines parallel evolution of human and nonhuman primates (8,18, 23,40,41,43,71,97,213,217,268,278,285,328). Cavalli-Sforza anticipates that the joint study from all these perspectives will be especially effective in a time when modern molecular techniques are bringing analysis of genetic variation to an unprecedented degree of resolution (316).

HLA antigens and other blood and serum factors display ethnic variation (Table 7) (298). Differences in HLA antigen frequencies can occur within a country under study. For example, Beckman and his collaborators (29,30) have shown distinct genetic differences between northern and southern Sweden. Albert et al. (4) demonstrated HLA phenotypic differences between Caucasians and blacks as well as the admixture studies by Allsopp et al. (8), Chakraborty et al. (71), and Reed (328). Russell and his group (336) point out that polygenic influences may be reflected in HLA variations among populations as evidenced in the difference between psoriatic HLA phenotypes of Caucasians and blacks, whereby the blacks present with a high frequency of HLA B17 and yet express a low frequency of psoriasis (250).

Anthropologists studying blood groups traced migration routes, isolation, and acculturation patterns in ethnic groups employing serological techniques (67,285,298,361,421). Today, the study of population genetics follows the spread of various populations throughout the world by using the varying frequency distributions of such groups as well as collating disease entities with associated HLA antigens (198,226,254,255,304,307,313,317,380,398,421).

Although matching data are becoming more available to correlate frequency rates of psoriasis with the "psoriatic antigen," HLA B13, 17, 37, Cw6, and DR7 vary among different racial groups. Also, some preliminary relationships can be seen in ethnic groups that lack one or more of these antigens. For example, the comprehensive dermatological survey of more than 25,000 Andean Indians revealed not one case of psoriasis (82). Clinical observations support similar findings in Native Americans of the United States and the Arctic area. Recent HLA determinations in many of these groups showed a lack or very low occurrences of either HLA B13 and/or B17: pure-stock Greenland Eskimo (216), Canadian Eskimo (101,102), Native Americans of the southwest—the Papago (314), Pima (356), and Zuni (386); Central America—Guatemalans (61,85); and South America—Chilean Aymara (390), Peruvian Quechuan (383), and Venezuelan Warao (213,231).

In general, psoriasis is more common in colder Northern climates than in tropical regions. African blacks from the hot, wet western central countries have been reported to be less affected than African blacks from milder, dry eastern central nations. As a rule, tropical races are less frequently and less severely affected than Caucasians (42,114,144,304,398).

In Middle and Central America, Canizares (59,60) reported that psoriasis is as common in Mexico as in other parts of the world. Failmezger (115) examined inhabitants in various Central and South American regions of white, black, and Indian ancestry and found that in an overall study population of 3140 persons with skin diseases, psoriasis was seen in 0.7% in Guatemala, 0.7% in Honduras, 0.996 in an urban site of Nicaragua, and 0.2% in a rural site in that country.

The Caribbean Islands form an arch from northern Venezuela to Cuba. Trinidad and Tobago are two island masses northeast of Venezuela with a population of 43% West Indians of African descent and 40% East Indians. Quamina (321) reported on an analysis of 4048 cases of skin disease, of which 256 (6%) were psoriatic.

Sachs (337) has found Nigerian HLA frequencies to be closest to those of the Caribbean St. Lucians and U.S. blacks as discussed below.

Table 7 Association Between HLA Antigens and Psoriasis in Selected Series (%)[a]

Ref.	Patients' ethnic origin	HLA specificities						
		B12	B13	B16	B17	B37	Cw6	DR7
336	NAC	23	27 (25)	NG (3)	23	NG (9)	NG	NG
370	EUC	NG	15	NG (4) [4]	36	NG (8) [7]	NG	NG
230	EUC	NG	26	NG (4)	31	NG (8)	NG	NG
341	EUC	13	23 (24)	NG (8)	22	NG (8)	NG	NG
225	NAC	16	9 (22)	22 (3)	31 (5)	NG (6)	NG	NG
235	EUC	6 (2)	NG	9 (1)	NG	NG	NG	NG
265[b]	NAC	NG	3	6	13	NG	NG[c]	NG
54	EUC	NG	23	NG	27	7	NG	NG
16	JAP	NG	NG	NG	NG	NG	9 (0)	NG
323	EUC	NG	18 (5) [4]	10 (9)	25 (6) [6]	3 (2)	40 (17) [4]	60 (21) [7]
381	EUC	8 (15)	35 (6)	NG	19 (4)	NG	46 (7)	28 (20)
72	CHIN	2 (3)	37 (19) [3]	NG	14 (14)	0 (1)	4 (6)	NG
330	ME	NG	0 (8)	NG	7 (12)	7 (19)	25 (18)	21 (28)
307	EUC	NG	93	NG (253) [6.08]	93	NG (253) [2.9]	NG	NG

[a]Controls are shown in parentheses; relative risk in brackets.
[b]DMA = 16/38.
[c]Cw7 = 19-28/33.
CHIN: Chinese; EUC: European Caucasian; JAP: Japanese; ME: Middle East; NAC: North American Caucasian; NG: not given
B17: Te57, Bw17; CT7: Cw6.

The tropical countries of South America have many different climates ranging from hot, humid sea level to the cool, raining Andes (339).

Although there are conflicting theories as to the population of the New World, it is accepted by many anthropologists that Amerindians (69) have a common Mongoloid ancestry originating along the western Siberian coast. Early mankind may have crossed the Bering Strait during the last North American ice age and dispersed from Alaska southward to the tip of South America (61). An absence of psoriasis has also been observed in the Amerindians in the remote villages of the Amazon-Orinoco forest (213). Layrisse et al. (231) reported that HLA B13 and B27 were lacking in the HLA profiles of the Warao and other Indian tribes in the Orinoco delta.

Based on HLA typing studies, Allsopp and collaborators have sketched the distribution and genetic distances of various populations of Western Africa and have placed the origins of American blacks intermediary between the coastal western Africans from Mali and the Gambiah and Nigerian populations (8).

Kenney (211,212) published reports on the occurrence of psoriasis in American blacks based on his private practice and found that in 3860 consecutive patients, 27 (0.7%) had psoriasis. At a later time, he examined 2400 records of American black patients in his practice in Washington, DC, which revealed 33 cases (1.4%) of psoriasis. These figures reflect the low frequency of psoriasis in the western African coast countries from which a high number of slaves were captured.

It has been reported that by 1518, the demand for slaves in the Spanish New World was so great that King Charles I of Spain sanctioned the direct transport of slaves from West Africa to the American colonies. By the 1530s, the Portuguese were also using African slaves in Brazil. From then until the abolition of the slave trade in 1870, at least 10 million Africans were forcibly brought to the Americas: about 47% to the Caribbean Islands and the Guianas, 38% to Brazil, 6% to mainland Spanish America, and approximately 4.5% to North America. The genetic admixture between African blacks and North American whites is estimated to be between 20% (328) and 25% (71).

In Central and Southeast Asia, the prevalence of psoriasis in India ranges from 0.5% to 1.5%. Malaysia is a federation of 13 states and occupies the greater part of the Malay Peninsula. Studies have reported the occurrence of psoriasis to be 4–5.5%. The tropical island of Singapore is located just north of the equator and south of Malaysia. In studying the HLA frequency rates in Singapore, Chan et al. (72–74) noted that the Chinese lack the HLA-Cw6 antigen, although it is highly associated with the white and Japanese populations (281).

Yip (425) compiled statistics on the prevalence in Hong Kong and various Chinese cities to the north. At the Hong Kong Government Skin Clinics, psoriasis was noted in 1.48% of 52,307 patients examined over a 2-year period.

The frequency of psoriasis in the white Australian resembles that of the Western world, approximately 2.6%, whereas no psoriasis has been found in the Australian Aborigines (90,167,168). The Aborigines have been in Australia for at least 30,000 years, originating in Southeast Asia. In HLA typing of 177 members, of the Walbiri tribe of the desert area of the Northwest Territory, HLA B17 is absent (23). In recent times, however, they have moved closer to the fringes of the European communities for economic opportunities, and admixture with whites has become common.

The line of reasoning for testing different ethnic groups is that if an association between an HLA allele and a disease susceptibility is established in several disease population groups, it would indicate that the disease susceptibility gene is most probably located in very close proximity to this specific HLA allele (9). In recent publications the Cw6 was been designated as that potential gene because of its high relative risk value as compared to the A and B loci (77,111–113,185,282,284,362,419). Several interesting reports deal with HLA C associated with psoriasis: one in Finland (195), another in Israel (330), and a third in Japan (16). In essence, coding sequences of the HLA-C molecule suggest that alanine at position 73 may have a significant role in susceptibility to the disease. Nakagawa et al. (280,281) HLA-typed 56 unrelated Japanese psoriasis patients and found significant increases in A1, A2, B39, Bw46, Cw6, Cw7, and Cw11. They observed that the most specific finding was the increase of Cw11, a recently recognized antigen that is always associated with Bw46 and occurs in East Asian populations. The authors indicated that in addition to Cw6 and Cw7, Cw11 has a strong association with Japanese patients suffering from psoriasis vulgaris, pointing up racial and ethnic difference among these patients.

Looking at another population, Pitchappan et al. (318) studied HLA antigen frequencies in 83 south India patients with psoriasis and compared them with 77 controls. HLA Bw57 (a split of B17) and DR7 were found elevated in the patients. The two sexes differed in their age-at-onset curves: females had a preponderance to early onset, while males had late onset.

Nini et al. (301) studied HLA frequency distributions in pediatric groups. They observed a close association of HLA B17, Cw6, and DR6 in the total psoriatic group and noticed high relative risk figures for A28, Cw6, and DR6 in children under 6 years: RR = 3.0, 2.9, and 2.5, respectively. In the older group (7–12 years) the relative risk figures were A30 and 31 = 3.4, B14 and B17 = 2.8; Cw6 = 4.4, and DR7 = 2.01.

Population geneticists may one day determine whether *lacking* a certain antigen (gene) or having a *lower frequency* of certain HLA antigens, such as HLA B8, than seen in the general population may serve as a protection against psoriasis (235,286).

GENES AND ENVIRONMENT

Low frequency of diabetes, myocardial infarction, autoimmune disorders, and a unique cancer pattern are among the traits characteristic of Eskimo noninfectious epidemiology. They are common to all circumpolar populations, whether Siberian, Alaskan, Canadian, or Greenland (180,181). It has been suggested that diet has an impact on the occurrence of various diseases.

The different groups that ranged from Alaska through Canada and Greenland to Siberia obtained land and marine animals as their primary food supply—seal, walrus, whale, bear, caribou, and musk ox as well as fish and birds (24,285). The traditional Eskimo diet was, therefore, very high in protein and fat and low in ascorbic acid and tocopherols. The fat of the Arctic marine animals is the most unsaturated found in the animal kingdom, being particularly rich in the long-chain fatty acids of the linolenic or n-3 class of essential fatty acids (EFAs). The dietary intake of the Eskimos has been studied over the last couple of decades by nutritionists to establish a base for investigating the Eskimo and their disease patterns.

Bates and his colleagues (24) have reported that one of the possible reasons for the low prevalence of cardiovascular disease and cancer in the Eskimo is the high intake of eiocosapentaenoic acid (EPA) and low arachidonic acid (AA) levels in Eskimo plasma. When on their traditional diet, Vancouver Island Indians (like the Eskimos) have high EPA and low AA levels in their plasma. It has been suggested that the low AA levels are probably genetically determined; therefore, the unusual disease patterns in these populations cannot be attributed entirely to diet. As stated earlier, dietary supplementation with fish oil alone for the treatment of psoriasis has not been shown to be clinically effective (355,430).

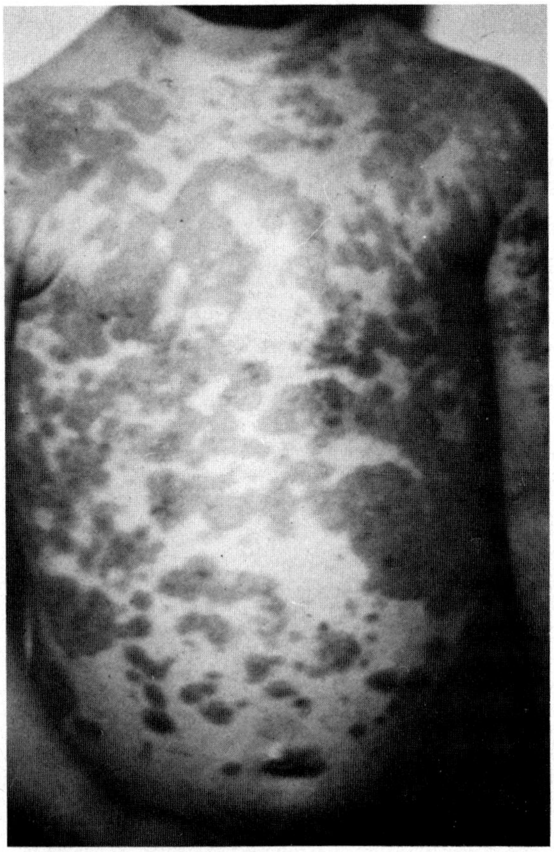

Figure 13 Guttate psoriasis in a 4-year-old boy following streptococcal throat infection. HLA Cw6 is greatly increased in guttate psoriasis.

VARIANTS OF PSORIASIS AND HLA FREQUENCY DISTRIBUTIONS

Guttate Psoriasis

This form of psoriasis has been discussed earlier (see Pediatric Psoriasis). Tonsillitis and upper respiratory infections occurring 1–3 weeks before acute guttate psoriasis are a significant association in childhood psoriasis (Fig. 13) (15,138,302,376). The pathogenesis of guttate eruption is not clearly understood, but with the use of HLA genetic markers, the relationship between streptococcal throat infection and guttate psoriasis is becoming clearer.

A plausible explanation for the association seemed to be emerging in the early 1970s (170) when the following reports were published. In 1970, Hirata and Terasaki (189) reported cross-reactions between M protein of beta-hemolytic group A streptococci and HLA antigens A1, 2, 3, 5, 7, and 9 in animal experiments. Later, Russell et al. (336) determined the frequency of HLA antigens in a series of psoriasis patients and noted a positive correlation between psoriasis and antigens HLA B13 and B17. Then Krain (219) found a significant association in patients with guttate psoriasis between the HLA B13 and a history of severe streptococcal infections. Bertrams et al. (35) observed that psoriatic patients who were positive for HLA B13 had significantly lower antistreptolysin-O titers than HLA B13–negative patients. From this observation, they suggested that the inability to produce normal amounts of antibody to streptolysin-O might be the reason streptococcal infections and HLA B13 positivity were correlated in guttate psoriasis.

In the late 1970s, Gross and his colleagues (174) questioned the interpretation made by Hirata and Terasaki of a cross-reaction between streptococcal antigens in tissue-typed patients with different forms of psoriasis. In their study, Gross et al. looked for evidence of an association between streptococcal antigen-induced lymphocyte activation, guttate psoriasis, and psoriasis-associated antigens of the HLA-B locus. They were not able to find evidence of such an association and stressed that their findings were in agreement with the results of detailed studies in humans by Tauber et al. (375), in which no cross-reaction between A-streptococcal antigens and HLA determinants could be demonstrated.

Pustular Psoriasis and Related Form

Pustular psoriasis includes a group of disorders that have in common recalcitrant, sterile, and pustular eruptions appearing in psoriasiform patches (Fig. 14). Pustular psoriasis may be either localized or generalized (136,320).

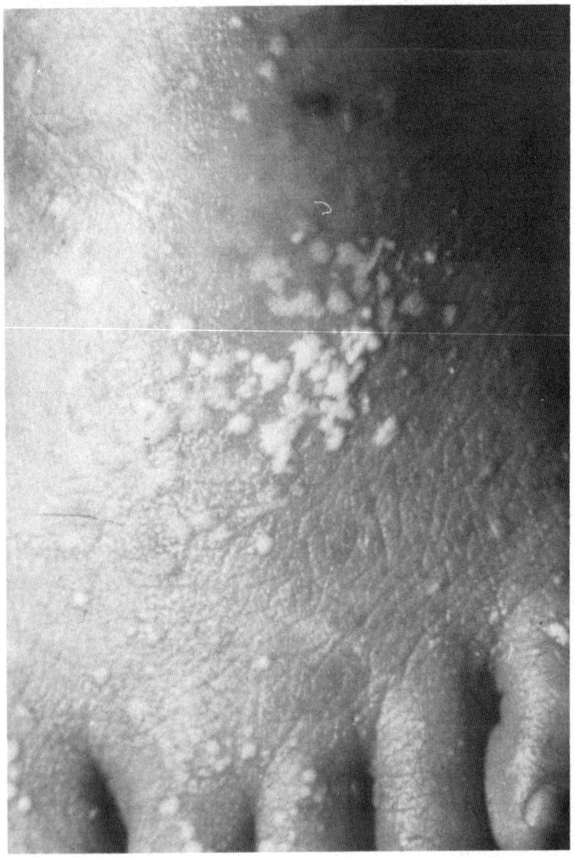

Figure 14 Pustular psoriasis of the foot. HLA antigens B13 and B17 are not associated with this form of psoriasis.

Scandinavian investigators (206–209,426,427) have studied this form of psoriasis as well as other forms with respect to HLA typing. Their findings reveal that HLA B13, B17, and B16 are not associated with pustular psoriasis, pustulosis palmaris et plantaris, or pustular psoriasis of the palms and soles (Fig. 15). The failure to find the usual HLA psoriasis antigens in persons with these diseases does not mean they are not forms of psoriasis. Indeed, HLA-linked factors may play some role in either limiting the disease to the palms and soles or generating pustules rather than keratotic plaques.

Persistent palmoplantar pustulosis, lacking the psoriasis antigens, may be an entity genetically distinct from psoriasis (209).

Erythrodermic and Flexural Psoriasis

Karvonen et al. (207) found that patients with erythrodermic psoriasis (Fig. 16) had a high frequency of HLA B13 and B17, which has been supported by the work of Economidou and co-workers (108). These antigens were rare in patients with flexural psoriasis. Again, it was proposed that a different genetic background for flexural and common psoriasis may exist.

Psoriasis and Arthritis

This relationship of psoriasis and arthritis is controversial (65,66) and is discussed elsewhere in this book. However, the HLA B13, B17, and B27 have been found in patients with psoriasis and arthritis (Fig. 17) (426).

TRADITIONAL EPIDEMIOLOGICAL METHODOLOGY

From the findings of large census investigations, twin, family, and HLA frequency studies, a multifactorial origin, in which both genetic and environmental components play a role in the onset and course of psoriasis, seems likely.

Family Studies

It is essential in interpreting research findings from family studies that the degree of relationship between the proband and the relatives be established. First-degree relatives include parents, siblings, and children; second-degree relatives include grandparents,

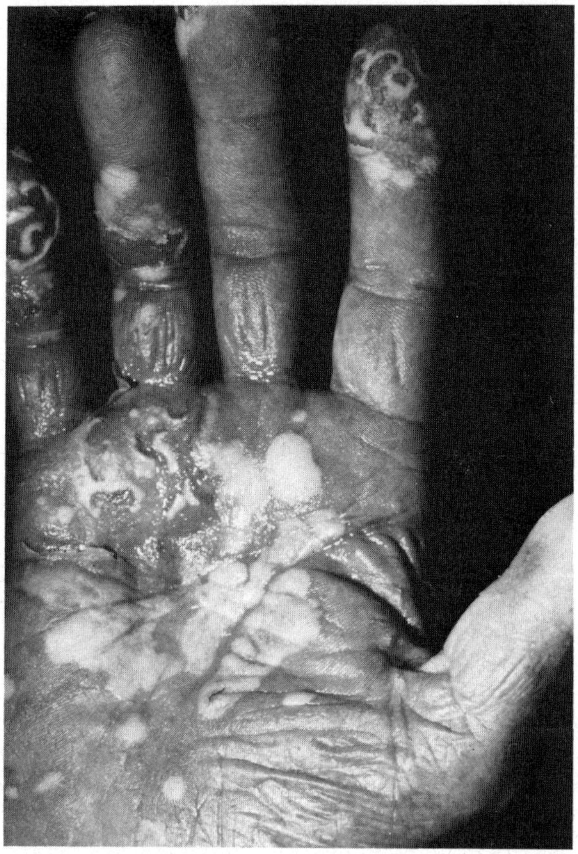

Figure 15 Psoriasis of the palms. HLA antigens B13 and B17 are lacking in pustular psoriasis of the palms and soles.

aunts, and uncles; and third-degree relatives include cousins.

A further indication that genetic factors play a role in the hereditary composition of psoriasis is the high occurrence of family cases. The percentages given by different authors vary, as widely as 4% to 91% familial aggregation (Table 8). Most investigators have found the family occurrence of psoriasis to be approximately 35%. The more thorough the examination of the blood relatives of the psoriasis probands, the higher the prevalence rate of family history of psoriasis.

In the Stanford study of familial occurrence of psoriasis (404), a questionnaire was sent to 698 patients who had indicated that one or more members of their families had psoriasis. Statistical analysis of these data (as given below) compared to those of a control of families of nonpsoriatic patients supported the hypothesis that psoriasis is a multifactorial disease requiring multiple genetic and environmental factors for its expression.

One of the criteria in testing for multifactorial inheritance (357) is the use of segregation ratio (sibanalysis) of affected and unaffected sibs. If affected sibs are more than 2.5 times more frequent in pedigrees with one affected parent than in pedigrees with two affected parents, the multifactorial model should be preferred. Here again, a ratio of less than 2.5 does not exclude multifactorial inheritance.

In trying to determine the mode of inheritance of psoriasis, Watson and colleagues (109,404) analyzed the proportion of the proband siblings affected according to whether either or both parents had psoriasis. There were 1140 sibs from families in which neither parent had psoriasis. Of these siblings determined from the 698 probands, 7.5% had psoriasis. When one parent had psoriasis, 15.6 of the siblings were affected. When both parents had the disease, 50% of the siblings were observed to have psoriasis (Fig. 18).

In attempting to fit these results into the frames of various modes of inheritance, the following steps were considered. If psoriasis were an autosomal recessive trait, 25% of the siblings would have been affected if neither parent had been affected; as indicated, Watson et al. (404) found only 7.5% affected. If psoriasis were an autosomal recessive trait, all of the siblings would have been affected when both parents had psoriasis; as seen by the investigators, only 50% of the siblings were affected. If psoriasis were inherited in an autosomal dominant pattern, 50% of the siblings would have been affected if one parent had psoriasis; the findings indicated 15.6% were involved.

Since these figures are much lower than would be expected in the simple autosomal dominance or recessivity models, Watson and co-workers concluded that the mode of inheritance was most likely dependent on both genes and environment for clinical manifestation: multifactorial inheritance.

Andressen and Henseler's study (12) is in concurrence with the Stanford findings. They predicted that children of parents without psoriasis have a 2% chance of developing the disease, whereas if one parent has psoriasis, the risk is 8.1%.

Krulig et al. (225) found only one of six families with enough affected members to support a useful genetic study. The pedigree of that family is shown in Figure 19. Psoriasis occurred in three generations, with all affected members having the HLA B17 antigen. Absence of the B17 antigen coincided with absence of psoriasis (with the exception of one subject,

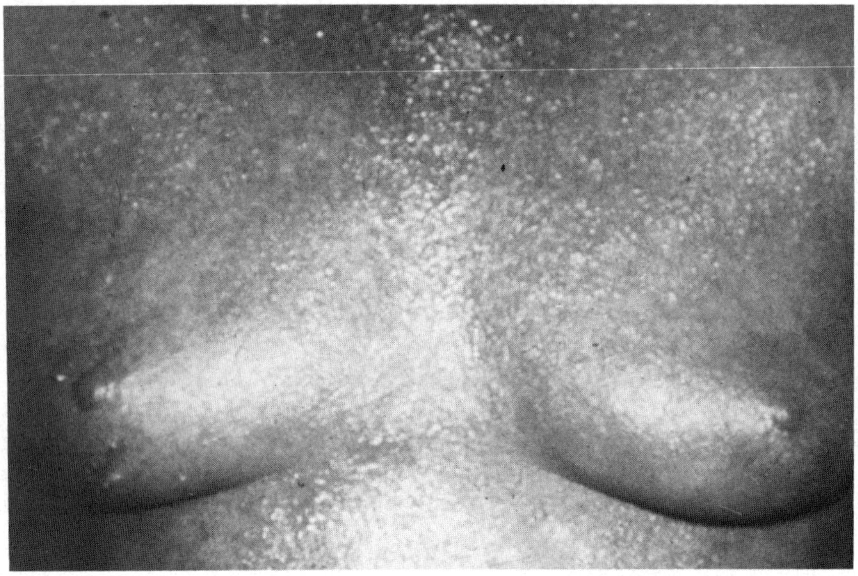

Figure 16 Erythrodermic psoriasis reflects high frequency of HLA B13 and B17.

age 13, who is now being followed for signs of early stages of the disease).

Twin Studies

Allen (7) has stated that use of twins as a research tool is still proving its worth both by the number of scientists engaged in twin research and by the significance of their results. Of current interest are the epidemiological studies made possible by the assembly of large numbers of twins in twin registries (47–52,64,81,155,193,205,222,295,296,411).

The twin method serves three purposes: (1) The difference in concordance between monozygotic (identical) and dizygotic (fraternal) twins can be used to determine whether genetic variability plays a role

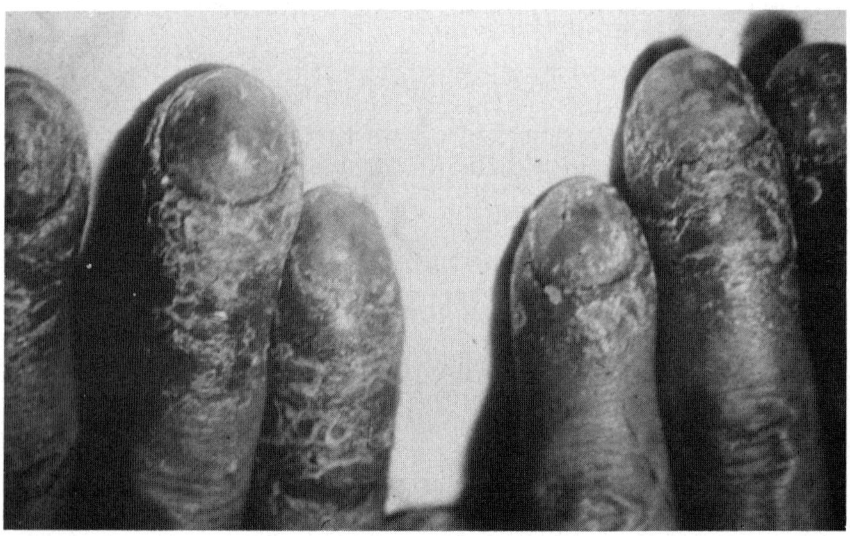

Figure 17 Psoriasis and arthritis occurring in the same patient reveal increased frequency of HLA B27 as well as B13, B17, and B37.

Table 8 Familial Occurrence of Psoriasis in Selected Series

Ref.	Year	No. probands	% Family members with psoriasis
163	1928	452	4
175	1978	1,366	8
297	1990	112	10
360	1935	6,768	10
423	1971	313	11
253	1982	3,500	12
2	1980	203	13
31	1977	162	14
17	1957	243	18
242	1982	336	24
5	1994	190	28
275	1969	314	32
53	1972	524	33
19	1969	452	33
94	1993	808	33
190	1931	154	34
124	1974	5,600	36
183	1967	758	36
374	1994	5,197	36
100	1997	312	40
272	1973	300	45
319	1982	406	49
302[a]	1975	245	59
15[a]	1971	100	64
243	1963	312	91

[a]Children.

in a given disease; (2) penetrance (i.e., that probability of manifestation of the disease) can be estimated; and (3) the conditions of manifestation can be examined (357).

The first use made of twins in the study of hereditary phenomenon dates back to the publication of Galton's work, "The History of Twins as a Criterion of the Relative Powers of Nature and Nurture," in 1875. Between 1910 and 1940 various European and American schools contributed to the formulation and application of the theoretical nature versus nurture models. During the last few decades twin data studies have been used extensively and found to be helpful in evaluating the role of genetic factors in the etiology of some diseases and in normal development (125).

One method in common use in analyzing and interpreting categorical twin data is the calculation of concordance rates among monozygotic and dizygotic twins, and based upon these rates, a heritability index indicating the relative influence of genetic and environmental factors evolves. Twin-pair techniques can be enhanced with the use of standard data-gathering methods.

In the Stanford twin study, Farber and co-workers (125), using a mailed questionnaire, investigated 61 monozygotic (Fig. 20) and dizygotic (Fig. 21) concordant and discordant twin pairs. The course of psoriasis in the 95 individual twin members was compared with a matched control group of singleton (nontwin) psoriatic patients. The findings indicated that twin members with psoriasis do not differ from psoriatic singletons in the general population with respect to the clinical manifestation of the disease.

Psoriasis in concordant monozygotic twin pairs tended to be similar with respect to age-onset, distribution pattern, severity, and course. This pattern was not found in concordant dizygotic twin pairs. The striking difference in the rate of concordance for psoriasis between monozygotic and dizygotic twin pairs indicated an inheritable contribution to the etiology of psoriasis. The fact that not all monozygotic twin pairs are concordant lends credence to the concept that environmental factors are also important and supports the theory of multifactorial inheritance of psoriasis.

In an Australian twin study (103), the investigators found that monozygotic twin pair concordance for confirmed psoriasis was 35% (12 of 34 pairs) and the dyzygotic twin concordance was 12% (5 of 43 pairs). The investigators concluded that from their case-control analysis of psoriasis-discordant twin pairs there was no evidence for the influence of alcohol or coffee intake, overweight, birth weight, or personality in the origin of psoriasis.

Table 9 is an analysis of 296 twin pairs with one or both members concordant for psoriasis. Literature data from 1924 to 1969 (125) as well as the statistics in the Stanford twin study are given. Also included in the tabulated data are two studies based on twin registries: one by Lynfield (248) utilizing the U.S. National Academy of Sciences–National Research Council's Follow-up Twin Panel of World War II male twins (193) and the other by Brandrup et al. (47–52) from the Danish registry of twins born between 1891 and 1920.

Pedigree Analysis

Many pedigrees (Fig. 22) demonstrate the distribution of psoriasis in a family. Although the pedigrees of two

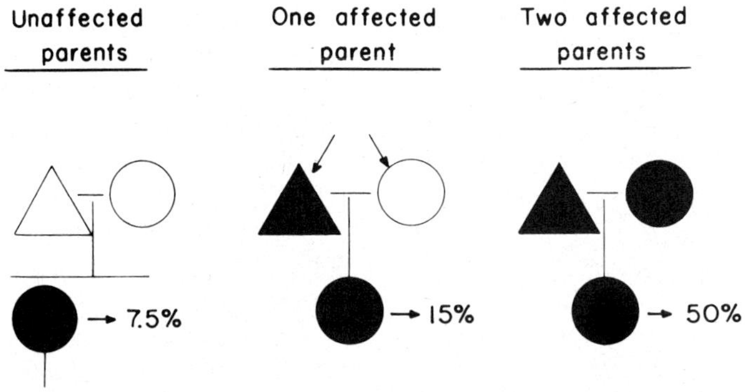

Figure 18 Sibship analysis in 698 psoriatic probands led to a suggested multifactorial inheritance mode.

large kindred in Utah (402) and North Carolina (1) were found to be consistent with autosomal dominance inheritance, Watson and his co-workers (404) observed that the pedigrees of the families of 698 probands in their genetic investigation showed great variation in the character of the familial distribution of affected and unaffected individuals; this did not substantiate the concept of a single simple mode of inheritance. Perhaps the suggested difference in the configuration of the pedigrees provides supporting evidence that the disease is genetically of multifactorial influence.

Conjugal Psoriasis

Conjugal psoriasis studies trace the occurrence of psoriasis in the offspring of two affected related parents (Fig. 23) and provide opportunities to examine modes of inheritance of the disease. In a questionnaire survey, Farber and associates (122) found that 2% of the 1609 married psoriasis patients in their sample of 2144 had spouses with psoriasis. Of these psoriasis patients, 18 had married cousins, none of whom had psoriasis. Slightly higher but similar figures were reported by Farber's group in a later study (124). None of these conjugal alliances had produced children with psoriasis at the time the two studies were conducted.

Lomholt (243) reported one case of conjugal psoriasis in his series from the Faroe Islands.

Aschner and co-workers (17) have reported two instances of marriages of two related psoriatics. In one, the children were still too young for investigators to

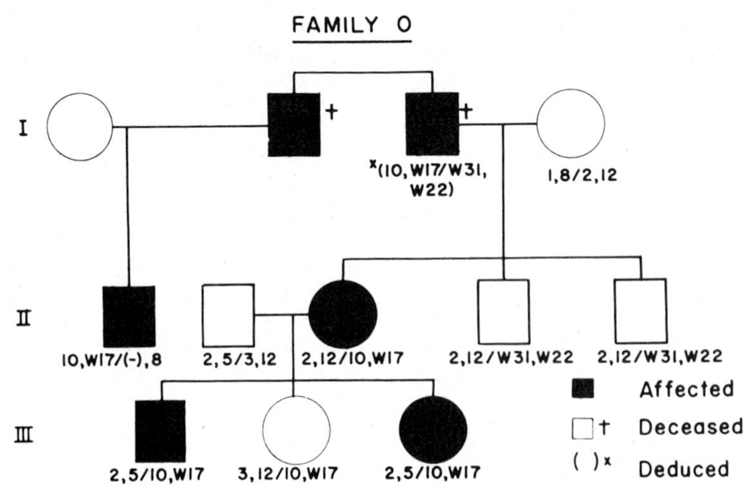

Figure 19 Psoriasis occurring in three generations with all affected members having HLA B17.

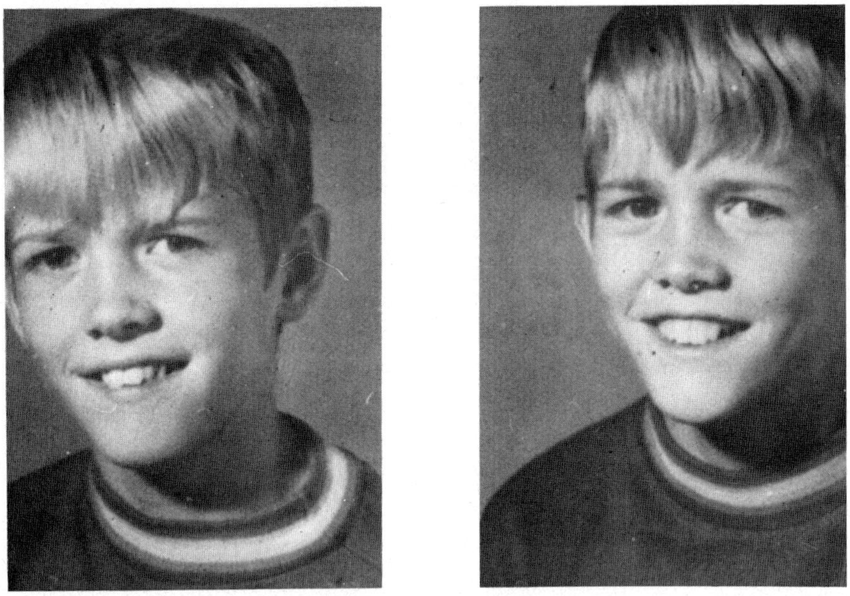

Figure 20 Monozygotic twins are as alike as "two peas in a pod."

observe the expression of the disease. In the other case, two of five children aged 22–35 years had acquired psoriasis, one in a severe generalized form. The authors posed the question of whether the severely affected patient represented the homozygous stage of a dominant gene.

In analysis of 2035 families of psoriasis probands, Andressen and Henseler (12) found 18 probands from marriages with conjugal psoriasis. Psoriasis was also found in 42 siblings. One such family had 17 of 18 (94%) siblings affected when both parents had psoriasis.

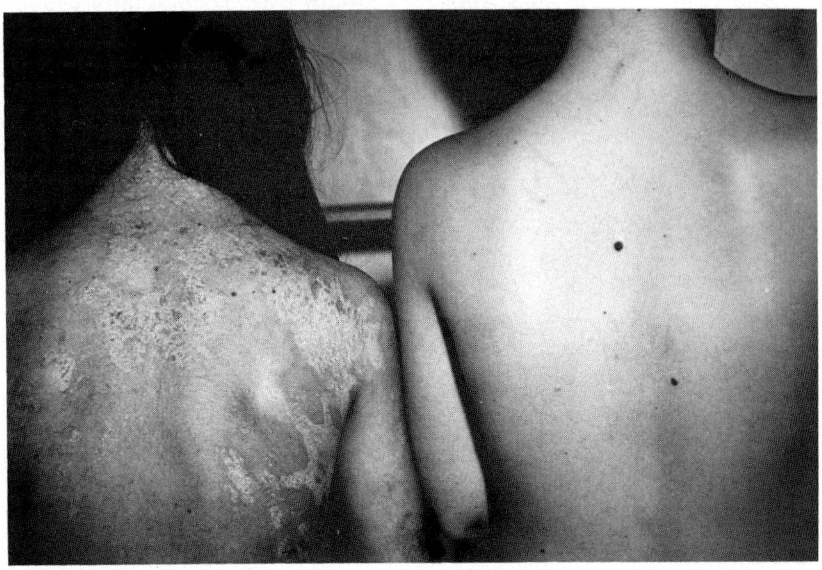

Figure 21 Dizygotic twins are as alike as ordinary siblings.

Table 9 Twin Pairs with Psoriasis ($n = 296$)

Reference	Sample	Mean age onset (years)	Monozygotic		Dizygotic		Total
			Concordant	Discordant	Concordant	Discordant	
125	Varied	Varied	28	14	10	30	82
125	USA	18	30	11	4	16	61
248[a]	USA	>50	2	2	2	4	10
47[a]	Denmark	>55	9	5	3	19	36
12	Germany	NG	1	5	7	17	30
103	Australia	NG	12	22	5	38	77
Total			82	59	31	124	296

[a]Twin registry.
NG: not given.

Half Sibships

In conjunction with full-sib and parental observations, half-sib analysis (Fig. 24) permits an estimation of the genetic and environmental variance as well as a partitioning of genetic variance into its additive dominance and epistatic components (295). The offspring of monozygotic twins are a unique class of human half-sibs who provide an unusual opportunity for researchers to resolve and measure several additional potentially important sources of human variation, including assortative mating, the influence of the in utero environment, and the impact of common environmental factors.

Corey and Nance (84) encourage the use of the monozygotic half-sib model as a tool for epidemiological research. The new approach utilizes the children of identical twins and provides a means of assessing genetic and environmental influences on qualitative traits as well as for resolving many of the controversies surrounding the etiology of certain multifactorial traits. By taking advantage of the unique relationship between identical twins, but not focusing on the twins themselves, this half-sib model circumvents many of the problems associated with classic twin and nuclear family studies.

The study of half-sibships may provide an idea of whether disease is recessive or dominant. If psoriasis occurs quite frequently among half-siblings, this favors dominant inheritance. In the event of single recessive inheritance, the disease would only affect half-siblings in exceptionally few cases (243).

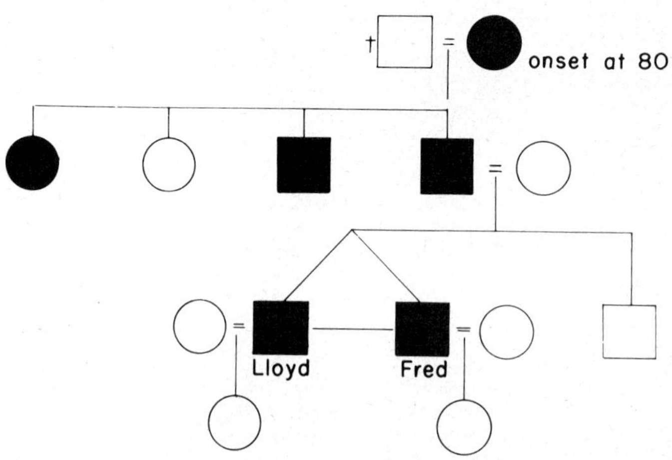

Figure 22 Example of a pedigree in which psoriasis affected three generations of family members. In the third generation there is a set of monozygotic twins.

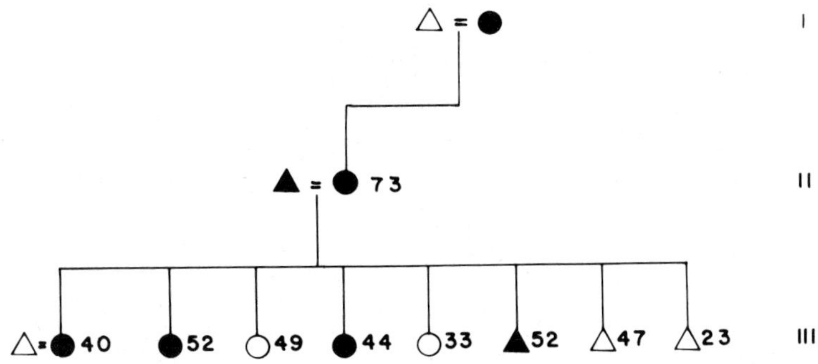

Figure 23 In conjugal psoriasis, offspring are the product of two related parents with psoriasis.

Hoede (190) published 15 cases of half-sibships. In two cases, the common parent was affected, and among the half-siblings one had psoriasis, whereas the other eight were unaffected. In 13 cases, the common parent was unaffected. Among the half-siblings there was one case of psoriasis among 35 healthy children.

Romanus (333) reported two cases in which the common parent had psoriasis. Among the half-siblings, there were three cases of psoriasis. The size of the sibship is not stated. There was no case of psoriasis among half-siblings whose common parent was unaffected. The number of these half-sibling relationships is not given.

Genetic Models

Various genetic models have been suggested to account for the heritability of psoriasis (264,361,397).

Autosomal Dominant Inheritance

The data of Hoede indicate that the frequency of psoriasis among siblings of the probands is 4.5% in families with unaffected parents and 11% when one of the parents had psoriasis. From this, Hoede (190) suggests that the distribution of psoriasis in these families was by autosomal dominant pattern. This mode of inheritance has been supported by a number of investigators, including Abele et al. (1), Montagnani and Rossi (276), and Marcusson et al. (255).

Recessive Inheritance

Steinberg et al. (359) found similar results, but interpreted their findings by negating the autosomal dominance hypothesis and selected double recessive genes as being responsible for the onset of psoriasis.

Cao et al. (63) investigated 34 psoriatic patients in 12 Chinese families and 21 healthy persons. The phenotype frequencies of HLA A-1, B13, B17, Cw4, and Cw6 in the patients were higher than those in the controls. The LOD score for six families showed that there was a close linkage between the gene of psoriasis and the HLA antigens, which prompted the investigators to consider that psoriasis may be controlled by a recessive gene(s) linked to the HLA zone.

In a large epidemiological study, Swanbeck and coworkers (374) inspected 5197 families with psoriasis. Psoriasis was present in the parents of about 36% of the probands. According to the authors, in families in which *one* or *both* parents have psoriasis, the occurrence of the disease among the siblings does not provide any information that can differentiate between a dominant and recessive mode of inheritance, but is compatible with both. In families with *neither* parent affected, the probability of the siblings suffering from psoriasis was close to 0.25, indicating a recessive mode of inheritance. The distribution of psoriasis among the parents of all probands, and among their children, was also compatible with the recessive mode of inheritance. Swanbeck et al. compared their data with that of Lomholt to underscore that the latter's data fit the recessive mode of inheritance: *psoriasis among parents*: Swanbeck, 18%, and Lomholt, 21%; *psoriasis among siblings*, Swanbeck, 16%, and Lomholt, 16%; and *psoriasis among children*, Swanbeck, 15%, and Lomholt, 12%.

Multifactorial Inheritance

As discussed earlier, in the multifactorial mode of inheritance, both genetic and environmental factors play a part in the expression of psoriasis (10,11). Multifactorial disorders may be distributed along a continuum. Figure 25 demonstrates a number of disorders in which both genetic and environmental factors contribute to the manifestation of psoriasis. They vary from

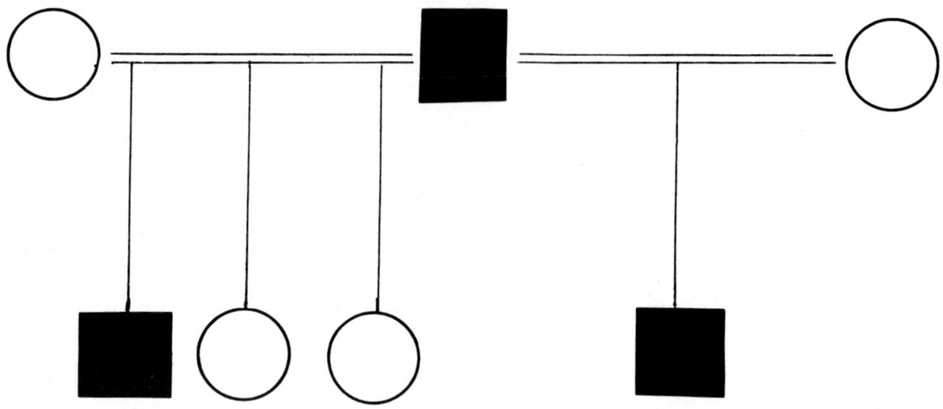

Figure 24 Half-sibships provide an opportunity to trace the mode of inheritance in two marriages in which the common partner has psoriasis.

phenylketonuria, which is caused by a single recessive gene influenced by diet, to duodenal ulcer, where there is a twofold risk in nonsecretors with blood group O as compared with the general population. From the studies of Watson and his group (404), inheritability of psoriasis was calculated to be 65%, which would place this disease toward the genetic end of the continuum.

In 1961, Vogel (396) suggested a multifactorial inheritance pattern for psoriasis. Farber et al. (404) have advocated this hypothesis. Falconer (117) and Edward (109) have developed methods for estimating quantitatively the relative importance of genetic and environmental factors in multifactorial settings. Falconer coined the term *heritability*, which he defined as the additive genetic variance to the environmental variance. The heritability estimates stemming from several genetic studies are given in Table 10.

Cann (62) has indicated that linkage analysis with batteries of efficient genetic markers of families with multiple affected individuals offers promise of locating one or more genes involved in psoriasis. Evidence of coinheritance of the phenotype and a marker can be interpreted as localizing one of the genes in the multifactorial process as being linked to the marker locus. Localization of a locus involved in multifactorial inheritance of a genetic disorder will be the first step in learning about its contribution to disease determination. Such an approach can be applied to psoriasis in an attempt to localize, in addition to an HLA-linked locus identified by population association, a second genetic locus involved in determination of this disease.

Through the identification of oncogenes, a great deal of insight has been gained into the mechanism of cancer. It has been proposed by Mansbridge and associates (252) that the mutations seen in psoriasis occur in a gene (or genes) analogous to oncogenes, and they coined the term "psoriagene" to express the

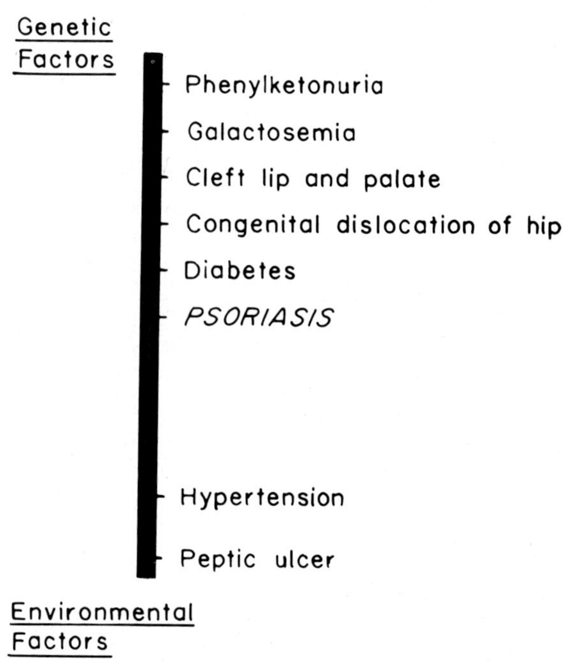

Figure 25 Multifactorial inheritance can be illustrated on a continuum with genetic and environmental factors at either end of a column. (From Ref. 264.)

Table 10 Estimates of Heritability for Psoriasis

Ref.	Geographic location	% Heritability
183	Sweden	52
277	Russia	60–70
242	China	63
404	USA	65
371	Sweden	69
243	Sweden	79
103	Australia	80
47	Denmark	90

gene(s) responsible for the onset and course of psoriasis.

CONCLUSIONS: FUTURE ROLE OF EPIDEMIOLOGY IN PSORIASIS RESEARCH

Unraveling the questions of the etiology of psoriasis is one of the most complex problems facing investigators in the field of psoriasis research today. Within the last decades advances in the knowledge of the biochemical, immunological, and genetic aspects of this disorder have brought us closer to the etiology of psoriasis, which in turn one day will lead to more effective therapeutic modalities for its control, and possibly its cure.

Epidemiologists, clinicians, and geneticists should be urged to concentrate their thinking toward the contribution that population genetics can make to epidemiology. In doing so, they will recognize that current epidemiological problems concerning diseases of unknown etiology can be fully elucidated only if genetic factors are considered and studied concurrently with environmental factors.

While the cause of psoriasis remains an enigma, certain triggers are known to increase its morbidity. Alertness to these factors can provide information to physician and patient that will help to lessen the morbidity (345) and prevent the worsening of the disease. The term "disability prevention" (80) means extending the services of physicians and others to deal systematically with two kinds of factors involved in disease development: the genetic and environmental components (128,413).

Epidemiology not only serves medical science by identifying determinants and distribution of disease, but it also provides the clinician with a profile of factors to better understand the etiology and management of a disorder. As the application of epidemiological methods to the study of psoriasis and other dermatoses of unknown cause and pathogenesis grows, data-gathering techniques will eventually become standardized.

When reviewing the items we had projected in the 1990 edition of this book for future psoriasis research, we find that each forecast has found its mark: (1) the development of biometric techniques for estimating extent and severity of psoriasis lesions (156–158,187,292,400), (2) employment of advanced computerized models for recording and displaying medical and pedigree information (251,288) and (3) the application of new mathematical methods for assessing patient outcome following therapy with the aim of improving life for psoriasis patients (157,158).

Now we look forward to the future of epidemiological research and its relationship to the clinical and experimental aspects of psoriasis. We suggest emphasizing the following:

1. For today: Through a multidisciplinary approach, consider controlling psoriasis through the concept of the Farber Regimen of Total Care, developed at the Psoriasis Research Institute (146). In addition to exemplary medical treatment, we include modification of the patient's everyday life-style encompassing nutrition, exercise, and stress-reduction programs, and recommend reading materials and audiovisual tapes for patient education (393). Adherence to a *Total Care* program over a period of time, making changes in life-style when relevant, and developing an understanding of the mind/body connection in a stress-related disease will yield a lowering of the morbidity of psoriasis (139,156).
2. Toward tomorrow: Continue the search for the psoriasis susceptibility gene(s). Psoriasis is a candidate disease that will be amenable to gene therapy using various delivery systems such as a gene "gun" or liposomes (172,215).
3. Underscoring the concept of *disability prevention* is a main function of epidemiology to prevent and control psoriasis as well as promoting attitudes of wellness (129).
4. Expand alternative/complementary medicine (153,199,263,308,428) as holistic approaches to healing are being studied empirically. The

availability of alternative therapies, for many health problems is a well-documented historical fact in both Western medicine and ethnomedicine. Table 11 is a selected listing of complementary and alternative forms of techniques.

At the Psoriasis Research Institute we are contemplating a preliminary clinical study on the application of stress-reduction techniques as adjunct therapies to traditional treatment modalities of psoriasis with the aim of inducing earlier clearing and longer remissions as well as lowering the costs of a lifelong disease (191).

5. Participate in the World Wide Web to bring scientific people and their research findings closer together. In so doing, standardized and uniform data collection techniques will be established and findings can be compared.

As a closing statement, we concur with colleague and fellow epidemiologist Robert Stern, who so succinctly places epidemiological research in its proper perspective in dermatology with these words: "Although there has been an explosion in information concerning the genetic immunology of psoriasis, epidemiological investigations are likely to be the source of much of the most important and clinically relevant information about psoriasis and its treatment. Well controlled epidemiological studies are essential in identification of risk factors for the development and exacerbation of psoriasis as well as for the assessment of the risks and benefits of therapy including the identification of the characteristics of patient subgroups, who are most likely to benefit from or are at highest risk of the adverse effects of a treatment" (362).

Table 11 Selected List of Forms of Complementary and Alternative Therapies

Acupuncture
Aromatherapy
Biofeedback
Centering
Chinese medicine
Chiropody
Conditioning
Guided imagery
Dance/movement therapy
Herbal medicine
Homeopathy
Massage therapy
Mediation
Music therapy
Native Indian medicine
Naturopathy
Progressive relaxation
T'ai Chi
Therapeutic touch
Yoga

REFERENCES

1. Abele, D.C., Dobson, R.L., and Graham, J.B. (1963). Heredity and psoriasis; study of a large family. *Arch. Dermatol.* 88:38–47.
2. Adam, B.A. (1980). Psoriasis in hospital population. *Med. J. Malaysia* 34:370–374.
3. Al'Abadie, M.S., Kent, G.G., and Gawkrodger, D.J. (1994). The relationship between stress and the onset of psoriasis and other skin conditions. *Br. J. Dermatol.* 130:199–203.
4. Albert, E.D., Mickey, M.R., and Terasaki, P.I. (1971). Genetics of four new HL-A specificities in the Causasian and Negro populations. *Transplant Proc.* 3: 95–100.
5. Al-Fouzan, A.B., and Nanda, A. (1994). A survey of childhood psoriasis in Kuwait. *Pediatr. Dermatol.* 11: 116–119.
6. Allen, A.M. (1978). Epidemiologic methods in dermatology, Part 1: Describing the occurrence of disease in human populations. *J. Int. Dermatol.* 3: 186–193.
7. Allen, G. (1976). Scope and methodology of twin studies. *Acta Genet. Med. Gemellol.* 25:79–85.
8. Allsopp, C.E.M., Harding, R.M., Taylor, C., Bunce, M., Kwiatkowski, D., Anstey, N., Brewster, D., McMichael, A.J., Greenwood, B.M., and Hill, A.V.S. (1992). Interethnic genetic differentiation in Africa: HLA class I antigens in The Gambia. *Am. J. Hum. Genet.* 50:411–421.
9. Amar, A., Rubinstein, N., Cohen, O., Hacham-Zadeh, S., Cohen, T., and Brautbar, C. (1984). HLA determinants in psoriasis vulgaris in Israel. *Tissue Antigens* 24:247–249.
10. Ananthakrishnan, R., Eckes, L., and Walter, H. (1973). On the genetics of psoriasis: an analysis of Hellgren's data for a model of multifactorial inheritance. *Arch. Dermatol. Forsch.* 247:53–58.
11. Ananthakrishnan, R., Eckes, L., and Walter, H. (1974). On the genetics of psoriasis: an analysis of Lomholt's data from Faroe Islands for a multifactorial mode of inheritance. *J. Genet.* 61:142–146.
12. Andressen, C., and Henseler, T. (1982). Erblichkeit der psoriasis: eine analyse von 2035 familienanamnesen. *Hautarzt* 33:214–217.

13. Aoki, T. (1971). Psoriasis in Japan. *Arch. Dermatol.* 104:328–329.
14. Armstrong, B.K., and Kricker, A. (1995). Skin cancer; dermatoepidemiology. *Dermatol. Clin.* 13: 583–594.
15. Asboe-Hansen, G. (1971). Psoriasis in childhood. In *Psoriasis: Proceedings of an International Symposium.* E.M. Farber and A.J. Cox (Eds.). Stanford University Press, Stanford, CA, pp. 53–59.
16. Asahina, A., Akazaki, S., Nakagawa, H., Kuwata, S., Tokunaga, K., Ishibashi, Y., and Juji, T. (1991). Specific nucleotide sequence of HLA-C is strongly associated with psoriasis vulgaris. *J. Invest. Dermatol.* 97:254–258.
17. Aschner, B., Cuth, H.O., and Gross, P. (1957). Genetic aspects of psoriasis. *Acta Genet. (Basel)* 7: 197–207.
18. Balner, H. (1971). The leukocyte antigens of rhesus monkeys and chimpanzees; current state and results of the First Primate Histocompatibility Workshop. In *Histocompatibility Testing.* J. Dausset and J. Colombani (Eds.) Munksgaard, Copenhagen, pp. 39–48.
19. Balyavichene, C.R. (1969). Psoriasis and heredity. *Vest. Dermatol. Vener.* 43:31–35.
20. Banerjee, B.N., and Datta, A.K. (1973). Prevalence and incidence patterns of skin diseases in Calcutta. *Int. J. Dermatol.* 12:41–47.
21. Baran, E. (1971). Some statistical data on psoriatics treated at the Department of Dermatology of the Medical Academy in Wroclaw from 1953 to 1968 in the light of the literature. *Przegl. Dermatol.* 58: 291–296.
22. Barisic-Drusko, V., Paljan, D., Kansky, A., and Vujasinovic, S. (1989). Prevalence of psoriasis in Croatia. *Acta Dermatol. Venereol. (Stockh.)* (Suppl.) 146: 178–179.
23. Bashir, H.V., MacQueen, J.M., Amos, D.B., Guinan, J.J., Johnston, J.M., Brotherton, J.V.M., Boettcher, B., and Ashton, G.J. (1973). A study of the HL-A system in an Australian Aboriginal population. In *Histocompatibility Testing 1972.* J. Dausset and J. Colombani (Eds.). Munksgaard, Copenhagen, pp. 311–316.
24. Bates, C., Van Dam, C., and Horrobin, D.F. (1985). Plasma essential fatty acids in pure and mixed race American Indians on and off a diet exceptionally rich in salmon. *Prostaglandins Leukotrienes Med.* 17: 77–84.
25. Baughman, R.D., Landee, R.H., Maloney, M.E., and Stern, R.S. (1982). Psoriasis and alcohol. In *Psoriasis. Proceedings of the Third International Symposium.* E.M. Farber, A.J. Cox, L. Nall, and P.H. Jacobs (Eds.) Grune & Stratton, New York, pp. 323–324.
26. Beales, A., and Farber, E.M. (1974). Unpublished data.
27. Beckman, G., Beckman, L., and Liden, S. (1980). Association between psoriasis and the alpha 1-antitrypsin deficiency gene Z. *Acta Dermatol. Venereol. (Stockh.)* 60:163–164.
28. Beckman, L. (1959). A contribution to the physical anthropology and population genetics of Sweden: variations of the ABO, Rh, MN and P blood groups. *Hereditas* 45:1–189.
29. Beckman, L., Bergdahl, K., Cedergren, B., and Liden, S. (1977). Genetic markers in psoriasis. Correlations to age at onset, continuity of symptoms, and the risk of developing the disease. *Acta Dermatol. Venereol. (Stockh.)* 57:247–251.
30. Beckman, L., and Frohlander, N. (1990). Heterozygosity effects in studies of genetic markers and disease. *Hum. Hered.* 40:322–329.
31. Bedi, T.R. (1977). Psoriasis in North India: geographic variations. *Dermatologica* 155:310–314.
32. Bell, L.M., Sedlack, R., Beard, C.M., Perry, O.P., Michet, C.J., and Kurland, L.T. (1991). Incidence of psoriasis in Rochester, MN, 1980–1983. *Arch. Dermatol.* 127:1184–1187.
33. Benacerraf, B. (1981). Role of MRC gene products in immune regulation. *Science* 213:1229–1238.
34. Berkson, J. (1946). Limitations of the application of fourfold table analysis to hospital data. *Biometrics Bull.* 1:47–53.
35. Bertrams, J., Lattke, C., and Kuwert, E. (1974). Correlation of antistreptolysin-O titer to HL-A 13 in psoriasis. *N. Engl. J. Med.* 291:631.
36. Beylot, C. (1991). Specific aspects of psoriasis in children. *Rev. Praticien* 41:2169–2173.
37. Bhate, S.M., Sharpe, G.R., Marks, J.M., Shuster, S., and Ross, W.M. (1993). Prevalence of skin and other cancers in patients with psoriasis. *Clin. Exp. Dermatol.* 18:401–404.
38. Binazzi, M., Calandra, P., and Lisi, P. (1975). Statistical association between psoriasis and diabetes: further results. *Arch. Dermatol. Res.* 254:43–48.
39. Bodmer, J.G., Marsh, S.G.E., Ekkehard, D.A., Bodmer, W.F., Bontrop, R.E., Charron, D., Dupont, B., Erlich, H.A., Mach, B., Mayr, W.F., Parham, P., Sasazuki, T., Schreuder, G.M.T., Strominger, J.L., Svejgaard, A., and Terasaki, P.I. (1995). Nomenclature for factors of the HLA system, 1995. *Tissue Antigens,* 46:1–18.
40. Bodmer, W.F. (1972). Evolutionary significance of the HL-A system. *Nature* 237:139–145.
41. Bodmer, W.F. (1978). The HLA system. *Br. Med. Bull.* 34:213–316.
42. Bortolini, M.C., Weimer, T.A., Franco, M.H., Salzano, F.M., Layrisse, Z., Schneider, H., Schneider, M.P., and Harada, ML. (1992). Genetic studies in three South American black populations. *Gene Geograph.* 6:1–16.
43. Bowcock, A.M., Kidd, J.R., Mountain, J.L., Hebert, J.M., Cartenuto, L., Kidd, K.K., and Cavalli-Sforza, L.L. (1991). Drift, admixture, and selection in human

evolution: a study with DNA polymorphisms. *Proc. Natl. Acad. Sci. USA* 88:839–843.

44. Bowker, N.C., Cross, K.W., Fairburn, E.A., and Wall, M. (1976). Sociological implications of an epidemiological study of eczema in the city of Birmingham. *Br. J. Dermatol.* 95:137–144.
45. Braathen, L.R., Botten, G., and Bjerkedal, T. (1989). Prevalence of psoriasis in Norway. *Acta Dermatol. Venereol. (Stockh.)* (Suppl.) 142:5–8.
46. Braathen, L.R., Botten, G., and Bjerkedal, T. (1989). Psoriatics in Norway. A questionnaire study on health status, contact with paramedical professions, and alcohol and tobacco consumption. *Acta Dermatol. Venereol. (Stockh.)* (Suppl.) 142:9–12.
47. Brandrup, F., Hauge, M., Henningsen, K., and Eriksen, B. (1978). Psoriasis in an unselected series of twins. *Arch. Dermatol.* 114:874–878.
48. Brandrup, F., and Green, A. (1981). Prevalence of psoriasis in Denmark. *Acta Dermatol. Venereol. (Stockh.)* 61:344–346.
49. Brandrup, F., Holm, N., Grunnet, N., Henningsen, K., and Hansen, H.E. (1982). Psoriasis in monozygotic twins: variations in expression in individuals with identical genetic constitution. *Acta Dermatol. Venereol. (Stockh.)* 62:229–236.
50. Brandrup, F. (1984). Psoriasis in first-degree relatives of psoriatic twins. *Acta Dermatol. Venereol. (Stockh.)* 64:220–226.
51. Brandrup, F. (1985). *Aetiological Studies of Psoriasis. A Survey.* Odense University Press, Odense, Denmark.
52. Brandrup, F. (1987). The use of twins in etiological studies of psoriasis. In *Psoriasis. Proceedings of the Fourth International Symposium.* E.M. Farber, L. Nall, V. Morhenn, and P.H. Jacobs (Eds.). Elsevier, New York, pp. 401–402.
53. Braun-Falco, O., Burg, G., and Farber, E.M. (1972). Psoriasis: eine Fragebogenstudie bei 536 Patienten. *Munch. Med. Wochenschr.* 114:1–15.
54. Brenner, W., Gschnait, F., and Mayr, W.R. (1978). HLA B13, W17, B37, and Cw6 in psoriasis vulgaris: association with the age of onset. *Arch. Dermatol. Res.* 262:337–339.
55. Buntin, D.M., Skinner, R.B., and Rosenberg, E.W. (1983). Onset of psoriasis at age 108. *J. Am. Acad. Dermatol.* 9:276–277.
56. Burch, P.R.J., and Rowell, N.R. (1965). Psoriasis: aetiological aspects. *Acta Dermatol. Venereol. (Stockh.)* 45:366–380.
57. Burch, P.F.J., and Rowell, N.R. (1981). Mode of inheritance in psoriasis. *Arch. Dermatol.* 117:251.
58. Burton, J.L., Savin, J.A., and Champion, R.H. (1994). Introduction, epidemiology, and historical bibliography. In *Rook/Wilkinson/Ebling Textbook of Dermatology.* 5th ed., Vol 1. R.H. Champion, J.L. Burton, and F.J.G. Ebling. Blackwell Scientific Publications, Oxford, pp. 4–9.
59. Canizares, O. (1961). Geographic dermatology: Mexico and Central America. *Arch. Dermatol.* 82: 870–893.
60. Canizares, O. (1982). *A Manual of Dermatology in Developing Countries.* Oxford University, Oxford.
61. Cann, H.M., Bodmer, J.G., and Bodmer, W.F. (1973). The HL-A polymorphism in Mayan Indians of San Juan La Laguna, Guatemala. In *Histocompatibility Testing* 1972. J. Dausett and J. Colomani (Eds.). Munksgaard, Copenhagen, pp. 367–375.
62. Cann H. (1987). Linkage mapping of the human genome. Relevance for genetic disease. In *Psoriasis. Proceedings of the Fourth International Symposium.* E.M. Farber, L. Nall, V. Morhenn, and P.H. Jacobs (Eds.). Elsevier, New York, pp. 283–293.
63. Cao, K., Song, F-J., Li, H-G., Hu, S-Y., Liu, Z-H, Su, X-han, and Wang, F-X. (1993). Association between HLA antigen and families with psoriasis vulgaris. *Chinese Med. J.* 106:132–135.
64. Carmelli, D., and Andersen, S. (1981). A longevity study of twins in the Mormon genealogy. In *Twin Research 3.* Part C. *Epidemiology and Clinical Studies.* Alan R. Liss, New York, pp. 187–200.
65. Cats, A. (1971). Psoriasis and arthritis. In *Psoriasis. Proceedings of an International Symposium.* E.M. Farber and A.J. Cox (Eds.). Stanford University Press, Stanford, CA, pp. 127–136.
66. Cats, A., van Romunde, L.K.J., Schreuder, I., Valkenburg, M.A., and Colenbrander, H. (1977). Arthritis and psoriasis. Recent findings. In *Psoriasis: Proceedings of the Second International Symposium.* E.M. Farber and A.J. Cox (Eds.). Yorke Medical Books, New York, pp. 155–162.
67. Cavalli-Sforza, L.L. (1975). Genetics of human populations. In *Biological Anthropology.* S.H. Katz (Ed.). W.H. Freeman, San Francisco, pp. 265–273.
68. Cavalli-Sforza, L.L. (1991). Genes, people, and languages. *Sci. Am.* Nov. 1991:104–110.
69. Cavalli-Sforza, L.L., Piazza, A., Menozzi, P., and Mountain, J. (1988). Reconstruction of human evolution: Bringing together genetic, archaeological, and linguistic data. *Proc. Natl. Acad. Sci. USA* 85: 6002–6006.
70. Cavalli-Sforza, L.L., Menozzi, P., and Piazza, A. (1994). *The History and Geography of Human Genes.* Princeton University Press, Princeton, N.J.
71. Chakraborty, R., Kamboh, M.I., Nwankwo, M., and Ferrell, R.E. (1992). Caucasian genes in American blacks. New data. *Am. J. Hum. Genet.* 50:145–155.
72. Chan, S.H. (1983). HLA and skin disease in the Chinese. *Ann. Acad. Med. (Singapore)* 12:3–5.
73. Chan, S.H., and Wee, G.B. (1979). Association of Bw46 and Cw1/Cw3 in the Chinese. *Tissue Antigens* 14:179–180.

74. Chan, S.H., Tan, T., Wee, G.B., Kamarudin, A., and Rajan, V.S. (1981). HLA and psoriasis in the Chinese. *Dermatologica* 163:348–352.
75. Chapel, H., and Haeney, M. (1993). *Essentials of Clinical Immunology.* Blackwell Scientific Publications, Oxford.
76. Chren, M-M. (1995). Dermatologic health services research. *Dermatol. Clin.* 13:689–694.
77. Christophers, E., and Henseler, T. (1987). Psoriasis of early onset is distinct from psoriasis of late onset. Characterization of type I and type II psoriasis. In *Psoriasis. Proceedings of the Fourth International Symposium.* E.M. Farber, L. Nall, V. Morhenn, and P.H. Jacobs (Eds.). Elsevier, New York, pp. 309–315.
78. Chuang, E.-Y., and Reizner, G.T. (1993). Dermatoepidemiology. Part 1. Epidemiologic methods. *Int. J. Dermatol.* 32:251–256.
79. Chua-Ty, G., Goh, C.L., and Koh, S.L. (1992). Pattern of skin diseases at the National Skin Centre (Singapore) from 1989–1990. *Int J. Dermatol.* 31:555–559.
80. Clark, D.W., and MacMahan, B. (1981). *Preventive and Community Medicine.* Little, Brown, Boston.
81. Clifford, C.A., and Hopper, J.L. (1986). The Australian NHMRC Twin Registry: a resource for the Australian scientific community. *Med. J. Aust.* 609:149.
82. Convit, J. (1963). Investigation of incidence of psoriasis among Latin American Indians. In *Proceedings of the 12th International Congress of Dermatology.* Washington 1962. Int Congress Series No. 55. Excerpta Medica Foundation, Amsterdam, pp. 196–199.
83. Coopman, S.A., Johnson, R.A., Platt, R., and Stern, R.S. (1993). Cutaneous disease and drug reactions in HIV infection. *N. Engl. J. Med.* 328:1670–1674.
84. Corey, L.A., and Nance, W.E. (1978). Monozygotic half-sib model: a tool for epidemiologic research. In *Twin Research. Proceedings of the Second International Congress on Twin Studies.* Aug. 29-Sept. 1, 1977. Part A: *Psychology and Methodology.* W.E. Nance, G. Allen, and P. Parisi (Eds.). Alan R. Liss, New York, pp. 201–209.
85. Corley, R.D., Spees, E.K., Cabrera, G.-M., Swanson, J.L., and Amos, D.B. (1973). HL-A antigens of the Guatemalan Ixils. In *Histocompatibility Testing* 1972. J. Dausset and J. Colomani (Eds.). Munksgaard, Copenhagen, pp. 351–357.
86. Crivellato, E., and Zacchi, T. (1985). Sistema HLA e psoriasi: uno studio de poplazione. *G. Ital. Dermatol. Venereol.* 120:103–108.
87. Crivellato, E., and Zacchi, T. (1985). Sistema HLA e psoriasi: uno studio su famiglie. *G. Ital. Dermatol. Venereol.* 120:247–254.
88. Crivellato, E., and Zacchi, T. (1986). Sistema HLA e psoriasi. Influenza di alcuni "antigeni psoriasici" sulle caratteristiche cliniche della malattia. *G. Ital. Dermatol. Venereol.* 121:173–178.
89. Crivellato, E., and Zacchi, T. (1987). Sistema HLA e psoriasi. Analisi delle interazioni tra antigeni HLA predisponenti. *G. Ital. Dermatol Venereol.* 122:25–28.
90. Cross, R.A., Alpers, M.P., York, T.J., Davey, M.G., Pollard, M., Kirk, R.L., Blake, N.M., McDermid, E.M., Law, W., and Morris, P.J. (1973). Studies of HL-A in Australian Aborigines. In *Histocompatibility Testing 1972.* J. Dausset and J. Colombina (Eds.). Munksgaard, Copenhagen, 1973, pp. 303–310.
91. Dahl, M.V. (1988). *Clinical Immunodermatology*, 2nd ed. Year Book Medical Publishers, Chicago, pp. 89–105.
92. Dausset, J. (1981). Major histocompatibility complex in man. *Science* 213:1469–1474.
93. Dausset, J., and Hors, J. (1975). Some contributions of the HL-A complex to the genetics of human diseases. *Transplant Rev.* 22:44–74.
94. del Toso-Depeder, Z. (1993). Prevalence of psoriasis in the Karlovac region. *Lijecnicki Vjesnik* 115:21–27.
95. del Toso-Depeder, Z. (1993). Familial aggregation in psoriasis. *Lijecnicki Vjesnik* 115:65–69.
96. Dick, H.M. (1978). HLA and disease: introductory review. *Br. Med. Bull.* 34:217–271.
97. Dorf, M.E., and Haber, J.A. (1972). Leukocyte antigens of primates. In *Primates in Medicine.* C. Kratochvil (Ed.). S. Karger, Basel, pp. 67–114.
98. Dorfman, R.A., Lubben, J.E., Mayer-Oakes, A., Atchison, K., Schweitzer, S.O., De Jong, F.J., and Matthias, R.E. (1995). Screening for depression among a well elderly population. *Social Work* 40:295–304.
99. Dorivitch, A., Cohen-Adad, G., Jabotinsky-Rubin, K., and Durst, R. (1994). Lithium-associated psoriasis. *Harefuah* 127:228–229, 287.
100. Dorn, H. (1957). Psoriasis als Erbleden unter besonderer berucksichtigung der mutationsrate. *Z. Haut.-Beschikr.* 22:110–119.
101. Dossetor, J.B., Howson, W.T., Schlaut, J., McConnachie, P.R., Alton, J.D.M., Lockwood, B., and Olson, L. (1973). Study of the HL-A system in two Canadian Eskimo populations. In *Histocompatibility Testing 1972.* J. Dausset and J. Colomani (Eds.). Munksgaard, Copenhagen, pp. 325–332.
102. Dossetor, J.B., Schlaut, J.W., Olson, L., Alton, J.M., Kovithavongs, T., and McConnachie, P.R. (1974). Histocompatibility studies on Canadian Inuit (Eskimo). In *Circumpolar Health.* J. Dausset and J. Colomani (Eds.). Munksgaard, Copenhagen, pp. 325–332.
103. Duffy, D.L., Spelman, L.S., and Martin, N.G. (1993). Psoriasis in Australian twins. *J. Am. Acad. Dermatol.* 29:428–434.
104. du Toit, E.D., MacGregor, K.J., Taljaard, D.G., and Oudshoorn, M. (1988). HLA-A, B, C, DR and DQ polymorphisms in three South African population groups: South African Negroes, Cape Coloureds and

South African Caucasoids. *Tissue Antigens* 31: 109–125.
105. Duvic, M., Johnson, T.M., Rapini, R.P., Freese, T., Brewton, G., and Rios, A. (1987). Acquired immunodeficiency syndrome-associated psoriasis and Reiter's syndrome. *Arch. Dermatol.* 123:1622–1632.
106. Eckes, L. (1978). Psoriasis und Lepro in Schicksal gemeinsamer Geschichte. *Hautartz* 29:331–336.
107. Eckes, L., Ananthakrishnan, R., and Walter, H. (1975). Zur geographischen Verteilung der Psoriasis. *Hautarzt* 26:563–567.
108. Economidou, J., Papasteriades, C., Varia-Leftherioti, M., and Stratigos, J. (1985). Human lymphocyte antigens A, B, and C in Greek patients with psoriasis: relation to age and clinical expression of the disease. *J. Am. Acad. Dermatol.* 13:578–582.
109. Edwards, J.H. (1969). Familial predisposition in man. *Br. Med. Bull.* 25:58–64.
110. El Zawahry, M. (1963). Psoriasis: its atypical clinical varieties. *J. Egypt. Med. Assoc.* 47:1213–1217.
111. Elder, J.T., Nair, R.P., and Voorhees, J.J. (1994). Epidemiology and the genetics of psoriasis. *J. Invest. Dermatol.* 102:24S–27S.
112. Elder, J.T., Henseler, T., Christophers, E., Voorhees, J.J., and Nair, R.P. (1994). Of genes and antigens: the inheritance of psoriasis. *J. Invest. Dermatol.* 103: 150S–153S.
113. Elder, J.T., Nair, R.P., Guo, S.-W., Henseler, T., Christophers, E., and Voorhees, J.J. (1994). The genetics of psoriasis. *Arch. Dermatol.* 130:216–224.
114. Emokpare, N.A. (1976). Psoriasis in Nigeria. *Int. Ps. Bull.* 3(1):1.
115. Failmezger, T.C. (1978). A clinical survey of skin diseases in selected Latin American countries. *Int. J. Dermatol.* 17:583–591.
116. Failmezger, T.C. (1992). Incidence of skin diseases in Cuzco, Peru. *Int. J. Dermatol* 31:560–561.
117. Falconer, D.S. (1965). The inheritance of liability to certain diseases estimated from the incidence among relatives. *Ann. Hum. Genet.* 29:51–76.
118. Falk, E.S. and Vandbakk, O. (1993). Prevalence of psoriasis in a Norwegian Lapp population. *Acta Dermatol. Venereol. (Stockh.)* (Suppl.) 182:6–9.
119. Farber, E.M. (1992). Ear psoriasis. *Cutis* 50:105–107.
120. Farber, E.M. (1992). Facial psoriasis. *Cutis* 50:25–28.
121. Farber, E.M., and Peterson, J.B. (1961). Variations in the natural history of psoriasis. *Calif. Med.* 95:6–11.
122. Farber, E.M., Bright, R.D., and Nall, M.L. (1968). Psoriasis. A questionnaire survey of 2,144 patients. *Arch. Dermatol.* 98:248–259.
123. Farber, E.M., Jacobs, P.H., and Nall, M.L. (1974) Relationship of mild to severe psoriasis. *Cutis* 13: 774–777.
124. Farber, E.M., and Nall, M.L. (1974). The natural history of 5,600 patients. *Dermatologica* 148:1–18.
125. Farber, E.M., Nall, M.L., and Watson, W. (1974). Natural history of psoriasis in 61 twin pairs. *Arch. Dermatol.* 109:207–211.
126. Faber, E.M., and Jacobs, A. (1977). Infantile psoriasis. *Am. J. Dis. Child.* 131:1255–1269.
127. Farber, E.M., and Nall, M.L. (1983). Epidemiology in psoriasis research. *Hawaii Med. J.* 41:430–442.
128. Farber, E.M., Nall, M.L. (1983). Symposium on etiology and pathogenesis: an overview. In *Proceedings of the XVI International Congress of Dermatology, May 23–28, 1982, Tokyo*. Kukilo, A., and M. Seiji (Eds.). University of Tokyo Press, Tokyo, pp. 363–380.
129. Farber, E.M., and Nall, L. (1983). An appraisal of measures to prevent and control psoriasis. *J. Am. Acad. Dermatol.* 10:511–517.
130. Farber, E.M., Mullen, R.H., Jacobs, A.H., and Nall. L. (1986). Infantile psoriasis. A follow-up study. *Pediatr. Dermatol.* 3:237–243.
131. Farber, E.M., and Nall, L. (1992). Natural history and treatment of scalp psoriasis. *Cutis* 49:396–400.
132. Farber, E.M., and Nall, L. (1992). Nail psoriasis. *Cutis* 50:174–178.
133. Farber, E.M., and Nall, L. (1992). Genital psoriasis. *Cutis* 50:263–265.
134. Farber, E.M., and Nall, L. (1992). Perianal and intergluteal psoriasis. *Cutis* 50:336–338.
135. Farber, E.M., and Nall, L. (1992). Nonpustular palmoplantar psoriasis. *Cutis* 50:407–410.
136. Farber, E.M., and Nall, L. (1993). Pustular psoriasis. *Cutis* 51:29–32.
137. Farber, E.M., and Nall, L. (1993). Erythrodermic (exfoliative) psoriasis. *Cutis* 51:79–82.
138. Farber, E.M., and Nall, L. (1993). Guttate psoriasis. *Cutis* 51:157–164.
139. Farber, E.M., and Nall, L. (1993). The office visit and the self-help concept in treating the patient with psoriasis: a strategy revisited. *Cutis* 51:236–240.
140. Farber, E.M., and Nall, L. (1993). Psoriasis: a stress-related disease. *Cutis* 51:322–326.
141. Farber, E.M., and Nall, L. (1993). Psoriasis associated with human immunodeficiency virus/acquired immunodeficiency syndrome. *Cutis* 52:29–35.
142. Farber, E.M., and Nall, L. (1993). Psoriasis and ultraviolet radiation. *Cutis* 52:145–152.
143. Farber, E.M., and Nall, L. (1994). Psoriasis and alcoholism. *Cutis* 53:21–26.
144. Farber, E.M., and Nall, L. (1994). Psoriasis in the tropics. Epidemiologic, genetic, clinical, and therapeutic aspects. *Dermatol. Clin.* 12:805–816.
145. Farber, E.M., and Nall, L. (1997). *Conquering Psoriasis*. Empowering Press, Hamilton, Ontario, Canada.
146. Farber, E.M., Raychauduri, S.P. (1997). Concept of total care: a third dimension in the treatment of psoriasis. *Cutis* 57:35–39.

147. Festenstein, H., Adams, E., Brown, J., Burke, J., Lincoln, P., Oliver, R.T.D., Rondiak, G., Sachs, J.A., Welch, S.G., and Wolf, E. (1973). The distribution of HLA antigens and other polymorphisms in Bantu-speaking Negroids living in Zambia. In *Histocompatibility Testing 1972*. J. Dausset and J. Colomina (Eds.). Munksgaard, Copenhagen, pp. 397–407.
148. Findlay, G.H. (1967). The age incidence of common skin diseases in the white population of the Transvaal. *Br. J. Dermatol.* 79:538–542.
149. Finlay, A.Y., and Kelly, S.E. (1987). Psoriasis—an index of disability. *Clin. Exp. Dermatol* 12:8–11.
150. Finlay, A.Y., Khan, G.K., Luscombe, D.K., and Salek, M.S. (1990). Validation of Sickness Impact Profile and Psoriasis Disability Index in psoriasis. *Br. J. Dermatol.* 123:751–756.
151. Fleischer, A.B., Rapp, S.R., Reboussin, D.M. Vanarthos, J.C., and Feldman, S.R. (1994). Patient measurement of psoriasis disease severity with a structured instrument. *J. Invest. Dermatol.* 102:967–969.
152. Fleischer, A.B., Feldman, S.R., and Bradham, D.D. (1994). Office-based physician services provided by dermatologists in the United States in 1990. *J. Invest. Dermatol.* 102:93–97.
153. Fleischer, A.B., Feldman, S.R., Rapp, S.R., Reboussin, D.M., Exum, M.L., and Clark, A.R. (1996). Alternative therapies commonly used with a population of patients with psoriasis. *Cutis* 58:216–220.
154. Friedman, G.D. (1976). Medical usage and abusage: "prevalence" and "incidence." *Ann. Intern. Med.* 84: 502–504.
155. Friedman, G.D., and Lewis, A.M. (1978). The Kaiser-Permanente twin registry. In *Twin Research. Proceedings of the Second International Congress on Twin Studies, Aug. 29-Sept. 1, 1977, Washington, D.C.* Part B: *Biology and Epidemiology*. W.E. Nance, G. Allen, and P. Parisi (Eds.). Alan R. Liss, New York, pp. 173–177.
156. Fries, J.F. (1972). Time-oriented patients records and a computer databank. *J.A.M.A.* 222:1536–1542.
157. Fries, J.F. (1983). Toward an understanding of patient outcome measurement. *Arthritis Rheum.* 26:697–704.
158. Fries, J.F., Spitz, P., and Young, D.Y. (1982). The dimensions of health outcomes: the Health Assessment Questionnaire, disability and pain scale. *J. Rheumatol.* 9:789–793.
159. Ganor, S. (1978). Diseases associated with psoriasis. *Int. J. Dermatol.* 17:715–716.
160. Goh, C.L., and Akarapanth, R. (1994). Epidemiology of skin disease among children in a referral skin clinic in Singapore. *Pediatr. Dermatol.* 11:125–128.
161. Goldman, J.N., and Goldman, M.G. (1981). What the clinician should know about the major histocompatibility complex. *J.A.M.A.* 246:873–876.
162. Goldsmith, L.A. (1981). Principles of genetics as applied to dermatologic diseases. *J. Am. Acad. Dermatol.* 4:255–256.
163. Gorbulew. (1928). Falle von Psoriasis vulgaris. *Vener. Dermatol.* 5:342.
164. Goudie, R.B., Spence, J.C., and MacKie, R. (1979). Vitiligo patterns simulating autoimmune and rheumatic diseases. *Lancet* 2:393–395.
165. Goudie, R.B., Goudie, D.R., Dick, H.M., and Ferguson-Smith, M.A. (1980). Unstable mutation in vitiligo, organ specific autoimmune disease, and multiple endocrine adenoma-peptic-ulcer syndrome. *Lancet* 2:285–287.
166. Goudie, R.B., Spence, J.C., and Scothorne, R.J. (1980). Do vascular clones determine developmental patterns? *Lancet* 1:570–572.
167. Green, A. (1973). Australian aborigines. *Int. Psoriasis Bull.* 1(2):40.
168. Green, A.C. (1984). Australian Aborigines and psoriasis. *Australasian J. Dermatol* 25:18–24.
169. Greenbaum, C.H., and Beerman, H. (1965). Epidemiology of diseases of the skin. *Am. J. Med. Sci.* 250: 459–471.
170. Greenberg, L.J., Gray, E.D., and Yunis, E.J. (1975). Association of HL-A 5 and immune responsiveness in vitro to streptococcal antigens. *J. Exp. Med.* 141: 935–943.
171. Greenberg, R. (1993). *Medical Epidemiology*. Appleton & Lange, Norwalk, CT.
172. Greenhalgh, D.A., Rothnagel, J.A., and Roop, D.R. (1994). Epidermis: an attractive target tissue for gene therapy. *J. Invest. Dermatol.* 103:63S–69S.
173. Griffiths, T.W., Christophers, E., Griffiths, M., and Voorhees, J.J. (1995). Immunopathogenesis and immunotherapy of psoriasis. *Dermatol. Clin.* 13: 739–749.
174. Gross, W.L., Packhauser, U., Hahn, G., Westphal, E., Christophers, E., and Schlaak, M. (1977). Lymphocyte activation by streptococcal antigens in psoriasis. *Br. J. Dermatol.* 97:529–536.
175. Gunawardena, D.A., Gunawardena, K.A., and Vasanthanathan, J.A. (1978). Psoriasis in Sri Lanka—a computer analysis 1,366 cases. *Br. J. Dermatol.* 98: 85–96.
176. Gupta, M.A., Schork, N.J., Gupta, A.K., and Ellis, C.N. (1993). Alcohol intake and treatment responsiveness of psoriasis: a prospective study. *J. Am. Acad. Dermatol* 28:730–732.
177. Hall, R., and Burrows, D. (1968). Diagnostic review of hospital dermatology in Northern Ireland 1954–1966. *Br. J. Dermatol.* 80:261–264.
178. Hammond, M.G., Reeve, C.E., Sargent, A.V., and Betuel, H. (1977). HLA and disease: psoriasis. *Histocompatibility Testing 1977*. W.F. Bodmer (Ed.). Munksgaard, Copenhagen, pp. 230–231.

179. Harris, D.W.S., Benton, E.C., and Hunter, J.A.A. (1990). The changing face of dermatology out-patient referrals in the south-east of Scotland. *Br. J. Dermatol.* 123:745–750.

180. Harvald, B.J. (1974). Current genetic trends in the Greenlandic population. In *Circumpolar Health. Proceedings of the Third International Symposium. Yellowknife, NWT.* R.J. Shephard, S. Itoh (Eds.). Toronto University Press, Toronto, Ontario, Canada, pp. 165–169.

181. Harvald, B. (1982). Eskimo disease pattern—genes or environment. *Acta Med. Scand.* 212:97–98.

182. Hawkins, B.R., Tiwari, J.L., Lowe, N., and Wolfish, P. (1980). HLA and psoriasis. In *Histocompatibility Testing 1980.* P.I. Terasaki (Ed.). UCLA Tissue Typing Laboratory, Los Angeles, CA, pp. 711–714.

183. Hellgren, L. (1967). *Psoriasis: The Prevalence in Sex, Age, and Occupational Groups in Total Populations in Sweden. Morphology, Inheritance, and Association with Other Skin and Rheumatic Diseases.* Almqvist & Wiksell, Stockholm.

184. Henan Dermatoses Survey Group (1982). An analysis of 487 cases of psoriasis in 100,000 natural population of Henan rural district. *Chinese J. Dermatol.* 15: 83–84.

185. Henseler, T., and Christophers, E. (1985). Psoriasis of early onset distinct from psoriasis of late onset. Characterization of type I and type II psoriasis. *J. Am. Acad. Dermatol.* 13:450–456.

186. Henseler, T., and Christophers, E. (1995). Disease concomitance in psoriasis. *J. Am. Acad. Dermatol.* 32:982–986.

187. Herron, R. (1972). Biostereometrics. *Yearbook Phys. Anthropol.* 16:80–121.

188. Higgins, E.M., and duVivier, A.W. (1994) Cutaneous disease and alcohol misuse. *Br. Med. Bull.* 50:85–98.

189. Hirata, A.A., and Terasaki, P.I. (1970). Cross-reactions between streptococcal M proteins and human transplantation antigens. *Science* 168: 1095–1096.

190. Hoede, K. (1931). Umwelt und erblichkeit bei der entstehung der schuppenflechte. Wurzburg, *Habilitationsschrift.* 127:211–254.

191. Hoffman, C., Rice, D., and Sung, H-Y. (1996) Persons with chronic conditions. Their prevalence and costs. *J.A.M.A.* 276:1473–1479.

192. Holgate, M.C. (1975). The age-of-onset of psoriasis and the relationship to parental psoriasis. *Br. J. Dermatol.* 92:443–448.

193. Hrubec, Z., and Neel, J.V. (1978). The National Academy of Sciences-National Research Council Twin Registry: Ten years of operation. In *Twin Research.* Part B. *Biology and Epidemiology.* W.E. Nance, G. Allen, and P. Parisi (Eds). Alan R. Liss, New York, pp. 153–172.

194. Ikaheimo, I., Silvennoinen-Kassinen, S., J. Karvonen, and A. Tiilikainen (1994). Alanine at position 73 of HLA-C is associated with psoriasis vulgaris in Finland. *Br. J. Dermatol.* 131:257–259.

195. Ingram, J.T. (1954). The significance and management of psoriasis. *Br. Med. J.* 2:823–828.

196. Jacobs, P.H., Farber, E.M., and Nall, M.L. (1977). Psoriasis and skin cancer. In *Psoriasis: Proceedings of the Second International Symposium.* E.M. Farber and A.J. Cox (Eds.). Yorke Medical Books, New York, pp. 350–352.

197. Jacyk, W.K. (1981). Psoriasis in Nigerians. *Trop. Geogr. Med.* 33:139–142.

198. Jeannet, M., Schapira, M., Gervasoni, C., Metaxas-Buhler, M. Butler, R., and VanLughem, E. (1973). Study of the HL-A system and other polymorphisms in the Tibetan population. In *Histocompatibility Testing 1972.* J. Dausset and J. Colomani (Eds.). Munksgaard, Copenhagen, pp. 241–250.

199. Jensen, P. (1990). Use of alternative medicine by patients with atopic dermatitis and psoriasis. *Acta Dermatol. Venereol. (Stockh.)* 70:421–424.

200. Johnson, K.G. (1969). Epidemiology. In *Human Ecology and Public Health.* E.D. Kilbourn and W.G. Smilie (Eds.). Macmillan, Toronto, Ontario, Canada, pp. 125–142.

201. Johnson, M.-L. (1986). Aging in the United States population. The dermatologic implications. *Dermatol. Clin.* 4:371–376.

202. Johnson, M.-L., and Stern, R.S. (1993). Prevalence and ecology of skin disorders. In *Dermatology in General Medicine.* 4th ed. T.B. Fitzpatrick, A.Z. Eisen, K. Wolff, I.M. Freedberg, and K.F. Austen (Eds.). McGraw-Hill, New York, pp. 3–7.

203. Johnson, M.-L., and Roberts, J. (1978). Skin conditions and related need for medical care among persons 1 to 74. United States, 1971–1974. Vital and Health Statistics, Series 11. Data from National Health Survey, No. 212. DHEW Publication No. (PHS) 79-1660. Government Printing Office, Washington, D.C.

204. Kalla, G., and Goyal, A.M. (1996). Juvenile generalized pustular psoriasis. *Pediatr. Dermatol.* 13: 45–46.

205. Kaprio, J., Sarna, S., Koskenvuo, M., and Rantasalo, I. (1978). The Finnish Twin Registry: formation and compilation, questionnaire survey, zygosity determination procedure, and research program. In *Twin Research.* Part B. *Biology and Epidemiology.* W.E. Nance, G. Allen, and P. Parisi (Eds.). Alan R. Liss, New York, pp. 179–184.

206. Karvonen, J. (1975). HL-A antigens in psoriasis with special reference to the clinical type, age of onset, exacerbation after respiratory infection and occurrence of arthritis. *Ann. Clin. Res.* 7:301–311.

207. Karvonen, J., Lassus, A., and Sievers, A. (1974). HL-A antigens in psoriatic arthritis. *Ann. Clin. Res.* 6: 304.
208. Karvonen, Jr., Tiilikainen, A., and Lassus, A. (1975). HL-A antigens in patients with persistent palmoplantar pustulosis and pustular psoriasis. *Ann. Clin. Res.* 7:112–115.
209. Kavli, G., Forde, O.H., Arnesen, E., and Stenvold, S.E. (1985). Psoriasis: familial predisposition and environmental factors. *Br. Med. J.* 291:999–1000.
210. Kavli, G., Stenvold, S.E., and Vandbakk, O. (1985). Low prevalence of psoriasis in Norwegian Lapps. *Acta Dermatol. Venereol. (Stockh.)* 65:262–263.
211. Kenney, J.A. (1965). Management of dermatoses peculiar to Negroes. *Arch. Dermatol.* 91:126–129.
212. Kenney, J. (1971). Psoriasis in the American black. In: *Psoriasis: Proceedings of an International Symposium on Psoriasis.* E.M. Farber and A.J. Cox (Eds.). Stanford University Press, Stanford, CA, pp. 49–51.
213. Kerdel-Vegas, F. (1971). Psoriasis in South America: geographic and racial factors. In *Psoriasis: Proceedings of an International Symposium on Psoriasis.* E.M. Farber and A.J. Cox (Eds.). Stanford University Press, Stanford, CA, pp. 35–39.
214. Khaleque, K.A., and Basit, A. (1968). Study on psoriasis cases in East Pakistan. *J. Trop. Med. Hyg.* 7: 20–23.
215. Khavari, P.A., and Krueger, G.G. (1997). Cutaneous gene therapy. *Dermatol. Clin.* 15:27–35.
216. Kissmeyer-Nielsen, F., Kjerbye, K.E., Lamm, L.U., Jorgensen, J., Petersen, G.B., and Gurtler, H. (1973). Study of the HL-A system in Eskimos. In *Histocompatibility Testing 1972.* J. Dausset and J. Colomani (Eds.). Munksgaard, Copenhagen, pp. 317–324.
217. Klein, J., O'hUigin, C., Figueroa, F., Mayer, W.E., and Klein, D. (1993). Different modes of MHC evolution in primates. *Mol. Biol. Evol.* 10:48–59.
218. Kononen, M., Torppa, J., and Lassus, A. (1986). An epidemiological survey of psoriasis in the Greater Helsinki Area. *Acta Dermatol. Venereol. (Stockh.)* (Suppl. 124)66:1–10.
219. Krain, L.S. (1974). Histocompatibility antigens: a laboratory and epidemiologic tool. *J. Invest. Dermatol.* 62:67–73.
220. Kraning, K.K., and Odland, G.F. (Eds.). (1979). Prevalence, morbidity, and costs of dermatological diseases. *J. Invest. Dermatol.* 73:395–401.
221. Kraning, K.K., and Odland, G.F. (Eds.). (1979). I. Psoriasis. *J. Invest. Dermatol.* 73:402–413.
222. Kringlen, E. (1978). Norwegian twin registers. In *Twin Research.* Part C. *Biology and Epidemiology.* W.E. Nance, G. Allen, and P. Parisi (Eds.). Alan R. Liss, New York, pp. 185–187.
223. Krowchuk, D.P., Bradham, D.D., and Fleishcer, A.B. (1994). Dermatologic services provided to children and adolescents by primary care and other physicians in the United States. *Clin. Lab. Invest.* 11:199–203.
224. Krueger, G.G., and Duvic, M. (1994). Epidemiology of psoriasis: clinical issues. *J. Invest. Dermatol.* 102: 14S–18S.
225. Krulig, L., Farber, E.M., Grumet, F.D., and Payne, R.O. (1975). Histocompatibiity (HL-A) antigens in psoriasis. *Arch. Dermatol.* 111:857–860.
226. Lamm, L.U., Kissmeyer-Nielsen, F., Kjerbye, K.E., Jorgensen, J., Petersen, G.B., Gurtler, H., and Tordarson,G. (1973). The HL-A in an Icelandic population. In *Histocompatibility Testing 1972.* J. Dausset and J. Colomani (Eds.). Munksgaard, Copenhagen, pp. 69–72.
227. Lamm, L.U., Friedrich, U., Petersen, G.B., Jorgensen, J. (1974). Assignment of the major histocompatibility complex to Chromosome No. 6 in a family with a pericentric inversion. *Hum. Hered.* 24:273–284.
228. Larko, O. (1995). Problem sites: scalp, palm and sole, and nail. *Dermatol. Clin.* 13:771–777.
229. Larsson, P.-A., and Liden, S. (1980). Prevalence of skin diseases among adolescents 12-16 years of age. *Acta Dermatol. Venereol. (Stockh.)* 60:415–423.
230. Lattke, C., Heitmann, H.J., Bertrams, J., Kuwert, F. (1974). Vorlaufige Kurzmitteilung Genetische Faktoren bei der Psoriasis vulgaris: Histokompatibilitats (HL-A)-Antigene. *Hautartz* 25:39.
231. Layrisse, Z., Terasaki, P., Wilbert, J., Heinen, H.D., Rodriguez, B., Soyano, A., Mittal, K., and Layrisse, M. (1973). Study of the HL-A system in the Warao population. In *Histocompatibility Testing 1972.* J. Dausset and J. Colomani (Eds.). Munksgaard, Copenhagen, pp. 377–385.
232. Lazar, A.P., and Roenigk, H.H. (1987). Psoriasis and acquired immune deficiency syndrome. In *Psoriasis. Proceedings of the Fourth International Symposium.* E.M. Farber, L. Nall, V. Morhenn, and P.H. Jacobs (Eds.). Elsevier, New York, pp. 417–418.
233. Lazar, A.P., and Roenigk, H.H. (1987). AIDS and psoriasis. *Cutis* 39:347–351.
234. Li, H.-C. (1982). Psoriasis in China. *Chinese Med. J.* 95:245–256.
235. Liden, S., Beckman, L., Bergdahl, K., Bronnestam, R., and Cedergren, B. (1977). Genetic markers in psoriasis. In *Psoriasis: Proceedings of the Second International Symposium.* E.M. Farber and A.J. Cox (Eds.). Yorke Medical Books, New York, pp. 127–133.
236. Lilienfeld, D.E. (1978). Definitions of epidemiology. *Am. J. Epidemiol.* 107:87–90.
237. Lilienfeld, D.E., and Stolley, P.D. (1994). *Fundamentals of Epidemiology*, 3rd ed. Oxford University Press, New York.
238. Lin, X.-R. (1993). Psoriasis in China. *J. Dermatol.* 15:11–13.

239. Lindegard, B. (1986). Diseases associated with psoriasis in a general population of 159,200 middle-aged, urban, native Swedes. *Dermatologica* 172:298–304.
240. Lindsten, J., Bredberg, A., and Iselius, L. (1981). Genetic aspects of psoriasis: mode of inheritance and the action of PUVA on DNA. *Acta Dermatol. Venereol. (Stockh.)* (Suppl.) 95:58–63.
241. Liu, S., Serdula, M.K., Byers, T., Williamson, D.R., Mokdad, A.H., and Flanders, W.D. (1996). Reliability of alcohol intake as recalled from 10 years in the past. *Am. J. Epidemiol.* 143:177–186.
242. Liu, X., and Rui, J.X. (1982). Study on the genetic trend in psoriasis vulgaris. *Chinese J. Dermatol.* 15: 11–13.
243. Lomholt, G. (1963). *Psoriasis: Prevalence, Spontaneous Course, and Genetics. A Census Study on the Prevalence of Skin Diseases in the Faroe Island.* GEC Gad, Copenhagen.
244. Lomholt, G. (1971). Environment and genetics in psoriasis. In *Psoriasis: Proceedings of an International Symposium.* E.M. Farber and A.J. Cox (Eds.). Stanford University Press, Stanford, CA, pp. 21–24.
245. Lomholt, G. (1971). Psoriasis in Uganda: a comparative study with other parts of Africa. In *Psoriasis: Proceedings of an International Symposium.* E.M. Farber and A.J. Cox (Eds.). Stanford University Press, Stanford, CA, pp. 41–48.
246. Lomholt, G. (1976). Environment and genetics in psoriasis. *Ann. Clin. Res.* 8:290–297.
247. Lomholt, G. (1977). Problems of tropical dermatology in Africa. *Int. J. Dermatol.* 16:284–286.
248. Lynfield, Y.L. (1974). Skin diseases in twins. *Arch. Dermatol.* 110:722–724.
249. Majumder, M. (1980). Dermatology in Perak, Malaysia. *Int. Ps. Bull.* 7(3–4):3.
250. Maliarik, M.J., Kost, J.A., Harrington, D.W., Popovich, J., Major, M.L., Rybicki, B.A., and Iannuzzi, M.C. (1995). Chromosome 6p microsatellite polymorphisms in African-Americans. *Hum. Hered.* 45: 90–97.
251. Mamelka, P. (1993). Pedigree drawing computer program. Southwest Foundation for Biomedical Research, Department of Genetics, San Antonio, TX.
252. Mansbridge, J., Reusch, M., Bohr, V., and Hanawalt, P. (1987). The wound-healing model for psoriasis, the "psoriagene," and rational approaches to therapy. In *Psoriasis: Proceedings of the Fourth International Symposium.* E.M. Farber, L. Nall, V. Morhenn, and P.H. Jacobs (Eds.). Elsevier, New York, pp. 294–301.
253. Mao, V.H. (1982). Analysis of 3,500 cases of psoriasis. Cited by Li (234).
254. Marcusson, J., Moller, E., and Thyresson, N. (1975). HL-A (17, 27, UPS) in psoriasis with special reference to patients with arthritic lesions. *Acta Dermatol. Venereol. (Stockh.)* 55:297–300.
255. Marcusson, J., Moller, E., and Thyresson, N. (1976). Penetration of HLA-linked psoriasis-predisposing gene(s): a family investigation. *Acta Dermatol. Venereol. (Stockh.)* 56:453–463.
256. Marcusson, J., Moller, E., and Thyresson, N. (1979). Genetic problems concerning psoriasis. *Acta Dermatol. Venereol. (Stockh.)* (Suppl.) 87:28.
257. Marcusson, J.A., and Moller, E. (1986). Further studies on psoriasis-associated HLA-DwDR7 using PLT cells primed against a familial psoriasis-linked HLA haplotype. *Tissue Antigens* 27:1–9.
258. Marks, R. (1987). *Skin Disease in Old Age.* J.B. Lippincott, Philadelphia.
259. Marks, R., and Burton, S.P. (1989). Assessment of disease progress in psoriasis. *Arch. Dermatol.* 125: 235–240.
260. Masawe, A.E.J. (1973) Psoriasis in Tanzania. *Int. Ps. Bull.* 1(2):1.
261. Mazzetti, M., Mozzetta, A., Saavi, G.C., Andreoli, E., Foglio Bonda, P.G., Paddu, P., and Decaminada, F. (1994). Psoriasis, stress, and psychiatry characteristics of stressors. *Acta Dermatol. Venereol.* (Suppl.) 186:62–64.
262. McDevitt, H.O., and Bodmer, W.F. (1974). HL-A immune response genes and disease. *Lancet* 1: 1269–1275.
263. McGinnis, L.S. (1991). Alternative therapies, 1990. An overview. *Cancer* 67:1788–1792.
264. McKusick, V.A. (1983). Mendelian inheritance in man. Catalogs of autosomal dominant, autosomal recessive, and x-linked phenotypes, 6th ed. The Johns Hopkins University Press, Baltimore.
265. McMichael, A.J., Morhenn, V., Payne, R., Sasazuki, T., and Farber, E.M. (1978). HLA C and D antigens associated with psoriasis. *Br. J. Dermatol.* 98: 287–292.
266. McPherson-Turner, C. (1980). Education for aging. *J. School Health* 50:314–317.
267. Melski, J.W., and Stern, R.S. (1981). Separation of susceptibility of psoriasis from age at onset. *J. Invest. Dermatol.* 77:474–477.
268. Metzgar, R.S., Ward, T.E., and Siegler, H.F. (1973). Study of the HLA system in chimpanzees. In *Histocompatibility Testing* 1972. J. Dausset and J. Colomani (Eds.). Munksgaard, Copenhagen, pp. 55–61.
269. Meyer, L.J. (1990). Psoriasis: The application of genetic technology and mapping. *J. Invest. Dermatol.* 95:5S–6S.
270. Mills, C.M., Srivastava, E.D., Harvey, I.M., Swift, G.L., Newcombe, R.G., Holt, P.J., and Rhodes, J. (1992). Smoking habits in psoriasis: a case-control study. *Br. J. Dermatol.* 127:18–21.
271. Mitchell, J.C. (1967). Proportionate distribution of skin diseases in a dermatological practice: enumeration by standard nomenclature of 12,578 cases from

clinic and private practice. *Can. Med. Assoc. J.* 97: 1346–1350.

272. Molin, L. (1973). Psoriasis: a study of the course and degree of severity of joint involvement, sociomedical conditions, general morbidity, and influences of selection factors among previously hospitalized psoriatics. *Acta Dermatol. Venereol. (Stockh.)* (Suppl. 72)53:1–123.
273. Monk, B.E., and Neill, S.M. (1986). Alcohol consumption and psoriasis. *Dermatologica* 173:57–60.
274. Monplaisir, N., Valette, I., Lepage, V., Dijon, V., Lavocat, E., Ribal, C., and Raffoux, C. (1985). Study of HLA antigens of the Martinican population. *Tissue Antigens* 26:1–11.
275. Montagnani, A., and Rossi, A. (1969). Considerazioni su alcuni alberi genealogici di famiglie psoriasiche. *Giorn. Min. Dermatol.* 44:317–322.
276. Montagnani, A., and Rossi, A. (1969). Considerazioni su alcuni alberi genealogici di famiglie psoriasiche. *Giorn. Min. Dermatol.* 44:323–327.
277. Mordovtsev, V.N., Sergeyev, A.S., and Alieva, P.M. (1981). Genetic factors in psoriasis. *Int. J Dermatol.* 20:99–101.
278. Mourant, A.E., Kopec, A.C., and Domaniewska-Sobczak, K. (1976). *The Distribution of the Human Blood Groups and Other Polymorphisms, 2nd ed.* Oxford University Press, London.
279. Nair, R.P., Guo, S.W., Jenisch, S., Henseler, T., Lange, E.M., Terhune, M., Westphal, E., Christophers, E., Voorhees, J.J., and Elder, J.T. (1995). Scanning chromosome 17 for psoriasis susceptibility: lack of evidence for a distal 17q locus. *Hum. Hered.* 45: 219–230.
280. Nakagawa, H., Asahina, A., Akazaki, S., Tokunaga, K., Matsuki, K., Ishibashi, Y., and Juji, T. (1990). Association of Cw11 in Japanese patients with psoriasis vulgaris. *Tissue Antigens* 36:241–242.
281. Nakamizo, Y., Kukita, A., Aso, K., Mori, S., and Psoriasis Research Group (1987). Statistical observation of psoriasis in Japan. In *Psoriasis. Proceedings of the Fourth International Symposium.* E.M. Farber, L. Nall, V. Morhenn, and P.H. Jacobs (Eds.). Elsevier, New York, p. 397.
282. Naldi, L. (1995). Psoriasis. *Dermatol. Clin.* 13: 635–647.
283. Naldi, L., Parazzini, F., Brevi, A., Peserico, A., Veller Fornasa, C., Grosso, G., Rossi, E., Marinaro, P., Polenghi, M.M., Finzi, A., Galbiati, G., Recchia, G., Cristofolini, M., Schena, D., and Cainelli, T. (1992). Family history, smoking habits, alcohol consumption and risk of psoriasis. *Br. J. Dermatol.* 127:212–217.
284. Naldi, L., Tognoni, G., and Cainelli, T. (1994). Analytic epidemiology in psoriasis. *J. Invest. Dermatol.* 102:19S–23S.
285. Nall, M.L. (1967). Application of blood grouping techniques to the study of population distribution (Arctic Eskimo). Stanford University, Department of Anthropology, Stanford, CA.
286. Nall, L. (1987). Epidemiology of psoriasis: a global view. In *Psoriasis. Proceedings of the Fourth International Symposium.* E.M. Farber, L. Nall, V. Morhenn, and P.H. Jacobs (Eds.). Elsevier, New York, pp. 265–293.
287. Nall, L. (1992). *Symposium on Problems of the Aging, Las Vega, NV (Feb. 21–25, 1992):* Self-help in diseases of the elderly, Epidemiology of aging populations; (Feb. 26–March 1, 1992) Helping the caregiver for the elderly.
288. Nall, L. (1994). Epidemiologic strategies in psoriasis research. *Int. J. Dermatol.* 33:313–319.
289. Nall, L. (1996). Dermatoepidemiology. Internet, URL: http://www_leland.stanford.edu/~lnall.
290. Nall, M.L., and Farber, E.M. (1977). World epidemiology of psoriasis. In *Psoriasis. Proceedings of the Second International Symposium.* E.M. Farber and A.J. Cox (Eds.). Yorke Medical Books, New York, pp. 331–333.
291. Nall, L., Farber, E.M., Jacobs, P.H., and Wallace, P. (1981). Psoriasis epidemiology: relationship of psoriasis to skin and internal cancers. Poster presentation. *Third International Symposium on Psoriasis*, Stanford University, July 13–17.
292. Nall, L., Wallace, P., and Farber, E.M. (1982). Biometry of psoriasis. In *Psoriasis. Third International Symposium.* E.M. Farber and A.J. Cox (Eds.). Grune & Stratton, New York, pp. 309–310.
293. Nall, L., and Marder, C. (1987). *Psoriasis.* A single entity or two? In *Psoriasis. Proceedings of the Fourth International Symposium.* E.M. Farber, L. Nall, V. Morhenn, and P.H. Jacobs (Eds.). Elsevier, New York, pp. 393–394.
294. Nagreb, D.S. (1980). Dermatology in Penang, Malaysia. *Int. Ps. Bull.* 7(3–4):2–3.
295. Nance, W.E. (1976). Genetic studies of the offspring of identical twins: A model for the analysis of quantitative inheritance in man. *Acta Genet. Med. Gemellol.* 25:103–113.
296. Nance, W.E. (1980). The value of population-based twin registries for genetic and epidemiologic research. In *Cancer Incidence in Defined Populations.* J. Cairns, J.L. Lyon, and M. Skolnick (Eds.). Cold Spring Harbor Laboratories, Cold Spring Harbor, N.Y., pp. 215–235.
297. Nanda, A., Kaur, S., Kaur, I., and Kumar, B. (1990). Childhood psoriasis: an epidemiologic survey of 112 patients. *Pediatr. Dermatol.* 7:19–21.
298. Nevanlinna, H.R. (1972). The Finnish population structure: a genetic and genealogical study. *Hereditas* 71:195–236.
299. Newcomer, V.C., and Young, E.M. (Eds.). (1989). *Geriatric Dermatology.* Igaku-Shoin, New York.

300. NIAAA (1983). Fifth Special Report to the U.S. Congress on Alcohol and Health from the Secretary of Health and Human Services. Public Health Service, Alcohol, Drug Abuse, and Mental Health Administration.
301. Nini, G., Bianchi, L., Iraci, S., Camplone, G., Spagnuolo, A., Adorno, D., and Papola, F. (1989). HLA antigens and infantile psoriasis. *Acta Dermatol. Venereol. (Stockh.)* (Suppl.) 146:59–62.
302. Nyfors, A., and Lemholt, K. (1975). Psoriasis in children: a short review and a survey of 245 cases. *Br. J. Dermatol.* 92:437–442.
303. Nyfors, A., and Svejgaard, A. (1976). The relation of HL-A antigens to liver histology in methotrexate-treated psoriatics. *Acta Dermatol. Venereol. (Stockh.)* 56:235–238.
304. Obasi, O.E. (1986). Psoriasis vulgaris in the Guinea Savanah region of Nigeria. *Int. J. Dermatol.* 25: 181–183.
305. Obasi, O.E. (1987). Epidemiology and treatment of psoriasis in Black Africa. In *Psoriasis. Proceedings of the Fourth International Symposium.* E.M. Farber, L. Nall, V. Morhenn, and P.H. Jacobs (Eds.). Elsevier, New York, pp. 395–396.
306. Obuch, M.L., Maurer, T.A., and Becker, B. (1992). Psoriasis and human immunodeficiency virus infection. *J. Am. Acad. Dermatol.* 27:667–673.
307. O'Donnell, B.F., O'Loughlin, S., Codd, M.B., and Powell, F.C. (1993). HLA typing in Irish psoriatics. *Irish Med. J.* 86:65–68.
308. Off Alt Med (1994). Functional description. National Institutes of Health, The Office of Alternative Medicine, Bethesda, MD. May 20, 1994.
309. Oliveira, A. de (1957). Notes on dermatology and venereology in two towns of Angola (Lobito and Benguela: 1954–1957). *J. Med. (Lisbon)* 34:597.
310. Ott, J. (1995). Linkage analysis with biological markers. *Hum. Hered.* 45:169–174.
311. Ozawa, A., Ohkido, M., and Tsuji, K. (1981). Some recent advances in HLA and skin diseases. *J. Am. Acad. Dermatol.* 4:205–230.
312. Ozawa, A., Ohkido, M., Inoko, H., Ando, A., and Tsuji, K. (1988). Specific restriction fragment length polymorphism on the HLA-C region and suceptibility of psoriasis vulgaris. *J. Invest. Dermatol.* 90: 402–405.
313. Payne, R., Kidd, K.K., Radvan, Y.R., and Perkins, H.A. (1973). HL-A and other polymorphisms of the Chinese of the Canton area. In *Histocompatibility Testing 1972.* J. Dausset, and J. Colomani (Eds.). Munksgaard, Copenhagen, pp. 197–201.
314. Perkins, H.A., Payne, R.O., Kidd, K.K., and Huestis, D.W. (1973). HL-A and Gm typing of Papago Indians. In *Histocompatibility Testing 1972.* J. Dausset and J. Colomani (Eds.). Munksgaard, Copenhagen, pp. 333–338.
315. Peter, J.B., and Hawkins, B.R. (1992). The new HLA. *Arch. Pathol. Lab. Med.* 116:11–15.
316. Piazza, A., Rendine, S., Minch, E., Menozzi, P., Mountain, J., and Cavalli-Sforza, L.L. (1995). Genetics and the origin of European languages. *Proc. Natl. Acad. Sci. USA* 92:5836–5840.
317. Pickbourne, P., Piazza, A., and Bodmer, W.F. (1977). Population analysis. *Histocompatibility Testing 1977.* W.F. Bodmer (Ed.). Munksgaard, Copenhagen, pp. 259–278.
318. Pitchappan, R.M., Koteeswaran, A., Kakkaniah, V.N., Manickasundari, M., Rajaram, V., Muthuveeralakshmi, V., and Brahmajothibai, V. (1989). HLA Bw57 and DR association with psoriasis vulgaris in south India. *Tissue Antigens* 34:133–137.
319. Powell, F., Young, M., and Barnes, J. (1982). Psoriasis in Ireland. *Irish J. Med. Sci.* 151:109–113.
320. Prystowsky, J.H., and Cohen, P.R. (1995). Pustular and erythrodermic psoriasis. *Dermatol. Clin.* 13: 757–770.
321. Quamina, D.B.E. (1975). Psoriasis in Trinidad and Tobago. *Int Ps. Bull.* 2(2):5.
322. Race, R.R., and Sanger, R. (1975) Blood Groups in Man, 6th ed. Blackwell Scientific, Oxford.
323. Raffoux, C., Streiff, F., Blum, F., et al (1980). HLA-DRw7 dans le psoriasis vulgaire. *C. R. Acad. Sci. (Paris)* 290:883–884.
324. Ramsey, D.L., and Fox, A.B. (1981). Ability of primary care physicians to recognize the common dermatoses. *Arch. Dermatol.* 117:620–622.
325. Ratnam, A.V., and Jayaraju, K. (1979). Skin diseases in Zambia. *Br. J. Dermatol* 101:449–453.
326. Ratzer, M.A. (1969). The incidence of skin diseases in west of Scotland. *Br. J. Dermatol.* 81:456–461.
327. Rea, J.N., Newhouse, M.L., and Halil, T. (1976). Skin disease in Lambeth: a community study of prevalence and use of medical care. *Br. J. Prev. Soc. Med.* 30: 107–114.
328. Reed, T.E. (1992). Issues in estimating Caucasian admixture in American blacks. *Am. J. Hum. Genet.* 51: 678–679 (letter).
329. Reinberg, A. (1968). Statistics. In *Psoriasis* Sidi, Zagula-Mally, and Hincky (Eds.). Charles C Thomas, Springfield, IL, pp. 279–285.
330. Roitberg-Tambur, A., Friedman, A., Tzfoni, E.E., Battal, S., Hammo, R.B., Safirman, M.S., Tokunaga, K., Asahina, A., and Brautbar, C. (1994). Do specific pockets of HLA-C molecules predispose Jewish patients to psoriasis vulgaris. *J. Am. Acad. Dermatol.* 31:964–968.
331. Roitt, I.M. (1994). *Essential Immunology.* Blackwell Scientific Publications, Oxford.
332. Romaguera, C., and Grimalt, F. (1980). Statistical and comparative study of 4,600 patients tested in Barcelona (1973–1977). *Contact Derm.* 6:309–315.

333. Romanus, T. (1947). Psoriasis in twins. *Hereditas* 33: 297–300.
334. Rosbotham, J.L., Trembath, R.C., Glover, M., Leigh, I., and Barker, J.N. (1994). An association between psoriasis and hereditary multiple exostosis: a clue for the mapping of a psoriasis susceptibility gene? *Br. J. Dermatol.* 130:671–674.
335. Ross, H.-G. (1971). Untersuchen uber das Entstehungsalter der Psoriasis vulgaris. *Methods Inf. Med.* 10:108–115.
336. Russell, T.J., Schultes, L.M., and Kuban, D.J. (1972). Histocompatibility (HL-A) antigens associated with psoriasis. *N. Engl. J. Med.* 287:738–740.
337. Sachs, J.A. (1989). HLA antigens in Nigerians and their relevance to transplantation in Afro-Americans. *Transplant. Proc.* 21:3884–3886.
338. Saint-Andre, P., and Louvet, M. (1976). Psoriasis chez le noir a Bamako. *Ann. Dermatol. Syphiligr. (Paris)* 103:666.
339. Sampaio, S.A.P. Psoriasis in Sao Paulo. *Int. Ps. Bull.* 2(2):5–6.
340. Schaller, K.F. (1962). Skin diseases in Ethiopia. *Hautarzt* 13:289.
341. Schoefinius, H.H., Braun-Falco, O., Schultz, S., Steinbauer-Rosenthal, I., Wank, R., and Albert, E.D. (1974). Histokompatibilitatsantigene (HL-A) bei Psoriasis. Untersuchungen an 104 univerwandten patienten. *Dtsch. Med. Wochenschr.* 99:440–444.
342. Schork, N.J., Boehnke, M., Terwilliger, J.D., and Ott, J. (1993). Two-trait-locus linkage analysis: a powerful strategy for mapping complex genetic traits. *Am. J. Hum. Genet.* 53:1127–1136.
343. Schrank, A.B., and Harman, R.R.M. (1966). The incidence of skin diseases in a Nigerian teaching hospital dermatologic clinic. *Br. J. Dermatol.* 78:235.
344. Schulz, E.J., Findlay, G.H., and Scott, F.P. (1962). Skin diseaes in the Bantu: a survey of 4,000 cases from the Transvaal and Orange Free State. *S. Afr. Med. J.* 36:199.
345. Schweicker, R.S. (1982). Disease prevention and health promotion. J. Med. Educ. 57:15–19.
346. Sehgal, V.N., Rege, V.L. and Kharangate, V.N. (1972). An interrogative study of 142 psoriasis patients. (Unpublished manuscript).
347. Selim, M.M.E.-D. (1973). The pattern of skin disease in Kuwait. *J. Kuwait Med. Assoc.* 7:253–261.
348. Shao, C.G., Zhang, F.W., and Wang, K.C. (1987). The distribution of psoriasis. A nationwide screening in the People's Republic of China, 1984. In *Psoriasis. Proceedings of the Fourth International Symposium.* E.M. Farber, L. Nall, V. Morhenn, and P.H. Jacobs (Eds.). Elsevier, New York, pp. 398–399.
349. Shao, C.G., Ye, G., Hu, C., and Zhang, F. (1992). Psoriatic research in China. *Int. J. Dermatol.* 31: 840–844.
350. Shellow, W.V. (1983). The skin in alcoholism. *Int. J. Dermatol.* 21:506–510.
351. Singleton, J.A., Tabnak, F., Kuan, J., and Rutherford, G.W. (1996). Human immunodeficiency virus disease in California: effects of the 1993 expanded case definition of the acquired immunodeficiency syndrome. *West. J. Med.* 164:122–129.
352. Smith, A.E., Kassab, J.Y., Rowland Payne, C.M.E., and Beer, W.E. (1993). Bimodality in age of onset of psoriasis, in both patients and their relatives. *Dermatology* 186:181–186.
353. Snell, G.D. (1981). Studies in histocompatibility. *Science* 213:172–178.
354. Song, F., Cheng, Y., Liu, Z., Hueigang, L., Li, H., Xu, S., Su, X., Yang, C., and Liu, Z. (1981). HLA antigens and psoriasis. *Chinese J. Dermatol.* 14: 191–194.
355. Soyland, E., Funk, J., Rajka, G., Sandberg, T., Thune, P., Rustad, L., Helland, S., Middelfart, K., Odu, S., and Falk, E.S. (1993). Effects of dietary supplementation with very long-chain n-3 fatty acids in patients with psoriasis. *N. Engl. J. Med.* 328:1812–1816.
356. Spees, E.K., Kostyu, D.D., Elston, R.C., and Amos, D.B. (1973). HL-A profiles of the Pima Indians of Arizona. In *Histocompatibility Testing 1972*. J. Dausset and J. Colomani (Eds.). Munksgaard, Copenhagen, pp. 345–349.
357. Stauffer, H. (1958). Beobachtungen an Psoriasis. *Dermatologica* 117:413–428.
358. Steinberg, A.G., and Wilder, R.M. (1950). A reconsideration of the phenomenon of anticipation in diabetes mellitus. *Proc. Mayo Clin.* 25:625–630.
359. Steinberg, A.G., Becker, S.W., Fitzpatrick, T.B., and Kierland, R.R. (1951). A genetic and statistical study of psoriasis. *Am. J. Hum. Genet.* 3:267–281.
360. Steinke, A. (1935). Stellungnahme zu unstrittenen fragen bei der Psoriasis. Dissertation, Berlin.
361. Stern, C. (1960). *Principles of Human Genetics*, 2nd ed. W.H. Freeman, San Francisco.
362. Stern, R.S. (1995). Epidemiology of psoriasis. *Dermatol. Clin.* 13:717–722.
363. Stroebel, M., Ndiaye, B., Diop, M., and Marchand, J.P. (1981). Le psoriasis au Senegal. *Dakar Med.* 26: 18–25.
364. Suarez-Almazor, M.E., and Russell, A.S. (1990). The genetics of psoriasis: haplotype sharing in siblings with the disease. *Arch. Dermatol.* 126:1040–1042.
365. Sulzberger, M.B. (1958). Multiple factors in the causation of diseases and the implications of this concept for their understanding and management. *Dermatologica* 117:407–413.
366. Sulzberger, M.B. (1980). Multiple factors in the elicitation of skin disease and how this concept must influence our approaches to etiology and management. *J. Dermatol.* 7:385–387.

367. Summons, J. (1955). The incidence of skin disease in Australia. *Aust. J. Dermatol.* 3:15–18.
368. Sun, Y., An, J., Li, S., Li, H., Chen, W., Sin, L., Xu, L., Lu, L., Yang, Q., Zhang, X., and Zhao, G. (1987). HLA antigen distribution and haplotype segregation in Chinese patients with psoriasis. *Chinese Med. J.* 100:236–241.
369. Susitaival, P., Husman, L., Hollmen, A., and Horsmanheimo, M. (1995). Dermatoses determined in a population of farmers in a questionnaire-based clinical study including methodology validation. *Scand. J. Work, Environ, Health* 21:30–35.
370. Svejgaard, A., Svejgaard, E., Staub-Nielsen, L., and Jacobsen, B. (1973). Some speculation on the association between HL-A and disease based on studies of psoriasis patients and their families. *Transplant. Proc.* 5:1797–1798.
371. Svejgaard, A., Jersild, C., Staub-Nielsen, L., and Bodmer, W.F. (1974). HL-A antigens and disease—statistical and genetical considerations. *Tissue Antigens* 4:95–105.
372. Svejgaard, A., Staub-Nielsen, L., Svejgaard, E., Kissmeyer-Nielsen, F., Hjortshoj, A., and Zachariae, H. (1974). HLA in psoriasis vulgaris and in pustular psoriasis—population and family studies. *Br. J. Dermatol.* 91:145–153.
373. Svejgaard, A., Hauge, M., Jersild, C., et al. (1975). The HLA System: An Introductory Survey. *Monogr. Hum. Genet.* 7:1–100.
374. Swanbeck, G., Inerot, A., Martinsson, T., and Wahlstrom, J. (1994). A population genetic study of psoriasis. *Br. J. Dermatol.* 131:32–39.
375. Tauber, J.W., Falk, J.A., Falk, R.E., and Zabriskie, J.B. (1976). Nonspecific complement activation by streptococcal structures. I. Reevaluation of HLA cytotoxicity inhibition. *J. Exp. Med.* 14:1341–1351.
376. Telfer, N.R., Chalmers, R.J., Whale, K., and Colman, G. (1992). The role of streptococcal infection in the initiation of guttate psoriasis. *Arch. Dermatol.* 128: 39–42.
377. Terris, M. (1975). Approaches to an epidemiology of health. *Am. J. Public Health* 65:1037–1045.
378. Theeuwes, M., and Leder, R.O. (1993). Hereditary insights in psoriasis. *Eur. J. Dermatol.* 3:335–341.
379. Thorsby, E. (1974). The major histocompatibility system. *Transplant Rev.* 18:51–129.
380. Tiilikainen, A., Eriksson, A.W., Macqueen, J.M., and Amos, D.B. (1973). The HL-A system in the Skolt Lapp population. In *Histocompatibility Testing 1972*. J. Dausset and J. Colomani (Eds.). Munksgaard, Copenhagen, pp. 85–92.
381. Tiilikainen, A., Lassus, A., Karvonen, J., Vartianen, P., and Julin, M. (1980). Psoriasis and HLA-Cw6. *Br. J. Dermatol.* 192:179–184.
382. Tiling-Grosse, S., and Rees, J. (1993). Assessment of area of involvement in skin disease: a study using schematic figure outlines. *Br. J. Dermatol.* 128: 69–74.
383. Tittor, W., Sobenes, J., Smith, G.S., Sturgeon, P., Zeller, E., and Walford, R.L. (1973). Distribution of HL-A antigens, and serum protein groups in Quechua Indians of Peru. In *Histocompatibility Testing 1972*. J. Dausset and J. Colomani (Eds.). Munksgaard, Copenhagen, pp. 387–390.
384. Tiwari, J.L., Lowed, N.J., Abramovits, W., Hawkins, B.R., and Park, M.D. (1982). Association of psoriasis with HLA-DR7. *Br. J. Dermatol.* 106:227–230.
385. Tomfohrde, J., Silverman, A., Barnes, R., Fernandez-Vina, M.A., Young, M., Lory, D., Morris, L., Wuepper, K.D., Stastny, P., Menter, A., and Bowcock, A. (1994). Gene for familial psoriasis susceptibility mapped to the distal end of human chromosome 17q. *Science* 264:1141–1145.
386. Troup, G.M., Harvey, R.L., Walford, R.L., Smith, G.S., and Sturgeon, P. (1973). Analysis of the HL-A, erthrocyte and gamma globulin antigen systems in the Zuni Indians of New Mexico. In *Histocompatibility Testing 1972*. J. Dausset and J. Colomani (Eds.). Munksgaard, Copenhagen, pp. 339–344.
387. Tsuji, K., Inouye, H., Nose, Y., Saszuki, T., Ozawa, A., and Ohkido, M. (1979). Further study on HLA-A, B, C, D, DR, and haplotype antigen frequencies in psoriasis vulgaris. *Acta Dermatol. Venereol. (Stockh.)* (Suppl.) 87:107–108.
388. Turowski, G., Kapinska-Mrowka, M., and Pietrzyk, J.J. (1980). HLA antigens in psoriasis. *Arch. Immunol. Ther. Exp. (Warsz.)* 28:119–126.
389. U.S. Dept. of Health and Human Services (1983). Incidence of nonmelanoma skin cancer in the United States. Public Health Service, National Institutes of Health, NIH Publication No. 83-2433, Washington, D.C.
390. van der Does, J.A., D'amaro, J., Van Leeuwen, A., Kahn, P.M., Bernini, L.F., Van Loghem, E., Nijenhuis, L., Van Der Steen, G., Van Rood, J.J., and Rubinstein, P. (1973). HL-A typing in Chilean Aymara Indians. In *Histocompatibility Testing 1972*. J. Dausset and J. Colomani (Eds.). Munksgaard, Copenhagen, pp. 391–395.
391. van Hecke, E., and Eugingo, G. (1980). Prevalence of skin disease in Rwanda. *Int. J. Dermatol.* 19: 526–529.
392. Vasey, F.B., Espinoza, L.R., Bocanegra, T.S., and Germain, B.F. (1982). The major histocompatibility complex. *Ann. Clin. Lab. Sci.* 12:16–22.
393. Venables, J. (1994). Knowledge needed to educate patients about psoriasis. *Nurs. Times* 90:32–35.
394. Verhagen, A.R.H.B., and Koten, J.W. (1967). Psoriasis in Kenya. *Arch. Dermatol.* 96:39–41.
395. Verhagen, A.R.H.B., Koten, J.W., Chaddah, V.K., and Patel, R.I. (1968). Skin disease in Kenya. *Arch. Dermatol.* 98:577.

396. Vogel, F. (1961). Formalgenetik des Menschen. Bedingungen und Grenzen der Erganganayse. Multifaktorialle Verebung. In *Lehrbuch der Allegemeinen Humangeneiik.* Springer-Verlag, Berlin, pp. 146–148.
397. Vogel, F., and Motulsky, A.G. (1979). *Human Genetics: Problems and Approaches.* Springer-Verlag, New York.
398. Vollum, D. (1973). An impression of dermatology in Uganda. *Trans. St. John's Hosp. Dermatol. Soc.* 59: 120–125.
399. Wahba, A., Dorfman, M., and Sheskin, J. (1980). Psoriasis and other common dermatoses in leprosy. *Int. J. Dermatol.* 19:93–95.
400. Wallace, A.B. (1951). The exposure treatment of burns. *Lancet* 1:501–504.
401. Walshe, N.M. (1968). Dermatology in Jamaica. *Trans. St. John's Hosp. Dermatol. Soc.* 54:46–53.
402. Ward, J.H., and Stephens, F.E. (1961). Inheritance of psoriasis in a Utah kindred. *Arch. Dermatol.* 84: 105–108.
403. Wassertheil-Smoller, S. (1995). *Biostatistics and Epidemiology. A Primer for Health Professionals*, 2nd ed. Springer-Verlag, New York.
404. Watson, W., Cann, H.M., Farber, E.M., and Nall, M.L. (1972). The genetics of psoriasis. *Arch. Dermatol.* 105:197–207.
405. Weinstock, M.A. (1995). Dermatoepidemiology. (Ed.). *Dermatol. Clin.* 13(3):505–716.
406. Wellsource, Inc. (1993). Personal Wellness Profile Questionnaire. Clarkamas, OR.
407. Welton, D.G. (1960). Inside dermatology, USA—from a national survey of private office practice. *South. Med.* 53:210–223.
408. Wendt, G.G. (1968). Blood groups, serum factors, and psoriasis vulgaris. *Dermatologica* 136:1–10.
409. White, R., and Lalouel, J.-M. (1988). Chromosome mapping with DNA markers. *Sci. Am.* 258:40–48.
410. White, S.H., Newcomer, V.D., Mickey, M.R., and Terasaki, P.I. (1972). Distribution of HL-A antigen. *N. Engl. J. Med.* 287:740–743.
411. W.H.O. (1966). The use of twins in epidemiological studies. *Acta Genet. Med. Gemellol.* 15:111–128.
412. W.H.O. (1984). Prevention and control of genetic diseases and congenital defects. Scientific Pub. No. 460. World Health Organization, Washington, D.C.
413. W.H.O.-I.U.I.S. Terminology Committee (1975). Nomenclature for factors of the HLA system. In *Histocompatibility Testing 1975.* F. Kissmeyer-Nielson (Ed.). Munksgaard, Copenhagen, pp. 5–8.
414. Whyte, H.J., and Baughman, R.D. (1964). Acute guttate psoriasis and streptococcal infection. *Arch. Dermatol.* 89:350.
415. Williams, H.C. (1994). Smoking and psoriasis. *Br. Med. J.* 308:428–429.
416. Wilson, A.G., Clark, I., Heard, S.R., Munro, D.D., and Kirby, J.D. (1993). Immunoblotting of streptococcal antigens in guttate psoriasis. *Br. J. Dermatol.* 128:151–158.
417. Woimant, F., Lesobre, B., Dehay, C., and Pieron, R. (1980). HL-A and -B typing in the Sarakole population of West Africa. *Tissue Antigens* 15:216–219.
418. Woodrow, J.C., Dave, V.K., User, N., and Anderson, J. (1975). The HL-A systemic and psoriasis. *Br. J. Dermatol.* 92:427.
419. Wuepper, K.D., Coulter, S.N., and Haberman, A. (1990). Psoriasis vulgaris: a genetic approach. *J. Invest. Dermatol.* 95:2S–4S.
420. Wysocki, A.B. (1996). Wound measurement. *Int. J. Dermatol.* 35:82–91.
421. Xia, J.-Z., et al. (1983). HLA and psoriasis. *J. Clin. Dermatol.* 12:3–4.
422. Yap, K.B., Siew, M.G., and Goh, C.L. (1990). Pattern of skin diseases in the elderly seen at the National Skin Centre (Singapore) 1990. *Singapore Med. J.* 35: 147–150.
423. Yasada, H., Kobayashi, H., and Ohkawara, A. (1990). A survey of the social and psychological effects of psoriasis. *Jpn. J. Dermatol.* 100:1167–1171.
424. Yasada, T., Ishikawa, E., and Mori, S. (1971).Psoriasis in the Japanese. In *Psoriasis. Proceedings of an International Symposium, 1971.* E.M. Farber and A.J. Cox (Eds.). Stanford University Press, Stanford, CA, pp. 25–34.
425. Yip, S.Y. (1984). The prevalence of psoriasis in the Mongoloid race. *J. Am. Acad. Dermatol.* 10:965–968.
426. Zachariae, H., Hjortschoj, A., Kissmeyer-Nielsen, F., Svejgaard, A., Svejgaard, E., and Zachariae, E. (1974). HLA antigens and psoriatic arthritis. *Acta Dermatol. Venereol. (Stockh.)* 54:443.
427. Zachariae, H., Overgaard-Petersen, H., Kissmeyer-Nielsen, F., and Lamm, L. (1977). HL-A antigens in pustular psoriasis. *Dermatologia* 154:73–77.
428. Zachariae, R., Oster, H., Bjerring, P., and Kragballe, K. (1966). Effects of psychologic intervention on psoriasis. A preliminary report. *J. Am. Acad. Dermatol.* 19:101–104.
429. Zhang, G.W., Shao, C.G., and Wang, K.C. (1987). The annual incidence of psoriasis and the age-liability to psoriasis in the People's Republic of China. A nationwide screening in 1984. In *Psoriasis: Proceedings of the Fourth International Symposium.* E.M. Farber, L. Nall, V. Morhenn, and P.H. Jacobs (Eds.). Elsevier, New York, p. 400.
430. Ziboh, V.A., Cohen, K.A., and Ellis, C.N. (1986). Effects of dietary supplementation of fish oil on neutrophil and epidermal fatty acids. *Arch. Dermatol.* 122: 1266–1282.

10

Psoriasis Type I and Type II as Subtypes of Nonpustular Psoriasis

Tilo Henseler and Enno Christophers
University of Kiel, Kiel, Germany

During the last 20 years a significant number of studies were conducted dealing with epidemiological aspects of psoriasis. Investigations on disease susceptibility in relation to geographic patterns revealed varying incidence rates in different countries. In addition, many reports have been published on total morbidity, onset age, heredity, as well as the association of psoriasis with certain HLA antigens (1–5).

Furthermore, in the past three decades, by studying HLA antigens in psoriasis, several authors have noted the close association of certain HLA antigens such as B57 (which is a subtype of B17), B13, and Cw6 in psoriasis patients (6–9). In addition, it was found that early disease onset is frequently associated with the HLA antigens Cw6 (10–12) or B57 (3,4). Recently, investigations in HLA class II antigens presented a linkage disequilibrium with so-called extended haplotypes (13–15).

The existence of two types of nonpustular psoriasis showing morphologically similar skin lesions was ascertained by defining onset age in association with HLA typing as well as family inheritance and clinical course of disease (12). These data were substantiated by studying an additional 256 patients together with 806 relatives (16,17). These as well as previous data will be discussed in this chapter.

AGE ONSET

As stated by Steinberg et al. (18) and reemphasized by Farber and Nall (19), there may be inaccuracies in establishing the age of disease onset by reporting the patient's own data. On the other hand, studies concerned with this special aspect of the disease are quite numerous (Table 1), and rather large patient cohorts have been analyzed in the past. Evidence for bimodality was first noted by Burch and Rowell, who investigated 1356 patients (20). These authors found a peak onset at puberty and another smaller peak at the 4th–5th decade of life.

In subsequent studies the majority of authors concluded that two subgroups exist showing early and late onset (Table 1).

On the other hand, in a large study on the natural history of psoriasis based on questionnaires from 5600 patients, Farber et al. (22) found no evidence for the existence of bimodality.

We investigated a total of 2147 psoriasis patients (12) and found evidence suggesting the existence of two age-onset subgroups, the majority (75%) of the patients showing an early disease onset with a peak at 22 (males) and 16 (females) years. The second peak was at the age of 57 (males) and 60 (females) years

Table 1 Age of Onset Analysis in Psoriasis Patients

Ref.	Year	No. of patients	No. of subgroups related to onset age	Peak age of onset (years)	
				M/F	M/F
Burch (20)	1965	1356	2	16/11	55/45
Ross (21)	1971	963	2	28/16	55/55
Farber (22)	1968	5544	1	13/12	
Woodrow (23)	1975	157	2	15/15	15/66
Gunawardena (24)	1978	1366	2	19	41
Powell (25)	1982	406	2	15/20	>55
Henseler (12)	1985	2147	2	22/16	57/60
Bell (26)	1991	132	1	37/35	
Swanbeck (27)	1994	2434	1	17/13	

and both patient cohorts showed a Gaussian distribution (Fig. 1).

Our findings substantiated previous data by Burch and Rowell (20), Ross (21), Gunawardena et al. (24), Woodrow et al. (23) as well as Powell et al. (25). In these reports the majority of patients showed the earliest signs of psoriasis during the second decade of life, whereas later onset occurred most often above the age of 55 years (Table 1). Interestingly, in these surveys comprising six separate studies, two distinct age-onset groups were found with nearly identical peak age values.

Recently, further studies of the onset of psoriasis investigated the correlation between onset and stress (28) and onset and alcohol consumption (29). Other distinct features were found to differ in the early- and late-onset groups. Alpha 1-proteinase inhibitor was reduced in the early-onset group (30). The Koebner (isomorphic) response in psoriasis patients was noted significantly more often in the young-onset group and was found even higher (in 75% of patients) when early-onset patients presented with a severe form of the disease (31). Joint symptoms were found in 10% of patients with skin lesions (32). In this investigation two-thirds of psoriasis patients had an onset age of less than 30 years (32). In contrast to these findings, Bell et al. (26) and Swanbeck and co-workers (27) were not able to identify two cohorts of different age of onset. Swanbeck et al. investigated 5197 families with psoriasis and "could neither confirm nor refute the concept of two types of non-pustular psoriasis." Because of the large cohort size investigated, two groups of onset would have been detected by taking the actual age of patients (see below) into account. In a subsequent study the authors investigated 11,366 patients indicating three types with onset ages before 16, between 20 and 35, and over 35 years (33).

In a population-based study during a 4-year period in a U.S. white population, Bell et al. (26) found the highest prevalence rate in the 60–69-year age group, whereas in a Norwegian population the highest prevalence was identified in the 30–49-year age group (34). In both studies the onset age was unimodal with a peak between 30 and 40 years. Investigations of childhood psoriasis conducted in India have shown a median onset age of 7 years, the most common trigger factor being an infection of the throat (35). This was further substantiated by an investigation of Rasmussen (36), who reported that acute guttate psoriasis was most often seen after streptococcal infection of the upper respiratory tract. Following treatment the disease recurs often as large plaque psoriasis.

Furthermore, several studies have shown that hereditary psoriasis is found in patients with early onset and nearly absent in patients with an onset age greater than 40 years. Taken together, today nearly all studies of onset age of psoriasis identify two different peaks in the onset of psoriasis. It is worth mentioning that, as we pointed out earlier (16), all studies of onset age should take into account the fact that a systematic bias will be made neglecting the actual age of the patients. Ideally, one should ask a very great cohort of very old people for the time of the onset of psoriasis.

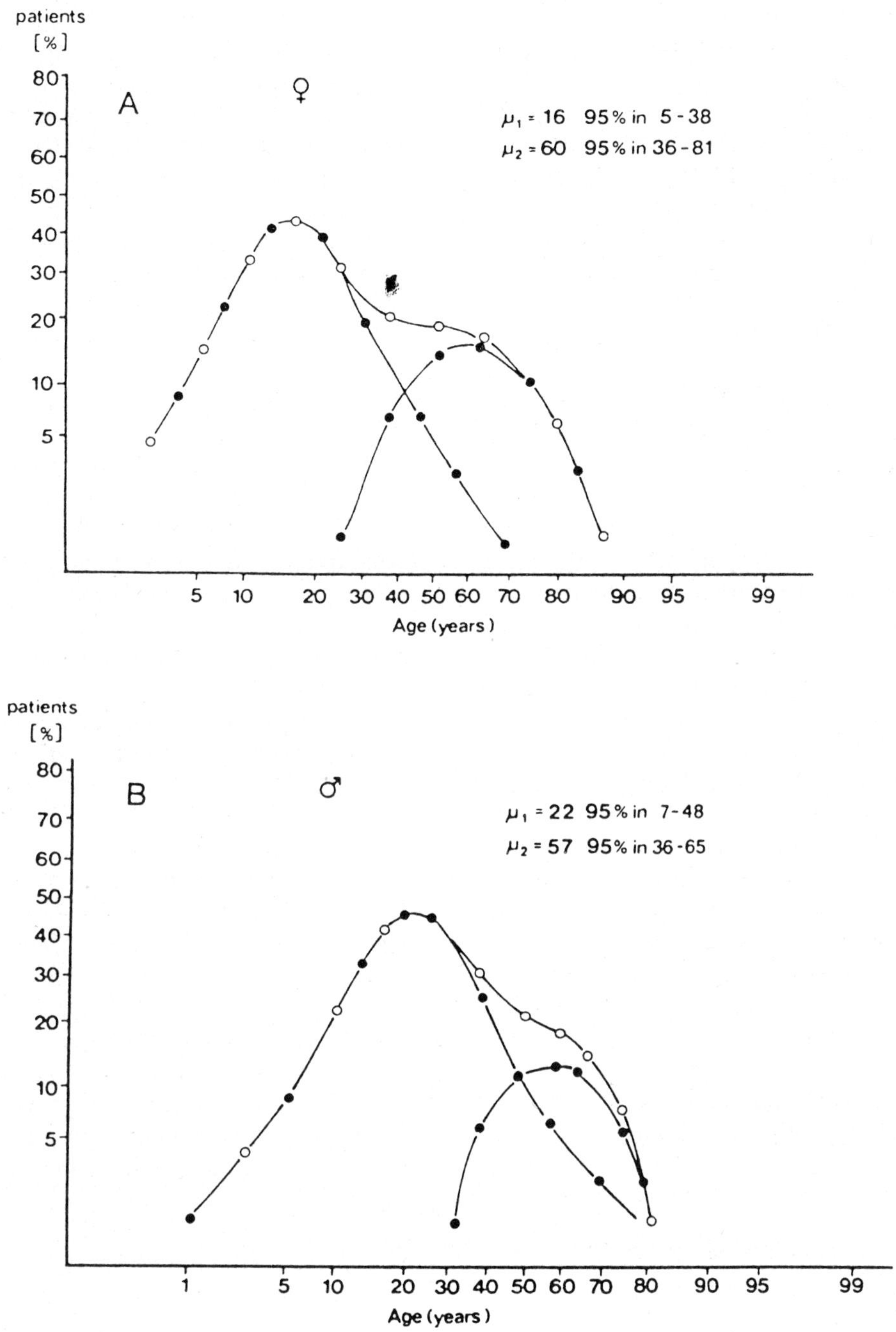

Figure 1 Age of onset in 1056 female (A) and 1091 male (B) patients with nonpustular psoriasis. The differences between both patient cohorts are significant ($p < .001$), the overlap between both curves being less than 15%. μ: Peak values with interval, in which 95% of patient cohort is found.

ASSOCIATION WITH HLA CLASS I ANTIGENS

Several studies have compared early and late onset in patients expressing HLA B13, B57 (which is identical in 93% to the formerly designated antigen B17), and Cw6 antigens. According to Farber and Nall (19), age onset appeared to be lower in patients positive for HLA B57 and B13. Also Brenner et al. (7) found significantly more HLA Cw6–positive patients with onset at young age. A more extensive analysis of the onset of psoriasis in HLA B17- and B57–positive patients was first provided by Karvonen (4) and subsequently by Hawkins et al. (11), Henseler and Christophers (12), and Economidou et al. (10). Data from these studies unanimously point toward a significant association between early onset and the expression of HLA B57, B13 (4) as well as Cw6 (12). So far the evidence provided by these five separate studies (Table 2) supports the idea of a higher frequency of HLA Cw6 and/or B57 as well as B13 antigens in patients with early onset.

Further data concerning the classification of clinical disease types were subsequently collected in 256 patients treated at the Department of Dermatology, University of Kiel (Table 3) (16). In this study complete phenotyping of the class I major histocompatibility complex (HLA A, B, C) was performed. Among a total of 43 antigens identified in each of the patients, six antigens were significantly more often expressed in psoriasis patients as compared to a healthy North German control group (comparing more than 2000 persons from the Department of Immunology, University of Kiel). These are listed in Table 3 and grouped according to age onset of these patients.

Table 3 shows that four antigens are present significantly more often in the early-onset age group (≤40 years, i.e., HLA Cw6, B13, Bw57, and A30). The antigen most frequently seen in this patient group is Cw6. The relative risk in these patients is 11 versus 1.8 in patients older than 40 years. Interestingly, the latter group of patients demonstrates an increased frequency of Cw2 as well as B27, raising the relative risk to 6.4 and 3.1, respectively (Table 3).

These data confirm previous findings on the association of HLA class I antigens, notably Cw6, with early-onset psoriasis [called type I psoriasis (12)]. On the other hand, a comparatively weak, although significant, association is seen for antigens Cw2 and B27 and late onset. The data demonstrate that the risk of acquiring late-onset psoriasis (beyond the age of 40) is 6.4 times higher when Cw2 is expressed and 2.3 times higher than normal when B27 is expressed.

Recently, further studies have confirmed these results and expanded these HLA antigens by other HLA and non-HLA markers:

1. Asahina and co-workers (37) investigated specific nucleotide sequences of HLA C. The authors found a coding region for Alanine at position 73 significantly increased in frequency in 75 Japanese patients compared with controls (relative risk = 4.7, $p <$ 0.0001). Alanine at position 73 is common to Cw4, Cw6, Cw7, and Cw12, Cw13 and Cw15. These authors suggest that Alanine at position 73 of HLA C molecules may play an important role in susceptibility to the disease.
2. Nakagawa et al. (38) studied HLA class I, class II, and complement genes (C2, C4A, C4B, and BF) in Japanese psoriatics and presented a so-called high-risk haplotype (supratype) HLA A2-Cw11-Bw46-C2C-BFS-C4A4-C4B2-DRw8. They suggested that this haplotype may indicate racial and ethnic differences among psoriatic patients.
3. Schmitt-Egenolf and co-workers (13) investigated the HLA type of patients with type I and type II psoriasis by means of genotyping using sequence-specific oligonucleotide probes. They detected a strong elevation of the HLA DRB1*0701/2, HLA DQA1*0201, and HLA DQB1*0303 extended haplotype in type I psoriasis.
4. In a further study (n = 64) of this high-risk haplotype it was shown by Ikäheimo and co-workers

Table 2 Studies on HLA Typing in Early- and Late-Onset Psoriasis (% patients)

	HLA Cw6			HLA B57		
Ref.	Early onset[a]	Late onset[a]	Normal Freq.	Early onset[a]	Late onset[a]	Normal Freq.
Svejgard (48)	87[b]		33.1	29[b]		8.0
Hawkins (11)	53.2	46.7	18.1	18.8	20.0	7.2
Henseler (12)	78.1	36.7	—	n.d.	n.d.	—
Economidou (10)	54.8	26.6	14.8	20.0	6.2	7.9
Henseler (17)	73.8	31.8	20.4	29.7	12.1	6.2

[a]Onset age ≤ 35 years or >35 years, in (11); ≤40 years or >40 years in (12) and (17); <25 years or ≥25 years in (10).
[b]Not classified according to age of onset.

Table 3 HLA Typing, Onset Age, and Relative Risk (RR) in 256 Patients with Nonpustular Psoriasis

HLA	Onset age ≤40 years %	RR	Onset age >40 years %	RR	Controls (European Caucasoids) (%)
Cw6	73.8	11.0	31.8	1.8*	20.4
B13	34.3	7.7	9.1	1.5*	6.4
Bw57	29.7	6.4	12.1	2.1*	6.2
A30	9.3	2.8	1.5	0.4*	3.6
Cw2	11.6	2.3*	27.3	6.4	5.5
B27	7.6	0.7*	25.8	3.1	10.1

$p \leq 0.01$; *n.s.

Table 4 Concurrent Skin Diseases in Psoriasis Patients (Relative Risk)

	Patient's age of onset ≤40 years	>40 years
Bacterial infections	0.38**	0.92
Viral infections	0.67*	0.93
Fungal infections	0.93	1.12

*$p < 0.001$; **$p < 0.0001$.

(14) that Cw6 and Cw6 DR7 DQA1 *0201 are closely associated with the heredity of psoriasis. The presence of Cw6 alone appeared sufficient to indicate a clinically significant risk for psoriasis. Recently Elder and co-workers confirmed this result in more than 100 psoriasis families with more than 800 family members (personal communication, 1996).

5. Suarez Almazor and Russell (39) studied 12 families with at least two siblings with psoriasis, comparing the HLA haplotypes in affected siblings of these families. All sib pairs shared at least one haplotype and 13 of the 15 were HLA identical. From these results they suggest that at least one, and probably more, genes are involved in psoriasis.

6. A gene designated S has been identified in the HLA class I region located 160 kilobases telomeric of HLA C (40). It has been shown that S-gene expression is restricted to differentiating keratinocytes. Furthermore, similarities were found in the amino acid sequences of the S gene and loricrin, keratin 1, and keratin 10, all major components of the granular-cell layer. It has been suggested that this gene may contribute to the pathogenesis of psoriasis.

To date, analyses of HLA haplotypes have provided evidence that psoriasis susceptibility is associated with the MHC class I and II region. However, no gene within the HLA region has been identified with genetic linkage with psoriasis. In addition, these studies

Table 5 Affected Family Members of 256 Patients with Psoriasis According to Type of Psoriasis

	Type I *N*	Affected	%	Type II *N*	Affected	%	*p*
Parents	264	37	14.0	100	5	5.0	0.05
Siblings	344	32	9.3	134	2	1.5	0.01
Children	145	21	14.5	75	2	2.7	0.01
Families with children	63	18	28.6	41	2	4.9	0.01

show that psoriasis, though clinically similar, in fact consists of two distinct disease types, type I and type II psoriasis, which differ in HLA haplotypes.

ASSOCIATED DISEASES IN EARLY-ONSET PSORIASIS

Recently we performed an investigation in which a total of 42,461 patients were studied for concomitant diseases (41).

The relative risk (RR) for disease from skin diseases with infectious causes, e.g., bacterial or viral agents, was lower in early-onset psoriasis patients. In contrast, susceptibility to bacterial or viral diseases in late-onset psoriasis is not different from that of nonpsoriatic control patients (Table 4). This difference is not due to the dissimilar actual age of patients investigated because the calculations were performed utilizing age- and sex-adjusting methods.

FAMILY MEMBERS AFFECTED IN TYPE I AND TYPE II PSORIASIS

Detailed analyses concerning the rate at which psoriasis is transmitted are given by several authors (42–46). In general, the data vary considerably and may range from high rates of psoriatic offspring, as found in the Lomholt study (43), to low transmittance rates (18). We evaluated first-degree relatives (17) of patients older than 60 years at the time the study was conducted. Thereby attempts were made to avoid erroneous family history data that may vary with the age of patients under study.

In Table 5 it is shown that familial aggregation is more frequently seen in type I as compared to type II. In fact, more that a quarter of patients (or families with offspring) of type I probands were affected as compared to those related to type II probands. This supports the overall notion that disease transmission is much stronger in the former type of psoriasis.

CONCLUSIONS

By simple means, e.g., recording patient data, age onset, family history as well as course of the disease, it became evident that nonpustular psoriasis with erythrosquamous lesions may not be one uniform disease but may present as subtypes indistinguishable by clinical inspection. Search for associated markers revealed that the HLA antigens (in addition to inheritance patterns and course of disease) indeed were instrumental in defining the psoriasis subsets.

The distinction between type I and type II psoriasis may have significant implications. To some extent it resembles the situation in diabetes mellitus or, as recently shown, multiple sclerosis (47). In both diseases two distinct subgroups with different HLA profiles exist. Furthermore, in both diseases as well as in others [e.g., rheumatoid arthritis (48)] significant associations between HLA genes and autoimmune pathomechanisms have been proposed (49). In fact, evidence is growing from genetic studies of autoimmunity that autoreactivity may be related to effects of genes that are located close to the HLA region and able to influence autoimmune responsiveness.

Also it has been observed that in some autoimmune diseases (e.g., rheumatic arthritis, diabetes type I) specific alleles of different loci tend to occur more often than expected (50,51). This linkage disequilibrium appears to be relevant to the genetic susceptibility to disease (50). As shown elsewhere (12), linkage disequilibrium appears to be present in type I psoriasis, and this is seen for Cw6, B13, A2, and Bw57 (16). Since erythrosquamous lesions are indistinguishable in type I and type II psoriasis, it is possible that different pathomechanisms are involved resulting in identical clinical lesions. As more evidence is accumulating in support of this idea, our findings certainly do not make it easier to understand psoriasis but add to the complexity of this disease.

REFERENCES

1. Russel, T.J., Schultes, L.M., and Kuban, D.J. (1972). Histocompatibility (HL-A) antigens associated with psoriasis. *N. Engl. J. Med.* 287:735–740.
2. Svejgaard, A., Svejgaard, E., Staub-Nielsen, L., and Jacobsen, B. (1973). Some speculation on the association between HL-A and disease based on studies of psoriasis patients and their families. *Transplant. Proc.* 5:1797–1798.
3. Svejgaard, A., Staub Nielsen, L., Svejgaard, E., Kissmeyer Nielsen, F., Hjortshoj, A., and Zachariae, H. (1974). HL-A in psoriasis vulgaris and in pustular psoriasis-population and family studies. *Br. J. Dermatol.* 91:145–153.
4. Karvonen, J. (1975). HL-A antigens in psoriasis with special reference to the clinical type, age of onset, exacerbation after respiratory infection and occurrence of arthritis. *Ann. Clin. Res.* 7:301–311.
5. Henseler, T., Koch, F., Westphal, E., Nair, R.P., Vorhees, J.J., Elder, J.T., and Christophers, E. (1992).

Presence of HLA-DR7 in type I psoriasis. *J. Invest. Dermatol.* 98:607.
6. Krulig, L., Farber, E., Grumet, F.C., and Payne, R.O. (1975). Histocompatibility (HL-A) antigens in psoriasis. *Arch. Dermatol.* 111:857–860.
7. Brenner, W., Gschnait, F., and Mayr, W.R. (1978). HLA B13, B17, B37, and Cw6 in psoriasis vulgaris: association with the age of onset. *Arch. Dermatol. Res.* 262:337–339.
8. Gaut, E., Brenner, S., Irfter, T., Orgad, S., Mizrachi, Y., and Krakowski, A. (1978). HLA antigens in patients with psoriasis. *Tissue Antigens* 12:195–199.
9. Tiilikainen, A., Lassus, A., Karvonen, J., Vartiainen, P., and Julin, M. (1980). Psoriasis and HLA-Cw6. *Br. J. Dermatol.* 102:179–184.
10. Economidou, J., Papasteriades, C., Varla Leftherioti, M., Vareltzidis, A., and Stratigos, J. (1985). Human lymphocyte antigens A, B, and C in Greek patients with psoriasis: relation to age and clinical expression of the disease. *J. Am. Acad. Dermatol.* 13:578–582.
11. Hawkins, B.R., Tiwari, J.L., Lowe, N., Wolfish, P., Pollock, C.A., Cho, Y.W., and Terasaki, P.I. (1980). HLA and psoriasis. In *Histocompatibility Testing 1980,* P.I. Terasaki (Ed.). Munksgaard, Copenhagen, pp. 711–714.
12. Henseler, T., and Christophers, E. (1985). Psoriasis of early and late onset: characterization of two types of psoriasis vulgaris. *J. Am. Acad. Dermatol.* 13:450–456.
13. Schmitt-Egenolf, M., Boehncke, W.H., Ständer, M., Eiermann, T.H., and Sterry, W. (1993). Oligonucleotide typing reveals association of type I psoriasis with the HLA-DRB1*0701/2, -DQA1*0201, -DQB1*0303 extended haplotype. *J. Invest. Dermatol.* 100:749–752.
14. Ikäheimo, I., Silvennoinen-Kassinen, S., Karvonen, J., Järvinen, T., and Tiilikainen, A. (1996). Immunogenetic profile of psoriasis vulgaris: association with haplotypes A2,B13,Cw6,DR7,DQA1*0201 and A1,B17, Cw6,DR7,DQA1*0201. *Arch. Dermatol. Res.* 188: 63–67.
15. Henseler, T., Westphal, E., Jenisch, S., Nair, R.P., Zavazava, N., Elder, J.T., Voorhees, J.J., and Christophers, E. (1993). Mechanism of linkage disequilibrium between Cw6 and DR7 in type I psoriasis: examples of inheritance in trans. *J. Invest. Dermatol.* 100:542.
16. Henseler, T. (1990). Bedeutung von Beginnalter, Vererbungsmuster und HLA- Typisierung bei Patienten mit nicht-pustulöser Psoriasis. 2nd Thesis, University of Kiel, Germany.
17. Henseler, T., and Christophers, E. (1988). Klassifizierung der nichtpustulösen Psoriasis. *Hautarzt* 39(Suppl. VIII):79–80.
18. Steinberg, A.G., Becker, S.W., Fitzpatrick, T.B., and Kierland, R.R. (1951). A genetic and statistical study of psoriasis. *J. Am. Hum. Genet.* 267–281.
19. Farber, E.M., and Nall, L. (1993). Psoriasis associated with human immunodeficiency virus/acquired immunodeficiency syndrome. *Cutis* 52:29–35.
20. Burch, P.R.J., and Rowell, N.R. (1965). Psoriasis: aetiological aspects. *Acta Derm. Venereol.* 45:366–380.
21. Ross, H.G. (1971). Untersuchungen über das Entstehungsalter der Psoriasis vulgaris. *Methods Inf. Med.* 10:108–115.
22. Farber, E.M., Forbes, E.M., Bright, R.D., and Nall, M.L. (1968). Psoriasis. A questionnaire survey of 2,144 patients. *Arch. Dermatol.* 98:248–259.
23. Woodrow, J.C., Dave, V.K., Usher, N., and Anderson, J. (1975). The HL-A system and psoriasis. *Br. J. Dermatol.* 92:427–436.
24. Gunawardena, D.A., Gunawardena, K.A., Vasanthananthan, N.S., and Gunawardena, J.A. (1978). Psoriasis in Sri-Lanka—a computer analysis of 1366 cases. *Br. J. Dermatol.* 98:85–96.
25. Powell, F., Young, M., and Barnes, J. (1982). Psoriasis in Ireland. *Irish J. Med. Sci.* 151:109–113.
26. Bell, L.M., Sedlack, R., Beard, C.M., Perry, H.O., Michet, C.J., and Kurland, L.T. (1991). Incidence of psoriasis in Rochester, MN, 1980–1983. *Arch. Dermatol.* 127:1184–1187.
27. Swanbeck, G., Inerot, A., Martinsson, T., and Wahlström, J. (1994). A population genetic study of psoriasis. *Br. J. Dermatol.* 131:32–39.
28. Al'Abadie, M.S., Kent, G.G., and Gawkrodger, D.J. (1994). The relationship between stress and the onset and exacerbation of psoriasis and other skin conditions. *Br. J. Dermatol.* 130:199–203.
29. Poikolainen, K., Reunala, T., Karvonen, J., Lauharanta, J., and Karkkainen, P. (1990). Alcohol intake: a risk factor for psoriasis in young and middle aged men? *Br. Med. J.* 300:780–783.
30. Glinski, W., Barszcz, D., Glinska Ferenz, M., Zarebska, Z., and Jablonska, S. (1989). Two subpopulations of patients with early and late onset of psoriasis differ regarding alpha 1-proteinase inhibitor activity. *Acta Derm. Venereol.* (Suppl.) 146:9–12.
31. Melski, J.W., Bernhard, J.D., and Stern, R.S. (1983). The Koebner (isomorphic) response in psoriasis. Associations with early age at onset and multiple previous therapies. *Arch. Dermatol.* 119:655–659.
32. Kononen, M., Torppa, J., and Lassus, A. (1986). An epidemiological survey of psoriasis in the greater Helsinki area. *Acta Derm. Venereol.* (Suppl.) 124:1–10.
33. Swanbeck, G., Inerot, A., Martinsson, T., Wahlström, J., Enerbäck, C., Enlund, F., and Yhr, M. (1995). Age at onset and different types of psoriasis. *Br. J. Dermatol.* 133:768–773.
34. Braathen, L.R., Botten, G., and Bjerkedal, T. (1989). Prevalence of psoriasis in Norway. *Acta Derm. Venereol.* (Suppl.) 142:5–8.

35. Nanda, A., Kaur, S., Kaur, I., and Kumar, B. (1990). Childhood psoriasis: an epidemiologic survey of 112 patients. *Pediatr. Dermatol.* 7:19–21.
36. Rasmussen, J.E. (1986). Psoriasis in children. *Dermatol. Clin.* 4:99–106.
37. Asahina, A., Akazaki, S., Nakagawa, H., Kuwata, S., Tokunaga, K., Ishibashi, Y., and Juji, T. (1991). Specific nucleotide sequence of HLA-C is strongly associated with psoriasis vulgaris. *J. Invest. Dermatol.* 97: 254–258.
38. Nakagawa, H., Akazaki, S., Asahina, A., Tokunaga, K., Matsuki, K., Kuwata, S., Ishibashi, Y., and Juji, T. (1991). Study of HLA class I, class II and complement genes (C2, C4A, C4B and BF) in Japanese psoriatics and analysis of a newly-found high-risk haplotype by pulsed field gel electrophoresis. *Arch. Dermatol. Res.* 283:281–284.
39. Suarez Almazor, M.E., and Russell, A.S. (1990). The genetics of psoriasis. Haplotype sharing in siblings with the disease. *Arch. Dermatol.* 126:1040–1042.
40. Zhou, Y., and Chaplin, D.D. (1993). Identification in the HLA class I region of a gene expressed late in keratinocyte differentiation. *Proc. Natl. Acad. Sci. U.S.A.* 90:9470–9474.
41. Henseler, T., and Christophers, E. (1995). Disease concomitance in psoriasis. *J. Am. Acad. Dermatol.* 32: 982–986.
42. Hoede, K. (1931). Umwelt und Erblichkeit bei der Entstehung der Schuppenflechte. *Würzburg. Abhandlung.* 27:212–254.
43. Lomholt, G. (1963). *Psoriasis. Prevalence, Spontaneous Course and Genetics: A Census Study on the Prevalence of Skin Diseases on the Faroe Islands.* G.E.C. Gad, Copenhagen.
44. Watson, W., Cann, H.M., Farber, E.M., and Nall, M.L. (1972). The genetics of psoriasis. *Arch. Dermatol.* 105: 197–207.
45. Andressen, C., and Henseler, T. (1982). [Inheritance of psoriasis. Analysis of 2035 family histories]. *Hautarzt* 33:214–217.
46. Wuepper, K.D., Coulter, S.N., and Haberman, A. (1990). Psoriasis vulgaris: a genetic approach. *J. Invest. Dermatol.* 95:2S–4S.
47. Van Lambalgen, R. (1985). Immunogenetic studies on multiple sclerosis and experimental allergic encephalomyelitis, Primate Center TNO. Rijswijk, The Netherlands.
48. Svejgaard, A., Hauge, M., Jersild, C., Platz, P., Ryder, L.P., Staub Nielsen, L., and Thomsen, M. (1979). The HLA System. An Introductory Survey. In *Monographs in Human Genetics*. L. Beckman, M. Hauge (Eds.). S. Karger, New York, pp. i–iii.
49. Batchelor, J.R. (1985). Genetic role in autoimmunity. In *Cyclosporin in Autoimmune Disease,* R. Schindler (Ed.). Springer, Heidelberg, pp. 16–23.
50. Vadheim, C.M., Rotter, J.I., Macleren, N.K., Riley, W.J., and Anderson, C.E. (1986). Preferential transmission of diabetic alleles within the HLA gene complex. *N. Engl. J. Med.* 315:1314–1318.
51. Köbberling, J. (1987). Genetik des Diabetes mellitus. *Internist* 28:210–217.

11

Population Genetics of Psoriasis

Gunnar Swanbeck, A. Inerot, T. Martinsson, and J. Wahlström
Göteborg University, Sahlgrenska University Hospital, Göteborg, Sweden

Psoriasis is a genetically determined disease with an intense and prolonged inflammatory reaction in the skin that does not seem to be self-limiting. The inflammatory reaction seems to need a triggering factor such as streptococcal throat infection or skin trauma to start. Psoriasis is highly variable between individuals but rather constant after onset within the individual. Some patients are severely affected by psoriasis while others have such minor skin lesions that they are hardly aware of having a skin disease. The age at onset of the disease also varies from earliest infancy to late age although the most common age at onset is in the second decade of life. These factors impose problems for population genetic studies. The penetrance of the genotype is thus dependent on age of the individual and a number of external factors. Primarily it is assumed that there is one specific psoriasis gene, but there may be several other genetic factors that influence the severity of the disease or the age at which it starts.

Following Mendelian concepts, we use relatively simple rules to describe the inheritance of different properties, namely, autosomal or sex-linked, and dominant or recessive inheritance. These rules make it possible to inform patients, in a simple and understandable way, about the risks for their children of getting a disease and to explain the distribution of the disease in the family. In the case of psoriasis these simple rules have been considered unable to describe the inheritance of the disease (1,5). The main purpose of this chapter is to show that this may not be the case.

Lomholt has made an admirable effort to study a large part of the population on the Faroe Islands with respect to the familial occurrence of psoriasis (1). His report has to some extent become the "psoriasis bible," the data of which have been reevaluated by other investigators (2). Hellgren (3) and Romanus (4) have also made significant efforts to collect representative Scandinavian data on psoriasis. The mode of inheritance has not emerged clearly from these studies. A multifactorial type of inheritance has been suggested (5). A recent reevaluation of Lomholt's data has made a single major gene for psoriasis probable (2). Other hypotheses on the inheritance of psoriasis with two types of psoriasis vulgaris (6) and genetic imprinting (7) have been put forward. We feel it is important to look critically at the epidemiology of psoriasis to determine which genetic models are needed to explain the epidemiological data. On the basis of available information, it is difficult to give information to patients regarding the risk of offspring developing psoriasis.

For a disease with a variable age at onset and different expressions of the disease, it is important to get as accurate information as possible about the relationship between the genotype and the phenotype of the disease. By penetrance of the genotype, we mean the quotient between the prevalence of the phenotype and of the genotype.

The prevalence of psoriasis in Scandinavia is considered to be slightly above 2% (1,3,10). This is the prevalence of the phenotype, which in the case of psoriasis is dependent on the age of the population studied. The prevalence of the phenotype, however, is of course lower than that of the genotype. A lower limit for the prevalence of the genotype can be estimated from the prevalence of the phenotype and data on the age at onset of psoriasis.

When we speak of age at onset, we also have to define what we mean by onset. A person with very minor psoriatic lesions, for instance on the scalp, may not be aware of having psoriasis until he gets skin lesions on other body areas, thereby reporting a later age at onset than if the first lesions had been recognized and diagnosed. Our definition of age at onset of psoriasis is the age at which the individual or relatives become aware that the individual has psoriasis.

The age at onset of a disease has to be corrected for the age of the population studied. In a general population, we will have an overrepresentation of younger ages in the age at onset distribution as the older group of the population contributes to onset at young age while the younger group cannot, of course, contribute to onset at old age. Therefore, the most relevant age-at-onset curve should be based on data only from the oldest part of the population.

Methods in population genetic studies generally assume random mating with respect to the property or disease being studied. In the case of skin diseases, it is not self-evident that random mating can be assumed. Efforts to check this are therefore important. Reporting of the presence of a skin disease among relatives of the proband may also vary with respect to sex and age.

We should stress that in virtually every human genetic analysis there are imperfections, such as incorrect reporting, lack of random mating, late onset of the disease, incomplete penetrance, or too little material. It is important that an analysis of possible errors is made. In material collected on the basis of case finding only, certain parts of the material will have some relevance in differentiating between dominant and recessive inheritance. Study of psoriasis among siblings of probands where no parent has the disease is relevant. Also relevant in this respect is study of the distribution of psoriasis among the parents but not among the children of the probands. Study of the children of probands and the other parent of the children is of importance for evaluating if random mating has occurred.

We have tried to get well-defined epidemiological material to be used to test the simplest possible hypothesis about the inheritance of psoriasis. A more extensive report has been given elsewhere (12).

METHODOLOGICAL CONSIDERATIONS

Our main purpose is to determine whether an autosomal dominant or an autosomal recessive mode of inheritance is compatible with population genetic data among first-degree relatives. As our material includes only first-degree relatives, any conclusion concerning multifactorial inheritance is speculative.

In the present study only data regarding psoriasis among first-degree relatives of probands with psoriasis have been analyzed. This includes data about psoriasis among parents, siblings, and, to some extent, children of the probands.

It is easy to understand that for probands with one or both parents having psoriasis the risk of the siblings of getting the disease does not differ significantly between a dominant and a recessive mode of inheritance. The majority of the probands have no parent with psoriasis. In this situation a dominant inheritance would mean a low penetrance of the genotype. A recessive mode of inheritance can be tested on this group with methods described by Emery (9). Using the formula $spn_s/(1\text{-}q^s)$, where s is the size of the sibship, n_s the number of sibships of size s, and $q = 1 - p$, the number of affected sibships can be obtained. This formula can also be used to calculate p from the data obtained.

For children of affected probands where the other parent is unaffected, there is a 50% risk of getting the disease with a dominant mode of inheritance, while with a recessive mode the risk is dependent on the gene frequency in the population.

The distribution of probands with both, one, or no parent having psoriasis may give an estimate of the gene frequency in the population, as is shown in the discussion.

By analyzing the oldest possible probands, the problem of late onset of the disease is minimized.

MATERIAL AND METHODS

Questionnaires were sent to about 22,000 members of the Swedish Psoriasis Association. The members, almost all of whom have psoriasis, were asked about age at onset of their psoriasis, number of siblings, number of siblings with psoriasis, and psoriasis among parents. The response rate was tested for the first 3333 questionnaires sent out—1578 responded promptly and 1022 after a reminder—giving a response rate of 78%. Among the 3333 first to receive the questionnaire we obtained information on 2434 who reported having psoriasis and 99 who did not have psoriasis (for instance, supporting members); 60 had moved to an unknown address, and 11 were dead. Six percent of those with psoriasis did not have reliable information on parents or siblings, for instance, adopted persons. The distribution of psoriasis among the parents of those responding to the first questionaire and to the reminder did not differ statistically significantly as judged by the chi-square test.

In all, data from 14,008 families with psoriasis were collected. In 11,366 families information about psoriasis among parents and siblings could be obtained. This material will be indicated with the roman figure (I) in the following. Only patients with psoriasis vulgaris have been included. Psoriatic arthritis has not been an exclusion criterion, but patients who never had psoriatic skin lesions have not been included, nor have patients with purely pustular diseases like pustulosis palmoplantaris been included.

To study psoriasis among the children of probands, questionnaires were sent to 1329 probands between the age of 50 and 70 to minimize the problem of too young children and late onset of the disease. The response rate was 89.9%.

The data are reported in Figure 1 and Tables 1, 2, 4, 5, and 8. Tables 6 and 7 are based on data from probands between 50 and 70 years of age. Table 1 is divided in two parts, one for probands under 40 years of age and one for those over 40 years of age.

To check the diagnosis given by the probands, 496 persons from 156 families were examined personally by one of us (AI).

The comparisons in Tables 1–3 with respect to the number of parents with psoriasis (0, 1, or 2) were performed by test for trend in contingency table (11). Chi-square test with Yates correction was used for comparison of proportions.

RESULTS

Accuracy of Diagnosis

Of 149 probands examined, the diagnosis of psoriasis could be verified in 146. Of 293 relatives of probands who were reported not to have psoriasis, 22 could be diagnosed as having psoriasis. In all relatives who were reported to have psoriasis, the diagnosis could be verified.

To compare reports from probands of different sex and age, data are given in Table 1 on psoriasis among the parents of male and female probands over and under 40 years of age.

The tendency for women to report a higher frequency of psoriasis is not statistically significant. The old group reported fewer parents with psoriasis than the young group among males ($p < 0.05$) and among females ($p < 0.05$).

The difference between males and females in reporting psoriasis among siblings is statistically significant ($p < 0.001$).

For 1329 probands between 50 and 70 years of age, the number of children, the number of children with psoriasis, and whether the other parent of the children has psoriasis were requested. A total of 1195 answered the questionnaire.

The data obtained about children of probands (further described below) indicate that women report a higher frequency of psoriasis than men, as shown in Table 3 ($p < 0.01$).

Age at Onset

Figure 1 gives the age at onset for probands over 55 years of age. It thus indicates the risk of getting psoriasis at a certain age for those having the genotype. Approximately 50% of those who get psoriasis have done so before age 25 and 90% before age 50.

Is a Monogenic Dominant or Recessive Inheritance Likely?

Psoriasis Among Parents

As is evident from Table 1, nearly two-thirds of the probands have parents who do not have psoriasis. For this to be compatible with a dominant inheritance, the penetrance of the gene must be lower than 50%. A recessive mode of inheritance is possible if the gene frequency is on the order of 25% (12).

Psoriasis Among Siblings

In all studies where the inclusion criterion for probands is having the disease, the families where no child has the disease are not included. This means that the distribution by number of affected children misses the term that corresponds to no affected child. We thus

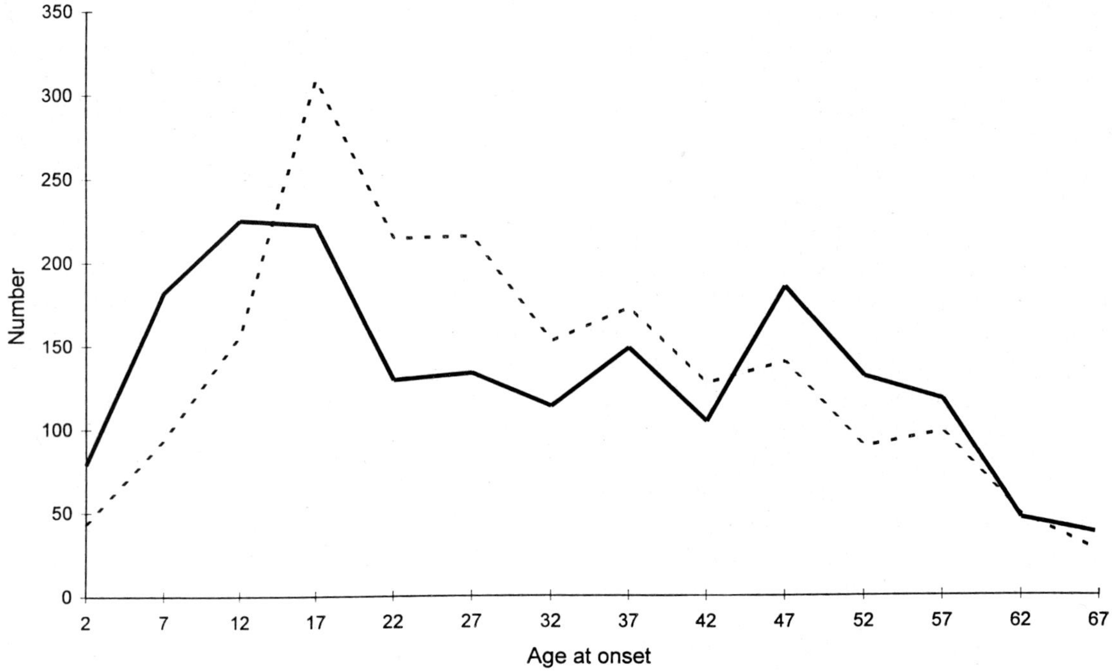

Figure 1 Age at onset for probands over 55 years of age. Midpoint of the 5-year age groups indicated on the abscissa. Solid line, female probands; broken line, male probands.

have a truncated binomial distribution. According to Hogben (8) [see also Emery (9)], the expected number of affected individuals for different size of sibships can be calculated. When one parent is affected, the probability of the offspring getting the disease is approximately $p = 0.5$, for both dominant and recessive inheritance; this segment of the population is very poorly differentiated between these two modes of inheritance.

To decrease the problem of late onset, Table 4 gives the expected and observed number of affected siblings for probands over 40 years of age. In Tables 4 and 5 penetrance refers to the quotient between observed and expected ($p = 0.5$) cases.

Table 4 tells us nothing about the mode of inheritance. An autosomal dominant and an autosomal recessive inheritance give approximately the same expected number of affected siblings when one parent has the disease and the proband is affected. However, if psoriasis is a monogenic disease, Table 4 tells us that the penetrance of the gene in this age group is relatively high.

Table 1 Comparison of Frequency of Reporting Psoriasis Among Parents for Male and Female Probands and for Probands Older and Younger than 40 Years of Age

Proband younger than 40 years					Proband older than 40 years				
Psoriasis among parents	Number		Percent		Psoriasis among parents	Number		Percent	
	M	F	M	F		M	F	M	F
Father	225	480	20.2	23.6	Father	812	1003	19.7	21.9
Mother	212	375	18.9	18.5	Mother	582	716	14.1	15.6
Both	25	44	2.2	2.2	Both	48	78	1.2	1.7
Neither	662	1132	58.7	55.7	Neither	2677	2788	65.0	60.8

Table 2 Comparison of Frequency of Reporting Psoriasis Among Siblings for Male and Female Probands

Male probands		Female probands	
No. of probands	5,375	No. of probands	6,696
No. of siblings	13,210	No. of siblings	15,962
No. with psoriasis	1,882	No. with psoriasis	2,695
% with psoriasis	14.3	% with psoriasis	16.9
No. sibs/probands	2.46	No. sibs/probands	2.38

Table 5 gives the observed and expected number of affected siblings for male and female probands if none of the parents have psoriasis and the inheritance is recessive, $p = 0.25$.

The average age of male probands is 51.14 and of female probands 47.70 years in the data recorded in Table 5.

The data of Table 5 strongly favor a recessive inheritance for psoriasis.

There are only 160 probands with both parents having psoriasis. If the corresponding calculations as in Table 4 and 5 are done on these, a penetrance of 58% is obtained when all siblings are expected to get the disease, as would be the case for a recessive mode of inheretance, and this figure would be about 75% for a dominant mode. The number of probands in this group is small, and this part of the data does not differentiate well between the two modes of inheritance.

The Mating of Probands

For 1329 probands between 50 and 70 years of age, information on the number of children, the number of children with psoriasis, and whether the other parent of the children has psoriasis was requested. A total of 1195 persons answered the questionnaire. Seventy-nine men and 83 women had no children. Of the men with children, 19 had a psoriatic mother for their children, and of the women, 25 had a psoriatic father for their children. There were 500 men with children whose mother did not have psoriasis and the corresponding number for women was 489. Of the male probands with children, the mother had psoriasis in 3.7% of the cases, and of the female probands with children, the fathers also had psoriasis in 4.9% of the cases. This indicates that mating was random with respect to having psoriasis or not, as these percentages are very similar to the prevalence of psoriasis in an adult population.

The children of the probands whose other parent does not have psoriasis might, in the case of recessive inheritance, have one parent with two psoriasis genes and the other parent with either no or one psoriasis gene. We thus have two populations of children, one group of children who will become heterozygotes and cannot get psoriasis and one with a 50% risk of getting the psoriasis genotype. In Table 6 the second population is represented in columns 1–5, while column 0 represents the first population plus children in the second population who belong to sibships without psoriasis.

Using the figures in the columns in Table 6 representing one to five children with psoriasis and the formula developed by Hogben (8) with $p = 0.5$, we get a penetrance of the genotype of 82%. Using $p = 0.41$ (0.5*0.82), we can calculate the contribution of the second population to the column representing zero children with psoriasis and thereby also the first population. The second population with one heterozygotic parent for psoriasis comprises 42% and the other 58%.

With random mating this is approximately what can be expected when we have a gene frequency of 0.25 and the distribution of psoriasis among the parents of the probands reported above.

Two Types of Psoriasis Vulgaris or Genetic Imprinting

Two types of psoriasis vulgaris has been proposed mainly on the basis of a peak on the age-at-onset curve at about 50 years of age. In our data (Fig. 2) this peak can only be seen for women and coincides with the menopause.

The higher incidence of psoriasis among children from psoriatic fathers than from psoriatic mothers has been the reason for suggesting genetic imprinting in psoriasis (7).

DISCUSSION

Are the members of the Swedish Psoriasis Association representative of psoriasis patients in general? Natu-

Table 3 Comparison of Frequency of Reporting Psoriasis Among Children for Male and Female Probands

Male probands		Female probands	
No. of children	1179	No. of children	1167
No. with psoriasis	151	No. with psoriasis	212
% with psoriasis	12.8%	% with psoriasis	18.2%
Aver. age of oldest child	32.3 year	Aver. age of oldest child	35.4
Children/probands	1.98	Children/probands	1.96

rally there is a selection of some kind, as in every dataset. The conclusions drawn in this study are therefore valid for this group. As shown below, our dataset is very similar to that of Lomholt (1), which is based on a population study on the Faroe Islands. We believe that psoriasis of very late onset may be slightly underrepresented in our material. Old people who get psoriasis may be less likely to become members of the patient organization.

Among the 149 probands checked, there were three for whom we could not find sufficient evidence in their skin status or in earlier medical records that they could be regarded as having psoriasis vulgaris. Of the 293 relatives who were reported not to have psoriasis, 22 had clinical signs of the disease, and of the 55 reported to have psoriasis, all were correctly diagnosed. Our impression is, therefore, that there is a small number of probands for whom we cannot be sure of their diagnosis and that there is a slight underreporting of psoriasis among relatives. The underreporting does not seem to be of such a magnitude that it severely disturbs the analysis but it has to be taken into account.

Table 1 indicates that females tend to report a higher frequency of psoriasis among parents than males do, and that younger probands report a higher frequency among their mothers than older probands do. Table 2 indicates that women report psoriasis about 20% more often among siblings than men. Table 3 shows that women report psoriasis among the children about 40% more often than men. Women may be more inclined to notice minor skin changes than men. We think it is likely that the difference in frequency of psoriasis among siblings and partly among parents of male and female probands is due to a difference in attitude and curiosity and not to a biological factor.

The relationship between the number of men and women in our material does not give any information about the same relationship in the whole population. However, the relationship of psoriasis among the parents may give information on this question, if we assume equal heredity of psoriasis from mothers and fathers. If we assume that women younger than 40 years of age are the most reliable reporters, 55% of the psoriatics would be men and 45% women. In a large epidemiological study of hand eczema among 20,000 individuals in Göteborg, Sweden, a question about psoriasis, not only on the hands, was also included. The population studied were between 20 and 65 years old and reported psoriasis among 4.5% of men and 3.7% of women (11). Romanus (4), Hellgren (3), and Brandrup and Green (10) reported a similar relationship of psoriasis in the two sexes. We are thus

Table 4 Number of Siblings Observed to Have Psoriasis in Sibships of Different Size When One Parent Has Psoriasis Compared with the Expected Number (for $p = 0.5$) as Calculated by the Method of Emery (9)

	Father has psoriasis		Mother has psoriasis	
Size of sibship	Observed	Expected	Observed	Expected
2	848	908	532	575
3	761	866	593	648
4	578	717	428	506
5	364	470	238	330
Sum	2551	2961	1791	2059
Penetrance	86.2%		87.0%	

Table 5 Number of Siblings Observed to Have Psoriasis in Sibships of Different Size When No Parent Has Psoriasis Compared with the Expected Number (for $p = 0.25$) as Calculated by the Method of Emery (9)

	Male probands		Female probands	
Size of sibship	Observed	Expected	Observed	Expected
2	1026	1055	1280	1278
3	857	932	1130	1187
4	618	689	763	802
5	422	500	489	538
Sum	2923	3176	3662	3805
Penetrance	92.0%		96.2%	

inclined to believe that psoriasis is slightly more common among men. As it is generally accepted that psoriasis is autosomally inherited, this would mean that a smaller fraction of women having the genotype of psoriasis will develop the disease than is the case for men.

The age-at-onset distribution of Figure 2 is to be regarded as reflecting the probability of getting psoriasis at a certain age in persons having the genotype. We find this more relevant than using the distribution of Figure 1.

The age-at-onset curve for men of Figure 2 shows that after the age of 20 the number of men getting psoriasis rapidly declines. This could mean that there are fewer individuals left with a psoriatic genotype who do not have symptoms of psoriasis. In other words, most men with a psoriasis genotype also get the disease. For women the age-at-onset curve looks different. A considerable number of women get psoriasis between 45 and 55 years of age. This peak in the age-at-onset curve coincides with menopause. This late onset of psoriasis has been interpreted as a special type II psoriasis by Henseler and Christophers (6).

The high frequency of HLA-Cw6 for those with an early onset may be regarded as a modifying factor favoring early onset, and not reflecting the primary gene of psoriasis. We may also look upon menopause as a triggering factor in women. The present report can neither reject nor confirm the concept of two types of nonpustular psoriasis.

The fact that as many as 60% of the probands have both parents without psoriasis led us to compare psoriasis among the siblings of probands in this situation with the expected result if a recessive gene was responsible for psoriasis. It is only psoriasis among siblings whose parents do not have psoriasis that can differentiate between the dominant and recessive mode of inheritance. The penetrance of the genotype would then be over 90%. The penetrance when one parent has the disease is between 80 and 90% and when both parents are affected, close to 60%. This is probably an effect of heterogeneity.

The reason why Lomholt (1) excluded a recessive mode of inheritance might have been that a very high gene frequency is required. As pointed out above, a gene frequency of 25% in the whole population would be needed. Our material is very similar to that of Lomholt. Table 8 gives overall data comparing the two materials.

The children in our material are older than in Lomholt's, which may explain the difference in the last column of Table 8; the lower percent of psoriasis among the parents in our material may indicate a lower degree of reporting. A comparison between the curves for accumulated age at onset in Lomholt's and our material shows practically identical values.

The prevalence of psoriasis is generally given for the whole population, children included. We estimate that the prevalence of psoriasis in a population of adults is about 1.7 times that of the whole population. This means around 4% in Scandinavia, which is in good agreement with the frequency found in the hand eczema study mentioned above. The fact that similar figures are obtained among spouses to probands as given above indicates that there is a random mating among psoriatics with respect to the partner having psoriasis or not.

Traupe et al. (7) propose a genetic mechanism called genetic imprinting to explain why, in Lomholt's data (1), the children seem to have psoriasis more often when the father has psoriasis than when the mother has the disease. Table 4 does not give any support for such an effect.

If we assume that nearly all men having the genotype of psoriasis also get the disease, the genotype frequency in the population is slightly over 6%. With

Table 6 Number of Families with Different Numbers of Children with Psoriasis in Sibships of Different Sizes Where One Parent Has Psoriasis (the proband)

Size of sibship	Number of children with psoriasis 0	1	2	3	4	5
1	164	29				
2	356	103	14			
3	150	48	21	3		
4	40	19	9	2	1	
5	12	2	1	1	1	0

an incomplete penetrance and/or a slight underreporting, the frequency will be higher. A frequency for the genotype between 6 and 8% therefore does not seem unrealistic. If we have a recessive monogeneic inheritance of psoriasis, a gene frequency of 25% would give 6.25% of the population having the psoriasis genotype.

In this study, we have shown that several types of independant data, namely, psoriasis among siblings with parents not having psoriasis, the distribution of psoriasis among parents of probands, psoriasis among children of probands, and the prevalence of psoriasis in the general population, all are compatible with the hypothesis that a single recessive gene with a gene frequency of about 0.25 causes the skin disease psoriasis. Although this does not prove that the hypothesis is true, the hypothesis may be used for genetic counseling. The following predictions will be in accordance with the present material of over 5000 families: if both parents have psoriasis the risk for the offspring of getting psoriasis is 75%; if one parent has psoriasis the risk for the children is 15% for getting psoriasis; and if none of the parents have psoriasis and one child has the disease, the risk for the siblings is 20%.

ACKNOWLEDGMENTS

This project has been supported by the Swedish Psoriasis Association and the Swedish Medical Research Council project No. B95-19C-11246-01A.

Table 7 Psoriasis Among Children of Male and Female Probands

	No. of probands	No. of children	No. of children with psoriasis	% with psoriasis
Male probands (father of the children)				
Mother has psoriasis	19	41	19	46.3
Mother does not have psoriasis	500	1132	131	11.6
Female probands (mother of the children)				
Father has psoriasis	25	46	16	34.8
Father does not have psoriasis	489	1117	195	17.5

Table 8 Comparison of the Present Material with That of Lomholt (1)

	Psoriasis among parents	Psoriasis among siblings	Psoriasis among children
The present material	18%	16%	15%
Lomholt's material	21%	16%	12%

REFERENCES

1. Lomholt, G. (1963). *Psoriasis; Prevalence, Spontaneous Course and Genetics; a Census Study on the Prevalence of Skin Diseases on the Faroe Islands.* GEC Gad, Copenhagen.
2. Iselius, L., and Williams, W.R. (1984). The mode of inheritance of psoriasis: evidence for a major gene as well as a multifactorial component and its implication for genetic counselling. *Hum. Genet.* 68:73–76.
3. Hellgren, L. (1967). *Psoriasis: The Prevalence in Sex, Age and Occupational Groups in Total Populations in Sweden. Morphology, Inheritance and Association with Other Skin and Rheumatic Diseases.* Almquist & Wiksells, Stockholm.
4. Romanus, T. (1945). Psoriasis from a prognostic and hereditary point of view. Dissertation, Uppsala.
5. Watson, E., Cann, H.M., Farber, E.M., and Nall, M.L. (1972). The genetics of psoriasis. *Arch. Dermatol.* 105: 197–207.
6. Henseler, T., and Christophers, E. (1985). Psoriasis of early and late onset: characterization of two types of psoriasis vulgaris. *J. Am. Acad. Dermatol.* 13:450–456.
7. Traupe, H., van Gurp, P.J., Happle, R., Boezeman, J., and van de Kerkhof, P.C. (1992). Psoriasis vulgaris, fetal growth, and genomic imprinting. *Am. J. Med. Genet.* 42:649–654.
8. Hogben, L. (1931). The genetic analysis of familial traits. I. Single gene substitutions. *J. Genet.* 25: 97–112.
9. Emery, A.E.H. (1976). *Methodology in Medical Genetics. An Introduction to Statistical Methods.* Churchill Livingstone, New York, p. 39.
10. Brandrup, F., and Green, A. (1981). The prevalence of Psoriasis in Denmark. *Acta Dermatovener (Stockh.)* 61:344–346.
11. Meding, B., and Swanbeck, G. Unpublished data.
12. Swanbeck, G., Inerot, A., Martinsson, T., and Wahlström, J. (1994). A population genetic study of psoriasis. *Br. J. Dermatol.* 131:32–39.

12

Genes in Psoriasis

Jayant Bhalerao and Anne M. Bowcock
University of Texas Southwestern Medical Center, Dallas, Texas

M. Alan Menter
Psoriasis Center, Baylor University Medical Center, Dallas, Texas

Alan K. Silverman
Professional Practice, Dallas Texas

Understanding the pathogenesis of psoriasis remains a significant challenge in dermatological research. A major thrust in recent research has been the clarification of the molecular basis for psoriasis and the relative importance of genetic and environmental factors in triggering it. Psoriasis appears to be a genetically heterogeneous disease with multiple and complex biological system abnormalities. Many attempts have been made to correlate these aberrant physiological findings with clinical features such as type of psoriasis (e.g., guttate, plaque), age of onset, trigger (Koebner) factors such as antecedent streptococcal infection, familial versus nonfamilial occurrence, and "permissive" HLA types. Theorizing that psoriasis is an autoimmune disorder has led to important advances in understanding the skin-associated immune system, the role of cytokines, and the remarkable biological flexibility of the keratinocyte.

However, the question of whether the different clinical forms of psoriasis (such as plaque, erythrodermic, etc.) are genetically distinct is unclear, as are the reasons for the wide variability in psoriasis prevalence among monozygotic twin pairs. Much research has been directed toward establishing genetic predisposition toward the disease. There are strong indicators, including twin and family studies, that show evidence of such a component. Results, however, remain inconclusive.

In 1980, Botstein et al. (1) proposed a systematic approach to finding and organizing markers on human chromosomes. A map consisting of such markers spaced throughout the chromosome could then be used to locate genes by correlating inheritance of the markers with inheritance of traits in families (linkage analysis). Linkage analysis is now widely used for tracking down disease genes by molecular geneticists. Accurate diagnosis is essential in linkage analysis, and in the case of psoriasis, it is not clear which phenotypic features should be graded as positive, for example, limited scalp dermatitis, nail pitting or onchocolysis, and eczematous dermatitis. Moreover, confounding factors that obscure the recognition of clearly defined inheritance patterns in psoriasis include the complex and phenotypic diversity of the disease, incomplete penetrance, the likelihood that several genes may be involved, and the role of environmental and other "triggering" factors.

One approach to determining the nature of the genetic component of the disease is to identify genes in altered biochemical pathways. To identify such predisposing genes, a researcher can do a linkage analysis with multiply affected families or sib-pairs followed by positional cloning. This chapter reviews historical aspects of psoriasis genetics research, summarizes our recent finding of a locus for psoriasis susceptibility on the long arm of chromosome 17 in a large U.S. family, and finally discusses mechanisms that might be involved in conferring psoriasis susceptibility.

BRIEF HISTORY

Although twin studies have shown a high concordance of psoriasis, there is no satisfactory explanation for the widely varying risk for psoriasis that has emerged out of multiple investigations. Factors such as incomplete penetrance (phentoypic expression of the trait is absent even though the disease genotype is present) and polygenic or multifactorial inheritance have been invoked as possible eplanations, as have environmental factors. The existence of different types of psoriasis, its variable age of onset, sporadic occurrences, and the lack of a clear correlation between clinical type of psoriasis and heritability have also confounded attempts to delineate a mode of inheritance for this disease.

In 1984, Ken Halprin (University of Miami) suggested that the National Psoriasis Foundation could provide the leadership for genetic studies of psoriasis, patterned along the lines of research for the Huntington's disease gene that was then in progress. The search for the Huntington's gene was greatly aided by the identification of a large, genetically isolated family in Venezuela by Americo Negrette, the sampling of individuals from that pedigree by Nancy Wexler, Jim Gusella, and colleagues, and the fortuitously rapid identification of a linkage between Huntington's disease and a locus on human chromosome 4 (2).

In 1987, the National Psoriasis Foundation (NPF) awarded Kirk Wuepper (Oregon Health Sciences University) a grant to facilitate collection of blood specimens from affected and unaffected first-degree relatives from highly informative families with psoriasis. This grant was also used to purchase supplies for isolation of DNA from these specimens. Wuepper defined highly informative families as those with unambiguous evidence of psoriasis in three or more generations, and he looked for large families with approximately six to 10 children. At the time, it was widely believed that psoriasis susceptibility was HLA-linked, so Wuepper initially planned to use DNA probes close to HLA in his linkage analyses. In his letter requesting funds, Wuepper wrote: "The significance of the work is that it allows one to search for genetic material close to or at a 'psoriasis gene.' This may be done without knowing the genetic product exactly. Nevertheless, it may represent less of a blind search than looking at complex mediator systems associated with cell proliferation, arachidonic acid metabolites and nucleotide-dependent second messenger systems." He also attempted to reinitiate contact with families previously identified in the literature (3) but was unsuccessful.

Wuepper established a genetics research program that successfully collected specimens from 10 informative families and, with an additional grant, began DNA studies. In 1989 he was unsuccessful in his application to NIAMS for a grant to characterize, sample, and store transformed cells from select families with psoriasis and (seronegative) psoriatic arthritis, proposing to ship cells to the American Type Culture Collection (ATCC) for immortalization and distribution in a public domain registry. However, the same year the NPF sponsored a basic research meeting in Deer Valley, Utah, out of which arose its commitment to develop a public gene bank for psoriasis. Requests for proposals were sent out in 1991 and the award was made in 1992, to the Dallas-based Baylor Hospital and Southwestern Medical Center. The NPF tissue bank, which is still expanding, opened in May 1994 with almost 200 cell lines.

The foresight of Wuepper and the commitment of the NPF were thus instrumental in mobilizing the academic community and led to more rapid progress in identifying genes involved in psoriasis internationally.

TWIN STUDIES

In some populations, monozygotic twins show a significantly higher concordance rate for psoriasis compared to dizygotic twins. Studies in Denmark using the Danish twin registry showed that 72% of monozygotic twins and 15% of dizygotic twins were concordant for psoriasis (4). The 2–3% prevalence of psoriasis in the Danish population gave a heritability of 90–100% (4–7). On the other hand, pedigree analysis elsewhere has not revealed a consistent pattern of inheritance. Thus a 40–65% concordance rate was observed in monozygotic twins in the United States, but only a 35% concordance rate in Australia (8). These studies again indicate that although defective genes are likely to be involved in the pathogenesis of psoriasis, environmental and other factors are important in allowing or triggering its clinical manifestations (9–14).

DEMOGRAPHIC AND EPIDEMIOLOGICAL STUDIES

Psoriasis is present more frequently in certain racial groups and geographic areas. For example, its prevalence is high in the Faroe Islands (14), moderately high in Sweden, Great Britain, Germany, and South America, and rare in Japan, North America (indigenous people), and West Africa. Reasons for these variations are likely to be both genetic and environmental (15).

In assessing the risk of developing psoriasis on the basis of family history, Lomholt studied families in the Faroe Islands (16) and reported an occurrence of 90% among first- and second-degree relatives. For siblings of affected probands the genetic risk of developing psoriasis was not constant, but depended on the family situation. Risk ranged from 12 to 14% when no parent was affected, but rose to 34–39% when one parent had psoriasis. Andressen and Henseler (17) found a risk of only 6.6% for a sibling of the index patient when no parent was affected: this risk rose to 14% when either the mother or the father had psoriasis. Other investigators have reported similar findings (18). In questionnaire studies or direct histories of patients in clinical situations, only about 30–50% of all patients with psoriasis indicated that they were aware of one or more affected first- or second-degree relatives (17).

Pedigrees of large families in the United States have suggested autosomal dominant inheritance or multifactorial inheritance with a strong genetic influence (3,9,19). On the other hand, a recent large population study of 5197 families in Sweden suggested a recessive mode of inheritance (20). Age at onset of psoriasis has been used as a means of delineating different types of the disease. Henseler and Christophers in 1985 (21) proposed that there are two types of psoriasis. Type I psoriasis, or the early-onset form, is usually more severe and appears to be familial, whereas type II psoriasis, the late-onset form, is sporadic.

Elder et al. (22) have bolstered support for the involvement of more than one gene in psoriasis (multilocus model) by reanalyzing previously collected epidemiological data. The data of Lomholt (16) and Hellgren in Sweden (23) were scrutinized by the method of Risch (24). λ_R-1 (where λ_R or *risk ratio* is defined as the risk of disease in a relative of degree R in relation to the population prevalence) was seen to decrease by factors greater than 2 with each degree of relationship, in both the populations, which is supportive of a multilocus model.

MARKERS FOR DISEASE GENE MAPPING

The concept of using markers for localizing disease genes was originally highlighted at a meeting on HLA and hematochromatosis in 1979 where it was realized that mapping of diseases such as hematochromatosis could be facilitated if there were sufficient DNA markers with the type of variation that is seen in the HLA cluster (25). This led to the proposal that DNA restriction fragment length polymorphisms (RFLPs) may serve as such markers (1), and the discovery in the same year of the first polymorphic locus, D14S1 (26). Since that time many important human disease genes have been localized with linkage analysis. These studies rely on cosegregation of a disease allele with non-disease-associated alleles at closely linked loci or, in other words, the coinheritance of a disease and a nearby marker as a mapping tool. Such linkage studies require large families in which the disease in question is segregating as a Mendelian trait, large numbers of small families, or even larger numbers of sib-pairs. In general, the greatest potential statistical support for linkage (usually measured by the LOD score) is obtained from large families with many affected members. However, these are not always easy to find and will not delineate most of the genes of heterogeneous and polygenic diseases. Many complex diseases are therefore now being evaluated with additional approaches such as genome-wide screens of large numbers of "sib-pairs" (see below).

One of the most important diseases to be first mapped with a "linkage" approach was the gene for Huntington's disease. This discovery was followed by the identification of other diseases with similarly clear-cut modes of Mendelian inheritance such as the gene for cystic fibrosis (27). However, even some genes for complex diseases such as familial breast cancer have now been isolated with an initial linkage approach (28,29). The subsequent isolation of many of these genes has been achieved with positional cloning approaches (30–33). Now that the genetic marker maps have reached an extremely high density, due to the development of a large number of PCR-based as well as RFLP-based markers (34–37), it is feasible to attempt to tackle a variety of other complex diseases with a linkage-based approach.

SEROLOGICAL STUDIES AND HLA ASSOCIATIONS

Alleles of the HLA (class I and II major histocompatibility complex locus) system on chromosome 6 have historically been associated with susceptibility to and resistance to the development of some autoimmune diseases. One of the most confounding and tantalizing factors in psoriasis research has been the observation of the association of psoriasis susceptibility with HLA. A variety of clinical forms of psoriasis, e.g., pustular (38–40), guttate (41), erythrodermic (42), and extent of body surface involvement have been shown to be associated with alleles of various HLA loci. Class I HLA types A1, B13, B17, and Cw6 and class II HLA types DR7 and DQw3 occur with increased frequency in patients with psoriasis compared to control populations (43–46). Type II psoriasis (late-onset) has been shown to be weakly associated with HLA Cw2 and B27 (47). The HLA B and DR alleles are in strong linkage disequilibrium with HLA Cw6 and can form extended haplotypes in different populations. It has also been postulated that HLA Cw6 is the factor primarily associated with susceptibility to psoriasis, and the multiple HLA associations are the result of linkage disequilibrium (48).

Table 1 summarizes some published HLA associations in different populations.

Psoriatic arthritis, which is classified in the seronegative spondyloarthropathies, is associated with HLA B27. Psoriatic arthritis also occurs in association with HLA B27, B38, B39, Cw6, DQ2, DR4, DR7 (57–59). These associations are sometimes weak and may be due to genetic and clinical heterogeneity.

Based on these studies, it was deduced that HLA would be tightly linked with disease susceptibility in psoriasis families. However, results of linkage studies are confusing and sometimes conflicting. When segregation of HLA antigens in families with at least two affected individuals was studied, the results were inconclusive (60,61). Other family studies provided evidence for an autosomal dominant mode of inheritance with penetrance values of 25% (62–64).

Only recently has it been seriously proposed that HLA-linked loci do not always play a role in psoriasis susceptibility in some multiply affected families (65,66). Failure to detect linkage in these families has been shown to be attributable to various factors: the small size of the families, so that support for linkage is minimal; because there is no linkage to be found; because HLA Cw6, which occurs in the normal Caucasoid population at a frequency of approximately 10%, can be inherited through both sides of the family including an unaffected parent. This abolishes the ability to detect cosegregation with a particular HLA-carrying chromosome (HLA allele) in affected family members only (67,68). Nevertheless, failure to detect HLA linkage in some families clearly indicates that factors in addition to certain HLA alleles can cause psoriasis.

ADDITIONAL GENES ASSOCIATED WITH PSORIASIS

In addition to HLA, some other gene variants have been proposed to be associated with psoriasis susceptibility. Beckman et al. (69) reported a significant increase in the z allele of the alpha$_1$-antitrypsin inhibitor gene. Jimenez-Nieto et al. (70) reported that the slow acetylator phenotype on chromosome 8 is a risk factor

Table 1 Published HLA Associations in Different Populations

HLA alleles	Country	Ref.
A1, B13, B17, Cw4, Cw6	China	49
Cw6, the haplotype: A2-Cw11-B46-DR8	Japan	50
Complement genes: C2C, C4A4, C4B2, BFS	Japan	51–53
DR9 in association with pustular hand and foot psoriasis	Japan	53, 54
A1, B17, Cw6	India	55
Cw6, Cw7	Israel	56
B13, B17	Ireland	57

for familial but not nonfamilial psoriasis. The validity of these associations still needs to be confirmed in additional patient populations.

COSEGREGATION OF PSORIASIS WITH OTHER DISEASES

A family was recently described where psoriasis was segregating with the autosomal dominant disorder, hereditary multiple exostoses (HME) (71). Loci linked to HME have previously been mapped to chromosomes 8q (72), 11p (73), and 19p (74) suggesting that these regions may harbor psoriasis susceptibility genes.

LINKAGE ANALYSES

Psoriasis shows many of the problems associated with genetic analyses of a common and complex disease. Some of these have been described elsewhere (28). When only a small proportion of cases are due to bona fide inherited susceptibility, some apparently familial cases may be present only because the disease is so common. Other factors that confound a linkage analysis are incomplete penetrance of the trait in susceptible individuals (phenotypic expression of the trait is absent even though the disease genotype is present) and variations in phenotypic expression of the trait [which may depend on age, gender, modifier genes, and environmental trigger factors such as antecedent streptococcal infection (75)]. The existence of more than one major gene accounting for psoriasis (genetic heterogeneity) is likely, again decreasing the ability to detect linkage by pooling LOD scores from different kindreds.

To detect cosegregating (linked) markers, one embarks on a fishing expedition with a set of DNA markers that span the genome. It has been estimated that approximately 300 markers, distributed at a resolution of 10 cM, are required, to be reasonably sure of localizing a simple Mendelian disease gene (1), and in the case of psoriasis, owing to its complexity, it has been suggested that it may be necessary to utilize markers at a resolution of 3 cM if sib-pairs are analyzed. Over the last few years the human genome has become saturated with highly variable DNA markers known as polymorphic microsatellites. These are usually di-, tri-, or tetranucleotide repeats of varying lengths present in the noncoding regions of the genome. They can be typed with PCR and require 100-fold less DNA than the Southern blots required for RFLP analyses. The combination of highly informative, easy-to-type markers and improved software for parametric and nonparametric analyses is now facilitating the identification of loci involved in complex diseases such as psoriasis.

MAPPING A PSORIASIS SUSCEPTIBILITY LOCUS TO CHROMOSOME 17q

With the aim of identifying loci in addition to HLA that predispose to psoriasis susceptibility, we identified eight psoriasis families with multiply affected members (66). A genome-wide search was undertaken for DNA markers cosegregating with a psoriasis susceptibility locus in these families with a total of 65 cases of psoriasis. The families, drawn from 15 states, were all Caucasian. Ascertainment was maximized by having a dermatologist obtain detailed medical histories and performing a complete body examination. All patients had plaque psoriasis. Blood was drawn from all family members and lymphoblastoid cell lines were established to make a permanent "in house" library representative of these individuals. These and other cell lines make up the National Psoriasis Tissue Bank. The Bank is managed by the National Psoriasis Foundation (Oregon), the Baylor Psoriasis Center (Dallas) (which is responsible for ascertainment of families and collection and correlation of clinical material and data), and the University of Texas Southwestern Medical Center at Dallas (where cell lines are established and maintained).

Genomic DNA was isolated from NPTC cell lines for genetic analyses. A set of polymorphic microsatellites spanning the genome (34,76) at an approximate resolution of 10 cM were selected with MultiMap (77) and used for genotyping.

Since no adequate model exists for the inheritance of psoriasis, the data were analyzed with both parametric and nonparametric approaches. All approaches ultimately yielded positive results supporting a psoriasis susceptibility locus at the end of the long arm of human chromosome 17 in the largest family in the study (66). Psoriasis susceptibility in this large family was inherited as an autosomal dominant trait with high penetrance. The LOD score for the D17S784 locus was 5.33 at a recombination fraction of 4%, which is well above the threshold value of 3.0 acceptable for linkage. All 20 affected individuals in this family carried the same segment containing the end of the long arm of human chromosome 17, and approximately 80% of the individuals who had inherited the susceptibility allele had been diagnosed with psoriasis. In addition to family PS1, two smaller families, PS2 and PS4, also showed evidence for linkage to the 17q locus.

This study also provided substantial evidence for genetic heterogeneity, with five of the other seven families being unlinked to the 17q locus. The admixture test as implemented in the HOMOG program (78) was significant when tested against multipoint LOD score data. Interestingly, no apparent differences in clinical presentation were observed between the linked and unlinked families, suggesting that several different causes may converge into a common pathogenic pathway in psoriasis. No association or linkage with HLA and psoriasis susceptibility in this large family was detected. However, among the unlinked families it appeared that the presence of HLA Cw6 allele may have contributed to the development of psoriasis in at least two, and possible three, of the families.

In studying complex diseases it is useful to refine the phenotype to enable analysis of only a class of affected members. One such phenotype may be psoriatic arthritis, which is defined as an inflammatory arthritis occurring during the course of psoriasis and characterized by negative rheumatoid factor (79). The incidence of psoriatic arthritis among psoriatic patients is 5–7% but can be as high as 30–40% in patients with severe psoriasis (80,81). The juvenile form of psoriatic arthritis appears before age 16 with a maximum occurrence around age 10 (82). The fact that there were several cases of psoriatic arthritis in the three families that show linkage to the 17q locus may suggest that the defective gene at 17q is part of a common pathogenic mechanism that links psoriasis and psoriatic arthritis. However, the alteration within the 17q locus resulting in high risk for psoriasis in the one large family does not appear to be responsible for many other familial cases of psoriasis since linkage to the 17q locus has not been seen in many of the other families studied by us and by other groups (83,84). Nevertheless, once this gene/locus is identified, it may highlight genes in specific biochemical pathways likely to be involved in the pathogenesis of the disease, and which could be altered in some way in psoriasis.

OTHER POSSIBLE LINKAGES

Several other groups recently described additional possible psoriasis susceptibility loci. Matthews et al. (85) reported linkage to D4S1535 on chromosome 4q in Irish and British families. In a study of 68 British families including 106 affected sibling pairs, Trembath et al. (86) found linkages on chromosomes 2 (D2S134), 8 (D8S284, near the gene for hereditary multiple exostosis) and 20 (D20S186). A major role for a gene in the MHC region on chromosome 6p21 was also proposed. In another study that involved 115 families including 86 nuclear and 29 extended families, Nair et al. (87) were able to confirm linkage to 17q, support the presence of a predisposing gene in the MHC region, and identify additional loci at 16q (D16S3110 near the Crohn's disease locus) and 20p (D20S851).

AFFECTED SIB-PAIR ANALYSIS

For a complex multifactorial and polygenic disease such as psoriasis, where the mode of inheritance is uncertain, nonparametric methods of genetic analysis such as the affected sib-pair method, which are not sensitive to specifications of modes of inheritance and penetrance, should also be used in inheritance studies. Pairs of siblings can share two, one, or no alleles transmitted from their parents. The expected frequency that any pair of siblings will share two, one, or no alleles at a given locus is 25%, 50%, and 25% respectively. If pairs of siblings affected with the same disease are examined, linkage will cause a shift in the sharing of loci, giving an excess of affected sib-pairs sharing one or two marker allele(s) identical by descent. This means that the affected siblings possess the "at risk" genotype, which is assumed to be the same in each pair (because they are siblings). The disease alleles should be identical by descent from the parents of the siblings except when the parents carry more than one copy of the disease alleles. When linkage has been established by a sib-pair method, the same data can also be used to suggest the mode of inheritance of the identified disease susceptibility gene (88).

Insulin-dependent diabetes mellitus (type I diabetes), like psoriasis, is an autoimmune disease with a multifactorial and multigenic etiology. Genome-wide linkage screens with affected sib-pairs from numerous families helped in the identification of at least 11 possible additional loci that could additively contribute to diabetes susceptibility (89). One region localized by sib-pair analysis that had previously been shown to confer susceptibility is the insulin gene on chromosome 11p, now termed IDDM2 (90–93). A range of specific allele sizes of a VNTR *(variable number of tandem repeats)* 5′ to the gene appears to confer increased susceptibility to diabetes (94). It is proposed that these alleles affect the levels of expression of insulin and other genes such as insulin-like growth factor II, present in the region (89).

By analogy, it would appear that similar sib-pair analyses of psoriasis families could help identify psoriasis susceptibility regions, and ultimately predisposing alleles.

GENE IDENTIFICATION

A logical approach in identifying disease-causing genes in linked regions is to screen for known "candidate genes" present within the region for disease-specific mutations. If these candidates cannot be shown to have mutations associated with the disease state, the disease-linked regions can be further screened to identify the disease-causing gene(s). The 17q susceptibility region identified in our studies spans a distance of approximately 11 cM, which would normally correspond to 11,000 kb in interstitial regions of the chromosome. However, at telomeres recombination is often inflated (95), and this distance may correspond to one-tenth of the estimated size (1100 kb). Such a chromosomal region can be isolated with physical mapping approaches such as cloning in a series of overlapping yeast artificial chromosomes (YACs), converting these to cosmids, and using these to select genes by a variety of approaches including direct hybridization to complementary DNA libraries, exon trapping (96,97), and direct selection (98,99). All newly identified genes in the region will need to be sequenced and examined for germline mutations in the affected individuals to isolate the psoriasis gene.

The genetic defect in psoriasis could be expressed in one of three cells, the T lymphocyte, an antigen-presenting cell (possibly the dermal dendritic cell), or the keratinocyte. The most likely site for the expression of a genetic defect is in the keratinocyte and in its response to cytokines. However, there is also evidence that the primary defect lies within the T cell: within lesions, there is a selective recruitment of CD4+ rather than CD8+ T cells, and treatment with monoclonal antibodies to CD4 antigen may result in clearance of psoriasis (100–102). Further evidence for the importance of T cells in the pathogenesis of psoriasis has been provided by the recent demonstration that targeted inhibition of activated T-lymphocyte growth can lead to a reversal of psoriatic lesions. The systemic administration of a fusion protein composed of IL-2 and the cytotoxic domain of diphtheria toxin resulted in a marked decrease in the number of T cells in the skin with clinical improvement in the majority of cases studied (103).

Once the susceptibility gene has been isolated, it would facilitate the understanding of the molecular pathways leading to psoriasis in familial and sporadic cases and in cases of psoriatic arthritis. The involvement of the gene in other dermatoses would also become clear. Ultimately, gene therapy methods to replace the defective gene in individuals with psoriasis using developing technologies such as bone marrow stem cell manipulation, and transplantation with genetically modified fibroblasts or keratinocytes (104), could be exploited as effective and possibly permanent treatments.

OTHER MECHANISMS THAT COULD ACCOUNT FOR PSORIASIS SUSCEPTIBILITY

Genetic analysis has become more sophisticated over time. Happle (18) suggested that somatic recombination in early development could produce cells homozygous for a psoriasis gene, and that this would be the stem cell of a clone proliferating in a linear pattern during development of the skin. For the ultimate manifestation of linear psoriasis, the presence of other predisposing genes as well as environmental factors would be necessary. Elder et al. pointed out that nevoid variants of psoriasis suggest somatic mutation of a single gene during development (22).

Recently genomic imprinting and microsatellite instability have been invoked to explain the variable risks reported in familial studies and the discordance in twin studies (105,106). Evidence for genomic imprinting as a causative agent in psoriasis included the following facts, (1) Birth weight of children from psoriatics was influenced by the sex of the psoriatic parent so that children from fathers with psoriasis were considerably heavier than children from mothers with psoriasis. (2) The disease manifestation (penetrance) depended in part on the sex of the psoriatic parent. Offspring from fathers with psoriasis and male gene carriers were significantly more often affected than offspring from mothers with psoriasis and female gene carriers. Of 91 grandchildren with psoriasis, 59 (65%) had an affected grandfather and 32 (35%) had a psoriatic grandmother. Traupe et al. proposed that modifications of a major predisposing gene in somatic tissues as a result of tissue-specific imprinting could cause differences in disease activity of psoriasis and could account for the often unpredictable clinical course of the disease (107).

Theeuwes and Morhenn reported that the preponderance of inheritance from the father over the mother was statistically significant, that a direct correlation existed between age of onset in affected siblings as well as age of onset in parent and child, and that age of onset in parents was greater than in offspring. They concluded that these findings were caused by allelic instability in mitosis (108).

As is the case in autoimmune diseases, it may be that the susceptibility for psoriasis is inherited, but that clinical expression of the psoriasis phenotype frequently requires other genetic (possibly HLA-associated) and environmental triggers. It is also possible that risks for psoriasis vary, depending on the predisposing allele, and that the variant allele on chromosome 17, predisposing to psoriasis in most family members, at a very early age, is sufficiently drastic to not require epistatic or environmental effects. What is fascinating is the degree to which this disease has withstood intensive investigative scrutiny and piece-by-piece dissection without yielding the secrets of its design. An important new development has been the formation in Dallas in October 1995 of an International Psoriasis Linkage Consortium. With efforts like this, the advances in genome technology and the rapid pace at which new genes are being identified, it seems likely that the answer to the genetic cause of psoriasis is not far away.

ACKNOWLEDGMENTS

We thank Colleen Campbell for secretarial assistance and Lisa Chu-Thielbar for valuable editorial comments. We also thank all the dermatologists nationwide who helped in the search for multiply affected families, making genetic analyses feasible. These studies were supported in part by the National Psoriasis Foundation and a grant from the National Institutes of Health (NIH Grant No. AR 43177).

REFERENCES

1. Botstein D., White R.L., Skolnick M., and Davis R.W. (1980). Construction of a genetic linkage map in man using restriction fragment length polymorphisms. *Am. J. Hum. Genet.* 32:314–331.
2. Gusella, J.F., Tanzi, R.E., Anderson, M.A., Hobbs, W., Gibbons, K., Raschtchian, R., Gilliam, T.C., Wallace, M.R., Wexler, N.S., and Conneally, P.M. (1984). DNA markers for nervous system diseases. *Science* 225:1320–1326.
3. Abele, D., Dobson R., and Graham, J. (1963). Heredity and psoriasis. Study of a large family. *Arch. Dermatol.* 88:38–47.
4. Brandrup, F., Hauge, M., Henningsen, J., and Eriksen, B. (1978). Psoriasis in an unselected series of twins. *Arch. Dermatol.* 114:874–878.
5. Brandrup, F., and Green, A. (1981). The prevalence of psoriasis in Denmark. *Acta Derm. Venereol. (Stockh.)* 61:344–346.
6. Brandrup, F., Holm, N., Grunnet, N., Henningsen, K., and Hansen, H. (1982). Psoriasis in monozygotic twins: variations in expression in individuals with identical genetic constitution. *Acta Derm. Venereol. (Stockh.)* 62:229–236.
7. Brandrup, F. (1987). The use of twins in etologic studies of psoriasis. In *Psoriasis: Proceedings of the Fourth International Symposium.* E. Farber, L. Nall, V. Morhenn, et al. (Eds.). Elsevier, New York, pp. 401–402.
8. Duffy, D.L., Spelman, L.S., and Martin, N.G. (1993). Psoriasis in Australian twins. *J. Am. Acad. Dermatol.* 29:428–434.
9. Watson, W., Cann, H. Farber, E., and Nall, M. (1972). The genetics of psoriasis. *Arch. Dermatol.* 105: 197–207.
10. Gottlieb, A. (1990). Immunologic mechanisms in psoriasis. *J. Invest. Dermatol.* 95:18S–19S.
11. Farber, E., Nall, M., and Watson, W. (1974). Natural history of psoriasis in 61 twin pairs. *Arch. Dermatol.* 109:207–211.
12. Farber, E., and Nall, M. (1974). The natural history of psoriasis in 5,600 patients. *Dermatologica* 148: 1–18.
13. Farber, E., Nall, L., and Watson, W. (1972). Natural history of psoriasis in 61 twin pairs. *Arch. Dermatol.* 105:197–207.
14. Farber, E., and Nall, L. (1982). Epidemiology in psoriasis research. *Hawaii Med. J.* 41:430.
15. Christophers, E., and Kruger, G. (1987). Psoriasis. In *Dermatology in General Medicine,* T. Fitzpatrick et al. (Eds.). New York. McGraw-Hill, pp. 465.
16. Lomholt G. (1963). In *Psoriasis: Prevalence, Spontaneous Course, and Genetics.* GEC GAD, Copenhagen, Denmark.
17. Andressen, C., and Henseler, T. (1982). Inheritance of psoriasis. Analysis of 2035 family histories. *Hautarzt* 33:214–217.
18. Happle, R. (1991). Somatic recombination may explain linear psoriasis. *J. Med. Genet.* 28:337.
19. Ward, J., and Stephens, F. (1961). Inheritance of psoriasis in a Utah kindred. *Arch. Dermatol.* 84:589–592.

20. Swanbeck, G., Inerot, A., Martinsson, T., and Wahlstrom, J. (1994). A population genetic study of psoriasis. *Br. J. Dermatol.* 131:32–39.
21. Henseler, T., and Christophers, E. (1985). Psoriasis of early and late onset: characterization of two types of psoriasis vulgaris. *J. Am. Acad. Dermatol.* 13: 450–456.
22. Elder, J.T., Nair, R.P., Guo, S.W., Henseler, T., Christophers, E., and Voorhees, J.J. (1994). The genetics of psoriasis. *Arch. Dermatol.* 130:216–223.
23. Hellgren L. (1967). In *Psoriasis.* Almqvist & Wiksell. Stockholm, Sweden.
24. Risch N. (1990). Linkage strategies for genetically complex traits. I. Multilocus models. *Am. J. Hum. Genet.* 46:222–228.
25. Kravitz, K., Skolnick, M., Cannings, C., Carmelli, D., Baty, B., Amos, B., Johnson, A., Mendell, N., Edwards, C., and Cartwright, G. (1979). Genetic linkage between hereditary hemochromotosis and HLA. *Am. J. Hum. Genet.* 31:601–619.
26. Wyman, A.R., and White, R. (1980). A highly polymorphic locus in human DNA. *Proc. Natl. Acad. Sci. U.S.A.* 77:6754–6758.
27. Tsui, L.-C., Buchwald, M., Barker, D., et al. (1985). Cystic fibrosis locus defined by a genetically linked polymorphic DNA marker. *Science* 230:104.
28. Hall J.M., Lee, M.K., Newman, B., Morrow, J.E., Anderson, L.A., Huey, B., and King, M.C. (1990). Linkage of early-onset familial breast cancer to chromosome 17q21. *Science* 250:1684–1689.
29. Wooster, R., Cleton-Jansen, A.M., Collins, N., Mangion, J., Cornelis, R.S., Cooper, C.S., Gusterson, B.A., von Deimling, A., Wiestler, O.D., et al. (1994). Instability of short tandem repeats (microsatellites) in human cancers. *Nature Genet.* 6:152–156.
30. Huntington's disease Collaborative Research Group (1993). A novel gene containing a trinucleotide repeat that is expanded and unstable on Huntington's disease chromosomes. *Cell* 72:971–983.
31. Rommens, J.M., Ianuzzi, M.C., Kerem, B., Drumm, M.L., Melmer, G., Dean, M., Rozmahel, R., Cole, J.L., Kennedy, D., Hidaka, N., Zsiga, M., Buchwald, M., Riordan, J.R., Tsui, L.-C., and Collins, F.S. (1989). Identification of the cystic fibrosis gene: chromosomal walking and jumping. *Science* 245:1059.
32. Miki, Y., Swensen, J., Shattuck-Eidens, D., Futreal, P.A., Harshman, K., Tavtigian, S., Liu, Q., Cochran, C., Bennett, L.M., and Ding, W. (1994). A strong candidate for the breast and ovarian cancer susceptibility gene BRCA1. *Science* 266:66–71.
33. Wooster, R., and Stratton, M.R. (1995). Breast cancer susceptibility: a complex disease unravels. *Trends Genet.* 11:3–5 (review).
34. Weissenbach, J., Gyapay, G., Dib, C., Vignal, A., Morissette, J., Millasseau, P., Vaysseix, G., and Lathrop, M. (1992). A second-generation linkage map of the human genome. *Nature* 359:794–801.
35. Gyapay G., Morssete J., Vignal A., et al. (1994). The 1993–94 Genethon human genetic map. *Nature Genet.* 7:246–339.
36. Sheffield, V.C., Nishimura, D.Y., and Stone, E.M. (1995). Novel approaches to linkage mapping. *Curr. Opin. Genet. Dev.* 5:335–341 (review).
37. Bowcock, A., Chipperfield, M.A., Ceverha, P., Yetman, E., and Phung, A. (1995). Report of the DNA committee. In Human Gene Mapping (a Compendium), The Johns Hopkins University Press, Baltimore and London, pp. 1454–1768.
38. Zachariae, H., Peterson, H., Kissmeyer-Nielsen, F., and Lamm L. (1977). HLA antigens in pustular psoriasis. *Dermatologica* 154:73–77.
39. Karvonen, J. (1975). HLA antigens in psoriasis with special reference to the clinical type, age of onset, exacerbations after respiratory infections and occurrence of arthritis. *Ann. Clin. Res.* 7:301–311.
40. Karvonen, J., Tilikainen, A., and Lassus, A. (1975). HLA antigens in patients with persistent palmoplantar pustulosis and pustular psoriasis. *Ann. Clin. Res.* 7: 112–115.
41. Raznatovsky, I., and Domeseva, T. (1978). On the morphology and immunology of parapsoriasis guttate. *Vestn. Dermatol. Venereol.* 616:17–20.
42. Lomholt, G. (1976). Environment and genetics in psoriasis. *Ann. Clin. Res.* 8:290–297.
43. Russell, T., Schultes, L., and Kuban, D. (1972). Histocompatibility (HLA) antigens associated with psoriasis. *N. Engl. J. Med.* 287:738–740.
44. White, S., Newcomer, V., Mickey, M., and Terasaki, P. (1972). Disturbance of HLA antigen frequency in psoriasis. *N. Engl. J. Med.* 287:740–743.
45. Ryder, L., and Svejgaard, A. (1977). B and T cells in immune recognition. In *Histocompatibility Associated Diseased.* F. Loor and E. Roelants (Eds.). Wiley, New York, pp. 437–456.
46. Batchelor, J., and Morris, P. (1977). Psoriasis. In *Histocompatibility Testing.* W. Bodmer (Ed.). Munksgaard, Copenhagen, pp. 230–231.
47. Christophers, E., and Henseler, T. (1991). Psoriasis type I and type II as subtypes of nonpustular psoriasis. In *Psoriasis.* H.H. Roenigk, Jr., and H.I. Maibach (Eds.). Marcel Dekker, New York, pp. 15–21.
48. Christophers, E., and Henseler, T. (1992). Psoriasis type I and II as subtypes of nonpustular psoriasis. *Semin. Dermatol.* 11:261–266 (review).
49. Kai, C., Fangji, S., Hui-gang, L., et al. (1993). Association between HLA antigens and families with psoriasis vulgaris. *Chin. Med. J. (Engl.).* 106: 132–135.
50. Zemmour, J., Gumperz, J.E., Hildebrand, W.H., Ward, F.E., March, S.G., Williams, R.C., and Parham, P. (1992). The molecular basis for reactivity of anti-

Cw1 and anti-Cw3 alloantisera with HLA-B46 haplotypes. *Tissue Antigens* 39:249–257.

51. Asahina, A., Akazakis, H., Nakagawa, S., Juwata, K., Tokunaga, Y., Ishibashi, Y., and Juji, T. (1991). Specific nucleotide sequence of HLA-C is strongly associated with psoriasis vulgaris. *J. Invest. Dermatol.* 97:254–258.
52. Nakagawa, H., Akazaki, S., Asahina, A., Tokunaga, K., Matsuki, K., Kuwata, S., Ishibashi, Y., and Juji, T. (1991). Study of HLA class I, class II and complement genes (C2, C4A, C4B and BF) in Japanese psoriatics and analysis of a newly-found high-risk haplotype by pulsed field gel electrophoresis. *Arch. Dermatol. Res.* 283:281–284.
53. Torii, H., Nakagawa, H., Ishibashi, Y., et al. (1992). Genetic polymorphisms in the fourth component of complement (C4) and in properdin factor B (BF) in Japanese patients with palmoplantar pustulosis. *J. Dermatol.* 19:353–355.
54. Torii, H., Nakagawa, H., Ishibashi, Y., et al. (1994). Genetic polymorphisms in HLA-A, -B, -C and -DR antigens in Japanese patients with palmoplantar pustulosis. *Dermatology* 188:290–292.
55. Chablani, U.A., Contractor, N.M., and Gadgil, R.B. (1992). HLA and complement C4 studies in psoriasis vulgaris. *Natl. Med. J. India* 5:8–11.
56. Roitberg-Tambur, A., Friedman, A., Tzfoni, E.E., Battat, S., Ben Hammo, R., Safirman, C., Tokunaga, K., Asahina, A., and Brautbar, C. (1994). Do specific pockets of HLA-C molecules predispose Jewish patients to psoriasis vulgaris? *J. Am. Acad. Dermatol.* 31:964–968.
57. O'Donnell, B.F., O'Loughlin, S., Codd, M.B., et al. (1993). HLA typing in Irish psoriatics. *Ir. Med. J.* 86: 65–68.
58. Woodrow, J., and Ilchysyn A., (1985). HLA antigens in psoriasis and psoriatic arthritis. *J. Med. Genet.* 22: 492–495.
59. Trabace, S., Cappellacci, S., Ciccarone, P., Liaskos, S., Polito, R., and Zorgin, L. (1994). Psoriatic arthritis: a clinical, radiological and genetic study of 58 Italian patients. *Acta Dermato-Venereol.* (Suppl.) 186: 69–70.
60. Svejgaard, A., Stahl-Nielsen, L. Svejgaard E., Kissmeyer-Nielsen, F., Mjortshoj, F., and Zachariae, H. (1974). HLA in psoriasis vulgaris and in pustular psoriasis: population and family studies. *Br. J. Dermatol.* 91:145–153.
61. Pietrzyk, J., Turowski, G., and Kapinska-Mrowka, M. (1982). Family studies in psoriasis. II. Inheritance of HLA genotypes. *Arch. Dermatol. Res.* 273:295–300.
62. Karvonen, J., Tilikainen, A., and Lassus, A. (1976). HLA antigens in psoriasis. A family study. *Ann. Clin. Res.* 8:298–304.
63. Civatte, J., Lazarovici, C., Ganas, P., Leon, S., Hors, J., Contu, L., et al. (1977). Le systeme HLA dans le psoriasis: étude de 31 families. *Ann. Dermatol. Venereol.* 104:525–532.
64. Espinoza, L., Bombardier, C., Gaylord, S., Lauter, S., Vasey, F., and Osterland, C. (1980). Histocompatibility studies in psoriasis vulgaris: family studies. *J. Rheumatol.* 7:445–452.
65. Lin, J.D., Auerbach, A.D., Auerbach, R., et al. (1991). Genetic linkage studies in psoriasis. *J. Invest. Dermatol.* 96:535A (abstract).
66. Tomfohrde, J., Silverman, A., Barnes, R., et al. (1994). Gene for familial psoriasis susceptibility mapped to the distal end of human chromosome 17q. *Science* 264:1141–1145.
67. Fernandez-Vina, M.A., Tomfohrde, J., Silverman, A., Barnes, R., Sang, S., Young, M., Lory, D., Morris, L., Wuepper, K.D., Menter, A., Bowcock, A., and Stasny, P. (1995). HLA genes in familial psoriasis vulgaris (pv): evidence for genetic heterogeneity. *Hum. Immunol.* 40 (suppl. 1):33, C-5.2.
68. Bowcock, A. (1995). Genetic locus for psoriasis identified. *Ann. Med.* 27:1883–186.
69. Beckman, G., Beckman, L., and Liden, S. (1980). Association between psoriasis and the alpha 1-antitrypsin deficiency gene z. *Acta Dermato-Venereol.* 60:163–164.
70. Jimenez-Nieto, L.C., Ladero, J.M., Fernandez-Gundin, M.J., and Robledo, A. (1989). Acetylator phenotype in psoriasis. *Dermatologica* 178:136–137.
71. Rosbotham, J.L., Trembath, R.C., Glover, M., Leigh, I., and Barker J.N.W.N. (1994). An association between psoriasis and hereditary multiple exostoses. A clue for mapping of a psoriasis susceptibility gene. *Br. J. Dermatol.* 130:671–674.
72. Cook, A., Raskind, W., Blanton, S.H., et al. (1993). Genetic heterogeneity in families with hereditary multiple exostoses. *Am. J. Hum. Genet.* 53:71–79.
73. Wu, Y.Q., Heutink, P., de Vriers, B.B.A., et al. (1994). Assignment of a second locus for multiple exostoses to the pericentromeric region of chromosome 11. *Hum. Mol. Genet.* 3:167–171.
74. Merrer, M.L., Legeai-Mallet, L., Jeannin, P.M., et al. (1994). A gene for hereditary multiple exostoses maps to chromosome 19p. *Hum. Mol. Genet.* 3: 717–722.
75. Baker, B.S., Bokth, S., Powles, A., et al. (1993). Group A streptococcal antigen-specific T lymphocytes in guttate psoriatic lesions. *Br. J. Dermatol.* 128: 493–499.
76. Beckmann, J., Tomfohrde, J., Barnes, R., Williams, M., Broux, O., Richard, I., Weissenbach, J., and Bowcock, A. (1993). A linkage map of human chromosome 15 with an average resolution of 2 cM and containing 54 polymorphic microsatellites. *Hum. Mol. Genet.* 2:2019–2030.
77. Matise, T.C., Perlin, M., and Chakravarti, A. (1994). Automated construction of genetic linkage maps us-

ing an expert system (MultiMap): a human genome linkage map. *Nature Genet.* 6:384–390.
78. Ott, J. (1991). *Analysis of Human Genetic Linkage,* 2nd ed. Johns Hopkins University Press, Baltimore.
79. Moll, J., and Wright, V. (1973). Psoriatic arthritis. *Semin. Arthritis Rheum.* 3:55–78.
80. Braun-Falco, O., and Ruzicka, T. (1994). Psoriatic arthritis. *Int. J. Dermatol.* 33:320–322.
81. Stern, R.S. (1987). The epidemiology of cutaneous diseases. In *Dermatology in General Medicine.* T. Fitzpatrick et al. (Eds.). McGraw-Hill, New York, pp. 6.
82. Shorte, A., and Ausell, B.M. (1982). Juvenile psoriatic arthritis: an analysis of 6 cases. *J. Pediatr.* 100: 529–535.
83. Nair, R.P., Guo, S.W., Jenisch, S., Henseler, T., Lange, E.M., Terhune, M., Westphal, E., Christophers, E., Voorhees, J.J., and Elder, J.T. (1995). Scanning chromosome 17 for psoriasis susceptibility: lack of evidence for a distal 17q locus. *Hum. Hered.* 45: 219–230.
84. Matthews, D., Fry, L., Powles, A., Weissenbach, J., and Williamson, R. (1995). Confirmation of genetic heterogeneity in familial psoriasis. *J. Med. Genet.* 32: 546–548.
85. Matthews, D., Fry, L., Powles, A., Weber, J., McCarthy, M., Fisher, E., Davies, K., and Williamson, R. (1996). Evidence that a locus for familial psoriasis maps to chromosome 4q. *Nature Genet.* 14:231–233.
86. Trembath, R.C., Lee Clough, R., Rosbotham, J.L., Jones, A.B., Camp, R.D.R., Frodsham, A., Browne, J., Barber, R., Terwilliger, J., Lathrop, G.M., and Barker, J.N.W.N. (1997). Identification of a major susceptibility locus on chromosome 6p and evidence for further disease loci revealed by a two-stage genome-wide search in psoriasis. *Hum. Mol. Genet.* 6: 813–820.
87. Nair, R.P., Henseler, T., Jenisch, S., Stuart, P., Bichakjian, C.K., Lenk, W., Westpahl, E., Guo, S-W., Christophers, E., Voorhees, J.J., and Elder, J.T. (1997). Evidence for two psoriasis susceptibility loci (HLA and 17q) and two novel candidate regions (16q and 20p) by genome-wide scan. *Hum. Mol. Genet.* 6: 1349–1356.
88. Cantor, R.M., and Rotter, J.I. (1992). Analysis of genetic data: methods and interpretations. In *The Genetic Basis of Common Diseases.* R.A. King, et al. (Eds.). Oxford University Press., Oxford, pp. 64–65.
89. Todd, J.A. (1995). Genetic analysis of type I diabetes using whole genome approaches. *Proc. Natl. Acad. Sci. U.S.A.* 92:8560–8565.
90. Bell, G.I., Horita, A., and Karam, J.H. (1984). A polymorphic locus near the human insulin gene is associated with insulin-dependent diabetes mellitus. *Diabetes* 33:176–183.
91. Thomson, G., Robinson, W.P., Kuhner, M.K., Joe, S., and Klitz, W. (1989). HLA and insulin gene associations with IDDM. *Genet. Epidemiol.* 6:155–160.
92. Julier, C., Hyer, R.N., Davies, J., Merlin, F., Soularue, P., Briant, L., Cathelineau, G., Deschamps, I., Rotter, J.I., Froguel, P., et al. (1991). Insulin-IGF2 region on chromosome 11p encodes a gene implicated in HLA-DR4-dependent diabetes susceptibility. *Nature* 354: 155–159.
93. Spielman, R.S., McGinnis, R.E., and Ewens, W.J. (1993). Transmission test for linkage disequilibrium: the insulin gene region and insulin-dependent diabetes mellitus (IDDM). *Am. J. Hum. Genet.* 52: 506–516.
94. Bennett, S., Lucassen, A., Gough, S., et al. (1995). Susceptibility to human type I diabetes at IDDM2 is determined by tandem repeat variation at the insulin gene minisatellite locus. *Nature Genet.* 9:284–292.
95. Hulten, M. (1974). Chiasma distribution at diakinesis in the normal human male. *Hereditas* 76:55–87.
96. Buckler, A., Chang, D., Graw, S., Brook, D., Haber, D., Sharp, P., and Housman, D. (1991). Exon amplification: a strategy to isolate mammalian genes based on RNA splicing. *Proc. Natl. Acad. Sci. U.S.A.* 88: 4005–4009.
97. Duyk, G.M., Kim, S.W., Myers, R.M., and Cox, D.R. (1990). Exon trapping: a genetic screen to identify candidate transcribed sequences in cloned mammalian genomic DNA. *Proc. Natl. Acad. Sci. U.S.A.* 87: 8995–8999.
98. Lovett, M., Kere, J., and Hinton, L. (1991). Direct selection: a method for the isolation of cDNAs encoded by large genomic regions. *Proc. Natl. Acad. Sci. U.S.A.* 88:9628–9623.
99. Parimoo S., Patanjali, S., Shukla, H., Chaplin, D., and Weismann, S. (1991). *Proc. Natl. Acad. Sci. U.S.A.* 88:9623.
100. Poizot-Martin, I., Oliver, C., Mawas, C., et al. (1991). Are CD4 antibodies and peptide T new treatments for psoriasis? *Lancet* 1:1477.
101. Prinz, J., Braun-falco, O., Meurer, M., et al. (1991). Chimaeric CD4 monoclonal antibody in treatment of generalised pustular psoriasis. *Lancet* 338:320–321.
102. Nicolas, J.F., Chamchick, N., Thivolet, J., et al. (1991). CD4 antibody treatment of severe psoriasis. *Lancet* 338:321.
103. Gottlieb, S.L., Gilleaudeau, P., Johnson, R., Estes, L., Woodworth, T.G., Gottlieb, A.B., and Krueger, J.G. (1995). Response of psoriasis to a lymphocyte-selective toxin (DAB_{389} IL-2) suggests a primary immune, but not keratinocyte, pathogenic basis. *Nature Med.* 1:442–447.
104. Krueger, G.G., Morgan, J.R., and Jorgensoen, C.M. (1994). Genetically modified skin to treat disease: potential and limitations. *J. Invest Dermatol.* (Suppl.) 103:76S-84S.

105. Traupe, H. (1995). The puzzling genetics of psoriasis. *Clin. Dermatol.* 13:99–103.
106. Zheng, G.J., Thomson, G., and Pen, Y.N. (1992). Allelic instability in mitosis can explain genome imprinting and other genetic phenomena in psoriasis. *Am. J. Med. Genet.* 51:163–164.
107. Traupe, H., Van Gurp, P.J., Happle, R., Boezeman, J., and van de Kerkhof, P.C. (1992). Psoriasis vulgaris, fetal growth, and genomic imprinting. *Am. J. Med. Genet.* 42:649–654.
108. Theeuwes, M., and Morhenn, V. (1995). Allelic instability in the mitosis model and the inheritance of psoriasis. *J. Am. Acad. Dermatol.* 32:44–52 (review).

Part III

PATHOGENESIS

13

Overview of Immunology

Hachiro Tagami and Setsuya Aiba
Tohoku University School of Medicine, Sendai, Japan

Psoriasis is a chronic skin disorder characterized by the formation of numerous scaly and erythematous plaques. There are a variety of clinical types, which form a spectrum from mild, localized sebopsoriasis of the scalp to generalized pustular psoriasis. In all lesions definite signs of inflammation can be found; clinically, erythematous changes can be observed and, much more easily, we can find inflammatory changes histopathologically. However, our attention tends to be drawn to the thick, silvery white scales covering the lesions and the histopathological features of epidermal proliferation associated with the characteristic elongation of the rete ridges and increased turnover. Thus, many dermatologists have considered psoriasis to be a dermatosis caused by epidermal hyperproliferation, rather than an inflammatory disease. The immunological approach to elucidating its pathogenesis began rather recently, about 20 years ago. However, the rapid progress of immunology has unexpectedly brought about great advances in our understanding of the pathophysiology of the disease.

INITIAL IMMUNOLOGICAL STUDIES ON PSORIASIS

The mid-1970s marked the beginning of a new era in the study of psoriasis. Three different research groups presented their data indicating that immunological changes take place in psoriatic lesions. First, Beutner et al. (1) suggested an autoimmune mechanism in psoriasis by demonstrating the presence of circulating anti–stratum corneum autoantibodies as well as the deposition of immunoglobulins and C3 in the lesional stratum corneum. Meanwhile, Cormane et al. (2), with the demonstration of antinuclear antibodies in the eluates of polymorphonuclear cells (PMNs) and lymphocytes of psoriatic patients, developed a theory implicating a delayed-type immune response at the basal cell layer as an initial step, and an Arthus-type reaction in the upper layers of the epidermis in a later stage of the disease process, with a keratinization disorder as a secondary phenomenon. In the same year, Tagami and Ofuji (3) demonstrated the presence of leukocyte chemotactic substances in lesional scale extracts, which they thought to be complement fragments due to the Arthus-type reaction that occurred at the subcorneal portion of the lesional stratum corneum. These findings, as well as the results of other immunological studies on psoriasis subsequently published in short succession, were compiled by Beutner in 1982 in a book entitled *Autoimmunity in Psoriasis* (4). Since then, a vast number of studies have been conducted on the immunology of psoriasis. They were comprehensively reviewed by Jablonska and Glinski in the previous edition of this book (5).

DIRECT EVIDENCE FOR PSORIASIS AS AN IMMUNE-MEDIATED DISEASE

It is not unusual for dermatologists to observe the development of pronounced inflammation in exacerbated cases of psoriasis, which may be accompanied by such systemic symptoms as fever, weakness, and arthralgia, together with pustulation of the skin, all of which are the features of generalized pustular psoriasis. Psoriasis is now thought to be an immune-mediated inflammatory skin disease.

The appearance or disappearance of psoriasis after bone marrow transplants clearly indicates that the cells of the immune system are involved in its pathogenesis (6,7). However, no specific immunodiagnostic hallmark such as the autoantibodies found in autoimmune bullous dermatoses has been found for psoriasis. It is noteworthy that, as in other autoimmune diseases such as systemic lupus erythematosus and rheumatoid arthritis, an abnormally reduced autologous mixed lymphocyte reaction, a reduced immunological response by CD4+ T cells to class II MHC antigens on autologous non-T cells such as B cells and monocytes, is also observed in psoriasis, indicating a perturbed immunoregulatory network (8).

Among various lines of evidence for the involvement of immune mechanisms in psoriasis, the most compelling one has emerged from the successful treatment with agents that suppress the activities of CD4+ T cells, i.e., newly developed immunosuppressive drugs such as cyclosporin, FK506 (tacrolimus) (9,10), and, particularly, anti-CD4 monoclonal antibody (11,12). These findings strongly suggested that psoriasis is a T-cell-mediated immune dermatosis that is associated with inflammation and, presumably, secondary epidermal hyperplasia. Even superficial inflammation such as that caused by stripping of the stratum corneum induces epidermal proliferation lasting for 10 days (13). Thus, we can easily imagine how the presence of chronic immune-mediated inflammation will affect the epidermis. Moreover, it was recently disclosed that lesional psoriatic T-lymphocyte clones are capable of enhancing keratinocyte proliferation in vitro by secreted products, most likely interferon (IFN)-γ (14,15).

In addition to these immunological characteristics, psoriasis shows a close association with certain HLA types (16,17). Thus, it is now considered an immune-mediated genetic dermatosis (18).

CHARACTERISTICS OF INFLAMMATION OBSERVED IN PSORIATIC SKIN LESIONS

The whole skin of psoriatic patients seems to be predisposed to the development of psoriatic lesions, which is known as the Koebner phenomenon. Histopathologically, even uninvolved portions of the skin in patients with psoriasis show a variable degree of dermal and epidermal mononuclear cell infiltration in addition to capillary dilatation, forming an intermediate between normal healthy skin and lesional psoriatic skin (19,20).

Clinically, psoriatic lesions may appear uniformly erythematous and scaly. However, experience has taught us that different areas in a single plaque lesion do not behave in a similar manner when treated. In general, the peripheral portions resolve more slowly than the central portions after topical application of potent steroids. We can appreciate much more readily the presence of such heterogeneity even in the same lesion by observing the development of the annular lesions of pustular psoriasis.

Histopathologically, there are portions of acute inflammation and of chronic inflammation within the same plaque lesion (21). Those areas with chronic inflammation respond quickly to treatment by potent topical steroids, whereas acutely inflamed areas are resistant to therapy (22).

BIPHASIC TYPE OF INFLAMMATION OBSERVED IN PSORIATIC LESIONS

As mentioned above, there are portions of acute inflammation and of chronic inflammation within the same plaque lesion (21). Only in the former can we observe a hallmark of the psoriatic tissue reaction, namely, squirting papillae, which is intermittent transepidermal migration of neutrophils from the tip of the dermal papillae toward the stratum corneum.

Chowaniec et al. (23) performed histopathological studies on prepinpoint lesions, the very early lesions of fine, erythematous papules at almost the skin level, which changed in the course of observation into typical pinpoint papules. In these lesions they found neutrophils penetrating into the epidermis, forming small focal accumulations in the stratum corneum. Hence, they speculated that neutrophil infiltration preceded mononuclear cell infiltration in psoriatic lesions. However, most authors think that mononuclear cell infiltration precedes neutrophil infiltration even in acutely inflamed lesions of pustular psoriasis. Although time course studies on pustular psoriasis are scarce, even those on pustulosis palmaris et plantaris indicate that, in the earliest phase, lymphocyte infiltration into the epidermis precedes that of neutrophils (24,25). Supporting these findings, there is a report that psoriasis can develop even in a patient without neutrophils and monocytes in the peripheral circulation; this finding strongly implicates T lymphocytes as having a crucial role in the initiation of psoriasis (26). The present authors also have studied a case of a rapidly developing annular-type psoriasis, which was clinically suggestive of pustular psoriasis. In the histological specimens of the skin lesions, we could find only a massive T-lymphocyte infiltration (27).

In the earliest pinpoint psoriatic lesions only the features of chronic dermatitis can be found, i.e., vasodilatation and edema of the upper dermis and, crowding around blood vessels, T lymphocytes and macrophages, which may migrate into mildly acanthotic epidermis with focal spongiosis (28). Subsequent pinpoint papules show acute inflammatory changes in the center, i.e., squirting papillae, which constitute a characteristic histological feature of the psoriasiform tissue reaction (29).

The transepidermal migration of leukocytes culminates in the formation of scattered Munro microabsesses in the stratum corneum or of Kogoj spongiform pustules in severely inflamed lesions. Although similar squirting papillae are also demonstrable in the lesions of seborrheic dermatitis, there is a distinct difference in the pathogenetic mechanisms of the psoriasiform tissue reactions observed in psoriasis compared with those in seborrheic dermatitis. No specific microorganism is involved in the former, whereas resident microorganisms such as *Malassezia furfur,* a potent activator of alternative complement pathway, play an important role in the induction of leukocyte chemotaxis toward the fungus-laden stratum corneum in the latter.

The histopathology of more developed plaque lesions shows the features of acute inflammatory spots scattered over chronic ones (21). All over the plaque lesions we can find the features of chronic inflammation consisting of a perivascular mononuclear cell infiltration and acanthotic epidermis characterized by regular elongation of the rete rides, and elongation and edema of the dermal papillae with thinning of the suprapapillary portions of the epidermis. The acute inflammatory changes characterized by the transepidermal migration of neutrophils with the formation of Munro microabsesses are found in localized areas, being scattered over the plaques but concentrating on the spreading edges. Accumulation of neutrophils in chronic plaque-type psoriasis was shown in 41% of skin biopsy specimens (30). The absence of neutrophils in the majority of skin biopsies suggests the cyclic pattern of the exocytosis of these cells.

In the lesions of pustular psoriasis, the acute inflammatory changes are predominant, occupying much larger areas of the epidermis with a massive accumulation of neutrophils beneath the stratum corneum, presenting the features of Kogoj spongiform pustules. The background inflammatory changes characterized by the mononuclear cell infiltrate are always observed in a much more exaggerated fashion.

BEHAVIOR OF IMMUNE CELLS AND INFLAMMATORY CELLS IN PSORIATIC SKIN

Uninvolved Skin

Even in uninvolved psoriatic skin, the absolute numbers of CD4+ and CD8+ T lymphocytes are significantly increased (19,20). The tendency of the uninvolved skin of psoriatic individuals to become lesional after tape-stripping trauma was reported to be associated with a predominance of CD4 over CD8+ T cells in the epidermis (31); in Koebner-positive patients, a larger proportion of helper T cells was found to result from a decrease in CD8+ cells rather than from an increase in CD4+ cells. There are small numbers of the HLA-DR+/CD1a-subclass of antigen-presenting cells which have an enhanced capacity to stimulate T cells (32,33).

Mast Cells

The studies performed in penicillin-induced acute eruptive psoriasis after throat infection showed that degranulation of resident dermal mast cells preceded the extravasation of mononuclear cells (34). Mast cells release their chemical mediators with degranulation to induce endothelial cell gaps and subsequent extravasation of mononuclear cells. T lymphocytes and monocytes were at first observed in the perivascular portion, predominantly in the papillary tips (35). Likewise, the observations made in the positive Koebner phenomenon showed a steady increase in the number of mast cells in the early psoriatic lesions induced experimentally by scratch (36). Another experimental study performed in early relapsing psoriatic lesions that were previously treated with potent topical steroids also demonstrated that degranulating mast cells as well as macrophages initiate the formation of the psoriatic-tissue alterations (37). The factors that activate mast cells remain unidentified.

T Lymphocytes

From its earliest stage of onset to the last point of regression, or in both acutely inflamed pustular lesions and chronic scaly plaques, chronic inflammatory changes characterized by an infiltration of CD4+ T lymphocytes and monocytes are consistently found in psoriatic lesional skin. Observations made in newly arising lesions demonstrated the extravasation of CD4+ T lymphocytes and monocytes in the upper dermis (20). T lymphocytes migrate toward and invade the epidermis, interacting with antigen-presenting cells to induce spongiotic changes. Monocytes also migrate toward the basement membrane and remain there lined up in close proximity to epidermal basal cells (38).

Sequential observation of the early events leading to the formation of a psoriatic skin lesion after tape stripping of uninvolved skin revealed an increased motility of Langerhans cells across the basement membrane as the earliest change occurring in the epidermis (39). It was observed as early as 2 min after stripping and remained until the development of clinical psoriasis, providing evidence of Langerhans cell–lymphocyte interaction and of increased Langerhans cell "activity." Further studies on intraepidermal dendritic cells disclosed a marked increase in the number of HLA-DR+/CD1a-dendritic cells and a slight decrease in the number of HLA-DR+/CD1a+ Langerhans cells in early psoriatic lesions (20,33). Moreover, as in contact sensitivity skin reactions, intraepidermal CD4+ T lymphocytes were observed in close apposition to HLA-DR+ dendritic cells (40).

Suction-blister fluid accumulates tissue fluid that contains various substances involved in ongoing biological events in the skin. In contrast, those contained in scale extracts of lesional skin reflect the past events that once occurred in the lesional epidermis. Because the levels of soluble CD4 and CD8 are significantly higher in the suction blister fluid and the scale extracts than in those from uninvolved or nonpsoriatic skin, both CD4+ and CD8+ T cells are thought to be activated in psoriatic lesions (41). Among these T lymphocytes, CD4+ T cells predominate in the dermis in both early and fully developed lesions (42). The efficacy of anti-CD4 therapy for psoriasis also strongly supports the crucial role played by CD4+ T cells (11,12,43).

From the cytokine production profile of lesional T lymphocytes, some researchers reported that there was no preferential shift to Th1- or Th2-type cells (44,45), while others found a shift to Th1-type cells that preferentially secreted interleukin (IL)-2, IL-2 receptors, IFN-γ, and IFN-γ-induced protein (IP-10) generated by keratinocytes, instead of IL-4 and IL-10 (46–48).

There is also a controversy concerning the T cells found in the lesional epidermis. Some authors found that they consisted primarily of helper T cells in early lesions, while CD8+ T cells became more prominent in spontaneously resolving lesions (49). Others claimed that CD8+ T cells predominated in the lesional epidermis (50,51).

Angiogenesis

Not only the epidermal hyperproliferation but also the elongation of edematous dermal papillae that contain dilated and tortuous blood vessels constitutes a characteristic histopathological architecture of psoriatic lesions. The keratinocytes composing the hyperplastic epidermis, whose proliferation is mainly stimulated by transforming growth factor (TGF)-α in an autocrine fashion, release a selective mitogen for dermal microvascular endothelial cells, i.e., vascular permeability factor, also known as vascular endothelial growth factor (VPF/VEGF) (52). It enhances vascular permeability to plasma proteins to produce perivascular edema and stimulates dermal angiogenesis (53). Additionally, T-cell-derived basic fibroblast growth factor (bFGF) is also thought to exert angiogenetic effects in psoriatic lesional skin where T-cell-mediated immune reactions take place (54).

Neutrophils (PMNs)

The cyclic transepidermal migration of PMNs seems to be associated with parakeratosis, because Munro microabscesses were found only in parakeratotic areas of the epidermis. However, parakeratosis seems to be secondary to PMN infiltration, because spongiform pustules found in the acute, inflammatory form of psoriasis are covered by an orthokeratotic stratum corneum (30). In vitro leukocyte adhesion tests show that prominent adhesion of leukocytes occurs in the lesional stratum corneum with subsequent activation of a respiratory burst (55), suggesting the trapping of active substances there. The adhesion of neutrophils to lesional psoriatic epidermis was also found to be strongly increased as compared with healthy skin. It was most pronounced in areas with the highest expression of intercellular adhesion molecule 1 (ICAM-1) (56).

The functional activities of peripheral blood neutrophils such as respiratory burst, enzyme release, and chemotaxis are generally enhanced in psoriatic patients (57,58), although some researchers found no differences from healthy individuals (59). Such functional analyses disclosed a transient, complete absence of PMN responses specifically to chemoattractant C5a in patients with pustular psoriasis as in acute infectious skin diseases (e.g., pyoderma, acne conglobata, and erysipelas) (60). This effect is apparently related to pronounced complement activation occurring in these diseases. Likewise, in patients with guttate psoriasis but not in stable psoriasis, in vitro degranulation of PMN enzymes in the presence of both FMLP and serum-activated zymosan that contain C5a was markedly reduced in patients with actively spreading guttate psoriatic lesions (61). These data showing a specific unresponsiveness suggest an in vivo activation of neutrophils in active inflammatory psoriasis that induces an unresponsiveness in these cells to subsequent in vitro stimulation or a migration of highly responsive neutrophils to skin lesions, which leaves in the circulation a subpopulation less reactive to chemotactic and phagocytic stimuli.

ANTIGENS

The psoriatic epidermal CD8+ T cells were reported to preferentially use restricted T-cell receptors, Vβ3 and/or Vβ13.1, suggesting that they are recruited and expanded in situ in response to antigen(s) in the skin (62). The persistence of these T cells in lesions that have not undergone resolution suggests their role as effector cells rather than as regulatory cells. However, the antigen recognizable by psoriatic lesional T cells has not been determined yet.

The only external trigger convincingly associated with the initiation and exacerbation of plaque-type psoriasis is throat infection with beta-hemolytic streptococci upper respiratory infection (63,64). Therefore, it is conceivable that streptococci contain antigenic substances that are recognized by psoriatic T cells. Indeed, altered responses of peripheral blood mononuclear cells from psoriatic patients to *Streptococcus* antigen in vitro were reported (65,66). Furthermore, T lymphocytes specific for group A streptococcal antigens can be consistently isolated from guttate psoriatic lesions (67). Thus, it is postulated that an abnormal expression of a skin determinant that cross-reacts with a conventional streptococcal antigen may be an essential part of the predisposition to psoriasis (68). Among the bacterial substances, M protein is a major pathogenic surface antigen in these streptococci. There is an extensive sequence homology between recombinant streptococcal M6 protein and the 50-kDa type I keratin (K14) (69), to which not only antibodies but also T cells are likely to cross-react. Valdimarsson et al. (68) implicated the homology between the 50-kDa keratin and the streptococcal M proteins in the process in which products of activated T cells can induce keratinocytes of psoriatic predisposition to express determinants that are recognized by T cells specific for epitopes on beta-hemolytic streptococci.

Recently, it has been reported that psoriasis may also be exacerbated by local skin infection with *Staphylococcus aureus* or *Candida albicans.* It was postulated that this exacerbation might be due to superantigens released locally from these organisms (70). The reported prevalence of certain Vβ-expressing families in psoriatic lesional T cells (62,70,71) suggests that Vβ3 and Vβ13.1 might represent the T-cell receptor predominantly used in psoriatic epidermis, while Vβ2 and Vβ6 dominate the dermal T-cell infiltrate (71). Therefore, these findings also suggest that autoantigen(s) or superantigen(s) stimulate lesional T cells (68).

ANTIGEN-PRESENTING CELLS

There are several kinds of antigen-presenting cells in the skin, i.e., epidermal Langerhans cells, dermal dendritic cells, and macrophages. In the skin lesions of psoriasis vulgaris CD1a+ Langerhans cells are decreased in number, but show enhanced expression of HLA class II molecules (HLA-DR, -DP, and -DQ) (72). Lesional psoriatic epidermis possesses an elevated alloantigen-presenting capacity (73) and an enhanced capacity to stimulate autologous T cells in the absence of exogenous antigens (33,74). This increased antigen-presenting capacity is suggested to be due to bone-marrow-derived non-Langerhans cells, which express HLA-DR antigen and macrophage marker (73).

Dermal dendrocytes, another population of dendritic cells that may serve as antigen-presenting cells, are strongly increased in number in psoriatic dermis, mainly within the papillary dermis and can also be found traversing the basement membrane (75).

Recently, in addition to these professional antigen-presenting cells, HLA-DR+ keratinocytes, which are often present in highly inflamed lesions of psoriasis (16,76), have been found to function as accessory cells in the stimulation of T cells by bacterial superantigens (77). It remains unclear how these cells contribute to the activation of T cells in psoriatic lesions.

ADHESION MOLECULES

Adhesion molecules expressed on endothelial cells and those expressed on the matrix protein and keratinocytes are important for the production of psoriatic lesions because they play an important role in the transendothelial and transepidermal migration of leukocytes toward the lesional stratum corneum.

Endothelial Cells

Endothelial cells in normal skin express only glycoprotein ICAM-1, which binds β2-integrin LFA-1 (CD11a/CD18) on neutrophils, lymphocytes, and monocytes. It is highly upregulated on psoriatic endothelial cells (78,79), preferentially on those in the papillary tips (80). However, a much slower movement of circulating blood cells is required for actual tight binding between them and endothelial cells. The endothelial cells in psoriatic lesional skin strongly express E-selectin (81), which binds sialylated carbohydrate moieties on neutrophils, monocytes, and memory T cells, as well as ICAM-1.

E-selectin slows the movement of inflammatory cells under the physiological shear force of the rapid blood circulation by inducing their rolling on the surface of endothelial cells, which facilitates the subsequent stronger binding between the inflammatory cell LFA-1 and endothelial cell ICAM-1. The LFA-1 and Mac-1 on inflammatory cells are enhanced by chemoattractants, enabling their transendothelial migration and subsequent movement in the direction of an increasing concentration of a chemoattractant that diffuses away from the site of its production. E-selectin is also an adhesion molecule for skin-homing memory T cells expressing a carbohydrate termed cutaneous lymphocyte-associated antigen (CLA), which have left the skin tissues after encountering antigen (82).

In contrast, VCAM-1, the ligand for VLA-4 on lymphocytes and monocytes, is not up-regulated as it is in allergic contact dermatitis (83). VCAM-1 expression is not a prerequisite for lymphocyte infiltration, because perivascular T-cell accumulation is observable around dermal endothelial cells strongly expressing E-selectin and ICAM-1, but not VCAM-1.

It is remarkable that the expression of E-selection and ICAM-1 is also up-regulated in psoriatic nonlesional skin, suggesting that even normal-looking psoriatic skin is constitutively in an activated state, which is in contrast to other inflammatory diseases such as allergic contact dermatitis (83). It is also the case even after successful treatment with cyclosporin and tacrolimus (84,85). Although ICAM-1 and E-selectin expression in active psoriatic plaques is significantly down-regulated with this treatment, it fails to return to that found in normal skin from healthy individuals. Thus, the dermal vessels in the skin of psoriatic patients seem to be primed for leukocyte extravasation, which may contribute to the development of the Koebner phenomenon and the rapid relapse of disease after clinically successful treatment.

Tissue Matrices and Epidermis

Once leukocytes emigrate across the vascular endothelium, movement through the dermal interstitium is in part mediated by chemoattractants and also by adhesion molecules. Fibronectin, which is present in high concentrations in psoriatic dermis and epidermis (86), may be important as a ligand of VLA-4, which is expressed on perivascular lymphocytes in psoriasis.

In psoriatic epidermis, keratinocyte ICAM-1 is focally expressed, especially in the region immediately overlying the dermal papillae; the ICAM-1 expressing keratinocytes are observed closely juxtaposed to infiltrating LFA-1 expressing lymphocytes (83,87). In addition, aberrant integrin expression (VLA-6 and VLA-3) is reported on lesional keratinocytes, as found in epidermal wound healing (88). In contrast, epidermotropic neutrophils appear to express CD11b/CD18 (MAC-1) rather than CD11a/CD18 (LFA-1) to interact with ICAM-1 and C3bi (89).

In vitro studies demonstrated that the expression of both of these adhesion molecules on the endothelial cells and keratinocytes is induced by proinflammatory cytokines that are demonstrable in psoriatic lesions; i.e., E-selectin is induced by IL-1 or TNF-α, whereas ICAM-1 on keratinocytes and endothelial cells is induced by TNF-α and IFN-γ (87).

BEHAVIOR OF PROINFLAMMATORY OR IMMUNOREGULATORY CYTOKINES IN LESIONAL SKIN

Those cells involved in pathophysiological processes release various cytokines that exert their effects on other cells in an autocrine, paracrine, or endocrine fashion in addition to those through direct cell-to-cell contact. The activities of individual cykokines are analyzed using various in vitro models. However, no single cytokine can explain a particular process as there are complex pathophysiological cytokine networks in psoriatic lesions. So far, the presence of individual cytokines in psoriatic skin has been mainly evaluated with two kinds of samples: suction blister fluid and horny tissue extract. Although the tissue fluid derived from suction blisters contains active substances that contribute to ongoing biological events, the detection of cytokines at the protein level is much easier with the scale extracts of lesional skin, which have accumulated various factors involved in the past events. Recently, the production of various cytokines by the cells involved in the immune-mediated inflammatory changes has also been analyzed at the mRNA level.

Most of the following multifunctional immunoregulatory cytokines found in psoriatic lesions are likely to affect both inflammatory cell functions and epidermal activation.

IL-1

Pleiotropic cytokine IL-1 can induce the skin inflammation and hyperproliferative epidermis that is found in inflammatory skin diseases (90). It is therefore reasonable to study its activity in psoriatic lesions. At first, scale extracts became a target of study because they retain various proinflammatory mediators involved in the preceding epidermal inflammatory changes. However, IL-1 activity was found to be decreased in psoriatic scale extracts when compared with the high activity detectable in normal stratum corneum (91). Both IL-1-α and -β are produced by psoriatic keratinocytes; IL-1-α is generated by psoriatic keratinocytes in quantities similar to those present in normal keratinocytes, whereas IL-1-β was found to be markedly increased in psoriatic epidermis, but in an inactive form (92). In regard to IL-1 activity, the balance between IL-1 receptor antagonist (ra) and IL-1-α may have an important influence on keratinocyte growth and/or differentiation, as well as on the inflammatory potential of IL-1 in psoriatic lesions. An elevated ratio of IL-1 ra to IL-1 prevails in extracts of psoriatic skin as compared with normal skin (93). These obtained data, however, do not completely exclude a possible role played by IL-1 in psoriatic lesions, because in vitro monitoring of short-term, nonstimulated cultures of freshly isolated psoriatic epidermal cells, which represent an ex vivo psoriasis model, demonstrated increased bioactive IL-1-β release (94).

IL-1 probably exerts its effects in an autocrine and paracrine manner. Meanwhile, decreased expression of the IL-1 receptor has been observed on psoriatic epidermal cells (95).

IL-6

IL-6 is another pleiotropic primary cytokine that is a major mediator of the host response to tissue injury and infection. In the skin it can stimulate keratinocyte growth and differentiation (96). Immunoreactive IL-6 levels were found to be increased in scale extracts and suction blisters, but no significant correlation was observed with the levels of immunoreactive IL-1 in these materials (97). In psoriasis, IL-6 is rather closely correlated to tumor necrosis factor (TNF)-α, as will be described below (98). Its increase was also demonstrated immunohistopathologically in psoriatic lesions (99). Dermal fibroblasts, probably together with the inflammatory infiltrate, are thought to represent a major source of IL-6 in psoriasis lesions in vivo (100), because cultured lesional keratinocytes express minimal levels of IL-6 mRNA and protein (94). IL-6 could directly contribute to the epidermal hyperplasia seen in psoriatic epithelium as well as affect the function of dermal inflammatory cells.

TNF-α

Another proinflammatory cytokine with multiple biological activities is TNF-α. Its immunoreactivity and bioactivity are increased in lesional skin, together with those of soluble TNF receptors (p55 and p75) (101). Lesional TNF-α levels, which were highly correlated with those of IL-6 in involved skin blister fluid, showed a significant correlation with the PASI scores of the patients, suggesting a direct relationship between these cytokines and the clinical manifestations of the disease (98). Immunohistologically, epidermal TNF-α expression did not differ from that observed in normal skin (102), suggesting that it has other immune cells as its major source. Because systemic administration of TNF-α induces beneficial effects in psoriasis (103,104), it is speculated that the immunological effects of local release of TNF-α may be quite different from those of its systemic injection (105).

IFN-γ

As already mentioned, the efficacy of anti-CD4 therapy for psoriasis also strongly supports the crucial role played by T cells. Reflecting their activation, scale extracts but not suction blister fluid from psoriatic lesions contain elevated IFN-γ activity (47). Furthermore, psoriatic lesional keratinocytes exhibit signs of exposure to IFN-γ such as the expression of IP-10 (46) and ICAM-1 (78), and HLA-DR whose expression, however, is not consistent but is observed only in actively inflamed portions such as the edges of spreading lesions and centers of pinpoint lesions (76,106).

Like IL-1 receptors, lesional psoriatic keratinocytes show decreased expression of IFN-γ receptors that are localized only to the lower epidermis (107), which may be responsible for the low HLA-DR expression in psoriatic lesions when compared with other inflammatory skin diseases.

GM-CSF

Granulocyte-macrophage colony-stimulating factor (GM-CSF), a product of activated T lymphocytes, macrophages, endothelial cells, fibroblasts, and keratinocytes, is thought to play an important role in inflammatory reactions by "priming" or enhancing the functions of neutrophils and macrophages. GM-CSF is not detected by ELISA in the suction blister fluid raised on normal, psoriatic uninvolved or involved skin. In contrast, immunoreactive GM-CSF is readily detected in most of the scale extracts from psoriasis and sterile pustular dermatoses (108). Its level was significantly higher than that from the controls, suggesting that, in psoriasis, GM-CSF may amplify and modulate inflammatory reactions and activated T cells. GM-CSF also functions as a potent keratinocyte mitogen (109).

Chemokines (IL-8 and Related Chemokines)

Psoriatic scale extracts contain a unique chemotactic peptide fraction that very likely is involved in the induction of rhythmic transepidermal leukocyte chemotaxis (3). Two unrelated chemotactic peptides are identified in this fraction, i.e., C5a/C5a des Arg and chemotactic cytokines (chemokines) such as IL-8 and MGSA/Gro (110). IL-8 is a chemotactic cytokine released by various skin cells including keratinocytes, fibroblasts, neutrophils, monocytes, and lymphocytes under the influence of proinflammatory primary cytokines such as IL-1, TNF-α (111,112), and IFN-γ (113,114), i.e., in situations that prevail in psoriatic lesions. Particularly, TNF-α and IFN-γ stimulate keratinocytes synergistically to produce IL-8 (113).

IL-8 is chemotactic for neutrophils and T lymphocytes, but also directly influences several keratinocyte functions such as HLA-DR expression (115) and growth (116). IL-8 mRNA was detected only in lesional psoriatic epidermis, and IL-8R-specific mRNA was found to be increased 10 times in lesional psoriatic epidermis. Type I IL-8R gene expression was found to be exclusively localized to the basal keratinocyte layer of psoriatic skin (117). These recent findings suggest that, in psoriatic skin, elevated IL-8 levels and markedly increased IL-8R expression may act in concert to induce the cardinal signs of psoriasis-epidermal hyperproliferation and leukocyte infiltration (118).

In regard to another related chemokine, MGSA/Gro, it was reported that the Gro-α gene is selectively overexpressed in psoriatic lesions and that there is a linear correlation between IL-8 and Gro-α mRNA levels (114,119).

The presence of dermal macrophages/dendrocytes in the papillary dermis and along the basement membrane of the elongated rete ridges leads to the assumption that monocyte-selective attractants are released in this area. Selective monocyte chemoattractant, monocyte chemotactic protein 1 (MCP-1), could be located to the proliferating basal keratinocytes at the tips of rete ridges (120). There is no evidence for the presence of other chemokines such as MCP-3 or RANTES.

Immunoregulatory Cytokines Involved in Epidermal Cell Hyperplasia

T lymphocytes activated in psoriatic lesions secrete cytokines that can induce epidermal hyperplasia. Isolated lesional T cells produce a heparin-binding epidermal growth factor–like growth factor (54) and secrete various Th1 and Th2 cell type cytokines (14,45,48,121). Bata et al. (15) demonstrated that the isolated T-cell clones secrete cytokines that augment the growth of a specific keratinocyte population with a stem cell phenotype that is in a hyperproliferative state in psoriatic lesions; they secreted high levels of GM-CSF and IFN-γ, low IL-3 and TNF-α, and variable amounts of IL-4, but only anti-IFN-γ antibody was able to neutralize the growth stimulatory activity of these supernatants on psoriatic lesional keratinocytes. It was demonstrated that GM-CSF and/or IL-3 converts IFN-γ from a growth-inhibitory lymphokine to a stem-cell growth-stimulating lymphokine when all are added together to psoriatic uninvolved epidermal cell culture (122).

IL-6 released by fibroblasts and inflammatory cells can stimulate keratinocyte growth and differentiation in the skin. GM-CSF released by various inflammatory cells as well as by keratinocytes also functions as a potent keratinocyte mitogen (109). Furthermore, IL-8 released by keratinocytes themselves induces cell growth in an autocrine fashion, like TGF-α (116).

Psoriatic skin grafts retain acanthosis and parakeratosis after transplantation to nude mice, despite the absence of the characteristic lymphocyte and neutrophil infiltration (123). However, even in this model, there occurs a considerable infiltrate of mouse lymphocytes suggestive of a low-grade rejection response against the human xenografts, which may release cytokines.

LEUKOCYTE CHEMOTACTIC FACTORS

The cyclic transepidermal migration of leukocytes toward the lesional stratum corneum from edematous dermal papillae is a hallmark of the psoriasiform tissue reaction. It suggests that the concentration of leukocyte chemotactic factors is highest at the subcorneal portion and that these substances are possibly trapped in the stratum corneum that is produced by such rapidly keratinizing lesional skin. In fact, there are substances that enhance the adhesion, phagocytosis, and respiratory burst of leukocytes in the lesional stratum corneum (55). Psoriatic leukotactic factor (PLF) was the first 12-kDa chemotactic peptide fraction isolated from psoriatic scale extracts and showed biological properties similar to those of C5a anaphylatoxin; that is, it enhances permeability of vascular walls and induces leukocyte chemotaxis (124). There was no difference in the anaphylatoxin levels between suction blister fluids from uninvolved skin of psoriatic patients and those from normal controls. However, significantly high anaphylatoxin levels were noted in fluids of suction blisters raised on lesional skin as compared with those produced on uninvolved skin in psoriatic patients, reflecting the ongoing complement activation taking place only in lesional skin (125), as in scale extracts that reflect the past inflammatory changes of lesional epidermis that involved complement activation (126). A recent study on complement fragments disclosed that the amount of C5a des Arg contained in psoriatic scales far exceeds that simply produced from the exudated plasma, suggesting the important role played by complement activation in psoriasis (127).

Epidermal keratinocytes produce C3, a key component of the complement system (128), and, as observed with IL-8 (113), its production is augmented by the presence of IFN-γ and TNF-α in vitro; thus the ongoing T-cell-mediated inflammation in psoriatic lesions seems to facilitate C3 production by keratinocytes (129). Analyses of the lesional skin with various methods indicate preferential complement activation via the alternative pathway (130–132). Probably, complement interacts with the stratum corneum, the target of leukocyte chemotaxis, to produce various bioactive substances in lesional skin via the alternative pathway (133).

As mentioned above, Schroder and Christophers (110) demonstrated the presence of another peptide fraction in psoriatic scale extracts, an anionic neutrophil-activating peptide (ANAP), which was confirmed to be identical to IL-8, a neutrophil chemotactic cytokine (chemokine) released by various cells including keratinocytes under the influence of proinflammatory primary cytokines such as IL-1, TNF-α, and IFN-γ (111–113). Subsequently, other chemokines such as Gro-α for neutrophils and MCAF/MCP-1 for monocytes and T cells were also found to be elevated in the lesional skin (119,134).

The concentrations of immunoreactive IL-8 were found to be consistently increased in the horny-tissue extracts from lesional skin and in cutaneous tissue fluid samples collected from suction blisters. However, the neutrophil chemotactic activity demonstrable in these samples correlated significantly with the levels of C5a/C5a des Arg in the scales rather than with IL-8. Based on these results, it was speculated that, although IL-8 may exert a synergistic effect with C5a/C5a des Arg in the induction of transepidermal leukocyte chemotaxis, it constitutes a proinflammatory cytokine that is involved in the production of the persistent inflammatory changes characterized by a T-lymphocyte infiltration (135).

As mentioned, the inflammation observed in psoriatic lesions is not uniform but heterogeneous (21). However, IL-8 is found to be consistently increased in the lesional scale extracts (135). In contrast, C5a des Arg shows large variation in its concentration in lesional skin (135). Such a fluctuation in the C5a des Arg concentration also suggests its pathogenetic role in the induction of cyclic transepidermal leukocyte chemotaxis. Moreover, IL-8 production by keratinocytes and fibroblasts is induced even in simply irritated skin (136). Therefore, although IL-8 and related chemokines may exert a synergistic effect with C5a anaphylatoxin in the induction of transepidermal leukocyte chemotaxis, they appear to act as proinflammatory cytokines that are involved in the production of the baseline inflammatory changes characterized by T-lymphocyte infiltration (135). Namely, C5a is important in the initiation of neutrophil tissue infiltration, whereas IL-8 and Gro-α together with some additional mediators, could be important in maintaining neutrophil migration into the tissue (114).

For the generation of C5a in the upper epidermis of psoriatic lesions, it is possible that C5 in tissue fluid is directly cleaved by serine proteinase (137), which is rich in upper lesional epidermis (138,139), as well as by enzymes released by infiltrating neutrophils. However, the presence of various complement fragments along with the terminal complex SC 5b-7 in lesional skin samples (140) suggests the complement activation in the lesional skin. The interaction between the stratum corneum and complement is the most plausible initiator of complement activation in the upper epidermis. The damages of the upper epidermal cells caused by the T-lymphocyte infiltration, which is prominent in the edematous suprapapillary portion of the lesional epidermis, may facilitate a direct exposure of the stratum corneum to the tissue fluid containing complement. Beutner et al. (1) hypothesized the activation of the classical complement pathway by the reaction between the stratum corneum antigen and anti–stratum corneum antibodies. However, the stratum corneum effectively activates complement via the alternative pathway to generate chemotactic C5a anaphylatoxin even under conditions that prevent activation of the classic complement pathway (133). Determination of complement fragments in scale extracts also indicates that the activation of the alternative complement pathway is a major mechanism for complement activation occurring in the psoriatic epidermis (132).

To facilitate the alternative complement pathway, its two key components, factor B and C3, are produced by human keratinocytes (128,141). Recently, we found that the C3 production occurs more effectively by differentiated keratinocyte such as those found in the upper epidermis than by actively proliferating keratinocytes composing the basal cell layer and that T-cell-derived cytokines such as IFN-γ and TNF-α synergistically enhance its generation (129). Thus, both proinflammatory cytokine IL-8 and C3 are produced in large amounts at the site of T-cell-mediated inflammation.

Other small molecular chemotactic substances such as leukotriene B4, the most potent arachidonic acid–derived lipid chemotactic factor, are also elevated in psoriatic lesions. However, they do not appear to be major ones (142) as abnormal production does not exist in psoriasis (114). The most likely source of the LTB4 detected in acute psoriatic lesions seems to be infiltrating neutrophils, because keratinocytes lack the ability to synthesize LTB4.

OTHER CLINICAL AND LABORATORY FINDINGS RELEVANT TO IMMUNE-MEDIATED DISEASE

Like other autoimmune diseases, psoriasis shows a close association with certain major histocompatibility complex genes (16,17). Moreover, it may not be simply a skin disease, but may involve other organs, though unnoticed by most patients. In fact, a significant proportion of patients develop chronic arthritis, either silent or manifest. Moreover, in the case of acute exacerbation, there definitely develop systemic symptoms such as fever, malaise, weakness, and joint pain accompanying generalized erythema with pustulation. Abnormal laboratory findings such as leukocytosis and an elevated erythrocyte sedimentation rate are also found, as observed in patients with generalized pustular psoriasis. This strongly suggests the involvement of organs other than the skin.

Circulating Complement-Derived Factors

Not only in lesional skin, but also in the circulating blood of psoriatic patients, there is evidence of ongoing inflammation association with complement activation (131,140,143–146). Plasma concentrations of C3a, C4a, iC3b, C4d, Bb fragments, and SC 5b-9 are all significantly increased, particularly in those with higher disease activity showing such inflammatory skin changes as erythrodermic pustular psoriasis, psoriatic arthritis, and Reiter's syndrome. This is much more prominent when compared with atopic dermatitis (144). Furthermore, there is an elevation in the plasma levels of regulatory factors for the alternative complement pathway activation, factor H, which inhibits the activities of C3b and the alternative pathway convertases C3bBb and PC3bBb, in addition to potentiating the inactivation of factor I, which cleaves and inactivates C3b in correlation with both the extent of skin changes and disease activity. All of these data suggest that complement activation chiefly via the alternative pathway takes place in psoriatic patients in correlation with the skin disease activity. This is considered to be derived mainly from skin lesions, but complement activation at other sites such as the joints cannot be ruled out.

Circulating Cytokines

The report of an induction or exacerbation of psoriasis by recombinant IFN-γ stresses their inductive role in this disease (147). Gomi et al. (148) found that IFN-γ levels were increased in the sera from patients and that these correlate with disease activity, whereas the mean serum levels of IL-1-α and TNF-α were not significantly different from those in controls. Or rather, they noted that serum levels of IL-1-α correlated negatively with the clinical disease severity and with the duration of psoriasis. In addition, an inverse correlation was noted between the IL-1-α levels and IFN-γ levels. Accordingly, they suggested that IL-1-α and IFN-γ might be relevant to the induction and perpetuation, respectively, of the inflammatory responses in psoriasis, and that these cytokines, which have similar biological properties, may strictly regulate each other's production in vivo.

Circulating Receptors and Adhesion Molecules

Serum interleukin-2 receptor (IL-2R) levels, which represent an early measure of T-cell activation, are significantly elevated in psoriatic patients (149,150). Likewise, increases in serum IL-2R, which may be due to T-cell activation in the dermis, are found during psoriatic inflammation. In addition, circulating forms of adhesion molecules such as cICAM-1, cICAM-3, E-selectin, and cTNF receptor 1 are elevated (151–153). The origin and function of these molecules in psoriasis remain to be defined except for E-selectin, which is derived from activated endothelial cells.

HIV-Associated Psoriasis

The well-documented exacerbation of psoriasis in human immunodeficiency virus (HIV)-infected individuals (154,155) appears contradictory from the hypothesis of psoriasis as a CD4+ T-cell-mediated disease. However, despite a decrease in the number of CD4+ T cells in the peripheral blood, an active recruitment of CD4+ T cells into lesional skin takes place as in HIV-negative psoriatic lesional skin (156). Moreover, HIV may act as superantigen (157) to activate T cells. Although no longitudinal studies on HIV-infected psoriatic patients have been conducted, psoriasis seems to improve during the terminal phase of HIV infection (158).

IMMUNOTHERAPY

Many drugs that have been introduced for the therapeutic armamentarium against psoriasis were originally targeted on hyperproliferative keratinocytes. However, it is now clear that most of them exert not only antimitotic activities against keratinocytes but also immunosuppressive effects.

Glucocorticoids and phototherapy with UVB and PUVA are all well-known immunosuppressants. Even in the case of methotrexate, which was initially introduced to effectively suppress epidermal proliferation, it has now been shown that proliferating lymphoid cells are a more likely cellular target than keratinocytes (159). However, it is the remarkable efficacy of cyclosporin that has totally revolutionized our ideas about the pathogenesis of psoriasis (160). It shows an effect not only on T lymphocytes, but also on epidermal accessory cell function (33) and vascular adhesion molecule expression of the dermis (161). To alleviate the side effects, various therapeutic modalities as well as combinations with other methods have been introduced. In the same fashion, tacrolimus, anti-CD3, and anti-CD4 monoclonal antibodies have also been tried clinically, confirming the effectiveness of immuosuppressive therapy targeting on CD4+ T cells, which play a key role in the pathogenesis of psoriasis (9–12).

In regard to the epidermal hyperproliferation in psoriasis, p53, a negative regulator of the cell cycle, expression in involved psoriatic skin is found to be decreased compared with skin from uninvolved areas, indicating that a loss of a growth-inhibitory activity is responsible for the hyperproliferative characteristics of the disease. Levels of p53 mRNA and protein are increased in cultured epidermal cells after treatment with tacrolimus (117).

CONCLUDING REMARKS

The present overview of various immunological studies on psoriasis has clearly shown that psoriasis is an inflammatory dermatosis resulting from activation of cellular immune responses in the skin and that immune-mediated activation of T cells can induce epidermal hyperplasia with a disturbed keratinization process together with lesional accumulation of neutrophils, probably through the concerted action of various secreted cytokines and humoral proinflammatory chemical mediators such as C5a des Arg. However, even such recently accumulated pieces are still fragmentary and the underlying complex pathophysiological processes have not fully been clarified yet. On the other hand, recent findings of oligoclonal T-cell subset expansion in lesional skin further suggest the possibility of a novel approach to psoriasis therapy such as T-cell-receptor-targeted immunotherapy, as well as the identification of thus far unknown antigens and elucidation of exact pathomechanisms.

ACKNOWLEDGMENT

This study was supported by Grants-in-aid for Scientific Research from the Ministry of Education, Science, and Culture, Japan.

REFERENCES

1. Beutner, E.H., Jablonska, S., Jarzabek, C.M., Marciejowska, E., Rzesa, G., and Chorzelski, T.P. (1975). Studies in immunodermatology. VI. IF studies of autoantibodies to the stratum corneum and of in vivo fixed IgG in stratum corneum of psoriatic lesions. *Int. Arch. Allergy Appl. Immunol.* 48:301–323.
2. Cormane, R.H., Hunyadi, J., and Hamerlinck, F. (1976). [The immunological mechanisms of psoriasis]. *Ann. Dermatol. Syphiligr. Paris* 103:567–572.
3. Tagami, H., and Ofuji, S. (1976). Leukotactic properties of soluble substances in psoriasis scale. *Br. J. Dermatol.* 95:1–8.
4. Beutner, E.H. (1982). *Autoimmunity in Psoriasis.* CRC Press, Boca Raton, FL.
5. Jablonska, S., and Glinski, W. (1991). Overview of immunology. In *Psoriasis,* 2nd ed., Revised and Expanded. H.H. Roenigk, Jr., and H.I. Maibach (Eds.). Marcel Dekker, New York, pp. 261–283.
6. Gardembas, P.M., Ifrah, N., Foussard, C., Boasson, M., Saint, A.J., and Verret, J.L. (1990). Psoriasis after allogeneic bone marrow transplantation. *Arch. Dermatol.* 126:1523 (letter).
7. Eedy, D.J., Burrows, D., Bridges, J.M., and Jones, F.G. (1990). Clearance of severe psoriasis after allogenic bone marrow transplantation. *Br. Med. J.* 300: 908.
8. Terui, T., Rokugo, M., Aiba, S., Kato, T., and Tagami, H. (1990). Autologous mixed lymphocyte reaction is reduced in patients with psoriasis. *Br. J. Dermatol.* 123:325–331.
9. Cooper, K.D., Voorhees, J.J., Fisher, G.J., Chan, L.S., Gupta, A.K., and Baadsgaard, O. (1990). Effects of cyclosporine on immunologic mechanisms in psoriasis. *J. Am. Acad. Dermatol.* 23:1318–1326.
10. Jegasothy, B.V., Ackerman, C.D., Todo, S., Fung, J.J., Abu, E.K., and Starzl, T.E. (1992). Tacrolimus (FK 506)—a new therapeutic agent for severe recalcitrant psoriasis. *Arch. Dermatol.* 128:781–785.
11. Prinz, J., Braun-Falco, O., Meurer, M., Daddona, P., Reiter, C., Rieber, P., and Riethmuller, G. (1991). Chimaeric CD4 monoclonal antibody in treatment of generalised pustular psoriasis. *Lancet* 338:320–321 (letter).
12. Nicolas, J.F., Chamchick, N., Thivolet, J., Wijdenes, J., Morel, P., and Revillard, J.P. (1991). CD4 antibody treatment of severe psoriasis. *Lancet* 338:321 (letter).
13. Rovee, D.T., Kurowski, C.A., Labun, J., and Downes, A.M. (1972). Effect of local wound environment on epidermal healing. In *Epidermal Wound Healing.* H. Maibach, and D.T. Rovee (Eds.). Year Book Medical Publishers, Chicago.
14. Prinz, J.C., Gross, B., Vollmer, S., Trommler, P., Strobel, I., Meurer, M., and Plewig, G. (1994). T cell clones from psoriasis skin lesions can promote keratinocyte proliferation in vitro via secreted products. *Eur. J. Immunol.* 24:593–598.
15. Bata, C.Z., Hammerberg, C., Voorhees, J.J., and Cooper, K.D. (1995). Kinetics and regulation of human keratinocyte stem cell growth in short-term primary ex vivo culture. Cooperative growth factors from psoriatic lesional T lymphocytes stimulate proliferation among psoriatic uninvolved, but not normal, stem keratinocytes. *J. Clin. Invest.* 95:317–327.
16. Gottlieb, A.B., and Krueger, J.G. (1990). HLA region genes and immune activation in the pathogenesis of psoriasis. *Arch. Dermatol.* 126:1083–1086.
17. Henseler, T., and Christophers, E. 1994. HLA and psoriasis. In *Psoriasis.* L. Dubertret (Ed). ISED, Brescia, Italy, pp. 10–13.
18. Tagami, H. (1993). Psoriasis—recent advances. In *Dermatology: Process and Perspectives. The proceedings of the 18th World Congress of Dermatology.* W.H.C. Burgdorf and S.I. Katz (Eds.). Parthenon Publishing, New York, pp. 78–90.
19. Baker, B.S., Swain, A.F., Fry, L., and Valdimarsson, H. (1984). Epidermal T lymphocytes and HLA-DR expression in psoriasis. *Br. J. Dermatol.* 110: 555–564.
20. Placek, W., Haftek, M., and Thivolet, J. (1988). Sequence of changes in psoriatic epidermis. Immunocompetent cell redistribution precedes altered expression of keratinocyte differentiation markers. *Acta Derm. Venereol. (Stockh.)* 68:369–377.
21. Soltani, K., and Van Scott, E.J. (1972). Patterns and sequence of tissue changes in incipient and evolving lesions of psoriasis. *Arch. Dermatol.* 106:484–490.
22. Griffin, T.D., Lattanand, A., and Van Scott, E.J. (1988). Clinical and histologic heterogeneity of pso-

riatic plaques. Therapeutic relevance. *Arch. Dermatol.* 124:216–220.
23. Chowaniec, O., Jablonska, S., Beutner, E.H., Proniewska, M., Jarzabek, C.M., and Rzesa, G. (1981). Earliest clinical and histological changes in psoriasis. *Dermatologica* 163:42–51.
24. Uehara, M., and Ofuji, S. (1974). The morphogenesis of pustulosis palmaris et plantaris. *Arch. Dermatol.* 109:518–520.
25. Bacharach, B.M., and Altmeyer, P. (1989). Pustulosis palmoplantaris. How initial ultrastructural alterations change into vesicles and pustules. *Acta Derm. Venereol. (Stockh.)* (Suppl.) 146:76–80.
26. Paslin, D. (1990). Psoriasis without neutrophils. *Int. J. Dermatol.* 29:37–40.
27. Terunuma, A., Takahashi, K., Sakakibara, A., Aiba, S., and Tagami, H. (1992). Annular psoriasiform eruption with lymphocytic infiltration of the epidermis: a variant of acute psoriasis? *Dermatology* 185: 156–159.
28. Ragaz, A., and Ackerman, A.B. (1979). Evolution, maturation, and regression of lesions of psoriasis. New observation and correlation of clinical and histologic findings. *Am. J. Dermatopathol.* 1:199–214.
29. Pinkus, H., and Mehregan, A.H. (1966). The primary histologic lesion of seborrheic dermatitis and psoriasis. *J. Invest. Dermatol.* 46:109–116.
30. van de Kerkhof, P.C.M., and Lammers, A.M. (1987). Intraepidermal accumulation of polymorphonuclear leukocytes in chronic stable plaque psoriasis. *Dermatologica* 174:224–227.
31. Baker, B.S., Powles, A.V., Lambert, S., Valdimarsson, H., and Fry, L. (1988). A prospective study of the Koebner reaction and T lymphocytes in uninvolved psoriatic skin. *Acta Derm. Venereol. (Stockh.)* 68: 430–434.
32. Cooper, K.D., Baadsgaard, O., Ellis, C.N., Duell, E., and Voorhees, J.J. (1990). Mechanisms of cyclosporine A inhibition of antigen-presenting activity in uninvolved and lesional psoriatic epidermis. *J. Invest. Dermatol.* 94:649–656.
33. Prens, E.P., Benne, K., van Joost, T., and Benner, R. (1991). The autologous mixed epidermal cell-T lymphocyte reaction is elevated in psoriasis: a crucial role for epidermal HLA-DR+/CD1a- antigen-presenting cells. *J. Invest. Dermatol.* 96:880–887.
34. Brody, I. (1984). Mast cell degranulation in the evolution of acute eruptive guttate psoriasis vulgaris. *J. Invest. Dermatol.* 82:460–464.
35. Brody, I. (1984). Dermal and epidermal involvement in the evolution of acute eruptive guttate psoriasis vulgaris. *J. Invest. Dermatol.* 82:465–470.
36. Toruniowa, B., and Jablonska, S. (1988). Mast cells in the initial stages of psoriasis. *Arch. Dermatol. Res.* 280:189–193.
37. Schubert, C., and Christophers, E. (1985). Mast cells and macrophages in early relapsing psoriasis. *Arch. Dermatol. Res.* 277:352–358.
38. Van den Oord, J., and De Wolf-Peeters, C. (1994). Epithelium-lining macrophages in psoriasis. *Br. J. Dermatol.* 130:589–594.
39. Heng, M.C., Kloss, S.G., Kuehn, C.S., and Chase, D.G. (1985). The sequence of events in psoriatic plaque formation after tape-stripping. *Br. J. Dermatol.* 112:517–532.
40. Heng, M.C., and Kloss, S.G. (1985). Cell interactions in psoriasis. *Arch. Dermatol.* 121:881–887.
41. Takematsu, H., and Tagami, H. (1991). Determination of released CD4 and CD8 antigens in the suction-blister fluid and horny-tissue extract in patients with psoriasis. *Br. J. Dermatol.* 124:550–554.
42. Bos, J.D., Hulsebosch, H.J., Krieg, S.R., Bakker, P.M., and Cormane, R.H. (1983). Immunocompetent cells in psoriasis. In situ immunophenotyping by monoclonal antibodies. *Arch. Dermatol. Res.* 275: 181–189.
43. Prinz, J., Braun-Falco, O., Meurer, M., Daddona, P., Reiter, C., Rieber, P., and Riethmuller, G. (1991). Chimaeric CD4 monoclonal antibody in treatment of generalised pustular psoriasis. *Lancet* 338:320–321 (letter).
44. Barna, M., Snijdewint, F.G., Van der Heijden, F.L., Bos, J.D., and Kapsenberg, M.L. (1994). Characterization of lesional psoriatic skin T lymphocyte clones. *Acta Derm. Venereol. (Stockh.)* (Suppl.) 186:9–11.
45. Vollmer, S., Menssen, A., Trommler, P., Schendel, D., and Prinz, J.C. (1994). T lymphocytes derived from skin lesions of patients with psoriasis vulgaris express a novel cytokine pattern that is distinct from that of T helper type 1 and T helper type 2 cells. *Eur. J. Immunol.* 24:2377–2382.
46. Gottlieb, A.B., Luster, A.D., Posnett, D.N., and Carter, D.M. (1988). Detection of a gamma interferon-induced protein IP-10 in psoriatic plaques. *J. Exp. Med.* 168:941–948.
47. Takematsu, H., and Tagami, H. (1990). Interleukin 2, soluble interleukin 2 receptor, and interferon-gamma in the suction blister fluids from psoriatic skin. *Arch. Dermatol. Res.* 282:149–152.
48. Schlaak, J.F., Buslau, M., Jochum, W., Hermann, E., Girndt, M., Gallati, H., Meyer, Z.B.K., and Fleischer, B. (1994). T cells involved in psoriasis vulgaris belong to the Th1 subset. *J. Invest. Dermatol.* 102: 145–149.
49. Onuma, S. (1994). Immunohistochemical studies of infiltrating cells in early and chronic lesions of psoriasis. *J. Dermatol.* 21:223–232.
50. Ros, A.M., and Wennersten, G. (1987). Photosensitive psoriasis—an immunohistochemical study after light provocation with UVA and UVB. *Photodermatology* 4:79–87.

51. Paukkonen, K., Naukkarinen, A., and Horsmanheimo, M. (1992). The development of manifest psoriatic lesions is linked with the invasion of CD8 + T cells and CD11c + macrophages into the epidermis. *Arch. Dermatol. Res.* 284:375–379.
52. Brown, L.F., Olbricht, S.M., Berse, B., Jackman, R.W., Matsueda, G., Tognazzi, K.A., Manseau, E.J., Dvorak, H.F., and Van, D.W.L. (1995). Overexpression of vascular permeability factor (VPF/VEGF) and its endothelial cell receptors in delayed hypersensitivity skin reactions. *J. Immunol.* 154:2801–2807.
53. Detmar, M., Brown, L.F., Claffey, K.P., Yeo, K.T., Kocher, O., Jackman, R.W., Berse, B., and Dvorak, H.F. (1994). Overexpression of vascular permeability factor/vascular endothelial growth factor and its receptors in psoriasis. *J. Exp. Med.* 180:1141–1146.
54. Blotnick, S., Peoples, G.E., Freeman, M.R., Eberlein, T.J., and Klagsbrun, M. (1994). T lymphocytes synthesize and export heparin-binding epidermal growth factor–like growth factor and basic fibroblast growth factor, mitogens for vascular cells and fibroblasts: differential production and release by CD4+ and CD8+ T cells. *Proc. Natl. Acad. Sci. U.S.A.* 91:2890–2894.
55. Tagami, H., Iwatsuki, K., and Takematsu, H. (1987). Psoriasis and leukocyte chemotaxis. *J. Invest. Dermatol.* 88(Suppl 3):18s–23s.
56. Barker, J.N.W.N., Groves, R.W., Allen, M.H., and Macdonald, D.M. (1992). Preferential adherence of T lymphocytes and neutrophils to psoriatic epidermis. *Br. J. Dermatol.* 127:205–211.
57. Schopf, R.E., Straussfeld, E., and Morsches, B. (1985). Changes in the chemiluminescence behavior of micro- and macrophages in psoriasis: more than just an epiphenomenon?. *Z Hautkr.* 60:797–798.
58. Jablonska, S., and Glinski, W. 1994. Neutrophils. In *Psoriasis.* L. Dubertret (Ed.). ISED, Brescia, Italy, pp. 56–62.
59. Kapp, A., and Schopf, E. (1986). Cellular reactivity of polymorphonuclear leukocytes in psoriasis and atopic dermatitis—measurement of lucigenin-dependent chemiluminescence. *Acta Derm. Venereol. (Stockh.)* 66:285–289.
60. Schroder, J.M., and Christophers, E. (1985). Transient absence of C5a-specific neutrophil function in inflammatory disorders of the skin. *J. Invest. Dermatol.* 85: 194–198.
61. Glinski, W., Tigalonowa, M., Jablonska, S., and Janczura, E. (1986). Decreased extracellular release of granule enzymes from in vitro-stimulated polymorphonuclear leukocytes in guttate psoriasis. *Inflammation* 10:99–108.
62. Chang, J.C., Smith, L.R., Froning, K.J., Schwabe, B.J., Laxer, J.A., Caralli, L.L., Kurland, H.H., Karasek, M.A., Wilkinson, D.I., Carlo, D.J., and et al. (1994). CD8+ T cells in psoriatic lesions preferentially use T-cell receptor V beta 3 and/or V beta 13.1 genes. *Proc. Natl. Acad. Sci. U.S.A.* 91:9282–9286.
63. Rosenberg, E.W., Noah, P.W., and Skinner, R.J. (1994). Psoriasis is a visible manifestation of the skin's defense against micro-organisms. *J. Dermatol.* 21:375–381.
64. Telfer, N.R., Chalmers, R.J., Whale, K., and Colman, G. (1992). The role of streptococcal infection in the initiation of guttate psoriasis. *Arch. Dermatol.* 128: 39–42.
65. Aiba, S., and Tagami, H. (1989). Proliferative responses of peripheral blood mononuclear cells from psoriatic patients to T lymphocyte-stimulating cytokines (IL-2, IL-3, IL-4, and granulocyte-macrophage colony-stimulating factor) and OK-432. *Arch. Dermatol. Res.* 281:310–315.
66. Baker, B.S., Powles, A.V., Malkani, A.K., Lewis, H., Valdimarsson, H., and Fry, L. (1991). Altered cell-mediated immunity to group A haemolytic streptococcal antigens in chronic plaque psoriasis. *Br. J. Dermatol.* 125:38–42.
67. Baker, B.S., Bokth, S., Powles, A., Garioch, J.J., Lewis, H., Valdimarsson, H., and Fry, L. (1993). Group A streptococcal antigen-specific T lymphocytes in guttate psoriatic lesions. *Br. J. Dermatol.* 128: 493–499.
68. Valdimarsson, H., Baker, B.S., Jonsdottir, I., Powles, A., and Fry, L. (1995). Psoriasis: a T-cell-mediated autoimmune disease induced by streptococcal superantigens? *Immunol. Today* 16:145–149.
69. McFadden, J., Valdimarsson, H., and Fry, L. (1991). Cross-reactivity between streptococcal M surface antigen and human skin. *Br. J. Dermatol.* 125:443–447.
70. Leung, D.Y., Walsh, P., Giorno, R., and Norris, D.A. (1993). A potential role for superantigens in the pathogenesis of psoriasis. *J. Invest. Dermatol.* 100: 225–228.
71. Menssen, A., Trommler, P., Vollmer, S., Schendel, D., Albert, E., Gurtler, L., Riethmuller, G., and Prinz, J.C. (1995). Evidence for an antigen-specific cellular immune response in skin lesions of patients with psoriasis vulgaris. *J. Immunol.* 155:4078–4083.
72. McGregor, J.M., Barker, J.N., Ross, E.L., and MacDonald, D.M. (1992). Epidermal dendritic cells in psoriasis possess a phenotype associated with antigen presentation: in situ expression of beta 2-integrins. *J. Am. Acad. Dermatol.* 27:383–388.
73. Baadsgaard, O., Gupta, A.K., Taylor, R.S., Ellis, C.N., Voorhees, J.J., and Cooper, K.D. (1989). Psoriatic epidermal cells demonstrate increased numbers and function of non-Langerhans antigen-presenting cells. *J. Invest. Dermatol.* 92:190–195.
74. Schopf, R.E., Hoffmann, A., Jung, M., Morsches, B., and Bork, K. (1986). Stimulation of T cells by autologous mononuclear leukocytes and epidermal cells in psoriasis. *Arch. Dermatol. Res.* 279:89–94.

75. Cerio, R., Griffiths, C.E., Cooper, K.D., Nickoloff, B.J., and Headington, J.T. (1989). Characterization of factor XIIIa positive dermal dendritic cells in normal and inflamed skin. *Br. J. Dermatol.* 121:421–431.
76. Terui, T., Aiba, S., Kato, T., Tanaka, T., and Tagami, H. (1987). HLA-DR antigen expression on keratinocytes in highly inflamed parts of psoriatic lesions. *Br. J. Dermatol.* 116:87–93.
77. Nickoloff, B.J., Mitra, R.S., Green, J., Zheng, X.G., Shimizu, Y., Thompson, C., and Turka, L.A. (1993). Accessory cell function of keratinocytes for superantigens. Dependence on lymphocyte function-associated antigen-1/intercellular adhesion molecule-1 interaction. *J. Immunol.* 150:2148–2159.
78. Griffiths, C.E., Voorhees, J.J., and Nickoloff, B.J. (1989). Characterization of intercellular adhesion molecule-1 and HLA-DR expression in normal and inflamed skin: modulation by recombinant gamma interferon and tumor necrosis factor. *J. Am. Acad. Dermatol.* 20:617–69.
79. Uyemura, K., Yamamura, M., Fivenson, D.F., Modlin, R.L., and Nickoloff, B.J. (1993). The cytokine network in lesional and lesion-free psoriatic skin is characterized by a T-helper type 1 cell-mediated response. *J. Invest. Dermatol.* 101:701–705.
80. Chin, Y.H., Falanga, V., and Cai, J.P. (1990). Lymphocyte adhesion to psoriatic dermal endothelium: mechanism and modulation. *J. Invest. Dermatol.* 95: 29s–31s.
81. Groves, R.W., and Barker, J.N. (1992). Pathophysiological aspects of psoriasis. *Eur. J. Med.* 1:166–172.
82. Picker, L.J., Kishimoto, T.K., Smith, C.W., Warnock, R.A., and Butcher, E.C. (1991). ELAM-1 is an adhesion molecule for skin-homing T cells. *Nature* 349: 796–799.
83. de Boer, O., Wakelkamp, I.M., Pals, S.T., Claessen, N., Bos, J.D., and Das, P.K. (1994). Increased expression of adhesion receptors in both lesional and non-lesional psoriatic skin. *Arch. Dermatol. Res.* 286: 304–311.
84. Horrocks, C., Duncan, J.I., Oliver, A.M., and Thomson, A.W. (1991). Adhesion molecule expression in psoriatic skin lesions and the influence of cyclosporin A. *Clin. Exp. Immunol.* 84:157–162.
85. Thomson, A.W., Nalesnik, M.A., Rilo, H.R., Woo, J., Carroll, P.B., and Van Thiel, D. (1993). ICAM-1 and E-selectin expression in lesional biopsies of psoriasis patients responding to systemic FK 506 therapy. *Autoimmunity* 15:215–223.
86. Fyrand, O. (1979). Studies on fibronectin in the skin. II. Indirect immunofluorescence studies in psoriasis vulgaris. *Arch. Dermatol. Res.* 266:33–41.
87. Griffiths, C.E., and Voorhees, J.J. (1992). Immunological mechanisms involved in psoriasis. *Springer Semin. Immunopathol.* 13:441–454.
88. Kellner, I., Konter, U., and Sterry, W. (1991). Overexpression of extracellular matrix receptors (VLA-3, 5 and 6) on psoriatic keratinocytes. *Br. J. Dermatol.* 125:211–216.
89. von den Driesch, P. (1993). Epidermotropic neutrophilic granulocytes express MAC-1 (CD1 1b/CD18) rather than LFA-1 (CD11a/CD18). *Arch. Dermatol. Res.* 285:444–446.
90. Ristow, H.J. (1987). A major factor contributing to epidermal proliferation in inflammatory skin diseases appears to be interleukin 1 or a related protein. *Proc. Natl. Acad. Sci. U.S.A.* 84:1940–1944.
91. Takematsu, H., Suzuki, R., Tagami, H., and Kumagai, K. (1986). Interleukin-1-like activity in horny layer extracts: decreased activity in scale extracts of psoriasis and sterile pustular dermatoses. *Dermatologica* 172:236–240.
92. Cooper, K.D., Hammerberg, C., Baadsgaard, O., Elder, J.T., Chan, L.S., Sauder, D.N., Voorhees, J.J., and Fisher, G. (1990). IL-1 activity is reduced in psoriatic skin. Decreased IL-1 alpha and increased nonfunctional IL-1 beta. *J. Immunol.* 144:4593–4603.
93. Hammerberg, C., Arend, W.P., Fisher, G.J., Chan, L.S., Berger, A.E., Haskill, J.S., Voorhees, J.J., and Cooper, K.D. (1992). Interleukin-1 receptor antagonist in normal and psoriatic epidermis. *J. Clin. Invest.* 90:571–583.
94. Debets, R., Hegmans, J.P., Troost, R.J., Benner, R., and Prens, E.P. (1995). Enhanced production of biologically active interleukin-1 alpha and interleukin-1 beta by psoriatic epidermal cells ex vivo: evidence of increased cytosolic interleukin-1 beta levels and facilitated interleukin-1 release. *Eur. J. Immunol.* 25: 1624–1630.
95. Prens, E., Debets, R., and Hegmans, J. (1995). T lymphocytes in psoriasis. *Clin. Dermatol.* 13:115–129.
96. Krueger, J., Ray, A., Tamm, I., and Sehgal, P.B. (1991). Expression and function of interleukin-6 in epithelial cells. *J. Cell Biochem.* 45:327–334.
97. Takematsu, H., and Tagami, H. (1994). Lack of correlation between interleukin 6 and interleukin 1 levels in psoriatic lesional skin. *Tohoku J. Exp. Med.* 172: 243–252.
98. Bonifati, C., Carducci, M., Cordiali, F.P., Trento, E., Sacerdoti, G., Fazio, M., and Ameglio, F. (1994). Correlated increases of tumour necrosis factor-alpha, interleukin-6 and granulocyte monocyte-colony stimulating factor levels in suction blister fluids and sera of psoriatic patients—relationships with disease severity. *Clin. Exp. Dermatol.* 19:383–387.
99. Grossman, R.M., Krueger, J., Yourish, D., Granelli, P.A., Murphy, D.P., May, L.T., Kupper, T.S., Sehgal, P.B., and Gottlieb, A.B. (1989). Interleukin 6 is expressed in high levels in psoriatic skin and stimulates proliferation of cultured human keratinocytes. *Proc. Natl. Acad. Sci. U.S.A.* 86:6367–6371.

100. Prens, E.P., Benne, K., van Damme, J., Bakkus, M., Brakel, K., Benner, R., and van Joost, T. (1990). Interleukin-1 and interleukin-6 in psoriasis. *J. Invest. Dermatol.* 95(Suppl 6):121s–124s.
101. Ettehadi, P., Greaves, M.W., Wallach, D., Aderka, D., and Camp, R.D. (1994). Elevated tumour necrosis factor-alpha (TNF-alpha) biological activity in psoriatic skin lesions. *Clin. Exp. Immunol.* 96:146–151.
102. Oxholm, A. (1992). Epidermal expression of interleukin-6 and tumour necrosis factor-alpha in normal and immunoinflammatory skin states in humans. *Apmis Suppl.* 24:1–32.
103. Takematsu, H., Ozawa, H., Yoshimura, T., Hara, M., Sakakibara, A., Oyama, J., and Tagami, H. (1991). Systemic TNF administration in psoriatic patients: a promising therapeutic modality for severe psoriasis. *Br. J. Dermatol.* 124:209–210 (letter).
104. Creaven, P.J., and Stoll, H.J. (1991). Response to tumor necrosis factor in two cases of psoriasis. *J. Am. Acad. Dermatol.* 24:735–737.
105. Sagawa, Y., Shiohara, T., Imanishi, K., and Nagashima, M. (1993). Is sustained production of tumor necrosis factor-alpha relevant to the development of pustular psoriasis? *Dermatology* 187:81–83.
106. Kaneko, F., Suzuki, M., Takiguchi, Y., Itoh, N., and Minagawa, T. (1990). Immunohistopathologic studies in the development of psoriatic lesion influenced by gamma-interferon and the producing cells. *J. Dermatol. Sci.* 1:425–434.
107. Scheynius, A., Fransson, J., Johansson, C., Hammar, H., Baker, B., Fry, L., and Valdimarsson, H. (1992). Expression of interferon-gamma receptors in normal and psoriatic skin. *J. Invest. Dermatol.* 98: 255–258.
108. Takematsu, H., and Tagami, H. (1990). Granulocyte-macrophage colony-stimulating factor in psoriasis. *Dermatologica* 181:16–20.
109. Hancock, G.E., Kaplan, G., and Cohn, Z.A. (1988). Keratinocyte growth regulation by the products of immune cells. *J. Exp. Med.* 168:1395–1402.
110. Schroder, J.M., and Christophers, E. (1986). Identification of C5des arg and an anionic neutrophil-activating peptide (ANAP) in psoriatic scales. *J. Invest. Dermatol.* 87:53–58.
111. Takematsu, H., Isono, N., Kato, T., and Tagami, H. (1990). Normal human epidermal keratinocyte-derived neutrophil chemotactic factor. *Tohoku J. Exp. Med.* 162:1–13.
112. Jinquan, T., and Thestrup-Pedersen, K. (1995). T lymphocyte chemotaxis and skin diseases. *Exp. Dermatol.* 4:281–290.
113. Barker, J.N., Sarma, V., Mitra, R.S., Dixit, V.M., and Nickoloff, B.J. (1990). Marked synergism between tumor necrosis factor-alpha and interferon-gamma in regulation of keratinocyte-derived adhesion molecules and chemotactic factors. *J. Clin. Invest.* 85: 605–608.
114. Schroder, J.M. (1995). Inflammatory mediators and chemoattractants. *Clin. Dermatol.* 13:137–150.
115. Kemeny, L., Kenderessy, A.S., Ocsovszky, I., Michel, G., Ruzicka, T., and Dobozy, A. (1995). Interleukin-8 induces HLA-DR expression on cultured human keratinocytes via specific receptors. *Int. Arch. Allergy Immunol.* 106:351–356.
116. Tuschil, A., Lam, C., Haslberger, A., and Lindley, I. (1992). Interleukin-8 stimulates calcium transients and promotes epidermal cell proliferation. *J. Invest. Dermatol.* 99:294–298.
117. Michel, G., Kemeny, L., Homey, B., and Ruzicka, T. (1996). FK506 in the treatment of inflammatory skin disease: promises and perspectives. *Immunol. Today* 17:106–108.
118. Schulz, B.S., Michel, G., Wagner, S., Suss, R., Beetz, A., Peter, R.U., Kemeny, L., and Ruzicka, T. (1993). Increased expression of epidermal IL-8 receptor in psoriasis. Down-regulation by FK-506 in vitro. *J. Immunol.* 151:4399–4406.
119. Kojima, T., Cromie, M.A., Fisher, G.J., Voorhees, J.J., and Elder, J.T. (1993). GRO-alpha mRNA is selectively overexpressed in psoriatic epidermis and is reduced by cyclosporin A in vivo, but not in cultured keratinocytes. *J. Invest. Dermatol.* 101:767–772.
120. Gillitzer, R., Wolff, K., Tong, D., Muller, C., Yoshimura, T., Hartmann, A.A., Stingl, G., and Berger, R. (1993). MCP-1 mRNA expression in basal keratinocytes of psoriatic lesions. *J. Invest. Dermatol.* 101: 127–131.
121. Barna, M., Snijdewint, F.G., van der Heijden, F.L., Bos, J.D., and Kapsenberg, M.L. (1994). Characterization of lesional psoriatic skin T lymphocyte clones. *Acta Derm. Venereol. (Stockh.)* (Suppl.) 186:9–11.
122. Nickoloff, B.J., Basham, T.Y., Merigan, T.C., and Morhenn, V.B. (1984). Antiproliferative effects of recombinant alpha- and gamma-interferons on cultured human keratinocytes. *Lab. Invest.* 51:697–701.
123. Baker, B.S., Brent, L., Valdimarsson, H., Powles, A.V., al, I.L., Walker, M., and Fry, L. (1992). Is epidermal cell proliferation in psoriatic skin grafts on nude mice driven by T-cell derived cytokines? *Br. J. Dermatol.* 126:105–110.
124. Tagami, H., and Ofuji, S. (1977). Characterization of a leukotactic factor derived from psoriatic scale. *Br. J. Dermatol.* 97:509–518.
125. Ohkohchi, K., Takematsu, H., and Tagami, H. (1986). Determination of anaphylatoxin concentrations in suction blisters in patients with psoriasis. *J. Invest. Dermatol.* 87:65–67.
126. Takematsu, H., Ohkohchi, K., and Tagami, H. (1986). Demonstration of anaphylatoxins C3a, C4a and C5a in the scales of psoriasis and inflammatory pustular dermatoses. *Br. J. Dermatol.* 114:1–6.

127. Bergh, K., Iversen, O.J., and Lysvand, H. (1993). Surprisingly high levels of anaphylatoxin C5a des Arg are extractable from psoriatic scales. *Arch Dermatol. Res.* 285:131–134.
128. Basset, S.N., Caughman, S.W., and Yancey, K.B. (1990). A-431 cells and human keratinocytes synthesize and secrete the third component of complement. *J. Invest. Dermatol.* 95:621–625.
129. Terui, T., Ishii, K., Ozawa, M., Tabata, N., Kato, T., and Tagami, H. (1997). C3 production of cultured human epidermal keratinocytes is enhanced by IFNg and TNFa through different pathway. *J. Invest. Dermatol.* 108:62–67.
130. Kaneko, F., Kawagishi, I., Miura, Y., Watanabe, M., Kishiyama, K., and Ohkawara, A. (1984). Immunocytochemical studies on inflammatory infiltrates in psoriasis. *J. Dermatol.* 11:73–79.
131. Rosenberg, E.W., Noah, P.W., Wyatt, R.J., Jones, R.M., and Kolb, W.P. (1990). Complement activation in psoriasis. *Clin. Exp. Dermatol.* 15:16–20.
132. Takematsu, H., and Tagami, H. (1992). Preferential activation of the alternative pathway of complement in psoriatic lesional skin. *Dermatology* 184:159–160 (letter).
133. Terui, T., Kato, T., and Tagami, H. (1989). Stratum corneum activation of complement through the antibody-independent alternative pathway. *J. Invest. Dermatol.* 92:593–597.
134. Schroder, J.-M. 1992. Generation of NAP-1 and related peptides in psoriasis and other inflammatory skin diseases. In *Interleukin-8 (NAP-1) and Related Chemotactic Cytokines.* M. Baggiolini, and C. Sorg (Eds.). Karger, Basel, pp. 54–76.
135. Takematsu, H., and Tagami, H. (1993). Quantification of chemotactic peptides (C5a anaphylatoxin and IL-8) in psoriatic lesional skin. *Arch. Dermatol.* 129: 74–80.
136. Nickoloff, B.J., and Naidu, Y. (1994). Perturbation of epidermal barrier function correlates with initiation of cytokine cascade in human skin. *J. Am. Acad. Dermatol.* 30:535–546.
137. Lazarus, G.S., Yost, F.J., and Thomas, C.A. (1977). Polymorphonuclear leukocytes: possible mechanism of accumulation in psoriasis. *Science* 198:1162–1163.
138. Dubertret, L., Bertaux, B., Fosse, M., and Touraine, R. (1982). Localization of proteolytic activity in psoriatic skin. *Br. J. Dermatol.* 107:499–504.
139. Dubertret, L., Bertaux, B., Fosse, M., and Touraine, R. (1984). Psoriasis: a defect in the regulation of epidermal proteases, as shown by serial biopsies after cantharidin application. *Br. J. Dermatol.* 110: 405–410.
140. Takematsu, H., and Tagami, H. (1992). Generation of terminal complement complexes in psoriatic lesional skin. *Dermatology* 185:246–250.
141. Yancey, K.B., Overholser, O., Domloge, H.N., Li, L.J., Caughman, S.W., and Bisalbutra, P. (1992). Human keratinocytes and A-431 cells synthesize and secrete factor B, the major zymogen protease of the alternative complement pathway. *J. Invest. Dermatol.* 98:379–383.
142. Takematsu, H., Terui, T., and Tagami, H. (1986). Demonstration of leukotriene B4 in the scale extracts of psoriasis and inflammatory pustular dermatoses. Correlation with leukocyte chemotactic activity and C5a anaphylatoxin. *Acta Derm. Venereol. (Stockh.)* 66:6–10.
143. Ohkohchi, K., Takematsu, H., and Tagami, H. (1985). Increased anaphylatoxins (C3a and C4a) in psoriatic sera. *Br. J. Dermatol.* 113:189–196.
144. Kapp, A., Wokalek, H., and Schopf, E. (1985). Involvement of complement in psoriasis and atopic dermatitis-measurement of C3a and C5a, C3, C4 and C1 inactivator. *Arch. Dermatol. Res.* 277:359–361.
145. Ohkohchi, K., Takematsu, H., and Tagami, H. (1986). Increased C5a anaphylatoxin in the sera of psoriatic patients and patients with inflammatory dermatoses. *J. Dermatol.* 13:266–269.
146. Ohkohchi, K., Torinuki, W., and Tagami, H. (1988). Increased plasma concentrations of complement modulating proteins (C1 inhibitor, C4-binding protein, factor H and factor I) in psoriasis. *Tohoku J. Exp. Med.* 154:315–321.
147. Fierlbeck, G., Rassner, G., and Muller, C. (1990). Psoriasis induced at the injection site of recombinant interferon gamma. Results of immunohistologic investigations. *Arch. Dermatol.* 126:351–355.
148. Gomi, T., Shiohara, T., Munakata, T., Imanishi, K., and Nagashima, M. (1991). Interleukin 1 alpha, tumor necrosis factor alpha, and interferon gamma in psoriasis. *Arch. Dermatol.* 127:827–830.
149. Kapp, A., Piskorski, A., and Schopf, E. (1988). Elevated levels of interleukin 2 receptor in sera of patients with atopic dermatitis and psoriasis. *Br. J. Dermatol.* 119:707–710.
150. Kapp, A., Neuner, P., Krutmann, J., Luger, T.A., and Schopf, E. (1991). Production of interleukin-2 by mononuclear cells in vitro in patients with atopic dermatitis and psoriasis. Comparison with serum interleukin-2 receptor levels. *Acta Derm. Venereol.* 71: 403–406.
151. Schopf, R.E., Naumann, S., Rehder, M., and Morsches, B. (1993). Soluble intercellular adhesion molecule-1 levels in patients with psoriasis. *Br. J. Dermatol.* 128:34–37.
152. Griffiths, C.M., Boffa, M.J., Gallatin, W.M., and Martin, S. (1996). Elevated levels of circulating intercellular adhesion molecule-3 (cICAM-3) in psoriasis. *Acta Derm. Venereol. (Stockh.)* 76:2–5.
153. Bonifati, C., Trento, E., Carducci, M., Sacerdoti, G., Mussi, A., Fazio, M., and Ameglio, F. (1995). Soluble

E-selectin and soluble tumour necrosis factor receptor (60 kD) serum levels in patients with psoriasis. *Dermatology* 190:128–131.
154. Duvic, M. (1991). Papulosquamous disorders associated with human immunodeficiency virus infection. *Dermatol. Clin.* 9:523–530.
155. Duvic, M. (1995). Human immunodeficiency virus and the skin: selected controversies. *J. Invest. Dermatol.* 9:523–530.
156. Ichihashi, N., Seishima, M., Takahashi, T., Muto, Y., and Kitajima, Y. (1995). A case of AIDS manifesting pruritic papular eruptions and psoriasiform lesions: an immunohistochemical study of the lesional dermal infiltrates. *J. Dermatol.* 22:428–433.
157. Laurence, J., Hodtsev, A.S., and Posnett, D.N. (1992). Superantigen implicated in dependence of HIV-1 replication in T cells on TCR V beta expression. *Nature* 358:255–259.
158. Colebunders, R., Blot, K., Mertens, V., and Dockx, P. (1992). Psoriasis regression in terminal AIDS. *Lancet* 339 (letter).
159. Jeffes, E.r., McCullough, J.L., Pittelkow, M.R., McCormick, A., Almanzor, J., Liu, G., Dang, M., Voss, K., Voss, J., Schlotzhauer, A., et al. (1995). Methotrexate therapy of psoriasis: differential sensitivity of proliferating lymphoid and epithelial cells to the cytotoxic and growth-inhibitory effects of methotrexate. *J. Invest. Dermatol.* 104:183–188.
160. Bos, J.D. (1988). The pathomechanisms of psoriasis; the skin immune system and cyclosporin. *Br. J. Dermatol.* 118:141–155.
161. Petzelbauer, P., Stingl, G., Wolff, K., and Volc, P.B. (1991). Cyclosporin A suppresses ICAM-1 expression by papillary endothelium in healing psoriatic plaques. *J. Invest. Dermatol.* 96:362–369.

14

The Polymorphonuclear Leukocytes

Peter C. M. van de Kerkhof
University of Nijmegen Hospital, Nijmegen, The Netherlands

Early and active psoriatic lesions are characterized by the intraepidermal penetration of polymorphonuclear leukocytes (PMNs). In pustular psoriasis, the accumulation of PMNs dominates the picture.

For many decades, studies on the functioning of PMNs have been focused on their capacity to serve as a defense against microbiological assault. In this light, the appearance of PMNs in the psoriatic lesion can be incriminated to be an epiphenomenon, as microorganisms do not play a role in the pathogenesis of psoriasis.

Contemporary immunologists and cell biologists have enlarged their view of the function of the PMNs by confirming a more recent hypothesis that PMN activation may be detrimental to the host. During the last decade the hypothesis that the PMN is of pathogenetic significance in psoriasis has been tested by many investigators. This chapter discusses some of the clinical observations and experimental data supporting the autoaggressive role of PMNs in psoriasis.

Mature PMNs participate as effector cells in a variety of inflammatory disorders, frequently being the first cells to migrate into tissue after injury. Mature PMNs are terminal, since they are incapable of further cell division and survive for only about 8 hr after their release to the peripheral vascular compartment. The following stages can be defined in the participation of PMNs in the psoriatic process:

1. The peripheral blood PMNs
   Production in bone marrow
   Chemotaxis and random migration
   Endothelial attachment
2. The behavior of PMNs in psoriatic skin
   Extravasation
   Interference with skin via release of
   a. Proteinases
   b. Mediators of inflammation
   c. Reactive oxygen intermediates

In this chapter, the studies on the peripheral blood PMNs will be reviewed first. In the second section, the behavior of the PMNs in the skin will be discussed.

THE CIRCULATING BLOOD PMNs

Several groups have studied the circulating blood PMNs as to functional and biochemical properties.

Chemotaxis and Random Migration

Chemotaxis is defined as the movement of PMNs, which results from the conversion of random directional changes into nonrandom ones. Random migration is defined as the integrated effect of migration across the surface in a straight line and periodic random changes in direction. Table 1 (1–13) summarizes the observations on chemotaxis and random migration of PMNs obtained from psoriatic patients.

Chemotactic responsiveness in psoriatics was found to be normal, increased, and decreased by various

Table 1 Chemotaxis and Random Migration of PMNs in Psoriatic Patients

Ref.	Chemoattractant	Chemotaxis	Random migration
1	Zymosan/serum	↑	
2	Casein	↑	
3	Zymosan/serum	↑	
4	Casein	↑	
5	Escherichia coli	↑	↑
6	C5a, f-FMLP	↑	
7	Shigella flexneri	↑	
8	LTB4/f-FMLP	↑	
9	Zymosan/serum Escherichia coli	=	
10	Endotoxin/casein	=	↑
11	f-FMLP	=	=
12	f-FMLP Zymosan/serum	=	
13	Zymosan/serum	↓	=

groups. Although the differences in observation could be explained partly by different methods, a more likely explanation is the variation as to the clinical activity of the psoriatic process in the patients investigated. Several investigations indicate that the activity of the psoriatic process dictates the chemotactic activity of the PMNs; patients with chronic stable plaque psoriasis having relatively low values, patients with actively spreading lesions having relatively high levels (4,8). The extent of the psoriatic lesions, however, was not correlated to PMN chemotaxis (4,7,8,12).

PMN Adherence

The movement of PMNs into tissue requires as a first step their attachment to endothelial walls within the tissue to be invaded. This process of attachment requires the alteration of endothelial surface and an alteration in the PMN cell surface even prior to attachment. MacGregor and his colleagues, in attempting to determine how PMNs are prepared for this process of attachment, developed an assay for PMN adherence (14) to be used in patients with systemic inflammatory disorders (15). It depends upon the passage of heparinized peripheral blood through nylon fiber columns, and the subsequent depletion of PMNs from their selective adherence to the nylon fibers. In vitro adherence in these studies has been strongly correlated with adherence of PMNs to endothelial cells in culture (16). Using this assay, Sedgwick and co-workers (17) demonstrated that mean PMN adherence in patients with psoriasis was significantly above that of control subjects. When the patients were classified according to the extent of their disease, there was a linear stepwise correlation between adherence and the three disease severities: minimal, moderate, and extensive. Whereas patients with minimal disease had normal values for PMN adherence, patients with moderate and extensive disease had significantly increased values.

To determine whether increased adherence might simply be a reflection of cutaneous inflammation, control patients were evaluated. Their mean PMN adherence was not different from that of normal control subjects, demonstrating specificity for increased PMN adherence in psoriasis. Csato et al. reported increased adherence of PMNs of psoriatic patients to plastic plates (3). In this study, the extent and activity of the psoriatic process was not specified.

Although these adherence assays are correlated to the attachment to endothelial cells in culture the in vivo situation is far more complex. Recently, surface glycoproteins on the PMNs and adhesion molecules on the endothelial cells proved to be crucial in the interaction (18). The expression of these surface molecules is modulated during the process of inflammation.

PMN Counts and Morphology

Peripheral blood PMN counts are elevated in untreated patients with psoriasis compared to healthy controls (11,17). Although significant in a statistical sense for psoriatic patients as a whole, this leukocytosis is often not out of the normal range for individual patients. Moreover, it is confined to the neutrophil series with no alteration in peripheral blood lymphocytes, monocytes, or other formed elements (17).

Peripheral blood smears from patients with psoriasis were found to have increased numbers of PMNs with irregular shapes and ruffled membranes (19,20). Such morphological changes in cell surface membranes reflect alterations which may contribute to PMN participation in the cutaneous lesions of psoriasis.

At the time of PMN activation, lysosomal granules fuse with phagosomes, forming phagolysosomes, and they fuse with the cell surface, releasing their contents to the extracellular space. Preissner and his associates examined degranulation sensitivity to C5a and f-MLP (6) and observed both a lower threshold for beta-glucaronidase release (azurophilic granules) as well as higher released amounts of the enzyme. Psoriatic PMNs are substantially more susceptible to lithium-stimulated degranulation (21). In this respect, it is of importance that lithium carbonate causes an exacerbation in psoriasis (22).

Molecular Biology of PMNs

A large repertoire of mediators of inflammation activate the PMNs. During the process of PMN activation oxygen-derived materials such as superoxide (O_2^-) play a central role. O_2^- is produced as a highly reactive intermediary by a one-electron reduction of molecular oxygen through a membrane enzyme system which includes a coupled oxidation of NAD(P)H (reduced nicotinamide adenine dinucleotide phosphate) to $NAD(P)^+$. Generated O_2^- is released in the extracellular space during activation. Extracellular O_2^- will interact directly with tissue components, and it has the capacity to injure tissue indirectly by the generation of even more reactive oxygen intermediates. Aggregated immunoglobulin and zymosan-induced generation of oxygen intermediates of PMNs of psoriatic patients have been reported to be increased (23), whereas normal opsonized zymosan-induced superoxide generation has been reported in psoriatic PMNs by another group (24). Patients in the latter investigation were described as being in a quiescent state of their psoriasis.

Most of the energy used during the process of PMN activation is supplied by glycolysis. The last step of glycolysis, namely, transfer of the phosphoryl residue (PO_3^{3-}) from phosphoenolpyruvate to adenosine diphosphate (ADP), which yields pyurvate and adenosine triphosphate (ATP), is catalyzed by pyruvate kinase. In one group of psoriatics, the activity of PMN pyruvate kinase proved to be significantly increased compared to normal controls, although patients in a phase of remission showed values slightly lower than the activity in healthy individuals (25).

The granule enzymes of the PMNs are released during the process of activation: neutral proteinases (cathepsin G and elastase), lysozymes, and myeloperoxidase. The enzymes are of relevance in modulating extracellular matrix proteins. In psoriatic PMNs, activities of these enzymes have been reported to be normal (11), decreased (26), and increased (21). Again, the activity of these enzymes proved to be related to disease activity: patients with actively spreading lesions showing increased activities, patients with guttate psoriasis showing normal activities, and patients with stationary plaque psoriasis showing decreased activities (26).

Inflammatory eicosanoids are released from the PMNs, and as such constitute an autoamplification loop in PMN chemotaxis. Although leukotriene B4 (LTB4) production by psoriatic PMNs has been reported to be normal by one group (27), other workers showed a higher production of LTB4 and higher omega-oxidation (= inactivation of LTB4) by psoriatic PMNs, resulting in the net release of normal amounts of LTB4 from these PMNs (28).

Psoriatic Sera and Modulation of PMN Functions

Several investigators have studied the interference of sera with PMN functions, and in particular whether psoriatic sera and sera from healthy volunteers show a difference in this respect. Breathnach demonstrated that serum from psoriatic patients did not confer altered chemokinetic or chemotactic activities on normal PMNs (10). Kawohl et al. (2), Fräki et al. (11), Silney et al. (1), and Sedgwick et al. (29) demonstrated increased chemotactic activity in the presence of psoriatic serum.

Casima and associates demonstrated that psoriatic sera caused a decreased response of stimulated PMNs as to lysozyme release and O_2^- generation (30). On the other hand, Schopf and Straussfeld could not show a significant difference between normal and psoriatic serum in this respect (23).

In serum of psoriatic patients increased levels of skin-associated antileukoprotease (SKALP) have been demonstrated (30a). It is attractive to speculate that SKALP is involved in the penetration of PMN into the skin.

From these investigations, it is not clear whether the activity of the psoriatic process might be responsible for the different observations.

Antipsoriatic Treatments and PMN Functions

Corticosteroids have been shown to inhibit the at-random migration and chemotaxis of PMN in vitro (31,32). Washing the granulocytes after incubation with hydrocortisone did not reverse the inhibitory effect of chemotaxis, indicating a direct cellular effect. It has been shown that corticosteroids inhibit the adhesion of PMNs to endothelial cells in vitro, which might reduce PMN passage into the skin (33).

Anthralin causes inhibition of at-random migration and chemotaxis of PMNs. In addition, PMNs pretreated with anthralin show a dose-dependent inhibition of superoxide anion generation (34). The authors showed that the effective dosages correspond to concentrations obtained in vivo after local application.

Treatment with PUVA (psoralen and ultraviolet A) has been reported to have no effect on the chemotactic responsiveness of the blood PMNs (1). However, another group reported an inhibition of the process by PUVA treatment (35). The leukocyte counts decreased in psoriatics during PUVA treatment (36). Grüner et al. reported a decreased activity of acid hydrolases of PMNs following PUVA treatment (37).

Inhibition of PMN chemotaxis by methotrexate has been reported by several groups (38,39). Those from psoriatic patients treated with methotrexate showed inhibition during 48 hr of chemotactic responsiveness during 48 hr after an oral dose of 7.5–15.0 mg. During the following days PMN chemotaxis recovered (30).

Aromatic retinoids (etretinate and acitretin) have been reported to inhibit PMN migration in vitro (40), although other groups could not demonstrate such an effect (41,42). A direct effect of retinoids on the microtubular cell system has been proposed as an explanation for the decreased directional migration of PMNs (43). On the other hand, Ellis and coworkers observed that etretinate therapy reduced the PMN chemotaxis-enhancing properties of psoriatic serum (42).

It has been suspected for some time that peritoneal dialysis and perhaps even hemodialysis would benefit some patients with psoriasis. This issue has been clarified recently by Whittier et al. in a double-blind cross-over study of peritoneal dialysis for refractory psoriasis (44). This paper demonstrates rather conclusively the effectiveness of this treatment. This conclusion adds relevance to the study by Glinski et al. (45), in which PMN function was assessed in patients undergoing peritoneal dialysis. Those patients experiencing greatest improvement also had the largest number of PMNs emerge in the dialysate (45,46). Equally striking was the observation that significantly increased amounts of neutral proteinase were found in the PMNs of patients with active psoriasis.

THE BEHAVIOR OF PMNs IN THE SKIN

The "Squirting Phenomenon"

The migration of PMNs through the skin was described more than 60 years ago (47), and this has been designated by Pinkus and Mehregan as the "squirting phenomenon" (48). The PMNs accumulate in the epidermis, forming so-called micropustules of Kogoj. These micropustules reveal a similar histology as the macropustules observed in pustular psoriasis. The morphogenesis of these pustules has been studied by Rupec (49). Before PMNs invade the epidermis, a perinuclear halo of the keratinocytes is seen at the sites of the pustule. These keratinocytes change into eosinophilic strands, forming a spongiform network. Subsequently, the PMNs adopt a fragmented pyknotic appearance and accumulate in the stratum corneum (microbascesses of Munro). It has been shown that these microabscesses always are localized within a zone of parakeratosis (50,51,51a).

Development of the Lesion

In prepinpoint papules, abundant infiltration of PMNs was seen in 78% and sporadic accumulation of PMNs in 91% of the lesions (52,53). In actively spreading psoriatic lesions, numerous and relatively large-sized microabscesses are present (54). Micro-abscesses were seen in 75% of such plaques and sporadic infiltration of PMNs into the epidermis was noticed in 95% of the lesions (55). In the margin zone of spreading psoriatic lesions, the accumulation of PMNs is more frequent and pronounced than in the central zone (56). In the central zone, the accumulation of PMNs is seen as "hot spots," intermingled with "cold spots" without any PMNs (57). In conclusion, the accumulation of PMNs in psoriasis is abundant in an early phase of the disease, whereas topographic heterogeneity is seen in the chronic lesion with maximal accumulation in the margin zone.

The question whether the PMN is the earliest infiltrate cell in the psoriatic lesions has not yet been answered conclusively. Chowaniec et al. stated that the PMN is the first infiltrate cell, appearing in prepinpoint lesions (58). However, Braun Falco and Christophers reported that mononuclear cells appear before

PMNs in pinpoint lesions (59). In the margin zone of psoriatic lesions, monocytes and mast cells are seen in the periphery, whereas PMN accumulation is seen more proximally (60). Following discontinuation of treatment with a potent corticosteroid a relapse occurs. Using this model, monocytes are seen before the invasion of PMNs in the incipient lesions (61). In pustular psoriasis, a similar dynamic has been observed: The accumulation of mononuclear cells precedes the accumulation of PMNs (62,63). The large body of evidence suggests that mononuclear cells appear before the invasion of PMNs in the psoriatic lesion, indicating that the PMN is not the initiator, but rather more an interphase in the pathogenesis of psoriasis (51a).

Epidermal growth and keratinization following the penetration of PMNs into the epidermis have been studied with different techniques (51a). Histological and histochemical studies in the margin zone of the psoriatic plaque showed in one study that the epidermal changes precede the inflammatory infiltrate (55); however, in pinpoint lesions inflammation dominates the picture (59). In studies with the monoclonal antibody Ki67, a marker for cycling cells recruited from the germinative population of keratinocytes, it was shown that the accumulation of PMNs in the lower regions of the epidermis is not associated with epidermal proliferation; however, when accumulations of PMNs in the stratum corneum were present, nuclear staining was markedly increased in the basal cell layers (63). This suggests that the infiltration of PMNs is not secondary to epidermal proliferation, but rather appears before overt epidermal changes. In the margin zone of spreading psoriatic lesions, parameters for epidermal growth (deoxyribonucleic acid [DNA] synthesis and glucose-6-phosphate dehydrogenase) were increased in the clinically uninvolved skin up to 4 mm outside the clinical boundary; however, the marker enzyme for the capillary infiltrate unit (alkaline phosphatase) appeared increased up to 1.2 cm outside the clinical lesion (64). Immunohistochemical studies with the Ki-67 antibody, keratinization markers, and inflammatory infiltrate markers suggest a multiphase transition between symptomless skin and psoriatic lesion (64a,b; M.J.P. Gerritesen, unpublished data). First, the extracellular matrix molecule tenascin is expressed and in this phase the endothelium is activated (increased activity of alkaline phosphatase). The second phase is the appearance of a mononuclear infiltrate together with suprabasal expression of keratin 16 consisting of T lymphocytes and macrophages. The third phase is recruitment of cycling epidermal cells (Ki-67) and abnormal keratinization (premature expression of involucrin and decreased expression of filaggrin). It is in the third phase that PMN appear in skin. In conclusion, in the actively spreading psoriatic lesion, epidermal proliferation and abnormal keratinization occur after the initiation of the inflammation.

MIGRATION OF PMNs THROUGH THE SKIN

In Vivo Models

The intraepidermal accumulation of PMNs can be studied in vivo using the skin as a natural diffusion chamber (51a). Advantages of the approach above in vitro work are:

- The PMNs which penetrate into the epidermis might well have properties distinct from the total population of blood PMNs (65). Csato and coworkers reported that PMNs collected from skin chambers display totally decreased chemotactic responsiveness compared to peripheral blood PMNs. Plastic surface adherence, nitroblue tetrazolium reduction, and the *Candida albicans*–killing activity is higher for skin PMNs (66).
- The study of migration of PMNs through the skin will give information on facilitating and inhibiting processes present in the skin itself. Modulation of the migration of PMNs by the skin itself has been shown by Colditz and Movat (67,68); local desensitization of the PMN inflammatory response has been observed following repeated injections of chemoattractants.

Skin Chambers

After removing the stratum corneum, skin chambers can be mounted on the skin (69). Skin chambers are filled with a medium containing a chemoattractant. In some studies, the epidermis is abraded (10,70), and in other studies, suction blistering is used to remove the epidermis (66,71,72). Another method is to strip off the stratum corneum by repeated application of cellophane tape (73). The advantage of this model is that the migrating PMNs can be collected and studied. The disadvantage is that this approach is rather unphysiological, as the release of mediators of inflammation and accumulation of PMNs is the consequence of wounding (74).

Epicutaneous Application of Leukotriene B4 (LTB4)

Polymorphonuclear leukocytes accumulation in the dermis and epidermis is induced by epicutaneous application of LTB4 (75). The concentration of LTB4 applied on the skin and the PMN accumulation, 24 hr later show a dose-response relationship. The PMN accumulation is well reproducible within the same subject (76,77). The interindividual variability is substantial. However, the response in this model is not confused by a response to trauma (model I), the PMN accumulation being the net result of the LTB4 application.

Standardized Injury

Standardized injury by repeated applications of cellophane tape is a standardized model for studies on psoriasis (78). It has been shown that a significant but modest intraepidermal accumulation of PMNs occurs after stripping with cellophane tape (79,80). Using elastase as a marker enzyme, an ultrasensitive method which permits the detection of as few as five PMNs per assay, the relatively low number of PMNs in stripped skin can be quantified reproducible (74).

PMN Infiltration in Normal Skin

In normal skin, a reproducible accumulation of PMN is induced by challenge with a chemoattractant.

1. Using skin chambers the accumulation of PMN after chemotactic challenge varies in time. After the first 48 hr, the accumulation of PMNs diminishes, indicating that some form of tachyphylaxis occurs (72).
2. Intradermal injection of LTB4 results promptly in extravasation of PMNs (81,82). Accumulation of PMNs occurs approximately 6 hr following epicutaneous application of LTB4, reaching a maximum after 18 hr. From that moment onward, PMN exocytosis declines (77). Repeated applications of LTB4 on the same skin area cause tachyphylaxis, resulting in profoundly decreased accumulation of PMNs (67,68,83).
3. Two hours after cellophane tape–stripping PMN accumulation is seen (74). After about 8 hr, the accumulation approaches maximum levels. An elastase inhibitor is induced from this moment onward. It is feasible that this inhibitor might limit the continuation of invasion of PMNs (84).

PMN Infiltration in Psoriatic Skin

Different models have been used for the investigation of migration of PMN through the skin in psoriatic patients. The results are summarized in Table 2.

1. Using skin chambers as a model most authors reported that PMN accumulation is decreased in clinically uninvolved skin of psoriatics compared to the response in normal controls (10,70,71). However, during the first 8 hr the accumulation has been reported to be normal or even increased.
2. Following epicutaneous application of LTB4, different groups agree that the intraepidermal accumulation of PMNs is decreased in the clinically uninvolved skin of psoriatic patients (83,85). In the lesional skin, LTB4-induced PMN accumulation is decreased substantially more (86). LTB4-induced PMN accumulation was decreased profoundly on different test sites in the involved and lesion-free skin of a patient with annular pustular psoriasis (61). As has been summarized in Figure 1, an inverse relationship has been shown between the production of LTB4 and the LTB4-induced PMN accumulation. Tachyphylaxis is induced by repeated applications of LTB4 (83).
3. Clinically uninvolved skin of psoriatics and normal skin show a similar PMN accumulation following cellophane tape–stripping (74). However, in patients with unstable psoriasis the accumulation of PMN following stripping is increased compared to the accumulation in patients with stable plaque psoriasis.

Antipsoriatic Therapies and PMN Infiltration

The migration of PMNs through the skin is modulated by a variety of antipsoriatic therapies. Table 3 (87–94) overviews these studies. It is striking that different treatment modalities such as corticosteroids, anthralin, UVB, PUVA, methotrexate, and retinoids have in common an inhibition of the movement of PMNs through the skin. The interference of these therapies with the different components of the "black box" of transdermal and epidermal migration of PMNs will be discussed below.

Cyclosporin is effective in the treatment of psoriasis (95). This treatment probably does not interfere with PMN functions (96). It has been established that the drug modulates functioning of activated T lymphocytes (97). Therefore, the interference of anti-

Table 2 PMN Accumulation In Vivo in Clinically Uninvolved Skin of Psoriatic Patients

	PMN accumulations			
Ref.	Total group	Extensive involvement	Unstable phase	Clinical models
10	⊜	↓ NS		Skin chamber, after abrasion
70	↓ NS			Skin chamber, after abrasion
71	↑ 0–8h ↓ 8–24h			Skin chamber, after suction blistering
73	↓ NS	↓ S	↑ S	Skin chamber, after skin stripping
83	↓ S			Epicutaneous application of LTB4
85	↓ S			Epicutaneous application of LTB4
74	⊜	⊜	↑ S	Tape-stripping

NS = not significant; S = statistically significant; ⊜ = equal; ↑ = increased; ↓ = decreased
Source: Ref. 51a.

psoriatic therapies is not restricted to modulation of the migration of the PMNs.

PMNs AND EPIDERMAL GROWTH

A statistical association between the degree of infiltration of PMNs and the degree of epidermal proliferation has been demonstrated in the psoriatic lesion (63). The relationship between both processes could either by interpreted as a direct cause-effect relation (PMN invasion causing subsequently epidermal proliferation) or two self-standing processes linked to one single cause with a more prompt responsiveness as to the accumulation of PMNs.

Experimental evidence for the induction of epidermal proliferation by the PMNs has been provided by the work of Ristow (98); a 100–170% increase of [^{3}H–TdR] incorporation of keratinocytes was shown after the addition of peripheral blood PMNs to an epidermal cell culture. A stimulation of DNA synthesis in cultures of keratinocytes has been shown after the addition of leukotrienes B4, C4, and D4 (99). 12-Hydroxyeicosatetraenoic acid (12-HETE) also stimulates DNA synthesis, being 100–1000 times less potent than LTB4 (100). Leukotrienes B4, C4, and D4 are released by the PMNs and could be an explanation for the effect of PMNs on epidermal growth.

Using an in vivo model a relationship between LTB4 and epidermal growth was shown (77). An increased DNA synthesis 72–120 hr after the application of LTB4 could be shown. Both a direct cause-effect relationship between LTB4 and epidermal growth, and an indirect cause-effect relationship via the accumulation of PMNs have been hypothesized.

THE PRODUCTION OF CHEMOATTRACTANTS

Several chemotactic factors have been identified in the clinically involved skin of psoriatic patients: C5a (101), arachidonic acid metabolites, including the chemoattractants LTB4 and 12-hydroxyeicosatetraenoic acid (12-HETE), platelet-activating factor and the chemokines IL-8, Gro-α, Gro-β, Gro-γ, NAP-2, and ENA-78 (101–108). The epidermis, dermis, and the invading infiltrate cells are the sources of these chemoattractants.

The increased formation rate of the arachidonic acid metabolite LTB4 in the clinically uninvolved skin of psoriatics is of major interest (64,109). Arachidonic acid is released from the plasma membrane and metabolized via the cyclooxygenase pathway to prostaglandins and via the lipoxygenase pathway to leukotrienes. Prostaglandins and the peptidoleukotrienes (LTC4 and LTD4) are vasoactive, and leukotriene B4 is the most potent chemoattractant. The activity of phospholipase A_2, the rate-limiting enzyme for arachidonic acid release, is increased as well as symptomless as in lesional skin (110,111).

Some arachidonic acid metabolites inhibit the chemotactic response of PMNs. The dermal lipoxygenase product 15-hydroxyeicosatetraenoic acid (15-HETE) is a potent inhibitor of LTB4-induced PMN accumulation (112). In this respect, it is of interest that intra-

	Lesional skin	Symtomless skin
$LTBM_4$ production	↑↑↑↑	↑
PMN accumulation by LTB_4	↓↓↓	
PMN accumulation after trauma	not done	⊜
"Spontaneous" PMN accumulation	↑	0

Figure 1 Leukotriene B4 production and PMN accumulation (spontaneous, LTB4-induced, and trauma-induced) in clinically involved and uninvolved skin of psoriatics. ↑ = increased, ↓ = decreased: — = equal; 0 = absent. (From Ref. 51a.)

lesional injections of 15-HETE improve the psoriatic lesion (113). Prostaglandin E_2, a strongly vasoactive substance, has been shown to inhibit LTB4-induced PMN accumulation in vivo (82).

The classic antipsoriatic therapies have been shown to modulate the synthesis of arachidonic acid metabolites. Topical corticosteroid treatment of psoriatic lesions resulted in a significant reduction of arachidonic acid and LTB4 (114). The formation and to a lesser extent the inactivation (omega-oxidation) of LTB4 is inhibited by anthralin (115). The release of [^{14}C]-arachidonic acid in human keratinocytes in culture is

Table 3 PMN Accumulation In Vivo During Antipsoriatic Treatments

Ref.	Treatment	PMN accumulation	Clinical models
87	Etretinate	↓S	Skin chamber, after suction blistering
76	Methotrexate	↓S	Epicutaneous application of LTB4
88	Methotrexate	↓S	Epicutaneous application of LTB4
89	Etretinate	↓S	Epicutaneous application of LTB4
90	Clobetasol 17 propionate	↓S	Epicutaneous application of LTB4
		↓S	Tape-stripping
91	UVB	↓S	Epicutaneous application of LTB4
		↓S	Tape-stripping
	PUVA	↓S	Epicutaneous application of LTB4
		↓S	Tape-stripping
92	Acitretin	↓S	Epicutaneous application of LTB4
93	Acitretin		Epicutaneous application of LTB4
94	Anthralin	↓S	Epicutaneous application of LTB4
		⊜	Tape-stripping

↓ = decreased; ⊜ = equal; S = statistically significant
Source: Ref. 51a.

modulated by UVB (116). The modulation of arachidonic acid metabolism by retinoids is debated: a reduction of 12-HETE and arachidonic acid has been reported by Wong et al. (117), whereas Ruzicka could not show a modulation of arachidonic acid metabolism by retinoids (118).

In the last decade, a mild therapeutic effect of dietary fish oil supplementation has been suggested (119,120). The rationale is the increased formation of leukotriene B5 from eicosapentaeonic acid at the expense of LTB4. Currently, new inhibitors of the lipoxygenase pathway are in different phases of toxicological investigation.

"ENDOTHELIAL GATE CONTROL"

The interaction between PMNs are the endothelium is a field of current inflammation research (51a, 120a). In vitro experiments have demonstrated that LTB4 enhances the adhesion between PMNs and endothelial cells. Reusch et al. reported that LTB4 and N-formyl-L-methionyl-L-leucyl-phenylalanine (f-MLP) significantly stimulated the adhesion of PMNs to dermal microvasculature endothelial cells (121). Hoover et al. reported an increased PMN-endothelial attachment following pretreatment of either endothelial cells or PMNs with chemoattractants (122).

Not the net surface charge, but high-affinity receptors are of relevance in this respect (123).

Trafficking of leukocytes across the vessels comprises a complex expression pattern of adhesion molecules. Selectins (in particular, E- and P-selectin), integrins (MAC-1, LFA-1, and P 150,95), and members of the immunoglobulin supergene family (in particular, ICMA-1 and VCAM-1) are of relevance in trafficking of PMN into the psoriatic lesion (120a–d). VCAM-1, ICAM-1, and E-selectin are released into the circulation and the levels of these adhesion molecules in serum correlate with disease activity (51f). Various cytokines have been shown to up-regulate the expression of E-selectin, ICAM-1, and VCAM-1. In this respect, it is of relevance that chronic intradermal administration of tumor necrosis factor-alpha and interferon-gamma may mimic a psoriatic lesion (123a–d). In patients with a deficiency of these glycoproteins, extravasation of leukocytes has been shown to be impaired (124,125). Blocking these adhesion molecules with monoclonal antibodies resulted in inhibition of leukocyte-endothelial cell binding (126). Binding between ICAM-1 and LFA-1, has been shown to be a critical event in the interaction of the PMNs with the endothelium (124). Surface receptors on PMNs and endothelium are an intriguing target for pharmacological development directed at inflammation control.

THE INDUCTION OF TACHYPHYLAXIS

Several observations indicate the existence of a homeostatic control system (51a), which counteracts the migration of PMNs through the skin:

1. In acute phases of the psoriatic lesion, PMNs are a dominating cell type, and in the chronic phase they are sparse (50,52,53).
2. A local tachyphylaxis to LTB4 occurs following repeated application of LTB4 (67,68,83).
3. In lesional and symptomless skin of psoriatics, a diminished intraepidermal LTB4-induced accumulation of PMNs occurs (85,86). The decreased responsiveness in psoriatics can be interpreted as an attempt to balance the biological effects of the increased generation of chemoattractants.
4. In psoriatic scales, chemotactic inhibitors have been demonstrated (127,128).

At which point is it that the molecular reality of this self-defense process is situated?

Cytochrome P_{450}

This enzyme system is involved in the inactivation of leukotrienes. Bösterling and Trudell showed that LTB4 is inactivated by this enzyme system via omega-oxidation (129). Bickers et al. reported increased inducibility of arylhydrocarbon hydroxylase in the clinically uninvolved skin of psoriatic patients. This enzyme is part of the cytochrome P_{450} system (130). Ultraviolet B and tar induce cytochrome P_{450} (131,132).

The Release of Mediators of Inflammation

Some mediators inhibit PMN migration such as prostaglandin E_2 and 15-HETE. Several antipsoriatic therapies are only effective if slight inflammation is induced: UVB, PUVA, anthralin. Indeed, UVB irradiation and the application of anthralin result in prostaglandin E_2 release (133,134). Prostaglandin E_2 inhibits LTB4-induced PMN chemotaxis (135). A fivefold increase of dermal lipoxygenase activity has been shown in the skin of mice treated with PUVA

(136). Normal human dermis metabolizes arachidonic acid mainly to 15-HETE, which component recently has been shown by Kragballe et al. to inhibit the LTB4-induced chemotaxis of PMNs in vitro (112).

Protease Inhibitors

Elastase is released during the process of extravasation, and this enzyme degrades collagen type IV, which is a major constituent of the basal lamina of the endothelium (137). Protease inhibitors are induced in the epidermis during acute inflammation such as cellophane tape-stripping (74). Elastase-inhibiting activity is present in various scaling disorders of the skin; a profound inhibition is present in diseases with a mixed infiltrate, including PMNs, such as psoriasis (138). Elastase-inhibiting activity has been characterized in the psoriatic lesion and in cultured keratinocytes (139–141). SKALP is an 11-kDa polypeptide that inhibits human leukocyte elastase, porcine pancreatic elastase, and proteinase-3.

The Interaction Between PMNs and Capillaries

A role of the PMN–endothelial cell interaction has been suggested to be of relevance for the process of tachyphylaxis (67). Studies on high-affinity receptors localized on the endothelial cells and PMNs, intercellular adhesion molecules, and the secretion of mediators of inflammation by the endothelial cells might provide new insights in inflammation control.

The phenomenon of tachyphylaxis in the migration of PMNs during chronic challenge with mediators of inflammation is an important target for future research on inflammation control.

CONCLUSIONS

From Civatte (1924) onward, the role of the PMNs in the pathogenesis of psoriasis has been discussed (1). What is the position of PMNs today?

The dynamics of the release of mediators of inflammation from the epidermis, causing the intraepidermal invasion of PMNs, resulting ultimately in epidermal proliferation and parakeratosis has been substantiated by several observations.

1. Psoriasis is characterized by intraepidermal invasion of PMNs, anticipated by the release of mediators of inflammation, followed by hyperproliferation and parakeratosis in a focal distribution.
2. The dynamics of the development of the psoriatic lesion reflects the dynamics of the corresponding histological changes in the dermal and epidermal compartment after challenging normal skin with a chemoattractant.
3. Direct interference with the migration of PMNs by peritoneal dialysis, Eskimo diet, 15-HETE results in an improvement of the psoriatic lesion. All classic antipsoriatic therapies inhibit the in vivo migration, and most antipsoriatic therapies diminish the in vitro migration of PMN.

Some observations indicate that this pathogenetic concept cannot in itself explain psoriasis:

1. In animals, the application of some tumor promoters results in inflammation, epidermal proliferation, and parakeratosis, indicating that this metabolic "hardware" is present in the animal kingdom. However, psoriasis is a disease restricted to the human species.
2. Leukotriene B4–induced intraepidermal accumulation of PMNs in humans never has resulted in overt psoriatic lesions.
3. No intrinsic abnormality of the circulating blood PMNs in psoriasis has been demonstrated convincingly.

Therefore, it is feasible that the PMNs, migrating into the epidermis is a trait d'union in the pathogenesis of psoriasis. Other processes, such as an immune reaction, changes of the plasma membrane, and abnormalities of endothelial cells or fibroblasts, might be more primarily involved in the pathogenesis of psoriasis. From a therapeutic point of view, the migration of PMNs into the skin remains an issue of central interest. Treatments modulating transdermal and transepidermal migration of PMNs might have important implications for psoriasis.

REFERENCES

1. Silny, W., Pehamberger, H., Zielinsky, C., and Gschnait, F. (1980). Effect of PUVA treatment on the locomotion of polymorphonuclear leukocytes and mononuclear cells in psoriasis. *J. Invest. Dermatol.* 75:187–188.
2. Kawohl, G., Szperalski, B., Schröder, J.M., and Christophers, E. (1980). Polymorphonuclear leuko-

cyte chemotaxis in psoriasis: enhancement by self activated serum. *Br. J. Dermatol.* 103:527–533.
3. Csato, M., Dobozy, A., Hunyadi, J., and Simon, N. (1983). Polymorphonuclear leukocyte function in psoriasis vulgaris. *Dermatol. Monatsschr.* 169: 238–242.
4. Lagner, A., Chorzelski, T.P., Fraczykowska, M., Jablonska, S., and Szymanczyk, J. (1983). Is chemotactic activity in polymorphonuclear leukocytes increased in psoriasis? *Arch. Dermatol. Res.* 275: 226–228.
5. Michaelsseon, G. (1980). Increased chemotactic activity of neutrophil leukocytes in psoriasis. *Br. J. Dermatol.* 103:351–356.
6. Preissner, W.C., Schröder, J.M., and Christophres, E. (1983). Altered polymorphonuclear leukocyte responses in psoriasis: chemotaxis and degranulation. *Br. J. Dermatol.* 109:1–8.
7. Whaba, A., Cohen, H.A., Bar-Eli, M., and Gallily, R. (1978). Enhanced chemotactic and phagocytic activities in leukocytes in psoriasis vulgaris. *J. Invest. Dermatol.* 73:186–188.
8. Ternowitz, T. (1986). Monocyte and neutrophil chemotaxis in psoriasis. *J. Am. Acad. Dermatol.* 15: 1191–1199.
9. Scheja, A., Bruze, M., and Forsgren, A. (1987). Leukocyte migration in vivo and in vitro in patients with psoriasis. *Acta Derm. Venereol. (Stockh.)* 67: 427–432.
10. Breathnach, S.M., Carrington, P., and Black, M.M. (1981). Neutrophil leukocyte migration in psoriasis vulgaris. *J. Invest. Dermatol.* 76:271–274.
11. Fräki, J.E., Laszlo, J., Davies, A.O., Lefkowitz, R.J., Schneiderman, R., and Lazarus, G.S. (1983). Polymorphonuclear leukocyte function in psoriasis: chemotaxis, chemokinesis, beta-adrenergic receptors, and proteolytic enzymes of polymorphonuclear leukocytes in the peripheral blood from psoriasis patients. *J. Invest. Dermatol.* 81:254–257.
12. Pease, C.T., Fennel, M., Staughton, R.C.D., and Brewerton, D.A. (1987). Polymorphonuclear leukocyte function in psoriasis. *Br. J. Dermatol.* 117: 161–167.
13. Pigatto, P.D., Riva, F., Altomare, G.F., Brugo, A.M., Morandotti, A., and Finzi, A.F. (1983). Effects of etretinate on chemotaxis on neutrophils from patients with pustular and vulgar psoriasis. *J. Invest. Dermatol.* 81:418–419.
14. MacGregor, R.R., Spangnuolo, P.J., and Lentnek, A.L. (1974). Inhibition of granulocyte adherence by ethanol, prednisone and aspirin, measured with an assay system. *N. Engl. J. Med.* 291:642–646.
15. MacGregor, R.R. (1976). The effect of anti-inflammatory agents and inflammation on granulocyte adherence. *Am. J. Med.* 61:597–607.
16. MacGregor, R.R., Macarak, E.J., Kefalides, N.A. (1978). Comparative adherence of granulocytes to endothelial monolayers and nylon fibers. *J. Clin. Invest.* 61:697–702.
17. Sedgwick, J.B., Bergstresser, P.R., and Hurd, E.R. (1980). Increased granulocyte adherence in psoriasis and psoriatic arthritis. *J. Invest. Dermatol.* 74:81–84.
18. Tonnesen, M.G. (1989). Neutrophil-endothelial cell interactions: mechanisms of neutrophil adherence to vascular endothelium. *J. Invest. Dermatol.* 93: 53S–58S.
19. Sedgwick, J.B., and Hurd, E.R., and Bergstresser, P.R. (1982). Abnormal granulocyte morphology in patients with psoriasis. *Br. J. Dermatol.* 107:165–172.
20. Cox, N.H. (1986). Morphological assessment of neutrophil leukocytes in psoriasis. *Clin. Exp. Dermatol.* 11:340–344.
21. Bloomfield, F.J., and Young, M.M. (1983). Enhanced release of inflammatory mediators from lithium-stimulated neutrophils in psoriasis. *Br. J. Dermatol.* 109:9–13.
22. Skoven, I., and Thormann, J. (1979). Lithium compound treatment and psoriasis. *Arch. Dermatol.* 115: 1185–1187.
23. Schopf, R.E., and Straussfeld, E. (1985). Stimulus-dependent increased generation of oxygen intermediates in monocytes and polymorphonuclear leukocytes in psoriasis. *J. Invest. Dermatol.* 84:73–76.
24. Geerdink, J.P.M., Troost, P.W., Schalkwijk, J., Joosten, L.A.B., and Mier, P.D. (1985). The metabolic burst in polymorphonuclear leukocytes from patients with quiescent psoriasis. *Br. J. Dermatol.* 112:387–392.
25. Wasik, F., Jedrezejak, J., and Miklaszewska, M. (1987). Granulocyte pyruvate kinase in psoriasis vulgaris and psoriasis anthropatica. *Br. J. Dermatol.* 116: 9–14.
26. Glinski, W., Barszcz, D., Janczcera, E., Zarebska, Z., and Jablonska, S. (1984). Neutral proteinases and other neutrophil enzymes in psoriasis, and their relation to disease activity. *Br. J. Dermatol.* 111: 147–154.
27. Ruzicka, T., Radspieler, H., Strasser, T., Przybilla, B., and Ring, J. (1985). Polymorphonuclear leukocytes 5-lipoxygenase activity in psoriasis. *Prostaglandins, Leukotrienes Med.* 18:313–319.
28. Stüning, M., Schultz-Ehrenburg, U., Altmeyer, P., Raulf, M., and König, W. (1987). Metabolism of ^{14}C arachidonic acid by polymorphonuclear leukocytes in patients with psoriasis. *Br. J. Dermatol.* 116:153–159.
29. Sedgwick, J.B., Bergstresser, P.R., and Hurd, E.R. (1981). Increased superoxyde generation by normal granulocytes incubated in sera from patients with psoriasis. *J. Invest. Dermatol.* 76:158–163.
30. Camisa, Ch., Kraut, E., and Jayanthi-Zvara, B. (1984). Psoriatic sera decrease responses of stimu-

lated granulocytes from normal and psoriatic subjects. *J. Invest. Dermatol.* 82:318–321.

30a. Alkemade, J.A.C., de Jongh, G.J., Arnold, W.P., van de Kerkhof, P.C.M., and Schalkwijk, J. (1995). Levels of skin-derived antileukoproteinase (SKALP/Elafin) in serum correlate with disease activity during treatment of severe psoriasis with cyclosporin A. *J. Invest. Dermatol.* 104:1-5.

31. Ketchel, M.M., Favour, C.B., and Sturgis, S.H. (1985). The in vitro action of hydrocortisone on leukocyte migration. *J. Exp. Med.* 58:211–218.

32. Shea, C., and Morse, E.D. (1978). Inhibition of human neutrophil chemotaxis by corticosteroids. *Ann. Clin. Lab. Sci.* 8:30–33.

33. Kjellström, B.T., and Risberg, B. (1985). High dose corticosteroids and cell-cell interactions. *Acta Chir. Scand.* 526:37–47.

34. Schröder, J.M., Kosfeld, U., and Christophers, E. (1985). Multifunctional inhibition by anthralin in nonstimulated and chemotactic factor stimulated human neutrophils. *J. Invest. Dermatol.* 85:30–34.

35. Lagner, A., and Christophers, E. (1977). Leukocyte chemotaxis after in vitro treatment with 8-methoxypsoralen and UVA. *Arch. Dermatol. Res.* 260:51–55.

36. Dahl, K.B., Nyfors, A., and Brodthagen, H. (1978). Decrease in neutrophils observed in vivo in psoriatics after PUVA therapy. *Arch. Dermatol. Res.* 262: 131–134.

37. Gruner, S., Diezel, W., Zwirner, A., Müller, G.M., von Baehr, R., and Sönnichesen, N. (1987). The effect of PUVA treatment on acid hydrolases in human polymorphonuclear leukocytes. *Br. J. Dermatol.* 116: 785–792.

38. Cream, J.J., and Pole, D.S. (1980). The effect of methotrexate and hydroxyurea on neutrophil chemotaxis. *Br. J. Dermatol.* 102:557–563.

39. Walsdorfer, U., Christophers, E., and Schröder, J.M. (1983). Methotrexate inhibits polymorphonuclear leukocyte chemotaxis in psoriasis. *Br. J. Dermatol.* 108: 451–456.

40. Bauer, R., Schütz, R., and Orfanos, C.E. (1984). Impaired motility and random migration of vital polymorphonuclears in vitro after therapy with oral aromatic retinoid in psoriasis. *Int. J. Dermatol.* 23: 72–77.

41. Camisa, C., Eisenstat, B., Ragaz, A., and Weissmann, G. (1982). The effect of retinoids on neutrophil functions in vitro. *J. Am. Acad. Dermatol.* 6:620–629.

42. Ellis, C.N., Kang, S., Grekin, R.C., Voorhees, J.J., and Silva, J. (1985). Etretinate therapy reduces polymorphonuclear leukocyte chemotaxis-enhancing properties of psoriatic serum. *J. Am. Acad. Dermatol.* 13:437–443.

43. Orfanos, C.E., and Bauer, R. (1983). Evidence for anti-inflammatory activities of oral synthetic retinoids: experimental findings and clinical experience. *Br. J. Dermatol.* 109 (Suppl. 25):55–60.

44. Whittier, F.C., Evans, D.H., Anderson, P.C., and Nolph, K.D. (1983). Peritoneal dialysis for psoriasis: a controlled study. *Ann. Intern. Med.* 79:165–168.

45. Glinski, W., Zarebska, A., Jablonska, S., Imiela, J., and Nosarzewski, J. (1980). The activity of polymorphonuclear leukocyte neutral proteinases and their inhibitors in patients with psoriasis treated with continuous peritoneal dialysis. *J. Invest. Dermatol.* 75: 481–487.

46. Glinski, W., Jablonska, S., Imiela, J., Nosarzewski, J., Jarzabek-Chorzelska, M., Haftek, M., and Obalek, S. (1979). Continuous peritoneal dialysis for psoriasis. I. Depletion of PMNL as a possible factor in clearing of psoriatic lesions. *Arch. Dermatol. Res.* 266: 337–341.

47. Civatte, A. (1924). Psoriasis and seborrhoeic eczema: pathological anatomy and diagnostic histology of the two dermatoses. *Br. J. Dermatol.* 36:461–476.

48. Pinkus, H., and Mehregan, A.H. (1966). The primary histologic lesion of seborrhoeic dermatitis and psoriasis. *J. Invest. Dermatol.* 46:109–116.

49. Rupec, M. (1970). Zur Ultrastruktur der spongiformen Pustel. *Arch. Klin. Exp. Dermatol.* 239:30–49.

50. Van de Kerkhof, P.C.M., and Lammers, A.M. (1987). Intraepidermal accumulation of polymorphonuclear leukocytes in chronic stable plaque psoriasis. *Dermatologica* 174:224–227.

51. Cox, A.J. (1981). Polymorphonuclear leukocytes in psoriasis. In *Psoriasis: Proceedings of the 3rd International Symposium.* E.M. Farber and A.J. Cox (Eds.). Grune & Stratton, New York, pp. 233–234.

51a. Van de Kerkhof, P.C.M., and Chang, A. Migration of polymorphonuclear leukocytes in psoriasis. *Skin Pharmacol.* 2:138–154.

52. Chowaniec, O., Jablonska, S., Beutner, E.H., Proniewska, M., Jarzabek-Chorzelska, M., and Rzesa, G. (1981). Earliest clinical and histological changes in psoriasis. *Dermatologica* 163:42–51.

53. Jablonska, S., Chowaniec, O., Beutner, E.H., Maciejowska, E., Jarzabek-Chorzelska, M., and Rzesa, G. (1982). Stripping of the stratum corneum in patients with psoriasis. *Arch. Dermatol.* 118:652–657.

54. Burks, J.W., and Montgomery, H. (1943). Histopathological study of psoriasis. *Arch. Dermatol. Syphilol.* 48:479–493.

55. Gordon, M., and Johnson, W.C. (1967). Histopathology and histochemistry of psoriasis. *Arch. Dermatol.* 95:402–407.

56. Soltani, K., and Van Scott, E.J. (1972). Patterns and sequence of tissue changes in incipient and evolving lesions of psoriasis. *Arch. Dermatol.* 106:484–490.

57. Griffin, T.D., Lattanaud, A., and Van Scott, E.J. (1988). Clinical and histological heterogeneity of

psoriatic plaques: Therapeutic relevance. *Arch. Dermatol.* 124:216–220.

58. Braun-Falco, O., and Christophers, E. (1974). Structural aspects of initial psoriatic lesions. *Arch. Derm. Forsch.* 251:95–110.
59. Braun-Falco, O. (1971). Dynamics of growth and regression in the psoriatic lesions: Alterations in the skin from normal into a psoriatic lesion and during regression of psoriatic lesions. In *Psoriasis: Proceedings of the 1st International Symposium.* E.M. Farber and A.J. Cox (Eds.). Stanford University Press, Stanford, Ca., pp. 215–237.
60. Schubert, C., Schlaak, H.E., Schröder, J.M., and Christophers, E. (1984). Ultrastructural sequences of papillary body changes in incipient psoriasis. *J. Invest. Dermatol.* 82:555.
61. Van de Kerkhof, P.C.M., and Lammers, A.M. (1988). Intraepidermal accumulation of polymorphonuclear leukocytes in annular pustular psoriasis. *Dermatologica* 176:282–287.
62. Schubert, C., and Christophers, E. (1987). Activated macrophages in pustular psoriasis. *J. Invest. Dermatol.* 89:335–336.
63. Beurskens, T., Chang, A., van Erp, P.E.J., and Van de Kerkhof, P.C.M. Epidermal proliferation and accumulation of polymorphonuclear leukocytes in the psoriatic lesions. *Dermatologica.* In press.
64. Van de Kerkhof, P.C.M., van Rennes, H., de Grood, R., Bauer, F.W., and Mier, P.D. (1983). Metabolic changes at the margin of the growing psoriatic lesion. *Br. J. Dermatol.* 108:647–652.

64a. de Mare, S., de Jong, E.M.G.J., van Erp, P.E.J., and van de Kerkhof, P.C.M. (1990). Markers for proliferation and keratinization in the margin of the active psoriatic lesion. *Br. J. Dermatol.* 122:469–475.

64b. de Jong, E.M.G.J., Schalkwijk, J., and van de Kerkhof, P.C.M. (1991). Epidermal proliferation and differentiation, composition of the inflammatory infiltrate and the extracellular matix of the spreading psoriatic lesions. *Eur. J. Dermatol.* 1:221–227.

65. Greaves, M.W. (1983). Neutrophil polymorphonuclears, mediators and the pathogenesis of psoriasis. *Br. J. Dermatol.* 109:115–118.
66. Csato, M., Dobozy, A., Raith, L., and Simon, N. (1985). The functions of polymorphonuclear leukocytes emigrating into the skin. *Acta Dermatol. Venereol (Stockh.)* 65:106–110.
67. Colditz, I.G., and Movat, H.Z. (1984). Desensitization of acute inflammatory lesions to chemotaxins and endotoxin. *J. Immunol.* 133:2163–2168.
68. Colditz, I.G., and Movat, H.Z. (1984). Chemotactic factor-specific densitization of skin to infiltration by polymorphonuclear leukocytes. *Immunol. Lett.* 8: 83–87.
69. Gange, R.W., Black, M.M., and Carrington, P. (1979). Defective neutrophil migration in granuloma annulare, necrobiosis lipoidica and sarcoidosis. *Arch. Dermatol.* 115:32–35.
70. Pigatto, P.D., Radaelli, A., Tadini, G., Polenghi, M.M., Brambilla, L., Altomare, G., and Carandente, F. (1985). Circadian rhythm of the in vivo migration of neutrophils in psoriatic patients. *Arch. Dermatol. Res.* 277:185–189.
71. Dubertret, L., Lebreton, C., and Touraine, R. (1982). Neutrophil studies in psoriatics: in vivo migration, phagocytosis and bacterial killing. *J. Invest. Dermatol.* 79:74–78.
72. Michel, L., Mencia-Huerta, J.M., Benveniste, J., Dubertret, L. (1987). Biological properties of LTB_4 and Paf-acether in vivo in human skin. *J. Invest. Dermatol.* 88:675–681.
73. Tigalonowa, M., Glinski, W., and Jablonska, S. (1983). In vivo mobilization of polymorphonuclear leukocytes in psoriasis: relationship to clinical parameters and serum inhibitory factors. *J. Invest. Dermatol.* 81:6–9.
74. Chang, A., de Jong, G.J., Mier, P.D., and Van de Kerkhof, P.C.M. (1988). Enzymatic quantification of polymorphonuclear leukocytes in normal and psoriatic skin following standardized injury. *Clin. Exp. Dermatol.* 13:62–66.
75. Camp, R., Russell Jones, R., Brain, S., Woodlard, P., and Greaves, M. (1984). Production of intraepidermal microabscesses by topical application of leukotriene B_4. *J. Invest. Dermatol.* 82:202–204.
76. Van de Kerkhof, P.C.M., Bauer, F.W., and Maassen-de Grood, R.M. (1985). Methotrexate inhibits the leukotriene B_4 induced intraepidermal accumulation of polymorphonuclear leukocytes. *Br. J. Dermatol.* 113: 251–255.
77. Bauer, F.W., van de Kerkhof, P.C.M., and Maassen-de Grood, R.M. (1986). Epidermal hyperproliferation following the induction of microabscesses by leukotriene B_4. *Br. J. Dermatol.* 114:409–412.
78. Pinkus, H. (1951). Examination of the epidermis by the strip method of removing horny layers. I. Observation on thickness of the horny layer and on mitotic activity after stripping. *J. Invest. Dermatol.* 16: 383–386.
79. Heng, M.C.Y., Kloss, S.G., Kuehn, C.S., and Chase, D.G. (1985). The sequence of events in psoriatic plaque formation after tape stripping. *Br. J. Dermatol.* 112:517–532.
80. Lammers, A.M., van de Kerkhof, P.C.M., Schalkwijk, J., and Mier, P.D. (1986). Elastase, a marker for polymorphonuclear leukocytes in skin infiltrates. *Br. J. Dermatol.* 115:181–186.
81. Camp, R.D.R., Coutts, A.A., Greaves, M.W., Kay, A.B., and Walport, M.J. (1983). Responses of human skin to intradermal injection of leukotrienes C_4, D_4 and B_4. *Br. J. Pharmacol.* 80:497–502.

82. Ruzicka, T., and Burg, G. (1987). Effects of chronic intracutaneous administration of arachidonic acid and its metabolities: Induction of leukocytoclastic vasculities by leukotriene B_4 and 12-hydroxyeicosatetraenoic acid and its prevention by prostaglandins E_2. *J. Invest. Dermatol.* 88:120–123.
83. Wong, E., Camp, R.D., and Graves, M.W. (1985). The responses of normal and psoriatic skin to single and multiple topical applications of leukotriene B_4. *J. Invest. Dermatol.* 84:421–423.
84. Briggamen, R.A., Schechter, N.M., Fraki, J., and Lazarus, G.S. (1984). Degradation of the epidermal-dermal junction by proteolytic enzymes from human skin and human polymorphonuclear leukocytes. *J. Exp. Med.* 160:1027–1042.
85. Lammers, A.M., and Van de Kerkhof, P.C.M. (1987). Response of polymorphonuclear leukocytes to topical leukotriene B_4 in healthy and psoriatic skin. *Br. J. Dermatol.* 116:521–524.
86. Lammers, A.M., and Van de Kerkhof, P.C.M. (1987). Leukotriene B_4 fails to induce the penetration of polymorphonuclear leukocytes in the psoriatic lesions. *Br. J. Dermatol.* 117:541–545.
87. Dubertret, l., Lebreton, C., and Touraine, R. (1982). Inhibition of neutrophil migration by etretinate and its main metabolite. *Br. J. Dermatol.* 107:681–685.
88. Lammers, A.M., van de Kerkhof, P.C.M., and Mier, P.D. (1987). Reduction of leukotriene B_4 induced intraepidermal accumulation of polymorphonuclear leukocytes by methotrexate in psoriasis. *Br. J. Dermatol.* 116:667–671.
89. Lammers, A.M., Mier, P.D., and Van de Kerkhof, P.C.M. (1987). Etretinate modulates the leukotriene B_4 induced intraepidermal accumulation of polymorphonuclear leukocytes. *Br. J. Dermatol.* 117:297–300.
90. Chang, A., and Van de Kerkhof, P.C.M. (1988). Topical application of clobetasol-17-propionate inhibits the intraepidermal accumulation of polymorphonuclear leukocytes. *Acta Derm. Venereol. (Stockh.)* 68: 57–60.
91. Chang, A., Alkemade, J.A.C., and Van de Kerkhof, P.C.M. (1988). PUVA and UVB inhibit the intraepidermal accumulation of polymorphonuclear leukocytes. *Br. J. Dermatol.* 119:281–287.
92. Van de Kerkhof, P.C.M., Chang, A., van Dooren-Greebe, R., Geiger, J.M., and Happle, R. Intraepidermal accumulation of polymorphonuclear leukocytes in persistent palmoplantar pustulosis during treatment with acitretin. *Acta Derm. Venereol. (Stockh.)* In press.
93. Van Dooren-Greebe, R., van de Kerkhof, P.C.M., Chang, A., and Happle, R. Acitretin in the treatment of acrodermatitis continua Hallopeau. *Acta Derm. Venereol. (Stockh.)* In press.
94. Chang, A., Alkemade, H., and Van de Kerkhof, P.C.M. Dithranol modulates the leukotriene B_4-induced intraepidermal accumulation of polymorphonuclear leukocytes. *J. Invest. Dermatol.* In press.
95. Mueller, W., and Hermann, B. (1979). Cyclosporin for psoriasis. *N. Engl. J. Med.* 301:555.
96. Weinbaum, D.L., Kaplan, S.S., Zdziarsky, U., et al. (1984). Human polymorphonuclear leukocyte interaction with cyclosporin A. *Infect. Immunol.* 43: 791–798.
97. Bos, J.D. (1988). The pathomechanisms of psoriasis; the skin immune system and cyclosporin. *Br. J. Dermatol.* 118:141–155.
98. Ristow, H.J. (1982). Stimulation of DNA synthesis in cultured mouse epidermal cells by human peripheral leukocytes. *J. Invest. Dermatol.* 79:408–411.
99. Kragballe, K., Desjarlais, L., and Voorhees, J.J. (1985). Leukotrienes B_4, C_4 and D_4 stimulate DNA synthesis in cultured human epidermal keratinocytes. *Br. J. Dermatol.* 113:43–52.
100. Kragballe, K., and Fallon, J.D. (1986). Increased aggregation and arachidonic acid transformation by psoriatic platelets: evidence that platelet derived 12-hydroxyeicosatetraenoic acid increases keratinocyte DNA synthesis in vitro. *Arch. Derm. Res.* 278: 449–453.
101. Ruzicka, A., and Printz, M.P. (1984). Arachidonic acid metabolism in skin: a review. *Rev. Physiol. Biochem. Pharmacol.* 100:122–160.
102. Greaves, M.W., and Camp, R.D.R. (1988). Prostaglandins, leukotrienes, phospholipase, platelet activating factor and cytokines: an integrated approach to inflammation of human skin. *Arch. Dermatol. Res.* 280:533–541.
103. Schröder, J.M., and Christophers, E. (1986). Identification of C5a des arg and an anionic neutrophil-activating peptide (ANAP) in psoriatic scales. *J. Invest. Dermatol.* 87:53–58.
104. Greaves, M.W., and Camp, R.D.R. (1988). Prostaglandins, leukotrienes, phospholipase, platelet activating factor, and cytokines: an integrated approach to inflammation of human skin. *Arch. Dermatol. Res.* 280(Suppl.):S33–S41.
105. Schröder, J.M. (1992). Interleukin 8. *Adv. Neuroimmunol.* 2:109–124.
106. Baggiolini, M., Dewald, B., and Moser, B. (1994). Interleukin 8 and related chemotactic cytokines—CXC and CC chemokines. *Adv. Immunol.* 55:97–179.
107. Schröder, J.M. (1995). Inflammatory mediators and chemoattractants. *Clin. Dermatol.* 13:137–150.
108. Mallet, A.I., and Cunningham, F.M. (1985). Structural identification of platelet activating factor in psoriatic scale. *Biochem. Biophys. Res. Commun.* 126: 192–198.
109. Ziboh, V.A., Tamara, L., Casebolt, B.S., Marcelo, C.L., and Voorhees, J.J. (1984). Biosynthesis of lipoxygenase products by enzyme preparations from

normal and psoriatic skin. *J. Invest. Dermatol.* 83: 426–430.

110. Forster, S., Ilderton, E., Summerly, R., and Yardley, H.J. (1983). The level of phospholipase A_2 activity is raised in the uninvolved epidermis of psoriasis. *Br. J. Dermatol.* 108:103–105.

111. Verhagen, A., Bergers, M., van Erp, P.E.J., Gommans, J.M., van de Kerkhof, P.C.M., and Mier, P.D. (1984). Confirmation of raised phospholipase A_2 activity in the uninvolved skin of psoriasis. *Br. J. Dermatol.* 110: 731–732.

112. Kragballe, K., Ternowitz, T., Fogh, K. (1987). 15-Hydroxyeicosatetraenoic acid (15-HETE) specifically inhibits LTB_4 induced chemotaxis of PMN. *J. Invest. Dermatol.* 89:325.

113. Fogh, K., Sogaard, H., Herlin, T., and Kragballe, K. (1988). Improvement of psoriasis vulgaris after intralesional injections of 15-hydroxyeicosatetraenoic acid (15-HETE). *J. Am. Acad. Dermatol.* 18:279–285.

114. Wong, E., Barr, R.M., Cunningham, F.M., Mistry, K., Woollard, P.M., Mallet, A.I., and Greaves, M.W. (1986). Topical steroid treatment reduces arachidonic acid and leukotriene B_4 in lesional skin of psoriasis. *Br. J. Clin. Pharmacol.* 22:627–632.

115. Schröder, J.M. (1986). Anthralin (1,8-dihydroxyanthrone) is a potent inhibitor of leukotriene production and LTB_4-oxidation by human neutrophils. *J. Invest. Dermatol.* 7:624–629.

116. Punnonen, K., Puustinen, T., and Jansén, C.T. (1986). UVB irradiation induces changes in the distribution and release of ^{14}C-arachidonic acid in human keratinocytes in culture. *Arch. Dermatol. Res.* 278: 441–444.

117. Wong, E., Barr, R.M., Brain, S.D., Greaves, M.W., Olins, L.A., and Mallet, A.I. (1984). The effect of etretinate on the cyclooxygenase and lipoxygenase products of arachidonic acid metabolism in psoriatic skin. *Br. J. Clin. Pharmacol.* 18:523–527.

118. Ruzicka, T. (1984). The effect of retinoids on arachidonic acid metabolism in human epidermis and polymorphonuclear leukocytes. In *Retinoids: New Trends in Research and Therapy.* Retinoid Symposium, Geneva, 1984. Karger, pp. 180–182.

119. Bittner, S.B., Cartwright, I., Tucker, W.F.G., and Bleehen, S.S. A double blind randomized placebo-controlled trial of fish oil in psoriasis. *Lancet* 1: 378–380.

120. Kettler, A.H., Baughn, R.E., Orengo, I.F., Black, H., and Wolf, J.E. (1988). The effect of dietary fish oil supplementation on psoriasis. *J. Am. Acad. Dermatol.* 18:1267–1273.

120a. Smith, C.H., and Barker, J.N.W.N. (1995). Cell trafficking and role of adhesion molecules in psoriasis. *Clin. Dermatol.* 13:151–158.

120b. Griffiths, C.E.M., Voorhees, J.J., and Nickoloff, B.J. (1989). Characterization of intercellular adhesion molecule-1 and HLA-DR expression in normal and inflamed skin: modulation by recombinant gamma-interferon and tumor necrosis factor. *J. Am. Acad. Dermatol.* 20:617–629.

120c. Grooves, R.W., Ross, E., Barker, J.N.W.N., and MacDonald, D.M. (1993). Vascular cell adhesion molecule-1 (VCAM-1): expression in normal and diseased skin and regulation in vivo by interferon-gamma. *J. Am. Acad. Dermatol.* 29:67–72.

120d. Thomson, A.W., Nalestrik, M.A., and Rilo, H.R. (1993). ICAM-1 and E. selectin expression in lesional biopsies of psoriasis responding to IK506 therapy. *Autoimmunity* 15:215–223

121. Reusch, M.K., Fullerton, S.H., Nickoloff, B.J., Glinski, W., and Karasek, M.A. (1988). Leukotriene B_4 enhances adherence of human polymorphonuclear leukocytes to dermal microvascular endothelial cells in vitro. *Arch. Dermatol. Res.* 280:194–197.

122. Hoover, R.L., Folger, R., Haering, W.A., Ware, B.R., and Karnovsky, M.Y. (1980). Adhesion of leukocytes to endothelium: roles of divalent cations, surface charge, chemotactic agents and substrate. *J. Cell. Sci.* 45:73–86.

123. Görög, P., and Born, G.V.R. (1982). Increased adhesiveness of granulocytes in rabbit ear-chamber blood vessels perfused by neuraminidase. *Microvasc. Res.* 23:380–384.

123a. Schopf, R.E., Naumann, S., Rekder, M., and Morsches, B. (1993). Soluble intercellular adhesion molecule-1 levels in patients with psoriasis. *Br. J. Dermatol.* 128:34–37.

123b. Groves, R.W., Ross, E., Barker, J.N.W.N., and MacDonald, D.M. (1992). Effect of acute and chronic administration of IFN-alpha in normal human skin (abstract). *J. Invest. Dermatol.* 98:510.

123c. Barker, J.N.W.N., Allen, M.H., and MacDonald, D.M. (1989). The effect on in vivo interferon-gamma on the distribution of LFA-1 and ICAM-1 in normal human skin. *J. Invest. Dermatol.* 93:439–442.

123d. Barker, J.N.W.N., Allen, M.H., and MacDonald, D.M. (1990). Alterations induced in normal human skin by in vivo interferon-gamma. *Br. J. Dermatol.* 122:451–458.

124. Berkinshaw, C.J., Weemaes, C.M.R., Roos, D., Tetteroo, P.A.T., and Weening, R.S. (1987). Congenital deficiency of leukocyte-adherence glycoproteins: a familial defect. *Neth. J. Med.* 31:158–170.

125. Schmalstieg, F.C. (1988). Leukocyte adherence defect. *Pediatr. Infect. Dis. J.* 7:876–872.

126. Haskara, D., Cavender, D., Beatty, T., et al. (1986). T lymphocyte adhesion to endothelial cells: mechanisms demonstrated by anti-LFA-1 monoclonal antibodies. *J. Immunol.* 137:2901–2906.

127. Grabbe, J., Overwien, B., and Czarnetzki, B.M. (1980). Identification and partial characterization of

chemotactic inhibitors in psoriatic scales. *Arch. Dermatol. Res.* 277:426.

128. Czarnetzki, B.M. (1988). Failure in neutrophils to migrate into psoriatic lesions. *Br. J. Dermatol.* 118: 733–734.
129. Bösterling, B., and Trudell, J.R. (1983). Leukotriene B_4 metabolism by hepatic cytochrome-450. *Biochem. Biophys.* Res. Commun. 114:850–854.
130. Bickers, D.R., Mukhtar, H., Dutta-Choudhury, T., Marcelo, C.L., and Voorhees, J.J. (1984). Aryl hydrocarbon hydroxylase, epoxide hydrolase and benzo(a)pyrene metabolism in human epidermis: comparative studies in normal subjects and patients with psoriasis. *J. Invest. Dermatol.* 83:51–56.
131. Merk, H., Rumpf, M., Bolsen, K., Wirth, G., and Goerz, G. (1984). Inducibility of arylhydrocarbon hydroxylase activity in human hair follicles by topical application of liquor carbonis detergens (coal tar). *Br. J. Dermatol.* 111:279–284.
132. Mukhtar, H., Benjamin, J., Matgouranis, P.M., Das, M., Asoken, P., and Bickers, D.R. (1986). Additive effects of ultraviolet B and crude coal tar on cutaneous carcinogen metabolism: Possible relevance to the tumor-genicity of the Goeckerman regimen. *J. Invest. Dermatol.* 87:348–353.
133. Warin, A.P. (1978). The ultraviolet erythema in man. *Br. J. Dermatol.* 98:473–476.
134. Kobza Black, A., Barr, R.M., Wong, E., Brain, S., Greaves, M.W., Dickinson, R., Shroot, B., and Hensby, C.N. (1985). Lipoxygenase products of arachidonic acid in human inflamed skin. *Br. J. Clin. Pharmacol.* 20:185–190.
135. Ruzicka, T., and Burg, G. (1987). Effects of chronic intracutaneous administration of arachidonic acid and its metabolites. Induction of leukocytoclastic vasculitis by leukotriene B_4 and 12-hydroxyeicosatetraenoic acid and its prevention by prostaglandin E_2. *J. Invest. Dermatol.* 88:120–123.
136. Ruzicka, T., Walter, J.P., and Printz, M.P. (1983). Changes in arachidonic acid metabolism in UV-irradiated hairless mouse skin. *J. Invest. Dermatol.* 81:300–303.
137. Bray, M.A., McKeran Smith, C., and Metz Virea, G. (1987). Stimulated release of neutral proteinase elastase and cathepsin G from inflammatory rat polymorphonuclear leukocytes. *Inflammation* 11:23–27.
138. Chang, A., Schalkwijk, J., Happle, R., and van de Kerkhof, P.C.M. (1990). Elastase-inhibiting activity in scaling skin disorders. *Acta. Derm. Venereol. (Stock.)* 70:147–151.
139. Schalkwijk, J., Chang, A., Janssen, P., de Jongh, G.J., and Mier, P.D. (1990). Skin derived antileukoproteinases ($SKALP_5$) characterization of two new elastase inhibitors from psoriatic epidermis. *Br. J. Dermatol.* 122:631–641.
140. Alkemade, H.A.C., Molhuizen, H.O.F., Ponec, M., Kempenaar, J.A., Zeeuwen, P.L.J.M., de Jongh, G.J., van Vlijmen-Willems, I.M.J.J., van Erp, P.E.J., van de Kerkhof, P.C.M., and Schalkwijk, J. (1994). SKALP/Elafin is an inducible proteinase inhibitor in human epidermal keratinocytes. *J. Cell. Sci.* 107: 2335–2342.
141. Molhuizen, H.O.F., Alkemade, H.A.C., Zeeuwen, P.L.J.M., de Jongh, G.J., Wieringa, B., and Schalkwijk, J. (1993). SKALP/Elafin: an elastase inhibitor from cultured human keratinocytes. Purification, CDNA sequence, and evidence for transglutaminase cross-linking. *J. Biol. Chem.* 268:12028–12032.

15

Keratinocyte Abnormalities and Signaling Pathways

Mark R. Pittelkow
Mayo Clinic and Mayo Medical School, Rochester, Minnesota

A host of cellular, biochemical, and molecular alterations have been identified in the active, lesional epidermis of psoriasis. The majority of these abnormalities have been implicated in the pathogenesis of this hyperproliferative skin disease, although the etiology of psoriasis remains elusive to date. This chapter presents an overview of the structural and functional aberrations of the psoriatic keratinocyte as well as representative cellular signal transduction pathways in the keratinocyte that mediate these phenotypic abnormalities. In addition, the seemingly diverse keratinocyte-related abnormalities will be correlated and integrated into several schemes that provide a framework for understanding the pathophysiology and eventually delineating the etiology of psoriasis. More specific aspects of disordered keratinocyte proliferation and differentiation, and perturbed epidermal biochemistry and metabolism as well as alterations in other cellular elements of the epidermis (e.g., Langerhans cells) and dermis (e.g., endothelium) will be reviewed more extensively in subsequent chapters. The detailed analysis of light microscopic and ultrastructural abnormalities identified in the epidermis and dermis at various stages of psoriasis will be elaborated in another chapter.

THE PSORIATIC EPIDERMIS AND KERATINOCYTE

The clinical features of psoriatic epidermis together with the histopathological and pathobiological changes summarized herein clearly demonstrate that many, if not virtually all of the cutaneous abnormalities are dependent on the biological potential of the keratinocyte to express the psoriatic phenotype. The spectrum of abnormalities identified in the epidermis and, in particular, the keratinocyte of psoriasis can be categorized by several criteria (Table 1). Each division of the classification system distinguishes particular structural or functional characteristics of the psoriatic keratinocyte. Though these alterations are wide ranging, it is possible to establish fundamental interrelationships among the abnormal attributes (Table 2). Cumulatively, these keratinocyte abnormalities represent the characteristic epidermal phenotype of psoriasis.

The role of the keratinocyte in the development of psoriasis, the specificity of the keratinocyte abnormalities for psoriasis, and the interactions of epidermis with mesenchymal cells, immune/inflammatory cells, and environmental factors are among the most significant, yet perplexing, aspects of this disease. Comparing psoriasis to other benign and malignant epidermal disease states, it is apparent that while the structural alterations may be instrumental in initiating or propagating the epidermal pathology, they are not necessarily to be regarded as unique markers of psoriatic epidermis. Further complexity in elucidating the pathogenesis of psoriasis is recognized at the functional level where diverse cell types and tissues interact to generate the psoriatic lesion.

Table 1 Summary of Epidermal Keratinocyte Abnormalities

Structural abnormalities	Ref.
Light microscopic	
Increased epidermal mitoses	1,2
Elongation, thickening and coalescence of rete ridges—regular acanthosis	2,3
Intercellular edema—exoserosis, spongiosis	
Increased epidermal cell volume—enlarged nuclei and nucleoli	1–6
Hyperkeratosis	
Reduction or absence of stratum granulosum	
Parakeratosis with variable foci and zones of orthokeratosis	2,7–9
Ultrastructural	
Prevalent epidermal mitoses	Chap. 26
Widened intercellular spaces, decreased desmosomes	10–13
Pinocytotic vesicles along basal portions of basal cells	
Basal cell herniations—basal lamina gaps	10,14–16
Decreased quantity and diameter of tonofilaments	10–12
Enlarged nuclei, abundant ribosomes, edematous cytoplasm	
Increased mitochondria	17
Microvillous plasma membrane projections with intertwining	13
Increased membrane-associated particles	18
Increased gap junctions	18
Dyskeratotic keratinocytes	10,11
Keratohyaline granules reduced in number, smaller or absent	
Decreased/absent keratohyaline-tonofilament associations	
Nuclear and cytoplasmic remnants and lipid drops within stratum corneum	10–12,19
Functional abnormalities, cellular, biochemical, molecular alterations	**Ref.**
Hyperproliferation	
Increased DNA labeling index, DNA synthesis, and cycling cells	20–25, Chap. 16
Expanded growth fraction and decreased population generation time	25,29–31
Recruitment of psoriatic stem cell proliferation by soluble factors of lesional T lymphocytes	32,33
Increased population of cells expressing proliferation associated antigens (4F2, Ki67, cyclin/PCNA, proliferin, etc.)	34–38
Accelerated epidermal cell transit	1,20,39
Increased cellular RNA content	30
Elevated ornithine decarboxylase (ODC) activity and polyamine production	40–43
Enhanced or perturbed activities of oxidative and energy-producing enzymes	5,44–46
Enhanced thioredoxin reductase activity	47
Cyclic nucleotide (cAMP, cGMP) perturbations	48–50
Misregulated eicosanoid production/metabolism	49–51,51–53
Calcium-calmodulin abnormalities	54–56
Elevated phosphorylase kinase activity	55–57
Increased proteinase and plasminogen activator activity	58–60
Enhanced activation of protein kinase C, phospholipase C, phospholipase A_2, inositol phospholipid cascade	61–65
Increased protein tyrosine kinase, phosphatidylinositol kinase, and phosphatase activity	66,67
Enhanced expression of TGF-α, amphiregulin and other mitogenic growth factors and growth factor receptors	68–71
Altered differentiation and cell activation	
Expression of hyperproliferative/wounding-induced keratins	72–74
Decreased and delayed expression of differentiated-type keratins	72–76
Increased expression of EGF receptor in upper stratified layers of epidermis	77,78, Chap. 22
Up-regulation of p21 WAF1/CIP1	79
Premature expression of involucrin and transglutaminase activity in supra-basal layers	80–82

Table 1 Continued

Functional abnormalities, cellular, biochemical, molecular alterations	Ref.
Premature expression of KF2 at cell periphery	82
Abnormal cross-linked envelope formation	83
Delayed and reduced filaggrin expression	82,84
Enhanced *ras* p21 expression	85
Increased interleukin (IL-1, IL-6, IL-8) expression, activation, or turnover and IL-1 receptor antagonist	86–92
Induction/enhancement of ICAM-1 (CD54), HLA DR (class II-MHC), CD36 (OKM5), CD16 (*leu* 11b), CD71 (OKT9, transferrin receptor), IP-10, interferons, and CD60 antigen expression	93–104
Enhanced MCP-1, MGSA/GRO and other chemokines	105–107
Diminished glycoprotein GP37 immunoreactivity	108
Reduced expression of KL_3, membrane associated differentiation antigen	109
Loss of HLK20, intercellular antigen expression	110
Altered HLK3, HLK7 expression	110
Expression of ψ3 antigen in stratifying epithelium	111, Chap. 18
Altered sugar residue/glycoprotein expression detected by lectin histochemistry and immunoreactivity	
Altered F_c receptor and IL 2 antibody binding	117–118
Expression of p27, retrovirus-associated major internal protein	119
Enhanced LDL receptor activity in upper epidermal layers	120
Up-regulation of elafin/SKALP protease inhibitor	121
Enhanced elastase activity	122
Enhanced plasminogen activator enzyme expression	123
Enhanced psoriasis, cystatin A, calgranulins and psoriasis-associated fatty acid binding protein	124
Enhanced or reduced expression of other undefined or incompletely characterized epidermal differentiation-associated antigens	125–127
Enhanced production of angiogenic factors, vascular endothelial growth factor (VEGF), IL-8, and thrombospondin-1	128–129
Enhanced expression of 65 and 72-kDa heat shock proteins	130
Increased manganese superoxide dismutase (MnSOD)	131
Expression of other inflammatory cytokines	132
Altered protooncogene expression	133,134

The epidermis is well known to be the primary target tissue in psoriasis. Extensive investigations have demonstrated misregulation of epidermal metabolic pathways including growth factor production, signal transduction, and enzymatic activation that are closely associated with expression of the epidermal psoriatic lesion. However, epidemiological and other biological research has revealed that genetic, immune/inflammatory, and dermal factors contribute prominently to the evolution of the psoriatic lesion (Fig. 1). In this regard, the psoriatic keratinocyte and epidermis function as cellular effectors that are genetically programmed to initiate a cascade of pathological responses following specific "triggering" or stimulatory events, contributing to the development and propagation of the psoriatic lesion (Fig. 2.). Hence, the epidermal keratinocyte is the principal target tissue of biochemical- and molecular-activating events that may be initiated or regulated within the epidermis itself and by the immune/inflammatory system and the subjacent dermis.

These schemes largely account for the multitude of clinical observations and pathological findings described in psoriasis. Specifically, the important features of psoriasis that are incorporated into these diagrams include:

1. Genetic factors
2. Trigger factors and the Koebner response
3. Immune and inflammatory factors
4. Dermal and microvascular factors
5. Epidermal hyperproliferation and altered differentiation

Table 2 The Psoriatic Epidermis. Morphological-Functional Correlates for Anatomical Compartments of the Epidermal Keratinocyte Population

	Morphological	Functional
Stratum basale	Acanthosis, elongated rete ridges, accentuated labeling index, increased cell mass, and mitotic figures Enlarged nuclei, increased ribosomes, and mitochondria	Keratinocyte hyperproliferation. Increased keratinocyte growth fraction and metabolism (enhanced growth factor expression, increased activity of enzyme pathways regulating oxidative metabolism, energy-production and signal transduction)
	Basal cell herniations—basal lamina gaps	Increased proteolytic activity, enhanced keratinocyte replication/migration, and transit from basal lamina
Stratum spinosum and granulosum (stratum intermedium)	Decreased tonofilaments, desmosomes, keratohyaline, and lamellar granules Widened intercellular spaces	Altered epidermal program of keratinocyte differentiation and activation. Delayed, absent, or premature expression of numerous differentiation-associated gene products
	Increased membrane associated particles, gap junctions, microvillous projections Dyskeratotic keratinocytes	Perturbed growth regulation, proliferation-differentiation coupling and intercellular communication
Stratum corneum	Hyperkeratosis and parakeratosis with nuclear/cytoplasmic remnants, lipid drops	Persistence and transmission of defects expressed in the stratum malpighii

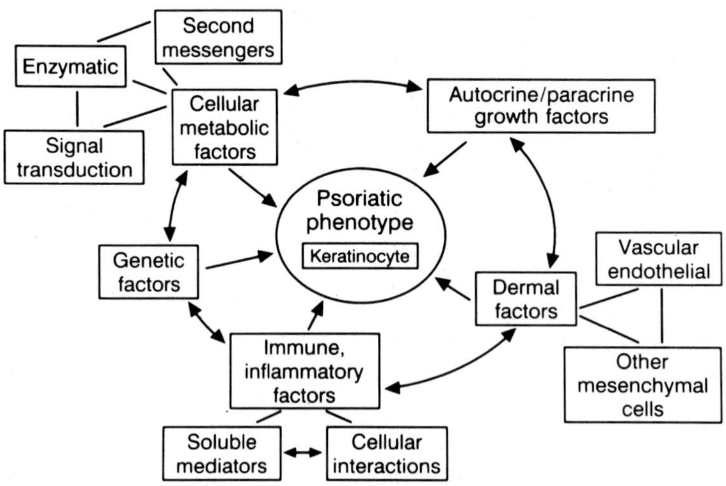

Figure 1 Genetic factors, biological components, and biochemical pathways that interact to create and modulate the psoriatic phenotype of epidermal keratinocytes.

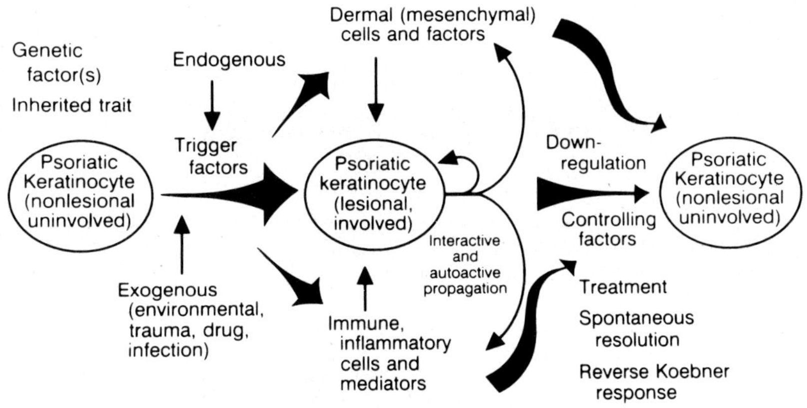

Figure 2 The psoriatic keratinocyte and major factors affecting the epidermal phenotype. Inherited trait and dynamic events regulate expression of psoriatic disease (lesional, involved keratinocyte) and the unstimulated/inhibited or "latent" psoriatic state (nonlesional, uninvolved keratinocyte).

6. Therapeutic responses (see sections in individual chapters on therapy and treatments)

CHARACTERIZATION AND REGULATION OF THE PSORIATIC KERATINOCYTE

The epidermis and keratinocytes of individuals destined to develop psoriasis are inherently different than their normal counterparts. Based on this premise, virtually all epidermal keratinocytes of psoriatic individuals could be expected to exhibit the psoriatic phenotype with elicitation of the most severe expression of the disease. However, individuals with psoriasis often exhibit more limited involvement of the body surface that fluctuates over time. Yet, over a lifetime, many cutaneous sites may express the psoriatic phenotype.

The psoriatic keratinocyte appears to be modulated by both inhibitory (controlling or restorative) factors and stimulatory (positive or initiating) factors (Fig. 3). The net effect of these opposing factors is expression of the "normal," nonlesional (uninvolved or symptom-free) epidermal phenotype or the psoriatic, lesional (involved or symptomatic) epidermal phenotype.

A continuous gradation of disease activity or a discrete, "all-or-none" epidermal response can be integrated into this diagrammatic representation if additional variables of activation threshold and "set point" abnormalities are defined for the psoriatic keratinocyte. As an example, the Koebner phenomenon has been regarded as an all-or-none response in psoriasis. By visual examination, the epidermis of patients with psoriasis appears to be either clinically "normal" (uninvolved, nonlesional) or involved (lesional). However, a growing number of experimental approaches have been adapted to examine the nonlesional, uninvolved epidermis from patients with psoriasis and have shown differences between this tissue and epidermis of individuals without psoriasis. This evidence points to psoriasis as a disease that is continuous in extent or degree and only becomes clinically manifest if the level of disease expression or activity is of sufficient severity. Furthermore, the overall activity of psoriasis, the severity of the active lesions, the extent of body involvement, and relative control of the disease may be factors that also place psoriasis on a continuous scale of disease expression.

Both gradational and discrete mechanisms of disease expression that regulate the keratinocyte abnormalities are likely operative in psoriasis. These alternative but interactive mechanisms may account for several significant and provocative findings that have been identified in psoriatic epidermis. If psoriasis is regulated exclusively by an all-or-none response, keratinocytes from nonlesional epidermis of psoriasis would be expected to exhibit biochemical markers, growth kinetic parameters, and differentiation indistinguishable from normal, nonpsoriatic skin. However, several independent approaches investigating nonlesional psoriatic epidermis have identified aberrations related to those in lesional, psoriatic epidermis (Table 3; cf. Table 1). The abnormalities in nonlesional psoriatic epidermis are usually less pronounced than in

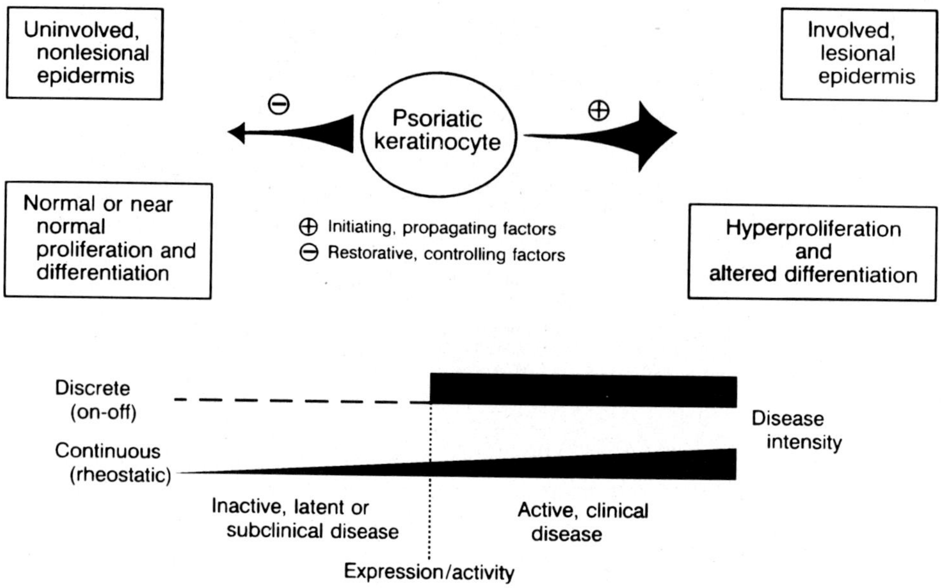

Figure 3 Clinical and pathological markers of disease activity, factors influencing disease activity, and representative modes of disease expression for the psoriatic keratinocyte. Specific aspects of psoriatic epidermal disease may be expressed on discrete and/or continuous bases. Invoking a continuous mode of disease activity may explain evidence of abnormal keratinocyte proliferation and differentiation in the absence of clinical observation of disease ("subclinical" or "latent" disease).

lesional psoriatic epidermis. Nonetheless, these detectable differences are, perhaps, the most intriguing and potentially important findings to delineate the etiology and identify the principal tissue defect of psoriasis.

Recognizing the apparent complexity of this disease and the technical sophistication of experiments required to detect subtle differences, it is not surprising that results of studies demonstrating abnormalities in nonlesional epidermis of psoriasis have been conflicting. Discrepancies may be based on numerous clinical and experimental variables of the research including (1) type and severity of psoriasis, (2) site of selection, (3) recent therapy and type of treatment, (4) sample preparation, (5) differing methods of assay, (6) sensitivity (detection threshold) and accuracy of assay, and (7) other uncontrolled endogenous and environmental factors influencing the epidermis. Also, if the all-or-none response operates in a selected manner by modulating specific biochemical and cellular processes, differences would unlikely be detected in these particular systems or activation pathways. Table 3 summarizes evidence illustrating that both unstimulated and stimulated, nonlesional epidermis of psoriasis exhibit selected abnormalities. Furthermore, epidermis and cultured keratinocytes from nonlesional psoriasis appear to express particular intrinsic defects. These abnormalities may represent the abnormal phenotype that can be elicited and perpetuated in the psoriatic keratinocyte (which can persist in the absence of nonepidermal, psoriatic genetic factors). Alternatively, the abnormalities may reflect the aberrant genotype that is inherited and expressed to variable degrees by the psoriatic keratinocyte in vivo and in vitro.

SPECIFIC KERATINOCYTE ABNORMALITIES, PATHOBIOLOGICAL MECHANISMS, AND DISEASE EXPRESSION

The cumulative body of data characterizing psoriatic epidermis is extensive and has revealed that a range of structural and functional abnormalities are involved in the pathology of psoriasis (see Table 1). Many of the structural alterations pertaining to lesional psoriatic epidermis are reviewed in the chapter on the histology and electron microscopy of psoriasis. Therefore, the major findings will be summarized only briefly to compare them with the functional aberrations.

Table 3 Comparison of Keratinocyte/Epidermis Abnormalities: Nonlesional Psoriatic vs. Normal Epidermis

	Ref.
In vivo	
Increased growth fraction and percentage of cycling cells (some studies)	25,26,34,36,38
Increase in tritiated thymidine-labeling indices (some studies)	20–22,24,25
Increased RNA content	30
Decreased cAMP levels and cAMP/cGMP ratios	48
Increased polyamine levels (some studies)	40,41,135
Calmodulin perturbations (some studies)	54–56
Increased phospholipase A_2 activity (some studies)	62,64,65,136
Increased and altered expression of HLK3 and HLK7 immunoreactivity	110
Increased germinative intermediate filament immunoreactive cells	36
Increased oxidative enzyme activity	5
Ultrastructural differences	137
No difference in epidermal wound healing	138
No differences in phosphatidylinositol kinase, protein tyrosine kinase, phosphoprotein phosphatase, plasminogen activator, and TGF-α levels	60–63,66–68,139,140
No differences in gap junctions and membrane-associated particles	18
No differences in select keratin antibody-reactive cells	38,141
In vivo-stimulated	
Increased DNA synthesis (tritiated thymidine-labeling index) and prolonged proliferative response following propranol, saline, or tape-stripping stimulation of nonlesional psoriatic epidermis	142–145
Ex vivo, in vitro, and grafting studies	
Increased oxygen consumption and CO_2 production	44
Increased proliferation (some studies)	146–149
Increased thioredoxin reductase activity (lesional vs. nonlesional vs. normal)	47
Increased inflammatory cytokines	132
Attenuated inhibition of proliferation by γ interferon	150
Decreased/altered sialoprotein and fucoprotein expression (some studies)	115,151–155
Altered ultrastructural features (some studies)	156,157
Nonlesional psoriatic epidermis mimics lesional epidermis following xeno-grafting	158,159
Nonlesional psoriatic epidermis similar to normal epidermis measuring proliferation in skin equivalent model	160
No differences in acantholytic changes during organ culture	161

Early macular and fully developed guttate lesions of psoriasis show characteristic alterations of the epidermal keratinocyte by light microscopy (2–4, 162,163). Though controversial, several reports have presented convincing evidence that epidermal changes of early psoriatic lesions precede the immune/inflammatory changes and microvascular alterations which characterize the histopathology of mature lesions of psoriasis (4,5,12,163). Furthermore, in resolving lesions of psoriasis, certain features of epidermal normalization such as granular layer reappearance are observed concomittant with capillary regression. Also, return of the arterial capillary component precedes the decrease in epidermal labeling index and acanthosis. Restoration of the intercellular integrity of endothelium ensues, but interestingly microvascular fenestrations are detected even in nonlesional skin of psoriasis (164,165; Chap. 25). Therefore, initiating factors in psoriasis, including those mediating vascular perturbations, appear to reside in the epidermis, though epidermal hyperplasia is dependent upon vascular proliferation during certain stages in the development and perpetuation of psoriasis.

Light microscopic findings of increased epidermal mitoses, prominent keratinocyte nuclei and nucleoli, and epidermal acanthosis are relatively nonspecific but parallel the ultrastructural and functional abnormalities detected in psoriatic epidermis. Hyperkeratosis and parakeratosis appear to reflect the structural and kinetic alterations observed in the germinative compartments of the psoriatic epidermis. However, an alternate hypothesis has suggested that altered differentiation is the primary defect in psoriasis which, in turn, induces the compensatory increase in the germinative compartment (29). Evidence for inefficient keratinization causing psoriasis may be derived from assessment of recent and potentially useful therapies. Several topical treatments for psoriasis may exert their effects by modulating or correcting the inefficient keratinization resulting in improvement of psoriasis. For example, occlusion creates a multifunctional barrier that minimizes trauma and transepidermal water loss. Occlusion may regulate differentiation by retaining products of desquamation that normalize keratinization. Repression of misregulated differentiation at the level of gene expression is another possible mechanism by which occlusion therapy as well as active forms of vitamin D or their analogues act topically. Once keratinization is normalized, growth control within the germinative compartment is reestablished by feedback mechanisms.

Histological evidence of variable parakeratosis, projected both in the horizontal and vertical axes, appear to correlate with mitotic figures and epidermal growth activity. Within active lesions of psoriasis, proliferation and differentiation of epidermal functional units or compartments are likely not uniform, and selected populations of keratinocytes are stimulated to express the psoriatic phenotype to variable degrees (2,7,162). This concept is supported by in vitro and in vivo studies that have characterized the regulation of normal keratinocyte growth and differentiation and by regional, dynamic abnormalities of proliferation that have been delineated for psoriatic epidermis in vivo (1,166–168).

Ultrastructural analysis of the pathology in psoriatic epidermis confirms the abnormalities of keratinocyte hyperproliferation and perturbed differentiation. Early, eruptive guttate lesions of psoriasis show evidence of epidermal hyperplasia and dyskeratotic keratinocytes with only a few mononuclear cells present in the dermis and epidermis (12). Dilation of the intercellular space of the epidermis is detected in early guttate lesions and in selected specimens of nonlesional epidermis (12,137).

The widened intercellular space is associated with a decrease in desmosomal contacts. Decreased epidermal cell attachments may create a microenvironment that signals keratinocyte proliferation by allowing a loss of contact inhibition of growth (13). Significant advances in our understanding of cellular growth control have emerged since the initial observations of contact inhibition of growth in vitro were implicated in the pathogenesis of psoriasis. A variety of biological molecules and regulatory factors, including growth factors, proto-oncogenes, signal pathways, intracellular messengers, the cytoskeleton, and extracellular matrix have been shown to play crucial roles in growth control of cells and regulation of normal tissue homeostasis in vivo (169–171). While the notion of loss of contact inhibition causing psoriatic epidermal hyperproliferation is presently overly simplistic, the concept has guided subsequent investigation into more contemporary research examining the cellular growth response in normal and psoriatic epidermis and keratinocytes. As the molecular mechanisms of cell proliferation and tissue renewal are better defined, our understanding of growth disturbances in the epidermis of psoriasis will undoubtedly become more clear.

Intercellular communication is another crucial function to maintain epithelial integrity and epidermal homeostasis. Though certain elements of structural integrity (e.g., desmosomal contacts) are disrupted in psoriatic epidermis, intercellular communication appears to be accentuated or altered (13,18). The increased numbers of membrane-associated particles and gap junctions may be the essential organelles in generating the organized, yet pronounced, hyperproliferation and altered differentiation of psoriatic epidermis. Gap junctions function as channels of communication within normal epidermis and facilitate transport of specific messenger molecules or other regulatory factors between keratinocytes and among other epidermal cells (172,173). The increased number of gap junctions in psoriasis may alter keratinocyte communication and induce or propagate the psoriatic epidermal phenotype.

Keratinocytes of the basal layer in psoriatic epidermis often develop cytoplasmic processes that protrude into the dermis through gaps in the basal lamina (15). These basal keratinocyte herniations are not found exclusively in psoriasis, but their formation may be related to epidermal proteolytic activity or to proteases released by inflammatory cells or activated dermal endothelial cells (15,16,174). The markedly enhanced keratinocyte replication and accelerated cell transit of psoriasis are propagated largely within the germinative basal layer, implying that the rate of detachment or uncoupling of keratinocytes from the basal lamina is increased. Epidermal plasminogen activator and other proteases, such as elastase and collagenase, are produced by replicating or migrating keratinocytes, in part, to effect their release from the basal lamina

(122,123,139,175). As a result, the basal lamina is interrupted and basal keratinocyte herniations may develop. A recent transgenic mouse model overexpressing collagenase in the epidermis demonstrates that increased proteolytic enzyme expression appears to contribute to the psoriatic phenotype as it induces scaly skin and histological evidence of acanthosis, hyperkeratosis, and epidermal hyperplasia (177).

The quantity and diversity of functional abnormalities identified in psoriatic epidermis challenge researchers to establish links among the defects and, hopefully, provide a framework to identify the pathogenic mechanisms in psoriasis. By cataloging the epidermal defects according to hyperproliferation or altered differentiation/cell activation, a unified and integrated format is developed that more clearly characterizes the psoriatic epidermal phenotype (see Table 1). Moreover, the current understanding of cell growth control and the coupling of growth arrest and differentiation indicates that abnormalities of epidermal proliferation can induce alterations in epidermal differentiation (166,167,176).

KERATINOCYTE SIGNAL TRANSDUCTION AND CELL REGULATION

The epidermal keratinocyte, as well as most nucleated cells such as lymphocytes, fibroblasts, endothelial cells, and other cell types involved in generating the psoriatic phenotype, are capable of transmitting biological messages within the cell via intricate and highly complex biochemical signaling pathways. The pathways link the extracellular environment to the cytoplasm and nucleus and mediate cellular communication to coordinate biological responses (178–180).

Only in the past few years have multiple signaling pathways in various epithelial and mesenchymal cell types been identified and begun to be assembled into functional cascades (Fig. 4). Growth factors, peptide hormones, and other extracellular factors that are collectively designated ligands bind to transmembrane receptors on the cell surface and initiate activation (or inhibition) events. Several classes of receptors include the receptor tyrosine kinases (RTK), which are phosphorylated on tyrosine residues following activation, and the seven-membrane-spanning receptor (SMSR) family or G-protein-coupled receptors that are activated by various peptide hormones or smaller molecular mass ligands. RTKs, for example, regulate the specificity and intensity of signals that are initiated following the binding growth factors such as the EGF-related ligands, the FGF family of growth factors, and insulin-like growth factor (IGF) (181,182). Cellular signals are amplified and modified by various intracellular adapter proteins as well as specific protein kinases and substrate-enzyme interactions that are functionally linked, and become activated within the cytoplasm following ligand-receptor binding.

Several representative signal transduction pathways are illustrated in Figure 4. The ras-raf-MEK pathway is one of the better characterized cascades that mediates nuclear events associated with cell replication. This series of protein kinases phosphorylates downstream mediators, including a family of cell-cycle-regulated proteins, the cyclins through activation of cyclin-dependent kinases (cdk) as well as activation of nuclear transcription factors that are coupled to proliferation. EGF receptor is one of several RTKs in keratinocytes that is activated by EGF-related ligands and stimulates cell proliferation. Keratinocytes express specific EGF-related growth factors that endow the cell with autocrine (self-growth) activity (182, 183). Another kinase signaling cascade expressed in a wide range of cell types is the Jak-STAT pathway(s), which is activated by interferon-α (IFN-α) and IFN-γ as well as EGF and other specific ligands. STATs (signaling transducers and activators of transcription) are transcription factors activated by Jaks (Janus kinases) that function in a condensed pathway to trigger nuclear activation and gene expression. A distinctive family of novel MAP (mitogen-activated protein) kinases are JNK (C-jun-amino terminal kinase)/SAPK (stress-activated protein kinase) that function as stress-induced signaling molecules following exposure to tumor necrosis factor-α (TNF-α), interleukin-1 (IL-1), ultraviolet radiation, and other mediators such as lipopolysaccharide (LPS) and heat shock. Phosphorylation of specific transcription factors, such as C-jun, is a downstream response to JNK activation. A separate kinase involved in a mitogen-stimulated signaling pathway is p70 ribosomal protein S6 kinase (S6K), which may be activated by phosphotidylinositol 3-kinase (PI3K) or a related kinase. Another activator of S6K appears to be a rapamycin-sensitive kinase called FRAP (FKBP-rapamycin-associated protein)/RAFT (rapamycin and FKBP targets), which interacts with the immunosuppressant FK 506, an agent with potent activity in psoriasis. In this regard, rapamycin, another immunosuppressant agent, may be an effective therapy for psoriasis since it has the potential to exert inhibitory activity on cell cycle checkpoints in both keratinocytes and lymphocytes.

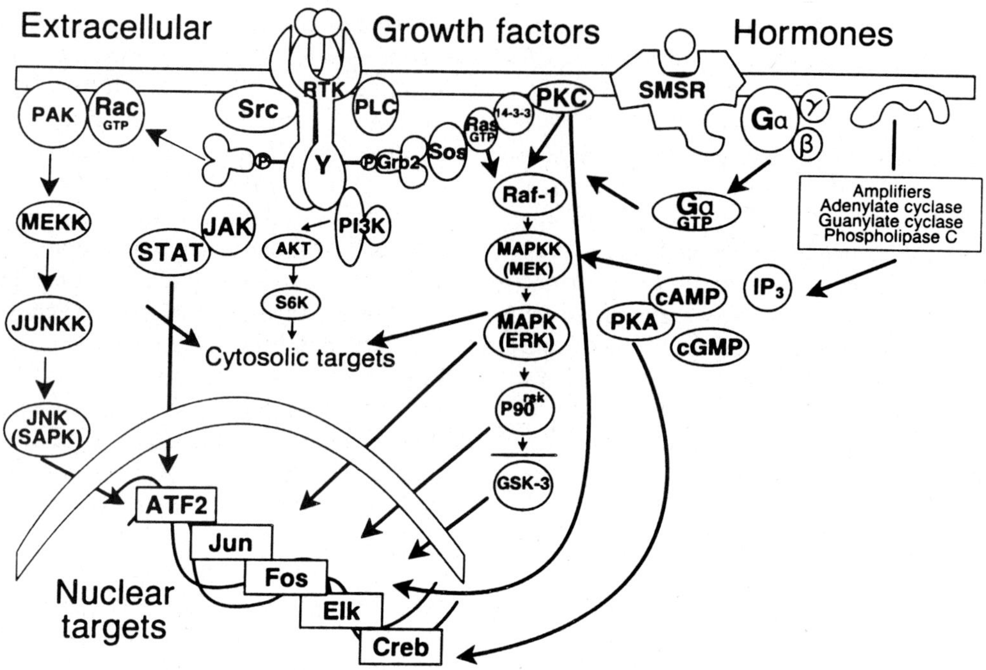

Figure 4 The main signaling cascades regulating cell proliferation and differentiation. Five main signaling pathways from the plasma membrane to the cytoplasm and nucleus are shown. The receptor tyrosine kinases (RTK) and seven-membrane-spanning receptors (SMSR) trigger activation of downstream phosphorylation events. For explanation of abbreviations, see text. The ras-raf-MEK, JNK, Jak-STAT, S6K, and G-protein-coupled receptor pathways are represented.

The SMSR/G protein-coupled signaling pathway interacts with several intracellular enzymes such as adenylate cyclase to generate crucial second messengers such as cAMP, cGMP, and inositol 1,4,5-trisphosphate (IP_3). Several classes of SMSR have been identified, including the rhodopsin/β-adrenergic receptors, secretin/vasoactive intestinal peptide, and metabotropic glutamate receptor subfamilies (179, 180). The heterotrimeric G proteins couple these specific cell surface receptors to intracellular signaling effectors including adenylate and guanylate cyclases, phospholipase C (PLC), and selected ion channels and downstream kinases such as protein kinase A (PKA). Composition of the β- and γ-subunits in conjunction with specific α-subunits of the multimember G-protein family also determines coupling specificity and response. As an example of the range of ligands that activate this signaling cascade, many neuropeptides are mediated through the SMSR/G protein pathway and may be of significant relevance to psoriasis.

Although these families of signal transduction molecules have been functionally linked together in specific cascades, there is clearly overlap and interaction among the pathways allowing greater diversity of response and a rheostatic, rather than a simple "on or off" level of cellular activity. Experimental evidence in keratinocytes supports these implications. Catecholamines and adenosine/adenine nucleotides mediate their activities, in part, through receptors linked to the G-protein pathway. These agonists regulate keratinocyte growth and differentiation (184,185). Physiological agonists or antagonists of receptors for growth factors, hormones, and small ligands, such as biogenic amines, purinergic substances, and neuropeptides, cooperate within the skin and epidermis to exert normal as well as pathological responses. It is likely that the phenotype of psoriasis is initiated and/or propagated through abnormal signaling pathway responses.

More recently, it has been shown that novel families of cell adhesion molecules (CAMs) including the cadherins and integrins are also involved in cell communication (186–189). Integrins are heterodimeric (α and β subunits) cell surface receptors that mediate attachment to the extracellular matrix (ECM) as well as functioning in cell-cell adhesive interactions. More than 20 different integrin receptors have been identified. Several, including $\alpha_2\beta_1$, $\alpha_3\beta_1$, $\alpha_5\beta_1$, $\alpha_2\beta_5$, and $\alpha_6\beta_4$, are expressed on keratinocytes and are abnormally regulated in psoriasis (190,191). Figure 5 outlines intracellular signaling pathways that are linked to the integrins and regulate cell communication and cell shape. Focal adhesion kinase (FAK) associates with integrins that form focal adhesions. Signaling molecules and cytoskeletal proteins, in turn, associate with FAK and create a network that can activate ras, a signaling substrate in the ras-raf-MEK pathway. Another small GTP-binding protein, Rho, is activated by integrin clustering and regulates downstream cytoskeletal changes controlled by vinculin, actin stress fibers, and other cytoskeletal components.

Integrin-mediated signaling alterations may also play an important role in the development of psoriasis. A recent animal model for psoriasis was developed using a transgenic approach in which α_2 or α_5 in conjunction with β_1 integrin was expressed in suprabasal epidermis of mouse (192). Epidermal hyperproliferation, aberrant keratinocyte differentiation, and skin inflammation were induced. Clearly, forced alteration of epidermal integrin expression results in disrupted cellular responses that are likely propagated by abnormal cytokine and growth factor expression. These factors may mediate hyperproliferation and abnormal differentiation of epidermis as well as trigger an immune/inflammatory reaction. This transgenic model should prove to be useful in further understanding epidermal pathobiology and psoriasis, in particular.

Cadherins are another class of CAMs expressed in epidermis. E-cadherin is expressed throughout the epidermis, and several desmosomal cadherins as well as newer cadherin members also are produced in epidermis. Cadherins are homophilic, calcium-dependent adhesion molecules that are linked to β-catenin or plakoglobin within the cytoplasm of the cell. Recent studies have demonstrated that signal transduction of cadherins is mediated partly through β-catenin (187). Also, β-catenin is a substrate for tyrosine kinases and has been found to associate with EGF receptor. Interestingly, intracellular activation of $\alpha_6\beta_4$ integrin via tyrosine phosphorylation and protein interactions with Shc and grb2 also has recently been shown to be suppressed by EGF, although $\alpha_6\beta_4$-dependent cell migration is up-regulated (193). Together, integrins and cadherins are additional receptor families that mediate signal transduction in the epidermis and interact with other well-known signaling pathways such as the RTK and G-protein-coupled receptors.

The majority of the abnormalities related to epidermal hyperproliferation directly involve biochemical and/or molecular pathways that regulate cell replication. Classification of these abnormalities is

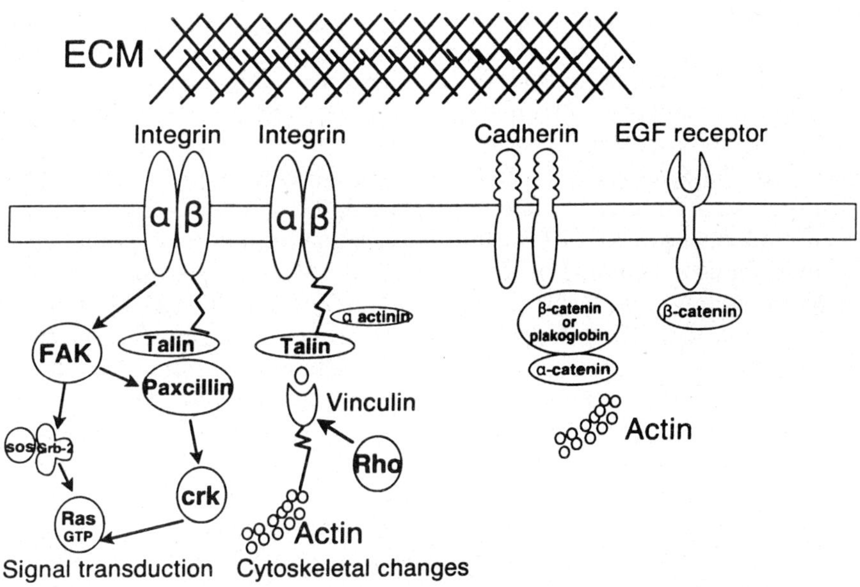

Figure 5 Integrin, cadherin, and EGF receptor (RTK) signaling pathways. Abbreviated scheme of components and cytoplasmic interactions mediating signal transduction and cytoskeletal changes within the cell following integrin, cadherin, and RTK activation. Extracellular matrix (ECM) is involved in integrin, and likely other signaling cascades. See text for explanation of abbreviations.

structured on the particular classes of molecules or component pathways that control the cellular biology of the keratinocyte. These include (1), growth factors [e.g., transforming growth factor α (TGF); amphiregulin and other EGF-related peptides]; (2) signal transduction (e.g., RTK and SMSR); (3) second messengers and intracellular mediators (e.g., cyclic nucleotides, inositol phospholipids, eicosenoids, calcium-calmodulin); (4) regulatory enzymes (e.g., phospholipase C, phospholipase A_2, protein phosphatases, proteases; (5) enzymes of oxidoreduction and intermediary metabolism (e.g., thioredoxin reductase, ornithine decarboxylase, β-glucuronidase, and succinic dehydrogenase); and (6) membrane, cytoplasmic, and nuclear proteins associated with deoxyribonucleic acid (DNA) synthesis and mitosis (e.g., 4F2, Ki67, cyclins, cyclin-dependent kinases (cdk) and proliferin). While each of these classes of biological molecules cooperates with other factors to stimulate cell cycle progression and cell division, several factors that act early or prominently in the mitogenic response will be reviewed here in greater detail. Subsequent chapters provide more extensive analyses of eicosenoid functions, plasma membrane activities, and neuropeptide regulation.

Polypeptide growth factors are among the most potent biological molecules in stimulating cell proliferation. They are mitogens and act as initiators of biochemical pathways or cascades that ultimately lead to nuclear activation, DNA synthesis, cellular duplication, and mitosis. Each polypeptide growth factor elicits potent, yet specific cellular responses and targets activities by binding to the relevant receptor on the cell surface (194,195). One of the first growth factors to be purified, named, and characterized was EGF (196; Chap. 22). Cohen first demonstrated the activity and potency of EGF for epidermal growth (197). Related members of the EGF family, including TGF-α, amphiregulin, and heparin-binding EGF (HB-EGF) are growth factors homologous to EGF and bind to the EGF receptor. TGF-α is one of several transforming growth factors isolated from virally transformed mesenchymal cell lines (198). This factor, similar to EGF, is a potent mitogen for human keratinocytes in culture, and has been implicated as an important regulator of epidermal hyperproliferation in psoriasis (199). Subsequent studies have shown that TGF-α as well as amphiregulin and HB-EGF are autocrine/paracrine growth factors in human keratinocytes and are expressed by normal epidermis (200). Additional investigations have confirmed the hypothesis that TGF-α and amphiregulin protein and messenger RNA are overexpressed in psoriatic epidermis (68). These EGF-related gene products appear to be among the major growth factors that are locally produced in epidermis and regulate keratinocyte proliferation and differentiation.

We have recently demonstrated that transgenic mice overexpressing amphiregulin targeted to epidermis exhibit cutaneous erythema and scaling that strongly resembles psoriasis (201). Histologic features of acanthosis, parakeratosis, spongiform pustules, and neutrophils in the stratum corneum were seen.

In addition, lymphocytic inflammation within the dermis and epidermal exocytosis were observed. The epidermis shows dramatic hyperproliferation and thickening. These findings indicate that growth factors such as amphiregulin have the potential to "activate" epidermal keratinocytes and induce inflammatory responses that produce a psoriatic phenotype.

Phorbol esters are potent epidermal hyperplastic agents when applied to skin, and active phorbol esters markedly enhance expression of TGF-α (202). Phorbol ester also activates protein kinase C and, with chronic exposure, causes downregulation of this enzyme involved in signal transduction. These findings have been related to psoriasis by demonstrating that protein kinase C activity is decreased in psoriatic epidermis (61).

Other specific families of growth factors stimulate keratinocyte replication. Members of the heparin-binding or fibroblast growth factor family (FGF), including KGF or FGF-7 are potent mitogens for keratinocytes and may be produced by epidermis or neighboring mesenchymal cells in normal and pathological states, including psoriasis (181,203).

Besides growth factors, epidermis contains a multitude of other biological factors that influence endocrine and immune function and cutaneous physiology (198,204). For example, psoriasis is closely associated with neovascularization of dermis subjacent to epidermis. Angiogenic factors have been isolated from normal and psoriatic epidermis, but not dermis (205,206). Specific factor(s) inducing vessel growth have been isolated, including VEGF and IL-8 (128,129), but TGF-α, amphiregulin, TGF-β, or other substances may also be released by activated epidermis and directly or indirectly stimulate vascular endothelium (69,207).

Epidermal proliferation depends on the appropriate cellular signals that must be initiated, received, and acted upon by the epidermis, adjacent dermis, and its cellular elements. The interactions of diverse biochemical factors as well as different tissues in the development of psoriatic epidermal hyperproliferation is a reflection of the requirements for these biological elements in normal epidermal growth control. The pivotal, if not etiological, factors in initiating and perpetuating the pathology of psoriatic epidermis may be discovered in new biochemical pathways or biological functions that have yet to be defined in normal epidermis.

Epidermal differentiation, like proliferation, is regulated by specific cellular and molecular processes that interact to generate a concisely ordered program of keratinization. The expression of each gene product during differentiation and its regulation temporally and spatially in the epidermis has the potential to be suppressed, enhanced, or misregulated by cutaneous disease. For example, specific keratin polypeptides produced during reepithelialization or by disruption of epidermal homeostasis (e.g., tape-stripping) also are expressed in psoriasis (72–74). A host of other structural proteins, enzymes, receptors, biological mediators, cell surface molecules, and undefined differentiation-associated antigens are modulated by the psoriatic state (see Table 1). Which of these are instrumental in creating the psoriatic epidermis is unknown.

Normal epidermal proliferation and differentiation appear to be integrated and regulated structurally and functionally by local expression of growth factors, such as TGF-α, amphiregulin or HB-EGF, and selective expression of the cognate receptor, the EGF receptor, within germinative layers of epidermis (208; Chap. 22). By contrast, psoriasis is associated with unbalanced proliferation and differentiation evidenced both by enhanced expression of TFG-α, amphiregulin or HB-EG and persistent expression of EGF receptor in the upper stratified layers of psoriatic epidermis (68,77). The fact that postmitotic, differentiating keratinocytes express EGF receptor and appear to synthesize or, at least, have ready accessibility to several EGF-related growth factors, indicates that activation of the EGF receptor in keratinizing cells may significantly modify expression of various gene products during differentiation. Other altered receptor-ligand interactions also appear to operate in psoriatic epidermis and would be expected to exert specific effects on the program of differentiation.

The lesional psoriatic keratinocyte differs markedly from its normal counterpart and is "activated" in the sense that a distinctive epidermal phenotype is expressed which can be readily identified by its characteristic set of structural and functional markers. One of the consequences of activation of the psoriatic keratinocyte is the development of epidermal hyperproliferation and altered differentiation. Of equal importance in understanding the overall pathology of psoriasis is the fact that the activated psoriatic kera-

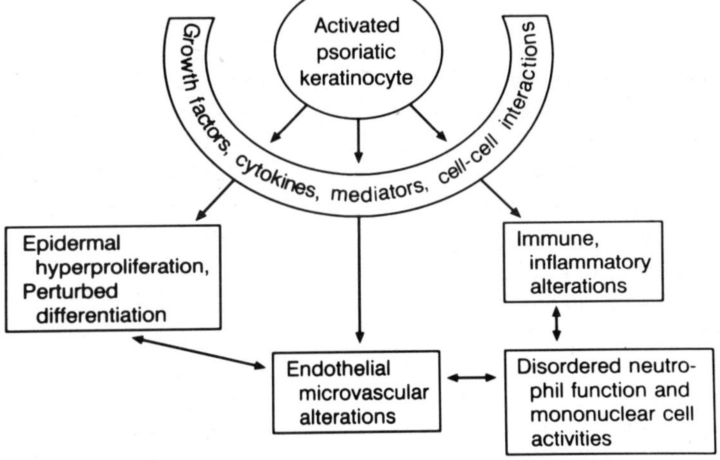

Figure 6 The cascade of growth factors, cytokines, other biological mediators, and direct celular interactions that result from activation or triggering of the psoriatic keratinocyte. Consequences of epidermal keratinocyte activation include altered keratinocyte proliferation and differentiation, dermal/endothelial changes, and perturbed immune/inflammatory reactivity. The sequence of pathological events and interdependence of these component systems in initiating and propagating the psoriatic lesion are not completely understood.

tinocyte has the capacity to express a variety of growth factors, cytokines, and other biological mediators with activities extending beyond the epidermal domain. These factors have the potential to affect vascular, immune, and inflammatory components of the skin and related systemic compartments (Fig. 6) (192,209–211). Primary alterations of vascular endothelium and immune/inflammatory cells induced by the psoriatic epidermis may orchestrate a variety of secondary responses, such as disordered neutrophil and mononuclear cell function (212–214). In this regard, therapeutic agents such as methotrexate that were initially considered to exert their effect primarily on epidermis are now recognized to have potent activities on lymphocytes (215). Similarly, although other newer therapies directed at the lymphocyte may ameliorate psoriasis, the ultimate roles of the epidermis and the immune system in this disease are still being dissected. Furthermore, direct cellular interactions between the activated psoriatic keratinocyte and adjacent epidermal cells (e.g., Langerhans cell), immune/inflammatory cells, and dermal cells likely occur because of their proximity within the cellular microenvironment and the recognized limitations of diffusable factors which are incapable of mediating certain pathological responses. An increasing number of effector molecules and specific cellular interactions regulated by the psoriatic keratinocyte have been characterized. Undoubtedly, many new biological and pathological factors of epidermis will be characterized and bear important discoveries for psoriasis.

Identification and characterization of keratinocyte abnormalities in psoriasis have generated considerable interest and fostered productive investigation over the past decade. An enlarging spectrum of structural and functional alterations have been recognized, not only in lesional psoriatic epidermis, but in unstimulated and stimulated, nonlesional epidermis of psoriasis. The mysteries of epidermal physiology and enigmas of psoriasis are steadily being transformed into a more complete understanding of epidermal growth control and keratinocyte differentiation in health and disease. The concept of the epidermal keratinocyte expressing the psoriatic phenotype has been extremely useful in understanding potential genotypic alterations that reside in the epidermis or adjacent tissues and recognizing the critical role of the epidermis and keratinocyte in initiating and propagating the psoriatic lesion.

REFERENCES

1. VanScott, E.J., and Ekel, T.M. (1963). Kinetics of hyperplasia in psoriasis. *Arch. Dermatol.* 88:373–381.
2. Montgomery, H. (1967). *Dermatopathology.* Vol. 1. Harper and Row, New York, pp. 309–326.
3. Lever, W.F., and Schaumburg-Lever, G. (1990). *Histopathology of the Skin.* 7th edition. Lippincott, Philadelphia, pp. 156–163.
4. Braun-Falco, O., and Christophers, E. (1974). Structural aspects of initial psoriatic lesions. *Arch. Dermatol. Forsch.* 251:95–110.
5. Gordon, M., and Johnson, W.C. (1967). Histopathology and histochemistry of psoriasis. *Arch. Dermatol.* 95:402–407.
6. Chapman, D., and Ross, J. (1988). Objective measurement of three epidermal parameters in psoriasis vulgaris and in dermatopathology in general. *Br. J. Dermatol.* 119:333–343.
7. Cox, A.J., and Watson, W. (1972). Histological variations in lesions of psoriasis. *Arch. Dermatol.* 106: 503–506.
8. Farber, E.M., and Cox, A.J. (1967). The biology of psoriasis. *J. Invest. Dermatol.* 49:348–357.
9. Fry, L., and McMinn, R.M.H. (1970). Observations on mitosis in psoriatic epidermis. *Br. J. Dermatol.* 82: 19–22.
10. Brody, I. (1962). The ultrastructure of the epidermis in psoriasis vulgaris. Parts 1–4. *J. Ultrastruct. Res.* 6: 304–367.
11. Brody, I. (1963). The ultrastructure of the epidermis in psoriasis vulgaris. Parts 5–7. *J. Ultrastruct. Res.* 8: 566–606.
12. Brody, I. (1978). Alterations in clinically normal skin in early eruptive guttate psoriasis. *J. Cutan. Pathol.* 5:219–233.
13. Orfanos, C., Schaumberg-Lever, G., Mahrle, G., and Lever, W. (1973). Alterations of cell surfaces as a pathogenetic factor in psoriasis. *Arch. Dermatol.* 107: 38–46.
14. Cox, A.J. (1969). The dermal-epidermal junction in psoriasis. *J. Invest. Dermatol.* 53:428–435.
15. Heng, M., Kloss, S., Kuehn, C., and Chase, D. (1986). Significance and pathogenesis of basal keratinocyte herniations in psoriasis. *J. Invest. Dermatol.* 87:362–366.
16. Kanerva, L. (1978). Basal keratinocyte herniation. *Acta Derm. Venereol. (Stockh.)* 67:254–257.
17. Lupulescu, A., Chadwick, J., and Downham, T., II (1979). Ultrastructural and cell surface changes of human psoriatic skin following Goeckerman therapy. *J. Cutan. Pathol.* 6:347–363.

18. Caputo, R., Innocenti, M., Gasparini, G., and Pelschetti, D. (1978). Plasma membranes in psoriatic cells. A freeze-fracture study. *J. Invest. Dermatol.* 71: 245–249.
19. Jahn, H., Nielson, E.H., Elberg, J., Ronne, M., and Brandrup, F. (1988). Ultrastructure of psoriatic epidermis. *AMPIS* 96:723–731.
20. Weinstein, G., and Van Scott, E. (1965). Autoradiographic analysis of turnover times of normal and psoriatic epidermis. *J. Invest. Dermatol.* 45:257–262.
21. Weinstein, G., and Frost, P. (1968). Abnormal cell proliferation in psoriasis. *J. Invest. Dermatol.* 50: 254–259.
22. Gelfant, S., Ozawa, A., Chalker, D., and Smith, J. (1982). Circadian rhythms and differences in epidermal and dermal cell proliferation in uninvolved and involved psoriatic skin *in vivo. J. Invest. Dermatol.* 78:58–62.
23. Grove, G. (1979). Epidermal cell kinetics in psoriasis. *Int. J. Dermatol.* 18:111–121.
24. Weinstein, G., McCullough, J., and Ross, P. (1985). Cell kinetic basis for pathophysiology of psoriasis. *J. Invest. Dermatol.* 85:579–583.
25. Wright, N., and Camplejohn, R. (Eds.). (1983). *Psoriasis: Cell Proliferation.* Churchill Livingstone, Edinburgh.
26. Galosi, A., Pullmann, H., and Steigleder, G. (1980). Abnormal epidermal cell proliferation on the elbow in psoriatic and normal skin. *Arch. Derm. Res.* 267: 105–107.
27. Goodwin, P., Hamilton, S., and Fry, L. (1976). The cell cycle in psoriasis. *Br. J. Dermatol.* 90:517–524.
28. Duffill, M., Wright, N., and Shuster, S. (1976). The cell proliferation kinetics of psoriasis examined by three *in vivo* techniques. *Br. J. Dermatol.* 94: 355–362.
29. Heenen, M., and Galand, P. (1984). On cell kinetics in psoriasis. *Br. J. Dermatol.* 110:241–245.
30. Staiano-Coico, L., Gottlieb, A., Barazini, L., and Carter, D.M. (1978). RNA, DNA and cell surface characteristics of lesional and non-lesional psoriatic skin. *J. Invest. Dermatol.* 88:646–651.
31. Van Neste, D., Staquet, M., Leroy, B., and DeCoster, W. (1988). Distribution pattern of psoriatic keratoblasts: computer-assisted image-analysis for combined evaluation of DNA synthesis and expression of 67 Kd keratin polypeptides in the epidermis of stable plaques of psoriasis. *J. Invest. Dermatol.* 90:382–386.
32. Prinz, J.C., Gross, B., Vollmer, S., Trommler, P., Strobel, I., Meurer, M., and Plewig, G. (1994). T cell clones from psoriasis skin lesions can promote keratinocyte proliferation in vitro via secreted products. *Eur. J. Immunol.* 24:593–598.
33. Bata-Csorgo, Z., Hammerberg, C., Voorhees, J.J., and Cooper, K.D. (1995). Kinetics and regulation of human keratinocyte stem cell growth in short-term primary ex vivo culture. Cooperative growth factors from psoriatic lesional T lymphocytes stimulate proliferation among psoriatic uninvolved, but not normal, stem keratinocytes. *J. Clin. Invest.* 95:317–327.
34. Bauer, F., Crombag, N., Boezeman, J., and DeGrood, R. (1981). Flow cytometry as a tool for the study of cell kinetics in skin. 2. cell kinetic data in psoriasis. *Br. J. Dermatol.* 104:271–276.
35. Patterson, J., Eisinger, M., Haynes, B., Berger, C., and Edelson, R. (1981). Monoclonal antibody 4F2 reactive with basal layer keratinocyte studies in the normal and a hyperproliferative state. *J. Invest. Dermatol.* 83:210–213.
36. Bauer, F., Boezeman, J., Engden, L., DeGrood, R., and Ramaekers, F. (1986). Monoclonal antibodies for epidermal population analysis. *J. Invest. Dermatol.* 87:72–75.
37. Miyagawa, S., Okada, N., Takasaki, Y., Iida, T., Kitano, Y., Yoshikawa, K., Sakamoto, K., and Steinberg, M. (1989). Expression of proliferating cell nuclear antigen/cyclin in human keratinocytes. *J. Invest. Dermatol.* 93:678–681.
38. Van Erp, P., Rijzewijk, J., Boezeman, J., Leenders, J., deMare, S., Schalkwijk, J., Van de Kerkhof, P., Ramaekers, F., and Bauer, F. (1989). Flow cytometric analysis of epidermal subpopulations from normal and psoriatic skin using monoclonal antibodies against intermediate filaments. *Am. J. Pathol.* 135: 865–870.
39. Rothberg, S., Crounse, R., and Lee, J. (1961). Glycine-^{14}C incorporation into the proteins of the normal stratum corneum and the abnormal stratum corneum of psoriasis. *J. Invest. Dermatol.* 37:497–505.
40. Russell, D., Combest, W., Duell, E., Stawiski, M., Anderson, T., and Voorhees, J. (1978). Glucocorticoid inhibits elevated polyamine biosynthesis in psoriasis. *J. Invest. Dermatol.* 77:177–181.
41. Lowe, N., Breeding, J., and Russell, D. (1982). Cutaneous polyamines in psoriasis. *Br. J. Dermatol.* 107: 21–26.
42. Laurahanta, J., Kousa, M., Kapyaho, K., Linnamaa, K., and Mustakallio, K. (1981). Reduction of increased polyanine levels in psoriatic lesions by retinoids and PUVA treatments. *Br. J. Dermatol.* 105: 267–272.
43. Lowe, N., Kaplan, R., and Breeding, J. (1982). Etretinate for psoriasis inhibits epidermal orithine decarboxylase. *J. Am. Acad. Dermatol.* 8:95–102.
44. Herdenstam, C. (1962). On the *in vitro* metabolism of labeled glucose in normal and psoriatic skin slices. *Acta Derm. Venereol. (Stockh.)* 42 (Suppl. 47):6–62.
45. Mahrle, G., and Orfanos, C. (1975). Ultrastructural localization and differentiation of membrane-bound ATP utilizing enzymes including adenyl cyclase in normal and psoriatic epidermis. *Br. J. Dermatol.* 93: 495–507.

46. Jones, W., Helwig, E., and Harman, L. (1964). Oxidative enzymes activity in the skin of patients with psoriasis. *J. Invest. Dermatol.* 44:189–195.
47. Schallreuter, K., and Pittelkow, M.R. (1987). Anthralin inhibits elevated levels of thioredoxin reductase in psoriasis. *Arch. Dermatol.* 123:1494–1498.
48. Marcelo, C., Duell, E., Stawiski, M., Anderson, T., and Voorhees, J. (1979). Cyclic nucleotide levels in psoriatic and normal keratomed epidermis. *J. Invest. Dermatol.* 72:20–24.
49. Voorhees, J. (1982). Psoriasis as a possible defect of the adenyl cyclase-cyclic AMP cascade. *Arch. Dermatol.* 118:862–868.
50. Iizuka, H., Matsuo, S., Tamura, T., and Ohkuma, N. (1988). Increased choleratoxin-, and forskolin-induced cyclic AMP accumulations in psoriatic involved versus uninvolved or normal human epidermis. *J. Invest. Dermatol.* 91:154–157.
51. Plummer, N., Hensky, C., Warin, A., Camo, R., and Greaves, M. (1978). Prostaglandin E_2, $F_2\alpha$ and arachidonic acid levels in irradiated and unirradiated skin of psoriatic patients receiving PUVA treatment. *Clin. Exp. Dermatol.* 3:367–369.
52. Hammerström, S., Hamberg, M., Samuelsson, B., Duell, E., Stawiski, M., and Voorhees, J. (1975). Increased concentrations of nonesterified arachidonic acid, 12L-hydroxy-5,8,10,14-eicosatetraenoic acid (HETE), prostaglandin E_2 and prostaglandin $F_2\alpha$ in epidermis of psoriasis: evidence of perturbed regulation of arachidonic acid levels in psoriasis. *Proc. Natl. Acad. Sci. (U.S.A.)* 72:5130–5134.
53. Camp, R., Mallet, A., Woolard, P., Brain, S., Black, A.K., and Greaves, M. (1983). Monohydroxy metabolites of arachidonic and linoleic acids in psoriatic skin. *J. Invest. Dermatol.* 80:359–360.
54. Mizumoto, T., Hashimoto, Y., Hirokawa, M., Ohkuma, N., Iizuka, H., and Ohkawara, A. (1985). Calmodulin activities are significantly increased in both uninvolved and involved epidermis in psoriasis. *J. Invest. Dermatol.* 85:45–452.
55. Fairley, J., Marcelo, C., Hogan, V., and Voorhees, J. (1985). Increased calmodulin levels in psoriasis and Low Ca^{++} regulated mouse epidermal keratinocytes. *J. Invest. Dermatol.* 84:195–198.
56. Wollina, U., Klinger, R., Wetzker, R., and Knopf, B. (1989). Increase of epidermal calmodulin precedes formation of a psoriatic lesion. *Arch. Dermatol. Res.* 281:73–74.
57. Heng, M.C., Song, M.K., and Heng, M.K. (1994). Elevated phosphorylase kinase activity in psoriatic epidermis: correlation with increased phosphorylation and psoriatic activity. *Br. J. Dermatol.* 130:298–306.
58. Mier, P., and Van den Hurk, M. (1976). Lysosomal hydrolases of the epidermis. 6. Changes in disease. *Br. J. Dermatol.* 95:271–274.
59. Fräki, J., Djupsund, B., and Hopsu-Havu, V. (1978). Plasminogen activators of psoriatic scale extracts. Separation of two plasminogen activators by isoelectric focusing. *Arch. Dermatol. Res.* 261:259–266.
60. Grondahl-Hansen, J., Ralfkiaer, E., Nielsen, L., Kristensen, P., Frentz, G., and Dano, K. (1987). Immunohistochemical localization of urokinase and tissue-type plasminogen activators in psoriatic skin. *J. Invest. Dermatol.* 88:28–32.
61. Horn, F., Marks, F., Fisher, G., Marcelo, C., and Voorhees, J. (1987). Decreased protein kinase C activity in psoriatic versus normal epidermis. *J. Invest. Dermatol.* 88:220–222.
62. Bartel, R., Marcelo, C., and Voorhees, J. (1987). Partial characterization of phospholipase C activity in normal, psoriatic uninvolved and lesional epidermis. *J. Invest. Dermatol.* 88:447–451.
63. Inohara, S., Tatsumi, Y., Tanaka, Y., Tateishi, H., and Sagami, S. (1988). Immunohistochemical identification of protein kinase C isozymes in normal and psoriatic epidermis. *Arch. Dermatol. Res.* 280:454–455.
64. Forster, S., Ilderton, E., Summerly, R., and Yardley, H. (1983). The level of phospholipase A_2 activity is raised in the uninvolved epidermis of psoriasis. *Br. J. Dermatol.* 108:103–105.
65. Bergers, M., Verhagen, D., Jongerius, M., Van de Kerkhof, P., and Mier, P. (1988). A unique phospholipase A_2 in human epidermis. Its physiologic function and its level in certain dermatoses. *J. Invest. Dermatol.* 90:23–25.
66. Gentleman, S., Martensen, T., Digiovanna, J., and Chader, G. (1984). Protein tyrosine kinase and protein phosphotyrosine phosphatase in normal and psoriatic skin. *Biochem. Biophys. Acta* 798:53–59.
67. Pike, M., Lee, C., Elder, J., Voorhees, J., and Fisher, G. (1989). Increased phosphatidylinositol kinase activity in psoriatic epidermis. *J. Invest. Dermatol.* 92: 791–797.
68. Elder, J., Fisher, G., Lindquist, P., Bennett, G., Pittelkow, M., Coffey, R., Ellingsworth, L., Derynck, R., and Voorhees, J. (1989). Overexpression of transforming growth factor α in psoriatic epidermis. *Science* 243:811–814.
69. Pittelkow, M., Coffey, R., and Moses, H. (1988). Keratinocytes produce and are regulated by transforming growth factors. In *Endocrine, Metabolic and Immunologic Functions of Keratinocytes. Ann. N.Y. Acad. Sci.* 548:211–224. L. Milstone and R. Edelson (Eds.).
70. Cook, P.W., Pittelkow, M.R., Keeble, W.W., Graves-Deal, R., Coffey, R.J., Jr., and Shipley, G.D. (1992). Amphiregulin messenger RNA is elevated in psoriatic epidermis and gastrointestinal carcinomas. *Cancer Res.* 52:3224–3227.
71. Krane, J.F., Gottlieb, A.B., Carter, D.M., and Krueger, J.G. (1992). The insulin-like growth factor I receptor is overexpressed in psoriatic epidermis, but is

differentially regulated from the epidermal growth factor receptor. *J. Exp. Med.* 175:1081–1090.
72. Baden, H., McGilvray, N., Cheng, C., et al. (1978). The keratin polypeptides of psoriatic epidermis. *J. Invest. Dermatol.* 70:294–297.
73. Weiss, R., Eichner, R., and Sun, T. (1984). Monoclonal antibody analysis of keratin expression in epidermal disease: a 48- and 56-K dalton keratin as molecular markers for hyperproliferative keratinocytes. *J. Cell. Biol.* 98:1397–1406.
74. Stoler, A., Kopan, R., Duvic, M., and Fuchs, E. (1989). Use of monospecific antisera and cRNA probes to localize the major changes in keratin expression during normal and abnormal epidermal differentiation. *J. Cell. Biol.* 107:427–446.
75. Skerrow, D., and Hunter, I. (1978). Protein modifications during the keratinization of normal and psoriatic human epidermis. *Biochem. Biophys. Acta* 537: 474–484.
76. Bernerd, F., Magnaldo, T., and Darmon, M. (1992). Delayed onset of epidermal differentiation in psoriasis. *J. Invest. Dermatol.* 98:902–910.
77. Nanney, L., Stoscheck, C., Magid, M., and King, L. (1986). Altered [^{125}I] epidermal growth factor binding and receptor distribution in psoriasis. *J. Invest. Dermatol.* 86:260–265.
78. Amagai, M., Ozawa, S., Ueda, M., Nishikawa, T., Abe, O., and Shimizu, N. (1988). Distribution of EGF receptor expressing and DNA replicating epidermal cells in psoriasis vulgaris and Bowen's disease. *Br. J. Dermatol.* 119:661–668.
79. Healy, E., Reynolds, N.J., Smith, M.D., Harrison, D., Doherty, E., Campbell, C., and Rees, J.L. (1995). Upregulation of p21WAF1/CIP1 in psoriasis and after the application of irritants and tape stripping. *J. Invest. Dermatol.* 105:274–279.
80. Bernard, B., Reano, A., Darmon, M., and Thivolet, J. (1986). Precocious appearance of involucrin and epidermal transglutaminase during differentiation of psoriatic skin. *Br. J. Dermatol.* 114:279–283.
81. Dover, R., and Watt, F. (1987). Measurement of the role of epidermal terminal differentiation. Expression of involucrin by S-phase keratinocytes in culture and in psoriatic plaques. *J. Invest. Dermatol.* 89:349–352.
82. Bernard, B., Asselineau, D., Schaffar-Deshayes, L., and Darmon, M. (1988). Abnormal sequence of expression of differentiation markers in psoriatic epidermis: inversion of two steps in the differentiation program? *J. Invest. Dermatol.* 90:801–805.
83. Michel, S., Schmidt, R., Shroot, B., and Reichert, U. (1988). Morphological and biochemical characterization of the cornified envelopes from human epidermal keratinocytes of different origin. *J. Invest. Dermatol.* 91:11–15.
84. Kanitakis, J., Ramirez-Bosca, A., Reano, A., Viac, J., Roche, P., and Thivolet, J. (1988). Filaggrin expression in normal and pathological skin: A marker of keratinocyte differentiation. *Virchows Arch.* [*A*] 412: 375–382.
85. Kobayashi, H., Yasuda, H., Ohkawara, A., Dosaka, H., Oda, A., Ogiso, Y., and Kuzumaki, N. (1988). Enhanced expression of ras products in psoriatic epidermis. *Arch. Dermatol. Res.* 280:259–263.
86. Camp, R., Fincham, N., Cunningham, F., Greaves, M., Morris, J., and Chu, A. (1986). Psoriatic skin lesions contain biologically active amounts of an interleukin 1-like compound. *J. Immunol.* 137:3469–3474.
87. Romero, L., Ikejima, T., and Pincus, S. (1989). *In situ* localization of interleukin-1 in normal and psoriatic skin. *J. Invest. Dermatol.* 93:518–522.
88. Oxhelm, A., Oxholm, P., Staberg, B., and Bendtzen, K. (1989). Interleukin-6 in the epidermis of patients with psoriasis before and during PUVA treatment. *Acta Derm. Venereol.* (*Stockh.*) 69:195–199.
89. Grossman, R., Krueger, J., Yourish, D., Granelli-Piperno, A., Murphy, D., May, L., Kupper, T., Sehgal, P., Gottlieb, A. (1989). Interleukin 6 is expressed in high levels in psoriatic skin and stimulates proliferation of cultured human keratinocytes. *Proc. Natl. Acad. Sci.* (*U.S.A.*) 86:6367–6371.
90. Gillitzer, R., Berger, R., Mielke, V. (1991). Upper keratinocytes of psoriatic skin lesions express high levels of NAP-1/IL-8 mRNA in situ. *J. Invest. Dermatol.* 97:73–79.
91. Paludan, K., Thestrup, P.K. (1992). Use of the polymerase chain reaction in quantification of interleukin 8 mRNA in minute epidermal samples. *J. Invest. Dermatol.* 99:830–835.
92. Hammerberg, C., Arend, W.P., Fisher, G.J., Chan, L.S., Berger, A.E., Haskill, J.S., Voorhees, J.J., and Cooper, K.D. (1992). Interleukin-1 receptor antagonist in normal and psoriatic epidermis. *J. Clin. Invest.* 90:571–583.
93. Morhenn, V., Abel, E., and Mahrle, G. (1982). Expression of HLA-DR antigen in skin from patients with psoriasis. *J. Invest. Dermatol.* 78:165–168.
94. Terui, T., Aiba, S., Kato, T., Tanaka, T., and Tagemi, H. (1987). HLA-DR antigen expression on keratinocytes in highly inflamed parts of psoriatic lesions. *Br. J. Dermatol.* 116:87–93.
95. Singer, K., Tuck, D., Sampson, H., and Hall, R. (1989). Epidermal keratinocytes express the adhesion molecule intercellular adhesion molecule-1 in inflammatory dermatoses. *J. Invest. Dermatol.* 92:746–750.
96. Lisby, S., Ralfkiaer, E., Rothlein, R., and Vejlsgaard, G. (1989). Intercellular adhesion molecule-1 (ICAM-1) expression correlated to inflammation. *Br. J. Dermatol.* 120:479–484.
97. Soyer, H., Smolle, J., and Kerl, H. (1989). Distribution patterns of the OKM5 antigen in normal and diseased human epidermis. *J. Cutan. Pathol.* 16:60–65.

98. Barker, J., Markey, A., Allen, M., and MacDonald, D. (1989). Keratinocyte expression of OKM5 antigen in inflammatory cutaneous disease. *Br. J. Dermatol.* 120:613–618.
99. Niedecken, H., Wehrmann, W., Bauer, R., and Kreysel, H. (1988). Reaction of human keratinocytes with the monoclonal antibody anti-Leu 11: An immunohistologic study. *J. Am. Acad. Dermatol.* 18:504–510.
100. Gottlieb, A., Luster, A., Posnett, D., and Carter, D.M. (1988). Detection of a γ interferon-induced protein IP-10 in psoriatic plaques. *J. Exp. Med.* 168:941–948.
101. Livden, J., Nilsen, R., Bjerke, J., and Matre, R. (1989). *In situ* localization of interferons in psoriatic lesions. *Arch. Dermatol. Res.* 281:392–397.
102. Iwata, M., Otsuka, F., Watanabe, S., Nogita, T., and Ishibashi, Y. (1988). Expression of transferrin receptor in normal human skin, psoriatic skin and various skin tumors. *J. Dermatol. (Jpn)* 15:208–211.
103. Baadsgaard, O., Fisher, G., Fox, D., Salvo, B., Cary, T., Marcelo, C., Voorhees, J., and Cooper, K. (1989). Conditioned medium from lesional psoriatic T-cell clones induces keratinocyte proliferation and expression of the surface activation molecule UM4D4. *J. Invest. Dermatol.* 92:398.
104. Paukkonen, K., Naukkarinen, A., and Horsmanheimo, M. (1995). The development of manifest psoriatic lesions is linked with the appearance of ICAM-1 positivity on keratinocytes. *Arch. Derm. Res.* 287: 165–170.
105. Gillitzer, R., Wolff, K., Tong, D., Muller, C., Yoshimura, T., Hartmann, A.A., Stingl, G., and Berger, R. MCP-1 mRNA expression in basal keratinocytes of psoriatic lesions. *J. Invest. Dermatol.* 101:127–131.
106. Schroder, J.M. (1992). Generation of NAP-1 and related peptides in psoriasis and other inflammatory skin diseases. *Cytokines* 4:54–76.
107. Tettelbach, W., Nanney, L., Ellis, D., King, L., and Richmond, A. (1993). Localization of MGSA/GRO protein in cutaneous lesions. *J. Cutan. Pathol.* 20: 259–266.
108. Zambruno, G., Reano, A., Meissner, K., and Thivolet, J. (1986). GP37 expression in normal and diseased human epidermis. A marker for keratinocyte differentiation. *Acta Derm. Venereol. (Stockh.)* 66:185–192.
109. Viac, J., Haftek, M., Staquet, M., Reano, P., Brochier, J., Thivolet, J. (1985). A monoclonal antibody labelling the keratinocyte membrane: A marker of epidermal differentiation. *Acta Derm. Venereol. (Stockh.)* 65:1–8.
110. McCullough, J., Weinstein, G., Ross, P., Barr, R., and Stanbridge, E. (1988). Identification of differentiation-specific antigens in psoriatic versus normal skin using monoclonal antibodies. *Int. J. Dermatol.* 27: 626–632.
111. Strefling, A., Knapp, A., and Mansbridge, J. (1985). Histologic distribution of staining by a monoclonal antibody ψ-3 in psoriasis and occurrence of ψ-3 antigen in other cutaneous diseases. *J. Invest. Dermatol.* 84:100–104.
112. Goggi, G., Bonelli, M., Bonoldi, E., and Viale, G., et al. (1984). Lectin histochemistry in psoriasis. *Acta Derm. Venereol. (Stockh.)* 113(Suppl.):80–84.
113. Schaumberg-Lever, G., Alroy, J., Ucci, A., Lever, W., and Orfanos, C. (1984). Cell surface carboxydrates in psoriasis. *J. Am. Acad. Dermatol.* 11:1087–1094.
114. Brysk, M., Miller, J., and Herberg, A. (1984). Conconavalin A distinguishes among diseases of altered epidermal differentiation. *J. Invest. Dermatol.* 82: 18–20.
115. Roelfzema, H., Bergers, M., Van Erp, P., Gommans, J., and Mier, P. (1981). Studies on the plasma membrane of normal and psoriatic keratinocytes. 4. characterization of glycoconjugates. *Br. J. Dermatol.* 105:509–516.
116. Saga, K., Takahashi, M. (1995). Localization of anionic sites in normal and psoriatic epidermis: the effect of enzyme digestion on these anionic sites. *Br. J. Dermatol.* 132:710–717.
117. Livden, J. (1988). Fcγ receptors on keratinocytes in psoriasis. *Arch. Dermatol. Res.* 280:12–17.
118. Dreno, B., Jacques, Y., Barriere, H., and Soulillou, J.-P. (1986). Monoclonal antiinterleukin 2 (15-2) antibody binding to granular layer keratinocytes of human skin. *J. Invest. Dermatol.* 86:359–362.
119. Iversen, O., Rodahl, E., and Dalen, A. (1985). Rabbit antibodies against major internal protein of a retrovirus-like particle bind to epidermal cells in psoriatic skin. *Arch. Virol.* 86:341–346.
120. Mommas-Kienhuis, A.-M., Grayson, S., Wijsman, M., Vermeer, B., and Elias, P. (1987). Low density-lipoprotein receptor expression on keratinocytes in normal and psoriatic epidermis. *J. Invest. Dermatol.* 89:513–517.
121. Nonomura, K., Yamanishi, K., Yasuno, H., Nara, K., and Hirose, S. (1994). Up-regulation of elafin/SKALP gene expression in psoriatic epidermis. *J. Invest. Dermatol.* 103:88–91.
122. Wiedow, O., Wiese, F., Streit, V. (1992). Lesional elastase activity in psoriasis, contact dermatitis, and atopic dermatitis. *J. Invest. Dermatol.* 99:306–309.
123. Spiers, E.M., Lazarus, G.S., Lyons, G.B. (1994). Expression of plasminogen activator enzymes in psoriatic epidermis. *J. Invest. Dermatol.* 102:333–338.
124. Madsen, P., Rasmussen, H.H., Leffers, H. (1992). Molecular cloning and expression of a novel keratinocyte protein (psoriasis-associated fatty acid-binding protein [PA-FABP]) that is highly up-regulated in psoriatic skin and that shares similarity to fatty acid-binding proteins. *J. Invest. Dermatol.* 99:299–305.
125. Saurat, J., Didierjean, L., and Habibi, B. (1981). Pr antigens in the skin: distinct localization linked to the

stage and the type of keratinocyte differentiation. *Br. J. Dermatol.* 105:25–38.

126. Kariniemi, A., Lehto, V., and Virtanen, I. (1984). Distribution of p230, an α-spectrin-related polypeptide in normal and psoriatic epidermis and in cultured human keratinocytes. *Br. J. Dermatol.* 111:139–145.

127. DiCicco, L., Fraki, J., and Mansbridge, J. (1987). The plasma membrane in psoriasis. *Int. J. Dermatol.* 26: 631–638.

128. Nickoloff, B.J., Mitra, R.S., Varani, J., Dixit, V.M., and Polverini, P.J. (1994). Aberrant production of interleukin-8 and thrombospondin-1 by psoriatic keratinocytes mediates angiogenesis. *Am. J. Pathol.* 144: 820–828.

129. Detmar, M., Brown, L.F., Claffey, K.P., Yeo, K.T., Kocher, O., Jackman, R.W., Berse, B., and Dvorak, H.F. (1994). Overexpression of vascular permeability factor/vascular endothelial growth factor and its receptors in psoriasis. *J. Exp. Med.* 180:1141–1146.

130. Puig, L., Fernandez-Figueras, M.T., Ferrandiz, C., Ribera, M., and de Moragas, J.M. (1995). Epidermal expression of 65 and 72 kd heat shock proteins in psoriasis and AIDS-associated psoriasiform dermatitis. *J. Am. Acad. Dermatol.* 33:985–989.

131. Lontz, W., Sirsjo, A., Liu, W., Lindberg, M., Rollman, O., and Torma, H. (1995). Increased mRNA expression of manganese superoxide dismutase in psoriasis skin lesions and in cultured human keratinocytes exposed to IL-1 beta and TNF-alpha. *Free Radical Biol. Med.* 18:349–355.

132. Yoshinaga, Y., Higaki, M., Terajima, S., Ohkubo, E., Nogita, T., Miyasaka, N., and Kawashima, M. (1995). Detection of inflammatory cytokines in psoriatic skin. *Arch. Derm. Res.* 287:158–164.

133. Elder, J.T., Klein, S.B., Tavakkol, A. (1990). Growth factor and proto-oncogene expression in psoriasis. *J. Invest. Dermatol.* 95:75–95.

134. Elder, J.T., Tavakkol, A., Klein, S.B. (1990). Protooncogene expression in normal and psoriatic skin. *J. Invest. Dermatol.* 94:19–25.

135. Bohlen, P., Grove, J., Beya, M., Koch-Weser, J., Henry, M., and Grosshans, E. (1978). Skin polyamine levels in psoriasis: the effect of dithranol therapy. *Eur. J. Clin. Invest.* 8:215–218.

136. Forster, S., Ilderton, E., Norris, J., Summerly, R., and Yardley, H. (1985). Characterization and activity of phospholipase A_2 in normal human epidermis and in lesion-free epidermis of patients with psoriasis or eczema. *Br. J. Dermatol.* 112:135–147.

137. Nagy-Vezekenyi, C., and Zs-Nagy, I. (1971). Studies on the ultrastructure of psoriasis and of the "normal" skin of psoriatics. *Acta Derm. Venereol. (Stockh.)* 51: 435–443.

138. Ortone, J., Schmitt, D., Bonnot, G., and Thivolet, J. (1982). Epidermal wound healing in psoriasis. In *Psoriasis: Proceedings of the Third International Symposium.* E. Farber, A. Cox, L. Nall, and P. Jacobs (Eds.). New York, Grune & Stratton, pp. 311–312.

139. Jensen, P., Baird, J., Morioka, S., Lessin, S., and Lazarus, G. (1988). Epidermal plasminogen activator is abnormal in cutaneous lesions. *J. Invest. Dermatol.* 90:777–782.

140. Takematsu, H., Fisher, G., and Voorhees, J. (1989). A novel histone-stimulated protein kinase in normal and psoriatic epidermis. *J. Invest. Dermatol.* 92: 385–390.

141. deMare, S., Van Erp, P., and van de Kerkhof, P. (1989). Epidermal hyperproliferation assessed by the monoclonal antibody K_S 8.12 on frozen sections. *J. Invest. Dermatol.* 92:130–131.

142. Wiley, H.E., and Weinstein, G.D. (1979). Abnormal proliferation of uninvolved psoriatic epidermis: differential induction by saline, propanol, and tape stripping *in vivo. J. Invest. Dermatol.* 73:545–547.

143. Grove, G. (1980). Proliferative response to fluid injection in psoriatic and normal human epidermis. *Br. J. Dermatol.* 102:281–284.

144. Van de Kerkhof, P., Van Rennes, H., De Grood, R., De Jongh, G., Bauer, F., and Mier, P. (1983). Response of the clinically uninvolved skin of psoriatic patients to standardized injury. *Br. J. Dermatol.* 109: 287–294.

145. Braun-Falco, O., Christophers, E., and Kurban, A. (1967). Abnormes verhalten der epidermalen regeneration bei patienten mit psoriasis vulgaris. *Arch. Klin. Exp. Dermatol.* 229:276–284.

146. Harper, R., Rispler, J., and Urbanek, R. (1978). DNA synthesis among uninvolved and involved psoriatic epidermal cells and normal epidermal cells *in vitro. J. Invest. Dermatol.* 70:254–256.

147. Kragbelle, K., Desjarlais, L., and Marcelo, C. (1985). Increased DNA synthesis of uninvolved psoriatic epidermis is maintained *in vitro. Br. J. Dermatol.* 112: 263–270.

148. Chopra, D., and Flaxman, B. (1974). Comparative proliferative kinetics of cells from normal human epidermis and benign epidermal hyperplasia (psoriasis) *in vitro. Cell Tissue Kinet.* 7:69–76.

149. Liu, S., and Parsons, S. (1983). Serial cultivation of epidermal keratinocytes from psoriatic plaques. *J. Invest. Dermatol.* 81:54–61.

150. Baker, B., Powles, A., Valdi Marsson, H., and Fry, L. (1988). An altered response by psoriatic keratinocytes to gamma interferon. *Scand. J. Immunol.* 28:735–740.

151. Mann, P., Williams, R., and Gray, G. (1980). Distribution of glycoproteins containing fucose in normal and psoriatic keratinocytes. *Br. J. Dermatol.* 102: 649–657.

152. Kariniemi, A., Lehto, V., and Virtanen, I. (1983). Surface glycoproteins of cultured human keratinocytes from normal and uninvolved psoriatic epidermis. *Br. J. Dermatol.* 109:531–537.

153. Roelfzema, H., Bergers, M., Van Erp, P., Gommans, J., and Mier, P. (1981). Studies on the plasma membrane of normal and psoriatic keratinocytes. 3. Uptake of labelled sugars and their incorporation into glycoconjugates. *Br. J. Dermatol.* 104:635–640.
154. Roelfzema, H., and Van Erp, P. (1983). Glycoprotein composition of psoriatic epidermis in relation to growth control. *J. Invest. Dermatol.* 80:20–23.
155. Roelfzema, H., and Van Erp, P. (1983). Studies on plasma membrane of normal and psoriatic keratinocytes, 6. Cell surface and shed glycoproteins. *J. Invest. Dermatol.* 80:24–26.
156. Lagerholm, B., and Frithz, A. (1964). Cellular changes in the psoriatic epidermis III studies on the submicroscopic organization of epidermal cells cultured *in vitro. Acta Derm. Venereol. (Stockh.)* 44: 385–398.
157. Nielsen, E., Elberg, J., Ronne, M., Jahn, H., and Bierring, F. (1987). Surface ultrastructure of cultures of affected psoriatic keratinocytes, unaffected psoriatic keratinocytes and normal keratinocytes. *AMPIS* 95: 303–308.
158. Fraki, J., Briggaman, R., and Lazarus, G. (1981). Uninvolved skin from psoriatic patients develops signs of involved psoriatic skin after being grafted to nude mice. *Science* 215:685–687.
159. Krueger, G., Chambers, D., and Shelby, J. (1981). Involved and uninvolved skin from psoriatic subjects: are they equally diseased? Assessment by skin transplanted to congenitally athymic (nude) mice. *J. Clin. Invest.* 68:1548–1557.
160. Saiag, P., Coulomb, B., Lebreton, C., Bell, E., and Dubertret, L. (1985). Psoriatic fibroblasts induce hyperproliferation of normal keratinocytes in a skin equivalent model *in vitro. Science* 230:669–672.
161. Iizuka, H., Ishida, A., Matsumoto, M., Koizumi, H., and Ohkawara, A. (1986). Acantholytic change of psoriatic-involved epidermis during organ culture *in vitro. Clin. Exp. Dermatol.* 11:345–351.
162. Braun-Falco, O. (1963). Zur morphogenese der psoriatischen haut reaktion. *Arch. Klin. Exp. Dermatol.* 216:130–154.
163. Braun-Falco, O. (1971). Dynamics of growth and regression in psoriatic lesions: alterations in the skin from normal into a psoriatic lesion, and during regression of psoriatic lesions in psoriasis. In *Psoriasis: Proceedings of the International Symposium.* E. Farber, A. Cox, and P. Jacobs (Eds.). Stanford University Press, Stanford, CA, pp. 215–237.
164. Braverman, I., and Sibley, J. (1982). Role of microcirculation in the treatment and pathogenesis of psoriasis. *J. Invest. Dermatol.* 78:12–17.
165. Braverman, I., and Yen, A. (1986). Three-dimensional reconstruction of endothelial cell gaps in psoriatic vessels and their morphologic identity with gaps produced by intradermal injection of histamine. *J. Invest. Dermatol.* 86:577–581.
166. Wille, J., Pittelkow, M., Shipley, G., and Scott, R. (1984). Integrated control of growth and differentiation of normal human prokeratinocytes cultured in serum-free medium: clonal analyses, growth kinetics and cell cycle studies. *J. Cell Physiol.* 121:31–44.
167. Pittelkow, M., Wille, J., Jr., and Scott, R. (1986). Two functionally distinct classes of growth arrest states in human prokeratinocytes that regulate clonogenic potential. *J. Invest. Dermatol.* 86:410–417.
168. Potten, C. (1981). Cell replacement in epidermis (keratopoiesis) via discrete units of proliferation. *Int. Rev. Cytol.* 69:271–318.
169. Lieberman, M., and Glaser, L. (1981). Density-dependent regulation of cell growth: an example of a cell-cell recognition phenomenon. *J. Membrane Biol.* 63:1–11.
170. Pardee, A. (1987). Molecules involved in proliferations of normal and cancer cells. *Cancer Res.* 47: 1488–1491.
171. Pardee, A. (1989). G_1 events and regulation of cell proliferation. *Science* 246:603–608.
172. Kam, E., Melvile, L., and Pitts, J. (1986). Patterns of junctional communication in skin. *J. Invest. Dermatol.* 87:748–753.
173. Solomon, D., Saurat, J.-H., and Meda, P. (1988). Cell-to-cell communication within intact human skin. *J. Clin. Invest.* 82:248–254.
174. Heng, M., Kloss, S., Kuehn, C., and Chase, D. (1985). Sequence of events in psoriatic plaque formation after tape stripping: a light and electron microscopic study. *Br. J. Dermatol.* 112:517–532.
175. Petersen, M., Woodley, D., Stricklin, G., and O'Keefe, E. (1987). Production of procollagenase by cultured human keratinocytes. *J. Biol. Chem.* 262: 835–840.
176. Eckert, R. (1989). Structure, function and differentiation of the keratinocyte. *Physiol. Rev.* 69:1316–1346.
177. D'Armiento, J., DiColandrea, T., Dalal, S.S., Okada, Y., Huang, M.-T., Conney, A.H., Chada, K. (1995). Collagenase expression in transgenic mouse skin causes hyperkeratosis and acanthosis and increases susceptibility to tumorigenesis. *Mol. Cell. Biol.* 15: 5732–5739.
178. Malarkey, K., Belham, C., Paul, A., Graham, A., McLess, A., Scott, P., Plerin, R. (1995). The regulation of tyrosine kinase signaling pathways by growth factors and G-protein-coupled receptors. *Biochem. J.* 309:361–375.
179. Milligan, G. (1995). Signal sorting by G-protein-linked receptors. *Adv. Pharmacol.* 32:1–29.
180. Strader, C., Fong, T., Tota, M., Underwood, D., Dixon, R. (1994). Structure and function of G protein coupled receptors. *Annu. Rev. Biochem.* 63:101–132.

181. Pittelkow, M.R. Growth factors in cutaneous biology and disease (1992). *Adv. Dermatol.* 7:55–81.
182. Pittelkow, M.R., Cook, P.W., Shipley, G.D., Derynck, R., and Coffey, R.J., Jr. (1993). Autonomous growth of human keratinocytes requires epidermal growth factor receptor occupancy. *Cell Growth Differ.* 4: 513–521.
183. Barnard, J.A., Graves-Deal, R., Pittelkow, M.R., DuBois, R., Cook, P., Ramsey, G.W., Bishop, P.R., Damstrup, L., and Coffey, R.J. (1994). Auto- and cross-induction within the mammalian epidermal growth factor-related peptide family. *J. Biol. Chem.* 269:22817–22822.
184. Schallreuter, K.U., Lemke, K.R., Pittelkow, M.R., Wood, J.M., Korner, C., and Malik, R. (1995). Catecholamines in human keratinocyte differentiation. *J. Invest. Dermatol.* 104:953–957.
185. Cook, P.W., Ashton, N.M., and Pittelkow, M.R. (1995). Adenosine and adenine nucleotides inhibit the autonomous and epidermal growth factor-mediated proliferation of cultured human keratinocytes. *J. Invest. Dermatol.* 104:976–981.
186. Koch, P., Franke, W. (1994). Desmosomal cadherins: Another growing multigene family of adhesion molecules. *Curr. Op. Cell Biol.* 6:682–687.
187. Gumbiner, B.M. (1995). Signal transduction by β-catenin. *Curr. Op. Cell Biol.* 7:634–640.
188. Parsons, J.T. (1996). Integrin-mediated signalling: Regulation by protein tyrosine kinases and small GTP-binding proteins. *Curr. Op. Cell Biol.* 8: 146–152.
189. Clark E.A., and Brugge, J.S. (1995). Integrins and signal transduction pathways: The road taken. *Science* 268:233–239.
190. Adams, J., Watt, F. (1991). Expression of β_1, β_2, β_4 and β_5 integrins by human keratinocytes and non-differentiating keratinocytes. *J. Cell. Biol.* 115:829–841.
191. Hertle, M.D., Kubler, M.D., Leigh, I.M., and Watt, F.M. (1992). Aberrant integrin expression during epidermal wound healing and in psoriatic epidermis. *J. Clin. Invest.* 89:1892–1901.
192. Carroll, J.M., Romero, M.R., and Watt, F.M. (1995). Suprabasal integrin expression in the epidermis of transgenic mice results in developmental defects and a phenotype resembling psoriasis. *Cell* 83:957–968.
193. Mainiero, F., Pepe, A., Yeon, M., Ren, Y., and Giancotti, F.G. (1996). The intracellular functions of $\alpha_6\beta_4$ integrin are regulated by EGF. *Cell Biol.* 134: 241–253.
194. Yarden, Y., and Ulrich, A. (1988). Growth factor receptor tyrosine kinases. *Annu. Rev. Biochem.* 57: 443–478.
195. Waterfield, M. (Ed.). (1989). Growth factors. *Br. Med. Bull.* 45:317–600.
196. Cohen, S. (1964). *Isolation and Biological Effects of an Epidermal Growth-Stimulating Protein in Metabolic Control Mechanisms in Animal Cells.* Monograph 13. W. Rutter (Ed.). National Cancer Institute, Bethesda, MD, pp. 13–27.
197. Cohen, S. (1965). The stimulation of epidermal proliferation by a specific protein (EGF). *Dev. Biol.* 12: 394–407.
198. Pittelkow, M., Coffey, R., and Moses, H. (1990). Transforming Growth Factor-β and Other Growth Factors. In *Biochemistry and Physiology of the Skin.* L. Goldsmith (Ed.). Oxford University Press, Oxford, England.
199. Pittelkow, M.R. (1987). Keratinocyte commitment to differentiation: Regulation by growth factors and calcium. In *Psoriasis: Proceedings of the Fourth International Symposium.* E. Farber, L. Nall, V. Morhenn, and P. Jacobs (Eds.). Elsevier Science Publishing Company, New York, pp. 87–95.
200. Coffey, R., Derynck, R., Wilcox, J., Bringman, T., Goustin, A., Moses, H., and Pittelkow, M. (1987). Production and autoinduction of transforming growth factor-α in human keratinocytes. *Nature* 328: 817–820.
201. Cook, P.W., Piepkorn, M., Clegg, C.H., Plowman, G.D., DeMay, J.M., Brown, J.R., Pittelkow, M.R. (1997). Transgenic expression of the human amphiregulin gene induces a psoriasis-like phenotype. *J. Clin. Invest.* (in press).
202. Pittelkow, M., Lindquist, P., Abraham, R., Graves-Deal, R., Derynck, R., and Coffey, R. (1989). Induction of transforming growth factor-α expression in human keratinocytes by phorbol esters. *J. Biol. Chem.* 264:5164–5171.
203. Shipley, G., Keeble, W., Hendrickson, J., Coffey, R., and Pittelkow, M. (1989). Growth of normal human keratinocytes and fibroblasts in serum-free medium is stimulated by acidic and basic fibroblast growth factor. *J. Cell. Physiol.* 138:511–518.
204. Milstone, L., and Edelson, R. (Eds.). (1988). Endocrine, metabolic and immunologic functions of keratinocytes. *Ann. N.Y. Acad. Sci.* 548.
205. Wolf, J., and Harrison, R. (1973). Demonstration and characterization of an epidermal angiogenic factor. *J. Invest. Dermatol.* 61:130–141.
206. Malhotra, R., Stenn, K., Fernandez, L., and Braverman, I. (1989). Angiogenic properties of normal and psoriatic skin associated with epidermis, not dermis. *Lab. Invest.* 61:162–165.
207. Folkman, J. (1972). Angiogenesis in psoriasis: Therapeutic implications. *J. Invest. Dermatol.* 59:40–43.
208. Nanney, L., McKanna, J., Stoscheck, C., Carpenter, G., and King, L. (1984). Visualization of epidermal growth factor receptors in human epidermis. *J. Invest. Dermatol.* 82:165–169.
209. Prober, J. (1988). Cytokine-mediated activation of vascular endothelium. *Am. J. Pathol.* 133:426–433.

210. Taniguchi, T. (1988). Regulation of cytokine gene expression. *Ann. Rev. Immunol.* 6:439–464.
211. Balkwill, F., and Burke, F. (1989). The cytokine network. *Immunol. Today* 10:299–304.
212. Dianzani, U., Malavasi, F. (1995). Lymphocyte adhesion to endothelium. *Crit. Rev. Immunol.* 15: 167–200.
213. Bevilacqua, M.P., Nelson, R.M., Mannori, G., Cecconi, O. (1994). Endothelial-leukocyte adhesion molecules in human disease. *Ann. Rev. Med.* 45:361–378.
214. Barker, J.N. (1995). Adhesion molecules in cutaneous inflammation. *Ciba Foundation Symposium* 189: 91–101.
215. Jeffes, E.W., III, McCullough, J.L., Pittelkow, M.R., McCormick, A., Almanzor, J., Liu, G., Dang, M., Voss, K., Voss, J., and Schlotzhauer, A. (1995). Methotrexate therapy of psoriasis: differential sensitivity of proliferating lymphoid and epithelial cells to the cytotoxic and growth-inhibitory effects of methotrexate. *J. Invest. Dermatol.* 104:183–188.

16

Cell Proliferation Kinetics

Gerald D. Weinstein, Ross S. Kaplan, and Jerry L. McCullough
University of California School of Medicine, Irvine, California

The clinical lesion of psoriasis is marked by extensive scaling and a thickened epidermis. Both characteristics have a clinicopathological correlation with the hyperplasia of the psoriatic epidermis that has been elucidated in the past 2 decades. The earliest suggestions of hyperproliferation in psoriasis were based on mitotic counts as a means of measuring cell and tissue renewal in involved epidermis compared to normal skin. In 1963, Van Scott suggested and quantitated the concept of "hyperplasia of psoriasis" based on the finding of 27 times as many mitoses per unit surface area in psoriatic epidermis (Ps) compared to normal-appearing uninvolved skin (UnPs) (1). Many studies have since confirmed the substantially higher mitotic counts in Ps, but without accurate measurement of the *duration* of the mitotic event, other kinetic parameters concerning the hyperplastic process cannot be obtained. Efforts to use mitotic activity (stathmokinetic studies) as a measure of cell proliferation have been explored utilizing mitosis-arresting drugs, but these have generally been unsuccessful (2).

Basic biological and cancer research has led to many conceptual and practical developments concerning cell and tissue renewal in living organisms. Foremost in this area have been methods to measure the rate of cell proliferation using factors such as cell cycle time, growth fractions, and labeling indices. The apparent differences in proliferative activity in normal and psoriatic epidermis suggested by Van Scott have led to many studies that attempt to define precisely if, where, and to what extent there are kinetic defects in psoriasis compared with normal skin. This chapter reviews the principal concepts and presents evidence for three proliferative defects in psoriasis: an eightfold shortening of the psoriatic cell cycle, a doubling of the proliferative cell population, and an approximate doubling of the growth fraction.

In recent years molecular markers have been identified that can now separate more precisely three populations of cells that are constituents of the proliferative epidermis: stem cells, transient amplifying cells (actively proliferating cells), and differentiating cells. This technology now supplements the earlier techniques utilizing mitotic cell activity and thymidine-labeled cells to understand the proliferative components of the psoriatic pathophysiology.

TRANSIT TIMES

The availability of radioactively labeled compounds has permitted a different and more sophisticated approach to the study of human epidermal regeneration in vivo. The amino acid [^{14}C]-glycine was used as a marker for protein synthesis to label epidermal protein and its appearance was then measured in the stratum corneum (3). Epidermal protein was found at the surface of psoriatic stratum corneum in only 2 days, whereas it took 13–14 days to appear in the surface stratum corneum of normal epidermis. These values were the first measurements of transit or turnover times in a human epidermal compartment; namely, stratum corneum. Using the [^{14}C[-glycine-derived transit times and mitotic counts, Van Scott (1) calculated turnover times of 27 and 4 days in normal and psoriatic epidermis, respectively.

The use of tritiated thymidine ([^{3}H]-thymidine) as a marker for deoxyribonucleic acid (DNA) synthesis together with autoradiography provided better techniques for the measurement of transit times. When [^{3}H]-thymidine is injected into normal epidermis, intermittent cell labeling is seen in the germinative cell compartment consisting of the first and second rows. Autoradiographs of biopsy specimens obtained 1 hr after injection show approximately 3% labeling of cells in the basal row. When multiple skin sites were injected with [^{3}H]-thymidine and biopsy specimens obtained sequentially over 16 days, labeled cells were found migrating distally (4,5). At 1 week, labeled cells were found in the midepidermis as a front of migrating cells. At 10–14 days, the first labeled cells were found at the granular cell layer just below the stratum corneum. These transit times measure the first cells leaving the germinative compartment as they move through the differentiated cell compartment in a reproducible manner for different skin conditions. Such a measurement reflects only the turnover time of the middle compartment of the epidermis and does not include, but does reflect in part, the proliferative activity of the germinative cell compartment.

The transit time in psoriatic epidermis was measured in the same manner. In the original study (4), labeled cells were found just below the stratum corneum at 48 hr and in subsequent subjects this occurred as early as 36 hr. In two patients, labeled nuclei were seen in the outermost layers of the parakeratotic stratum corneum at 96 hr (4). It thus appears that the mean transit times of labeled cells through the viable differentiated cell compartment are 12.0 and 1.75 days in normal and psoriatic epidermis, respectively. Some question has been raised as to whether these are minimum or average transit times. Unfortunately, no direct experimental approaches at this time clarify that point, but based on the total evidence of available cell kinetic data and the models presented below, we believe these to be mean transit times.

Several studies using isotopic-labeled compounds or fluorescent compounds have provided evidence that normal stratum corneum has a transit time of about 14 days with some values to 21 days (7,8). These numbers vary depending on the body location for sampling, routine skin care that might remove surface scale, and/or experimental manipulations that can provoke a hyperproliferative response. In the psoriatic stratum corneum, the transit time appears to be 2 days (4). An interesting but unexplained parallel is the finding of approximately equal transit times in the viable and nonviable differentiated compartments of both normal and psoriatic epidermis.

CELL CYCLE ANALYSIS

What is responsible for the shorter transit time of cells through the obviously thicker epidermis of psoriasis? Several theories have been proposed, including a shortened cell cycle time, different growth fractions, and/or an increased cell population in psoriasis. The best available information indicates that each of these three factors plays a role in the hyperplasia of psoriasis, with the alterations in cell cycle times being the predominant factor. The movement of cells through the epidermis appears to be the result of cell proliferation in the germinative compartment that is continually producing new cells by mitosis. With the underlying dermis providing a firm barrier, each new daughter cell must force another cell (or itself) out of the germinative compartment and into the differentiated cell compartment. Likewise, a cell must migrate upward from the differentiated to the stratum corneum compartment, forcing a concurrent loss of a cell at the surface. In this manner a constantly renewing epidermis of the same size is maintained with kinetic homeostasis. The rate of cell proliferation in the germinative compartment is a critical factor in understanding the pathophysiology of psoriasis.

Availability of tritiated thymidine made possible a more detailed study of the life cycle of germinative cells. The cell cycle can be divided into four main phases: G_1 phase; the S, or DNA synthesis phase; the G_2 or "resting" phase; and the M, or mitotic phase (Fig. 1). The classic cell cycle also includes the possibility for a G_0 population. The G_0 population represents *potential* proliferative cells in a resting or inactive position that can be induced to enter into the active cycling state by specific stimuli. Until recently, G_0 cells could not be identified by available histological techniques, and thus be separated from G_1 cells. Recent advances in cell receptor molecular identification techniques allow for cells in the G_0 phase to be studied. Based on analysis of integrins, molecules involved in cell-to-cell adhesion, keratinocytes in the different stages of the cycle can now be identified with a measure of certainty (55). If G_0 cells are present

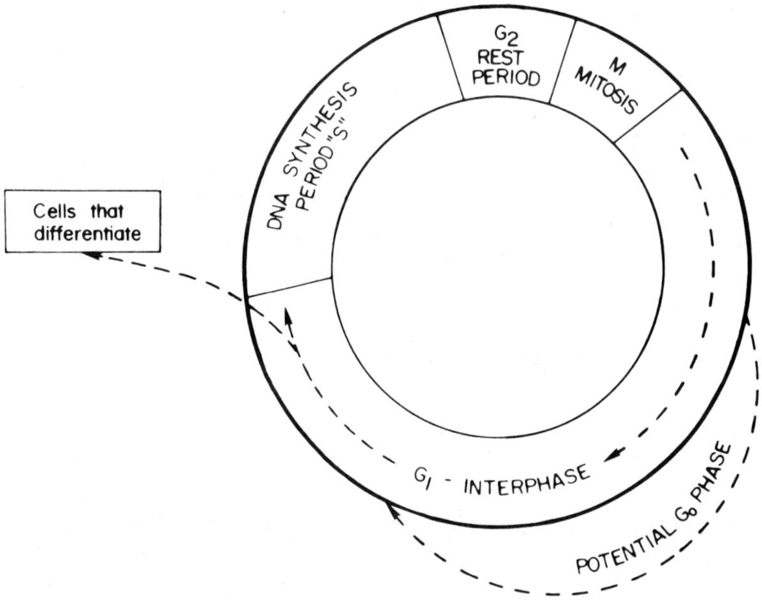

Figure 1 The proliferative (germinative) cell cycle. The cell cycle is divided into four phases described in the text. The G_0 phase represents a potential population of cells in a "resting" state that can be stimulated to reenter the cell cycle by various triggers. On the average, one of every two daughter cells of mitosis must leave the germinative cell cycle to differentiate.

within a defined germinative cell population, then the growth fraction (GF) will be less than unity (100%). The GF is the ratio of actively proliferating cell per total number of cells in the defined proliferative compartment, that is, the basal row. Earlier studies of epidermal kinetics presumed that all basal cells were actively proliferating, but current studies now suggest a growth fraction of 60% in normal epidermis (see below).

The proliferative (or germinative) cell population has generally been considered to be a relatively homogeneous keratinocyte population (excluding melanocytes) in the basal layer and to a lesser extent in the second row where there is an admixture with differentiating cells. In recent years, there has been the suggestion that there may be two kinetically separate subpopulations which consist of stem cells and transient amplifying cells (46,47). In the deep rete ridges of monkey palm epidermis higher labeling was found in the suprabasal layers, thought to be transient amplifying cells, compared to the basal layer "stem cells" (46). Since the deep rete ridge really reflects a relative area of acanthosis, the higher labeling index may be simply required to supply more differentiated cells in that "column" of epidermal cells. In human skin, there is no evidence that these two cell subpopulations are really present or in monkey epidermis that there is a kinetic difference in their proliferative behavior. In human epidermis, most labeling (approximately 70%) is in the basal layer as contrasted to the monkey palm epidermis. The kinetic discussions of normal and psoriatic epidermis in this paper will assume that the proliferative cells are inhomogeneous populations. The mean values may reflect some heterogeneity from variations in the duration of cell cycle compartments of individual cells.

Several experimental approaches allow analysis of the cell cycle depending on the type of cell population, whether animal or human, in vivo or in vitro, location on or in the body, and other variables. In human epidermis, the earliest technique utilized mitotic counts with or without mitotic inhibitors. Van Scott's classic description of the hyperplasia of psoriasis was based on mitotic count information. Absolute time components of the cell cycle could not be obtained with reproducible accuracy with this method.

To determine absolute time parameters for the cell cycle, tritiated thymidine, incorporating as a precursor of new DNA formation, is used. [^{3}H]-Thymidine was injected into both normal and psoriatic skin with sequential biopsy specimens obtained at 3-hr intervals (10). The labeling index from the 1-hr pulse injections provides a measure of the number of cells in DNA synthesis at any time. The germinative labeling index

(LI) is the percentage of labeled basal cells per 100 basal cells. When different tissues are compared, the LI can be considered a crude measurement of proliferative activity subject to several variables, including the duration of the S period, the growth fraction, and the delineation of the proliferative (germinative) cell compartment.

Further information on cell cycle parameters is obtained by following the cells moving as a labeled cohort around the cell cycle through its different phases. Specimens are obtained at sequential times after [^{3}H]-thymidine injections. A fraction of labeled mitoses (FLM) curve is obtained by counting the percentage of labeled mitoses/total mitoses at 3-hr intervals (Fig. 2). If adequate sequential specimens can be obtained, then it is sometimes possible to obtain a second peak on the FLM curve resulting from the labeled cell cohort cycling a second time. Although the double-peaked FLM curve has been shown in many animal and tissue culture experiments, psoriasis is the only human study demonstrating such a curve. The distance between the two peaks in a double-peaked FLM curve equivalent to the cell cycle time is the most direct and the preferred technique for quantitating the cell cycle duration. The double-peaked psoriatic FLM curve in Figure 2 provides a cell cycle duration for psoriasis of approximately 36 hr. A double-peaked curve for normal epidermis has not yet been obtained because of the large number of biopsy specimens and amount of isotope injection required. The cell cycle duration for normal epidermis has been obtained in the past by the "stage-duration method" utilizing the following equation:

$$\frac{N_s}{N_{gc} \times \mathrm{GF}} = \frac{T_s}{T_c}$$

where N_s is the number of cells in DNA synthesis, N_{gc} is the total number of proliferative cells, and N_s/N_{gc} is the labeling index. T_s and T_c represent the duration of the S period and total germinative cycle, respectively. N_s, N_{gc}, and T_s can be determined experimentally, from which T_c can be calculated. In the past, assumptions have included a GF of 100% and a rectangular age distribution (12). If the GF is less than 100%, the T_c would be proportionally decreased.

NORMAL EPIDERMIS

In normal epidermis, the labeling index varied from 2.2 to 3.8% (13–15). The LI obtained from 23 normal subjects in our studies is 2.7 ± 1.2% and is used in the computations below. The only direct measurement of T_s available from FLM data is 14 hr (14,28). A growth factor of approximately 60% has been found in normal skin by the continuous administration of intravenous [^{3}H]-thymidine to patients with multiple myeloma (16). Whether the malignant disease process or prior chemotherapy has influenced epidermal kinetics is not known; this study provides the only human in vivo data on the epidermal growth fraction. The GF of 60% is supported by studies of normal human skin transplanted to nude mice that have produced GF values ranging from 55 to 100% (12,17,18). Additional studies that back up high epidermal GF values in the 80–100% range are found in swine and mouse epidermis (28,49). Swine epidermis is a very good model for human epidermal kinetics with similar proven values for transit times (50) and LI. The T_c for normal epidermal cells, calculated by the stage duration method, is 311 hr using the values of LI = 2.7%; T_s = 14 hr; GF = 60%, incorporated into the above equation.

Bauer et al. have studied the GF in normal epidermis by the "nonphysiological" technique of cutaneous tape-stripping (48). Using flow cytometry, they estimate the GF to be 20–40%. Even if one uses the midpoint value of 30% as the GF, it would reduce the T_c of normal epidermal cells from 311 hr to 155 hr using the above equation. The latter value would still reflect a substantially different or fourfold longer cell cycle time than psoriasis. The difficulty with a tape-stripping stimulus, just like ultraviolet and other traumatic stimuli to the skin, is that G_0 and/or G_1 cells may be induced rapidly into proliferation and subsequent mitosis. Thus, the physiological mechanisms of the skin are being significantly altered and, therefore, not providing a true picture of the homeostasis in normal epidermal kinetics.

UNINVOLVED SKIN IN PSORIASIS

The uninvolved skin of psoriatic patients has become an increasingly interesting area for investigation of biological and/or biochemical abnormalities possibly related to the psoriatic process. Several abnormalities involving proliferation kinetics have been reported. Using adhesive tape-stripping of normal and UnPs, Braun-Falco et al. (19) found a differential increase in the LI of the UnPs. Wiley and Weinstein (20) used intradermal propranolol and found a sixfold increase in LI selectively induced in UnPs. We found the LI about 50% higher in UnPs (4.2% ± 0.9) than in nor-

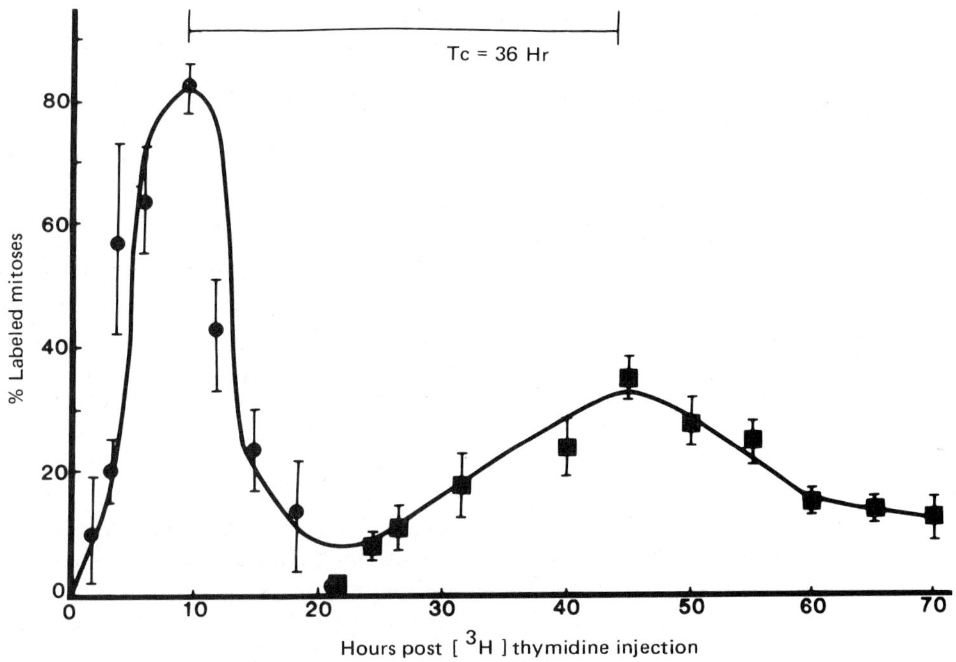

Figure 2 Frequency of labeled mitoses (FLM) curve obtained from two groups of patients. The group of patients represented in the first peak provided the T_s = 8.5 hr and T_{G2} = 4 hr (10). The second group of six patients was studied between 20 and 75 hr after [^{3}H]-thymidine injection (28). The distance between the two peaks represents the direct approach to determine the duration of the psoriatic cell cycle. (From Ref. 28.)

mal skin (14), and other investigators have made similar observations (21,22).

In an innovative approach two groups of investigators transplanted N_s, UnPs, and Ps to nude mice and obtained labeling indices (23,24). While the LI of N_s remained at the low pretransplantation levels, the LI of UnPs increased to that of the Ps skin (which decreased slightly). The kinetic behavior of UnPs resembles that of Ps rather than N_s in an environment outside of the human subject; the reasons for this are not known (see below). Aside from the LIs there is no experimental information available to determine either the T_c or GF in UnPs. The one direct measurement of T_s by an FLM curve includes few patients and time points, but suggests a T_s of 12.5 hr, which is not different from the value for N_s noted above (21). It appears that the kinetic behavior of UnPs should be considered comparable to N_s on the basis of clinical, histological, and LI similarities. The GF ratio, based on the G_1/G_0 fraction value of approximately 60%, is supported by recent studies (55), which can stain for β-integrin positive cells (corresponding to G_0 phase), and accurately differentiate the two populations for numerical analysis.

In uninvolved (nonlesional) skin from patients with psoriasis there is an altered response to immune stimulation. The stem cells, identified as β-integrin+, K1/K10-, keratinocytes, are hyperresponsive in their reaction to T-cell-produced lymphokines, relative to stem cells from patients without the disease. Clinically, this is reflected in what is known as the Koebner phenomenon; where uninvolved skin can be seen to react with psoriatic hyperplasia to a traumatic insult.

PSORIASIS

The cell cycle duration (T_c) of psoriatic proliferative cells, which generally occupy the lower two or three rows of the epidermis, has been measured by both the stage-duration and the direct FLM method. The in vivo LI determined initially for psoriasis was 22.7%, which included a 1.4 correction factor (10). Although these results were subject to criticism by Gelfant (25), he subsequently confirmed a high LI of 21.2 ± 1.0% for psoriasis using a long autoradiographic exposure, which has a similar net effect to the 1.4 correction factor (22). Utilization of the correction factor by

Weinstein and Frost (10) led to a close approximation of the FLM-derived T_c. Two other groups have found lower LIs in psoriasis of 10.3% and 11.0% using intradermal [^{3}H]-thymidine (26,27). Technical differences in these studies may account for the lower LIs (28).

The T_s for psoriasis obtained by the FLM method in our studies was 8.5 hr (10). Similar values of 9.8 and 7.7 hr have been found with the direct FLM method by Goodwin et al. and Duffil et al. (26,27). Utilizing our values of LI = 22.7% and T_s = 8.5 hr, the T_c of psoriasis was calculated to be 37.5 hr by the stage-duration method (10). A GF of 100% was assumed for psoriatic epidermis.

The optimal approach for quantitating the T_c of a proliferating cell population is to obtain the second peak in the FLM curve. Based on the consistency of the first FLM peak in three separate studies of psoriasis, a search for a second FLM peak in another series of psoriatic patients was carried out (28). In six additional patients [^{3}H]-thymidine-injected sites were biopsied sequentially from 27 to 70 hr later. The time range for the study was estimated from the previously determined T_s of 37.5 hr. A double-peaked curve was obtained by combining the FLM results of the first study (10) with the new information (see Fig. 2). The second peak was found at 45 hr, reaching a level of approximately 40% labeled mitoses. As in most other animal studies, the second peak is damped, indicating some dispersion of cell cycle times as a result of asynchronous movement of the labeled cohort of cells. The distance between the two peaks provides a direct measurement of the mean T_c of 36 hr. This value confirms the previously determined T_c of 37.5 hr by the stage-duration method. The combined data of this FLM curve has also been computer analyzed by Dr. M. Mendelsohn (Lawrence Livermore Laboratories, University of California). The results of this analysis resemble the hand analysis. The coefficient of variation (standard deviation expressed as a percentage of the mean) for the psoriatic T_c is 0.28 and indicates only a small difference in the rates at which individual cells move around the cell cycle. The cell cycle parameters for normal and psoriatic epidermis are summarized in Table 1.

Table 1 Cell Cycle: Normal and Psoriatic Epidermis

	Duration (hr)				
	S	G_2	M	G_1	CC
Normal	14	10	1	286	311
Psoriatic	8.5	4	0.3	23	36

GROWTH FRACTION

The initial stage-duration method analysis assumed a GF of 100%. The first study aimed at defining the proliferative cell population by measuring the GF used the pharmacological effects of methotrexate followed by [^{3}H]-thymidine. Since methotrexate blocks DNA synthesis for at least 12 hr after intradermal administration, it was injected into psoriatic sites three times at 12-hr intervals to produce a cumulative 36-hr drug effect (29). In this manner cells already in the S phase when first exposed to methotrexate and those cells subsequently arriving at the S phase during the 36 hr should be blocked in that phase. Subsequently injection of [^{3}H]-thymidine at 36 hr should label all those cells sequestered in the S phase. If the T_c is approximately 36 hr and the GF is 100%, then all the cells in the proliferative compartment should be labeled. As seen in Figure 3, essentially 100% of the cells were labeled in the area designated as the proliferative compartment: the bottom three to four rows in the acanthotic areas which contain the mitotic figures, the thymidine-labeled cells, and the cells with relatively greater nuclear/cytoplasmic ratios. The results of this experiment showed (1) the location and demarcation of the proliferative cell compartment; (2) the T_c to be approximately 36 hr or less; and (3) the GF to be approximately 100%. The demarcation of the proliferative compartment occurred because methotrexate, by inhibiting DNA synthesis, which blocks cell division, prevents upward migration of proliferative cells and left all the accumulated (labeled) S-phase cells in their initial compartment.

Since methotrexate, as a chemotherapeutic agent, could possibly pharmacologically alter the epidermal kinetics, an additional study was performed using four repeated intradermal [^{3}H]-thymidine injections at 12-hr intervals over 36-hr (12). (Ideally, continuous intravenous thymidine infusion for at least 2 days would be the preferable method to obtain a GF in psoriasis, but this type of experiment is unlikely in patients with benign disease.) Control areas were injected with saline × 3 followed by a single injection of [^{3}H]-thymidine. The LI of the proliferative compartment approximates 100%, whereas in the control psoriatic

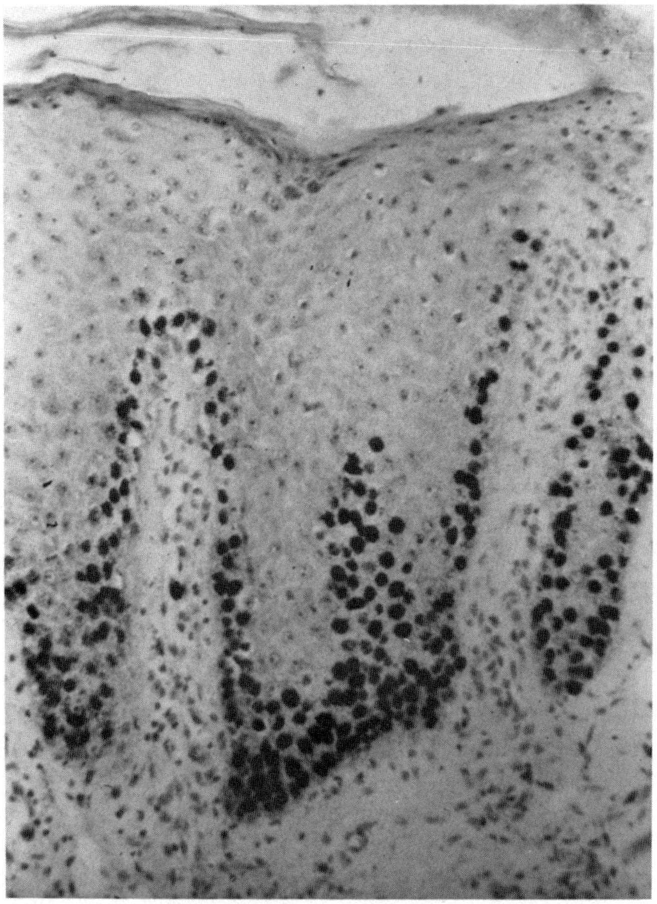

Figure 3 The proliferative cell population of the psoriatic epidermis is demonstrated by [^{3}H]-thymidine labeling of all putative proliferative cells (see text). This suggests that the growth fraction in psoriasis approximates 100%. In this experiment methotrexate was injected intradermally into the same patch of psoriasis three times at 12-hr intervals, followed by a single injection of [^{3}H]-thymidine. (From Ref. 29.)

site the LI is approximately 30%, a little above the normal psoriatic LI. It appears that the multiple intradermal injections did not stimulate a significant number of potential G_0 cells into the active cycling phase. In this GF experiment, in contrast to the methotrexate GF study, cell division continues with upward migration of labeled cells through the differentiated compartment. Labeled cells are seen just below the stratum corneum at 36 hr, which is similar to when only a single [^{3}H]-thymidine injection is used 36 hr earlier to obtain a transit time. A third approach that confirms the 100% GF in psoriasis is based on mathematical calculations relating to the age distribution of psoriatic cells in the cell cycle. This information is discussed in detail elsewhere (12).

KINETIC MODEL FOR NORMAL AND PSORIATIC EPIDERMAL PROLIFERATION

It is now possible to develop a kinetic model of cell proliferation for the epidermis in the normal and psoriatic state. The epidermis, as a constantly renewing cell population, must maintain a kinetic equilibrium involving its three major cell compartments: the proliferative, viable differentiated, and stratum corneum compartments. The rate of birth/entry, transit, and/or loss of keratinocytes in each compartment must be of the same order of magnitude to maintain both kinetic and physiological homeostasis in the epidermis. Kinetic information developed from separate studies on all compartments can be interrelated in a model that helps to confirm the values of the component parts. This model requires information on the number of cells and rate of cell movement in each compartment.

While cell counts can be obtained relatively easily from histological sections, identifying whether individual cells are in the proliferative or differentiated compartments is more difficult. In normal epidermis, the distribution of labeled and mitotic cells is mainly in the first or basal row and, to a lesser extent, in the second row. As measured in a detailed three-dimensional study of normal skin autoradiographs, 68% of all labeled cells are in the basal row and the remaining 32% are in the second row (39). From data on the LI of the first and second rows and the percentage of suprabasal labeled cells (30), we have calculated that 72% of the cells in the second row belong to the proliferative compartment in addition to those in the basal row (14). The remaining cells in the second row (28%) plus all viable cells in the distal rows (stratum malpighii) are considered the viable differentiated cell compartment. Cell counts were obtained from microphotographs of epidermis and extrapolated to values per square millimeter of surface length. The values are expressed in a schematic representation of epidermis (Fig. 4) and show an almost equal number of cells in the proliferative and differentiated cell compartments: 270 and 268 cells, respectively (14).

On examining epidermis microscopically, the cells of these compartments differ in size, which must be taken into consideration to obtain absolute cell counts. On a three-dimensional basis, the average diameter of a proliferative cell is 10.1 $\mu \pm 0.84$ (SD) and of a differentiated cell is 16.2 $\mu \pm 2.4$. These numbers can be combined with the cell counts above to get the number of cells under 1 mm^2 of surface area (SA) for each compartment (12). In the proliferative compartment under 1 mm^2 SA there would be 100 slices 10 μ thick, each containing 270 cells, totaling 27,000 cells in the proliferative compartment. The total viable cell count (proliferative and differentiated compartments) adds up to 44,000 cells/mm^2 SA (see Fig. 4), which is almost identical to the value of 47,000 cells found by Bergstresser and Taylor (31) using different methodology.

A similar approach is used to quantitate cells in the psoriatic epidermis. Using the definition of the psoriatic proliferative compartment described earlier, the proliferative cell population is calculated to have 52,000 cells/mm^2 SA (twice normal) and an almost equal number of differentiated cells; 47,000 (see Fig. 4).

The rate of cell movement (birth or transit rate) per day in each compartment can be quantitated using the cell counts, cell cycles or transit times, and growth fractions. In the normal proliferative compartment, there are 16,200 cells (60% of 27,000) actively cycling. With a cell cycle duration of 311 hr (13 days) the birth rate/day (BR/d) is 1246 cells (16,200/13) (Fig. 5). Equilibrium within the germinative compartment can only be maintained if a similar number of postmitotic daughter cells exit, presumably on a random basis, into the differentiated cell compartment. In the viable differentiated cell compartment the mean transit time (TT) was earlier shown to be 12 days. From the independent measurements of 17,000 cells/mm^2 surface area and the 12-day TT for the differentiated compartment, a transit rate/day of 1417 cells (17,000/12) is obtained. The stratum corneum compartment has been computed to have a cell loss/day of 1490 cells/mm^2 SA (31). The similarities of the "turnover" rates in the three compartments independently derived strongly confirm the proposed kinetic model of epidermal homeostasis.

The turnover time of the normal epidermis in its entirety consists of the sum of the turnover (cell cycle or transit) times of the individual compartments. The stratum corneum TT is approximately 14 days (4,7). The mean epidermal turnover time is, therefore, 39 days: 13 days for the proliferative compartment, 12 days for the viable differentiated cells, and 14 days for the stratum corneum.

A kinetic model for psoriasis can be established in a similar manner. In psoriasis, the BR/d is 35,000 cells and the TT/d is 27,000 cells (see Fig. 5). Considering the accuracy of the experimental procedures, these rates are remarkably similar, indicating a kinetic equilibrium for these two compartments. For the stratum corneum compartment the transit time appears to be approximately 2 days (4), but no information is available on a cell count to obtain a transit rate through the cornified layers. From the data presented in Figure 5, the rate of cell proliferation in psoriasis is 28-fold greater than in normal epidermis (35,000 new cells/mm^2/day vs 1246 cells/mm^2/day). This vast increase in cell production must bear the major responsibility for the hyperkeratosis and extensive scaling of the clinical lesion.

Wright (32) and Gelfant (25) hypothesized that the development of the rapidly proliferating psoriatic lesion results from a presumed low GF in normal epidermis changing to a 100% GF in psoriasis. They suggest that there is little or no difference in the cell cycles of normal and psoriatic skin. These hypotheses

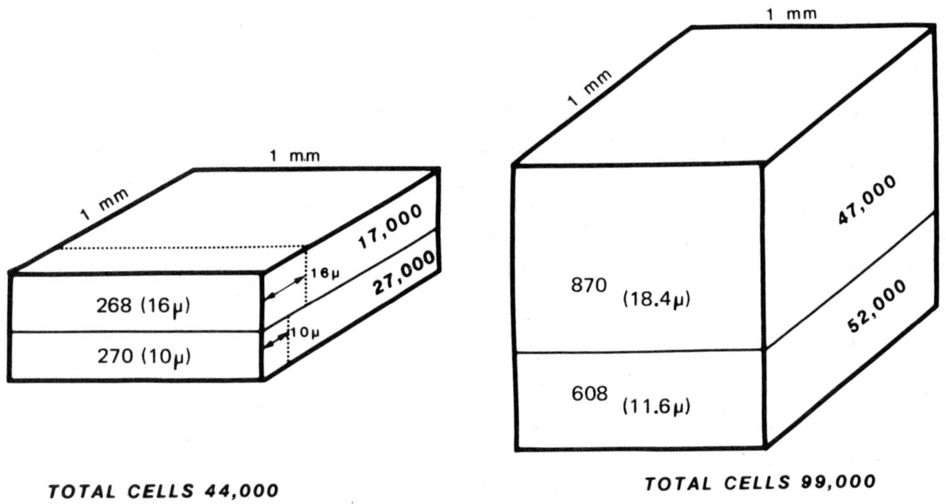

Figure 4 Cell populations of the proliferative and viable differentiated (stratum malpighii) compartments. The numbers on the front of each box (normal epidermis on left) are the cell counts/mm surface length obtained microscopically. The numbers on the side are extrapolated, based on the average cell diameter/compartment, to provide total numbers of cells under 1 mm^2 of surface area. Normal epidermis has approximately half the total number of cells present in psoriasis (see text).

cannot be substantiated by the facts presented above, since the opposite conclusion is obtained. The cell kinetics picture shows an eightfold difference or shortening of the normal T_c from 311 to 36 hr. Furthermore, using Gelfant's data (16) and nude mice experimental results for the normal epidermal GF, the proliferative capacity is shown to increase less than twice, with the change in GF from 60 to 100% accounting for only a small part of the tremendous increase in psoriatic cell production.

The kinetic alterations in transforming "normal" to psoriatic epidermis are summarized in Figure 5. This cell kinetic model contains the three proliferative alterations that have been found: the major kinetic dif-

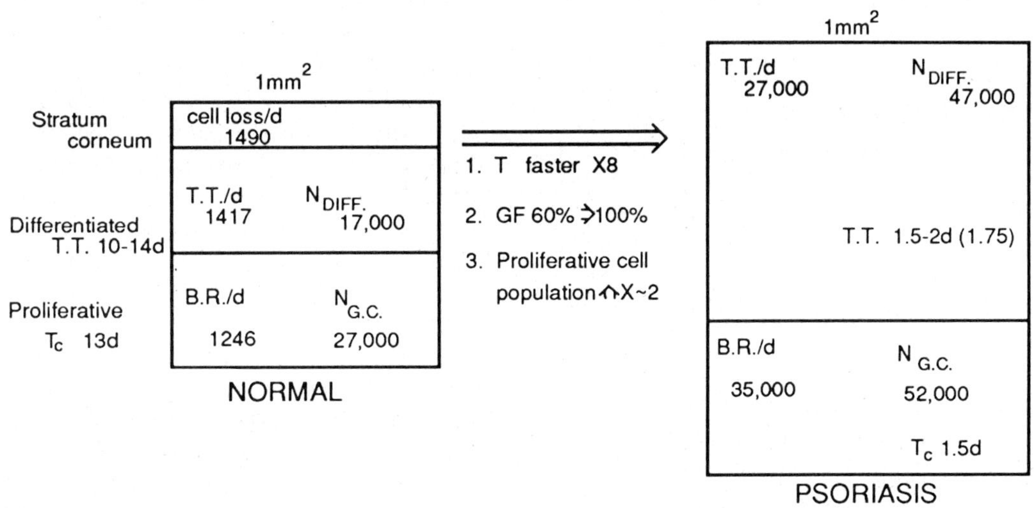

Figure 5 A model of cell proliferation kinetics for normal and psoriatic epidermis. The birth rates or transit rates for each compartment show that a kinetic equilibrium is present in each tissue. The major proliferative defect in psoriasis is accounted for by the eightfold shortening of the cell cycle compared to normal.

ference from the eightfold shortening of T_c, and the two smaller kinetic alterations, an increase in the GF from 60 to 100% and an approximate doubling of the germinative population from 27,000 to 52,000 cells. The calculated birth rate/day of 35,000 cells (52,000/1.5) in psoriasis is obviously adequate to provide the estimated 27,000 cells required in the differentiated compartment. If, however, as proposed by Wright and Gelfant, there is no change in the T_c (if it remains the normal 13 days), then the birth rate in the psoriatic proliferative compartment would only be 4000 cells/day (52,000/13), which is hardly enough to supply the differentiated compartment.

The kinetic model described above is based on information from normal human epidermis and not from the uninvolved epidermis in psoriasis. As described earlier, the UnPs may proliferate at a rate somewhat faster than in N_s, but the only current kinetic information available concerns labeling indices. Based on these LIs, mitotic counts, and histological behavior, it is likely that a complete kinetic picture of UnPs will be similar to that presented using normal skin.

The rapid psoriasis cell cycle has also been used as the basis for the common methotrexate schedule of three doses at 12-hr intervals each week (51). Tissue-drug exposure for 36 hr would theoretically affect the entire population of psoriatic cells, whereas only partially affecting other proliferating tissues with a longer cell cycle, i.e., bone marrow. In this manner, a relative selectively for psoriasis vs other tissues can be obtained by considering just cycle parameters. The pharmacological rationale is discussed in greater detail elsewhere (33). This dosage schedule is used by 74% of dermatologists surveyed (52).

OTHER STUDIES OF NORMAL/PSORIATIC CELL KINETICS

In vitro single- and double-labeling studies have also been utilized to study normal and psoriatic epidermal kinetics. In vitro labeling techniques are subject to potential difficulties, including nonphysiological conditions, questionably adequate penetration of isotope throughout the tissue, and altered enzyme activities and cell substrate pools, any or all of which have led to results somewhat in conflict with those obtained in vivo (12). Born and Kalkoff found fewer grains/labeled cells in psoriasis compared to UnPs and concluded that the T_s and T_c of psoriasis were consequently prolonged (35). This technique is based on [^{3}H]-thymidine grain counts being proportional to the rate of DNA synthesis, and assumes that enzymatic activities and substrate pool sizes are the same in both cell types. Evidence suggests that the de novo pathway is more active in psoriasis for thymidine availability, whereas the opposite is present in normal cells (12). The double-labeling method, when used in vitro, requires physiological incorporation of [^{14}C] and [^{3}H]-thymidine over incubation times of 2–3 hr. The influence of in vitro conditions is seen with an average LI in psoriatic patients of 10.2 ± 3.3%, which is much lower than in vivo values (12,34). The data presented by Galosi et al. using in vitro double-labeling technique give shorter T_s values in normal skin (7.2–9.0 hr) and longer values in psoriatic epidermis (10.5–13.6 hr) (36). The computations from this study produce a reversal of T_s values compared to direct in vivo methods presented elsewhere in this chapter. The large variations in LIs and the combined use of [^{14}C] and [^{3}H]-thymidine incubations in skin specimens raise serious questions about the validity of these values. It is apparent that the in vitro techniques producing prolonged cell cycles in psoriasis compared to normal do not fit the in vivo kinetic models presented.

Heenen et al. have developed a mathematical model of cell renewal suggesting that the psoriatic lesion cannot be induced only by an increase in the turnover rate of the germinative cell population (53). They postulate that a reduced transit time in the differentiated cell compartment leading to a less functional stratum corneum and premature shedding of these cells provides for the stimulus to increased proliferative cell production. This would appear to be the conundrum of the chicken or egg question—Which comes first? While the question of the trigger site in the pathophysiological process in psoriasis, proliferative or differentiated cell compartments, is still unresolved, many other biochemical or cytokine systems are being investigated for their possible influence on one or both of these epidermal cell compartments. Furthermore, one cannot easily compare other "hyperproliferative" diseases such as epidermolytic hyperkeratosis and pityriasis rubra pilaris for the relative sizes of their proliferative and differentiated cell compartments versus psoriasis. There must be other inherent pathological abnormalities for each of these conditions above and beyond the parameters of cell proliferation and differentiation.

KINETICS OF CELL PROLIFERATION UTILIZING MOLECULAR MARKERS

Molecular Differentiation of the Stem Cell Population

Based on studies of the structural, morphological, and anatomical location of regenerative cells in the skin, they can be classified into separate populations. There appear to be at least three types (phases) of keratinocytes: stem cells, transient amplifying cells, and committed cells.

Stem cells are highly self-regenerative, capable of undergoing replication many times. These are the cells thought to be in the G_0 phase of the cell cycle and are in a resting or quiescent state. Transit amplifying cells are the daughters of stem cells, capable of one to five rounds of division, and produce mostly committed cells (1). Committed cells are terminally differentiated. These cells have detached from the basement membrane and are in transit, as a result of cell turnover to the cornified surface of the skin. As the cells move their physical location in the strata and change in their morphology, molecular markers found on the cell surface, as well as those produced by the keratinocyte, are useful in separating and studying the varying subpopulations. Initially, the lack of reliable markers to distinguish the different cell populations hindered attempts to correlate cell cycle analysis to psoriasis. Radiolabeling studies using tritiated thymidine could be used to identify the proliferating cell population. However, there was no way to study the nonproliferating "stem" cell population. With the development of molecular staining techniques (monoclonal antibodies), we can now isolate the different populations of keratinocytes and study their behavior in disease states.

β-Integrins

Stem cells are found in the basal layers of the skin, connected both to the basement membrane and to one another. The class of cell-to-cell adhesive molecules known as β-integrins is found in an abundance in the stem cell population (55). Using fluorescent monoclonal antibodies to these integrins, these cells can now be elucidated. Cells abundant in β-integrins are well correlated to the histological localization of the stem cells.

Keratin Expression

Stem cells are in a state of high potential for regeneration and are thus less differentiated than cells found higher in the stratum. This correlates with the lack of differentiated keratins found in these cells. Staining techniques for keratins show stem cells to be $K1^-/K10^-$ (based on monoclonal antibody staining of keratin subsets).

PCNA Expression

While β-integrins and keratin expression are markers of cell differentiation that can be used to isolate stem cell populations, another marker, PCNA, can be used as an indicator of cell proliferation. Proliferating cell nuclear antigen (PCNA) can be used both to identify the stem cell populations and to study the dynamics of their recruitment. Stem cells are $PCNA^-$ (57). PCNA is a DNA polymerase molecule appearing early in G_1, when it becomes positive, becomes more abundant during S phase, and then diminishes during G_2 and M phase. Initially, stem cells are $PCNA^-$; however, once the cycle of proliferation begins, regardless of the source of stimulus, the PCNA expression is upregulated ($PCNA^+$), and can be followed as an indicator of proliferation. A portrait of the stem cell population emerges for cells identifiable by the molecular marker systems:

Stem cells: β-integrin$^+$, $K1/K10^-$ $PCNA^-$

Transient amplifying cells, and committed cells, are distinguished from the stem cell population in the respect of diminishing β-integrin expression, with increased positive K1/K10 and PCNA expression.

Stem Cell Activation and Proliferation

Since stem cells are a resting population of cells, they can be viewed as a reserve population, waiting for specific signals to increase their proliferative activity and undergo differentiation. When these quiescent cells (G_0, diploid DNA, $PCNA^-$, thymidine$^3H^-$), are activated, they undergo the transition from G_0 to G_1. Stem cells are usually slowly cycling. Studies indicate that 95% of β-integrin$^+$ cells are in the G_0 phase and do not express K1/K10 antigens because they remain, for the most part, undifferentiated. Recruitment of the stem cells from the G_0 to G_1 phase involves stimulation by direct injury, or immune mechanisms.

Lymphokine Stimulation of Keratinocytes

A growing body of information points to the evidence that products of lymphatic cells, cytokines, serve to initiate activation and proliferation of keratinocytes. In vitro experimentation with T-cell factors, IL-3, and

GM-CSF showed a pronounced stimulatory effect on keratinocyte colony formation and growth. In the same in vitro experiments, IFN-γ was shown to be an *inhibitor* of proliferation. When the same experiments were conducted on keratinocytes from psoriatic individuals, the in vivo results were the opposite. IFN-γ, in the presence of IL-3 and GM-CSF, acts as a *stimulator* of growth (56). The induction of quiescent cells into the proliferating cycle is localized in β-intergrin$^+$, K1/K10$^-$ populations of keratinocytes, which are recruited into action by the combination of lymphokines. Quiescent (G_0) cells, when exposed to the T-cell factors, can be studied by staining for these markers and PCNA expression, which actually precedes the up-regulation of β-integrin$^+$ cells into G_1.

The Role of Lymphocyte Activation in Psoriatic Cell Cycle Analysis

The role of the stem cells in normal or uninvolved epidermis, a population in which the majority (95%) are resting in G_0, may be to provide a source of additional cells for the rapid reaction of skin to injury. With the identification of a quiescent population of cells as stem cells, the disease of psoriasis may be related to the aberrant response of this group of reserve cells. The altered role of lymphokines or an exaggerated response may be involved, as evidenced by the interleukin studies. However, the common denominator in the psoriatic response seems to be the conversion of the stem cell population from a predominantly resting one to a population with the majority of its constituents in the proliferative (G_1) state. Increased cell cycle entry of the normally quiescent population by lymphocyte activation seems to be a plausible explanation of this phenomenon and is consistent with the clinical observation of the improvement that immunosuppressive agents provide.

Recruitment of the Stem Cell Population in Psoriasis

In studies using radiolabeled thymidine, it was found that approximately 60% of normal epidermal basal cells were located in the "proliferating" compartment (16). It was then inferred that there was a resting (G_0), stem cell population that accounted for the remaining 40% of the basal keratinocytes. The recent advances in molecular staining techniques have allowed researchers to also demonstrate the existence of the stem cell population and to accurately estimate their percentage of the basal population in normal epidermis at approximately 40%. This confirms the calculated estimates based on the previous radiolabeling studies. Recent studies have shown that it is the stem cell population, identified by its molecular markers (β-integrin$^+$, K1/K10$^-$) which is recruited from essentially no activity, as measured by PCNA, to nearly 100% activation. The addition of the stem cell compartment to the normally proliferative compartment accounts for much of the increase (of the total proliferative compartment) seen in the disease state of psoriasis.

CYTOPHOTOMETRIC ANALYSES

Deoxyribonucleic acid cytophotometry has been used to study epidermal cell kinetics. With this technique the DNA content of individual cells can be determined to categorize these cells into the G_1, S, or G_2/M phases of the cell cycle. Cytophotometry can be utilized with microscopic methods allowing individual cells in tissue sections or smears to be examined, or by measuring individual cells in a suspension as they *flow* through the spectrophotometer. Grove, using the microspectrophotometric method with Feulgen staining of cellular DNA, found that in normal and psoriatic epidermis, 7.8 and 26.6% of cells were in S phase, respectively (37). These values were similar to the [^{3}H]-thymidine LIs found by Weinstein and Frost (10). Grove converted the spectrophotometric data into estimates of cell cycle times (T_c) and obtained values of 33 hr for psoriasis vs 270 hr for normal epidermis (38), which is close to our present values of 36 and 311 hr.

When epidermal suspensions are used for flow cytophotometric analyses the technique cannot experimentally separate proliferative from differentiated cells, whereas microspectrophotometry can visualize exactly where the cells are from; specifically basal row, mid-stratum-malpighii, etc. As discussed below, our estimate of the ratio of proliferative to viable differentiated cells is approximately 1:1. Using flow cytophotometry, Bauer et al. found 9.7% of total nucleated psoriatic epidermal cells in S phase vs 2.7% in normal epidermis (39,40). If those data are analyzed in light of the 1:1 ratio, then these values would not seem substantially different from the reported in vivo LIs. Additional information on cytophotometric studies is reviewed by Grove (38), McCullough and Weinstein (41), and Bauer et al. (40). The results obtained by these cytophotometric studies all support the concept of a rapid T_c in psoriasis compared to normal.

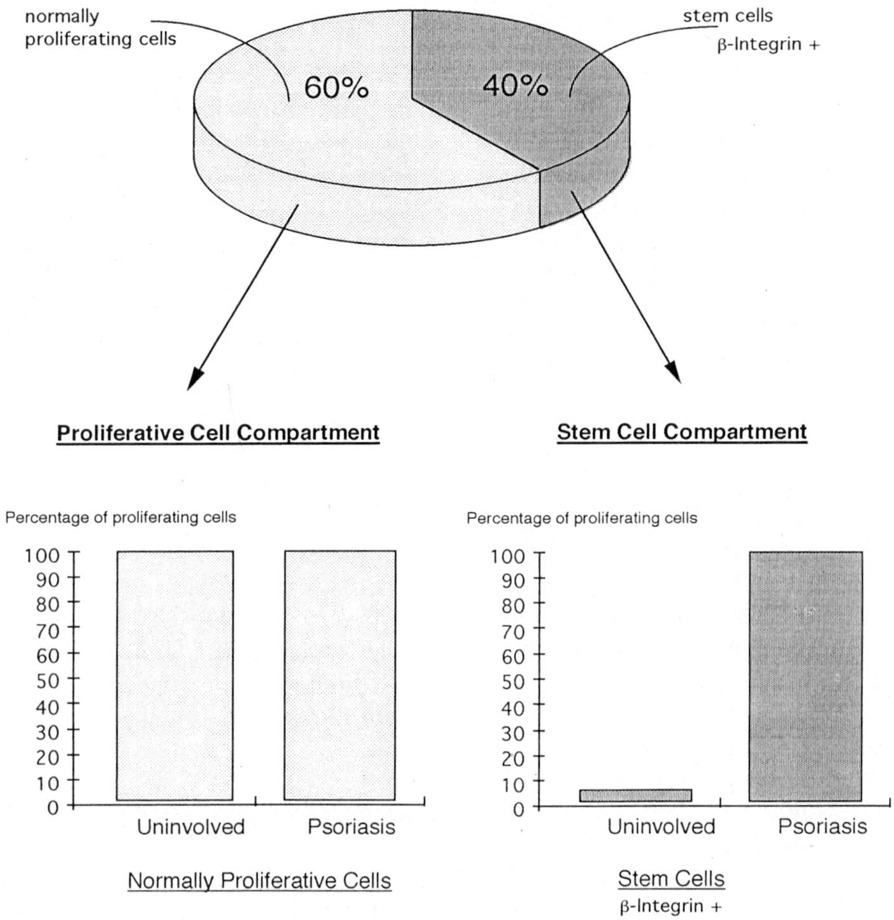

Figure 6 The basal layer is comprised of a ratio of *normally proliferating cells* (β-integrin$^-$, K1/K10$^+$, PCNA$^+$) to *stem cells* (β-integrin$^+$, K1/K10$^-$, PCNA$^+$) of 60% to 40%. In the disease state of psoriasis, the normally proliferating cell group continues to utilize nearly its entire population subgroup. However, the stem cell population mobilizes from only 5% of its members actively proliferating to nearly 100% activity (57).

TISSUE CULTURE AND ANIMAL STUDIES OF CELL KINETICS IN PSORIASIS

Normal and psoriatic epidermal cells have defied most efforts to grow them with classic cell culture techniques. Using short-term outgrowth cultures, Chopra and Flaxman (42) found that normal and psoriatic cells proliferate at similar rates, in the range of 50–60 hr. Liu and Parsons have serially cultivated large quantities of keratinocytes from N_s, UnPs, and Ps (43). They were unable to detect differences in cell proliferation in these three cell types or evidence of hyperproliferation as seen in situ. Harper et al., studying 8- to 10-day-old epidermal outgrowth cultures, found no apparent proliferative differences between UnPs and Ps cells in vitro, although psoriatic epidermal cells did proliferate at a greater rate than normal cells (44).

Another approach to psoriatic kinetics utilized the athymic nude mouse model. Krueger et al. (24) and Fraki et al. (23), transplanting N_s, UnPs, and Ps to nude mice, found that the LIs in UnPs increased significantly toward the psoriatic levels *without comparable increases in normal skin controls.* These animal and in vitro results suggest that when UnPs is removed from its human host in situ it behaves hyperproliferatively. With the exception of Chopra and Flaxman's study (42), normal skin retains a proliferative pattern in these experimental situations as seen in the human subject. The reason(s) for the apparent increased proliferation in the uninvolved epidermis when outside of the human host is not known, but raises interesting questions about cell proliferation controls. One speculation is that there is a systemic or humoral physiological controlling factor normally present but when the tissue is removed it proliferates at the "native or wild" state for keratinocytes (12,24). We have suggested that this "native" state might be the maximum proliferative rate for keratinogenic cells as found in normal hair matrix cells (T_c = 38.8 hr) (45) and in psoriatic cells (T_c = 36 hr). If the normal controlling factors were removed or inactivated locally the result would be a speeding up of the proliferative process and result in the development of a lesion. These possibilities are outlined in Table 2.

The commonly accepted working hypothesis is that the normal cell proliferation rate is indeed the "native" state. Thus, psoriasis, as a hyperplastic disease with a shortened cell cycle, would result from a proliferative *stimulation* of the slowly cycling normal cells.

Paus and Link have also noted the cell cycle similarities of psoriasis and the anagen hair (54). Other observations are also considered such as the parallel effects of systemic steroids and cyclosporine on improving psoriasis and producing hypertrichosis. They suggest there may be common "switch on" mechanisms that should be explored for new insights into epithelial-mesenchymal interactions.

SUMMARY

The kinetics of normal and psoriatic epidermal proliferation are presented. The rapid psoriatic cell cycle duration (36 hr) is confirmed with the first double-peaked FLM curve obtained in human subjects. In contrast to psoriasis, the mean T_c for normal cells is 311 hr, assuming a growth fraction of 60%.

Uninvolved epidermal cells may proliferate slightly faster than normal epidermal cells by virtue of a 50% increase in the LI over normal. These are inadequate data, however, for the other kinetic parameters (GF and FLM curves) in UnPs to obtain its absolute cell kinetic values. Studies using molecular markers confirm the evidence of a stem cell population of 40% as previously estimated by the radiolabeling studies.

A kinetic model is described that interrelates available information on the three compartments of normal and psoriatic epidermis and shows a kinetic equilibrium within each tissue. The psoriatic epidermis produces 35,000 new cells/mm^2 per day in a proliferative compartment containing 52,000 cells, whereas the parallel values in normal epidermis are 1246 new cells/mm^2 per day and 27,000 cells.

Psoriasis appears to involve at least three proliferative defects in the transformation of normal to psoriatic epidermis. The most significant kinetic change is the reduction of cell cycle duration from 311 to 36 hr. The other two changes are a doubling of the proliferative cell population and an increase in the GF from 60 to 100%. From a consideration of other available kinetic information obtained from experimental situations, speculations are suggested on the nature of proliferative cell controls in psoriasis.

Table 2 Cell Proliferation Controls in Normal and Psoriatic Epidermis

	Epidermal cells	
	Normal	Psoriasis
Cell cycle in vivo (hr)	311	36
Effect of controls	(1) inhibitory or (2) "wild type"	"wild type" stimulatory

Source: Ref. 12.

ACKNOWLEDGMENTS

This study was supported in part by NIH Grant No. 5 R01 AM27110 and by the Southern California Dermatology Foundation.

REFERENCES

1. Van Scott, E.J., and Ekel, T.M. (1963). *Arch. Dermatol.* 88:373–381.
2. Wright, N.A., and Appleton, D.R. (1980). *Cell Tissue Kinet.* 13:643–663.
3. Rothberg, S., Crouse, R.G., and Lee, J.L. (1961). *J. Invest. Dermatol.* 37:497–505.
4. Weinstein, G.D., and Van Scott, E.J. (1965). *J. Invest. Dermatol.* 45:257.
5. Epstein, W., and Maibach, H. (1965). *Arch. Dermatol.* 92:462–468.
6. Grove, G. L. (1979). *Int. J. Dematol.* 18: 123–129.
7. Baker, H., and Kligman, A.M. (1967). *Arch. Dermatol.* 95:408–411.
8. Finlay, A.Y., Marshall, R.J., and Marks, R. (1982). *Br. J. Dermatol.* 107:35–42.
9. Weinstein, G.D., Ross, P., McCullough, J., and Colton, A. (1983). *J. Invest. Dermatol.* 80:360–361.
10. Weinstein, G.D., and Frost, P. (1965). *J. Invest. Dermatol.* 50:254–258.

11. Quastler, H. (1963). In *Cell Proliferation.* L.F. Lamberton and R.J.M. Fry (Eds.). F.A. Davis, Philadelphia, pp. 18–34.
12. Weinstein, G.D., Ross, P., McCullough, J.L., and Colton, A. (1983). In *Psoriasis: Cell Proliferation.* N. Wright and R. Camplejohn (Eds.). Churchill Livingstone, Edinburgh, pp. 34–44.
13. Lachapelle, J.M., and Gillman, T. (1969). *Br. J. Dermatol.* 81:603–616.
14. Weinstein, G., McCullough, J., and Ross, P. (1984). *J. Invest. Dermatol.* 82:623–628.
15. Allegra, F., and DePanfilis, G. (1974). *Acta Dermatol.* 54:87–90.
16. Gelfant, S. (1982). *Cell Tissue Kinet.* 15:393–397.
17. Briggaman, R.A., and Kelly, T. (1982). *J. Invest. Dermatol.* 78:359.
18. Krueger, G. (1983). Personal communication.
19. Braun-Falco, O., Christophers, E., and Kurban, A. (1967). *Arch. Klin. Exp. Dermatol.* 229:276–284.
20. Wiley, H.E., and Weinstein, G.D. (1979). *J. Invest. Dermatol.* 73:545–547.
21. Goodwin, P., and Fry, L. (1977). *Clin. Exp. Dermatol.* 2:259–264.
22. Gelfant, S., Ozawa, A., Chalker, D.K., and Smith, J.G. (1982). *J. Invest. Dermatol.*78:58–62.
23. Fräki, J.E., Briggaman, R.A., and Lazarus, G.S. (1982). *Science* 215:685–687.
24. Krueger, G.G., Chambers, D.A., and Shelby, J. (1981). *J. Clin. Invest.* 68:1548–1557.
25. Gelfant, S. (1976). *Br. J. Dermatol.* 95:577–590.
26. Duffill, M., Wright, N., and Shuster, S. (1976). *Br. J. Dermatol.* 94:355–362.
27. Goodwin, P., Hamilton, S., and Fry, L. (1974). *Br. J. Dermatol.* 90:517–524.
28. Weinstein, G.D., Colton, A., and McCullough, J.L. (1983). In *Psoriasis: Cell Proliferation.* N. Wright and R.S. Camplejohn (Eds.), Churchill Livingstone, Edinburgh, pp. 189–208.
29. Weinstein, G.D. (1971). *Ann. N.Y. Acad. Sci.* 186: 452–466.
30. Penneys, N.S., Fulton, J.E., Jr., Weinstein, G.D., and Frost, P. (1970). *Arch. Dermatol.* 101:323–328.
31. Bergstresser, P.R., and Taylor, J.R. (1977). *Br. J. Dermatol.* 96:503–509.
32. Wright, N.A. (1980). *Recent Advances in Dermatology.* 5th Edition. A Rook and J. Saven (Eds.). Churchill Livingstone, Edinburgh.
33. McCullough, J.L., and Weinstein, G.D. (1983). In *Psoriasis: Cell Proliferation.* N.A. Wright and R.S. Camplejohn (Eds.). Churchill Livingstone, Edinburgh, pp. 347–354.
34. Steigleder, G.K., and Pullman, H. (1979). *Acta Derm. Venereol. (Stockh.)* 87(Suppl.):64–66.
35. Born, W., and Kalkoff, K.W. (1969). *Arch. Klin. Exp. Dermatol.* 236:43–52.
36. Galosi, A., Pullman, H., and Steigleder, G.K. (1980). *Arch. Dermatol. Res.* 267:105–107.
37. Grove, G.L., Anderton, R.L., and Smith, J.G. (1976). *J. Invest. Dermatol.* 66:236–238.
38. Grove, G.L. (1979). *Int. J. Dermatol.* 18:111–121.
39. Bauer, F.W., Crombag, N.H., DeGrood, R.M., and Jongh, G.J. (1980). *Br. J. Dermatol.* 102:629–639.
40. Bauer, F.W., Crombag, N.H., Boezeman, J.B., and DeGrood, R.M. (1980). *Br. J. Dermatol.* 104:271–276.
41. McCullough, J.L., and Weinstein, G.D. (1979). *J. Pharmacol. Ther.* 7:601–615.
42. Chopra, D.P., and Flaxman, B.A. (1974). *Cell Tissue Kinet.* 7:69–105.
43. Liu, S.C., and Parsons, C.S. (1983). *J. Invest. Dermatol.* 81:54–61.
44. Harper, R.A., Rispler, J., and Urbanek, R.W. (1978). *J. Invest. Dermatol.* 70:254–256.
45. Weinstein, G.D., and Mooney, K. (1980). *J. Invest. Dermatol.* 74:43–46.
46. Lavker, R., and Sun, T. (1983). *J. Invest. Dermatol.* 81:121s–127s.
47. Potten, C.S. (1983). In *Psoriasis: Cell Proliferation.* N. Wright and R.S. Camplejohn (Eds.). Churchill Livingstone, Edinburgh, pp. 149–162.
48. Bauer, F.W. (1986). In *Textbook of Psoriasis.* P.D. Mier (Ed.). Churchill Livingstone, Edinburgh, pp. 100–112.
49. Potten, C.S. (1981). In *Normal Epidermis. The Epidermis in Disease.* J.B. Lippincott, Philadelphia, pp. 171–191.
50. Weinstein, G.D. (1965). *J. Invest. Dermatol.* 44:413.
51. Weinstein, G.D., and Frost, P. (1971). *Arch. Dermatol.* 103:33–38.
52. Peckham, P.E., Weinstein, G.D., and McCullough, J.L. (1987). *Arch. Dermatol.* 123(10):1303–1307.
53. Heenen, M., Galand, P., de Maertelaer, V., and Heenen, P.H. (1987). *Cell Tissue Kinet.* 20:561–570.
54. Paus, R., and Link, R. (1988). *Yale J. Biol. Med.* 61: 467–476.
55. Jones, P.H., Harper, S., and Watt, F.M. (1995). Stem cell patterning and fate in human epidermis. *Cell* 80(1):83–93.
56. Bata-Csorgo, Z., Hammerberg, C., Voorhees, J.J., and Cooper, K.D. (1995). Intralesional T-lymphocyte activation as a mediator of psoriatic epidermal hyperplasia. *J. Invest. Dermatol.* 105(Suppl. 1):89S–94S.
57. Bata-Csorgo, Z., Hammerberg, C., Voorhees, J.J., and Cooper, K.D. (1995). Kinetics and regulation of human keratinocyte stem cell growth in short-term primary ex vivo culture. Coopertive growth factors from psoriatic lesional T lymphocytes stimulate proliferation among psoriatic uninvolved, but not normal, stem keratinocytes. *J. Clin. Invest.* 95(1):317–327.
58. Bata-Csorgo, Z., Hammerberg, C., Voorhees, J.J., and Cooper, K.D. (1993). Flow cytometric identification of proliferative subpopulations within normal human epidermis and the localization of the primary hyperproliferative population in psoriasis. *J. Exp. Med.* 178(4): 1271–1281.

17

The Langerhans Cell

Marek Haftek
Edouard Herriot Hospital, Lyon, France

BIOLOGY OF THE LANGERHANS CELL

Origin

Langerhans cells are a subpopulation of dendritic cells residing in the epidermis, and they represent approximately 2–4% of all epidermal cells. Unlike ectoderm-derived keratinocytes, the Langerhans cells are of bone marrow origin (1), and belong to the macrophage-monocyte-histiocyte lineage deriving from CD34+ progenitor cells (2,2a,2b). The cells which disappear from the epidermis during physiological or pathological processes may, therefore, be replaced by the putative precursors from the circulating pool. Mitoses of normal human Langerhans cells were reported in skin xenografts to athymic, "nude" mice (3) and in enriched epidermal Langerhans cell suspensions after 24-hr culture (4), indicating the cell's self-reproducing capacity in situ. Cell division may, therefore, be an alternative way of compensating for the cell loss of the evolutive epidermal Langerhans cell population.

Distribution

Typically, Langerhans cells reside in the midepidermis and are evenly distributed (Fig. 1). Some regional variations in the density of the Langerhans cell population can be observed (5), but are often irregular and partially due to factors influencing Langerhans cell expression; e.g., sun exposure. There are fewer Langerhans cells in the hyperkeratotic epidermis of the palms and soles, and they are more numerous in the fundibular portion of the hair follicle than in the interadnexial epidermis (6). In normal conditions, Langerhans cells are virtually absent from the papillary dermis. Their appearance in this region is an indication of cell migration related to their functional role.

Morphology

The dendritic appearance of Langerhans cells is one of the most characteristic, although not specific, features of these cells and the explanation for this most probably lies in their function. The dendrites of Langerhans cells penetrate the interkeratinocyte spaces, thereby creating a zone of influence composed of several neighboring epidermal cells.

The ultrastructural hallmark of the Langerhans cell is its cytoplasmic organelle—the Birbeck granule. It is specific to Langerhans cells and, by definition, determines whether a cell can be called a Langerhans cell or not (7). The number and size of Birbeck granules depend on the stage of cell activity. These sandwichlike organelles, composed of closely apposed membranes, may be formed by cell membrane endocytosis, and therefore were proposed to be of importance for the antigen-processing function (8). Until recently, the only reliable method of checking for the presence of Birbeck granules has been by electron microscopy. It is, however, conceivable that even examination of serial ultrathin sections of an entire cell may sometimes yield false negative results in the case

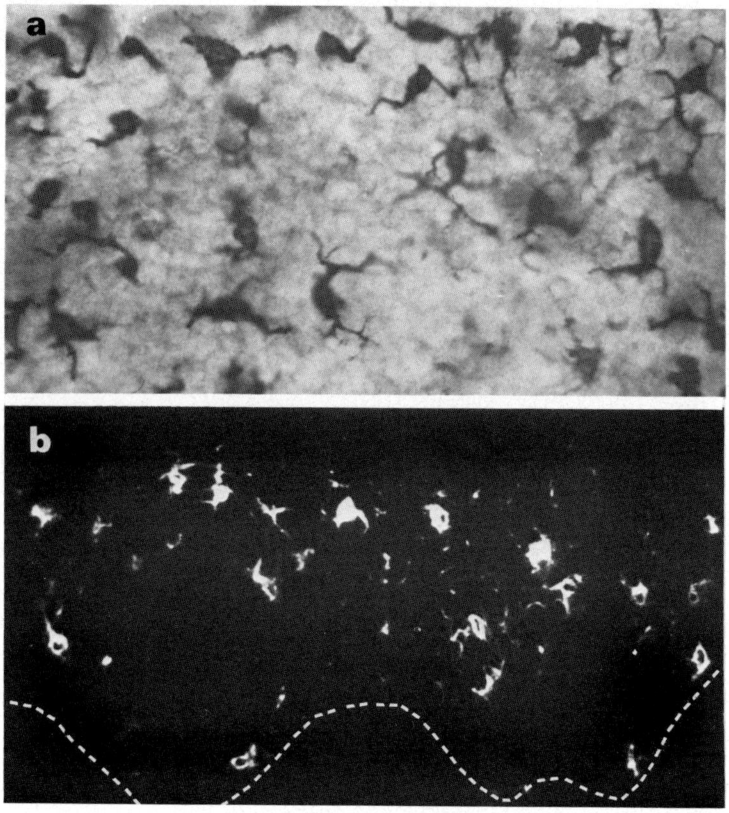

Figure 1 (a) Normal Langerhans cells visualized in an epidermal sheet by ATPase staining method. Note the regular distribution of histochemically labeled dendritic cells forming an intraepidermal "net." (b) Cross-section of an uninvolved human skin labeled with a monoclonal antibody to CD1a antigen in an indirect immunofluorescence method. The CD1a-expressing Langerhans cells are clearly visible in the midepidermis. No staining can be observed in the dermis. Broken line = dermo-epidermal junction.

of Langerhans cells that are marginally poor in the specific organelle. Detection of a Birbeck granule-related antigen, the role of which remains obscure, may potentially help in such studies (8a).

Since the devleopment of fine tools for immunological and immunocytochemical studies such as monoclonal antibodies, much progress has been made in studying the surface proteins of Langerhans cells. A specific immunophenotypic repertoire expressed by Langerhans cells allows these cells to be distinguished not only from other epidermal cells (keratinocytes, melanocytes, Merkel cells), but also from other members of the family of bone marrow–derived dendritic cells (9,10). In normal human epidermis, resting Langerhans cells are characterized by the expression of cell surface antigens, which are detailed in Table 1. Some of the proteins which can be detected on the Langerhans cell surface (e.g., major histocompatibility complex class II molecules, adhesion (costimulatory receptors) are important for the cell function. Most Langerhans cell surface markers, however, do not seem to play any relevant physiological role. Cytoplasmic protein S-100 and vimentin cytoskeleton (both of them expressed also by melanocytes and endothelial cells) are intracellular markers of Langerhans cells recognizable by specific monoclonal antibodies. Although definition of the Langerhans cell immunophenotype may facilitate cell identification in tissues, immunocytochemical studies are often inadequate in this respect owing to the variability of the surface antigen expression pattern related to the cell's functional state (11). Indeed, various modifications of the Langerhans cell phenotype occur during cell differentiation and in cell activation stages, as indicated by studies in skin pathology and in vitro experiments.

Table 1 Some of the Most Important Cell Surface Antigens Observed on Normal Human Langerhans Cells

Antigens	Specificity
CD1a	Expressed exclusively by cortical thymocytes and virtually all Langerhans cells; diminished expression upon activation, in the "functionally mature" antigen-presenting cells
CD4	Antigens occurring on thymus-dependent lymphocytes; expressed in small quantities also by Langerhans cells
CD49a-f (α1-6)/CD29 (β_1), CD11a-c($\alpha_{L,M,X}$)/CD18 (β_2)	Surface glycoprotein complexes which, although not restricted to hemopoietic lineages, are preferentially expressed by early hemopoietic cells, T lymphocytes, and monocytes; heterodimers of the β_1(VLA) and β_2 integrin families involved in mediating cellular adhesion; help guide the Langerhans cell migration (on laminin, fibronectin) and cell-cell recognition during cell-mediated immune responses, respectively
CD54 (ICAM 1), CD50 (ICAM 3), CD58 (LFA 3)	Accessory adhesion molecules stablizing Langerhans cell–T cell interaction; the lymphocyte countereceptor for ICAMs is CD11a/CD18 (LFA 1) and for LFA 3 - CD2
CD80 (B7-1), CD86 (B7-2)	Costimulatory molecules involved in intercellular signaling during the initiation and maintenance phases of primary T-cell responses; their lymphocyte ligand is CD28
E-cadherin	Transmembraneous glycoprotein involved in homotypic binding with identical molecules expressed on other cells (mostly epithelial cells); possibly required for maintaining Langerhans cells in intraepithelial position
FcγRII, FcϵRI, receptor for C_3 fraction of complement	The antigens shared by the freshly isolated LC and monocytes-macrophages; one can speculate that these receptors for the Fc fragments of γ and ϵ immunoglobulins and for C_3 may promote interaction of Langerhans cells during humoral immune responses
CD45	The leukocyte common antigen
"Common" class I antigens of the major histocompatibility complex	Individual-specific, present on virtually all cell types, expressed in relatively low quantities on Langerhans cells
Major histocompatibility complex class II antigens (HLA-DR, -DQ, and -DP)	Besides Langerhans cells, characteristic of B and activated T lymphocytes, macrophages/histiocytes, and some other dendritic cells of lymphoid organs; play an essential role in the process of antigen presentation and thus prove indispensable for transmission of the antigen-related information between "immunocompetent" cells

CD = cluster of differentiation [as defined by the International Conference on Human Leukocyte Differention Antigens; *Leukocyte Typing IV*, Knapp, W., et al. (Eds.), 1989, Oxford University Press, Oxford].

Function

Langerhans cells have many phenotypic characteristics in common with macrophages, but their phagocytic potential is much lower than that of a typical macrophage. Nevertheless, Langerhans cells are capable of selective uptake of antigens and contact allergens. Epidermal Langerhans cells are potent antigen-presenting cells, much more efficient than their circulating monocyte/macrophage homologues. Affinity of the Langerhans cell membrane for "foreign" molecules, its capacity for specific ligand-mediated endocytosis, and the particular distribution of these dendritic cells in the epidermis make these skin histiocytes a veritable trap for antigens (12). Activation of the T helper lymphocytes in cell-mediated immune responses requires "antigen presentation" by specialized accessory cells (e.g., dendritic cells, macrophages). This process consists of co-recognition by T lymphocytes of the given antigen along with one of the major histocompatibility complex class II determinants present on the surface of an antigen-presenting cell. The T lymphocyte–dendritic cell interaction is further stabilized by various molecules, some of them fulfilling a supplementary role of costimulators (12a). In normal conditions, Langerhans cells and their Birbeck granule—lacking counterparts, called indeterminate cells, are the only epidermal cells expressing class II molecules on the cell surface and possessing the antigen presenting function (13). Acrosyryngium keratinocytes, which are also HLA DR positive, are not believed to exert the accessory cell function. In vitro studies of highly enriched Langerhans cells have demonstrated that an increase in HLA DR (class II) expression observed in these cell suspensions is paralleled by an enhancement of their immunostimulatory capacities (14). HLA DR antigen expression may be modulated by several factors such as ultraviolet radiation, various pharmacological treatments, and mediators of inflammatory reaction. Cytokines, such as the granulocyte/macrophage colony-stimulating factor (GM-CSF), are produced not only by sensitized T lymphocytes, but also by keratinocytes, fibroblasts, and endothelial cells in tissue sites where there is some stimulus for their release (e.g., antigen deposition). They may be responsible for local amplification of the accessory function of Langerhans cells (15). The latter produce interleukin 1, the soluble factor necessary for further lymphocyte attraction, proliferation, maturation, and their lymphokine secretion (16). Keratinocytes, which are the major source of the epidermal T cell-activating factor (ETAF, a cytokine which is very similar if not identical to interleukin 1), seem also to be involved in this process (17). Sensitized T lymphoblasts (produced in lymphoid organs) release interferon γ, a lymphokine responsible for the expression of HLA DR molecules by keratinocytes in the foci of inflammatory reactions (18,19). This indicates that close functional interactions between various cell types take place in the epidermis during cell-mediated immune reactions in health and in disease. The local induction of class II antigens may ensure that most class II–restricted T cells are retained and function in the inflammatory site (20).

According to the currently available data, the Langerhans cells mediate the transfer to the immune system of information about antigens (haptens) appearing intraepidermally. Langerhans cells are capable of presenting chemical allergens, bacterial, fungal, viral, and virus-associated tissue antigens, neoantigens, and other modified tissue antigens. Another important function of Langerhans cells is antigen processing, which consists of endocytosis of complicated molecules, their intracellular digestion, and reexpression of representative fragments (peptides) on the cell surface in an immunologically recognizable form (20).

Apart from antigen "processing" and its "presentation," Langerhans cells which become locally activated (and fully operative) perform the "sensitization" function with regard to circulating nonactivated and memory lymphocytes. This activity is unique to dendritic cells (other accessory cells like macrophages or B lymphocytes, although capable of class II—restricted antigen presentation, act only on recently sensitized lymphoblasts). The sensitization process requires interleukin 1 and is severalfold amplified by GM-CSF cytokine (20).

During the "sensitization" phase, the Langerhans cells carrying antigens leave the epidermis and migrate via dermis and lymph ducts to the peripheral lymph nodes, where they interact with helper lymphocytes and induce proliferation of T cells. During migration, the Langerhans cells change phenotype; they progressively lose CD1a membrane receptors and Birbeck granules and express increased quantities of HLA DR as well as the adhesion molecules like ICAM-1, LFA3, and B7-1. According to their morphology, they are called "veiled cells" when migrating through lymphatic vessels and "interdigitating cells" in the T-cell zones of lymph nodes (20a).

In the efferent limb of the immune response, activated, "foreign" antigen-bearing Langerhans cells may serve as targets for the homing effectory T lymphocytes (21). This function does not require Langerhans cell migration to lymph nodes. The antigen presentation and stimulation of a specific clone of "memory" lymphocytes takes place in the reexposed skin. Such a mechanism can be partially responsible for the local degenerative changes in the epidermis, probably caused by the interacting antigen-specific infiltrate cells.

Several bacterial toxins and viral proteins possess a faculty of circumventing the regular process of antigen presentation. Binding to both the major histocompatibility complex class II molecules and particular T-cell receptors, they crosslink, in a nonspecific way, the antigen-presenting cells and lymphocytes, leading to polyclonal T-cell activation. Such superantigens do not require intracellular processing and are capable of activating as much as 20% of both helper and supressor T lymphocytes (compared to approximately 0.1% of the total T-cell population activated by conventional antigens). It is therefore not surprising that the clinical results of superantigen action are widespread and violent (21a).

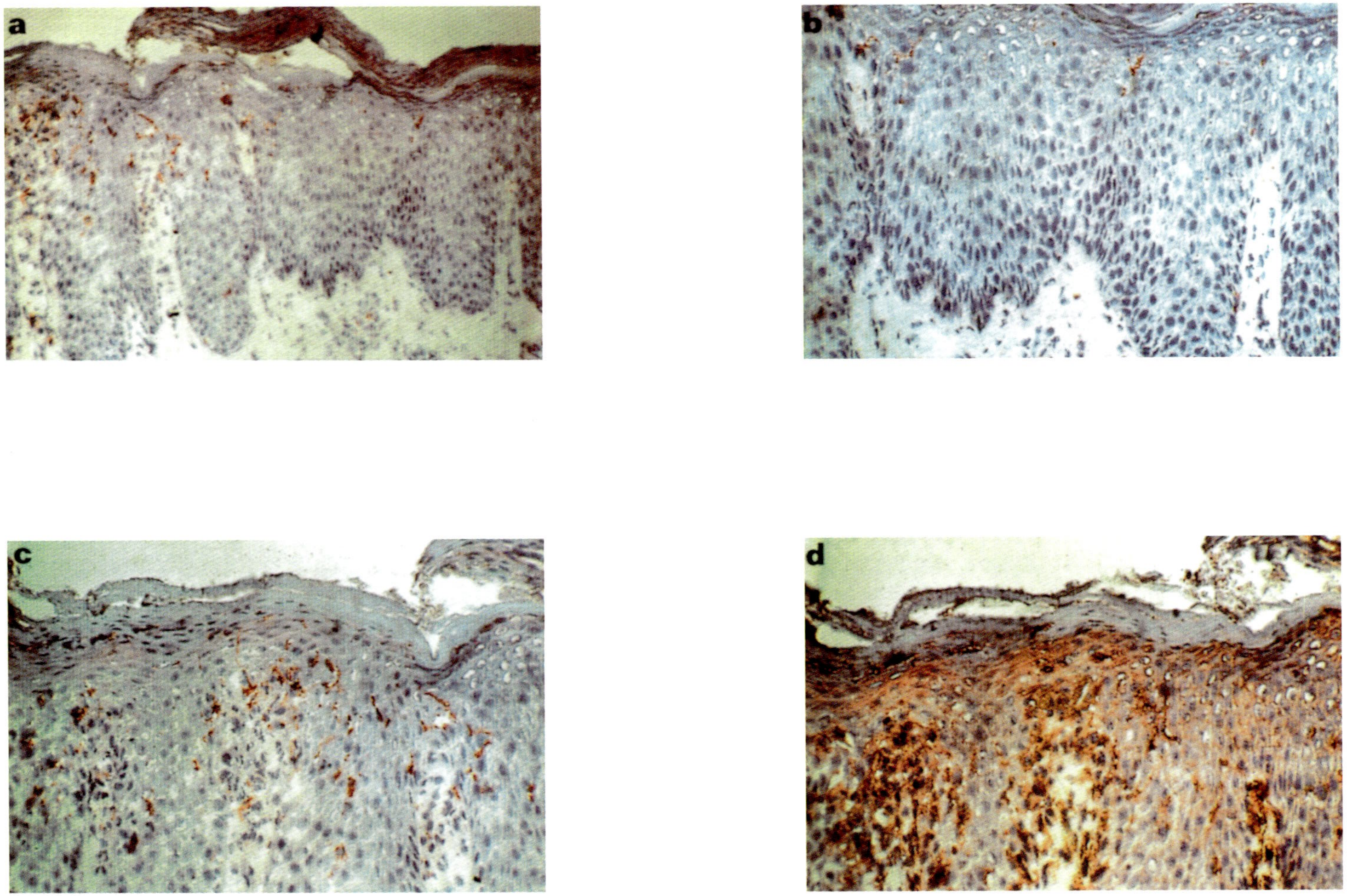

Figure 2

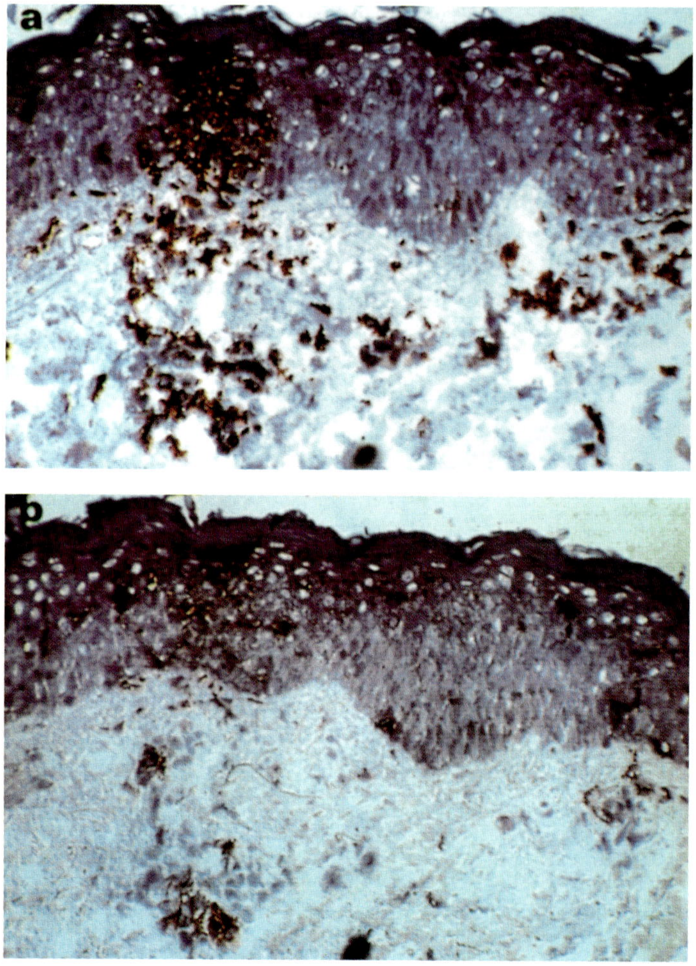

Figure 4

Observations of the Langerhans cell distribution in oral epithelium (22) as well as studies on normal and hair-plucking-induced hyperplastic epidermis led Potten and Allen (23) to formulate the concept of the "epidermal proliferative unit" whereby dendritic Langerhans cells would appear to occupy the central position both morphologically and functionally. It has been suggested that Langerhans cells could be involved in the process of the control of epidermal proliferation. Schweizer and Marks (24) reported on a particular Langerhans cell distribution pattern in mouse tail epidermis, supporting the idea of this cell's involvement in the control of keratinocyte differentiation. In fact, in these anatomical regions naturally composed of the ortho- and parakeratotic epidermis, Langerhans cells can be observed in the orthokeratotic zones exclusively, as if they were necessary for the induction of normal keratinization. The hypothesis of the Langerhans cell–mediated down-regulation of epidermal proliferation and its involvement in the control of keratinocyte differentiation has to be considered with caution, since the evidence is mostly circumstantial and no direct proof can yet be presented. The possibility that it is rather the Langerhans cell population which undergoes the influence of the local keratinocyte environment and not vice versa is an interesting counter hypothesis.

METHODS OF STUDIES OF LANGERHANS CELLS

Studies on Cell Distribution

A classic method of staining the Langerhans cell consists of revealing by histochemistry its ectoenzyme activity, the ATPase (25). It results in a dark brownish black staining, which unfortunately may be confounded with the black-colored, dendritic melanocytes in the pigmented skin showing also some cell membrane ATPase activity (25). Further, the technique often does not permit an even staining of all the Langerhans cells in a given sample, and the enzymatic reactivity is rather labile and liable to be influenced by several physical factors; e.g., ultraviolet light (26). More specific markers of the Langerhans cell are its immunocytochemically distinguishable surface antigens (27,28). The remarkable regularity of coexpression of the CD1a antigen and Birbeck granule in cells other than cortical thymocytes places this membrane antigen in a privileged position for Langerhans cell labeling. However, it must be borne in mind that the expression of even such a "sure" marker may be modified in certain pathological conditions or during experimental procedures (29).

Another frequently used Langerhans cell marker, the HLA DR antigen, is also expressed by B lymphocytes, macrophages, and activated T lymphocytes. For this reason, the anti–HLA DR antibody is specific for Langerhans cells (and indeterminate dendritic cells) only in normal epidermis. The dermis and pathological epidermis invaded by a cellular infiltrate contain also HLA DR–positive cells that are different from Langerhans cells. Furthermore, a focal and diffuse expression of HLA DR antigen by lesional keratinocytes has been reported in several inflammatory diseases characterized by intraepidermal lymphocyte infiltrate (30–32).

Langerhans cells visualized with the various aforementioned methods may be studied qualitatively and quantitatively. Their position in the epidermis and their presence in the dermis are best assessed on vertical skin sections, whereas the regularity of their distribution, eventual clustering, and average length of the dendrites are better observable in split epidermis preparations.

The quantitative approach requires the choice of an appropriate method depending on the type of specimen studied (33,34). Cell counting in separated pathological epidermal sheets, especially from acanthotic lesions with pronounced clubbing, is often very difficult. In these conditions, the best information is obtained from well-oriented vertical sections. Modes of expression of the Langerhans cell number—per unit of epidermal section length and per unit of epidermal section area—help to evaluate, respectively, the density of the cell distribution irrespective of the epidermal thickness, and the relationship between the Langerhans cell number and the volume of the epidermis which they inhabit (34–36).

Studies on Antigen Expression

A recent study demonstrated that all the CD1a positive epidermal Langerhans cells express simultaneously class II, HLA D antigens (37). Flow cytometric analysis of double-stained human epidermal cell suspensions preenriched with Langerhans cells did not reveal the presence of HLA DR$^+$ CD1a or HLA DR$^-$ CD1a subsets (38), the existence of which has been postulated by some authors on the basis of double labeling studies. Therefore, the previously reported numerical differences between the CD1a and HLA DR$^+$ epidermal dendritic cells were most probably due to the insufficient DR-antigen detectability with the immunohistochemical methods used. Semiquantitative results of the ultrastructural immunogold labeling studies on CD1a and HLA DR, DP, DQ antigen expression revealed the presence in normal epidermis of two subpopulations of Langerhans cells: 25% of the population was strongly DR positive, whereas the remaining 75% showed a low density of surface DR sites (39).

Studies on Cell Function

The in vitro model of immune interactions between epidermal cells and the circulating immune system cells, mixed epidermal-lymphocyte reaction, has been extensively used to investigate the role of Langerhans cells in generating immune responses. Experiments on rodent Langerhans cells established that these cells do indeed function as specialized epidermal antigen-presenting cells, since they induce allogenic and antigen-specific T cell activation and proliferation in vitro (40). Similar studies with human cells confirmed these findings (41). A modification of the mixed culture method has been successfully used for the demonstration of Langerhans cell-mediated generation of cytotoxic T cells in an antigen-specific response to the murine hapten-modified (42) or human allogenic (43) epidermal cells. One apparently unique feature of dendritic cells is their ability to aggregate the antigen-reactive T lymphocytes during immune reactions in culture (44). The mechanisms underlying dendritic/T cell cluster formation represent an interesting field of in vitro research (45). Another intriguing question, that of the role of the Birbeck granule in antigen processing, can also be studied in vitro using ultrastructural immunocytochemistry and time-course experiments on the antigen internalization in highly enriched populations of Langerhans cells (8).

In vivo experiments with common topical sensitizers (such as dinitrofluorobenzene, DNFB) have helped to gain a better understanding of the influence of the Langerhans cell number and distribution in the skin on the induction of contact allergy. Application of allergens or alloantigens to the skin regions either depleted of Langerhans cells with physicochemical agents (ultraviolet and gamma radiation, tape-stripping, corticosteroids) or naturally deficient in Langerhans cells (hamster cheek pouch, mouse tail) resulted in significantly decreased immune responses (46–48).

Since both the Langerhans cell distribution (or their surface antigen detectability) and the cell function can be influenced by various pharmacological and physical agents, the results of these treatments studied with the above-mentioned methods may also contribute to our knowledge of the role of Langerhans cells in health and disease. The in vivo model of human skin xenograft on the athymic (nude) mouse is particularly interesting in this respect. The human Langerhans cells persist in the grafts (49), but cannot be replaced by the precursors from the circulation in the case of definitive cell destruction. Furthermore, the graft being cut off from the human environment, the usual interactions with the immune system are no longer possible. This results in a "pure" experimental model for studies on normal and pathological skin.

LANGERHANS CELLS IN PSORIASIS

Skin lesions of psoriasis are characterized, besides the epidermal hyperproliferation and signs of incomplete keratinocyte differentiation, by an inflammatory infiltrate penetrating the lesional epidermis. Known functional interactions between the epidermal accessory cells, T lymphocytes, and keratinocytes have rendered particularly interesting the studies on the fate and role of Langerhans cells in psoriasis. Since there are various clinical forms of psoriasis which vary considerably according to the disease activity, the findings on the Langerhans cells also have to be related to the type and stage of development of psoriatic lesions.

Plaque Psoriasis

The stationary, chronic form of skin lesions is the most commonly studied type of psoriasis. In 1971, using the ATPase histochemical staining of frozen skin sections, Muller et al. (50) described the marked decrease in the density of the Langerhans cell population in psoriatic plaques. The rarefaction of epidermal Langerhans cells in the acanthotic lesions in general and in chronic psoriasis in particular has also been reported by Lisi (51). These findings have been confirmed with more specific immunohistochemical methods using monoclonal antibody anti-CD1a antigen (36,52). The number of CD1a positive Langerhans cells proved particularly decreased (three- to fivefold vs noninvolved epidermis of the same patients) when the quantitation results were expressed in a manner relating the labeled cell number to the epidermal volume (considerably increased in the psoriatic acanthotic plaques) (35,36,54). Otherwise, the population of CD1a positive epidermal cells in relation to the skin surface area was reported to be of normal density [epidermal sheets (53); counts per linear length of skin section (35,55)] or even increased (56). Flow cytometry analysis of single-cell suspensions from the plaque epidermis indicated unchanged percentages of CD1a positive cells when compared to the normal values (57). Whatever the method of staining used, the lesional Langerhans cells were irregularly distributed in the lesional epidermis, often occurred aggregated in small clusters, most frequently situated in the vicinity of hair follicles and over the top of elongated dermal papillae (36,50,52,58,59) (Fig. 2). They appeared less dendritic (36,51,52) except at the limits of the peripherally spreading psoriatic plaques.

Exacerbated lesions of psoriasis vulgaris (52) and the periphery of spreading psoriatic plaques (36) are infiltrated by the polymorphonuclears and the mononuclear HLA DR–positive cells. As demonstrated by in situ immunocytochemistry, the latter cells appear to be mostly "activated" T lymphocytes (32,52,58,60); the observation is further supported by the cytofluorimetric analysis of dermal infiltrates (61). Since these cells invade the epidermis and squeeze into the epithelial intercellular spaces, they may circumstantially acquire a "dendritic" appearance and be taken for Langerhans cells when labeled with the anti-HLA DR antibody. Focal HLA DR-positive staining of lesional keratinocytes in active psoriasis has also been reported (31,32). It was apparently independent of the presence of lymphocytic infiltrate or CD1a positive Langerhans cells. Therefore, apart from the immunoelectron microscope studies, the CD1a antigen seems best suited for Langerhans cell detection in psoriatic lesions. Considerable amounts of the dendritic CD1a positive cells have been observed in the papillary dermis of exacerbated lesions, but not in inactive stationary plaques (32,36,52). These cells frequently co-express surface antigens characteristic of interdigitating cells of the lymphoid organs (62), which supports the concept of close histogenic and functional links between the two kinds of antigen-presenting cells. Furthermore, close cell-cell apposition of epidermal Langerhans cells with infiltrating lymphocytes has been demonstrated ultrastructurally in psoriatic plaques (63). These cell interactions were noted mainly in active untreated lesions, irrespective of the extent of the skin involvement. The lymphocytes present in the epidermis of persistent and exacerbated plaque lesions were predominantly of the T suppressor/cytotoxic immunophenotype (52,64,65).

Desquamation of many remnants of Langerhans cells was seen in the psoriatic stratum corneum by Muller et al. (50). This tended to be patchy and centered primarily over the dermal papillae. This finding was confirmed by Shelley (66) using the same ATPase technique but on psoriatic stratum corneum sheets, and can also be observed with the specific anti-CD1a staining on epidermal sections (see Figs. 2a and 3). Shelley hypothesized that Langerhans cells may be eliminated from the lesional epidermis owing to the highly increased turnover of keratinocytes. Indeed, such may be so on the condition that the lesional Langerhans cells are so altered that they are unable to maintain their physiological position among viable keratinocytes.

Guttate Psoriasis

Light and electron microscope studies on the earliest changes occurring in the skin of patients with acute eruptive guttate psoriasis either following or not associated with a streptococcal infection were performed by Brody (67,68). They revealed the punctiform spongiotic areas involving the stratum basale and lower stratum spinosum in the epidermis of 2-day-old lesions. The intraepidermal edema was situated ex-

Figure 2 Immunoperoxidase staining of a peripherally spreading psoriatic plaque. Anti-CD1a monoclonal antibody (a,b,c) labels few dendritic epidermal cells situated over the top of elongated dermal papillae. On a consecutive section (d), HLA DR–positive cells fill the papillary dermis and penetrate the suprapapillary epidermis at places where the Langerhans cells are visualized in (c). The left part of the section in (a), seen at a higher magnification in (c), is the plaque periphery, where the Langerhans cells are more numerous and more dendritic than in the plaque center (the right part of a and b). Rare CD1a-positive cells can be observed in the dermal papillae at the periphery of the lesion (c). Note a focal reactivity of the parakeratotic stratum corneum with an anti-CD1a monoclonal antibody (a). (Published in part in Ref. 59.)

Figure 4 Two consecutive cryostat sections of uninvolved skin from a patient with eruptive psoriasis stained with (a) anti-HLA DR and (b) anti-CD1a monoclonal antibodies by the indirect avidin-biotin-immunoperoxidase labeling method. In the epidermis and dermis focally infiltrated by DR-positive inflammatory cells, CD1a-positive Langerhans cells display blurred outlines. The epidermis of this subclinical lesion does not show any acanthosis or irregularity of the dermo-epidermal junction. (Published in part in Ref. 59).

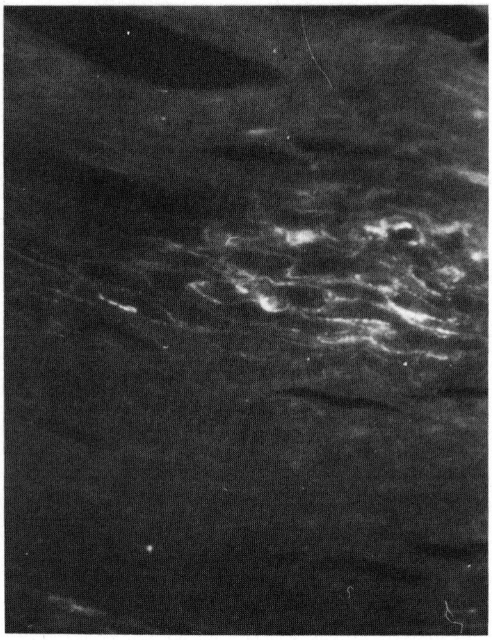

Figure 3 Evidence for a focal deposition of CD1a-positive debris in the interkeratinocyte spaces of the parakeratotic stratum corneum in a psoriatic plaque. A close view of the indirect immunofluorescence labeling with an anti-CD1a monoclonal antibody.

actly in the center of the lesion and was accompanied by a moderately strong dermal inflammatory reaction with vasodilatation. Ultrastructurally, the inflammatory infiltrate in the upper dermis contained mostly mononuclear cells and only a few polymorphonuclear leukocytes. The exocytosis of mononuclears into the epidermis and the presence of intraepidermal macrophages, lymphocytes, and single polymorphonuclears were the constant features. Occasional Langerhans cells, migrating through the basement membrane could also be observed. As the lesions developed, the Langerhans cells became less apparent in the hyperplastic epidermis and were only seldom found in the 2- and 3-week-old lesions.

On the basis of results obtained with a double-staining immunofluorescent technique, Baker et al. reported on the presence of HLA DR-positive but CD1a-negative dendritic cells in the lesional epidermis of psoriasis (69) and other inflammatory dermatoses characterized by a predominating HLA DR-positive T helper lymphocyte subpopulation in the infiltrate (70). They speculated that such cells could be of the Langerhans cell lineage and represent immature cells which have been recruited at an abnormally rapid rate into the epidermis (71). Consequently, these authors incriminated the mediator-secreting activated T helper lymphocytes as being responsible for the influx of the Langerhans cell precursors into the psoriatic epidermis, and suggested that this mechanism may be a part of a possible pathogenic pathway common to a variety of T cell-mediated skin diseases. The existence of such $CD1a^-$, DR^+ Langerhans cells could not, however, be proved on immunoelectron microscopy, since all of the Birbeck granule-bearing cells were more or less reactive with the OKT6 (anti-CD1a) monoclonal antibody (70). This opens up the possibility that the $CD1a^-$, DR^+ cells with the "dendritic" appearance observed intraepidermally by immunofluorescence were infiltrating macrophages or "activated" T lymphocytes. Difficulties encountered in assessing the double-label immunofluorescence of epidermis may well be illustrated by the fact that the same group of researchers observed the occasional (but unlikely) expression of CD1a antigen by keratinocytes in both normal and psoriatic (lesional and uninvolved) skin (69).

The characteristic clustering of the epidermal HLA DR-positive dendritic cells has been described in guttate psoriatic lesions of less than 2 mm in diameter, and was further accentuated in late guttate psoriasis (more than 1 cm in diameter) (69). The increase in the epidermal DR-positive dendritic cell number in the early guttate lesions was not statistically significant compared with uninvolved skin. This and the further augmentation of these cell numbers in a later phase of the evolution of guttate lesions (quantified per 100 high-power microscopic fields, thus per epidermal section length) may be related to the increasing epidermal acanthosis. Epidermal T helper lymphocytes, some of them DR positive, appeared in the early lesions (less than 1 week old), but the balance was reversed after 3–12 weeks of evolution when T suppressor cells predominated (many DR positive). The dermis of guttate lesions showed an increase in T cell infiltration involving both helper and suppressor cells, with the great majority of DR-positive lymphocytes being of the T helper subset. Dermal DR- and CD1a-positive cells were observed in uninvolved skin and early lesions, and increased twofold in the late lesions.

Eruptive Psoriasis and Koebner Phenomenon

Our own studies on the sequence of events occurring in the earliest phases of the development of psoriatic lesions indicate that the Langerhans cells become involved in the pathological process at a very early stage (59,72). Foci of the HLA DR-positive infiltrate cells penetrating the clinically uninvolved epidermis could be observed in patients with eruptive psoriasis. In these localizations, CD1a-positive Langerhans cells appeared more dendritic, but often displayed blurred outlines by the indirect immunoperoxidase method (Fig. 4). The CD1a-positive cells were also observed in the dermal parts of these focalized infiltrates. Our results fit well with the light and electron microscope findings of Brody (67,68), who described the punctate spongiotic areas in the stratum basale and lower stratum spinosum in the regions of uninvolved skin of patients with acute guttate eruptions. Concomitant with these early epidermal changes were hypertrophy of postcapillary venule endothelium and dermal mastocyte degranulation, followed by a slight perivascular inflammatory infiltrate and intraepidermal exocytosis of mononuclear cells. Langerhans cells crossing the dermoepidermal junction and numerous examples of Langerhans cell–mononuclear cell apposition were also noted, but no cell damage was discerned.

Further support for the thesis of early Langerhans cell involvement was obtained from the prospective studies we performed in such patients with an extremely active form of psoriasis (72). The first clinical changes observed in the noninvolved skin were erythematous pinpoint spots similar to the "prepinpoint" lesions described by Chowaniec and Jablonska (73). When studied with immunohistochemistry and electron microscopy, the punctate erythemas displayed the same kind of immunocompetent cell redistribution as the subclinical changes observed previously. Additionally, ultrastructural signs of the Langerhans cell involvement could also be observed (Fig. 5) (72). Some of these cells presented signs of cell damage with discharge of the cytoplasmic contents into the dilated interkeratinocyte spaces. Most frequently, however, the observed numerous mitochondria and ribosomes, well-developed often enlarged ergastoplasmic reticulum, and abundant Birbeck granules were suggestive of the increased metabolic activity of Langerhans cells. Frequent anatomical interactions between Langerhans cells and keratinocytes and, occasionally, between Langerhans cells and intraepidermal lymphocytes were noted. This observation confirmed the findings of Heng and Kloss (63) and Heng et al. (74a), who reported on the intimate apposition of the plasma membranes and on the characteristic contacts via cytoplasmic processes between the three cell types in active (Koebner-induced) psoriatic plaques.

Further, we observed the constant presence of organelle-free, cell membrane–delimited rounded blebs in the Langerhans cell vicinity (Fig. 6). These structures were of keratinocyte origin and resembled the basal keratinocyte herniations occurring in psoriatic lesions, probably under the influence of proteolytic enzymes (74). The association of keratinocyte herniations and Langerhans cells showing either increased cytoplasmic activity or cell damage was suggestive of the influence of these latter cells on the epidermal environment. Interestingly, none of the initial changes observed in the clinically noninvolved skin and the earliest clinical lesions of eruptive psoriasis were accompanied by the structural skin modifications characteristic of psoriasis. The altered expression of epidermal differentiation antigens and the appearance of the histological signs of psoriasis could be observed in the developed lesions only.

In their elegant study on the Koebner phenomenon, Eyre and Krueger (75) demonstrated that the reaction is of the all-or-none type, and that the patients in whom psoriasis did not recur after removal of a lesion ("reverse" Koebner) had less skin involvement in the follow-up, and thus a better prognosis. The experiments of Jablonska et al. (76) and the observations of Heng and Kloss (63) also suggested that the Koebner reaction is incompatible with spontaneously resolving or successfully treated psoriasis, thus relating the phenomenon to the active stage of disease. Systemic factors responsible for generation of the Koebner phe-

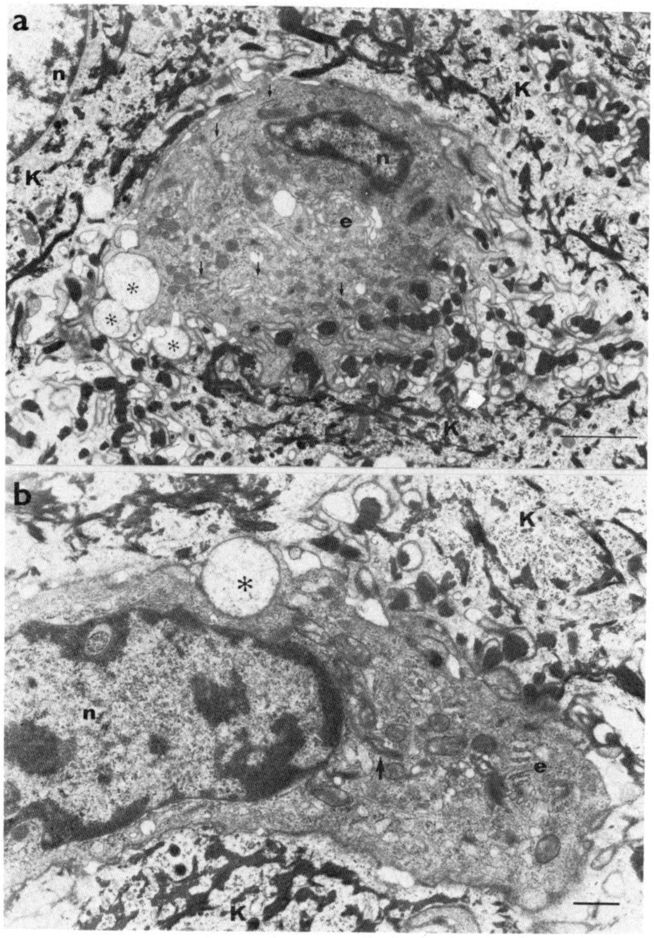

Figure 5 Electron microscopy of the earliest, minute epidermal lesions in a patient with eruptive psoriasis. (a, b) Two Langerhans cells in the spinous layer with (a) numerous cytoplasmic protrusions penetrating between the desmosome-joined keratinocytes (K). Note highly convoluted keratinocyte membranes, numerous mitochondria and signs of cytoplasmic activity in the Langerhans cells, and electron-lucid blebs (asterisks) between the cells in the vicinity of the Langerhans cells. n = nucleus; e = well-developed ergastoplasmic reticulum; arrows point to the Birbeck granules. Bars = 1 μm.

nomenon have been proposed on the grounds that all skin regions of a given individual react to the injury in the same manner (75). Baker et al. (77) noted the predominance of CD4 (T helper) lymphocytes in the uninvolved epidermis of patients with chronic plaque psoriasis who later responded with the Koebner phenomenon to skin injury (tape-stripping and punch biopsy). No significant difference in the CD4/CD8 (helper/suppressor) lymphocyte ratio between Koebner-positive and -negative subjects could be found in the dermal infiltrates. The influx, activation, and resulting imbalance in the distribution of intraepidermal T cell populations in the uninvolved skin of psoriatic patients were proposed as factors contributing to the reactivity to injury. The same authors reported no quantitative difference in the CD1a-positive epidermal Langerhans cell number between the two groups of patients studied (77). However, interactions of the Langerhans cells with keratinocytes and infiltrating lymphocytes occurred mostly in psoriatic lesions induced by the Koebner phenomenon (63). Tape-stripping of clinically uninvolved psoriatic skin provoked a very rapid Langerhans cell depletion from the traumatized epidermis, when compared with the simultaneously studied nonpsoriatic controls (74). A movement of the Langerhans cells across the basement membrane was observed and this increased Langerhans cell mobility along with ultrastructural signs of enhanced cytoplasmic activity was noticed exclusively in patients who later developed the Koebner

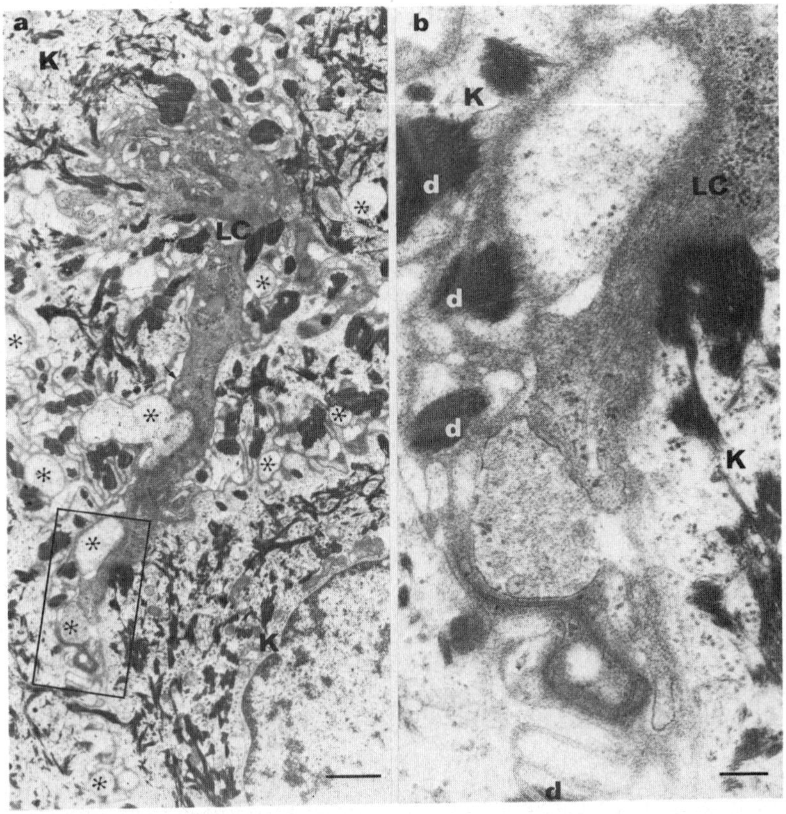

Figure 6 Ultrastructural evidence of Langerhans cell–keratinocyte interactions in a minute eruptive lesion of psoriasis. (a) Langerhans cell (LC) dendrite penetrating between keratinocytes (K). Numerous rounded, organelle-free, membrane-delimited structures (asterisks) can be seen in the intercellular spaces around the dendrite. An arrow points to a Birbeck granule. Bar = 1 μm. (b) Higher magnification of the zone delimited in (a). The Langerhans cell dendrite (LC) is closely appositioned to keratinocytes (K) and to the blebs displaying the electron density and structure similar to the keratinocyte cytoplasm. d = desmosomes. Bar = 200 nm.

reaction. Biopsies of Koebner-positive patients were characterized by interactions between keratinocytes, epidermal lymphocytes, and macrophages, suggestive of cell activation and cytotoxicity (74a).

These observations further implicate the Langerhans cell in the chain of events related to the development of psoriatic lesions.

Pustular Psoriasis

The most striking feature in this form of psoriasis is the massive intraepidermal influx of polymorphonuclear (neutrophil) leukocytes which accumulate in the upper epidermis and constitute aseptic spongiform pustules. Here again, the apposition of epidermal Langerhans cells and infiltrating mononuclear and polymorphonuclear cells has been reported in both the generalized (78) and palmoplantar (79) types. The ultrastructural evidence of cell destruction and of deposition of the cellular debris in the interkeratinocyte spaces was suggestive of local cellular interactions involving Langerhans cells. The resulting microscopic changes rapidly become macroscopic due to the amplificatory effect exerted by proteinase-rich neutrophils. Quantification of Langerhans cells in the localized pustular psoriasis of the palms and soles showed an increase of the cell number in the nonpustular areas when the results were expressed per length unit of the biopsy section (80).

Uninvolved Psoriatic Skin

Quantitation of Langerhans cells in the uninvolved epidermis yields less conflicting results than the studies of the psoriatic lesions. Here, epidermal Langerhans cell counts are not influenced by the histological features inherent to the pathological epidermis, irrespective of the method of quantification or mode of expression of the results. According to most authors, there is no or only a slight modification in the Langerhans cell population density in the uninvolved skin of psoriatic patients (53,57,77). However, a statistically significant decrease in Langerhans cell number has also been reported (36,81). Once again, this variability may depend on the phase of the disease activity in which the studies were performed.

Effect of the Treatments Resulting in Clinical Improvement

All investigators dealing with the treatment of psoriasis know that a simple occlusion of a psoriatic lesion may have a beneficial therapeutic effect. Although electron microscopic signs of the epidermal Langerhans cells alteration have been reported in occluded skin (82), the recently published quantitative data did not indicate numerical changes of this cell population ($CD1a^+$; DR^+) during prolonged occlusion (83a). Also, dithranol failed to induce any quantitative changes in the CD1a positive epidermal cell population both in lesional and in unaffected psoriatic skin during the treatment resulting in clinical resolution (53,64). However, prominent ultrastructural signs of both Langerhans cell activation and degeneration were reported in normal human skin after 24 hr of occlusion with 0.2% dithranol in petrolatum (84). Similar fine structural changes and repopulation of the healing epidermis with Langerhans cells were reported in topical tar-treated psoriatic lesions (85).

Several experimental studies demonstrated that the topical application of glucocorticosteroids to normal human skin results in a marked decrease in the Langerhans cell number demonstrable with various staining methods (48,86–88). Also, in psoriatic plaques and uninvolved psoriatic skin the treatment caused a decrease in epidermal DR-positive (64) and both epidermal and dermal CD1a-positive dendritic cells (65). The degree of the Langerhans cell depletion correlated well with the anti-inflammatory action of topical steroids and was associated with a dose-dependent reduction of Langerhans cell-dependent T lymphocyte activation, as tested in vitro (48,87). Thus, the influence of steroids on the immunologically important class II antigen expression (86,88a) and on the cell function is a more probable mode of action on Langerhans cells than a direct killing effect.

Ultraviolet B and photochemotherapy (PUVA) are other modalities that are effective in the treatment of psoriasis and which simultaneously influence Langerhans cells. Both treatments were demonstrated to deplete the Langerhans cell surface markers in a dose-dependent manner (89). ATPase staining proved the most sensitive to ultraviolet irradiation (89,90), whereas CD1a and HLA DR antigens persisted even after ultraviolet light doses transiently inhibiting the Langerhans cell function (91a). Within the dose range normally used for PUVA therapy, the ATPase-positive cells disappeared from the epidermis still containing ultrastructurally recognizable Langerhans cells and reappeared after cessation of the treatment (92–94). Variable degrees of reduction of the Langerhans cell number during PUVA treatment were assessed with CD1a and/or DR immunocytochemical markers employed in various quantitation methods (53,56,57,65). The Langerhans cell morphology was considerably modified (95,96) and its function could also be impaired, as indicated by the depressed cell-mediated immune responses (97,98).

Aromatic retinoid proved to be effective in the treatment of psoriasis. We quantified the CD1a and HLA DR-expressing epidermal cells in peripherally spreading psoriatic plaques and found that etretinate therapy resulted in a gradual correction of the initially decreased cell number (36). Systemic retinoid treatment had practically no influence on the normal frequency of Langerhans cells in uninvolved epidermis (36,99). These findings were later confirmed semiquantitatively by others (100). The increase in the number of epidermal Langerhans cells in psoriasis treated with aromatic retinoid is accompanied by a similar increase in the dermal Langerhans cell frequency (101), and by a growing peripheral blood monocyte count (102). These data, although only morphological, suggest that aromatic retinoid may stimulate differentiation of monocyte precursors to mature Langerhans cells and promote their migration to the epidermis. A clinically obvious regulatory influence of retinoids on epidermal keratinization, when paralleled by the retinoid-induced repopulation of the healing lesions with fresh, immunologically intact (unprimed) Langerhans cells, may result in restoration of the local physiological balance. Furthermore, observations of the treatment efficiency and duration of the remission periods indicate that better results can be obtained with the combination retinoid-PUVA therapy. Also, this treatment results in a more rapid normalization of the Langerhans cell distribution and number in the healing psoriatic lesions (80,103). The previously summarized data on PUVA-induced changes and the retinoid-PUVA influence on Langerhans cells suggest that the more complete "recycling" of the Langerhans cells and keratinocytes accompanied by suppression of the inflammatory infiltrate may be at the origin of the dramatic clinical efficacity of the combined treatment. In general, rupture of the vicious circle of cellular/humoral feedbacks that perpetuate the inflammatory changes with the resulting metabolic keratinocyte dysfunction could be the possible underlying mechanism of any successful antipsoriatic therapy* (85).

Although these various treatments for psoriasis appear to influence the population of epidermal Langerhans cells, they are also equally or even more effective in their action on other immunocompetent cell types present in the psoriatic skin (56,64,97,98,101). This is also the case of cyclosporin A, an immunosuppressive drug used in the treatment of severe psoriasis (104,105). Cyclosporin A exerts its effect by interfering with the functional activation of T helper lymphocytes. Its beneficial influence on psoriasis speaks for the important role of this cell subpopulation in the disease. However, a further explanation for the drug's effectiveness in psoriasis may be its inhibitory action on the antigen-presenting capacity of Langerhans cells (106,107a). Impairment of interleukin 1 and interleukin 2 production (108) by cyclosporin A may also inhibit lymphokine-mediated induction of class II antigen expression, and thus additionally decrease local immunological reactivity (109). Clinically successful treatment of psoriasis, both intralesional (110) and general (111,112a), results in an improvement-correlated increase in the originally reduced CD1a-positive epidermal cells and in the normalization of their distribution pattern. Langerhans cell numbers in uninvolved psoriatic skin remain virtually unchanged by cyclosporin A treatment (71); however, some investigators have observed the drug-induced depletion of epidermal Langerhans cells, which equaled that seen with UVB or PUVA (112b).

A decade ago, vitamin D_3 analogs, which inhibit proliferation and increase differentiation of several cell types, were introduced as a new treatment of psoriasis. This family of drugs acts through the interaction with a specific nuclear receptor (VDR) forming heterodimers with the receptors for retinoids, which suggests that both compounds may act synergistically as they use similar signaling pathways. Although topical calcipotriol does not seem to influence directly the number of epidermal Langerhans cells, even a moderate improvement of psoriatic plaques after 2-week treatment was associated with an increase in CD1a+ cell population (112c).

*Haftek, M. A possible role of Langerhans cells in the pathogenesis of psoriasis. Lecture presented at the Meeting of the Swedish Dermatological Society (Western Section), Göteborg, May 27, 1983.

CURRENT HYPOTHESES OF THE PATHOGENSIS OF PSORIASIS AND A POSSIBLE ROLE OF LANGERHANS CELLS IN THE DEVELOPMENT OF PSORIATIC LESIONS

A defect of the mechanism(s) responsible for the control of keratinocyte proliferation and differentiation is the most obvious, though disappointingly vague, hypothesis attempting to account for the pathomechanism of psoriasis. It provides an explanation for the histological, immunocytochemical, biochemical, and cell cycle (cytodynamic) features observed in psoriasis. For this reason, various groups of researchers agree that some kind of dysregulation of the process of keratinocyte proliferation and differentiation must take place in the psoriatic lesions, and the first question they try to answer is whether the putative defect is primary or secondary. Krueger et al. (113) observed that monocytes/macrophages from patients with psoriasis appear "activated." The increased cell chemotaxis persisted in remission, indicating the possibility of a constitutional defect. Since epidermal Langerhans cells have most probably circulating monocyte/macrophage precursors, Mier et al. (114) speculated that these cells are also functionally abnormal in psoriasis. The authors indicated that the Langerhans cell distribution in psoriatic plaques was reported to be disturbed and that such a decrease in the Langerhans cell density is often associated with epidermal hyperproliferations (51) and a parakeratotic type of keratinization (115). The idea has received further indirect support from Krueger (49), who reported that after grafting to athymic mice the density of Langerhans cell distribution in lesional epidermis is the same as in clinically uninvolved skin grafts. Although uninvolved psoriatic skin grafts were reported to display some of the characteristics of psoriatic lesions, such as an increased rate of mitoses (49) and plasminogen activator synthesis (116), we could demonstrate that several histological hallmarks of psoriasis disappear from the lesional skin 1 month after grafting (117).

There is no more intraepidermal infiltrate, normal granular layer reappears, and even the typical clubbing of the dermoepidermal junction can be observed in only 60% of grafts. Thus, a possible direct influence of the Langerhans cells or, more precisely, their lack of control in the psoriatic epidermis (23,115) could be retained as a plausible physiopathological cause. Today, both humoral and cellular interactions directly or indirectly involving Langerhans cells are still a matter of discussion. However, our knowledge of these interrelationships has considerably evolved during the last decade and the theories implicating these mechanisms have changed accordingly.

Morhenn (118) proposed a general model for the regulation of keratinocyte proliferation in wound healing and skin diseases. The model predicts the existence of at least two kinds of dermatoses as regarded from the keratinocyte mitotic activity viewpoint. One group is characterized by the expression of class II antigens by slowly or normally growing lesional keratinocytes (e.g., lichen planus, polykilodermatous form of mycosis fungoides). The other type, possibly represented by psoriasis, displays keratinocyte hyperproliferation associated with little, if any, HLA DR production by keratinocytes. Since the HLA DR expression on keratinocytes may result from the influence of high concentrations of interferon γ (of T lymphocyte origin) (19), and since such elevated interferon γ levels exert an inhibitory effect on keratinocyte growth (119), the absence of the diffuse epidermal HLA DR expression in psoriatic lesions may testify to the absence of the growth regulatory mechanism mediated by interferon γ. Indeed, no or only focal expression of HLA DR antigen on lesional keratinocytes has been found in psoriasis by most of the researchers studying this problem (31,36,69, 120,120a,120b). The contrary, however, has been reported by Gottlieb et al. (32), who found 7–84% of the lesional keratinocytes to be HLA DR positive in 8 out of 20 patients studied. These authors observed a close correlation between keratinocyte DR antigen expression and the severity of the disease; namely, the presence of psoriatic arthritis. Additionally, keratinocyte HLA DR expression may be limited in time, as demonstrated in studies of human delayed-type hypersenstivitiy reactions in vivo (121), and this would further explain discrepancies between the cited findings. Interferon γ production by activated T lymphocytes may be downregulated by normal keratinocytes through the decrease of interleukin 2 production mediated by secretion of prostaglandin E_2 and the keratinocyte-derived lymphocyte inhibitory factor (122,123). In this context, it is particularly interesting to recall that cyclosporin A impairs secretion of interleukins 1 and 2, and that a clinical relapse of psoriasis in its erythrodermic form can be induced by a general interleukin 2 treatment (124). Whether psoriatic individuals are deficient in one or several feedback mechanisms involved in the inhibition of keratinocyte growth after regeneration of the damaged epidermis has been completed remains to be studied. A recent report by Bata-Csorgo et al. (124a) provides evidence that psoriatic noninvolved keratinocyte stem cell proliferation may be induced by soluble factors secreted by lesional T helper lymphocyte clones. Interestingly, normal keratinocyte stem cells exhibit no such growth stimulation.

Valdimarsson et al. (125) proposed that homeostasis in psoriatic epidermis is disturbed when the intraepidermal influx of T helper lymphocytes overrides the influence of T suppressor cells, which are a predominating lymphocyte subpopulation in normal and noninvolved psoriatic epidermis. It has been suggested that a humoral factor produced by such activated T helper lymphocytes could stimulate keratinocyte proliferation.

Other researchers (78,126–129), have reported that proteolytic enzymes released in the epidermis by infiltrating polymorphonuclear leukocytes are likely to alter the keratinocyte surfaces (130,131) and interfere with the function of membrane-bound enzymes (132, 133), the two factors which may be implicated in the control of epidermal proliferation.

Numerous inflammatory dermatoses can be aggravated by stress, and psoriasis is no exception in this respect. Farber et al. (134) observed that exacerbations and remissions of psoriatic lesions are often affected by such general factors as stress under its various forms. They proposed that neuropeptides released from the peripheral sensory nerve endings contribute to the inflammatory reaction in the psoriatic lesion (neurogenic inflammation). These neural transmitters (e.g., substance P) would appear to exert their influence through binding to the receptors on mast cells, and by induction of degranulation, resulting in the release of numerous mediators of inflammation. Whereas there is no evidence in the current data that this mechanism could be responsible for initiation of new lesions, the mast cell degranulation has been reported as an early event in initial eruptive lesions of nonstreptococcal guttate psoriasis (135) and an increased number of neurofilament- and substance P–positive nerves has been observed in the developed psoriatic plaques (but not in the uninvolved skin)

(136). While considering the role of Langerhans cells in psoriasis, it is interesting to mention that intimate associations between these cells and intraepidermal nerve fibers were observed in normal human skin ultrastructurally and with laser confocal scanning microscope (136a). The majority of the CD1a+ Langerhans cell bodies appeared to be the destination of the sensory nerve endings expressing calcitonin gene-related neuropeptide (CGRP). Functional assays suggest that CGRP, which can be coexpressed in mammalian peripheral neurons with either substance P or somatostatin, is able to downregulate antigen presentation by macrophages and epidermal Langerhans cells and inhibit interleukin-2 production and T-cell proliferation (136b). On the other hand, as a potent vasodilator, it may be an important factor in neurogenic inflammation (136c), as is substance P, which was reported to bind to and stimulate both T lymphocytes (137,138) and macrophages (139).

Whatever the final effectory mechanism leading to the local keratinocyte hyperproliferation in psoriasis, the initial steps of the pathological process may have the same origin: an immune reaction taking place in the skin and mediated by the major epidermal antigen-presenting cell population, i.e., the Langerhans cells. Interleukin-1 secreted by Langerhans cells (16) is highly chemotactic for T lymphocytes, which in turn become "activated" after recognition of the foreign antigen and synthesize surface HLA DR antigen, interleukin-2 and interferon-γ. The interactions between antigen-presenting Langerhans cells and homing T lymphocytes take place mainly in the dermis, where activated Langerhans cells migrate and are easily accessible to the circulating immunocompetent cells. In this afferent limb of the cell-mediated immune response, the antigen-bearing Langerhans cells, which serve as a target for the homing antigen-specific cytotoxic lymphocytes, most probably perish in this ultimate interaction. Lymphokines released during this phase of the immune response and the proteolytic enzymes discharged from the destroyed cells may be responsible for several secondary mechanisms resulting in the local epidermal changes:

1. Factor(s) stimulating keratinocyte proliferation directly (124a,125) or indirectly—through the interleukin-1–mediated dermal fibroblast activation and somatomedin C production (140,141)—have been proposed. A possible positive feedback loop may subsequently take place since the proliferating keratinocytes synthesize epidermal T-cell-activating factor (ETAF), which is closely related to interleukin-1 (17), and because the cytokines amplify the presentation and sensitization functions of accessory cells (20) as well as the expression of several adhesion molecules on immunocompetent and endothelial cells important in cell interaction and trafficking (141a).
2. Chemoattraction of polymorphonuclear leukocytes to the epidermis can also be provoked directly by cytokines or through the secretion of the inflammation mediators (129,142,143) resulting in the additional proteinase release and initiation of the self-perpetuating process of maintenance and spreading of psoriatic lesions (127,128).

Several antigens potentially can be recognized as "foreign" by Langerhans cells and, therefore, may serve as the starting factors in a psoriatic relapse. These include the putative viral (144–146) and bacterial proteins (147), the altered native proteins or unmasked but otherwise inaccessible tissue antigens (148) resulting from widely understood "physicochemical traumas." Langerhans cells may play the role of a link between these various antigens recognized as "foreign" and the rest of the immune system. In this context, the presence of HLA DR antigen on a great proportion of T lymphocytes infiltrating psoriatic lesions is of particular interest since it is a sign of the specific T-cell activation (149). An immune reaction taking place in the skin in the areas where a hypothetic antigen was recognized, captured, and presented to the circulating lymphocytes may explain the irregular distribution of psoriatic lesions. Superantigens of bacterial origin may circumvent this antigen-specific interaction and are probably responsible for the multifocal induction of highly inflammatory "guttate" psoriasis lesions during infections (21a,21b).

Mechanisms regulating the local immune response in the skin comprise a cytokine-controlled amplification of accessory cell function (20) and adhesion molecule–dependent cell trafficking (141a).

The most important cytokine involved in Langerhans cell maturation is GM-CSF (15), which may be released from many cell types including sensitized T cells, keratinocytes, fibroblasts, endothelial cells, and smooth muscle cells. Thus, local release of GM-CSF, interleukin-1, and interferon-γ results in the mobilization of active accessory cells and in the local induction of HLA D antigens on epithelia, endothelia, and fibroblasts ensuring the retention of most of the class II–restricted cells in the inflammatory site. Indeed, the increased numbers of lesional Langerhans cells in psoriasis coexpress surface antigens of lymphoid interdigitating cells, which are known to be mature, very potent antigen-presenting cells (62,150). In vitro assays of autologous mixed epidermal cell–T lymphocyte reaction (MECLR) showed that the epidermis from psoriatic patients contained a population of HLA DR+, CD1a− cells with singularly strong stimulatory properties (107a,150a). These psoriatic antigen-presenting cells displayed a functional phenotype typical of isolated Langerhans cells maintained in a short-term culture (107a). It is now admitted that such a phenotype corresponds in vivo to the "mature" stimulatory state of Langerhans cells, acquired after migration to the peripheral lymph nodes and compatible with induction of major histocompatibility antigen class II–restricted lymphocyte proliferation (150b). The fact that healthy controls and contact allergy patients do not present stimulatory faculty in autologous MECLR (150a) and that the "mature" state of epidermal antigen-presenting cells in psoriasis may precede the appearance of active skin lesions, as it is detected also in uninvolved skin (107a), indicates that the abnormality in psoriatic Langerhans cell function may be important in the expression of keratinocyte pathology. In vitro release of unspecified leukocyte migration-inhibition factor(s) observed in cocultures of psoriatic epidermal cells with autologous peripheral blood mononuclear cells (151) also points to the possibility that cell-mediated immune mechanisms are significant in the physiopathology of the disease.

Another important factor regulating immunocompetent cell interaction are surface receptors permitting migration, reciprocal adhesion, and stabilization of cells during various phases of the immune response. Expression of an E-selectin ligand, sialyl Lewis X, involved in cell migration through endothelia and inducible by interferon-γ, can be observed on "cultured" Langerhans cells and is characteristic of the Langerhans cells in psoriasis (151a). Lymphokine-induced up-regulation of several adhesion molecules, e.g., ICAM-1, β_2 integrins, on immunocompetent and endothelial cells observed in psoriasis contributes to the leukocyte trafficking and enhanced accessory/T-cell interaction (151a,151b,151c).

IMPLICATIONS FOR FURTHER RESEARCH

More functional studies are needed, especially as concerns Langerhans cell interactions with other populations of skin cells that are possibly involved in the pathological psoriatic process. In vitro autologous epidermal cell–leukocyte assays represent recent examples of such an experimental approach (107a, 150a,151). A cautionary note should, however, be sounded. First, not all the complicated cell interactions can be reliably reproduced in vitro. Second, certain functional features observed in the cells, which are isolated, enriched, and thus modified due to the extraction from their natural environment, may not physiologically occur in situ.

Observations on the modification of the natural course of psoriasis related to the coexisting diseases are another way to acquire valuable information. Challenging questions can be raised concerning Langerhans cell and T helper lymphocyte role in the pathogenesis of psoriasis because of the reported "induction" of psoriatic lesions in AIDS patients with no past history of psoriasis and several cases of exacerbation of psoriatic skin lesions resulting in severe involvement correlated with aggravation in the course of AIDS (152,153). The Langerhans cells can be infected by HIV virus (154,155) and they tend to express less HLA DR antigen and ATPase activity during the initial stages of AIDS (156). A decrease in the Langerhans cell population density could be observed in AIDS patients at stages III and IV, and the Langerhans cell involvement could be correlated with the degree of reduction in the absolute number of circulating T helper lymphocytes (157). Comparison between HIV-1-positive and -negative psoriatic patients demonstrated a reduction in the number of protein S-100-expressing suprabasal cell population (putative Langerhans cells) in both involved and clinically normal epidermis of the former (157a). Fine regulatory mechanisms (both humoral and cellular) essential for the immunological homeostasis within skin are most probably perturbed in AIDS. A few cases of clearing of the psoriatic lesions were observed in AIDS patients treated with peptide-T, a synthetic molecule that is identical to the viral envelope glycoprotein gp120 (158). The peptide binds to the T4 receptor on leukocytes, which is thought to be the first step leading to the HIV penetration. It is conceivable that the beneficial effect of peptide-T on psoriasis is due to the interference with the function of T4-positive helper lymphocytes and Langerhans cells. Indeed, in a recent report, Wang et al. (158a) describe normalization of S-100 immunoreactive (Langerhans) cell distribution and number in HIV-negative psoriatic patients successfully treated with peptide-T. Prospective studies of psoriatic patients becoming HIV-positive would greatly help to define the prevalence of exacerbation of psoriasis in AIDS. Moreover, they would help to demonstrate possible cases with improvement of psoriasis and with prolongated remissions.

There is no doubt that studies on the influence of various pharmacological and physicochemical treatments, which prove to be clinically efficient, on the different cellular components of the skin and the immune system and on their functional interactions will also be of primary importance. A number of new, often experimental treatments have been observed to influence favorably psoriatic lesions, e.g., cyclosporin A (159), FK 506 (159a), peptide-T (158), interferon-γ (160), vitamin D_3 (161,162) or to worsen and even induce them, e.g., interleukin-2 (124), interferon-α (163,164). As these same treatments are likely to modulate local and general immune responses, further studies of their action on the Langerhans cell function and distribution in normal and psoriatic skin would be justified and could supply further clues to our comprehension of the physiopathology of psoriasis.

The use of new tools in immunocytochemistry, such as still more raffined monoclonal antibodies to cellular and humoral factors and components, in situ hybridization technique, and quantitative image/data analysis methods, combined with the possibilities of three-dimensional image reconstruction, also opens up further perspectives in morphological studies on the evolution of psoriatic lesions and the Langerhans cells involvement in the process.

Over a decade ago, Gerald G. Krueger (49) mentioned that "the complexity of the interaction of the humorally borne cellular/noncellular factors with one another is nearly overwhelming. If such factors also participate in the regulation of proliferation and differentiation of organs such as the skin, the magnitude of the problem seems incomprehensible. Despite such an unpalatable possibility, it appears that a complete understanding of psoriasis lies in the dissection of such interactions." Today, as we steadily progress in comprehension of these complicated cellular and humoral interactions, it seems that the announced "promised land" of complete understanding of psoriasis gets ever closer.

REFERENCES

1. Katz, S.I., Tamaki, K., and Sachs, D.H. (1979). Epidermal Langerhans cells are derived from cells originating in bone marrow. *Nature* 282:324–326.
2. Tamaki, K., Stingl, G., and Katz, S.I. (1980). The origin of Langerhans cells. *J. Invest. Dermatol.* 74: 309–311.

2a. Caux, C., Dezutter-Dambuyant, C., Schmitt, D. Banchereau, J. (1991). GM-CSF and TNFα cooperate in the generation of dendritic Langerhans cells. *Nature* 360:258–261.

2b. Reid, C.D.L., Stackpoole, A., Meager, A., and Tikerpae, J. (1992). Interactions of tumor necrosis factor with granulocyte-macrophage colony stimulating factor and other cytokines in the regulation of dendritic cell growth in vitro from early bipotent CD34 + progenitors in human bone marrow. *J. Immunol.* 149: 2681–2688.

3. Czernielewski, J.M., and Demarchez, M. (1987). Further evidence for the self-reproducing capacity of Langerhans cells in human skin. *J. Invest. Dermatol.* 88:17–20.
4. De Fraissinette, A., Staquet, M.J., Dezutter-Dambuyant, C., Schmitt, D., and Thivolet, J. (1988). Langerhans cells in S-phase in normal skin detected by simultaneous analysis of cell surface antigen and BrdU incorporation. *J. Invest. Dermatol.* 91:603–605.
5. Horton, J.J., Allen, M.H., and MacDonald, D.M. (1984). An assessment of Langerhans cell quantification in tissue sections. *J. Am. Acad. Dermatol.* 11: 591–593.
6. Thomas, J.A., Biggerstaff, M., Sloane, J.P., and Easton, D.F. (1984). Immunological and histochemical analysis of regional variations of epidermal Langerhans cells in normal human skin. *Histochem. J.* 16: 507–519.
7. Wolff, K. (1967). The fine structure of the Langerhans cell granule. *J. Cell Biol.* 35:468–477.
8. Ray, A., Schmitt, D., Dezutter-Dambuyant, C., Fargier, M.C., and Thivolet, J. (1989). Reappearance of CD1a antigenic sites after endocytosis on human Langerhans cells evidenced by immunogold re-labelling. *J. Invest. Dermatol.* 92:217–224.

8a. Kashihara, M., Ueda, M., Horiguchi, Y., Furukawa, F., Hanaoka, M., and Imamura, S. (1987). A monoclonal antibody specifically reactive to human Langerhans cells. *J. Invest. Dermatol.* 87:602–607.

9. Stingl, G., Romani, N., and Wolff, K. (1987) Langerhans cells: a distinctive member of bone marrow–derived dendritic cells. *Adv. Dermatol.* 2: 269–281.
10. Dezutter-Dambuyant, C. (1988). Membrane antigens and Birbeck granules of human Langerhans cells. In *The Langerhans Cell.* Colloques INSERM Vol.172. J. Thivolet and D. Schmitt (Eds.) John Libbey Eurotext, Montrouge, pp. 87–97.
11. Groh, V., Gadner, H., Radaszkiewicz, T., Rappersberger, K., Konrad, K., Wolff, K., and Stingl, G. (1988). The phenotypic spectrum of histiocytosis X cells. *J. Invest. Dermatol.* 90:441–447.

12. Shelley, W.B., and Juhlin, L. (1976). Langerhans cells form a reticulo-epithelial trap for external contact antigens. *Nature* 261:46–47.
12a. Caux, C., Vanbervliet, B., Massacrier, C., Azuma, M., Okumura, K., Lanier, L.L., and Banchereau, J. (1994). B70/B7-2 is identical to CD86 and is the major functional ligand for CD28 expressed on human dendritic cells. *J. Exp. Med.* 180:1841–1847.
13. Katz, S.I., Cooper, K.D., Tijima, M., and Tsuchida, T. (1985). The role of Langerhans cells in antigen presentation. *J. Invest. Dermatol.* 85:96s–98s.
14. Picut, C.A., Lee, C.S., Dougherty, E.P., Anderson, K.L., and Lewis, R.M. (1988). Immunostimulatory capabilities of highly enriched Langerhans cells in vitro. *J. Invest. Dermatol.* 90:201–206.
15. Heufler, C., Koch, F., and Schuler, G. (1988). Granulocyte/macrophage colony-stimulating factor and interleukin 1 mediate the maturation of murine epidermal Langerhans cells into potent immunostimulatory dendritic cells. *J. Exp. Med.* 167:700–705.
16. Sauder, D.N., Dinarello, C.A., and Morhenn, V.B. (1984). Langerhans cell production of interleukin-1. *J. Invest. Dermatol.* 82:605–607.
17. Luger, T.A., Stadler, B.M., Katz, S.I., and Oppenheim, J.J. (1981). Epidermal cell (keratinocyte)–derived thymocyte-activating factor (ETAF). *J. Immunol.* 127:1493–1498.
18. Preble, O.T., and Friedman, R.M. (1983). Interferon-induced alterations in cells: relevance to viral and nonviral diseases. *Lab. Invest.* 49:4–18.
19. Basham, T.Y., Nickoloff, B.J., Merigan, T.C., and Morhenn, V.B. (1984). Recombinant gamma interferon induces HLA DR expression on cultured human keratinocytes. *J. Invest. Dermatol.* 83:88–90.
20. Steinman, R.M. (1988). Cytokines amplify the function of accessory cells. *Immunol. Lett.* 17:197–202.
20a. Steinman, R.M. (1991). The dendritic cell system and its role in immunogenicity. *Annu. Rev. Immunol.* 9: 271–296.
21. Silberberg, I., Baer, R.L., and Rosenthal, S.A. (1976). The role of Langerhans cells in allergic contact hypersensitivity. A review of findings in man and guinea pigs. *J. Invest. Dermatol.* 66:210–217.
21a. Leung, D.Y.M., Walsh, P., Giorno, R., and Norris, D. (1993). A potential role for superantigens in the pathogenesis of psoriasis. *J. Invest. Dermatol.* 100: 225–228.
21b. Skov, L. and Baadsgaard, O. (1995). Superantigens. Do they have a role in skin diseases? *Arch. Dermatol.* 131:829–832.
22. Sagebiel, R.W., Clarke, M.A., and Hutchens, L.H. (1971). Dendritic cells in oral epithelium. In *Current Concepts of the Histology of Oral Mucosa.* C.A. Squier and J. Meyer (Eds.). Charles C Thomas Publisher, Springfield, IL, p. 143.
23. Potten, C.S., and Allen, T.D. (1976). A model implicating the Langerhans cell in keratinocyte proliferation control. *Differentiation* 5:43–47.
24. Schweizer, J., and Marks, F. (1977). A developmental study of the distribution and frequency of Langerhans cells in relation to formation of patterning in mouse tail epidermis. *J. Invest. Dermatol.* 69:198–204.
25. Juhlin, L., and Shelley, W.B. (1977). New staining techniques for the Langerhans cell. *Acta Derm. Venereol.* 57:289–296.
26. Miyazaki, H., Kawada, A., Takaki, Y., Sato, T., and Masutani, M. (1974). Effects of ultraviolet light on epidermal dendritic cells of hairless mice. In *Sunlight and Man.* M.A. Pathak, L.H. Harber, M. Seiji, and A. Kukita (Eds.). University of Tokyo Press, Tokyo, pp. 217–229.
27. Schmitt, D., Faure, M., Dezutter-Dambuyant, C., and Tuffery, D. (1984). Ultrastructural immunogold labelling of human Langerhans cells enriched epidermal cell suspension. *Arch. Dermatol. Res.* 276:27–32.
28. Thivolet, J. and Schmitt, D. (1987). Langerhans cell and T cell subset identification using monoclonal antibodies: immunocytochemical methods in light and electron microscopy applied on human skin. In *Immunopathology of the Skin.* E.H. Beutner, T.P. Chorzelski, and V. Kumar (Eds.). Wiley, New York, pp. 125–150.
29. Dezutter-Dambuyant, C., Schmitt, D., Staquet, M.J., Zambruno, G., Frappaz, A., Boumsell, L., and Thivolet, J. (1988). CD1 antigens on human epidermal Langerhan cells: alteration of cell-surface CD1a molecule by proteolysis. In *The Langerhans Cell.* Colloques INSERM Vol.172. J. Thivolet and D. Schmitt (Eds.). John Libbey Eurotext, Montrouge, pp. 125–138.
30. Lampert, I.A. (1984). Expression of HLA DR (Ia-like) antigen on epidermal keratinocytes in human dermatoses. *Clin. Exp. Immunol.* 57:93–100.
31. Gomes, M., Schmitt, D., Dezutter-Dambuyant, C., Capra, J.D., and Thivolet, J. (1986). Expression des antigènes HLA de classe II (HLA DR, DQW1, DQW3) au niveau de la peau normale et en pathologie cutanée. *Pathol. Biol.* 34:157–164.
32. Gottlieb, A.B., Lifshitz, D., Fu, S.M., Staiano-Coico, L., Wang, C.Y., and Carter, D.M. (1986). Expression of HLA DR molecules by keratinocytes, and presence of Langerhans cells in the dermal infiltrate of active psoriatic plaques. *J. Exp. Med.* 164:1013–1028.
33. Haftek, M. and Thivolet, J. (1984). Quantitation of epidermal dendritic cells. *J. Invest. Dermatol.* 83:78 (letter).
34. Bieber, T., Ring, J., and Braun-Falco, O. (1988). Comparison of different methods for enumeration of Langerhans cells in vertical cryosections of human skin. *Br. J. Dermatol.* 118:385–392.

35. Haftek, M., Schmitt, D., Brochier, J., Faure, M., and Thivolet, J. (1982). A specific method of Langerhans cell quantification in human epidermis. Difference in expression of HLA DR and T6 antigens. *J. Invest. Dermatol.* 78:332.
36. Haftek, M., Faure, M., Schmitt, D., and Thivolet, J. (1983). Langerhans cells in skin from patients with psoriasis: quantitative and qualitative study of T6 and HLA DR antigen-expressing cells and changes with aromatic retinoid administration. *J. Invest. Dermatol.* 81:10–14.
37. Sontheimer, R.D., Stasny, P., and Nunez, G. (1986). HLA-D region antigen expression by human Langerhans cells. *J. Invest. Dermatol.* 87:707–710.
38. Cooper, K.D., Breathnach, S.M., Caughman, S.W., Palini, A.G., Waxdal, M.J., and Katz, S.I. (1985). Fluorescence microscopic and flow cytometric analysis of bone marrow-derived cells in human epidermis: a search for the human analogue of the murine dendritic Thy-1+ epidermal cell. *J. Invest. Dermatol.* 85: 546–552.
39. Dezutter-Dambuyant, C., Cordier, G., Schmitt, D., Faure, M., Laquoi, C., and Thivolet, J. (1984). Quantitative evaluation of two distinct cell populations expressing HLA DR antigens in normal human epidermis. *Br. J. Dermatol.* 111:1–11.
40. Stingl, G., Katz, S.I., Clement, L., Green, I., and Shevach, E.M. (1978). Immunologic functions of Ia-bearing epidermal Langerhans cells. *J. Immunol.* 121: 2005–2013.
41. Braathen, L.R. and Thorsby, E. (1980). Studies on human epidermal Langerhans cells. I. Alloactivating and antigen presenting capacity. *Scand. J. Immunol.* 11:401–408.
42. Pehamberger, H., Stingl, L.A., Pogantsch, S., Steiner, G., Wolff, K., and Stingl, G. (1983). Epidermal cell-induced generation of cytotoxic T lymphocyte responses against alloantigens or TNP-modified syngeneic cells: requirement for Ia-positive Langerhans cells. *J. Invest. Dermatol.* 81:208–211.
43. Faure, M., Frappaz, A., Schmitt, D., Dezutter-Dambuyant, C., and Thivolet, J. (1984). Role of HLA DR bearing Langerhans and epidermal indeterminate cells in the in vitro generation of alloreactive cytotoxic T cells in man. *Cell. Immunol.* 83:271–279.
44. Inaba, K. and Steinman, R.M. (1984). Resting and sensitized T lymphocytes exhibit distinct stimulatory (antigen-presenting cell) requirements for growth and lymphokine release. *J. Exp. Med.* 160:1717–1735.
45. Inaba, K. and Steinman, R.M. (1987). Monoclonal antibodies to LFA-1 and to CD4 inhibit the mixed leukocyte reaction after the antigen-dependent clustering of dendritic cells and T lymphocytes. *J. Exp. Med.* 165:1403–1417.
46. Streilein, J.W. and Bergstresser, P.R. (1981). Langerhans cell function dictates induction of contact hypersensitivity or unresponsiveness to DNBF in Syrian hamsters. *J. Invest. Dermatol.* 77:272–277.
47. Austad, J. and Braathen, L.R. (1985). Effects of UVB on alloactivating and antigen-presenting capacity of human epidermal Langerhans cells. *Scand. J. Immunol.* 21:417–423.
48. Ashworth, J., Booker, J., and Breathnach, S.M. (1988). Effect of topical corticosteroid therapy on Langerhans cell antigen presenting function in human skin. *Br. J. Dermatol.* 118:457–469.
49. Krueger, G.G. (1981). Psoriasis: current concepts of its etiology and pathogenesis. In *Year Book of Dermatology.* R.L. Dobson and R.H. Thiers (Eds.). Year Book Medical Publishers, Chicago, pp. 13–70.
50. Muller, S.A., Winkelman, R.K., and Vanderstein, P.R. (1971). Langerhans cells and cutaneous nerves in psoriasis: a histochemical study. In *Psoriasis. Proceedings of the First International Symposium.* E.M. Farber and A.J. Cox (Eds.). Stanford University Press, Stanford, pp. 187–202.
51. Lisi, P. (1973). Investigation on Langerhans cells in pathological human epidermis. *Acta Derm. Venereol. (Stockh.).* 53:425–428.
52. Bos, J.D., Hulsebosch, H.J., Krieg, S.R., Bakker, P.M., and Cormane, R.H. (1983). Immunocompetent cells in psoriasis. In situ immunophenotyping by monoclonal antibodies. *Arch. Dermatol. Res.* 275: 181–189.
53. Czernielewski, J., Juhlin, L., Shroot, S., and Brun, P. (1985). Langerhans cells in patients with psoriasis: effect of treatment with PUVA, PUVA bath, etretinate and anthralin. *Acta Derm. Venereol. (Stockh.)* 65: 97–101.
54. Torinuki, W., Mauduit, G., Haftek, M., and Thivolet, J. (1987). Effects of PUVA and mechlorethamine treatment of psoriatic patients on epidermal Langerhans cells. *Acta Derm. Venereol. (Stockh.)* 67: 532–535.
55. Ashworth, J. and MacKie, R.M. (1986). A quantitative analysis of the Langerhans cell in chronic plaque psoriasis and effects of treatment. *Clin. Exp. Dermatol.* 11:594–599.
56. Baker, B.S., Swain, A.F., Griffiths, C.E.M., Leonard, J.N., Fry, L., and Valdimarsson, H. (1985). Epidermal T lymphocytes and dendritic cells in chronic plaque psoriasis: the effects of PUVA treatment. *Clin. Exp. Immunol.* 61:526–534.
57. Gommans, J.M., Van Hezik, S.J.T.M., and Van Huystee, B.E.W.L. (1987). Flow cytometric quantification of CD1a-positive cells in psoriatic epidermis after PUVA and methotrexate therapy. *Br. J. Dermatol.* 116:661–666.
58. Morhenn, V.B., Abel, E.A., and Mahrle, G. (1982). Expression of HLA DR antigen in skin from patients with psoriasis. *J. Invest. Dermatol.* 78:165–168.

59. Placek, W., Haftek, M., and Thivolet, J. (1988). Sequence of changes in psoriatic epidermis: immunocompetent cell redistribution precedes altered expression of keratinocyte differentiation markers. *Acta Derm. Venereol. (Stockh.)* 68:369–377.
60. Bjerke, J.R. and Matre, R. (1983). Demonstration of Ia-like antigens on T lymphocytes in lesions of psoriasis, lichen planus and discoid lupus erythematosus. *Acta Derm. Venereol. (Stockh.)* 63:103–107.
61. Lange-Wantzin, G., Larsen, J.K., Christensen, I.J., Ralfkiaer, E., Tjalve, M., Lund-Kofoed, M., and Thomsen, K. (1985). Activated and cycling lymphocytes in benign dermal lymphocytic infiltrates including psoriatic skin lesions. *Arch. Dermatol. Res.* 278: 92–96.
62. Alegre, V.A., MacDonald, D.M., and Poulter, L.W. (1986). The simultaneous presence of Langerhans cell and interdigitating cell antigenic markers on inflammatory dendritic cells. *Clin. Exp. Immunol.* 64: 330–333.
63. Heng, M.C.Y. and Kloss, S.G. (1985). Cell interactions in psoriasis. *Arch Dermatol.* 121:881–887.
64. Baker, B.S., Swain, A.F., Griffiths, C.E.M., Leonard, J.N., Fry, L., and Valdimarsson, H. (1985). The effects of topical treatment with steroids or dithranol on epidermal T lymphocytes and dendritic cells in psoriasis. *Scand. J. Immunol.* 22:471–477.
65. Bos, J. D. and Krieg, S.R. (1985). Psoriasis infiltrating cell immunophenotype: changes induced by PUVA or corticosteroid treatment in T cell subsets, Langerhans cells and interdigitating cells. *Acta Derm. Venereol. (Stockh.)* 65:390–397.
66. Shelley, W.B. (1971). Adenosine triphosphatase activity as evidence for persistence of Langerhans cell in psoriatic scales. *Acta Derm. Venereol. (Stockh.)* 51: 101–106.
67. Brody, I. (1978). Alterations of clinically normal skin in early eruptive guttate psoriasis. A light- and electron-microscopic study. *J. Cutan. Pathol.* 5:219–233.
68. Brody, I. (1984). Dermal and epidermal involvement in the evolution of acute eruptive guttate psoriasis vulgaris. *J. Invest. Dermatol.* 82:465–470.
69. Baker, B.S., Swain, A.F., Fry, L., and Valdimarsson, H. (1984). Epidermal T lymphocytes and HLA DR expression in psoriasis. *Br. J. Dermatol.* 110: 555–564.
70. Baker, S.B., Lambert, S., Powels, A.V., Valdimarsson, H., and Fry, L. (1988). Epidermal DR+ CD1a− dendritic cells in inflammatory skin diseases. *Acta Derm. Venereol. (Stockh.)* 68:209–217.
71. Baker, B.S., Griffiths, C.E.M., Lambert, S., Powles, A.V., Leonard, J.N., Valdimarsson, H., and Fry, L. (1987). The effects of cyclosporin A on T lymphocyte and dendritic cell subpopulations in psoriasis. *Br. J. Dermatol.* 116:503–510.
72. Haftek, M., Placek, W., and Thivolet, J. (1989). Modifications of immunocompetent cells precede altered expression of epidermal differentiation antigens in psoriatic epidermis. *Acta Derm. Venereol. (Stockh.)* (Suppl. 146):20–25.
73. Chowaniec, O. and Jablonska, S. (1979). Pre- pinpoint papules. Changes preceding pin-point lesions of psoriasis. *Acta Derm. Venereol. (Stockh.)* (Suppl. 85): 39–45.
74. Heng, M.C.Y., Kloss, S.G., Kuehn, C.S., and Chase, D.G. (1985). The sequence of events in psoriatic plaque formation after tape-stripping. *Br. J. Dermatol.* 112:517–532.
74a. Heng, M.C.Y., Allen, S.G., Haberfelde, G., and Song, M.K. (1991). Electron microscopic and immunocytochemical studies of the sequence of events in psoriatic plaque formation following tape-stripping. *Br. J. Dermatol.* 125:548–556.
75. Eyre, R.W. and Krueger, G.G. (1982). Response to injury of skin involved and uninvolved with psoriasis, and its relation to disease activity: Koebner and "reverse" Koebner reactions. *Br. J. Dermatol.* 106: 153–159.
76. Jablonska, S., Chorzelski, T.P., Beutner, E.H., Jarzabek-Chorzelska, M., Chowaniec, O., Maciejowska, E., and Rzesa, G. (1977). Autoimmunity in psoriasis. II. Immunohistologic studies on various forms of psoriasis and the Koebner phenomenon. In *Psoriasis. Proceedings of the Second International Symposium.* E.M. Farber and A.J. Cox (Eds.). Yorke Medical Books, New York, pp. 73–80.
77. Baker, B.S., Powles, A.V., Lamberts, S., Valdimarsson, H., and Fry, L. (1988). A prospective study of the Koebner reaction and T lymphocytes in uninvolved psoriatic skin. *Acta Derm. Venereol. (Stockh.)* 68: 430–434.
78. Dubertret, L. and Touraine, R. (1977). The role of neutrophil leukocytes in the psoriatic epidermal process: preliminary results. In *Psoriasis. Proceedings of the Second International Symposium.* E.M. Farber and A.J. Cox (Eds.). Yorke Medical Books, New York, pp. 371–374.
79. Bacharach-Buhles, M. and Altmeyer, P. (1989). Pustulosis palmo-plantaris: how the initial ultrastructural alterations change into vesicles and pustules. *Acta Derm. Venereol. (Stockh.)* (Suppl. 146):76–80.
80. Rosän, K., Jontell, M., Mobacken, H., and Rosdahl, I. (1988). Epidermal Langerhans cells in patients with pustulosis palmoplantaris treated with etretinate or etretinate + methoxalen photochemotherapy. *Acta Derm. Venereol. (Stockh.)* 68:218–223.
81. Oxholm, A., Oxholm, P., and Staberg, B. (1987). Reduced density of CD1a-positive epidermal Langerhans cells in uninvolved skin of patients with psoriasis. *Acta Derm. Venereol. (Stockh.)* 67:8–11.

82. Lindberg, M. and Forslind, B. (1981). The effects of occlusion of the skin on the Langerhans cells. *Acta Derm. Venereol. (Stockh.)* 61:201–205.
83. Nieboer, C., Bruynzeel, D.P., and Broosma, D.M. (1987). The effect of occlusion of the skin with transdermal therapeutic system on Langerhans cells and the induction of skin irritation. *Arch. Dermatol.* 123: 1499–1502.
83a. Griffiths, C.E. Tranfaglia, M.G., Kang, S. (1995). Prolonged occlusion in the treatment of psoriasis: a clinical and immunohistologic study. *J. Am. Acad. Dermatol.* 32:618–622.
84. Kanerva, L., Ranki, A., and Lauharanta, J. (1984). Langerhans cells show greater fine structural changes than keratinocytes in normal skin after occlusion with dithranol. *Acta Derm. Venereol. (Stockh.)* (Suppl. 113):57–59.
85. Haftek, M. (1987). Langerhans cells in psoriasis. In *Psoriasis. Proceedings of the Fourth International Symposium.* E.M. Farber, L. Nall, V. Morhenn, and P.H. Jacobs (Eds.). Elsevier, Amsterdam, pp. 368–369.
86. Berman, B., France, D.S., Martinelli, G.P., and Hass, A. (1983). Modulation of expression of epidermal Langerhans cell properties following in situ exposure to glucocorticosteroids. *J. Invest. Dermatol.* 80: 168–171.
87. Braathen, L.R. and Hirschberg, H. (1984). The effect of short-term corticosteroid incubation on the alloactivating and antigen-presenting capacity of human epidermal Langerhans cells. *Br. J. Dermatol.* 111: 295–302.
88. Krueger, G.G. and Emam, M. (1984). Biology of Langerhans cells: analysis by experiments to deplete Langerhans cells from human skin. *J. Invest. Dermatol.* 82:613–617.
88a. Mommaas, A.M. (1993). Influence of glucocorticoids on the epidermal Langerhans cell. *Curr. Probl. Dermatol.* 21:67–72.
89. Koulu, L. and Jansén, C.T. (1988). In vivo PUVA and UVB sensitivity of various human epidermal Langerhans cell markers (ATPase, HLA DR and CD1a). Dose-response and time-sequence studies. *Clin. Exp. Dermatol.* 13:173–176.
90. Aberer, W., Schuler, G., Stingl, G., Hönigsmann, H., and Wolff, K. (1981). Ultraviolet light depletes surface markers of Langerhans cells. *J. Invest. Dermatol.* 76:202–210.
91. Czernielewski, J., Vaigot, P., Asselineau, D., and Prunièras, M. (1984). In vitro effect of UV radiation on immune function and membrane markers of human Langerhans cells. *J. Invest. Dermatol.* 83:62–65.
91a. Mommaas, A.M., Mulder, A.A., and Vermeer, B.J. (1993). Short-term and long-term UVB-induced immunosuppression in human skin exhibit different ultrastructural features. *Eur. J. Morphol.* 31:30–34.
92. Tjerdlund, U. and Juhlin, L. (1982). Effect of UV-irradiation on immunological and histochemical markers of Langerhans cells in normal appearing skin of psoriatic patients. *Arch. Dermatol. Res.* 272: 171–176.
93. Friedmann, P.S., Ford, G., Ross, J., and Diffey, B.L. (1983). Reappearance of epidermal Langerhans cells after PUVA therapy. *Br. J. Dermatol.* 109:301–307.
94. Koulu, L., Söderström, K.O., and Jansén, T. (1984). Relation of antipsoriatic and Langerhans cell depleting effects of systemic psoralen photochemotherapy: a clinical, enzyme histochemical, and electron microscopic study. *J. Invest. Dermatol.* 82:591–593.
95. Juhlin, L. and Shelley, W.B. (1979). Giant Langerhans cells induced by psoralen and ultraviolet radiation. *Arch. Dermatol. Res.* 266:311–314.
96. Ree, K. (1982). Reduction of Langerhans cells in human epidermis during PUVA therapy: a morphometric study. *J. Invest. Dermatol.* 78:488–492.
97. Morhenn, V.B., Benike, C.J., and Engelman, E.G. (1980). Inhibition of cell mediated immune responses by 8-methoxypsoralen and long-wave ultraviolet light: a possible explanation for the clinical effects of photoactivated psoralen. *J. Invest. Dermatol.* 75: 249–252.
98. Moss, C., Friedmann, P.S., and Shuster, S. (1981). Impaired contact hypersensitivity in untreated psoriasis and the effects of photochemotherapy and dithranol/UV-B. *Br. J. Dermatol.* 105:503–508.
99. Koulu, L. and Jansén, C.T. (1982). Epidermal Langerhans cell number and morphology during oral retinoid treatment. *Arch. Dermatol. Res.* 272:135–137.
100. Ranki, A., Lauharanta, J., and Kanerva, L. (1984). Effect of etretinate on the distribution of Langerhans cells and T lymphocytes in psoriatic skin. *Arch. Dermatol. Res.* 276:102–104.
101. Tsambaos, D. and Orfanos, C.E. (1981). Ultrastructural evidence suggesting an immunomodulatory activity of oral retinoid. Its effect on dermal components in psoriasis. *Br. J. Dermatol.* 104:37–45.
102. Orfanos, C.E., Mahrle, G., Goerz, G., Happle, R., Hofbauer, M., Landes, E., and Schimpf, A. (1979). Laboratory investigations in patients with generalized psoriasis under oral retinoid treatment. A multicenter study of computerized data. *Dermatologica* 159: 62–70.
103. Kanerva, L., Lauharanta, J., Niemi, K.M., and Lassus, A. (1982). Light and electron microscopy of psoriatic epidermis before and during retinoid (Ro 10-9359) and retinoid-PUVA treatment. *J. Cutan. Pathol.* 9: 175–188.
104. Ellis, C.N., Grosulowsky, D.C., Hamilton, T.A., Billings, J.K., Brown, M.D., Haedington, J.T., Cooper, K.D., Baadsgaard, O., Duell, E.A., Annesley, T.M., Turcotte, J.G., and Voorhees, J.J. (1986). Cyclospor-

ine improves psoriasis in a double-blind study. *J.A.M.A.* 256:3110–3116.

105. Van Joost, Th., Heule, F., Stotz, E., and Beukers, R. (1986). Short-term use of cyclosporin A in severe psoriasis. *Br. J. Dermatol.* 114:615–620.

106. Varey, A.M., Champion, B.R., and Cooke, A.K. (1986). Cyclosporine affects the function of antigen presenting cells. *Immunology* 57:111–114.

107. Furue, M. and Katz, S.I. (1988). Cyclosporine A inhibits accessory cell and antigen-presenting cell functions of epidermal Langerhans cells. *Transplant. Proc.* 20 (Suppl. 2):87–91.

107a. Demidem, A., Taylor, J.R., Grammer, S.F., and Steilein, J.W. (1991). T lymphocyte-activating properties of epidermal antigen-presenting cells from normal and psoriatic skin: evidence that psoriatic epidermal antigen-presenting cells resemble cultured normal Langerhans cells. *J. Invest. Dermatol.* 97:454–460.

108. Bunjes, D., Hardt, C., Röllinghoff, M., and Wagner, H. (1981). Cyclosporin A mediates immunosuppression of primary cytotoxic T cell responses by impairing the release of interleukin 1 and interleukin 2. *Eur. J. Immunol* 11:657–661.

109. Halloran, P.F., Wadgymar, A., and Autenried, P. (1986). Inhibition of MHC product induction may contribute to the immunosuppressive action of ciclosporin. In *Ciclosporin. Progress in Allergy*, vol. 38. J.F. Borel (Ed.). Karger, Basel, pp. 258–268.

110. Powles, A., Baker, B., Valdimarsson, H., and Fry, L. (1989). Intradermal cyclosporin in psoriasis. *Acta Derm. Venereol. (Stockh.)* (Suppl. 146):148–150.

111. Finzi, A.F., Mozzanica, N., Pigatto, P.D., and Chiappino, G. (1989). Cyclosporin for psoriasis: clinical and immunological studies. *Acta Derm. Venereol. (Stockh.)* (Suppl. 146):137.

112. Tigalonowa, M., Bjerke, J.R., and Matre, R. (1989). Immunological changes following treatment of psoriasis with ciclosporin. *Acta Derm. Venereol. (Stockh.)* (Suppl. 146):142–146.

112a. Mozzanica, N., Pigatto, P.D., and Finzi, A.F. (1993). Cyclosporin in psoriasis: pathophysiology and experimental data. *Dermatology* 187(Suppl. 1)3–7.

112b. Petzelbauer, P. and Wolff, K. (1992). Effects of cyclosporin A on resident and passenger immune cells of normal human skin and UV-induced erythema reactions. *Br. J. Dermatol.* 127:560–565.

112c. Mozzanica, N., Cattaneo, A., Schmitt, E., Diotti, R., and Finzi, A.F. (1994). Topical calcipotriol for psoriasis - an immunohistologic study. *Acta Derm. Venereol. (Stockh.)* (Suppl. 186):171–172.

113. Krueger, G.G., Jederberg, W.W., Ogden, B.E., and Reese, D.L. (1978). Inflammatory and immune cell function in psoriasis: II. Monocyte function, lymphokine production. *J. Invest. Dermatol.* 71:195–201.

114. Mier, P.D., Gommans, J.M., and Roelfzema, H. (1980). On the aetiology of psoriasis. *Br. J. Dermatol.* 103:457–460.

115. Schweizer, J. (1981). Langerhans cells, epidermal growth control mechanisms and type of keratinization. In *The Epidermis in Disease.* R. Marks, and E. Christophers (Eds.). MTP Press, Lancaster, pp. 481–499.

116. Fraki, J.E., Briggaman, R.A., and Lazarus, G.S. (1983). Transplantation of psoriatic skin onto nude mice. *J. Invest. Dermatol.* 80:31s–35s.

117. Haftek, M., Ortonne, J.P., Staquet, M.J., Viac, J., and Thivolet, J. (1981). Normal and psoriatic human skin grafts on "nude" mice: morphological and immunochemical studies. *J. Invest. Dermatol.* 76:48–52.

118. Morhenn, V.B. (1988). Keratinocyte proliferation in wound healing and skin diseases. *Immunol. Today* 9: 104–107.

119. Nickoloff, B.J., Basham, T.Y., Merigan, T.C., and Morhenn, V.B. (1984). Antiproliferative effects of recombinant α- and γ-interferons on cultured human keratinocytes. *Lab. Invest.* 51:697–701.

120. Aiba, S. and Tagami, H. (1984). HLA DR antigen expression on the, keratinocyte surface in dermatoses characterized by lymphocyte exocytosis (e.g., pityriasis rosea). *Br. J. Dermatol.* 111:285–294.

120a. Verga, M. and Braverman, I.M. (1991). The use of immunohistologic analysis in differentiating cutaneous T cell lymphoma from psoriasis and dermatitis. *Arch. Dermatol.* 127:1503–1510.

120b. De Boer, O.J., Van der Loos, C.M., Hamerlinck, F., Bos, J.D., and Das, P.K. (1994). Reappraisal of in situ immunophenotypic analysis of psoriasis skin: interaction of activated HLA DR+ immunocompetent cells and endothelial cells is a major feature of psoriatic lesions. *Arch. Dermatol. Res.* 286:87–96.

121. Kaplan, G., Witmer, M.D., Nath, I., Steinman, R.M., Laal, S., Prasad, H.K., Sarno, E.N., Elvers, U., and Cohn, Z.A. (1986). Influence of delayed immune reactions on human epidermal keratinocytes. *Proc. Natl Acad. Sci. U.S.A.* 83:3469–3473.

122. Nickoloff, B.J., Basham, T.Y., Merigan, T.C., Torsetth, J.W., and Morhenn, V.B. (1986). Human keratinocyte-lymphocyte reactions in vitro. *J. Invest. Dermatol.* 87:11–18.

123. Nicholas, J.F., Kaiserlian, D., Dardenne, M., Faure, M., and Thivolet, J. (1987). Epidermal cell-derived lymphocyte differentiating factor (ELDIF) inhibits in vitro lymphoproliferative responses and interleukin-2 production. *J. Invest. Dermatol.* 88:161–166.

124. Lee, R.E., Gaspari, A.A., Lotze, M.T., Chang, A.E., and Rosenberg, S.A. (1988). Interleukin 2 and psoriasis. *Arch. Dermatol.* 124:1811–1815.

124a. Bata-Csorgo, Z., Hammerberg, C., Voorhees, J.J., and Cooper, K.D. (1995). Kinetics and regulation of human keratinocyte stem cell growth in short-term primary ex vivo culture. Cooperative growth factors from psoriatic lesional T lymphocytes stimulate proliferation among psoriatic uninvolved, but not normal, stem keratinocytes. *J. Clin. Invest.* 95:317–327.

125. Valdimarsson, H., Baker, B.S., Jonsdottir, I., and Fry, L. (1986). Psoriasis: a disease of abnormal keratinocyte proliferation induced by T lymphocytes. *Immunol. Today* 7:256–259.
126. Glinski, W., Zarebska, Z., Jablonska, S., Imiela, J., and Nosarzewski, J. (1980). The activity of polymorphonuclear leukocyte neutral proteinases and their inhibitors in patients with psoriasis treated with a continuous peritoneal dialysis. *J. Invest. Dermatol.* 75: 481–487.
127. Jablonska, S., Chowaniec, O., and Maciejowska, E. (1982). Histology of psoriasis: the role of polymorphonuclear neutrophils. In *Autoimmunity in Psoriasis.* E.H. Beutner (Ed.). CRC Press, Boca Raton, FL, pp. 21–36.
128. Beutner, E.H., Dabski, K., Jablonska, S., Glinski, W., and Kumar, V. (1983). Stratum corneum antigens, their role in psoriasis and in the autoimmune repair mechanisms. In *Stratum Corneum.* R. Marks and G. Plewig (Eds.). Springer-Verlag, Berlin, pp. 92–111.
129. Greaves, M.W. (1983). Neutrophil polymorphonuclears, mediators and the pathogenesis of psoriasis. *Br. J. Dermatol.* 109:115–118.
130. Mercer, E.H. and Maibach, H.I. (1968). Intercellular adhesion and surface coats of epidermal cells in psoriasis. *J. Invest. Dermatol.* 51:215–221.
131. Orfanos, C.E., Schaumburg-Lever, G., and Lever, W.F. (1973). Alterations of cell surfaces as a pathogenetic factor in psoriasis. Possible loss of contact inhibition of growth. *Arch. Dermatol.* 107:38–46.
132. Voorhees, J. and Buell, E.A. (1971). Psoriasis as a possible defect of the adenyl cyclase-cyclic AMP cascade: A defective chalone mechanism? *Arch. Dermatol.* 104:352–358.
133. Wright, R.K., Mandy, S.H., Halprin, K.M., and Hsia, S.L. (1973). Defects and deficiency of adenyl cyclase in psoriatic skin. *Arch. Dermatol.* 107:47–53.
134. Farber, E.M., Nickoloff, B.J., Recht, B., and Fraki, J.E. (1986). Stress, symmetry, and psoriasis: Possible role of neuropeptides. *J. Am. Acad. Dermatol.* 14: 305–311.
135. Brody, I. (1984). Mast cell degranulation in the evolution of acute eruptive guttate psoriasis vulgaris. *J. Invest. Dermatol.* 82:460–464.
136. Naukkarinen, A., Nickoloff, B.J., and Farber, E.M. (1989). Quantification of cutaneous sensory nerves and their substance P content in psoriasis. *J. Invest. Dermatol.* 92:126–129.
136a. Hosoi, J., Murphy, G.F., Egan, C.L., Lerner, E.A., Grabbe, S., Asahina, A., and Granstein, R.D. (1993). Regulation of Langerhans cell function by nerves containing calcitonin gene-related peptide. *Nature* 363:159–163.
136b. Asahina, A., Hosoi, J., Grabbe, S., and Granstein, R.D. (1995). Modulation of Langerhans cell function by epidermal nerves. *J. Allergy Clin. Immunol.* 96: 1178–1182.
136c. Olsen, J. (1991). Calcitonin gene-related peptide, neurokinin A and substance P: effects on nociception and neurogenic inflammation in human skin and temporal muscle. *Peptides* 12:333–337.
137. Payan, D.G., Brewster, D.R., and Goetzl, E.J. (1983). Specific stimulation of human T lymphocytes by substance P. *J. Immunol.* 131:1613–1615.
138. Payan, D.G., Brewster, D.R., Missirian-Bustian, A., and Goetzl, E.J. (1984). Substance P recognition by a subset of human T lymphocytes. *J. Clin. Invest.* 74: 1532–1539.
139. Hartung, H.P., Wolters, K., and Toyka, K. (1984). Binding of substance P to macrophages: Stimulation of the release of proinflammatory and immunomodulating compounds. *Neurosci. Lett.* 18 (Suppl.):S101.
140. Nickoloff, B.J., Misra, P., Morhenn, V.B., Hintz, R.L., and Rosenfeld, R.G. (1988). Further characterization of the keratinocyte somatomedin-C/insulin-like growth factor I (SM-C/IGF-I) receptor and the biological responsiveness of cultured keratinocytes to SM-C/IGF-I. *Dermatologica* 177:265–273.
141. Saiag, P., Coulomb, B., Lebreton, C., Bell, E., and Dubertret, L. (1985). Psoriatic fibroblasts induce hyperproliferation of normal keratinocytes in a skin equivalent model in vitro. *Science* 230:669–672.
141a. Smith, C.H. and Barker, J.N. (1995). Cell trafficking and role of adhesion molecules in psoriasis. *Clin. Dermatol.* 13:151–160.
142. Voorhees, J.J. (1983). Leukotrienes and other lipoxygenase products in the pathogenesis and therapy of psoriasis and other dermatoses. *Arch. Dermatol.* 119: 541–547.
143. Camp, R. (1987). Mediators of inflammation in psoriasis. In *Psoriasis. Proceedings of the Fourth International Symposium.* E.M. Farber, L. Nall, V. Morhenn, and P.H. Jacobs (Eds.). Elsevier, Amsterdam, pp. 113–118.
144. Guilhou, J.J., Meynadier, J., and Clot, J. (1978). New concepts in the pathogenesis of psoriasis. *Br. J. Dermatol.* 98:585–592.
145. Stanbridge, E.J. (1981). A possible viral etiology for psoriasis. In *Psoriasis. Proceedings of the Third International Symposium.* E.M. Farber and A.J. Cox (Eds.). Grune & Stratton, New York, pp. 67–70.
146. Bjerke, J.R., Haukenes, G., Livden, J.K., Matre, R., and Degré, M. (1983). Activated T lymphocytes, interferon, and retrovirus-like particles in psoriatic lesions. *Arch. Dermatol.* 119:955–956 (letter).
147. Swerlick, R.A., Cunningham, M.W., and Hall, N.K. (1986). Monoclonal antibodies cross-reactive with group A streptococci and normal and psoriatic human skin. *J. Invest. Dermatol.* 87:367–371.
148. Beutner, E.H., Binder, W.L., Jablonska, S., and Kumar, V. (1981). Nature of stratum corneum autoanti-

bodies, antigens and antigen conversion and their role in healing and in psoriasis. In *The Epidermis in Disease.* R. Marks and E. Christophers (Eds.). MTP Press, Lancaster, England, pp. 333–357.

149. Reinherz, E.L. and Schlossman, S.F. (1982). The characterization and function of human immunoregulatory T lymphocyte subsets. *Pharmacol. Rev.* 34: 17–22.

150. Bos, J.D., Van Garderen, I.D., Krieg, S.R., and Poulter, L.W. (1986). Different in situ distribution patterns of dendritic cells having Langerhans (T6+) and interdigitating (RFD1+) cell immunophenotype in psoriasis, atopic dermatitis, and other inflammatory dermatoses. *J. Invest. Dermatol.* 87:358–361.

150a. Prens, E.P., Benne, K., Van Joost, T., and Benner, R. (1991). The autologous mixed epidermal cell-T lymphocyte reaction is elevated in psoriasis: a crucial role for epidermal HLA DR+/CD1a− antigen-presenting cells. *J. Invest. Dermatol.* 96:880–887.

150b. Peguet-Navarro, J., Dalbiez-Gauthier, C., Dezutter-Dambuyant, C., and Schmitt, D. (1993). Dissection of human Langerhans cells' allostimulatory function: the need for an activation step for full development of accessory function. *Eur. J. Immunol.* 23:376–382.

151. Steinmuller, D., Zinsmeister, A.R., and Rogers, R.S. (1988). Cellular autoimmunity in psoriasis and lichen planus. *J. Autoimmun.* 1:279–298.

151a. Ross, E.L., Barker, J.N., Allen, M.H., Chu, A.C., Groves, R.W., and MacDonald, D.M. (1994). Langerhans cell expression of the selectin ligand, sialyl Lewis x. *Immunology* 81:303–308.

151b. DeBoer, O.J., Wakelkamp, I.M., Pals, S.T., Claessen, N., Bos, J.D., and Das, P.K. (1994). Increased expression of adhesion receptors in both lesional and nonlesional psoriatic skin. *Arch. Dermatol. Res.* 286: 304–311.

151c. McGregor, J.M., Barker, J.N., Ross, E.L., MacDonald, D.M. (1992). Epidermal dendritic cells in psoriasis possess a phenotype associated with antigen presentation: in situ expression of beta 2 integrins. *J. Am. Acad. Dermatol.* 27:383–388.

152. Johnson, T.M., Duvic, M., Rapini, R.P., and Rios, A. (1985). AIDS exacerbates psoriasis. *N. Engl. J. Med.* 313:1415 (letter).

153. Fisher, B.K. and Warner, L.C. (1987). Cutaneous manifestations of the acquired immunodeficiency syndrome. *Int. J. Dermatol.* 26:615–630.

154. Rappersberger, K., Gartner, S., Schenk, P., Stingl, G., Groh, V., Tschachler, E., Mann, D.L., Wolff, K., Konrad, K., and Popovic, M. (1988). Langerhans cells are an actual site of HIV-1 replication. *Intervirology* 29: 185–194.

155. Gielen, V., Schmitt, D., Dezutter-Dambuyant, C., and Thivolet, J. (1989). AIDS and Langerhans cells: CD4 antigenic site density modification evidenced by single-cell immunogold labeling. *Regional Immunol.* 2:7–13.

156. Belsito, D.V., Sanchez, M.R., Baer, R.L., Valentine, F., and Thorbecke, G.J. (1984). Reduced Langerhans cell Ia antigen and ATPase activity in patients with the acquired immunodeficiency syndrome. *N. Engl. J. Med.* 310:1279–1282.

157. Dréno, B., Milpied, B., Bignon, J.D., Stalder, J.F., and Litoux, P. (1988). Prognostic value of Langerhans cells in the epidermis of HIV patients. *Br. J. Dermatol.* 118:481–486.

157a. Zemelman, V., Van Neer, F., Roberts, N., Patel, P., Langtry, J., and Staughton, R.C. (1994). Epidermal Langerhans cells, HIV 1 infection and psoriasis. *Br. J. Dermatol.* 130:307–311.

158. Marcusson, J.A. and Wetterberg, L. (1989). Peptide-T and psoriasis. *Acta Derm. Venereol. (Stockh.)* (Suppl. 146):117–121.

158a. Wang, L., Hilliges, M., Talme, T., Marcusson, J.A., Wetterberg, L., and Johansson, O. (1995). Rearrangement of S-100 immunoreactive Langerhans cells in human psoriatic skin treated with peptide T. *J. Dermatol. Sci.* 9:20–26.

159. Bos, J.D. (1988). The pathomechanism of psoriasis; the skin immune system and cyclosporin. *Br. J. Dermatol.* 118:141–155.

159a. Thomson, A.W., Nalesnik, M., Abu-Elmagd, K., and Starzl, T.E. (1991). Influence of FK506 on T lymphocytes, Langerhans cells and the expression of cytokine receptors and adhesion molecules in psoriatic skin lesions: a preliminary study. *Transplant. Proc.* 23:3330–3331.

160. Morhenn, V.B., Pregerson-Rodan, K., Mullen, R.H., Wood, G.S., Nickoloff, B.J. Sherwin, S.A., and Farber, E.M. (1987). Use of recombinant interferon gamma administrated intramuscularly for the treatment of psoriasis. *Arch Dermatol.* 123:1633–1637.

161. Kato, T., Rokugo, M., Terui, T., and Tagami, H. (1986). Successful tratment of psoriasis with topical application of active vitamin D_3 analogue, 1α,24-dihydroxycholecalciferol. *Br. J. Dermatol.* 115: 431–433.

162. Holick, M.F., Smith, E., and Pincus, S. (1987). Skin as the site of vitamin D synthesis and target tissue for 1,25-dihydroxyvitamin D_3. Use of calcitriol (1,25-dihydroxyvitamin D3) for treatment of psoriasis. *Arch. Dermatol.* 123:1677–1683.

163. Quesada, J.R. and Gutterman, J.U. (1986). Psoriasis and alpha-interferon. *Lancet* 1:1466–1468.

164. Shiohara, T., Kobayashi, M., Abe, K., and Nagashima, M. (1988). Psoriasis occurring predominantly on warts: possible involvement of interferon alpha. *Arch. Dermatol.* 124:1816–1821.

18

The Cell Membrane in Psoriasis

Jonathan Mansbridge
Advanced Tissue Sciences, La Jolla, California

Vera B. Morhenn
University of California, San Diego, California

The plasma membrane is the interface between the cell and its environment. As such, it detects and provides the initial response to cytokines and other factors through receptors. The response to ligands is an active process, involving not only binding and transmission of the signal to the interior of the cell, but also exposure, desensitization, and degradation of receptors.

Since much intercellular control operates through the cell membrane, discussion of its properties has ramifications for many aspects of cellular physiology, which will be referred to in passing in this discussion. It must be borne in mind that the receptors feed into a complex intracellular control system that includes in its activities modification of receptors as well as control of growth and differentiation. Thus, we may expect response to a ligand to be dependent both on the differentiation state of the cell and on the presence of other cytokines.

Recently, the great importance of one particular group of membrane receptors that react with ligands that are insoluble or bound to the extracellular matrix has become evident. These receptors, the integrins, are a complex group of dimeric molecules that, in their ligand-activated form, are generally connected to cytoskeletal structures inside the cell and to matrix molecules such as collagen, laminin, or fibronectin outside the cell. They are capable both of transmitting information modifying cell behavior from extracellular structures and of modifying the external matrix through cell activities. In addition, their ability to bind ligands at all may be under cellular control.

Keratinocytes are particularly active in the exchange of intercellular signals, secreting and responding to a number of factors (1). These cytokines are especially important in conditions in which the homeostasis of the skin is disturbed, such as following injury, infection, or in pathological states such as psoriasis.

This chapter begins with a brief overview of membrane properties and then deals with changes that have been observed in psoriasis, with particular reference to the keratinocyte and Langerhans cell membranes. Rather than attempt to cover all aspects of all membranes in psoriasis, this review will concentrate on a few areas that have advanced in the last few years or have not been summarized recently.

OVERVIEW OF THE CELL MEMBRANE

Our view of cell membranes has steadily matured since Davson first proposed the lipid bilayer as the basic structure. The membrane provides a barrier between the interior of the cell and the external medium through which nutrients and signals may be filtered by a variety of transport and transducing proteins. In the last few years, the structures of a variety of representative membrane proteins have been determined, permitting an understanding of the control systems governing the selective mechanisms.

The Membrane Skeleton

The lipid bilayer, with its proteins, is supported on a cytoskeletal structure composed of spectrin/fodrin (2–4). This system, which was first demonstrated in the red blood cell, has since been shown to be common to most cell types, including the keratinocyte (5). Attachment of this protein network to components on the internal cytoskeleton enables the cell to control its shape through the actin system (6–8). The actin system is also attached at the cell membrane through structures that provide adhesion to the basement membrane, composed of various combinations of integrins that react with various types of matrix-bound ligand. Examples include the $\alpha_6\beta_4$ integrin in hemidesmosomes and the $\alpha_5\beta_1$ integrin that provides attachment to fibronectin. In addition, various structures attach one cell to another, in particular desmosome gap junctions, and, under certain circumstances, tight junctions.

Membrane Lipids

Membrane lipids are important not only as structural components of the plasma membrane but also, as is increasingly becoming evident, as active control elements. The hydrolysis of phosphatidyl inositol diphosphate by phospholipase C to give inositol triphosphate and diacyl glycerol is critical to the activation of protein kinase C (9–11). It has recently become evident that sphingolipids have an important inhibitory effect on this same enzyme system (12) and will inhibit ornithine decarboxylase activity (13). Membrane phospholipids are also the source of arachidonic acid, the starting point for prostaglandin and leukotriene synthesis. The hydrolytic release of arachidonic acid, mainly through phospholipase A_2, one form of which is increased in psoriasis (14), but also possibly involving other enzymes (15), is the rate-limiting step in this pathway. This system is the subject of detailed discussion elsewhere in this volume, but it may be noted in passing that it has been demonstrated to be an intimate component of signal transduction systems generally thought of as operating through other mechanisms such as tyrosine phosphorylation. An example is the EGF receptor system (16,17). It is becoming evident that many of the signal transduction systems that have been studied separately, such as those originating from the tyrosine phosphorylation-, G-protein-, and calcium channel–linked receptors, are interconnected within an integrated cellular signal interpretation system (18).

Membrane Proteins

A variety of types of membrane proteins are known to exist, which differ in their attachment systems. The range extends from proteins that are totally immersed in the membrane, the protein spanning the lipid bilayer, to proteins attached only by a fatty acid modification. A representative selection is listed below, but these are only known proteins and we can expect the list to be extended.

1. Proteins with a single membrane traversing amino acid sequence, with a large extracellular domain and a small (e.g., MHC proteins) or large (e.g., many growth factor receptors) intracellular domain (19). The membrane domain of these proteins may be as short as 10 residues, but is frequently longer. In these cases, a signal is transmitted across the membrane from the extracellular ligand-binding site to the intracellular domain, frequently a tyrosine kinase (20), by a mechanism that frequently involves receptor dimerization, resulting in mutual phosphorylation (21).
2. Proteins containing multiple membrane-traversing domains. One group, characterized by seven such α-helical domains, are often receptors that associate with guanosine triphosphate (GTP)-binding control proteins, termed G-proteins, which act as intermediate carriers in signal transduction. The most fully studied of these is rhodopsin (22), but the β-adrenergic receptors are also of this type (23). A second group are the ion channel proteins, such as the ion-sensitive sodium and calcium channel proteins which have 24 α-helical domains that cross the membrane repeatedly (24,25).
3. Proteins bound to the membrane by a fatty acyl chain, reviewed in Ref. 26. These include proteins myristilated at their N-terminals, such as the membrane tyrosine kinase *c*-src, palmitoylated proteins, including the G-protein ras, and a group of proteins carrying a C-terminal glycosyl-phosphatidyl-inositol modification, including alkaline phosphatase and acetyl cholinesterase (27). Fatty acid modifications also

occur elsewhere than at the terminals of the molecules, as in the case of major histocompatibility complex (MHC) antigens, which are acylated on cysteine residues (28).

Membrane Glycoproteins

The extracellular domains of membrane proteins are generally glycosylated. Two broad types of glycosylation occur: N-glycosylation on asparagine residues, usually in a sequence of the type Asn-Xaa-Ser-Thr, and O-glycosylation, which occurs on serine and threonine residues.

Oligosaccharide side chains of the N-glycosylation type are added to glycoproteins in a posttranslational process that occurs by stages in the rough endoplasmic reticulum and Golgi region of the cell. The first step involves transfer of a $Glc_3Man_9GlcNAc_2$ unit from dolichol pyrophosphate to an asparagine residue in the nascent peptide on the luminal surface of the endoplasmic reticulum. The protein is then transported successively by a vesicle-dependent mechanism to the *cis*-Golgi, medial Golgi, and *trans*-Golgi, being modified along the way, unless diverted to a specific alternative route. In the *cis*-Golgi, the outer four mannose residues of the original oligosaccharide may be removed. *N*-Acetyl glucosamine residues are added in the medial Golgi and galactose and sialic acid residues in the *trans*-Golgi. These reactions are not dependent on dolichol derivatives and use nucleoside diphosphate sugars. Sulfation may also occur at this stage. The *trans*-Golgi is also a major site of protein sorting for transport to different parts of the cell. These systems have been well reviewed by Pfeffer and Rothman (29) and Hirschberg and Snider (30).

An indication of the complexity and fascinating ramifications of glycoconjugates may be found in the review by Rademacher et al. (31). At this stage, few generalizations can be made. Most glycoproteins generally have several glycosylation sites, each of which carries a single type of side chain, one of a small, restricted class or any of a wide range (site heterogeneity), even when the protein is made by a single cell type, such as a hybridoma. However, even with a substantial site heterogeneity, the pattern is reproducible in any given cell and not random. Different proteins may show different glycosylation patterns depending on the state of differentiation or transformation of the cell in which it is made (32,33), but the pattern is cell type and species specific. In a single cell type, a variety of proteins may carry the same range of oligopeptide structures.

The carbohydrate moieties of O-glycosylated proteins contain sulfated repeating disaccharide units and may reach considerable length. Examples of such proteins that are membrane-bound include betaglycan, the TGF-β type III receptor, CD44, and the syndecans. The repeating disaccharide side chains contain binding sites for heparin-binding growth factors such as members of the FGF family and TGF-β. Some of these interactions are essential in the activity of the bound growth factor (34,35). CD44 occurs in several splice variants that differ in their ability to present HBEGF to the EGF receptor through its heparan sulfate chain. The variant expressed by keratinocytes, which contains the V3 exon, is active in this regard (36). CD44 is associated with epithelial proliferation (37), but lost in association with leukocyte invasion as seen in psoriasis (38).

The physiological importance of this variety of molecules remains largely a matter for speculation, but N-glycosylation has been reported to affect thermal stability, protease sensitivity, aggregation, and hormonal and enzymatic properties (31). For instance, the proportion of high-affinity epidermal growth factor (EGF) receptors has been shown to be correlated with reduced *N*-acetyl galactosamination of surface proteins in A431 squamous cell carcinoma cells (39). Thus, while glycosyl side chains are infrequently the prime mechanism of an interaction, they may well play an important role in preventing access or providing a secondary control system regulating a primary interaction.

Cytokine-Binding Receptors

An important function of many of the membrane proteins is signal transduction. A ligand bound to a receptor on the surface of the cell causes activation of a second-messenger system within the cell. At least six systems of this type have been characterized, although it is clear that others exist.

1. The adenylate and guanylate cyclase systems, which cause the production of cyclic adenosine monophosphate (cAMP) and cyclic guanosine monophosphate (cGMP)
2. The phospholipase C system, causing the release of diacyl glycerol and inositol triphosphate, which activates protein kinase C, and the transport of calcium from intracellular sources (9,11)
3. A series of tyrosine kinases such as the EGF receptor (19,20)

4. Ion, particularly calcium, transport systems
5. Serine/threonine kinases, such as the TGF-β receptors (40–42)
6. Receptors that, when activated, bind tyrosine kinases such as *fyn*, *Yes*, focal adhesion kinase, and *src*

Cell-Binding Receptors of Inflammatory Systems

Another group of receptors that have come into prominence recently are concerned with binding of cells, particularly lymphocytes and inflammatory cells (43–45). These have been well characterized on the high endothelial venules of lymph nodes, but it is evident that the microvascular endothelium of the skin carries a specific set of lymphocyte-binding receptors (46,47). The mechanisms involved in selecting particular types of inflammatory cells for invasion in particular tissues such as psoriatic skin are reviewed in Butcher and Picker (48).

In psoriasis, capillaries show a characteristic tortuous morphology and resemble high endothelial venules in their ability to bind lymphocytes and in the presence of tannic acid–stainable material (49). The binding of lymphocytes to frozen sections in vitro shows specificity, CD4+ (helper) cells being bound more strongly than CD8+ (suppressor/cytotoxic) T cells. The process is energy and Ca^{2+}-dependent and involves receptors distinguishable from those of lymph node, tonsillar, or Peyer patch endothelium (47).

Receptors capable of binding lymphocytes can be induced on keratinocytes by interferon-γ (50,51). Binding to keratinocytes appears to involve the LFA-1 receptor of T lymphocytes (52) and intercellular adhesion molecule 1 (ICAM-1) (53) on the keratinocytes (51). Within subclasses of lymphocytes, keratinocyte adhesion shows some bias toward CD8+ cytotoxic/suppressor cells, as is shown in the epidermis of the psoriatic plaque (54,55).

ICAM-1 is clearly expressed by keratinocytes in psoriatic plaques (56) and ICAM-1 and E-selectin are even more markedly increased on endothelial cells (57–60). This reflects a general activation of endothelial cells (61,62) that includes some increase in VCAM. The changes are restricted to the psoriatic plaque and are much less pronounced in nonlesional skin (63). These adhesion molecules, particularly E-selectin, are released into the serum in psoriatic patients, causing an increase in concentration that has been correlated with the severity of the disease (64–67). However, although significant, the changes are not very large (64). The implication of these studies, that the emigration of inflammatory cells from the circulation into the skin plays a critical role in psoriasis, has given rise to attempts to correlate treatment regimens with measurements of the concentrations of adhesion molecules and to control psoriasis by reducing their expression (68). The results have been equivocal. In several instances, psoriasis treatment resulted in reduction in ICAM expression, as in the cases of dimethyl fumarate (69), calcipotriol (70), and FK506 (71). In other cases, following cyclosporin (72) or anthralin treatment (73), it did not. Although it is likely that these adhesion molecules play an important role in the inflammatory process in psoriasis, it appears unlikely that they cause the disease.

Integrins

The integrins are an important group of cell adhesion receptors involved in adherence, migration, and signal transduction. The field is complex and developing rapidly; for details, the reader is recommended to consult a recent review such as Ref. 74. Several integrins are capable of organizing intracellular structures connected to cytoskeletal molecules such as the actin system in the case of focal adhesion plaques and the intermediate filament system in the case of hemidesmosomes. Through these mechanisms, the integrins are able to transmit information from the extracellular matrix to the cell. The cell is also able to control the activity of integrin receptors themselves and to use them to modify the extracellular matrix. The integrins thus form a critical, bidirectional link between the cell and its environment. In keratinocytes, there is strong evidence that commitment to terminal differentiation is controlled through the $\alpha_5\beta_1$ fibronectin receptor (75). Integrins have been found to control apoptosis in several cell systems (76), and the terminal differentiation process of keratinocytes may be considered a modified apoptotic program. Further, cells with high proliferative potential, among them stem cells, can be identified through increased expression of β_1 integrin (77).

Integrins are heterodimeric molecules, composed of an α and a β chain, each of which comes from a large family of similar molecules. Most cell types express a limited range, in the case of keratinocytes $\alpha_1\beta_1$; $\alpha_2\beta_1$, primarily a collagen receptor; $\alpha_3\beta_1$, a laminin/laminin 5 receptor; $\alpha_5\beta_1$, a fibronectin receptor; $\alpha_6\beta_4$, a laminin 5 receptor involved in hemidesmosomes; $\alpha_v\beta_5$, a vitronectin receptor; and $\alpha_v\beta_6$, a fibronectin and tenascin receptor (78,79). The $\alpha_1\beta_1$ and $\alpha_5\beta_1$ receptors are absent from normal adult skin. In general, the expression of these integrins changes little at early stages of wound healing and during the keratinocyte migration phase of reepithelialization (80). However, at about 7 days, strong suprabasal staining for $\alpha_2\beta_1$, $\alpha_3\beta_1$, and α_6, presumably as $\alpha_6\beta_1$, is seen (80), and $\alpha_v\beta_6$ is induced (79). The synthesis of α_2 integrin is stimulated by activation of the EGF receptor (81).

Juxtacrine Ligands

While the cell membrane receptors are able to respond to soluble growth factors, several such ligands have been detected in an active form on the surface of cells (82). In these cases receptor/ligand interaction, termed juxtacrine, occurs on cell contact. TGF-α, HBEGF, and amphiregulin, which are thought to play major roles in controlling keratinocyte proliferation, are important examples of this mechanism (83–88). Others, which may also play a role in psoriasis, include IL-1α and TNF-α (89). The potential importance of these "private" communications between cells has been little studied in comparison with the "broadcast" signals of diffusible receptors, but may well, ultimately, prove at least as important.

THE KERATINOCYTE MEMBRANE

Keratinocytes possess a variety of known receptors, which probably represents a small fraction of the total. They include low-density lipoprotein (LDL) (90,91), Fcγ (92), β-adrenergic (93), IL-1 (94), EGF/TGF-α (95–97), KGF (98, 99), insulin (100,101), insulin-like growth factor 1 (IGF_1) (102), TGF-β (103), leukotriene C4 (104), PGE_2 (105), interferon-γ (106), transferrin (97), the hyaluronic acid receptor CD44 (38), the thrombospondin receptor CD36, CD16 (61), the 55 k TNF receptor, although not the 75 k receptor (107), and class I MHC proteins. Some of these, notably β-adrenergic, PGE_1, and protein kinase C (the phorbol ester receptor), are down-regulated in psoriasis, whereas others, such as the EGF receptor, the Fcγ receptor, and the LDL receptor, show either induction or a lack of the down-regulation seen in normal skin. In the case of EGF and interferon-γ, receptors are found in a suprabasal position not seen in normal skin (108). A few receptors have been shown not to occur on keratinocytes, including leukotriene B4 (104), IL-2 (109), CD11b, CD15, and CD33. Receptors have been inferred for prostaglandins (105,110,111), interferon-α (112), and other ligands by their biological activities. Basal keratinocytes have been reported to carry an intercellular lectin (113).

THE PSORIATIC KERATINOCYTE MEMBRANE

The importance of the cell membrane in signal transduction has given rise to a number of membrane-based hypotheses for the etiology of psoriasis. These include hypotheses based on cytokine receptors, abnormalities in the transduction mechanism itself, defects in the structure or chemistry of the membrane, and presentation of antigens. The cell membrane both of keratinocytes and of other cells has been reported to show a large number of changes in psoriasis, summarized in Ref. 114.

Ultrastructural Features of the Membrane of the Psoriatic Keratinocyte

Orfanos et al. (115,116) observed a decrease in desmosomes and a markedly microvillar appearance to keratinocytes in psoriasis. Gommans et al. (117), using freshly dispersed keratinocytes, showed that in normal skin the larger, and presumably more mature, keratinocytes lost the microvilli prominent in basal cells, but this was not the case in psoriasis. Differences in the cell surface were carried into the stratum corneum where they were presumed to play a role in the lack of cohesiveness of psoriatic corneocytes.

Desmosomes

Cells are connected by three major types of junctional structure: tight junctions, gap junctions, and desmosomes. Of these, the most prevalent in epidermis are desmosomes. Desmosomes are transmembrane structures that are linked to the intermediate filament (keratin) cytoskeleton within the cells (118) and from one cell to another through homotypic interactions. Despite their structurally rigid appearance, the proteins that form the structure, E-cadherin, catenins, desmoplakins, desmocollins, and desmogleins, can exist in a dissociated form within the cell but can assemble into desmosomes within minutes of application of a suitable signal such as increased calcium (119). It may be noted that calcium causes rigidification and dimerization of E-cadherin, forming an integral part of the molecular structure (120). The composition of desmosomes changes with keratinocyte differentiation (121).

Desmosome structures are reported to show ultrastructural alterations in psoriasis, although their overall number does not change significantly. Changes in the morphology of the desmosomes may be related to the known qualitative changes in keratin synthesis that occur in psoriasis (122,123). Soluble E-cadherin can be detected in serum and its concentration in psoriasis patients has been reported to correlate with the severity of the disease (124).

Gap Junctions

Gap junctions allow communication between cells in the form of low-molecular-weight, diffusible metabolites. They are composed of connexin subunits, hexamers of which form pores that allow diffusion of low-molecular-weight substances (125). They are of special interest in psoriasis as their loss has been associated with a breakdown in the control of proliferation in cancer and dysplasia (126,127). Furthermore, transmission of low-molecular-weight substances between normal and tumor cells has been reported to inhibit the growth of the transformed cell. Treatment of mouse skin with the tumor promoter 12-tetradecanoylphorbol-13-acetate causes loss of gap junctions, associated with a psoriasiform hyperplasia (126). Gap junctions have been suggested as the basis of a mechanism of control of growth and differentiation and are known to change during wound healing (128). This area has been reviewed by Pitts et al. (129).

In human skin, Salomon et al. (130), using Lucifer Yellow diffusion, have shown that connections between keratinocyte in human epidermis are somewhat more extensive than in mouse skin (131), extending to a few dozen cells, but not as extensive as in the dermis. There is no diffusion of Lucifer Yellow between the dermal and epidermal cells in vivo, although transfer of dye from keratinocytes to fibroblasts and other cells is easily demonstrated in culture (132,133). In nonplaque skin from psoriatic patients, Salomon et al. (130) found no significant difference in the extent of intercellular connections. So far, however, experiments on connectivity using diffusible dyes have been confined to nonplaque skin. It would be interesting to know whether the increase in the rate of cell replacement in psoriatic skin is associated with a decrease in the extent of Lucifer Yellow diffusion.

Mahrle has investigated turnover of desmosomes and gap junctions in normal and psoriatic epidermis by electron microscopic methods (134). He observed gap junctions incorporated into annular membrane structures in psoriasis, which he attributed to an increase in degradation by an endocytotic mechanism. The phenomenon was most prominent in the upper layers of psoriatic epidermis. This change may reflect increased turnover resulting from the mobility of keratinocytes in psoriasis.

Tight Junctions

Tight junctions are rarely found in normal epidermis, mainly in the granular layer, and never form an occluding band as in ductal or glandular epithelium (135). Tight junctions occur in human keratinocyte explant cultures, where Katajima et al. reported observing them between the most superficial cells of an outgrowing sheet (136). Cultures of this kind are a good model for wound healing. It would be of interest to determine whether tight junctions occur in a similar location in injury in vivo and, by extension, in psoriasis.

Hemidesmosomes

The membrane of the basal surface of the keratinocyte carries hemidesmosomes that are involved with attachment to the basement membrane through several molecular links. Major components of the hemidesmosome are $\alpha_6\beta_4$ integrin, which binds to laminin 5, and the bullous pemphigoid antigens, with molecular weights of 180,000 and 240,000. The 180-kDa molecule contains a large transmembrane collagenous domain (137).

Proteins

Changes in Cell Surface Glycosylation in Psoriasis

The possible importance of the glycocalyx was first suggested by Orfanos et al. (115,116) on the basis of electron microscopic observations. They noted a nearly complete absence of the glycoprotein-rich surface coat in the suprabasal layers. The loss of glycocalyx confirmed similar observations using light microscopy of PAS and Alcian Blue–stained sections.

The tissue distribution of glycosylation patterns can be easily characterized by histological techniques using suitably labeled lectins. The lectins are a series of proteins from a variety of plant and animal sources that bind particular oligosaccharide side chains specifically (138). Certain lectins, such as PNA, are specific for O-linked carbohydrate side chains, while many others bind to N-linked oligosaccharides. In the case of lectins labeled with fluorescent dyes, the tissue distribution of the corresponding oligosaccharide may be determined very simply by incubating frozen or, in many cases, paraffin sections with the lectin, and examining by epi-illuminated fluorescence microscopy. Important controls for these experiments are companion incubations with the sugar corresponding to the lectin-binding site, which will inhibit adsorption (139–141).

An alternative approach to examination of oligosaccharides is the use of ABH blood group antibodies. The epitopes involved include α-D-*N*-acetylgalactosamine (A), α-D-galactose (B), and α-L-fucose (H) (142,143). This system has been used successfully by Dabelsteen et al. to demonstrate changes in glycosylation during terminal differentiation in oral mucosa (144). Schaumberg-Lever et al. demonstrated similar findings in human skin, in which she correlated the patterns with the blood groups of the biopsy donors. She was able to demonstrate considerable individual variation in glycosylation patterns and alterations in skin diseases (142,143). Recently, glycoconjugate immunohistochemistry has been extended to monoclonal antibodies that recognize specific carbohydrate structures (145). An oligosaccharide structure, recognized by an anti-GM3 antibody and normally found in the stratum corneum, was found to be absent in psoriasis.

The initial mannose/glucose oligosaccharide structure, discussed above, is recognized by concanavalin A (Con A) and *Lens culinaris* agglutinin (LCA), which therefore bind to most glycoproteins destined for the cell surface at some stage of their synthesis and stain most cell types. Other lectins, in general, bind to secondarily modified oligosaccharides, and it is these structures which vary with cellular differentiation and in psoriasis.

Lectins react with carbohydrate structures on both lipids and proteins and both types of conjugates contribute to lectin binding to epidermis. The relative contribution of the two types of molecules may be determined in several ways. Nemanic et al. (146) and Mansbridge and Knapp (147) used extraction with chloroform/methanol to demonstrate that part of the staining by UEA, RCA 1, Con A, and HPA was contributed by lipids, whereas staining by PNA and WGA was not. Of particular interest in this context was the observation that UEA binding, whose staining pattern changes dramatically in psoriasis, went from 40% extractable in normal to 97% extractable in psoriatic epidermis. This indicates a major reduction in UEA-reactive glycoprotein in psoriasis, and that a major reason for the change in staining pattern is that a different class of cellular products is being detected.

The pattern of binding of lectin to skin cells varies with the animal species and also shows individual variation (143,148) without apparent clinical consequences. There thus appears to be no clear and absolute requirement for particular glycosylation patterns in keratinocyte differentiation.

In the skin, the glycosylation pattern of keratinocyte surface proteins alters with differentiation (139–141,143,146). By and large, basal cells show a distinctive pattern that is lost as the cells move into the suprabasal layer. This is followed by a progressive increase in the surface density of complex oligosaccharides as judged by increases in the intensity or staining by lectins binding to secondarily modified oligosaccharide side chains, such as SBA, SJA, HPA, WGA, and in a rather extreme form with UEA in the case of human epidermis. This is most likely to reflect accumulation of maturation products, both glycoproteins and glycolipids, with modified side chains. On cornification, keratinocytes lose the ability to bind lectins.

Basal cells display a different set of oligosaccharide side chains from those in suprabasal layers. Staining of the basal layer with HPA, PNA, SJA is dependent on treatment with neuraminidase, in contrast to the suprabasal layers (140). The number of cell layers showing this property is increased in psoriatic epidermis, along with the increase in the number of germinative layers. Roelfzema and van Erp have provided evidence that the size of the oligosaccharide side chains differs little in basal and suprabasal layers and suggest that the differences may be largely attributable to sialylation (149). Thus, modification by sialylation appears to be an important process in the germinative cells that is lost on commitment to terminal differentiation. Similar changes occur in rat skin, when the basal layer, but not the suprabasal, is stained with BSA II (148).

In sharp contrast, the normal human stratum corneum contains very little free oligosaccharide side chains (146). This loss of lectin staining in the stratum corneum has been attributed to two processes. Elias and his group, concentrating on glycolipids, have emphasized the importance of glycosidases, which they have demonstrated to be present in the stratum granulosum (146). Thus, they suggest the ceramides, derived from sphingolipids by hydrolysis in the stratum granulosum, contribute to the lipids of the intercorneocyte lamellae.

In addition to this mechanism, Brysk et al. have demonstrated the existence of an endogenous lectin in the stratum corneum (150), which contributes to corneocyte adhesion and is responsible for at least part of the loss of reactivity to lectins binding to amino sugar–containing oligosaccharides. They have observed clear binding of Con A, WGA, and SBA to ether- or detergent-dispersed corneocytes (151). Moreover, they were able to demonstrate lectin- and sugar-sensitive reaggregation of corneocytes. In conjunction with the lack of binding by these lectins to native stratum corneum, these results indicate that a lectin-like adhesion system plays a role in corneocyte coherence in the stratum corneum. The lectins involved included WGA, which was the most effective, Con A, and SBA. The most effective sugar inhibiting the aggregation was *N*-acetyl neuraminic acid, followed by *N*-acetyl glucosamine and mannose. Fucose and galactose were not involved.

Lectin-Staining Patterns in Psoriasis

A number of groups have independently investigated the surface glycosylation patterns in psoriasis using lectin stains and other methods. This has generated a plethora of data and hypotheses, especially involving fucose- and UEA-binding sites (149,152,153). We will summarize the data and then discuss them in terms of our current understanding of glycosylation.

Kariniemi et al. found that the distribution of staining with FITC-UEA I in psoriatic epidermis was much more extensive than in normal skin (152). The binding of UEA I is normally restricted to the granular layer and the most superficial layers of the epidermis, but in psoriasis expression of the UEA-binding site starts much earlier in the maturation process, very much as in wound healing (123). Schaumberg-Lever et al. noted that the distribution of UEA staining was largely intracellular and attributed this to a defect in the transport of fucose-containing glycopeptides to the surface (153). It was not, however, determined in this study whether the UEA binding was to glycoprotein or glycolipid. Other evidence suggests that a much larger proportion of the UEA staining of psoriatic skin is extractable by lipid solvents than is the case in normal skin (147) and, therefore, represents quite a different class of membrane components.

The most extensive study of the surface glycosylation of psoriatic keratinocytes was that of the Nijmegen group (149,154–159). They first determined the frequency of lectin-binding sites on normal keratinocytes by trypsinization of biopsy specimens. In freshly dispersed cells, they observed about 10^7 specific sites for HPA and PNA and about 10^8 specific sites for Con A, WGA, and UEA, with specific association constants of about 10^6 L/mol. These sites were 40–85% trypsin sensitive, with the exception of UEA, which was only 25% sensitive (154).

Interpretation of measurements of binding sites on cells freshly dispersed with trypsin is limited because of possible proteolytic degradation and fractionation of the cell population (154). In an attempt to overcome the first of these problems, Gommans et al. incubated the dispersed cells for 22 hr in vitro. Under these conditions, the number of Con A sites increased eightfold and WGA sites, nearly 20-fold. However, in the case of Con A, the increase continued in an approximately linear fashion for 6 days. During this time, keratinocyte differentiation changes markedly from the normal epidermal pathway (122), which may explain the increase of glycosylation. Comparison between preparations depends on the assumption that the amount of trypsin degradation is comparable in each case (154,160).

In psoriasis, Gommans et al. found that binding of HPA, PNA, and UEA was essentially unchanged, although Con A and WGA increased by factors of about 2 and 3, respectively (157). In the case of Con A, this was largely attributable to nonpolygonal cells, i.e., basal cells and cells recently committed to terminal differentiation. Polygonal cells showed a fourfold decrease in Con A binding. They also observed a similar, although smaller, increase in Con A, but not WGA, binding in unfractionated cells from tape-stripped skin. It may be noted that a difference in the association constant of UEA binding was detected between normal and psoriatic skin, supporting a qualitative change in the binding sites (157).

In a separate series of experiments, Roelfzema et al. showed that the rates of incorporation of a variety of sugars were increased in psoriasis (156). Most precursors showed a small, although significant increase, but *N*-acetyl glucosamine increased about threefold. The incorporation rates into keratinocytes from normal skin increased during 22-hr culture, whereas in psoriatic lesional cells, they fell, perhaps because of the limited viability of these cells. The initial increase in fucose uptake in psoriatic lesional keratinocytes agrees with the conclusion of Mann et al. (161) using electron microscope radioautographic methods. This group, however, found that a greater proportion was retained in an intracellular location.

In a more detailed characterization of the glycoconjugates Roelfzema et al. showed that for a variety of oligosaccharide precursors the proportion of incorporated sugar found in the glycolipid fraction increased in psoriatic lesions by comparison with normal (156). In the case of fucose, the increase was not as dramatic as might have been expected from data on the extractability of UEA-binding sites from histological sections with chloroform methanol. The most likely explanation of this finding is that much of the fucose incorporated into glycoprotein in psoriasis is not detected by UEA for structural reasons, as discussed below. The proportion of incorporated radioactivity to be found in lipid was not dependent on the size of the keratinocytes except in the case of galactose where a correlation was found. This presumably reflects a disproportionate accumulation of galactose-containing lipids during terminal maturation in psoriasis.

Of particular interest in this study was the observation that the size distribution of fucose-labeled oligosaccharide fragments derived from glycoproteins was altered in psoriasis. The analysis was carried out by Sephadex G-50 chromatography of papain fragments. The earliest peak eluted from the column, of high molecular weight, was labeled mainly with galactose and *N*-acetyl glucosamine and was thought to be composed mainly of fragments derived from O-linked sugar chains reactive with PNA. The asparagine-linked chains were eluted within the molecular-weight-sensitive range of the column. Fucose-labeled oligosaccharides of this type from psoriatic skin showed a marked increase in molecular weight, and presumably in complexity, by comparison with normal, caused by addition of further oligosaccharide chains (from biantennary to tri- or higher). Glycopeptides of this type were predominantly found in a fraction that did not bind to Con A Sepharose.

The Con A–unbound fraction, in which the primary oligosaccharide chains have been completely replaced, represents fully modified glycoproteins, which carry the most complex side chains. Con A binds to the initial oligosaccharide transferred onto the nascent protein by dolichol phosphate, which is subsequently modified in the *trans*-Golgi to structures that react with other lectins. The size of the modified fraction is greater in keratinocytes derived from psoriatic lesions than in normal. The extensive modification of the structure of these chains in psoriasis may also account for the loss of their reaction with UEA.

In a comparison of the complexities of oligosaccharide structures in shed, presumably secreted, and bound glycoproteins, Roelfzema and van Erp (159) showed that the higher-molecular-weight glycopeptides were derived from nonsecreted proteins. Proteins secreted from the surface of keratinocytes form a specific group, which may be induced or repressed by cytokines, including fibronectin, thrombospondin, and a wide variety of growth and differentiation factors (1). It is remarkable that the glycosylation of these proteins appears to be unaffected, whereas that of keratinocyte surface proteins is altered. The result implies specificity in the keratinocyte glycosylation process, and it is only those proteins that remain on the keratinocyte surface that show alterations in psoriasis associated with differentiation.

The evident complexity of glycosylation limits the amount of information that can be obtained from lectin-binding experiments. Further progress will depend on structural characterization of individual molecules. A start on characterizing glycoproteins and changes in them during differentiation and in disease has been made by several groups (160–167).

Kariniemi et al. (164) used periodate oxidation followed by [^{3}H]borohydride reduction to investigate changes in surface glycoproteins in nonplaque keratinocytes cultured from psoriatic patients. They observed that a protein with an M_r of 63,000 was found in keratinocytes from nonpsoriatic individuals, but not in those from patients. This protein was apparently induced in psoriatic nonplaque keratinocytes by etretinate.

Brysk and Snider (163) and Bonnefoy et al. (165) have exploited ^{125}I-labeled lectins to stain glycoproteins separated by electrophoresis in polyacrylamide gels. Using cultured rat keratinocytes, staining with concanavalin A showed at least eight major and a number of minor bands. The relative intensities of these bands changed on the induction of maturation by calcium switching. In particular, an 85,000-M_r peak became dominant. WGA and RCA stained only three proteins, which matched Con A proteins in molecular weight. It appeared, however, that the second-stage modification of glycoproteins in keratinocytes was protein specific and changed on differentiation (162).

Bonnefoy et al. (165), using extracts from freshly dispersed human keratinocytes stained with Con A, was also able to show a marked difference between patterns of glycoproteins dispersed from the epidermis by trypsin and those remaining with the stratum corneum, presumably the most mature. In particular, the most mature cells showed an increase in a 40,000-M_r molecule. The pattern changed on culture, with the loss of the 40,000-M_r protein and the appearance of higher-molecular-weight species.

In psoriasis, Brysk et al. found a considerable alteration in the Con A–staining pattern (166). In particular, the 40,000-M_r protein, later termed desquamin (168), found in normal epidermis, was much reduced, whereas a 50,000-M_r protein was considerably increased. They suggested that the 50,000-M_r protein is a marker for the abnormal differentiation seen in psoriasis and other skin diseases.

Morrison et al. (167) investigated the proteins that bind peanut lectin. Two very diffuse bands of M_r 110,000 and 250,000 were identified. While fluoresceinated PNA binding increases with keratinocyte maturation in normal human epidermis, a polyclonal antibody against the proteins bound equally throughout the epidermis, implying that the increase in PNA binding with differentiation reflects changes in the glycosylation of a protein found in all layers. In culture, the PNA-binding protein showed a striking change in distribution following induction of terminal differentiation with calcium. The specificity of PNA is for galactose in O-linked oligosaccharide chains (169). These chains are frequently much longer than asparagine-linked oligosaccharides, which is consistent with the high molecular weight of [^{14}C] galactose-labeled glycopeptides obtained from human epidermal keratinocytes by Roelfzema et al. (155).

The findings of these studies may be summarized as follows:

1. The glycosylation pattern of keratinocyte glycoconjugates changes on commitment of basal cells to terminal differentiation. In human skin, this is shown particularly in reduced sialylation. Surface glycoproteins with secondarily modified side chains accumulate during terminal maturation.
2. The pattern of glycosylation of keratinocytes derived from psoriatic plaques differs from that found in normal skin. The differences have the following features:
   a. A higher rate of glycosylation occurs as estimated by the rate of incorporation of radioactive sugars into glycoconjugates.
   b. A greater proportion of the glycoconjugates are glycolipids, especially in the case of UEA-binding molecules.
   c. Oligosaccharide side chains on keratinocyte surface proteins are more highly modified. This is reflected both in a reduction in the proportion of molecules carrying unmodified Con A–binding structures and in the proportion of Con A–binding molecules carrying triantennary or higher side chains. These alterations appear not to affect secreted keratinocyte proteins.

The changes in lectin binding are not directly related to keratinocyte proliferation. No correlation could be found between the kinetics of changes in glycosylation and proliferation in tape-stripped skin, all alterations taking place in cells in the G_1 phase of the cell cycle (149).

The changes in glycosylation seen in psoriasis are distinguishable from those seen in a number of other skin diseases (142,166,170), but show some similarity to those seen in culture (123). Psoriasis shows a number of characteristics in common with wound healing and culture and has been discussed as an abnormality of the control of the normal epidermal response to injury (123). The distribution of UEA binding in many psoriatic patients does, however, differ in detail from wound healing (123). In wound healing, UEA binding extends further into the epidermis from the most superficial layers than in normal skin, as in psoriasis, but retains its pericellular distribution and resistance to chloroform/methanol extraction. In most studies, UEA binding in psoriasis is intracellular (153,171,172) and largely extractable (147), although Kariniemi reported a largely pericellular distribution very much like wound healing (123,152).

The changes in keratinocyte glycosylation patterns, especially those involving fucose, have given rise to considerable speculation as to their possible importance in the pathogenesis of psoriasis (143,157,161). Since both UEA staining and [^{3}H]fucose incorporation show a far more intracellular distribution in psoriatic epidermis than in normal skin, a defect in the transport of fucosylated glycoconjugates has been proposed. It may be noted, however, that the overall incorporation of [^{3}H]fucose is increased in psoriasis (156,161). An increased proportion of the radioactivity is extractable by lipid solvents (155), although the overall incorporation into glycoprotein still seems to be increased. UEA binding to sections, however, is almost completely extractable (147). An explanation based on nonreactivity with UEA of the fucosylated oligosaccharide side chains found on glycoproteins in psoriasis seems more likely than one based on a lack of transport. This is consistent with evidence on the increase in the size of the oligopeptides (155) and the lack of alteration in the glycosylation of secreted proteins (159). Fucosidase activity is increased over normal in the psoriatic plaque, but is not changed in nonplaque skin (158). Moreover, the changes in oligosaccharide composition cannot be correlated with proliferation (156). It seems simplest to consider the changes in glycosylation to reflect differentiation of the keratinocyte, as is seen during commitment to terminal differentiation and in a variety of tumor cells in which differentiation is abnormal (32).

The use of lectins to fractionate and identify oligosaccharides has evolved to new heights of sophistication since most of these experiments were carried out (169,173–176). It would be valuable at this point to characterize the changes in glycosylation on specific proteins with differentiation in terms of specific glycosylation reactions. It is possible that a minor change in enzyme activities in the Golgi system may give rise to dramatic changes in lectin staining as has been observed.

The Envelope

Formation of the cornified envelope, consisting of proteins crosslinked by isopeptide bonds (between γ-carboxyl of glutamate and ϵ-amino of lysine), is an important function of the keratinocyte (177). The reaction is carried out by transglutaminase, of which three isoenzymes occur in the skin. One is membrane bound, specific to the keratinocyte and responsible for envelope formation, whereas another is common to several cell types (178–180).

A number of proteins have been recognized as envelope components. In cultured cells, the most important is involucrin (181), but this is a minor component in envelopes formed by simian virus 40 (SV40)-transformed human keratinocytes (182). A much smaller protein, with a molecular weight of 36,000 by gel filtration or 6000 by electrophoresis, was identified by Buxman et al. (183) and termed keratolinin. It has been suggested by Petersen et al. that this protein might be relatively more important in normal epidermis, whereas involucrin plays a greater role in wound healing, tissue culture, and psoriasis (184). It is clear that a variety of proteins are incorporated into envelopes under culture conditions, a number of which have been characterized by Kubilus and Baden's group (185–187) and Simons and Green (188).

More recently, a deoxyribonucleic acid (DNA) sequence has been cloned from an epidermal complementary DNA (cDNA) library that coded for a protein with an amino acid composition very similar to envelopes derived from normal stratum corneum and called loricrin (189). This is the major envelope protein of the normal epidermal differentiation pathway in association with a series of smaller proteins, small proline-rich (SPR) proteins 1 and 2 and elafin (190,191). These proteins are incorporated into the envelope in a well-defined manner and associate with keratins (191), through the formation of isopeptide bonds involving transglutaminases 1 and 3 (192).

Expression of loricrin, characteristic of orthokeratosis, is reduced in psoriasis (193), while that of cornifin, which is characteristic of squamous differentiation, is increased (194). Synthesis of involucrin and SPR-1 is also markedly increased (184,190). The envelope proteins show interesting responses to retinoic acid. Loricrin synthesis is repressed, as are the differentiation keratins, but involucrin synthesis is not (195). SPR-1 is slightly repressed.

The envelope formed in psoriasis differs markedly from that from normal skin. Michel et al. (196) showed that the electrophoretic pattern of cyanogen bromide–cleaved peptides from the cornified envelopes from normal skin differs markedly from that obtained from psoriatic scales, particularly in the frequency of low-molecular-weight peptides. Envelopes from cultured keratinocytes also showed many low-molecular-weight peptides, but the pattern differed in detail from that seen in psoriasis. The conclusion of the authors was that, when it is activated, the membrane-bound transglutaminase crosslinks whatever proteins are in its vicinity. These proteins appear to be quite different in normal skin and the psoriatic plaque.

The overall picture is that the envelope formed by psoriatic keratinocytes differs from normal in its composition of both protein and lipids (197,198). Specialized proteins of the normal epidermal envelope, such as loricrin and the 40-kDa glycoprotein, are reduced, whereas involucrin and cornifin are increased. On activation by the cornification process, the membrane-bound transglutaminase of psoriatic skin appears to incorporate any available proteins to form an apparently somewhat makeshift envelope.

Adhesion between corneocytes is brought about by lipid and lectin interactions (199). Both these systems are disrupted in psoriasis and may contribute to the scaling phenotype characteristic of the disease. Expression of the protease-resistant, glycoprotein lectin desquamin (168) is sensitive to cytokines (200) and is reduced in psoriasis (166). In addition, a chemokinetic 30k glycoprotein that is normally restricted to the stratum corneum is expressed throughout the epidermis in psoriasis (201).

Receptors

β-Adrenergic Receptor

The possibility that β-adrenergic receptors might be involved in the pathogenesis of psoriasis has long been attractive because certain β-blocking drugs are known to exacerbate psoriasis (202). The mechanism is, however, obscure. Keratinocytes carry adrenergic receptors (203), the major type being β_2 (204), which stimulate adenyl cyclase via a GTP-binding G_s-protein (205).

The adenlyate cyclase response for keratinocytes freshly isolated from psoriatic plaques to epinephrine is reduced by comparison with normal, although their cyclic adenosine monophosphate (cAMP) content on a DNA basis is not very different from that of normal skin (206,207). The β-adrenergic receptors are desensitized following stimulation by an agonist. The process involves an early change in sensitivity, which probably results from impairment of the interaction between the receptor and G_s, possibly involving phosphorylation. This may be followed by sequestration of the receptor in a nonplasma membrane vesicle and finally down-regulation. Recovery from down-regulation may or may not require protein synthesis depending on the cell type (208). In psoriasis, the frequency of β-adrenergic receptors is reduced, apparently on a long-term basis. Whether this is related to stimulation or to a general desensitization of receptor transduction systems is not known. Down-regulation of the PGE_2 receptor and protein kinase C system has been reported (110,209).

Propranalol, an antagonist of epinephrine that exacerbates psoriasis, has been reported to have no effect on the proliferation of keratinocytes (210). As an alternative mechanism, it has been pointed out that epinephrine inhibits some lymphocyte functions, and that the epinephrine antagonists might allow activation of the immune component of psoriasis, leading to stimulation of the pathogenic mechanism. In support of this view, Czernielewski et al. (211) demonstrated an increase in anti-HLA DR antibody staining of plaque epidermis from patients taking β-blocking drugs and a correlation between staining and the severity of psoriasis.

Epidermal Growth Factor Receptor

The epidermal growth factor (EGF) system is important in the epidermis. Keratinocytes cultured in defined medium are absolutely dependent on activation of the EGF receptor for growth (212,213), and the frequency of its receptor has been related to epithelial cell growth in the skin and its appendages (214). The EGF receptor also binds transforming growth factor α (TGF-α) (219), heparin-binding EGF-like growth factor (36), and β-cellulin (215–217). While in low-density cultures ligand for the EGF receptor must be added, as, for instance, EGF, as the culture becomes denser, this function may be fulfilled by autocrine or juxtacrine mechanisms (213), such as those involving TGF-α, HBEGF, or amphiregulin (218–220). The activity of amphiregulin, which can account for 75% of the autocrine growth of keratinocyte cultures, is, however, dependent on binding to heparan sulfate proteoglycan. As a consequence, autocrine keratinocyte proliferation is sensitive to inhibitors of heparan sulfate synthesis such as chlorate or hexadimethrine (221,222). Remarkably, the activity of heparin-binding EGF-like growth factor was not sensitive to chlorate. These observations raise the possibility of further, extracellular mechanisms of control of EGF receptor activation and keratinocyte proliferation. An example of a heparan sulfate–modified proteoglycan that might be involved in this process in the epidermis is the splice variant of CD44 containing exon V3 that is expressed by keratinocytes (36). This protein is locally depleted in psoriatic epidermis, apparently in relation to invasion by inflammatory cells (38).

Synthesis of TGF-α is controlled by a positive feedback autocrine system that is activated in psoriasis (223,224). The EGF receptor also shows stimulation-dependent desensitization involving endocytosis and degradation (225–227) through a mechanism requiring protein phosphorylation on tyrosine residues (228). Simulation studies (J. N. Mansbridge, unpublished data) have shown that a system of this type amplifies weak stimuli into a standardized response, so that keratinocyte activation changes by only 20% for a 50-fold change in the size of the activating stimulus. The same study has also shown that the critical feature controlling the magnitude of the response is receptor down-regulation. Increasing the gain in the autocrine feedback loop by a factor of 10 does not cause activation of the keratinocytes to lock on, but reduction in ligand-dependent receptor degradation does. Early attempts to cause abnormal growth by introducing plasmids that overproduce TGF-α into cells were not successful, despite demonstrated overproduction of the cytokine (229) in accord with the prediction. TGF-α-overexpressing mice, although showing epidermal hyperplasia, show no increased skin tumor incidence (230) and TGF-α has been shown not to be involved in *ras*-linked tumors (231). Abnormalities in the receptor, however, such as overproduction, lack of ligand-dependent down-regulation, or mutation, are known to give rise to tumors (232–238). The

EGF receptor, indeed, has given rise to the *erbB* oncogene (239).

In contrast with the β-adrenergic receptors, the frequency of EGF receptors in psoriatic skin is elevated (240). In normal epidermis, EGF receptors are largely confined to the basal layer, but in psoriatic skin, they have been detected throughout the living layers by in situ autoradiographic labeling of histological sections with ^{125}I-labeled EGF. The receptors in psoriatic skin grafted to nude mice have been shown to be responsive to EGF in terms of down-regulation and modification of the immunohistological distribution of phospholipase Cγ (241). One possible explanation for this observation is derived from the rapidity of transit of keratinocytes through the epidermis in psoriasis. Since keratinocyte maturation time is reduced from about 14 days in normal skin to about 2 days in psoriatic plaque, an EGF receptor half-life of 105 hr would account for the results observed (L. E. King, personal communication).

The distributions of EGF receptors in normal skin detected by ^{125}I-EGF and by antibody raised against the extracellular domain of the receptor give different patterns (242). While binding of the labeled hormone is restricted to the basal layer of normal skin, the antibody detects immunoreactive material throughout the epidermis. One explanation is that the receptor is present in suprabasal layers but desensitized and no longer able to bind EGF. It is, perhaps, the desensitization that is abnormal in psoriasis. An alternative explanation relates to the changes in protein glycosylation discussed above. A number of EGF-reactive antibodies are directed against glycosyl side chains. The point is interesting in view of the relationship between cellular glycosylation and the properties of the EGF receptor observed in experimental systems (39).

Signal transduction from the EGF receptor is thought to be initiated largely through dimerization (243–246) that allows mutual autophosphorylation on tyrosine residues, although other mechanisms may be involved (247,248). This results in the assembly of many proteins through SH2 domains and other interactions, including Grb2, hSos Ras, and phospholipase Cγ (249), that initiate further stages of information processing that lie outside the scope of this discussion.

A number of mechanisms of control of the activity of the EGF receptor that affect both ligand affinity and tyrosine kinase activity are known. First, the receptor phosphorylates itself at several tyrosine residues, the major one being position 1173 (250). This reaction is required for biological activity, presumably through phosphorylation of other proteins, including receptor down-regulation and endocytosis (228,251). Second, it may be phosphorylated by protein kinase C, predominantly at position threonine 654 (252–254). Phosphorylation at this position also occurs in response to platelet-derived growth factor (PDGF) by a protein kinase C–independent mechanism and reduces the affinity of the receptor for EGF (254). Other phosphorylation reactions occur on serine 1046 and serine 1047 by the calcium-calmodulin-dependent protein kinase, which are involved in inactivation and internalization following stimulation by EGF (255), and on threonine 669 by a specific IL-1-activated protein kinase (256). Third, sphingosine increases the affinity of the receptor for EGF and the maximal rate of tyrosine phosphorylation in a manner independent of protein kinase C and may also be involved in its control (12). Fourth, *N*-acetyl galactosamine transferase activity is correlated with the proportion of high-affinity receptors (39). The first of these mechanisms is ligand related, whereas the others are presumably part of the internal cell control mechanism.

In psoriasis, TGF-α is transcribed at a high level, and it is inferred that the autocrine loop is active (224). It is, therefore, surprising that the EGF receptor is not down-regulated, but rather persists in the suprabasal layers. The discrepancy warrants a detailed examination of the properties of the EGF-receptor desensitization system in psoriatic keratinocytes. The ability of TGF-α to function as a juxtacrine ligand may well affect its desensitization properties as it is not clear how a receptor may be internalized while bound to a ligand attached to a cell or a solid support.

The expression of the EGF receptor on keratinocytes has been shown to be reduced by calcium (257), an inducer of terminal maturation in cultured keratinocytes, as discussed below (119,258). A similar induction of maturation occurs on treatment of cultures with phorbol esters (259) or exogenous phospholipase C (260), and Jaken and Yuspa (261) have provided evidence that the protein kinase C system plays a central role in this process. Such activation of protein kinase C may also be the mechanism of desensitization of the EGF receptor in suprabasal keratinocytes. In psoriasis, protein kinase C activity is significantly lower than normal (209). It is possible that this is causally related to the retention of active EGF receptor in the suprabasal layers in psoriatic epidermis. Epidermal growth factor is itself able to cause the hydrolysis of phosphatidyl inositol to inositol triphosphate and diacyl glycerol through phospholipase C (262), presumably representing a negative feedback loop that may well be inactive in psoriasis.

Protein Kinase C

The protein kinase C family of proteins constitute a group of at least nine members that phosphorylate targets on serine and threonine residues. Characterized by structural similarities, they are, in general, activated by diacyl glycerol and are frequently calcium dependent. They are components of a signal transduction pathway involving phospholipase C on the input side and a variety of target proteins and calcium influx on the output. They are classified into calcium dependent (protein kinases C-α, -β, and -γ) and calcium independent groups (protein kinases, C-δ, -ϵ, -ζ -η, θ, λ, and μ). Members of the group found prominently in epidermis are protein kinases C-α, -β, -λ, -ϵ, -ζ, and -η (263–265). Protein kinase C-α is found largely in basal cells and -ζ and -η in suprabasal layers. Protein kinase-η is associated with differentiation and increases toward the granular layer (266). Protein kinase C-β, which represents two-thirds of the protein kinase C activity in the epidermis, is largely found in Langerhans cells.

The phospholipases C constitute a family of at least 10 proteins activated by a variety of receptors (10,267). Mechanisms of activation include phosphorylation of tyrosine residues by association through SH2 domains (activation of phospholipases C-γ by EGF receptor) and through GTP-binding G-proteins (phospholipase C-β) (268–270). The preferred substrate of phospholipase C is phosphatidyl inositol 4,5-diphosphate, which is hydrolyzed to diacyl glycerol and inositol 1,4,5-triphosphate. The inositol triphosphate stimulates calcium release from intracellular stores and the diacyl glycerol stimulates protein kinase C (10,11).

One mechanism for the control of the response of protein kinase C to ligands is its relocation from the plasma membrane to cytoplasmic vesicles. Phospholipase C and its receptors lie in the plasma membrane and produce diacylglycerol, which remains in the membrane. Removal of protein kinase C to a nonmembrane location thus prevents activation. This process is inhibited by ceramide, a hydrolysis product of sphingosine (271). Localization of protein kinase C to the cell membrane represents an early example of a phenomenon that is becoming a general mechanism for the control of enzymes involved in signal transduction pathways. For instance, it has been suggested that the major function of Ras is to attach the protein kinase Raf to the cell membrane (272–275). Likewise, a major function of receptor activation is to assemble a membrane-bound structure (249) and of integrins to assemble a membrane- and cytoskeleton-associated structure, the focal adhesion plaque that also includes growth factor receptors (276).

The protein kinases C are the major target for phorbol esters (277), which stimulate terminal differentiation in keratinocyte cultures (260) and cause a psoriasiform hyperplasia in mouse skin in vivo. They have, therefore, become the center of considerable interest in the study of psoriasis. Protein kinase C activity shows an overall decrease in psoriasis, which is mainly attributable to a marked loss of protein kinase C-β in Langerhans cells (278). Protein kinase C-α shows a slight decrease while protein kinase C-ζ shows about a twofold increase. The others are unchanged. The changes in soluble protein are not reflected in mRNA levels and it is thought that the decreases seen in protein kinases C-α and -β reflect activation with consequent down-regulation (265,278). Activation of protein kinase C in Langerhans cells has been associated with their emigration from the epidermis (279).

As discussed above, the protein kinase C system has been implicated in the control of the induction of terminal differentiation in keratinocytes (259–261). The view is supported by the observation of Gupta et al. (280) that phorbol ester effects can be inhibited by sphingosine, a known inhibitor of protein kinase C activation (reviewed in Ref. 12). In mouse keratinocytes, high concentrations of calcium (about 1 mM) cause an increase in inositol phosphates, apparently through activation of phospholipase C (281). Hydrolysis of phosphatidyl inositol by exogenous bacterial phospholipase C leads to cornification of cultured keratinocytes, very similar to that caused by phorbol esters. Squamous cell carcinoma-derived cell lines that show a resistance to the differentiation-inducing effects of calcium and phorbol esters are similarly resistant to phospholipase C (260). In mouse, protein kinase C activation by phorbol ester or Harvey *ras* transformation inhibits expression of keratins 1 and 10, which are characteristically synthesized in the spinous layer, and induces loricrin and filaggrin, which are granular layer markers (282,283). This result shows similarities to the phenotype seen in psoriasis (repression of keratins 1 and 10 synthesis) and differences (elevation of loricrin synthesis). In view of the concept that protein kinase C is important in keratinocyte differentiation, it is particularly interesting that the major epidermal activation of protein kinase C in psoriasis appears to be in Langerhans cells.

In psoriatic plaques, epidermal phospholipase C activity is elevated (284) and colocalized with EGF receptor (285). Protein kinase C is depressed by comparison with normal or nonplaque skin (209). Fibroblasts, which have been implicated in the psoriatic process (286), show elevated protein kinase C (287). An interesting possible consequence of the increase in phospholipase C in psoriasis arises from its ability to release glycosyl-phosphatidyl-inositol-anchored proteins from the cell membrane. Indeed, it has been shown that four such proteins, CD16, CD55, CD58, and CD59, are specifically depleted in psoriasis and not in other inflammatory diseases (288).

Among the consequences of stimulation of this system is activation of the release of arachidonic acid from phospholipids, by mechanisms outside the scope of this discussion (15,289). The reaction is important in psoriasis as it is the rate-limiting step in the synthesis of neutrophil chemotactic eicosanoids, such as 12-hydroxyeicosatetraenoic acid (12-HETE) and leukotriene B4, which are elevated in the psoriatic plaque.

Changes in Keratinocyte Integrins in Psoriasis

In psoriasis, the earliest observations of suprabasal expression of basal keratinocyte membrane markers used VM1 and VM2 monoclonal antibodies, produced using psoriatic keratinocytes as the immunogen, that were subsequently shown to react with α_2 and α_3 integrin subunits (Morhenn, unpublished results; 290). These results have been confirmed and extended using antibodies known to be directed against integrins (80,291). In addition, it has been noted that normal cellular integrin distribution is disrupted. The $\alpha_2\beta_1$ and $\alpha_3\beta_1$ integrins are normally found on the nonbasal surfaces of keratinocytes, $\alpha_5\beta_1$ is diffusely distributed, and $\alpha_6\beta_4$ occurs in hemidesmosomes (78). The roles of the $\alpha_2\beta_1$ and $\alpha_3\beta_1$ integrins are not clear as their known ligands have been shown to be absent above the basal layer of the epidermis (80), although it has been suggested that they may be involved in cell-cell interactions (8,292). In psoriasis, however, all these integrins are distributed on all surfaces of the basal keratinocytes and show no polarity, even in noninvolved skin (291). In culture on 3T3 feeder layers, normal keratinocytes adhere through $\alpha_6\beta_4$ structures that are not related to the actin cytoskeleton. Keratinocytes from psoriatic patients, whether derived from lesional or nonlesional skin, show adhesion plaques associated with microfilaments and containing α_2, α_3, β_1, and β_4 integrins. The change in the adhesive mechanisms used by keratinocytes is further substantiated by the demonstration that attachment of normal keratinocytes to matrigel can be inhibited by neutralizing antibodies to β_4 subunits but not β_1 while psoriatic keratinocyte attachment is inhibited by both anti-β_1 and anti-β_4 antibodies (291). The data are broadly consistent with the similarity between psoriasis and wound healing (78,123) and also indicate an abnormality in nonlesional skin. This abnormality reflects a fundamental alteration in a major signal transduction system in the keratinocyte that interprets information from structures surrounding the cell and is related to the control of differentiation.

Recently, the development of transgenic mice overexpressing integrins in differentiated keratinocytes controlled by the involucrin promoter has provided further evidence supporting the close relationship between these membrane receptors and psoriasis (293). Mice transgenic for the involucrin-driven β_1 integrin construct alone or in combination with α_2 or α_6 integrin constructs showed suprabasal expression of the expected integrin and a phenotype that, among other features, resembled psoriasis extraordinarily closely.

Thus, a series of observations has related integrins to psoriasis.

1. A psoriasis-like condition can be induced in transgenic mice by abnormalities in integrin expression.
2. Integrin expression shows abnormalities in cellular and tissue distribution in psoriasis.
3. The observed changes in integrin expression imply consequent changes in keratinocyte signal transduction.
4. Signal transduction from integrins is closely related to the control of differentiation.

Taken together, these data suggest that investigation of genetic and phenotypic abnormalities of the control of integrin expression, activation, signal transduction, and relationship to differentiation may be crucial to the understanding of psoriasis.

THE LANGERHANS CELL (LC) MEMBRANE IN PSORIASIS

Langerhans cells are bone-marrow-derived, epidermal dendritic cells that act as specialized macrophages and are involved in antigen presentation (294). They are increased significantly in wounded skin (295). That psoriasis is a lymphoid cell-mediated autoimmune disease has been suggested repeatedly (296,297), which raises the possibility of Langerhans cell involvement. It is of interest that the ICAM-3 expressed on Langerhans cell membranes is reduced in psoriasis (298) and the protein kinase C most affected in psoriasis, protein kinase CβII, is localized in Langerhans cells (265).

By analogy to macrophages, LC may be able to synthesize EGF and nitric oxide. The enzyme nitric oxide synthase catalyzes the synthesis of NO from L-arginine, a process that is inhibited by glucocorticoids and EGF (299). It has been shown recently that purinoreceptors on the surface of macrophages regulate the inducible nitric oxide synthase production of nitric oxide (300). Furthermore, these purinoreceptors also can mobilize Ca^{2+}, an important ion in the regulation of keratinocyte differentiation (see above). Nitric oxide stimulates guanylate cyclase, an enzyme found in many cell types including keratinocytes. Guanylate cyclase promotes the synthesis of cGMP and this cyclic nucleotide has been reported to be associated with keratinocyte proliferation (301).

Macrophages, of which Langerhans cells form a subclass, express both α_2 and β_2 adrenergic receptors (302,303). Idazoxan, an antagonist of the α_2 receptor, reduces nitrite accumulation in these cells whereas both propranalol, an antagonist of the β_2 receptor, and idazoxan can inhibit superoxide production. This suggests that a negative cross-feedback loop exists in this cell type (303). Furthermore, activation of β-adrenergic receptors inhibits the lipopolysaccharide-induced TNF release (304).

METHODS FOR STUDYING THE KERATINOCYTE MEMBRANE IN PSORIASIS

Information on alterations in the keratinocyte membrane in psoriasis have come from a number of sources—glycosylation patterns, studies of receptors in keratinocytes themselves and in other cell types, and studies of membrane structure. To date, little has come from a direct analysis of membrane proteins. Using lactoperoxidase labeling, Brysk and Snider were able to show numerous differences in the surface proteins of normal and transformed cultured human keratinocytes (305). DiCicco et al., using similar methods, were able to show differences between the surface proteins of keratinocytes cultured from nonpsoriatic and psoriatic individuals, but were not able to relate the changes to psoriasis (114). This may be contrasted with the experiments of Kariniemi et al., using a more selective labeling method, who did find a consistent difference (164). A method of purifying keratinocyte membranes has been published, which may provide the means of examining the gamut of keratinocyte surface proteins by direct chemical means (306). A summary of the available methods may be found in Ref. 307. Application of the newer techniques or oligosaccharide analysis (169,173–176) together with HPLC analysis on electrophoretically separated proteins will greatly enhance the precision of the analysis.

CONCLUSIONS

The complexities of the receptor control systems, in terms of both their actions on cell metabolism and the control of their expression by cellular mechanisms, are just beginning to be elucidated. A major function of the cell membrane is receipt of molecular information from the cellular environment and its transmission to the intracellular signal transduction systems. Many of the known agents that have been studied hitherto have been soluble growth factors, but it is likely that when our understanding of cellular communication matures, the majority of signals will be found to be from juxtracrine or from insoluble, matrix-bound ligands. Currently known examples of insoluble ligands include the integrin interaction with matrix molecules, juxtacrine signaling through TGF-α and the EGF receptor, and the widespread association of molecules such as KGF, HBEGF, and amphiregulin with extracellular matrix molecules. Such signals have not only activity but also localization and direction. The importance of this in terms of the polarity of basal keratinocytes has been demonstrated in integrins, but is likely to prove general in tissues composed of adherent cells.

More differences between the properties of receptors on normal epidermal and psoriatic keratinocytes and Langerhans cells will be found. The question, as always, will be whether such changes are fundamental in the pathogenesis of the disease, as the direct consequence of a basic pathogenic abnormality, or merely reflect the differentiation and inflammatory changes that are such prominent features of the psoriatic plaque.

REFERENCES

1. Milstone, L.M. (1988). Effector functions of keratinocytes. *Ann. N.Y. Acad. Sci.* 548:1–3.
2. Houslay, M.D., and Stanley, K.K. (1982). Dynamics of biological membranes; influence on structure, synthesis and function. In *Asymmetry in Biological Membrane.* Wiley, New York, pp. 152–205.
3. Lazarides, E., and Meon, R.T. (1984). Assembly and topogenesis of the spectrin based membrane skeleton and erythroid development. *Cell* 37:354–356.
4. Siman, R., Baudry, M., and Lynch, G. (1985). Regulation of glutamate receptor binding by the cytoskeleton protein fodrin. *Nature* 313:225–228.
5. Mutha, S., Langston, A., Bonifas, J., and Epstein, Jr. EH (1989). Identification of formalin and protein 4.1 in human epidermis. *J. Invest. Dermatol.* 92:487.
6. Bhatanagar, G., and Santana, H. (1980). Immunofluorescence staining of myosin, actin, and actinin in normal epidermis and cultured human epidermal cells. *J. Invest. Dermatol.* 74:258.
7. Lehto, V., Vartio, T., and Virtanen, I. (1980). Enrichment of a 140 KD glycoprotein in adherent, detergent-resistant cytoskeletons of human fibroblasts. *Biochem. Biophys. Res. Commun.* 95:909–916.
8. Carter, W. (1982). The cooperative role of the transformation sensitive glycoproteins GP140 and fibronectin in cell attachment and spreading. *J. Biol. Chem.* 257:3249–3257.
9. Berridge, M. (1984). Inositol triphosphate and diacylglycerol as second messengers. *Biochem. J.* 220: 345–360.
10. Berridge, M., and Irvine, R. (1984). Inositol triphosphate, a novel second messenger in cellular signal transduction. *Nature* 312:315–321.
11. Berridge, M. (1987). Inositol triphosphate and diacylglycerol: two interacting second messengers. *Annu. Rev. Biochem.* 56:159–193.
12. Hannun, Y., and Bell, R. (1989). Functions of sphingolipids breakdown products in cellular recognition. *Science* 243:500–507.
13. Arnold, W.P., Glade, C.P., Mier, P.D., and van de Kerkhof, P.C. (1993). Effects of sphingosine, isoquinoline and tannic acid on the human tape-stripping model and the psoriatic lesion. *Skin Pharmacol.* 6: 193–199.
14. Andersen, S., Sjursen, W., Laegreid, A., Volden, G., and Johansen, B. (1994). Elevated expression of human nonpancreatic phospholipase A2 in psoriatic tissue. *Inflammation* 18:1–12.
15. Levine, L., Xiao, D., and Little, C. (1987). Increased arachidonic acid metabolites from cells in culture after treatment with the phosphatidylcholine hydrolyzing phospholipase C from *Bacillus cereus. Prostaglandins* 34:633–642.
16. Handler, J.A., Danilowicz, R.M., and Eling, T.E. (1990). Mitogenic signaling by epidermal growth factor (EGF), but not platelet-derived growth factor, requires arachidonic acid metabolism in BALB/c 3T3 cells. *J. Biol. Chem* 265:3669–3673.
17. Peppelenbosch, M.P., Tertoolen, L.G.J., den Hertog, J., and de Laat, S.W. (1992). Epidermal growth factor activates calcium channels by phospholipase A_2/5-lipoxygenase-mediated leukotriene C_4 production. *Cell* 69:295–303.
18. Daub, H., Weiss, F.U., Wallasch, C., and Ullrich, A. (1996). Role of transactivation of the EGF receptor in signaling by G-protein-coupled receptors. *Nature* 379:557–560.
19. Carpenter, G. (1987). Receptors for epidermal growth factor and other polypeptide mitogens. *Annu. Rev. Biochem.* 56:881–914.
20. Yarden, Y., and Ullrich, A. (1988). Growth factor receptor tyrosine kinases. *Annu. Rev. Biochem.* 57: 443–478.
21. Honegger, A.M., Schmidt, A., Ullrich, A., and Schlessinger, J. (1990). Evidence for epidermal growth factor (EGF)-induced intermolecular autophosphorylation of the EGF receptors in living cells. *Mol. Cell. Biol* 10:4035–4044.
22. Stryer, L. (1987). The molecules of visual excitation. *Sci. Am. 257* (July):42–50.
23. Dohlman, H., Bouvier, M., Benovic, J., Caron, M., and Lefkovitz, R. (1987). The multiple membrane spanning topography of the beta-2-adrenergic receptor. Localization of the sites of binding, glycosylation by limited proteolysis. *J. Biol. Chem.* 262:14282–14288.
24. Noda, M., Ikeda, T., Kayano, T., Suzuki, H., Takeshima, H., Kurasaki, M., Takahashi, H., and Numa, S. (1986). Existence of distinct sodium channel messenger RNAs in rat brain. *Nature* 320:188–192.
25. Tanabe, T., Takeshima, H., Mikami, A., Flockerzi, V., Takahashi, H., Kangawa, K., Kojima, M., Matsuo, H., Hirose, T., and Numa, S. (1987). Primary structure or the receptor for calcium channel blockers from skeletal muscle. *Nature* 328:313–318.
26. Sefton, B., and Buss, J. (1987). The covalent modification of eukaryote proteins with lipid. *J. Cell Biol.* 101:1449–1453.
27. Ferguson, M., and William, A. (1988). Cell-surface anchoring of proteins via glycosylphosphatidylinositol structures. *Annu. Rev. Biochem.* 57:285–320.
28. Kaufman, J., Krangel, M., and Strominger, J. (1984). Cysteines in the transmembrane region of major histocompatibility complex antigens are fatty acylated via thioester bonds. *J. Biol. Chem.* 259:7230–7238.
29. Pfeffer, S., and Rothman, J.E., (1987). Biosynthetic protein transport and sorting by the endoplasmic reticulum and Golgi. *Annu. Rev. Biochem.* 56:829–852.

30. Hirschberg, C., and Snider, M. (1987). Topography of glycosylation in the rough endoplasmic reticulum and Golgi apparatus. *Annu. Rev. Biochem.* 56:63–87.
31. Rademacher, T., Parekh, R., and Dwek, R. (1988). Glycobiology. *Annu. Rev. Biochem.* 57:785–838.
32. Yamashita, K., Tachibana, Y., Obkura, T., and Kobata, A. (1985). Enzymatic basis for the structural changes of asparagine-linked sugar chains of membrane glycoproteins of baby hamster kidney cells induced by polyoma transformation. *J. Biol. Chem.* 260: 3963–3969.
33. Yamashita, K., Hitoi, A., Irie, M., and Kobata, A. (1986). Fractionation by lectin affinity chromatography indicates that the glycosylation of most ribonucleases in human viscera and body fluids is organ specific. *Arch. Biochem. Biophys.* 250:263–266.
34. Aviezer, D., Hecht, D., Safran, M., Eisinger, M., David, G., and Yayon, A. (1994). Perlecan, basal lamina proteoglycan, promotes basic fibroblast growth factor-receptor binding, mitogenesis and angiogenesis. *Cell* 79:1005–1013.
35. Spivak-Kroizman, T., Lemmon, M.A., Dikic, I., Ladbury, J.E., Pinchasi, D., Huang, J., Jaye, M., Crumley, G., Schlessinger, J., and Lax, I. (1994). Heparin-inducible oligomerization of FGF molecules is responsible for FGF receptor dimerization, activation, and cell proliferation. *Cell* 79:1015–1024.
36. Bennett, K.L., Jackson, D.G., Simon, J.C., Tanczos, E., Peach, R., Modrell, B., Stamenkovic, I., Plowman, G., and Aruffo, A. (1995). CD44 isoforms containing exon V3 are responsible for the presentation of heparin-binding growth factor. *J. Cell Biol.* 128:687–698.
37. Alho, A.M., and Underhill, C.B. (1989). The hyaluronate receptor is preferentially expressed on proliferating epithelial cells. *J. Cell Biol.* 108:1557–1565.
38. Tammi, R., Paukkonen, K., Wang, C., Horsmanheimo, M., and Tammi, M. (1994). Hyaluronan and CD44 in psoriatic skin. Intense staining for hyaluronan on dermal capillary loops and reduced expression of CD44 and hyaluronan in keratinocyte-leukocyte interfaces. *Arch. Dermatol. Res.* 286: 21–29.
39. Defize, L., Arndt-Jovin, D., Jovin, T., Boonstra, J., Meisenhelder, J., Hunter, T., Jey, H., and de Laat, S. (1988). A431 cell variants lacking the blood group A antigen display increased high affinity epidermal growth factor receptor numbers protein-tyrosine kinase activity and receptor turnover. *J. Cell Biol.* 107: 939–949.
40. Lin, H.Y., and Moustakas, A. (1994). TGF-beta receptors: structure and function. *Cell Mol. Biol. (Noisy-le-grand)* 40:337–349.
41. Miyazono, K., ten Dijke, P., Yamashita, H., and Heldin, C.H. (1994). Signal transduction via serine/threonine kinase receptors. *Semin. Cell Biol.* 5:389–398.
42. Chen, F., and Weinberg, R.A. (1995). Biochemical evidence for the autophosphorylation and transphosphorylation of transforming growth factor beta receptor kinases. *Proc. Natl. Acad. Sci. U.S.A.* 92:1565–1569.
43. Springer, T., Dustin, M., Kishimoto, T., and Marlin, S. (1987). The lymphocyte function-associated LFA-1, CD2 and LFA-3 molecules: cell adhesion receptors of the immune system. *Annu. Rev. Immunol.* 5: 223–252.
44. Streeter, P., Berg, E., Rouse, B., Bargatze, R., and Butcher, E. (1988). A tissue specific endothelial cell molecule involved in lymphocyte homing. *Nature* 331:41–46.
45. Stoolman, L. (1989). Adhesion molecules controlling lymphocyte migration. *Cell* 56:907–910.
46. Clayberger, C., Uychara, T., Hardy, B., Eaton, J., Karasek, M., and Krensky, A. (1985). Target specificity and cell surface structures involved in the human cytolytic T-lymphocyte response to endothelial cells. *J. Immunol.* 135:12–18.
47. Sackstein, R., Falanga, V., Streilein, W., and Chin, Y.-H. (1988). Lymphocyte adhesion to psoriatic dermal endothelium is mediated by tissue-specific receptor-ligand interaction. *J. Invest. Dermatol.* 91:423–428.
48. Butcher, E.C., and Picker, L.J. (1996). Lymphocyte homing and homeostasis. *Science* 272:60–66.
49. Heng, M.C.Y., Allen, S., and Chase, D. (1988). High endothelial venules in involved and uninvolved psoriatic skin: recognition by homing receptors on cytotoxic T-lymphocytes. *Br. J. Dermatol.* 118:315–326.
50. Nickoloff, B., Lewisohn, D., and Butcher, E. (1987). Enhanced binding of peripheral blood mononuclear leukocytes to gamma interferon treated cultured keratinocytes. *Am. J. Dermatopathol.* 9:413–418.
51. Nickoloff, B., and Mitra, R. (1988). Phorbol ester treatment enhances binding of mononuclear leukocytes to autologous and allogeneic gamma-interferon-treated keratinocytes. *J. Invest. Dermatol.* 90:684–689.
52. Nickoloff, B., Lewinsohn, D., Butcher, E., Krensky, A., and Clayberger, C. (1988). Recombinant gamma interferon increases the binding of peripheral blood mononuclear leukocytes and Leu-3+ T lymphocyte clone to cultured keratinocytes and to a malignant cutaneous squamous carcinoma cell line that is blocked by antibody against the LFA-1 molecule. *J. Invest. Dermatol.* 90:17–22.
53. Dustin, M., Singer, K., Tuck, D., and Springer, T. (1988). Adhesion of T-lymphoblasts to epidermal keratinocytes is regulated by interferon γ and is mediated by intercellular adhesion molecule 1 (ICAM-1). *J. Exp. Med.* 167:1323–1340.

54. Bos, J., Hulsebosch, H., Kreig, S., Bakker, P., and Cormane, R. (1983). Immunocompetent cells in psoriasis. *Arch. Dermatol. Res.* 275:181–189.
55. Hammar, H., Gu, S., Johannesson, A., Sundkvist, K., and Biberfeld, P. (1984). Subpopulations of mononuclear cells in microscope lesions of psoriatic patients. Selective accumulations of suppressor/cytotoxic T cells in epidermis during the evolution of the lesion. *J. Invest. Dermatol.* 83:416–420.
56. Paukkonen, K., Naukkarinen, A., and Horsmanheimo, M. (1995). The development of manifest psoriatic lesions is linked with the appearance of ICAM-1 positivity on keratinocytes. *Arch. Dermatol. Res.* 287: 165–170.
57. Elias, A.N., Goodman, M.M., and Rohan, M.K. (1993). Serum ICAM-1 concentrations in patients with psoriasis treated with antithyroid thioureylenes. *Clin. Exp. Dermatol.* 18:526–529.
58. Das, P.K., de Boer, O.J., Visser, A., Verhagen, C.E., Bos, J.D., and Pals, S.T. (1994). Differential expression of ICAM-1, E-selectin and VCAM-1 by endothelial cells in psoriasis and contact dermatitis. *Acta Derm. Venereol. (Stockh.)* (Suppl.) 186:21–22.
59. de Boer, O.J., Wakelkamp, I.M., Pals, S.T., Claessen, N., Bos, J.D., and Das, P.K. (1994). Increased expression of adhesion receptors in both lesional and non-lesional psoriatic skin. *Arch. Dermatol. Res.* 286: 304–311.
60. Veale, D., Rogers, S., and Fitzgerald, O. (1995). Immunolocalization of adhesion molecules in psoriatic arthritis, psoriatic and normal skin. *Br. J. Dermatol.* 132:32–38.
61. Hunyadi, J., Simon, M., Jr., Kenderessy, A.S., and Dobozy, A. (1993). Expression of monocyte/macrophage markers (CD13, CD14, CD68) on human keratinocytes in healthy and diseased skin. *J. Dermatol.* 20:341–345.
62. Lee, M.L., To, T., Nicholson, E., and Schrieber, L. (1994). Endothelial cell adhesion molecules in psoriasis. *Australas. J. Dermatol.* 35:65–70.
63. Petzelbauer, P., Pober, J.S., Keh, A., and Braverman, I.M. (1994). Inducibility and expression of microvascular endothelial adhesion molecules in lesional, perilesional, and uninvolved skin of psoriatic patients. *J. Invest. Dermatol.* 103:300–305.
64. Schopf, R.E., Naumann, S., Rehder, M., and Morsches, B. (1993). Soluble intercellular adhesion molecule-1 levels in patients with psoriasis. *Br. J. Dermatol.* 128:34–37.
65. Ameglio, F., Bonifati, C., Carducci, M., Alemanno, L., Sacerdoti, G., and Fazio, M. (1994). Soluble intercellular adhesion molecule-1 and procollagen III peptide are reliable markers of disease severity in psoriasis. *Acta Derm. Venereol (Stockh.)* (Suppl.) 186: 19–20.
66. Kowalzick, L., Neuber, K., Weichenthal, M., Kohler, I., and Ring, J. (1994). Elevated serum-soluble ELAM-1 levels in patients with severe plaque-type psoriasis. *Arch. Dermatol. Res* 286:414–416.
67. Bonifati, C., Trento, E., Carducci, M., Sacerdoti, G., Mussi, A., Fazio, M., and Ameglio, F. (1995). Soluble E-selectin and soluble tumour necrosis factor receptor (60 kD) serum levels in patients with psoriasis. *Dermatology* 190:128–131.
68. Caproni, M., Palleschi, G.M., Falcos, D., Papi, C., and Lotti, T. (1995). Pharmacologic modulation by cetirizine of some adhesion molecules expression in psoriatic skin lesions. *Int. J. Dermatol.* 34:510–513.
69. Sebok, B., Bonnekoh, B., and Mahrle, G. (1994). IL-1 alpha-induced expression of ICAM-1 on cultured hyperproliferative keratinocytes: suppression by antipsoriatic dimethyl-fumarate. *Int. J. Dermatol.* 33: 367–370.
70. Cagnoni, M.L., Ghersetich, I., Lotti, T., Pierleoni, M., and Landi, G. (1994). Treatment of psoriasis vulgaris with topical calcipotriol: is the clinical improvement of lesional skin related to a down-regulation of some cell adhesion molecules? *Acta Derm. Venereol. (Stockh.)* (Suppl.) 186:55–57.
71. Thomson, A.W., Nalesnik, M.A., Rilo, H.R., Woo, J., Carroll, P.B., and Van Thiel, D.H. (1993). ICAM-1 and E-selectin expression in lesional biopsies of psoriasis patients responding to systemic FK 506 therapy. *Autoimmunity* 15:215–223.
72. Edwards, B.D., Andrew, S.M., O'Driscoll, J.B., Chalmers, R.J., Ballardie, F.W., and Freemont, A.J. (1993). Changes in numbers of epidermal cell adhesion molecules caused by oral cyclosporin in psoriasis. *J. Clin. Pathol.* 46:713–717.
73. Kowalzick, L., Bildau, H., Neuber, K., Kohler, I., and Ring, J. (1993). Clinical improvement in psoriasis during dithranol/UVB therapy does not correspond with a decrease in elevated serum soluble ICAM-1 levels. *Arch. Dermatol. Res.* 285:233–235.
74. Akiyama, S.K., Olden, K., and Yamada, K.M. (1995). Fibronectin and integrins in invasion and metastasis. *Cancer Metastasis Rev.* 14:173–189.
75. Adams, J.C., and Watt, F.M. (1989). Fibronectin inhibits the terminal differentiation of human keratinocytes. *Nature* 340:307–309.
76. Bates, R.C., Lincz, L.F., and Burns, G.F. (1995). Involvement of integrins in cell survival. *Cancer Metastasis Res.* 14:191–203.
77. Jones, P.H., and Watt, F.M. (1993). Separation of human epidermal stem cells from transit amplifying cells on the basis of differences in integrin function and expression. *Cell* 73:713–724.
78. De Luca, M., Pellegrini, G., Zambruno, G., and Marchisio, P.C. (1994). Role of integrins in cell adhesion and polarity in normal keratinocytes and human skin pathologies. *J. Dermatol.* 21:821–828.

79. Haapasalmi, K., Zhang, K., Tonnesen, M., Olerud, J., Sheppard, D., Salo, T., Kramer, R., Clark, R.A.F., Uitto, V.-J., and Larjava, H. (1996). Keratinocytes in human wounds express αvβ6 integrin. *J. Invest. Dermatol.* 106:42–48.
80. Hertle, M.D., Kubler, M.-D., Leigh, I.M., and Watt, F.M. (1992). Aberrant integrin expression during epidermal wound healing and in psoriatic epidermis. *J. Clin. Invest.* 89:1892–1901.
81. Chen, J.D., Kim, J.P., Zhang, K., Sarret, Y., Wynn, K.C., Kramer, R.H., and Woodley, D.T. (1993). Epidermal growth factor (EGF) promotes human keratinocyte locomotion on collagen by increasing the alpha 2 integrin subunit. *Exp. Cell Res.* 209:216–223.
82. Bosenberg, M.W., and Massagué, J. (1993). Juxtacrine cell signaling molecules. *Curr. Opin. Cell Biol.* 5:832–838.
83. Brachmann, R., Lindquist, P.B., Nagashima, M., Kohr, W., Lipari, T., Napier, M., and Derynck, R. (1989). Transmembrane TGF-α precursors activate EGF/TGF-α receptors. *Cell* 56:691–700.
84. Anklesaria, P., Teixido, J., Laiho, M., Pierce, J.H., Greenberger, J.S., and Massague, J. (1990). Cell-cell adhesion mediated by binding of membrane-anchored transforming growth factor alpha to epidermal growth factor receptors promotes cell proliferation. *Proc. Natl. Acad. Sci. U.S.A.* 87:3289–3293.
85. Ono, M., Raab, G., Lau, K., Abraham, J.A., and Klagsbrun, M. (1994). Purification and characterization of transmembrane forms of heparin-binding EGF-like growth factor. *J. Biol. Chem.* 269: 31315–31321.
86. Higashiyama, S., Iwamoto, R., Goishi, K., Raab, G., Taniguchi, N., Klagsbrun, M., and Mekada, E. (1995). The membrane protein CD9/DRAP 27 potentiates the juxtacrine growth factor activity of the membrane-anchored heparin-binding EGF-like growth factor. *J. Cell Biol.* 128:929–938.
87. Nakamura, K., Iwamoto, R., and Mekada, E. (1995). Membrane-anchored heparin-binding EGF-like growth factor (HB-EGF) and diphtheria toxin receptor-associated protein (DRAP27)/CD9 form a complex with integrin alpha 3 beta 1 at cell-cell contact sites. *J. Cell Biol.* 129:1691–1705.
88. Salomon, D.S., Normanno, N., Ciardiello, F., Brandt, R., Shoyab, M., and Todaro, G.J. (1995). The role of amphiregulin in breast cancer. *Breast Cancer Res. Treat.* 33:103–114.
89. Schmid, E.F., Binder, K., Grell, M., Scheurich, P., and Pfizenmaier, K. (1995). Both tumor necrosis factor receptors, TNFR60 and TNFR80, are involved in signaling endothelial tissue factor expression by juxtacrine tumor necrosis factor alpha. *Blood* 86: 1836–1841.
90. Ponec, M., Havekes, L., Kempenaar, J., Lavrisen, S., Wijsman, M., Boonstra, J., and Vermeer, B. (1985). Calcium-mediated regulation of the low density lipoprotein receptor and intracellular cholesterol synthesis in human epidermal keratinocytes. *J. Cell Physiol.* 125:98–106.
91. Mommaas-Kienhuis, A.-M., Grayson, S., Wijsman, M., Verneer, B., and Elias, P. (1987). Low density lipoprotein receptor expression on keratinocytes in normal and psoriatic epidermis. *J. Invest. Dermatol.* 89:513–517.
92. Livden, J. (1988). Fcγ receptors on keratinocytes in psoriasis. *Arch. Dermatol. Res.* 280:12–17.
93. Gazith, J., and Reichert, U. (1982). High affinity membrane receptors in cultured human keratinocytes. 1. The β-adrenergic receptor. *Br. J. Dermatol.* (Suppl 23):125–133.
94. Kupper, T., Lee, F., Birchall, N., Clark, B., and Dower, S. (1988). Interleukin 1 binds to specific receptors on human keratinocytes and induces granulocyte macrophage colony-stimulating factor mRNA and protein. *J. Clin. Invest.* 82:1787–1792.
95. Green, N., Basketry, D., Coachman, J., and Reps, D. (1983). Distribution and number of epidermal growth factor receptors in skin is related to epithelial cell growth. *Dev. Biol.* 100:506–512.
96. Boonstra, J., de Laat, S., and Ponec, M. (1985). Epidermal growth factor receptor expression related to differentiation capacity in normal and transformed keratinocytes. *Exp. Cell Res.* 161:421–433.
97. Taylor, A., Hog, B., and Watt, F. (1985). Biosynthesis of EGF receptor, transferrin receptor and collagen by cultured human keratinocytes and the effect of retinoic acid. *Exp. Cell Res.* 159:47–54.
98. Werner, S., Smola, H., Liao, X., Longaker, M.T., Krieg, T., Hofschneider, P.H., and Williams, L.T. (1994). The function of KGF in morphogenesis of epithelium and reepithelialization of wounds. *Science* 266:819–822.
99. Marchese, C., Chedid, M., Dirsch, O.R., Csaky, K.G., Santanelli, F., Latini, C., LaRochelle, W.J., Torrisi, M.R., and Aaronson, S.A. (1995). Modulation of keratinocyte growth factor and its receptor in reepithelializing human skin. *J. Exp. Med.* 182:1369–1376.
100. Verrando, P., and Ortone, J.-P. (1984). Insulin receptors in cultured human keratinocytes. *Br. J. Dermatol.* 111:232–234.
101. Verrando, P., and Ortone, J.-P. (1985). Insulin binding properties of normal and transformed human epidermal keratinocytes. *J. Invest. Dermatol.* 85:328–332.
102. Misra, P., Nickoloff, B., Morhenn, V., Hintz, R., and Rosenfeld, R. (1986). Characterization of insulin-like growth factor-I/somatomedin-C receptors on human keratinocyte monolayers. *J. Invest. Dermatol.* 87: 264–267.
103. Fisher, G., Elder, J., Voorhees, J., Kowalki, J., Petersen, C., Derynck, R., and Ellingsworth, L. (1988). Transforming growth factor β mRNA is expressed in

normal and psoriatic epidermis and has similar biological effects on normal psoriasis keratinocytes. *J. Invest. Dermatol.* 90:558.

104. Muller, A., Michel, L., Basset-Sequin, N., Modat, G., Dubertret, L., and Bonne, C. (1988). Characterization of specific leukotriene C4 binding sites on cultured human keratinocytes. *Br. J. Dermatol.* 119:275–280.
105. Lord, J., and Ziboh, V. (1979). Specific binding of prostaglandin E_2 to membrane preparations form human skin: receptor modulation by UVB-irradiation and chemical agents. *J. Invest. Dermatol.* 73:373–377.
106. Nickoloff, B. (1987). Binding of ^{125}I-gamma interferon to cultured human keratinocytes. *J. Invest. Dermatol.* 89:132–135.
107. Kristensen, M., Chu, C.Q., Eedy, D.J., Feldmann, M., Brennan, F.M., and Breathnach, S.M. (1993). Localization of tumour necrosis factor-alpha (TNF-alpha) and its receptors in normal and psoriatic skin: epidermal cells express the 55-kD but not the 75-kD TNF receptor. *Clin. Exp. Immunol.* 94:354–362.
108. van den Oord, J.J., De Ley, M., and De Wolf-Peeters, C. (1995). Distribution of interferon-gamma receptors in normal and psoriatic skin. *Pathol. Res. Pract.* 191: 530–534.
109. Gaspari, A., Lotze, M., Rosenberg, S., Stern, J., and Katz, I. (1987). Dermatologic changes associated with interleukin-2 administration. *J.A.M.A.* 258: 1624–1629.
110. Adachi, K., Yoshikawa, K., Halprin, K., and Levine, V. (1975). Prostaglandins and cyclic AMP in epidermis. *Br. J. Dermatol.* 92:381–388.
111. Wilkinson, D., and Orenberg, E. (1979). Effects of prostaglandins on cyclic nucleotide levels in cultured keratinocytes. *Prostaglandins* 17:419–429.
112. Mansbridge, J., Nickoloff, B., and Morhenn, V. (1987). Induction of new proteins by γ-interferon in cultured human keratinocytes. *J. Invest. Dermatol.* 88:602–610.
113. Madsen, P., Rasmussen, H.H., Flint, T., Gromov, P., Kruse, T.A., Honore, B., Vorum, H., and Celis, J.E. (1995). Cloning, expression, and chromosome mapping of human galectin-7. *J. Biol. Chem.* 270: 5823–5829.
114. DiCicco, L., Fraki, J., and Mansbridge, J. (1987). Membrane polypeptides of keratinocytes. *Int. J. Dermatol.* 26:631–638.
115. Orfanos, C., Schaumberg-Lever, G., Mahrle, G., and Lever, W. (1973). Alterations of cell surfaces as a pathogenetic factor in psoriasis. *Arch. Dermatol.* 107: 38–46.
116. Orfanos, C., Mahrle, G., and Runne, U. (1976). Vertailungsstorung oberflachlicher Glycoconjugate der psoriatischen Zellmembran. *Arch. Dermatol. Res.* 256:39–51.
117. Gommans, J., Bergers, M., van Erp, P., van der Hurk, J., Meir, P., and Roelfzema, H. (1979). Studies on the plasma membrane of normal and psoriatic keratinocytes. 1. Preparation of material and morphological characterization. *Br. J. Dermatol.* 101:407–412.
118. Kouklis, P.D., Hutton, E., and Fuchs, E. (1994). Making a connection: direct binding between keratin intermediate filaments and desmosomal proteins. *J. Cell Biol.* 127:1049–1060.
119. Hennings, H., Michael, D., Cheng, C., Steinert, P., Holbrook, K., and Yuspa, S. (1980). Calcium regulation of growth and differentiation of mouse epidermal cells in culture. *Cell* 19:245–254.
120. Nagar, B., Overduin, M., Ikura, M., and Rini, J.M. (1996). Structural basis of calcium induced E-cadherin rigidification and dimerization. *Nature* 380: 360–364.
121. King, I.A., Tabiowo, A., Purkis, P., Leigh, I., and Magee, A.I. (1993). Expression of distinct desmocollin isoforms in human epidermis. *J. Invest. Dermatol.* 100:373–379.
122. Mansbridge, J. (1987). Changes in keratinocyte maturation in psoriasis. In *Psoriasis: Proceedings of the 4th International Symposium*, E.M. Farber, A.J. Cox, L. Nall, and P.H. Jacobs (Eds.). Elsevier Science, New York, pp. 347–348.
123. Mansbridge, J., and Knapp, A. (1987). Changes in keratinocyte maturation during wound healing. *J. Invest. Dermatol.* 89:253–263.
124. Matsuyoshi, N., Tanaka, T., Toda, K., Okamoto, H., Furukawa, F., and Imamura, S. (1995). Soluble E-cadherin: a novel cutaneous disease marker. *Br. J. Dermatol.* 132:745–749.
125. Yeager, M. (1995). Electron microscopic image analysis of cardiac gap junction membrane crystals. *Microsc. Res. Tech.* 31:452–466.
126. Kalimi, G., and Sirsat, S. (1984). The relevance of gap junctions to stage 1 tumour promotion in mouse epidermis. *Carcinogenesis* 5:1671–1677.
127. Trosko, J. (1987). Mechanisms of tumor promotion: possible role of inhibited intercellular communication. *Eur. J. Cancer Clin. Oncol.* 23:599–601.
128. Goliger, J.A., and Paul, D.L. (1994). Wounding alters epidermal connexin expression and gap junction-mediated intercellular communication. *Mol. Biol. Cell* 6:1491–1501.
129. Pitts, J., Kam, E., Melville, L., and Watt, F. (1986). Patterns of junctional communication in animal tissues. In *Ciba Foundation Symposium 125* Wiley, Chichester, UK, pp. 140–153.
130. Salomon, D., Saurat, J.-H., and Meda, P. (1988). Cell-to-cell communications within intact human skin. *J. Clin. Invest.* 82:248–254.
131. Kam, E., Melville, L., and Pitts, J. (1986). Patterns of junctional communication in skin. *J. Invest. Dermatol.* 87:748–753.

132. Cavato, F., and Flaxman, B. (1972). Communication between normal human epidermal cell in vitro. *J. Invest. Dermatol.* 59:370–374.
133. McKay, I., and Taylor-Papadimitriou, J. (1982). The non-selective junctional communication phenotype of normal and transformed human epidermal keratinocytes in vitro. *Exp. Cell Res.* 141:171–180.
134. Mahrle, G. (1982). Domain turnover of junctional membrane areas in the epidermis. *Arch. Dermatol. Res.* 274:993–999.
135. Caputo, R., and Peluchetti, D. (1977). The junctions of normal epidermis. *J. Ultrastruct. Res.* 61:44–61.
136. Katajima, Y., Eguchi, K., Ohno, T., Mori, S., and Yaoita, H. (1983). Tight junctions of human keratinocytes in primary culture: a freeze fracture study. *J. Ultrastruct. Res.* 82:309–313.
137. Giudice, G.J., Emery, D.J., Zelickson, B.D., Anhalt, G.J., Liu, Z., and Diaz, L.A. (1993). Bullous pemphigoid and herpes gestationis autoantibodies recognize a common non-collagenous site on the BP180 ectodomain. *J. Immunol.* 151:5742–5750.
138. Goldstein, I., and Hayes, C. (1979). The lectins: carbohydrate binding proteins of plants and animals. *Adv. Carbohydr. Chem. Biochem.* 35:127–340.
139. Nieland, M. (1973). Epidermal intercellular staining with flourescein-conjugated phyto-hemagglutinin. *J. Invest. Dermatol.* 60:61–66.
140. Mahrle, G. (1981). Cell interactions and cell surface membranes in psoriasis. In *Psoriasis: Proceedings of the 3rd International Symposium*, E.M. Farber, A.J. Cox, L. Nall and P.H. Jacobs (Eds.). Grune & Stratton, New York, pp. 43–52.
141. Reano, A., Fauré, M., Jacques, Y., and Reichert, U. (1982). Use of lectins for the study of human epidermal differentiation. *Br. J. Dermatol.* 107:143–146.
142. Schaumberg-Lever, G., Alroy, J., Gavris, V., and Ucci, A. (1984). Cell-surface carbohydrates in proliferative epidermal lesions. *Exp. Dermatopathol.* 6: 583–589.
143. Schaumberg-Lever, G., Alroy, J., Ucci, A., and Lever, W. (1984). Distribution of carbohydrate residues in normal skin. *Arch. Dermatol. Res.* 276:216–223.
144. Dabelsteen, E., Vedtofte, P., Hakomori, S.-I., and Young, W. (1982). Carbohydrate chains specific for blood group antigens in differentiation of human oral epithelium. *J. Invest. Dermatol.* 79:3–7.
145. Paller, A., Siegel, J., Spalding, D., and Bremer, E. (1989). Absence of a stratum corneum antigen in disorders of epidermal cell proliferation: detection with an anti-ganglioside GM3 antibody. *J. Invest. Dermatol.* 89:240–246.
146. Nemanic, M., Whitehead, J., and Elias, P. (1983). Alterations in membrane sugars during epidermal differentiation. *J. Histochem. Cytochem.* 31:887–897.
147. Mansbridge, J., and Knapp, A. (1984). The binding of *Helix pomatia* and *Ulex europeus* agglutinins to normal and psoriatic skin. *J. Invest. Dermatol.* 82: 170–175.
148. Brabec, R., Peters, B., Bernstein, I., Gray, R., and Goldstein, I. (1980). Differential lectin binding to cellular membranes in the epidermis of newborn rat. *Proc. Natl. Acad. Sci. U.S.A.* 77:477–479.
149. Roelfzema, H., and van Erp, P. (1983). Glycoprotein composition of psoriatic epidermis in relation to growth control. *J. Invest. Dermatol.* 80:20–23.
150. Brysk, M., Rajaraman, S., Penn, P., and Barlow, E. (1986). Endogenous lectin from terminally differentiated epidermal cells. *Differentiation* 32:230–237.
151. Brysk, M., Rajaraman, S., Penn, P., and Barlow, E. (1988). Glycoproteins modulate adhesion of terminally differentiated keratinocytes. *Cell Tissue Res.* 253:657–663.
152. Kariniemi, A.-L., Holthofer, H., Miettinen, A., and Virtanen, I. (1983). Altered binding of *Ulex europeus* I lectin to psoriatic epidermis. *Br. J. Dermatol.* 109: 523–529.
153. Schaumberg-Lever, G., Alroy, J., Ucci, A., Lever, W., and Orfanos, C. (1984). Cell surface carbohydrates in psoriasis. *J. Am. Acad. Dermatol.* 11:1087–1094.
154. Gommans, J., and van der Hurk, J. (1981). Lectin binding studies on suspensions of isolated epidermal keratinocytes. *Br. J. Dermatol.* 104:641–648.
155. Roelfzema, H., Bergers, M., van Erp, P., Gommans, J., and Mier, P. (1981). Studies on the plasma membrane of normal and psoriatic keratinocytes. 4. Characterization of glycoconjugates. *Br. J. Dermatol.* 105:509–516.
156. Roelfzema, H., Bergers, M., van Erp, P., Gommans, J., and Mier, P. (1981). Studies on the plasma membrane of normal and psoriatic keratinocytes. 3. Uptake of labeled sugars and their incorporation in to glycoconjugates. *Br. J. Dermatol.* 104:635–640.
157. Gommans, J., van den Hurk, J., Bergers, M., van Erp, P., Mier, P., and Roelfzema, H. (1982). Studies on the plasma membrane of normal and psoriatic keratinocytes. 5. Lectin binding. *Br. J. Dermatol.* 106: 317–322.
158. Meir, P., van Rennes, H., van Erp, P., and Roelfzema, H. (1982). Alpha-L-fucosidase in normal and psoriatic epidermis. *Br. J. Dermatol.* 106:367–368.
159. Roelfzema, H., and van Erp, P. (1983). Studies on the plasma membrane of normal and psoriatic keratinocytes. *J. Invest. Dermatol.* 80:24–26.
160. DiCicco, L., Fraki, J., and Mansbridge, J. (1985). Cell membrane polypeptides on keratinocytes from normal and psoriatic skin. *Arch. Dermatol. Res.* 278: 337–339.
161. Mann, P., Williams, R., and Gray, G. (1980). Distribution of glycoproteins containing fucose in normal and psoriatic keratinocytes. *Br. J. Dermatol.* 102: 649–657.

162. Brysk, M., and Snider, J. (1982). The effect of the state of differentiation on labeling of epidermal cell surface glycoproteins. *J. Invest. Dermatol.* 78: 366–370.
163. Brysk, M., and Snider, J. (1982). Concanavalin A binding to glycoproteins of epidermal cells. *J. Invest. Dermatol.* 79:193–197.
164. Kariniemi, A., Lehto, V., and Virtanen, I. (1983). Surface glycoproteins of cultured human keratinocytes from normal and uninvolved psoriatic epidermis. *Br. J. Dermatol.* 109:531–537.
165. Bonnefoy, J., Reano, A., Ledger, P., and Thivolet, J. (1984). Concanvalin (Con A) reactive human epidermal glycoproteins. *Acta Derm. Venereol. (Stockh.)* 64: 459–465.
166. Brysk, M., Miller, J., and Hebert, A. (1984). Concanavalin A distinguishes among diseases of altered epidermal differentiation. *J. Invest. Dermatol.* 82:18–20.
167. Morrison, A., Keeble, S., and Watt, F. (1988). The peanut lectin-binding glycoproteins of human epidermal keratinocytes. *Exp. Cell Res.* 177:247–256.
168. Brysk, M.M., Bell, T., and Rajaraman, S. (1991). Sensitivity of desquamin to proteolytic degradation. *Pathobiology* 59:109–112.
169. Osawa, T., and Tsuji, T. (1987). Fractionation and structural assessment of oligosaccharides and glycopeptides by use of immobilized lectins. *Annu. Rev. Biochem.* 56:21–42.
170. Wollina, U., Funfstuck, V., Hipler, C., and Knopf, B. (1988). Alterations in epidermal lectin binding sites in acute contact dermatitis. *Contact Derm.* 19: 109–115.
171. Wollina, U., Hipler, C., Schaarschmidt, H., Henkel, U., and Knopf, B. (1985). Enfluss neutraler Losungmittel auf die Lektinbindung gesunder und psoriatischer Epidermis. *Z. Hautker* 61:1379–1382.
172. Wollina, U., Hipler, C., Schaarschmidt, X., and Knopf, B. (1985). Untersuchungen zur Lektinbindung psoriatischer Haut. *Z. Hautkr* 61:1241–1249.
173. Nilsson, B. (1994). Analysis of protein glycosylation by mass spectrometry. *Mol. Biotechnol.* 2:243–280.
174. Dennis, R.P. (1995). A review of the biological significance of carbohydrates on glycoproteins and methods for their analysis. *Adv. Exp. Med. Biol.* 376: 1–11.
175. Wong, S.Y. (1995). Neoglycoconjugates and their applications in glycobiology. *Curr. Opin. Struct. Biol.* 5:599–604.
176. Kakehi, K., and Honda, S. (1996). Analysis of glycoproteins, glycopeptides and glycoprotein-derived oligosaccharides by high-performance capillary electrophoresis. *J. Chromatogr. A* 720:377–393.
177. Rice, R., and Green, H. (1977). The cornified envelope of terminally differentiated keratinocytes consists of cross-linked protein. *Cell* 11:417–422.
178. Thacher, S., and Rice, R. (1985). Keratinocyte specific transglutaminase of cultured human epidermal cells: relation to cross-lined envelope formation and terminal differentiation. *Cell* 40:685–695.
179. Thacher, S. (1989). Purification of keratinocyte transglutaminase and its expression during squamous differentiation. *J. Invest. Dermatol.* 92:578–584.
180. Rice, R.H., Mehrpouyan, M., O'Callahan, W., Parenteau, N.L., and Rubin, A.L. (1992). Keratinocyte transglutaminase: differentiation marker and member of an extended family. *Epithelial Cell Biol.* 1:128–137.
181. Rice, R., and Green, H. (1979). Presence in human epidermal cells of a soluble protein precursor of the cross-linked envelope: activation of the cross-linking by calcium ions. *Cell* 18:681–694.
182. Schmidt, R., Michel, S., Shroot, B., and Reichert, U. (1988). Transglutaminases in normal and transformed human keratinocytes in culture. *J. Invest. Dermatol.* 90:475–479.
183. Buxman, M., Lobitz, C., and Wuepper, K. (1980). Epidermal transglutaminase: identification and purification of a soluble substrate with studies of in vitro cross-linking. *J. Biol. Chem.* 255:1200–1203.
184. Petersen, L., Zettergren, J., and Wuepper, K. (1983). Biochemistry of transglutaminase and cross-linking in the skin. *J. Invest. Dermatol.* 81:95s–100s.
185. Baden, H., Kubilus, J., and Phillips, S. (1987). Characterization of monoclonal antibodies generated to the cornified envelope of human cultured keratinocytes. *J. Invest. Dermatol.* 89:454–459.
186. Baden, H., Kubilus, J., Phillips, S., Kvedar, J., and Tahan, S. (1987). A new class of soluble basic protein precursors of the cornified envelope of mammalian epidermis. *Biochem. Biophys. Acta* 925:63–73.
187. Kubilus, J., Kvedar, J., and Baden, H. (1987). Identification of new components of the cornified envelope of human and bovine epidermis. *J. Invest. Dermatol.* 89:44–50.
188. Simons, M., and Green, H. (1985). Enzymatic cross-linking of involucrin and other proteins by keratinocyte particulates in vitro. *Cell* 40:677–683.
189. Hohl, D., Mehra, T., Lichti, U., Yuspa, S., Roop, D., and Steinert, P. (1989). Loricrin–the human glycine-rich cornified envelope precursor–isolation and characterization of a cDNA clone encoding a major component of the human cornified envelope. *J. Invest. Dermatol.* 92:445.
190. Hohl, D., de Viragh, P.A., Amiguet-Barras, F., Gibbs, S., Backendorf, C., and Huber, M. (1995). The small proline-rich proteins constitute a multigene family of differentially regulated cornified cell envelope precursor proteins. *J. Invest. Dermatol.* 104:902–909.
191. Steinert, P.M., and Marekov, L.N. (1995). The proteins elafin, filaggrin, keratin intermediate filaments, loricrin, and small proline-rich proteins 1 and 2 are

isodipeptide cross-linked components of the human epidermal cornified cell envelope. *J. Biol. Chem.* 270: 17702–17711.

192. Candi, E., Melino, G., Mei, G., Tarcsa, E., Chung, S.I., Marekov, L.N., and Steinert, P.M. (1995). Biochemical, structural, and transglutaminase substrate properties of human loricrin, the major epidermal cornified cell envelope protein. *J. Biol. Chem.* 270: 26382–26390.
193. Hohl, D. (1993). Expression patterns of loricrin in dermatological disorders. *Am. J. Dermatopathol.* 15: 20–27.
194. Fujimoto, W., Marvin, K.W., George, M.D., Celli, G., Darwiche, N., De Luca, L.M., and Jetten, A.M. (1993). Expression of cornifin in squamous differentiating epithelial tissues, including psoriatic and retinoic acid-treated skin. *J. Invest. Dermatol.* 101:268–274.
195. Brown, L.J., Geesin, J.C., Rothnagel, J.A., Roop, D.R., and Gordon, J.S. (1994). Retinoic acid suppression of loricrin expression in reconstituted human skin cultured at the liquid-air interface. *J. Invest. Dermatol.* 102:886–890.
196. Michel, S., Schmidt, R., Shroot, B., and Reichert, U. (1988). Morphological and biochemical characterization of the cornified envelopes from human epidermal keratinocytes of different origin. *J. Invest. Dermatol.* 91:11–15.
197. Wertz, P., Madison, K., and Downing, D. (1989). Covalently bound lipids of human stratum corneum. *J. Invest. Dermatol.* 92:109–111.
198. Motta, S., Monti, M., Sesana, S., Caputo, R., Carelli, S., and Ghidoni, R. (1993). Ceramide composition of the psoriatic scale. *Biochim. Biophys. Acta* 1182: 147–151.
199. Brysk, M.M., and Rajaraman, S. (1992). Cohesion and desquamation of epidermal stratum corneum. *Prog. Histochem. Cytochem.* 25:1–53.
200. Brysk, M.M., Bell, T., Hoida, C., Tyring, S.K., and Rajaraman, S. (1991). Interferon-gamma modulates terminal differentiation and the expression of desquamin in cultured keratinocytes. *Exp. Cell Res.* 197: 140–147.
201. Rajaraman, S., Schmalsteig, F.C., Brysk, M.M., Hendrick, S.J., and Solomon, A.R. (1987). Aberrant expression of a chemokinetic glycoprotein in psoriatic skin. *J. Clin. Lab. Immunol.* 23:39–43.
202. Abel, E., DiCicco, L., Orenberg, E., Fraki, J., and Farber, E. (1986). Drugs in exacerbation of psoriasis. *J. Am. Acad. Dermatol.* 15:1002–1007.
203. Gazith, J., and Reichert, U. (1982). High affinity membrane receptors in cultured human keratinocytes. 1. The β-adrenergic receptor. *Br. J. Dermatol.* 10: 125–133.
204. Orenberg, E., and Wilkinson, D. (1983). Characterization of α- and β-adrenergic agonist stimulation of adenylate cyclase in human epidermal keratinocytes in vitro. *J. Invest. Dermatol.* 83:503–507.
205. Cavey, M., Cavey, D., Shroot, B., Reichert, U., and Gazith, J. (1986). Receptor-linked adenylate cyclase in the membranes of cultured human epidermal keratinocytes. *Arch. Dermatol. Res.* 278:293–297.
206. Gommans, J., Bergers, M., van Erp, P., van den Hurk, J., van de Kerkhof, P., Mier, P., and Roelfzema, H. (1979). Studies on the plasma membrane of normal and psoriatic keratinocytes 2. Cyclic AMP and its response to hormonal stimulation. *Br. J. Dermatol.* 101: 413–419.
207. Royer, E., Chaintreul, J., Maynadier, J., Michel, B., Guilhou, J., and Crastes de Paulet, A. (1982). Cyclic AMP and cyclic GMP production in normal and psoriatic epidermis. *Dermatologia* 165:533–543.
208. Fishman, P., and Perkins, J. (1988). Receptor desensitization. *Adv Second Messenger Phosphoprotein Res.* 21:25–32.
209. Horn, F., Marks, F., Fisher, G., Marcelo, C., and Voorhees, J. (1987). Decreased protein kinase C activity in psoriatic versus normal epidermis. *J. Invest. Dermatol.* 88:220–222.
210. Orenberg, E., and Wilkinson, D. (1982). Effect of β-adrenergic receptor blockade or refractoriness induced by isoproterenol on growth of keratinocytes in vitro. *Br. J. Dermatol.* 107:119–124.
211. Czernielewski, J., Schalla, W., Desbas, C., and Brun, P. (1986). Beta-blockers induce class II MHC antigens on psoriatic keratinocytes. *Lancet* 1(8484) 808.
212. Boyce, S., and Ham, R. (1986). Normal human epidermal keratinocytes. *In Vitro Models Cancer Res. Carcinomas Mammary Gland Uterus Skin* 3:245–274.
213. Pittelkow, M.R., Cook, P.W., Shipley, G.D., Derynck, R., and Coffey, R.J., Jr. (1993). Autonomous growth of human keratinocytes requires epidermal growth factor receptor occupancy. *Cell Growth Differ.* 4: 513–521.
214. Green, M., Basketter, D., Couchman, J., and Rees, D. (1983). Distribution and number of epidermal growth factor receptors in skin is related to epithelial cell growth. *Dev. Biol.* 100:506–512.
215. Barnard, J. (1993). Betacellulin: newest addition to the epidermal growth factor family. *J. Pediatr. Gastroenterol. Nutr.* 17:343–344.
216. Sasada, R., Ono, Y., Taniyama, Y., Shing, Y., Folkman, J., and Igarashi, K. (1993). Cloning and expression of cDNA encoding human betacellulin, a new member of the EGF family. *Biochem. Biophys. Res. Commun.* 190:1173–1179.
217. Riese, D.J.n., Bermingham, Y., van Raaij, T.M., Buckley, S., Plowman, G.D., and Stern, D.F. (1996). Betacellulin activates the epidermal growth factor receptor and erbB-4, and induces cellular response patterns distinct from those stimulated by epidermal

growth factor or neuregulin-beta. *Oncogene* 12: 345–353.
218. Plowman, G.D., Green, J.M., McDonald, V.L., Neubauer, M.G., Disteche, C.M., Todaro, G.J., and Shoyab, M. (1990). The amphiregulin gene encodes a novel epidermal growth factor-related protein with tumor-inhibitory activity. *Mol. Cell. Biol.* 10: 1969–1981.
219. Cook, P.W., Mattox, P.A., Keeble, W.W., Pittelkow, M.R., Plowman, G.D., Shoyab, M., Adelman, J.P., and Shipley, G.D. (1991). A heparin sulfate-regulated human keratinocyte autocrine factor is similar or identical to amphiregulin. *Mol. Cell. Biol.* 11: 2547–2557.
220. Barnard, J.A., Graves-Deal, R., Pittelkow, M.R., DuBois, R., Cook, P., Ramsey, G.W., Bishop, P.R., Damstrup, L., and Coffey, R.J. (1994). Auto- and cross-induction within the mammalian epidermal growth factor–related peptide family. *J. Biol. Chem.* 269:22817–22822.
221. Piepkorn, M., Lo, C., and Plowman, G. (1994). Amphiregulin-dependent proliferation of cultured human keratinocytes: autocrine growth, the effects of exogenous recombinant cytokine, and apparent requirement for heparin-like glycosaminoglycans. *J. Cell Physiol.* 159:114–120.
222. Cook, P.W., Ashton, N.M., Karkaria, C.E., Siess, D.C., and Shipley, G.D. (1995). Differential effects of a heparin antagonist (hexadimethrine) or chlorate on amphiregulin, basic fibroblast growth factor, and heparin-binding EGF-like growth factor activity. *J. Cell Physiol.* 163:418–429.
223. Coffey, R., Derynk, R., Wilcox, J., Bringman, T., Goustin, A., Moses, H., and Pittelkow, M. (1987). Production and auto-induction of transforming growth factor-α in human keratinocytes. *Nature* 328: 827–829.
224. Elder, J., Fisher, G., Lindquist, P., Bennett, G., Pittelkow, M., Coffey, R.J., Ellingsworth, L., Derynck, R., and Voorhees, J. (1989). Overexpression of transforming growth factor α in psoriatic epidermis. *Science* 243:811–814.
225. Krupp, M., Connolly, D., and Lane, M. (1982). Synthesis, turnover, and down-regulation of epidermal growth factor receptors in human A431 epidermoid carcinoma cells and skin fibroblasts. *J. Biol. Chem.* 257:11489–11496.
226. Beguinot, L., Lyall, R., Willingham, M., and Pastan, I. (1984). Down-regulation of the epidermal growth factor receptor in KB cells is due to receptor internalization and subsequent degradation in lysosomes. *Proc. Natl. Acad. Sci. U.S.A.* 81:2384–2388.
227. Stoscheck, C., and Carpenter, G. (1984). Characterization of the metabolic turnover of epidermal growth factor receptor protein in A431 cells. *J. Cell Physiol.* 120:296–302.
228. Glenney, J.J., Chen, W., Lazar, C., Walton, G., Zokas, L., Rosenfeld, M., and Gill, G. (1988). Ligand-induced endocytosis of the EGF receptor is blocked by mutational inactivation and anti-phosphotyrosine antibodies. *Cell* 52:675–684.
229. Finzi, E., Fleming, T., Segatto, O., Pennington, C., Bringman, T., Derynck, R., and Aaronson, S. (1987). The human transforming growth factor type α coding sequence is not a direct acting oncogene when overexpressed in NIH 3T3 cells. *Proc. Natl. Acad. Sci. U.S.A.* 84:3733–3737.
230. Jhappan, C., Takayama, H., Dickson, R.B., and Merlino, G. (1994). Transgenic mice provide genetic evidence that transforming growth factor alpha promotes skin tumorigenesis via H-ras-dependent and H-ras-independent pathways. *Cell Growth Differ.* 5: 385–394.
231. Dlugosz, A.A., Cheng, C., Williams, E.K., Darwiche, N., Dempsey, P.J., Mann, B., Dunn, A.R., Coffey, R.J., Jr., and Yuspa, S.H. (1995). Autocrine transforming growth factor alpha is dispensable for v-*ras*^{Ha}- induced epidermal neoplasia: potential involvement of alternate epidermal growth factor receptor ligands. *Cancer Res.* 55:1883–1893.
232. Wrann, M., and Fox, C. (1979). Identification of epidermal growth factor receptors in a hyperproducing human epidermoid carcinoma cell line. *J. Biol. Chem.* 234:8083–8086.
233. Liu, C., Chen, W., Kruiger, W., Stolarsky, L., Weber, W., Evans, R., Verma, I., Gill, G., and Rosenfeld, M. (1984). Expression cloning of human EGF receptor complementary DNA: gene amplification and three related messenger RNA in A431 cells. *Science* 224: 843–848.
234. Ullrich, A., Coussens, L., Hayflick, J., Dull, T., Gray, A., Tam, A., Lee, J., Yarden, Y., Libermann, T., Schlessinger, J., Downward, J., Mayes, E., Whittle, N., Waterfield, M., and Seeburg, P. (1984). Human epidermal growth factor receptor cDNA sequence and aberrant expression of the amplified gene in A431 epidermoid carcinoma cells. *Nature* 309:418–425.
235. Cowley, G., Smith, J., and Gusterson, B. (1986). Increased EGF receptors on human squamous carcinoma lines. *Br. J. Cancer* 53:223–229.
236. Yamamoto, T., Kamata, N., Kawano, H., Shimizu, S., Kuroki, T., Toyoshima, I., Rikimaru, K., Nomura, N., Ishizaki, R., and Pastan, I. (1986). High incidence of amplification of epidermal growth factor receptor gene in human squamous carcinoma lines. *Cancer Res.* 46:414–416.
237. Paolo Di Fiore, P., Pierce, J., Fleming, T., Hazan, R., Ullrich, A., King, C., Schlessinger, J., and Aaronson, S. (1987). Overexpression of the human EGF receptor confers an EGF-dependent transformed phenotype to NIH 3T3 cells. *Cell* 51:1063–1070.

238. Haeder, M., Rotsch, M., Bepler, G., Hennig, C., Havemann, K., Heimann, B., and Moelling, K. (1988). Epidermal growth factor receptor expression in human lung cancer cell lines. *Cancer Res.* 48: 1132–1136.
239. Kris, R., Lax, I., Gullick, W., Waterfield, M., Ullrich, A., Fridkin, M., and Schlessinger, J. (1985). Antibodies against a synthetic peptide as a probe for the kinase activity of the avian EGF receptor and v-erbB protein. *Cell* 40:619–625.
240. Nanney, L., Stoscheck, C., and King, L. (1985). Active psoriatic lesions contain increased levels of epidermal growth factor (EGF) receptors. *J. Invest. Dermatol.* 84:290.
241. Nanney, L.B., Yates, R.A., and King, L.J. (1992). Modulation of epidermal growth factor receptors in psoriatic lesions during treatment with topical EGF. *J. Invest. Dermatol.* 98:296–301.
242. Green, M., and Couchman, J. (1985). Differences in human skin between the epidermal growth factor receptor distribution detected by EGF binding and monoclonal antibody recognition. *J. Invest. Dermatol.* 85: 239–245.
243. Zhou, M., Felder, S., Rubinstein, M., Hurwitz, D.R., Ullrich, A., Lax, I., and Schlessinger, J. (1993). Real-time measurements of kinetics of EGF binding to soluble EGF receptor monomers and dimers support the dimerization model for receptor activation. *Biochemistry* 32:8193–8198.
244. Brown, P.M., Debanne, M.T., Grothe, S., Bergsma, D., Caron, M., Kay, C., and MD, O.C.-M. (1994). The extracellular domain of the epidermal growth factor receptor. Studies on the affinity and stoichiometry of binding, receptor dimerization and a binding-domain mutant. *Eur. J. Biochem.* 225:223–233.
245. Fan, Z., Lu, Y., Wu, X., and Mendelsohn, J. (1994). Antibody-induced epidermal growth factor receptor dimerization mediates inhibition of autocrine proliferation of A431 squamous carcinoma cells. *J. Biol. Chem.* 269:27595–27602.
246. Gadella, T.W., Jr., and Jovin, T.M. (1995). Oligomerization of epidermal growth factor receptors on A431 cells studied by time-resolved fluorescence imaging microscopy. A stereochemical model for tyrosine kinase receptor activation. *J. Cell Biol.* 129:1543–1558.
247. Carraway, K.L., and Cerione, R.A. (1993). Inhibition of epidermal growth factor receptor aggregation by an antibody directed against the epidermal growth factor receptor extracellular domain. *J. Biol. Chem.* 268:23860–23867.
248. Hazan, R., Krushel, L., and Crossin, K.L. (1995). EGF receptor-mediated signals are differentially modulated by concanavalin A. *J. Cell Physiol.* 162:74–85.
249. Carraway, K.L., and Carraway, C.A. (1995). Signaling, mitogenesis and the cytoskeleton: where the action is. Bioessays 17:171–175.
250. Downward, J., Parker, P., and Waterfield, M. (1984). Autophosphorylation sites on the epidermal growth factor receptor. *Nature* 311:483–485.
251. Chen, W., Lazar, C., Poenie, M., Tsien, R., Gill, G., and Rosenfeld, M. (1987). Requirement for intrinsic protein tyrosine kinase in the immediate and late actions of the EGF receptor. *Nature* 324:820–823.
252. Hunter, T., Ling, N., and Cooper, J. (1984). Protein kinase C phosphorylation of the EGF receptor at a threonine residue close to the cytoplasmic face of the plasma membrane. *Nature* 311:480–483.
253. Davis, R., and Czech, M. (1986). Inhibition of the apparent affinity of the epidermal growth factor receptor caused by phorbol esters correlates with phosphorylation of threonine-654 but not at other sites on the receptor. *Biochem. J.* 233:435–441.
254. Davis, R., and Czech, M. (1987). Stimulation of epidermal growth factor receptor threonine 654 phosphorylation by platelet-derived growth factor in protein kinase C–deficient human fibroblasts. *J. Biol. Chem.* 262:6832–6841.
255. Countaway, J.L., Nairn, A.C., and Davis, R.J. (1992). Mechanism of desensitization of the epidermal growth factor receptor protein-tyrosine kinase. *J. Biol. Chem.* 267:1129–1140.
256. Kracht, M., Shiroo, M., Marshall, C.J., Hsuan, J.J., and Saklatvala, J. (1994). Interleukin-1 activates a novel protein kinase that phosphorylates the epidermal-growth-factor receptor peptide T669. *Biochem. J.* 302:897–905.
257. Boonstra, J., de Laat, S., and Ponce, M. (1985). Epidermal growth factor receptor expression related to differentiation capacity in normal and transformed keratinocytes. *Exp. Cell Res.* 161:421–433.
258. Boyce, S., and Ham, R. (1983). Calcium-regulated differentiation of normal human epidermal keratinocytes in chemically defined clonal culture and serum-free serial culture. *J. Invest. Dermatol.* 81:33s–40s.
259. Hawley-Nelson, P., Stanley, R., Schmidt, J., Gullino, M., and Yuspa, S. (1982). The tumor promoter, 12-*O*-tetradecanoylphorbol-13-acetate accelerates keratinocyte differentiation and stimulates growth of an unidentified cell type in cultured human epidermis. *Exp. Cell Res.* 137:155–167.
260. Parkinson, E. (1987). Phospholipase C mimics the differential effects of phorbol-12-myristate-13-acetate on the colony formation and cornification of cultured normal and transformed human keratinocytes. *Carcinogenesis* 8:857–860.
261. Jaken, S., and Yuspa, S. (1988). Early signals for keratinocyte differentiation: role of Ca^{++}-mediated inositol lipid metabolism in normal and neoplastic epidermal cells. *Carcinogenesis* 9:1033–1038.
262. Moscat, J., Molley, C., Fleming, T., and Aaronson, S. (1988). Epidermal growth factor activates phospho-

inositide turnover and protein kinase C in BALB/MK keratinocytes. *Mol. Endocrinol.* 2:799–805.
263. Fisher, G., Harris, V., and Voorhees, J. (1987). Purification and characterization of calcium/phospholipid-dependent kinase from adult human epidermis. *J. Invest. Dermatol.* 89:484–488.
264. Inohara, S., Tatsumi, Y., Tanaka, Y., Tateishi, H., and Sagami, S. (1988). Immunohistochemical identification of protein kinase C isozymes in normal and psoriatic epidermis. *Arch. Dermatol. Res.* 280:454–455.
265. Fisher, G.J., Tavakkol, A., Leach, K., Burns, D., Basta, P., Loomis, C., Griffiths, C.E., Cooper, K.D., Reynolds, N.J., Elder, J.T., *et al.* (1993). Differential expression of protein kinase C isoenzymes in normal and psoriatic adult human skin: reduced expression of protein kinase C-beta II in psoriasis. *J. Invest. Dermatol.* 101:553–559.
266. Koizumi, H., Kohno, Y., Osada, S., Ohno, S., Ohkawara, A., and Kuroki, T. (1993). Differentiation-associated localization of PKC-η, a Ca^{++}-independent protein kinase C, in normal human skin and skin diseases. *J. Invest. Dermatol.* 101:858–863.
267. Hokin, L. (1985). Receptors and phosphoinositide-generated second messengers. *Annu. Rev. Biochem.* 54:205–235.
268. Foster, D.A. (1983). Intracellular signaling mediated by protein-tyrosine kinases: networking through phospholipid metabolism. *Cell Signal* 5:389–399.
269. Lee, S.B., and Rhee, S.G. (1995). Significance of PIP2 hydrolysis and regulation of phospholipase C isozymes. *Curr. Opin. Cell Biol.* 7:183–189.
270. Noh, D.Y., Shin, S.H., and Rhee, S.G. (1995). Phosphoinositide-specific phospholipase C and mitogenic signaling. *Biochim. Biophys. Acta* 1242:99–113.
271. Jones, M.J., and Murray, A.W. (1995). Evidence that ceramide selectively inhibits protein kinase C-alpha translocation and modulates bradykinin activation of phospholipase D. *J. Biol. Chem.* 270:5007–5013.
272. Leevers, S.J., Paterson, H.F., and Marshall, C.J. (1994). Requirement for Ras in Raf activation is overcome by targeting Raf to the plasma membrane. *Nature* 369:411–414.
273. Stokoe, D., Macdonald, S.G., Cadwallader, K., Symons, M., and Hancock, J.F. (1994). Activation of Raf as a result of recruitment to the plasma membrane [published erratum appears in *Science* (1994) 16; 266(5192):1792–1793]. *Science* 264:1463–1467.
274. Wartmann, M., and Davis, R.J. (1994). The native structure of the activated Raf protein kinase is a membrane-bound multi-subunit complex. *J. Biol. Chem.* 269:6695–6701.
275. Marais, R., Light, Y., Paterson, H.F., and Marshall, C.J. (1995). Ras recruits Raf-1 to the plasma membrane for activation by tyrosine phosphorylation. *EMBO J.* 14:3136–3145.
276. Plopper, G.E., McNamee, H.P., Dike, L.E., Bojanowski, K., and Ingber, D.E. (1995). Convergence of integrin and growth factor receptor signaling pathways. *Mol. Biol. Cell* 6:1349–1365.
277. Nishizuka, Y. (1984). The role of protein kinase C in cell surface signal transduction and tumor production. *Nature* 308:693–698.
278. Reynolds, N.J., Yi, J.Y., Fisher, G.J., Cooper, K.D., Voorhees, J.J., and Griffiths, C.E. (1995). Down-regulation of Langerhans cell protein kinase C-beta isoenzyme expression in inflammatory and hyperplastic dermatoses. *Br. J. Dermatol.* 133:157–167.
279. Halliday, G.M., and Lucas, A.D. (1993). Protein kinase C transduces the signal for Langerhans' cell migration from the epidermis. *Immunology* 79:621–626.
280. Gupta, A., Fisher, G., Elder, J., Nickoloff, B., and Voorhees, J. (1988). Sphingosine inhibits phorbol ester-induced inflammation, ornithine decarboxylase activity, and activation of protein kinase C in mouse skin. *J. Invest. Dermatol.* 91:486–491.
281. Galey, C., Ziboh, V., Marcelo, C., and Voorhees, J. (1985). Modulation of phospholipid metabolism in murine keratinocytes by tumor promoter 12-*O*-tetradecanoylphorbol-13-acetate. *J. Invest. Dermatol.* 85.
282. Dlugosz, A.A., and Yuspa, S.H. (1993). Coordinate changes in gene expression which mark the spinous to granular cell transition in epidermis are regulated by protein kinase C. *J. Cell Biol.* 120:217–225.
283. Dlugosz, A.A., Cheng, C., Williams, E.K., Dharia, A.G., Denning, M.F., and Yuspa, S.H. (1994). Alterations in murine keratinocyte differentiation induced by activated rasHa genes are mediated by protein kinase C-alpha. *Cancer Res.* 54:6413–6420.
284. Bartel, R., Marcelo, C., and Voorhees, J. (1987). Partial characterization of phospholipase C activity in normal, psoriatic, and lesional epidermis. *J. Invest. Dermatol.* 88:447–451.
285. Nanney, L.B., Gates, R.E., Todderud, G., King, L.J., and Carpenter, G. (1992). Altered distribution of phospholipase C-gamma 1 in benign hyperproliferative epidermal diseases. *Cell Growth Differ.* 3: 233–239.
286. Saiag, P., Coulomb, B., Lebreton, C., Bell, E., and Dubertret, L. (1985). Psoriatic fibroblasts induce hyperproliferation of normal keratinocytes in a skin equivalent model in vitro. *Science* 230:669–672.
287. Nagao, S., Seishima, M., Mori, S., and Nozawa, Y. (1988). Increased protein kinase C activity in fibroblasts membranes from psoriatic patients. *J. Invest. Dermatol.* 90:406–408.
288. Venneker, G.T., Das, P.K., Meinardi, M.M., van Marle, J., van Veen, H.A., Bos, J.D., and Asghar, S.S. (1994). Glycosylphosphatidylinositol (GPI)-anchored membrane proteins are constitutively down-regulated in psoriatic skin. *J. Pathol.* 172:189–197.

289. Fürstenberger, Rogers, M., Faberman, J., Ganss, M., Richter, H., and Marks, F. (1987). Effects of the phorbol ester TPA and of the ionophore A23187 on phospholipase A_2 and C activities in the mouse epidermal cell line HEL-30. *J. Cancer Res. Oncol.* 113:310–318.
290. Kaufmann, R., Frosch, D., Westphal, C., Weber, L., and Klein, C.E. (1989). Integrin VLA-3: ultrastructural localization at cell-cell contact sites of human cell cultures. *J. Cell Biol.* 109:1807–1815.
291. Pellegrini, G., De Luca, M., Orecchia, G., Balzac, F., Cremona, O., Savoia, P., Cancedda, R., and Marchisio, P.C. (1992). Expression, topography, and function of integrin receptors are severely altered in keratinocytes from involved and uninvolved psoriatic skin. *J. Clin. Invest.* 89:1783–1795.
292. Larjava, H., Peltonen, J., Akiyama, S.K., Yamada, S.S., Gralnick, H.R., Uitto, J., and Yamada, K.M. (1990). Novel function for the β_1 integrins in keratinocyte cell-cell interactions. *J. Cell Biol.* 110:803–815.
293. Carroll, J.M., Romero, M.R., and Watt, F.M. (1995). Suprabasal integrin expression in the epidermis of transgenic mice results in developmental defects and an phenotype resembling psoriasis. *Cell* 83:957–965.
294. Katz, S.I., Tamaki, K., and Sachs, D. (1979). Epidermal Langerhans cells are derived from and are repopulated by mobile precursor cells which originate in bone marrow. *Nature* 282:324–326.
295. Reusch, M.K., Mansbridge, J.N., Nickoloff, B.J., and B., M.V. (1991). Immunophenotyping of skin cells during healing of suction blister injury. *Dermatologica* 183:179–184.
296. Morhenn, V.B. (1984). Is psoriasis a disease of the immune system? *Cutis* 34:223–225.
297. Valdimarsson, H., Baker, B. s., Jonsdottir, I., Powles, A., and Fry, L. (1995). Psoriasis: a T-cell mediated autoimmune disease induced by streptococcal superantigens. *Immunol. Today* 16:145–149.
298. Griffiths, C.E., Railan, D., Gallatin, W.M., and Cooper, K.D. (1995). The ICAM-3/LFA-1 interaction is critical for epidermal Langerhans cell alloantigen presentation to CD4+ T cells. *Br. J. Dermatol.* 133: 823–829.
299. Heck, D.E., Laskin, D.L., Gardner, C.R., and Laskin, J.D. (1992). Epidermal growth factor suppresses nitric oxide and hydrogen peroxide production by keratinocytes. *J. Biol. Chem.* 267:21277–21280.
300. Denlinger, L.C., Fisette, P.L., Garis, K.A., Kwon, G., Vasquez-Torres, A., Simon, A.D., Nguyen, B., Proctor, R.A., Bertics, P.J., and Corbett, J.A. (1996). Regulation of inducible nitric oxide synthase expression by macrophage purinoreceptors and calcium. *J. Biol. Chem.* 271:337–342.
301. Wilkinson, D.I., Liu, S.C., and Orenberg, E.K. (1981). Cyclic nucleotide content of passaged keratinocytes in culture during various growth stages. *J. Invest. Dermatol.* 77:385–388.
302. Barnes, P.J. (1993). Beta-adrenoceptors on smooth muscle, nerves and inflammatory cells. *Life Sci.* 52: 2101–2109.
303. Shen, H.M., Sha, L.X., Kennedy, J.L., and Ou, D.W. (1994). Adrenergic receptors regulate macrophage secretion. *Int. J. Immunopharmacol.* 16:905–910.
304. Monastra, G., and Secchi, E.F. (1993). Beta-adrenergic receptors mediate in vivo the adrenaline inhibition of lipopolysaccharide-induced tumor necrosis factor release. *Immunol. Lett.* 38:127–130.
305. Brysk, M., and Snider, J. (1982). Lactoperoxidase-catalyzed iodination of membrane proteins in normal and neoplastic epidermal cells. *J. Invest. Dermatol.* 78:24–27.
306. Schmidt, R., Pautrat, G., Michel, S., Cavey, M., Gazith, J., Dalbiez, and Reichert, U. (1985). High-yield purification of plasma membranes from transformed human keratinocytes in culture. *J. Invest. Dermatol.* 85:50–53.
307. McName, M. (1989). Isolation and characterization of cell membranes. *Biotechniques* 7:466–475.

19

Pathogenic Interactions of Keratinocytes and T Lymphocytes in Psoriasis

James G. Krueger
The Rockefeller University, New York, New York

The formation, as well as persistence, of focal psoriatic skin lesions is tightly linked to skin infiltration by T lymphocytes. Recent evidence suggests that CD8+ lymphocytes that express Vβ3 or Vβ13.1 T-cell receptors are clonally activated in psoriatic lesions and that these cells accumulate selectively in lesional epidermis. This chapter reviews evidence that psoriasis is largely a programmed "regenerative" reaction of the epidermis that is stimulated by intraepidermal T lymphocytes, particularly those of the CD25+CD8+ subset. The hypothesis that keratinocyte-lymphocyte interactions are critical in the pathogenesis of psoriasis stems from (1) laboratory and clinical experiments that demonstrate that some immune-derived cytokines are potent mitogens for epidermal keratinocytes and (2) clinical studies that show that selective immunosuppressive or immunodepleting therapies reverse keratinocyte hyperproliferation and pathological epidermal differentiation.

This chapter is organized into sections that explain (1) key pathological differences between "normal" and lesional skin of psoriatic patients; (2) responses of psoriatic cells to immune-modulating therapies; and (3) pathogenic mechanisms that relate T-lymphocyte and keratinocyte interactions in psoriasis.

CELLULAR AND PATHOLOGICAL CHARACTERISTICS OF "NORMAL" VERSUS LESIONAL SKIN OF PSORIATIC PATIENTS

Activated T Lymphocytes Accumulate in Psoriatic Lesions

Psoriasis, which varies considerably in its clinical presentation, is defined as a unique skin disease through characteristic histopathological alterations that are present in different clinical variants. Psoriasis is characterized by changes in growth and architecture of resident skin cells (epidermal hyperplasia, rete elongation, "regenerative" epidermal differentiation, and vascular alterations) that appear concurrently with tissue infiltration by blood leukocytes (1,2). Activated leukocytes found in psoriatic skin lesions include T lymphocytes, neutrophils, and dendritic (antigen-presenting) cells. From the standpoint of disease pathogenesis, the T lymphocyte appears to be the most important leukocyte cell type. The eruption of new psoriatic skin lesions is closely associated with an influx of T lymphocytes into affected skin lesions (2) and worsening or chronicity of psoriasis vulgaris is associated with quantitative increases in lymphocytic infiltration (3). Since specific cellular immune responses are initiated and orchestrated by T lymphocytes, it is appropriate to focus on T lymphocytes in the psoriatic lesion.

As illustrated in Figure 1, one of the most characteristic differences between uninvolved and lesional skin is the marked accumulation of T lymphocytes in psoriatic plaques. Unaffected skin of psoriatic patients contains only a few T lymphocytes and these cells are mostly located in the dermis in a perivascular location (Fig. 1). Migration of dermal T lymphocytes into the epidermis is apparently a rare event, as intraepidermal T lymphocytes are rarely visualized in unaffected epidermis of psoriatic patients (this is also the case in normal skin of nonpsoriatics). In striking contrast, lesional psoriatic skin is heavily infiltrated with T lymphocytes, which are present in both the epidermis and dermis of psoriatic lesions (Fig. 1). Although not illustrated in Figure 1, CD4+ and CD8+ T-lymphocyte subsets are concentrated in different regions of the psoriatic plaque: CD8+ T cells are highly concentrated in psoriatic lesional epidermis, while CD4+ T cells are located principally in the papillary and superficial reticular dermis (4–6). Quantitative studies have shown that, on the average, psoriatic epidermis contains about twice as many CD8+ T cells as CD4+ T cells, a ratio that is inverted from the normal 1:2 ratio of CD8+/CD4+ cells in the blood circulation or in dermal inflammatory infiltrates (4–6). Furthermore, the number of CD8+ T lymphocytes in psoriatic lesional epidermis is higher than in a number of other inflammatory cutaneous disorders (4). Hence, one of the fundamental pathological characteristics of psoriasis is the presence of large numbers of CD3+ lymphocytes in psoriatic plaques and particularly the accumulation of CD8+ lymphocytes within the epidermis.

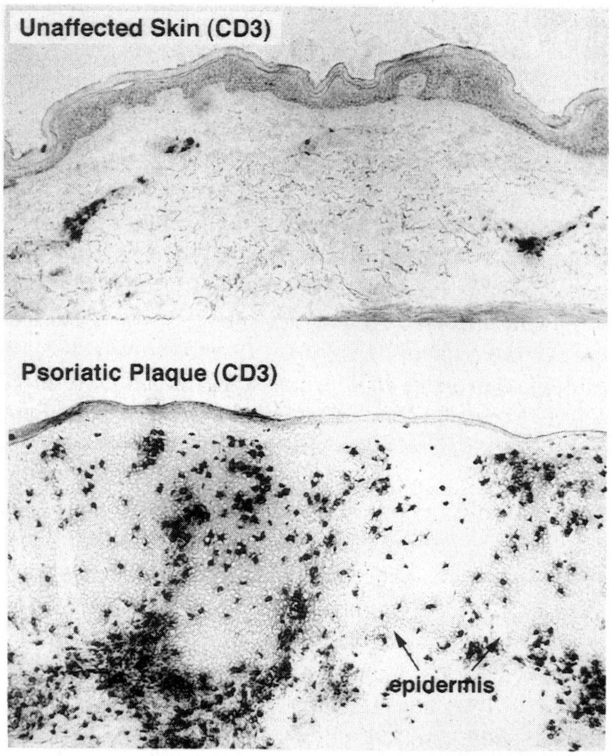

Figure 1 Immunohistochemical detection of T lymphocytes in unaffected skin or lesional skin of a psoriatic patient. Cryostat skin sections were reacted with CD3 monoclonal antibodies to detect T lymphocytes. Note the large number of T lymphocytes in lesional epidermis of the psoriatic plaque.

One of the most important questions concerning the prevalence of T cells in psoriatic lesions is whether these cells arise in skin lesions through specific immune (antigenic or superantigenic) activation or whether T cells are nonspecifically recruited to sites of cutaneous inflammation. Accumulated work from several research groups now suggests that specific immune activation occurs in psoriatic lesions. However, many T lymphocytes and most other leukocytes in psoriatic lesions probably arise through increased cellular trafficking and relatively less specific immune mechanisms. Specific immune activation in psoriatic lesions was first suggested by the identification of T lymphocytes bearing activated IL-2 receptors (7). Subsequently, memory T lymphocytes were identified in the psoriatic infiltrate (4), suggesting an amnestic response. Dermal dendritic cells in psoriatic lesional skin display marked increases in B7 proteins that are costimulatory signals for T-cell activation and these cells are potent inducers of T-lymphocyte proliferation in autologous reactions (8). Antigen presentation to T lymphocytes from dermal dendritic cells could underlie ongoing T-cell activation in psoriatic lesions, as dendritic cells found in uninvolved skin regions do not have potent T-lymphocyte-stimulating effects (8). The combined finding of activated dendritic cells, their T-cell-activating properties, and high numbers of proliferatively activated, memory T lymphocytes in psoriatic lesions provides circumstantial evidence of ongoing specific immune activation in lesional skin sites.

The strongest evidence for specific T-cell activation in psoriatic lesions comes from recent molecular analysis of T-cell-receptor usage. Using PCR amplification of T-cell-receptor β-chain isoforms expressed in isolated CD4+ and CD8+ lymphocytes from psoriatic lesional tissue, two recent studies have found selective increases in Vβ3 and Vβ13.1 gene families in CD8+ lymphocytes (9,10). Sequence analysis of specific lymphocyte clones derived from this analysis showed highly restricted clonality of expressing T cells. Cells expressing clonal usage of Vβ3 or Vβ13.1 genes belonged to the CD25+CD8+ T-cell subset, suggesting clonal expansion of only cytotoxic lymphocytes in lesional skin (9,10). It is unlikely that clonality detected in CD8+ T cells was a chance finding, as the same CD8+ clone could be identified in tissue samples taken from the same individual months apart or in different psoriatic lesions of the same person (10). In contrast, no consistent amplification of Vβ genes within CD4+ cells could be identified in these individuals. Selective activation of CD8+ T lymphocytes in psoriatic tissue fits neatly with prior identification of increased risk for psoriasis in certain HLA class I backgrounds (11,12) (antigens presented on HLA class I molecules would specifically activate CD8+ T cells) and with selective accumulations of CD8+ lymphocytes in psoriatic epidermis. Selective gene usage in Vβ2 and Vβ6 gene families, along with clonality in T-cell populations, has been found by other investigators using similar molecular approaches (13), and these data support the general concept of specific antigenic activation of T lymphocytes in psoriatic lesions. However, in these studies, T cells were not fractionated into CD4+ or CD8+ subsets, so it is not clear which T-cell subsets were clonally amplified. Analysis of Vβ-gene usage in guttate psoriasis using somewhat different molecular or antibody-based typing approaches has also identified selective use of specific Vβ genes, supporting a role for antigenic or superantigenic activation of T cells in this psoriasis variant (14,15). Some investigators consider guttate psoriasis to be a disease mediated by activated CD4+ lymphocytes (16), and substantial clinical differences in the clinical presentation and course of guttate and vulgaris forms of psoriasis might be based on T-cell activation triggered by different antigens or by involvement of different T-cell subsets in the guttate form. Hence, until potential disease differences are better resolved, data derived for guttate versus vulgaris forms of psoriasis should be clearly distinguished. It is the primary intent of this chapter to discuss psoriasis vulgaris, and readers are referred elsewhere for current views on the pathogenesis of guttate psoriasis (16).

"Regenerative" Epidermal Activation Is Characteristic of Psoriasis

Epidermal growth and differentiation alterations in psoriatic plaques produce much of the clinically visible disease, i.e., scaling and increased skin thickness. Epidermal changes are also the most conspicuous histopathological feature of psoriasis. Accumulated evidence now suggests that these epidermal changes are a manifestation of "regenerative" or "alternate" epidermal differentiation, a genetic program that is normally activated for repair of epidermal wounds. In psoriasis, regenerative epidermal growth appears to be triggered by T lymphocytes infiltrating diseased skin areas, and it is potentially reversible (so that homeostatic epidermal growth is restored) by treatments that deplete T lymphocytes from psoriatic lesions. Unaffected skin in psoriatic patients is effectively "normal" based on specific cellular or molecular markers that distinguish homeostatic from regenerative epidermis. This view of pathogenesis, which might be termed "reactive hyperplasia," does not require that keratinocyte growth/differentiation responses in psoriasis are intrinsically abnormal (see below). Instead, characteristic disease-defining histopathological features could arise from chronic activation of a programmed wound-repair pathway in the setting of a sustained immune trigger.

Regenerative Epidermal Differentiation: A Reactive Growth State

The growth and maturation of epidermal keratinocytes normally occurs in either (1) the homeostatic pathway or (2) the "regenerative" pathway (also termed the "alternate" pathway). Characteristic features of these alternative growth states are considered below, while Table 1 summarizes some of the key distinguishing features.

Homeostatic Differentiation

In the homeostatic pathway, keratinocyte proliferation is restricted to the basal layer and the proliferative cell cycle is quite long, with basal keratinocytes undergoing division at about 2-week intervals. Endogenous growth regulatory elements such as growth factor receptors and activating ligands are confined to the basal epidermis or expressed at low levels. Epidermal differentiation proceeds in a slow and progressive fashion with a sharp transition between the basal and spinous epidermis in suprabasal keratinocytes. The onset

Table 1 Characteristics of Homeostatic Versus Regenerative Epidermal Differentiation

	Homeostasis	Regeneration
Keratinocyte proliferation features		
Location	Basal	Basal and suprabasal
Mitotic rate	Low	High
Cell cycle duration	Long (~14 days)	Short (~2 days)
IGF-1 receptor	Basal	Basal and suprabasal
EGF receptors	Low (EGF binding)	High (EGF binding)
TGF-α and amphiregulin	Low	High
Keratinocyte differentiation features		
Integrins ($\alpha 3$, $\beta 1$, and others)	Basal	Basal and suprabasal
Keratins 6 and 16	Absent	Expressed
ψ-3 protein	Absent	Expressed
Filaggrin	Granular layer	Spinous and granular layer
Involucrin	Granular layer	Spinous and granular layer
Transglutaminase	Granular layer	Spinous and granular layer
Granular layer	Well defined	Diffuse
Parakeratosis	Absent	Often present
Epidermal transit time (basal layer to desquamation)	Slow	Fast
Epidermal patterning		
Acanthosis	Absent	Present
Rete elongation	Absent	Often present
Other		
Fibroblast activation	Low	↑KGF synthesis ↑PDGF receptors
Vascular activation	Low	↑PDGF receptors ↑ICAM-1, ELAM
Epidermal neutrophils	Absent	Often present
T lymphocytes	Few	Many in acute wounds, few in chronic wounds

of homeostatic differentiation above the basal layer is marked by loss of cell surface IGF-1 receptors (with associated loss of proliferative potential) and loss of several integrins expressed by basal keratinocytes (Table 1). Keratinocytes differentiate progressively, but precisely, as they rise through defined epidermal layers over a period of 2–4 weeks. Spinous differentiation is best characterized by the synthesis of keratins 1 and 10 by suprabasal cells and no synthesis of keratins 6 and 16. Keratinocyte terminal differentiation occurs in a sharp transition between the granular and cornified layer, producing a thin, orthokeratotic stratum corneum. This epidermal growth state is associated with relatively short dermal capillary loops, with a relative absence of adhesion molecules for leukocytes on vascular endothelium, and with a low abundance of leukocytes in the epidermis and dermis. In normal individuals, the growth of skin is usually restricted to this homeostatic program, but can be transiently activated into the regenerative program following wounding or biochemical manipulation (17–20).

Regenerative Differentiation

The epidermis and other skin regions undergo a series of complex changes in response to wounding. The epidermal reaction to wounding has been termed "regenerative maturation" or "alternate differentiation," terms meant to encompass complex, but consistent alterations in growth and differentiation of epidermal keratinocytes following wounding (17–19). It is now clear that the regenerative growth program can be activated by manipulations outside the arena of physical injury, e.g., by dietary deprivation of essential fatty acids, by topical application of retinoic acid, by direct administration of epidermal-activating cytokines, or by engineered expression of cytokine transgenes (21–25). In each of these settings, the epidermis undergoes proliferative activation and altered differentiation, but the magnitude of proliferative responses and epidermal thickening can vary. Depending on the extent of injury or inducing stimulus, the regenerative program will self-terminate within a few days or it can persist for years, as is the case in epidermis adjacent to chronic skin ulcers. Regenerative epidermal growth has some features, such as increased keratinocyte proliferation and altered keratinocyte differentiation, that are consistently observed (see Table 1) and other features that vary depending on the inducing stimulus and its chronicity.

The regenerative program permits rapid expansion of the number of available keratinocytes though mitotic activation, which consists of more cells recruited into the proliferative pool and in a shortened cell cycle time (1). Expression of growth-regulating cytokines and receptors is rapidly increased in regenerative growth (Table 1). Keratinocyte differentiation in regenerative growth differs in two general respects from homeostatic growth: (1) Keratinocyte differentiation is accelerated to restore stratum corneum function as rapidly as possible. Differentiation products normally expressed only in the granular layer become expressed in the mid- to lower spinous layer and corneocytes can be formed without a well-defined granular layer, resulting in parakeratotic cells in the newly formed corneum. (2) Unique proteins are synthesized by regenerative keratinocytes. Keratins 6 and 16 and the Ψ-3 protein are among uniquely synthesized regenerative proteins (Table 1). Lower spinous keratinocytes synthesize keratins 6 and 16 in regenerative epidermis, while synthesis of keratins 1 and 10 is often delayed or reduced. Regenerative keratinocytes also have migratory potential if epidermal continuity is lost through injury (17,19). Complex dermal and inflammatory changes are also initiated by regenerative activation. Over a period of hours to days following regenerative activation, dermal cells including fibroblasts and vascular elements may become proliferatively activated, vascular endothelial cells increase synthesis of leukocyte adhesion molecules, and leukocytes migrate into activated skin regions (Table 1). Overall, the regenerative response in rapidly healing acute wounds can appear remarkably similar to psoriasis, and parallels are particularly apparent when keratinocyte proliferation is maximally stimulated by wounding and high concentrations of cytokines (26) or by chronic regenerative activation (27,28).

Regenerative Growth Is Activated in Lesional Psoriasis, but Homeostatic Growth Persists in Unaffected Skin

We propose that psoriasis vulgaris is a focus of regenerative skin growth that is triggered and maintained though the actions of T lymphocyte subsets infiltrating localized skin regions. In contrast, unaffected skin of psoriatic patients maintains its growth within the homeostatic program and is phenotypically "normal" according to the criteria listed in Table 1. In effect, psoriasis may be an example of chronic, immune-associated regenerative epidermal growth.

Figure 2 illustrates unaffected or lesional skin in the same psoriatic patient after immunohistochemical reaction with antibodies to Ki67 (a protein expressed in proliferating cells) and to keratin 16. In unaffected epidermis, a small fraction of basal layer keratinocytes have nuclear staining for the Ki67 protein, indicating active cell cycling in positive cells. Epidermal keratinocytes in unaffected epidermis do not synthesize keratin 16. In contrast, the number of Ki67-reactive keratinocytes is much higher in lesional psoriasis vulgaris, with a high fraction of basal keratinocytes in cycle and with many suprabasal proliferating keratinocytes. Keratin 16 is uniformly expressed by spinous keratinocytes in active psoriatic lesions. Other markers of homeostatic versus regenerative epidermal growth that are listed in Table 1 have been studied in unaffected and lesional skin biopsies from a large number of psoriatic patients. Unaffected skin of psoriatic patients consistently displays a homeostatic growth phenotype, while lesional skin consistently displays a regenerative phenotype. As discussed in the next section, immune-depleting therapies convert regenerative growth to the homeostatic program, establishing the potential reversibility of "pathological" psoriatic alterations. The reversibility of psoriatic regenerative growth, in particular, suggests it is a physiologically regulated growth pattern and not a fixed growth response programmed into disease-associated keratinocytes.

Is Keratinocyte Growth Genetically Abnormal in Psoriasis?

While keratinocyte growth reactions that define psoriasis are inducible and potentially reversible, it is possible that the genetic element affected in psoriasis could alter transient or conditional keratinocyte growth responses. Three experimental observations

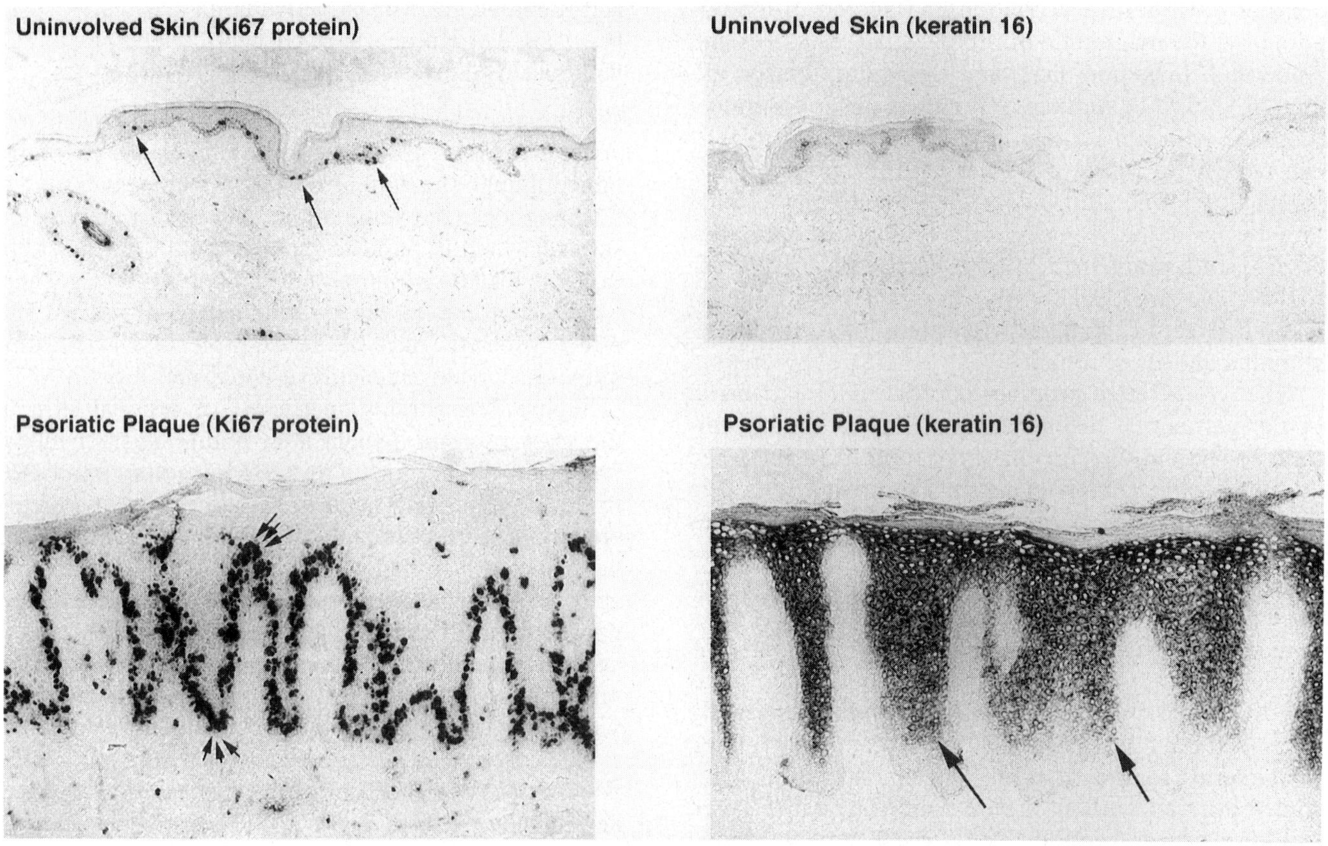

Figure 2 Immunohistochemical detection of proliferating cells and keratin 16 in uninvolved or lesional skin of psoriatic patients. Proliferating keratinocytes express the Ki67 nuclear protein (small arrows at left). Keratin 16 is not detected in uninvolved skin, but is highly expressed in lesional epidermis (large arrows at right).

are potentially related to this issue: (1) Unaffected skin of psoriatic patients becomes abnormally acanthotic when transplanted onto nude mice (29,30), (2) keratinocytes cultured from uninvolved psoriatic skin show increased proliferative responses to cytokines released from psoriatic T-lymphocyte clones (31), and (3) adult mice harboring a TGF-α transgene have a normal-appearing epidermis, but keratinocyte proliferative responses to wounds are exaggerated and may fail to self-terminate (23). In each experimental system, psoriatic or genetically altered keratinocytes display increased growth responses during wound repair or after exposure to growth-activating cytokines. Hence, one needs to consider the possibility that psoriatic genes might either produce increased growth responses of keratinocytes to activating stimuli or interfere with normal signals that eventually down-regulate or terminate regenerative growth responses. In conceptual terms, sustained regenerative activation in psoriatic lesions is more "pathological" and disease-defining than individual alterations in specific growth-regulating cytokines, keratinocyte differentiation, or tissue patterning that exists in psoriatic lesions. Recently, a state of chronic regenerative activation in the epidermis of mice was attained by overexpression of human integrin transgenes, and the overall tissue phenotype resembles psoriasis (32). If one assumes that the integrin transgenes are not immunogenic, this study serves as a clear example of how dysregulated expression of keratinocyte genes may contribute to sustained regenerative epidermal growth.

EFFECTS OF THERAPY ON CELLULAR ACTIVATION IN PSORIASIS

Many therapies have been developed for psoriasis without a clear understanding of cellular targets. Fortunately, continued research into cellular effects of different therapeutic agents has greatly advanced the understanding of the cellular basis of pathogenesis, as well as our understanding of specific pharmacological mechanisms relevant to psoriasis. Through mechanistic cellular studies, which are considered in more detail below, some generalizations can now be stated: (1) "pathological" cellular activation can be reversed so that a normal (homeostatic) growth program is attained in the epidermis; (2) complete reversal of psoriatic cellular pathology is attained when intraepidermal lymphocytes are depleted; and (3) numerous antipsoriatic therapies are directly immune-modulating, having direct effects to decrease T-lymphocyte activation or to induce apoptosis in activated T cells. In fact, antipsoriatic actions of most therapies may be generally related to immunomodulatory properties.

Regenerative Epidermal Activation in Psoriasis Can Be Reversed by T-Lymphocyte-Depleting Therapies

As discussed above, there is abundant evidence to suggest that activated T lymphocytes (as well as other types of activated leukocytes) accumulate in psoriatic lesional skin. In fact, the presence of large numbers of lymphocytes infiltrating psoriatic skin is an invariant feature of this disease. However, neither HLA disease associations nor phenotypic characteristics of immune cells in psoriatic tissue establish whether leukocytes contribute directly to disease pathogenesis. A potential pathogenic role for infiltrating lymphocytes is suggested from demonstrated mitogenic actions of immune-derived cytokines on epidermal keratinocytes (22,33–36). More direct evidence that cellular immunity contributes directly to the pathogenesis of psoriatic lesions is derived from study of specific immune-modulating therapies. In addition, the therapeutic actions of UVB and PUVA can probably be traced to selective cytotoxic effects of these agents on lymphocytes infiltrating psoriatic skin lesions.

For the purposes of this pathogenic discussion, therapeutic agents that restore regenerative epidermal growth to the normal, homeostatic program will be termed "remittive," and agents that produce disease improvements by modulating growth within the regenerative pathway will be termed "suppressive." DAB_{389}IL-2, UVB, and PUVA treatments produce remittive outcomes, whereas cyclosporin and etretinate generally produce suppressive outcomes.

DAB_{389}IL-2

This agent is a fusion toxin (or hybrid protein) in which a single polypeptide chain has been engineered by molecular technology to encode both human interleukin-2 (IL-2) sequences and a portion of the diphtheria toxin molecule that contains membrane-translocating and enzymatic (toxin) domains. This agent is a selective toxin for cells bearing high-affinity IL-2 cell surface receptors (chiefly activated T lymphocytes), and it has no intrinsic actions on epidermal keratinocytes, as this cell type expresses no IL-2 receptors (37). In initial phase I/II clinical trials, intracutaneous T-lymphocyte depletion was produced in several patients (37). Importantly, detailed examination of resolved psoriatic lesions by a panel of immunohistochemical markers of regenerative epidermal activation, as well as by routine histopathology, showed complete reversal of disease-defining markers and acquisition of normal, homeostatic epidermal growth (37). In cases where only moderate reductions in T lymphocytes were achieved, modest clinical improvements were noted and these were reflected in modest histopathological scores (using quantitative and qualitative disease markers). No instances were seen in which DAB_{389}IL-2 produced lymphocyte depletion in psoriatic tissue without accompanying reductions in epidermal disease features (an outcome that might have been attained if disordered epidermal growth is responsible for maintaining the disease phenotype). These data may be taken as evidence that a regenerative epidermal growth response is maintained by actions of T lymphocytes infiltrating defined skin regions. Furthermore, as the uptake of DAB_{389}IL-2 occurs selectively in cells having high-affinity IL-2 receptors (defined by the presence of the IL-2 receptor α-chain or the CD25 antigen), these data indicate that CD3+CD25+ T cells are important to the pathogenesis of psoriasis. The studies with DAB_{389}IL-2 do not directly address whether CD4+ or CD8+ T lymphocyte subsets are most important in pathogenesis, but disease improvements were most closely linked to elimination of intraepidermal CD8+ lymphocytes in these studies (37).

UVB

UVB is one of the most common treatments for psoriasis. The ability of UVB to suppress cutaneous T-cell-mediated hypersensitivity reactions in animals and humans has led to the assumption that its primary mode of action in psoriasis is through immunosuppression. However, the effects of clinically relevant, repetitive UVB exposure on T lymphocytes in psoriatic lesions have been investigated only recently (38). In this study, Goeckerman treatment (UVB combined with tar-containing emollients) produced a striking reduction in T lymphocytes located in lesional epidermis, but the number and activation state of dermal T lymphocytes were minimally affected. This type of UVB treatment was sufficient to produce a remittive outcome, as regenerative epidermal growth was restored to the normal, homeostatic program (38). Furthermore, parallel studies using cultured lymphocytes or keratinocytes showed that pharmacologically relevant doses of UVB induced cytotoxic outcomes in irradiated lymphocytes (with cellular death through apoptosis), but epidermal keratinocytes were quite resistant to UVB-induced apoptosis (38). If one considers the clinical and histopathological results together with the cell culture studies, it can be concluded that therapeutic actions of UVB may be based on its ability to selectively kill lymphocytes that are located in the uppermost portion of the psoriatic lesion. Hence, intraepidermal CD8+ lymphocytes are implicated as the disease-sustaining subset, as they are concentrated in the UVB-responsive zone. Lymphocytes located in the dermis are not depleted by UVB, presumably because UVB penetration is sharply diminished at the level of the dermoepidermal junction and therefore sufficient energy is not delivered to directly deplete activated lymphocytes. Relatively long-lasting remission of psoriasis following Goeckerman treatment (5) suggests that the dermal infiltrate, composed primarily of CD4+ lymphocytes, contains few lymphocytes that are immediately pathogenic. The probable pathogenicity of CD8+ lymphocytes is supported by TCR Vβ restrictions and T-cell clonality, which has been observed only in CD8+ lymphocytes derived from psoriatic lesions (9), as discussed previously.

PUVA

Treatment of psoriatic lesions with PUVA leads to marked depletion of lymphocytes from epidermal and dermal zones and to a reversal of remittive epidermal growth (5). Recent laboratory studies suggest that PUVA treatment selectively induces apoptosis in T lymphocytes when 8-methoxypsoralen and UVA are delivered in pharmacologically relevant doses (39). In contrast, keratinocytes appear to be quite resistant to PUVA-induced apoptosis (39). Hence, PUVA treatment may act primarily as a cytotoxic treatment for skin-infiltrating lymphocytes in psoriatic lesions, and relatively long-lasting remissions attained by this treatment might be best attributed to induced apoptosis in specific lymphocyte clones that are resident in psoriatic lesions (5,39).

Cyclosporin

This agent produces clinical resolution of psoriasis in a high percentage of patients (40). Its primary pharmacological action is to inhibit T lymphocyte activation and thereby decrease production of proinflammatory cytokines (41), but cyclosporin also has direct effects on epidermal keratinocytes to decrease proliferation (42) and to increase TGF-α production (43,44). The net effect of cyclosporin in psoriatic lesions is to decrease infiltrating T lymphocytes by 50–60% after 2 months of treatment, to decrease production of inflammation-associated molecules such as HLA-DR and ICAM-1, and to improve epidermal acanthosis and differentiation (44). However, in most patients with clinical clearing after 2 months of therapy, regenerative epidermal growth is not shut off (44), an outcome that defines a "suppressive response" to therapy. Overall results with cyclosporin suggest that activated T cells contribute significantly to the clinical psoriatic phenotype, but some controversy exists with respect to its relative pharmacological effects on lymphocytes versus activated keratinocytes in psoriatic lesions (45).

Etretinate

Retinoids produce significant, but rarely complete, clinical improvements in psoriasis (46,47). Retinoids have widespread effects on different cell types and, hence, antipsoriatic effects cannot be precisely ascribed to a single pharmacological action. A recent study established that acitretin (the pharmacologically active metabolite of etretinate) directly inhibited growth of epidermal keratinocytes in a dose-dependent fashion and that keratinocyte proliferation was suppressed in psoriatic lesions treated with systemically administered etretinate (48). In this context, expression of inflammation-associated epidermal proteins (ICAM-1 and HLA-DR) was greatly diminished and T-cell infiltration of lesional tissue was suppressed by about 50% (48). Surprisingly, epidermal differentiation was markedly enhanced by etretinate treatment in all patients. However, regenerative differentiation persisted in 80% of patients after treatment for 2 months (48). The sum of these findings is that etretinate exerts some unexpected properties to decrease T-cell-mediated inflammation and to improve epidermal features of psoriasis. It is a clear example of a disease-suppressive agent that could have direct effects on both leukocytic and epidermal cell types in psoriatic lesions (48).

Other Immune-Modulating Agents

Clear-cut clinical improvements in psoriasis have been produced by treatment with a number of relatively specific immune-modulating agents, e.g., CD3 or CD4 monoclonal antibodies (49,50), FK506 (51), or 2-chlorodeoxyadenosine (52). Improvements observed with each of these agents may be taken as prima facie evidence of a significant contribution of T lymphocytes to the psoriatic disease phenotype.

IMMUNE-MEDIATED PATHOGENESIS: POTENTIAL CELLULAR MECHANISMS

Cellular immune elements could contribute to the pathogenesis of psoriasis in at least two ways:

1. *Nonspecifically recruited and disease-contributing.* Leukocytes could be recruited into skin regions as a consequence of preceding epidermal keratinocyte activation, which increases elaboration of immune-trafficking or -activating cytokines (21,53). Leukocyte-derived cytokines or other molecules might then amplify keratinocyte proliferation and induce "inflammatory" changes in the epidermis; e.g., T-cell-derived γ-interferon would induce expression of HLA-DR, ICAM-1, and IP-10 proteins in epidermal keratinocytes (36,54). Under these circumstances, leukocytes would play an important, but secondary role in pathogenesis, as the initiating stimulus arises initially in the keratinocyte.
2. *Immune-activated and disease-mediating.* Keratinocytes could be unactivated at the time of T-lymphocyte entry into skin. T-cell activation in skin would arise as a result of antigenic or superantigenic stimuli presented by cutaneous dendritic cells. Keratinocyte regenerative activation would follow in response to cytokines elaborated from activated T lymphocytes. Under these circumstances, psoriasis would be induced by T-lymphocyte-mediated effector immune mechanisms (see below), while much of the overall phenotype would be due to regenerative epidermal activation. In this scheme, some disease features might be produced by leukocytes that are nonspecifically recruited to sites of cutaneous inflammation.

A role for specific immune activation of T lymphocytes in psoriatic lesions is suggested from (1) identification of dendritic cells in psoriatic lesions that have up-regulated expression of B7-1 and B7-2 costimulatory molecules (8,55), (2) demonstration that dendritic cells from skin lesions can activate resting peripheral blood T lymphocytes (8), and (3) identification of specific T-cell-receptor amplifications in lesional lymphocytes, as well as clonal populations in activated T lymphocytes (9,10,13–15). Based on these observations, as well as the responsiveness of psoriatic epidermal activation to immune-modulating therapies, one can hypothesize that psoriatic pathogenesis may proceed along the following pathways:

1. The initial event would be antigen or superantigen activation of T lymphocytes. Given the identification of clonality in CD8+ T lymphocytes, T-cell activation through HLA-A, -B, or -C molecules (MHC class I molecules) seems most likely. This possibility is also supported by the association of type I psoriasis with inheritance of specific MHC class I haplotypes, particularly HLA-Cw6 (11). Clonal expansion of T lymphocytes would occur focally in skin lesions, although some dendritic cells or T cells might also traffic to lymph nodes to recruit or expand additional memory T cells.
2. T-lymphocyte activation would be accompanied by release of TH1 cytokines (IL-2, γ-interferon, IL-6, GM-CSF, TNF-α, etc.). In turn, lymphocyte-derived cytokines would (i) mitogenically activate keratinocytes, (ii) modulate expression of immune-trafficking adhesion molecules on vascular endothelium to increase nonspecific leukocyte accumulations into skin, and (iii) enhance recruitment and activation of macrophages in psoriatic dermis, an event that would further enhance elaboration of "effector" cytokines from activated macrophages (36,56). In effect, nonspecific leukocyte recruitment and macrophage activation would produce an immune environment dominated by effector cytokines (a DTH-like response).
3. However, specific immune activation would produce "effector" lymphocyte clones that might be directly pathogenic. In particular, CD8+ lymphocyte clones, which accumulate selectively in psoriatic lesional epidermis, may directly induce "regenerative" epidermal acti-

vation by damaging the epidermis and its basement membrane. Epidermal disrupting effects would arise as a direct consequence of intraepidermal trafficking of CD8+ lymphocytes, by release of toxic cytokines, or by a combination of these mechanisms. Furthermore, migration of polymorphonuclear leukocytes into the epidermis would also disrupt epidermal structure and thus amplify the regenerative response. Experimental support for these concepts is provided by induction of a regenerative response in normal human epidermis following trafficking of neutrophils into the epidermis in response to topical LTB_4 application (57).

4. Activated keratinocytes synthesize and release a number of proinflammatory cytokines that might further stimulate keratinocyte proliferation or increase local trafficking of damaging leukocytes (21,53). For example, keratinocyte-derived IL-6 or GM-CSF could augment keratinocyte proliferative responses and/or further stimulate actions of inflammatory leukocytes (22,35). IL-8, which is synthesized by highly differentiated keratinocytes, might serve as the initial signal for neutrophil accumulations into lesional epidermis (58). Thus, specific immune mechanisms could result in overall amplification of tissue inflammation by a number of self-regulating cytokine circuits and nonspecific recruitment of other leukocyte types.
5. In most skin lesions, specific T-lymphocyte activation proceeds without self-termination. Hence, individual psoriatic lesions tend to persist, unless treated by therapy. The precise stimulus for ongoing, intracutaneous immune activation is not known, but is presumably "driven" by an antigen (or antigens) that persists in affected skin regions and is presented to T cells by activated, cutaneous dendritic cells. The putative psoriatic antigen could be derived from an exogenous pathogen that is not eliminated by available effector immune mechanisms or it could be derived from a "self" antigen. Thus psoriasis could be an "immune-appropriate" response to an unidentified pathogen or it could be an autoimmune reaction to a normal human protein. In either event, therapeutic intervention, particularly with lymphocyte cytotoxic agents, would reduce or remove effector T-cell clones from affected skin regions and thus remove the inciting stimulus for the regenerative epidermal response.

ACKNOWLEDGMENTS

This research was supported in part by a General Clinical Research Center grant (M01-RR00102) from the National Center for Research Resources at the National Institutes of Health; by a FIRST Award (CA54215) from the National Institutes of Health; by Grant GM42461 from the National Institutes of Health; by a training grant (T32 AR07525) from the National Institutes of Health (NIAMS) to the Laboratory for Investigative Dermatology and to the Department of Dermatology at Cornell University Medical Center; by a small instrumentation grant (ISI5-GM45521-01) from the National Institutes of Health to The Rockefeller University, the Carl J. Herzog Foundation, the American Skin Association, and the Carson Family Charitable Trust; and by a gift from Ms. Sue Weil.

REFERENCES

1. Weinstein, G.D., and Krueger, J.G. (1993). An overview of psoriasis. In *Therapy of Moderate-to-Severe Psoriasis*, G.D. Weinstein and A.B. Gottlieb (Eds). National Psoriasis Foundation, Portland, OR, pp. 1–22.
2. Paukkonen, K., Naukkarinen, A., and Horsmanheimo, M. (1992). The development of manifest psoriatic lesions is linked with the invasion of CD8+ T cells and CD11c+ macrophages into the epidermis. *Arch. Dermatol. Res.* 284:375–379.
3. Onuma, A. (1994). Immunohistochemical studies of infiltrating cells in early and chronic lesions of psoriasis. *J. Dermatol.* 21:223–232.
4. Bos, J.D., Hagenaars, C., Das, P.K., Krieg, S.R., Voorn, W.J., and Kapsenberg, M.L. (1989). Predominance of "memory" T cells (CD4+, CDw29+) over "naive" T cells (CD4+, CD45R+) in both normal and diseased human skin. *Arch. Dermatol. Res.* 281:24–30.
5. Vallat, V.P., Gilleaudeau, P., Battat, L., Wolfe, J., Nabeya, R., Heftler, N., Hodak, E., Gottlieb, A.B., and Krueger, J.G. (1994). PUVA bath therapy strongly suppresses immunological and epidermal activation in psoriasis: a possible cellular basis for remittive therapy. *J. Exp. Med.* 180:283–296.
6. Jones, J.L., Berth-Jones, J., Fletcher, A., and Hutchinson, P.E. (1994). Assessment of epidermal dendritic cell markers and T-lymphocytes in psoriasis. *J. Pathol.* 174:77–82.
7. Gottlieb, A.B., Lifshitz, B., Fu, S.M., Staiano-Coico, L., Wang, C.Y., and Carter, D.M. (1986). Expression of HLA-DR molecules by keratinocytes and presence of Langerhans cells in the dermal infiltrate of active psoriatic plaques. *J. Exp. Med.* 164:1013–1028.

8. Nestle, F.O., Turka, L.A., and Nickoloff, B.J. (1994). Characterization of dermal dendritic cells in psoriasis. Autostimulation of T lymphocytes and induction of Th1 type cytokines. *J. Clin. Invest.* 94:202–209.
9. Chang, J.C.C., Smith, L.R., Froning, K.J., Schwabe, B.J., Laxer, J.A., Caralli, L.L., Kurland, H.H., Karasek, M.A., Wilkinson, D.I., Carlo, D.J., and Brostoff, S.W. (1994). CD8+ T cells in psoriatic lesions preferentially use T-cell receptor Vβ3 and/or Vβ13.1 genes. *Proc. Natl. Acad. Sci. U.S.A.* 91:9282–9286.
10. Chang, J.C.C., Smith, L.R., Froning, K.J., Schwabe, B.J., Laxer, J.A., Caralli, L.L., Kurland, H.H., Karasek, M.A., Wilkinson, D.I., Carlo, D.J., and Brostoff, S.W. (1995). CD8+ T-cells in psoriatic lesions preferentially use T-cell receptors Vβ3 and/or Vβ13.1 genes. *Ann. N.Y. Acad. Sci.* 756:370–381.
11. Henseler, T., and Christophers, E. (1985). Psoriasis of early and late onset: characterization of two types of psoriasis vulgaris. *J. Am. Acad. Dermatol.* 13:450–456.
12. Baadsgaard, O., Fisher, G., Voorhees, J.J., and Cooper, K.D. (1990). The role of the immune system in the pathogenesis of psoriasis. *J. Invest. Dermtol.* 95: 32S–34S.
13. Menssen, A., Trommler, P., Vollmer, S., Schendel, D., Albert, E., Guertler, L., Riethmueller, G., and Prinz, J.C. (1995). Evidence for an antigenic-specific cellular immune response in skin lesions of patients with psoriasis vulgaris. *J. Immunol.* 155:4078–4083.
14. Leung, D.Y., Travers, J.B., Giorno, R., Norris, D.A., Skinner, R., Aelion, J., Kazemi, L.V., Kim, M.H., Trumble, A.E., Kotb, M., and Schlievert, P.M. (1995). Evidence for a streptococcal superantigen-driven process in acute guttate psoriasis. *J. Clin. Invest.* 96: 2106–2112.
15. Lewis, H.M., Baker, B.S., Bokth, S., Powles, A.V., Garioch, J.J., Valdimarsson, H., and Fry, L. (1993). Restricted T-cell receptor Vβ gene usage in the skin of patients with guttate and chronic plaque psoriasis. *Br. J. Dermatol.* 129:514–520.
16. Valdimarsson, H., Baker, B.S., Jonsdottir, I., Powles, A., and Fry, L. (1995). Psoriasis: a T-cell-mediated autoimmune disease induced by streptococcal superantigens? *Immunol. Today* 16:145–149.
17. Mansbridge, J.N., and Knapp, A.M. (1987). Changes in keratinocyte maturation during wound healing. *J. Invest. Dermatol* 89:253–263.
18. Hertle, M.D., Kubler, M-D., Leigh, I.M., and Watt, F.M. (1992). Aberrant integrin expression during epidermal wound healing and in psoriatic epidermis. *J. Clin. Invest.* 89:1892–1901.
19. McKay, I.A., and Leigh, I.M. (1995). Altered keratinocyte growth and differentiation in psoriasis. *Clin. Dermatol.* 13:105–114.
20. Weinstein, G.D. (1987). Epidermal cell kinetics. In *Dermatology in General Medicine*. T.B. Fitzpatrick, A.Z. Eisen, K. Wolff, I.M. Freedberg, and K.F. Austen (Eds.). McGraw-Hill, New York, pp. 154–165.
21. Wood, L.C., Jackson, S.M., Elias, P.M., Grunfeld, C., and Feingold, K.R. (1992). Cutaneous barrier perturbation stimulates cytokine production in the epidermis of mice. *J. Clin. Invest.* 90:482–487.
22. Braunstein, S., Kaplan, G., Gottlieb, A.B., Schwartz, M., Walsh, G., Abalos, R.M., Fajardo, T.T., Guido, L.S., and Krueger, J.G. (1994). GM-CSF activates regenerative epidermal growth and stimulates keratinocyte proliferation in human skin in vivo. *J. Invest. Dermatol.* 103:601–604.
23. Vassar, R., and Fuchs, E. (1991). Transgenic mice provide new insights into the role of TGF-alpha during epidermal development and differentiation. *Genes Dev.* 5:714–727.
24. Guo, L., Yu, Q-C., and Fuchs, E. (1993). Targeting expression of keratinocyte growth factor to keratinocytes elicits striking changes in epithelial differentiation in transgenic mice. *EMBO J.* 12:973–986.
25. Choi, Y., and Fuchs, E. (1990). TGF-β and retinoic acid: regulators of growth and modifiers of differentiation in human epidermal cells. *Cell Regul.* 1:791–809.
26. Staiano-Coico, L., Krueger, J.G., Rubin, J.S., D'limi, S., Vallat, V.P., Valentino, L., Fahey, T., III, Hawes, A., Kingston, G., Madden, M.R., Mathwich, M., Gottlieb, A.B., and Aaronson, S.A. (1993). Human keratinocyte growth factor effects in a porcine model of epidermal wound healing. *J. Exp. Med.* 178:865–878.
27. Krueger, J.G., Staiano-Coico, L., Smoller, B., Anzilotti, M., Vallat, V.P., Gilleaudeau, P., and Gottlieb, A.B. (1995). Endogenous growth factor pathways may regulate epidermal hyperplasia in chronic venous wounds: modulation by hydrocolloid dressings. In *Wound Healing and Skin Physiology*. P. Altmeyer et al. (Ed.). Springer-Verlag, Berlin, pp. 285–302.
28. Hodak, E., Gottlieb, A.B., Anzilotti, M., and Krueger, J.G. (1996). The IGF-1 receptor is expressed by epithelial cells with proliferative potential in human epidermis and skin appendages: correlation of increased expression with regenerative epidermal growth. *J. Invest. Dermatol.* 106:564–570.
29. Krueger, G.G., Chambers, D.A., and Shelby, J. (1981). Involved and uninvolved skin from psoriatic subjects: are they equally diseased? Assessment by skin transplanted to congenitally athymic (nude) mice. *J. Clin. Invest.* 68:1548–1557.
30. Krueger, G.G., Manning, D.D., Malouf, J., and Ogden, B. (1975). Long-term maintenance of psoriatic human skin on congenitally athymic (nude) mice. *J. Invest. Dermatol.* 64:307–312.
31. Bata-Csorgo, Z., Hammerberg, C., Voorhees, J.J., and Cooper, K.D. (1995). Kinetics and regulation of human keratinocyte stem cell growth in short-term primary ex vivo culture. *J. Clin. Invest.* 95:317–327.

32. Carroll, J.M., Romero, M.R., and Watt, F.M. (1995). Suprabasal integrin expression in the epidermis of transgenic mice results in developmental defects and a phenotype resembling psoriasis. *Cell* 83:957–968.
33. Strange, P., Cooper, K.D., Hansen, E.R., Fisher, G., Larsen, J.K., Fox, D., Krag, C., Voorhees, J.J., and Baadsgaard, O. (1993). T-lymphocyte clones initiated from lesional psoriatic skin release growth factors that induce keratinocyte proliferation. *J. Invest. Dermatol.* 101:695–700.
34. Prinz, J.C., Gross, B., Vollmer, S., Trommler, P., Strobel, I., Meurer, M., and Plewig, G. (1994). T cell clones from psoriasis skin lesions can promote keratinocyte proliferation in vitro via secreted products. *Eur. J. Immunol.* 24:593–598.
35. Grossman, R.M., Krueger, J., Yourish, D., Granelli-Piperno, A., Murphy, D.P., May, L.T., Kupper, T.S., Sehgal, P.B., and Gottlieb, A.B. (1989). Interleukin-6 (IL-6) is expressed in high levels in psoriatic skin and stimulates proliferation of cultured human keratinocytes. *Proc. Natl. Acad. Sci. U.S.A.* 86:6367–6371.
36. Krueger, J.G., and Gottlieb, A.B. (1994). Growth factors, cytokines and eicosanoids. In *Psoriasis.* L. Dubertret (Ed.). ISED, Brescia, Italy, pp. 18–28.
37. Gottlieb, S.L., Gilleaudeau, P., Johnson, R., Estes, L., Woodworth, T.G., Gottlieb, A.B., and Krueger, J.G. (1995). Response of psoriasis to a lymphocyte-selective toxin (DAB_{389}IL-2) suggests a primary immune, but not keratinocyte, pathogenic basis. *Nature Med.* 1:442–447.
38. Krueger, J.G., Wolfe, J.T., Nabeya, R.T., Vallat, V.P., Gilleaudeau, P., Heftler, N.S., Austin, L.M., and Gottlieb, A.B. (1995). Successful ultraviolet B treatment of psoriasis is accompanied by a reversal of keratinocyte pathology and by selective depletion of intraepidermal T cells. *J. Exp. Med.* 182:2057–2068.
39. Johnson, R., Staiano-Coico, L., Austin, L., Cardinale, I., Nabeya-Tsukifuji, R., and Krueger, J.G. (1996). PUVA treatment selectively induces a cell cycle block and subsequent apoptosis in normal and malignant T-lymphocytes. *Photochem. Photobiol.* 63:566–571.
40. Ellis, C.N., Fradin, M.S., Messana, J.M., Brown, M.D., Siegel, M.T., Hartley, A.H., Rocher, L.L., Wheeler, S., Hamilton, T.A., Parish, T.G., Ellis-Madu, M., Duell, E., Annesley, T.M., Cooper, K.D., and Voorhees, J.J. (1991). Cyclosporine for plaque-type psoriasis. Results of a multidose, double-blind trial. *N. Engl. J. Med.* 324:277–284.
41. Wong, R.L., Winslow, C.M., and Cooper, K.D. (1993). The mechanisms of action of cyclosporin A. in the treatment of psoriasis. *Immunol. Today* 14:69–74.
42. Khandke, L., Ashinoff, R., Krueger, J.G., Krane, J., Staiano-Coico, L., Grossman, R., Murphy, D., Delaney, R., and Gottlieb, A.B. (1990). Effect of cyclosporin A on the regulation of signal transduction mechanisms in cultured keratinocytes. *J. Invest. Dermatol* 94:541 (abstract).
43. Khandke, L., Ashinoff, R., Krane, J.F., Staiano-Coico, L., Granelli-Piperno, A., Luster, A.D., Carter, D.M., Krueger, J.G., and Gottlieb, A.B. (1991). Cyclosporine in psoriasis treatment: inhibition of keratinocyte cell-cycle progression in G1 independent of effects on transforming growth factor-alpha/epidermal growth factor receptor pathways. *Arch. Dermatol.* 127: 1172–1179.
44. Gottlieb, A.B., Grossman, R.M., Khandke, L., Carter, D.M., Sehgal, P.B., Fu, S.M., Granelli-Piperno, A., Rivas, M., Barazani, L., and Krueger, J.G. (1992). Studies of the effect of cyclosporine in psoriasis in vivo: combined effects on activated T lymphocytes and epidermal regenerative maturation. *J. Invest. Dermtol.* 98: 302–309.
45. Petzelbauer, P., Stingl, G., Wolff, K., and Volc-Platzer, B. (1991). Cyclosporin A suppresses ICAM-1 expression by papillary endothelium in healing psoriatic plaques. *J. Invest. Dermatol.* 96:362–369.
46. Rosenbach, T., and Czarnetzki, B.M. (1994). Retinoids. In *Psoriasis.* L. Dubertret (Ed.). ISED, Brescia, Italy, pp. 151–161.
47. Gollnick, H., Bauer, R., Brindley, C., Orfanos, C.E., Plewig, G., Wokalek, H., and Hoting, E. (1988). Acitretin versus etretinate in psoriasis. *J. Am. Acad. Dermatol.* 19:458–469.
48. Gottlieb, S.L., Hayes, E., Gilleaudeau, P., Cardinale, I., Gottlieb, A.B., and Krueger, J.G. (1996). Cellular actions of etretinate in psoriasis: enhanced epidermal differentiation and reduced cell-mediated inflammation are unexpected outcomes. *J. Cutan. Pathol.* 23: 404–418.
49. Rizova, H., Nicolas, J.-F., Morel, P., Kanitakis, J., Demidem, A., Revillard, J.-P., Wijdenes, J., Thivolet, J., and Schmitt, D. (1994). The effect of anti-CD4 monoclonal antibody treatment on immunological changes in psoriatic skin. *J. Dermatol. Sci.* 7:1–13.
50. Weinshenker, B.G., Bass, B.H., Ebers, G.C., and Rice, G.P.A. (1989). Remission of psoriatic lesions with uromonab-CD3 (Orthoclone OKT3) treatment. *J. Am. Acad. Dermatol.* 20:1132–1133.
51. Ackerman, C., Abu-Elaqd, K., Venkataramanan, K., Fung, J., Todo, S., Starzl, T., and Jegasothy, B. (1991). Recalcitrant psoriasis and pyoderma gangrenosum treated with Fk506. *J. Invest. Dermatol.* 96:536.
52. Eibschutz, B., Baird, S.M., Weisman, M.H., Amox, D.G., Spellman, M., Piacquadio, D., Carrera, C.J., and Carson, D.A. (1995). Oral 2-chlorodeoxyadenosine in psoriatic arthritis. A preliminary report. *Arthritis Rheum.* 38:1604–1609.
53. Nickoloff, B.J., and Naidu, Y. (1994). Perturbation of epidermal barrier function correlates with initiation of cytokine cascade in human skin. *J. Am. Acad. Dermatol.* 30:535–546.

54. Gottlieb, A.B., and Krueger, J.G. (1994). Role of T-lymphocytes. In *Psoriasis.* L. Dubertret (Ed.). ISED, Brescia, Italy, pp. 63–71.
55. Mitra, R.S., Judge, T.A., Nestle, F.O., Turka, L.A., and Nickoloff, B.J. (1995). Psoriatic skin-derived dendritic cell function is inhibited by exogenous IL-10. Differential modulation of B7-1 (CD80) and B7-2 (CD86) expression. *J. Immunol.* 154:2668–2677.
56. Nickolff, B.J., and Griffiths, C.E.M. (1990). Lymphocyte trafficking in psoriasis: a new perspective emphasizing the dermal dendrocyte with active dermal recruitment mediated via endothelial cells followed by intra-epidermal T-cell activation. *J. Invest. Dermatol.* 95:35S–37S.
57. de Jong, E.M.G., van Erp, P.E.J., van Vlijmen, I.M.J.J., and van de Kerkhof, P.C.M. (1992). The inter-relation between inflammation and epidermal proliferation in normal skin following epicutaneous application of leukotriene-B4—an immunohistochemical study. *Clin. Exp. Dermatol.* 17:413–420.
58. Gillitzer, R., Berger, R., Mielke, V., Muller, C., Wolff, K., and Stingl, G. (1991). Upper keratinocytes of psoriatic skin lesions express high levels of NAP-1/IL-8 mRNA in situ. *J. Invest. Dermatol.* 97:73–79.

20

Chemokines

Jens-Michael Schröder
University of Kiel, Kiel, Germany

Neutrophils constitute one of the most conspicuous cellular elements in the epidermal cellular infiltrate that characterizes psoriasis. This histological observation led to numerous studies in the past, where attempts were made to explain why neutrophils appear in the epidermal layer of active psoriatic lesions. Originally it was discussed whether chemotaxis is abnormal in psoriasis, but chemotactic migration of blood-derived neutrophils is only one part of the whole story. An understanding of data concerning chemotaxis of neutrophils in psoriasis requires at least a partial understanding of how neutrophil migration occurs in vivo.

Today we know that the first step of neutrophil tissue infiltration is the adherence of rolling neutrophils in postcapillary venules to the luminal side of the vessels. This process depends on the activation and expression of adhesion molecules of neutrophils near the locus of emigration. The next step is diapedesis followed by stimulated migration within the tissue directly toward the inflammatory focus. This can occur by real chemotactic migration along a gradient of soluble chemotactic and/or chemokinetic factors. On the other hand and possibly more likely, haptotactic migration is responsible for tissue immigration. Haptotaxis defines a stimulated migration along solid-phase gradients of chemoattractants (1). Finally, neutrophils would reach the locus where the stimulus is generated—in psoriasis, the upper epidermal layers.

CHEMOATTRACTANTS IN PSORIASIS

The presence of blood-borne neutrophils in the affected epidermis of psoriasis lesions implicates that within the epidermis attractants for neutrophils are generated. The original experiments by Langhof and Müller, who mixed psoriatic scales with fresh serum, revealed that under these conditions strong neutrophil chemotactic activity was indeed present (2). Later it was recognized that apart from the activity generated in serum after adding psoriatic scales, scale extracts exhibited heat-stable proteinaceous chemotactic activity, which derived from $C5a_{des\ arg}$ (3,4). Apart from $C5a_{des\ arg}$ lipid-like neutrophil attractants were reported to be present in lesional psoriatic scale material: The quantitatively dominating arachidonic acid–derived neutrophil attractant is 12-HETE (5). Interestingly, the 12(R)-isomer seems to represent the most prominent 12-HETE isomer in psoriasis (6). Since it has been shown to be more potent than 12(S)-HETE, it seems to be of importance in psoriasis. Apart from 12-HETE, the arachidonate 5-lipoxygenase product leukotriene B_4 (LTB_4) is also present in active psoriatic lesions as biologically active lipid (7,8). Furthermore, another structurally not characterized, lipid-like neutrophil attractant has been found ("compound X") in lesional psoriatic scales (9). Its significance for neutrophil recruitment as yet is speculative. All of these neutrophil chemotactic factors and activities are known to attract also other leukocytes, i.e., monocytes, eosinophils, and T lymphocytes. Thus these panleukotactic factors seem not to be solely responsible for neutrophil infiltration into the lesional epidermis of active psoriasis.

IDENTIFICATION OF NOVEL PROTEINACEOUS NEUTROPHIL ATTRACTANTS IN PSORIATIC SCALE EXTRACTS

The conclusion that panleukotactic factors cannot explain the appearance solely of neutrophils in the affected psoriatic skin led to the search for additional, rather neutrophil-selective attractants.

Originally IL-1 was suggested to be a neutrophil attractant (10,11). With the failure to demonstrate significant PMN-chemotactic activity in purified recombinant IL-1 preparations (12) and the development of modern analytical biochemical methods, it became clear that natural IL-1 or "ETAF" preparations were contaminated by a PMN attractant(s), which up to that time was not characterized.

By the use of gel chromatography together with PMN-chemotaxis and -degranulation assays, it could be shown that in extracts obtained from lesional psoriatic scales, apart from $C5a_{des\ arg}$, another proteinaceous attractant(s) was present (4,13). This was proven to be distinct from $C5a_{des\ arg}$ because responses to this chemotaxin, which was tentatively termed "anionic neutrophil activating peptide, ANAP" because of its relatively more anionic behavior than that of $C5a_{des\ arg}$, could not be desensitized by pretreatment with C5a indicating its cellular activation via a separate receptor (4). Similarly, it was shown that this activity could be separated from IL-1 activity by reversed-phase chromatography (13). Attempts to characterize the molecular nature of ANAP originally failed. However, biochemical behavior greatly resembled another and at that time novel proteinaceous neutrophil attractant, which was discovered in 1987 by several groups (14–16). This neutrophil chemotaxin, which was later termed interleukin-8, has been shown to have the unique property to preferentially attract neutrophils (14–16) and lymphocytes (17), but not monocytes and eosinophils (14,15).

Therefore, as a working hypothesis it was believed that ANAP obtained from lesional psoriatic scale could be identical with IL-8.

To test this working hypothesis directly we tried to biochemically purify ANAP by the use of modern HPLC techniques. Together with the use of neutrophil-chemotaxis assay systems to screen fractions and following the biological activity during all the purification steps, this systematic investigation should decrease the possibility of overlooking important biologically active neutrophil chemotactic proteins.

Indeed, in the beginning each HPLC fraction was screened for PMN-chemotactic activity at various dilutions ($1{:}5$–$1{:}10^6$), which guaranteed we would not overlook PMN attractants active only at very low concentrations and at restricted doses.

With this technique, using cation-exchange HPLC of crude extracts as the first step for purification, we identified several peaks of activity tentatively termed α-ANAPs and β-ANAPs (Fig. 1) (18).

After purification to homogeneity with several different reversed-phase-HPLC techniques (19), we could isolate three major 8–9-kDa polypeptides in sufficient amounts for amino-terminal sequencing.

THE CHEMOKINES IL-8 AND Gro_α ARE THE MAJOR NEUTROPHIL ATTRACTANTS IN LESIONAL PSORIATIC SCALES

Amino-terminal sequencing of purified ANAPs (Table 1) revealed that the predominant neutrophil attractant is β_1-ANAP. β_1-ANAP is identical with the 69 residues containing a form of IL-8 starting with glutaminic acid (single letter code: E) as amino-terminal amino acid (20). The 72 residues containing a form of IL-8 (so-called "monocyte-derived IL-8") starting with serine (single letter code: S) is usually present in smaller amounts (20). Apart from these two forms of IL-8, there is evidence that C-terminal truncation products are also present (19). These compounds show less biological potency and apparently represent degradation products of IL-8 (19). Interestingly, both $[\text{Ser-IL-8}]_{72}$ and $[\text{Glu-IL-8}]_{69}$ retain full biological activity (20). This is believed to be due to the presence of the Glu-Leu-Arg motif in the amino-terminus, which seems to contribute importantly to the neutrophil-chemotactic activity of IL-8. A loss of this motif or parts of it drastically reduces the biological activity of IL-8 (21).

Thus IL-8 can be isolated as a biologically active form from psoriatic lesions.

The catabolism of IL-8 in psoriatic lesions as yet is not well studied. The presence of high amounts of biologically active material in psoriatic lesions makes it likely that either production of IL-8 is high or catabolism is low or both. There is some evidence that

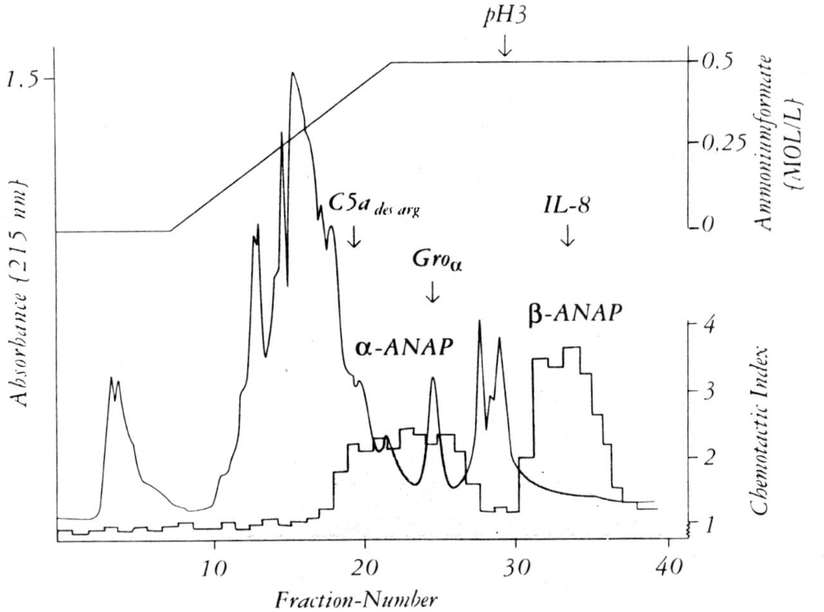

Figure 1 Identification of neutrophil-chemotactic chemokines by cation exchange HPLC of psoriatic scale extracts. Neutrophil chemotactic activity was determined in each fraction of the CM-cation-exchange-HPLC column. Peaks were indicated by the tentative terms α-ANAP and β-ANAP. For comparison elution positions for authentic $C5a_{des\ arg}$, Gro_α and $[Ser\text{-}IL\text{-}8]_{72}$ are indicated.

indeed the catabolism of IL-8 seems to be low. Treatment with several proteolytic enzymes including elastase does not destroy biological activity, although some truncation occurs (22).

Interestingly, an aminopeptidase seen in the plasma of patients with familial mediterranean fever is capable of cleaving IL-8 and destroying its activity (23). Whether this aminopeptidase is important in psoriasis as yet is unknown. Nevertheless a combination of affinity chromatography, HPLC analyses, and electrospray ionization mass spectrometry (ESI-MS) revealed that products bind to the anti-IL-8 column with low affinity. Upon SDS-PAGE, these products revealed M_r's near 4–5 kDa. N-terminal sequencing was not successful, indicating a blocked amino-terminus (our unpublished results). ESI-MS analyses revealed masses, which are in accordance with IL-8 fragments being N-terminally and C-terminally truncated, containing opened disulfide bridges and acetate at the N-terminus (A.I. Mallet and J.-M. Schröder, unpublished observation). Further studies are necessary to prove the hypothesis that these compounds represent degradation products of IL-8.

Apart from the different forms of IL-8, another 8-kDa proteinaceous neutrophil attractant termed α_2-ANAP was purified from lesional psoriatic scale extracts to homogeneity. Its N-terminal sequence showed similarity but not identity with that of IL-8 (Table 1). Comparison with sequences reported in the EMBL data bank revealed identity with so-called "melanoma growth stimulatory activity, MGSA" (24)

Table 1 N-Terminal Sequence Analysis and Relative Molecular Masses of Psoriatic Scale-Derived Extracts

Chemokine	Sequence[a]	M_r[b]
β_1-ANAP	ELRXQX	8.0
β_{2a}-ANAP	SAKELRXQX	8.5
β_{2b}-ANAP	AVLPRSAKELR	9.0
β_3-ANAP	ELRXQXL	6.0
β_4-ANAP	SAKELRXQXL	6.5
$[Ala\text{-}IL\text{-}8]_{77}$	AVLPRSAKELRCQCL. . .	9.0
α_{1a}-ANAP	ASVATELRXQXL. . .	8.0
α_{1b}-ANAP	ASVATELRXQXL. . .	8.1
α_2-ANAP	XXVATELRXQXL. . .	8.0
Gro_α	ASVATELRCQCL. . .	8.1

[a]The single-letter code for amino acids was used.
[b]M_r's were determined by high-resolution SDS-PAGE analysis as described (20,28,41).

as well as the gene product of the oncogene Gro_α (25). MGSA/Gro_α in addition to IL-8 is a member of the C–X–C chemokine family. This chemokine also contains the ELR motif in the amino-terminus and therefore it was expected to be a neutrophil attractant (26). In the MGSA/Gro_α form we isolated from psoriatic scales we could not identify the first two amino acids (20). Similarly, in a so-called "16-kDa form of MGSA" both N-terminal amino acids could not be characterized (27). Therefore, we believe that both forms are identical—despite the difference of the M_r. This might be due to known aggregation of chemokines, which often occurs when lyophilized samples are used in an usual SDS-PAGE system instead of the Tricene/Tris system (20,28).

More recently we purified two additional ANAPs to homogeneity. These ANAPs, termed α_{1a}-ANAP and α_{ab}-ANAP, were found to have identical biological behavior as seen for α_2-ANAP = 16-kDa MGSA. Indeed, microsequencing revealed that both forms showed an identical N-terminal sequence reported for Gro_α (Table 1). Unlike α_2-ANAP, both N-terminal amino acids could be identified as alanine and serine. Therefore, three biochemically different forms of Gro_α are present in pooled lesional scales. Upon SDS-PAGE analysis, all three forms of Gro_α show M_r's near 8 kDa. Therefore, C-terminal truncation of Gro_α seems not to be a reason for these phenomena. ESI-MS analyses of these three purified psoriasis-derived Gro_α forms revealed differences in mass, which cannot be explained by simple C-terminal truncation, whereas a single species could be detected by identity of its mass with that expected theoretically. Others show masses that cannot be explained simply by C-terminal truncation and/or 0-derivatization (A.I. Mallet and J.-M. Schröder, unpublished results). It cannot be excluded that a genetic polymorphism of Gro_α does exist, which is visible for us owing to the use of pooled lesional psoriatic scales.

ROLE OF OTHER α-CHEMOKINES AS NEUTROPHIL ATTRACTANTS IN PSORIASIS

Apart from IL-8 and Gro_α in its various forms, other neutrophil-attracting chemokines such as Gro_β, Gro_γ, ENA-78, NAP-2, and GCP-2 (for structures see Fig. 2) could be of relevance in psoriatic lesions.

In attempts to identify these chemokines in lesional psoriatic scale extracts, we first depleted these extracts from IL-8 by the use of an anti-IL-8 affinity column.

We then separated these IL-8-depleted extracts by a heparin-HPLC column. Chemokines are well known to bind to heparin (29), and therefore with this approach it should be possible to identify minor heparin-binding neutrophil-attracting chemokines. After preparative reversed-phase HPLC, apart from neutrophil-chemotactic activity coming from traces of remaining IL-8, an additional broad peak of activity was seen. This activity could be separated into three distinct peaks by analytical RP-HPLC all giving the identical sequence of Gro_α (Fig. 3). In the case of Gro_β or Gro_γ one would have expected different amino acids at positions 2, 3, and 4, respectively (see Fig. 2).

So far we have no evidence for secretion of Gro_β and Gro_γ in biologically significant amounts. This finding contrasts with molecular biological studies using RT-PCR techniques: In that case overexpression of both Gro_β and Gro_γ mRNA has been seen in psoriatic lesions (30). Obviously translation of these genes is not efficient in psoriatic lesions.

Because no other heparin-binding attractants are detectable, it is concluded that neither ENA-78 nor NAP-2 and GCP-2 are important for neutrophil attraction in psoriasis.

ENA-78 originally was detected in a lung epithelial cell line (31) and later in lung diseases (32). NAP-2 represents a truncation product of platelet basic protein (33). We have no evidence for release of platelet proteins in lesional epidermal skin of psoriatics. Therefore, the failure to identify NAP-2 in psoriatic skin is not unexpected.

GCP-2 so far has been isolated only from a tumor cell line (34). As yet there is no evidence for its involvement in neutrophil accumulation in diseases.

CELLULAR ORIGIN OF NEUTROPHIL-ACTIVATING CHEMOKINES IN PSORIASIS

The presence of huge amounts of biologically active IL-8 and Gro_α in psoriatic scales points toward its cellular origin within the epidermis. The most likely cellular source appears to be keratinocytes. This is proven by in situ hybridization experiments using both IL-8 and Gro_α riboprobes: When IL-8 mRNA expression was investigated in biopsies from active psoriasis lesions, a marked focal expression of IL-8 mRNA was seen in the upper parts of the epidermis (35). In some cases IL-8 mRNA expression is visible exactly where microabscesses are located. This finding can be interpreted by secretion of IL-8 by keratinocytes together

```
                        1     10         20         30          40          50        60         70
IL-8          AVLPRSAKELRCQCIKTYSKPFHP-KFIKELRVIES-GPHCANTEIIVKL-SDGRELCLDPKENWVQR-VVEKFLKRAENS
NAP-2                AELRCMCIKTTSG-IHP-KNIQSLEVIGK-GTHCNQVEVIATL-KDGRKICLDPDAPRIKK-IVQKKLAGDESAD
MGSA/gro α      ASVATELRCQCLQTLQG-IHP-KNIQSVMVKSP-GPHCAQTEVIATL-KNGRKACLNPASPIVKK-IIEKMLNSDKSN
Gro ß           ASPL ——————————— L —————K ——————————————————— Q ————————M ———————— KNG ——
Gro γ           ASVA———————————— L ———————R ————————————————— K ——————— MVQ————————ILNKGSTN
ENA 78        AGPAAAVLRELRCVCLQTTQG-VHP-KMISNLQVFAI-GPQCSKVEVVASL-KNGKEICLDPEAPFLKKVIQKILDGGNKEN
GCP-2         GPVSAVLTELRCTCLRVTLR...
IP-10           VPLSRTVRCTCISISNQPVNP-RSLEKLEIIPA-SQFCPRVEIIATMKKKGEKRCLNPESKAIKN-LL-KAVSKEMSKRSP
MIG             TPVVRKGRCSCISTNQGTIHL-QSLKDLKQFAP-SPSCEKIEI-IATLKNGVQTCLNPDSADVKELIKKWEKQVSQK...
PF-4           EAEEDGDLQCLCVKTTSQ-VRP-RHITSLEVIKA-GPHCPTAQLIATL-KDGRKICLDLQAPLYKK-II-KKLLES


MIP-1α            ADTPTAC-CFSYTSRQI-PQNFIAD-Y-FETSSQ-CSKP-GVIFLTKRSRQVCADPSEEWVQKYV--SDLELSA
MIP-1ß         APMGSDPPTSC-CFSYTARKL-PHNFVVD-Y-YETSSL-CSQP-AVVFQTKRGKQVCADPSESWVQEYV--YDLELN
MCP-1/MCAF     QPDAINAPVTC-CYNFTNRKI-SVQRLAS-YRRITSSK-CPKE-AVIFKTIVAKEICADPKQKWVQDSM--DHLDKQTQTPKT
MCP-2          QPDSVSIPITC-CFNVINRKI-PIQRLES-YTRITNIQ-CPKE-AVIFKT--GKEVCADPKERWVRDSMKHLDQIFQNLKP
MCP-3          QPDSVSIPITC-CFNVINRKI-PKQRLES-YRRTTSSH-CPRE-AVIF-K--DKEICADPTQKWVQDFMKHLDKKTQTPKL
Eotaxin        GPASV--PTTC-CFNLANRKI-PLQRLES-YRRITSGK-CPQK-AVIFKTKLAKDICADPKKKWVQDSMKYLDQKSPTPKP
RANTES          SPYSSDTTPC-CFAYIARPL-PRAHIKE-Y-FYTSGK-CSNPAVVF-VTRKNRQVCANPEKKWVREYI--NSLEMS
```

Figure 2 Amino acid sequences of α-chemokines and β-chemokines. The single letter code of amino acids was used.

with attraction of PMN toward the focus. Alternatively, PMN itself can represent a cellular origin of IL-8 mRNA.

This hypothesis is supported by recent observations that neutrophils can indeed produce their own attractant (36). Although amounts are low compared to other cellular sources, its significance could be high due to accumulation of masses of PMNs in the tissue.

Most likely we have IL-8 mRNA expression in psoriasis lesions by both keratinocytes and PMN. Whether both cell types secrete IL-8 is as yet speculative.

Apart from immediate IL-8 synthesis after gene expression, there is some evidence that in normal epidermis IL-8-like immunoreactivity is stored, which is released in active psoriatic lesions (37). The exact molecular nature of this IL-8 immunoreactivity is not yet well characterized but we have some evidence that it is stored in a high-molecular-weight complexed form lacking PMN-chemotactic activity. Possibly by enzymatic processes under inflammatory conditions biologically active IL-8 is released.

Similar to IL-8 mRNA of Gro_α is overexpressed in psoriatic lesions and localized focally in upper parts of the epidermal layer in active psoriasis (38). When serial specimens of a single biopsy were investigated for IL-8 and Gro_α mRNA expression, it became clear that both are colocalized, indicating that both chemokines are synthesized by identical cellular sources (38). Whether preformed Gro_α also exists in normal skin is as yet speculative, although some evidence supports this hypothesis (39).

The amounts of IL-8 and Gro_α present in psoriatic scale extracts are similar. Approximately 3 ng/mg scale of both biologically active chemokines was found when HPLC plus bioassay was used for estimation (20). When supernatants of appropriately stimulated monocytes (26), endothelial cells (40), or fibroblasts (41) were analyzed for the presence of both IL-8 and Gro_α, in all cases approximately 10-fold higher amounts of IL-8 than that of Gro_α were found. Although normal keratinocytes can produce IL-8 upon appropriate stimulation, it is difficult to detect biologically active Gro_α under these conditions (42). Therefore, in psoriasis lesions either particular conditions do exist, which preferentially activate Gro_α gene expression and release, or preferential liberation of preformed material occurs. Further studies are necessary to clarify this point.

Maximum stimulation of normal keratinocytes to produce IL-8 occurs with phorbolesters (42).

Although cytokines such as TNF-α or IL-1 induce IL-8 gene expression in normal keratinocytes (43,44), there is only sparse release of biologically active protein. Therefore, it needs to be determined whether other endogenous mediators exist, which, similar to phorbolester, induce a massive production of IL-8 and possibly also of Gro_α.

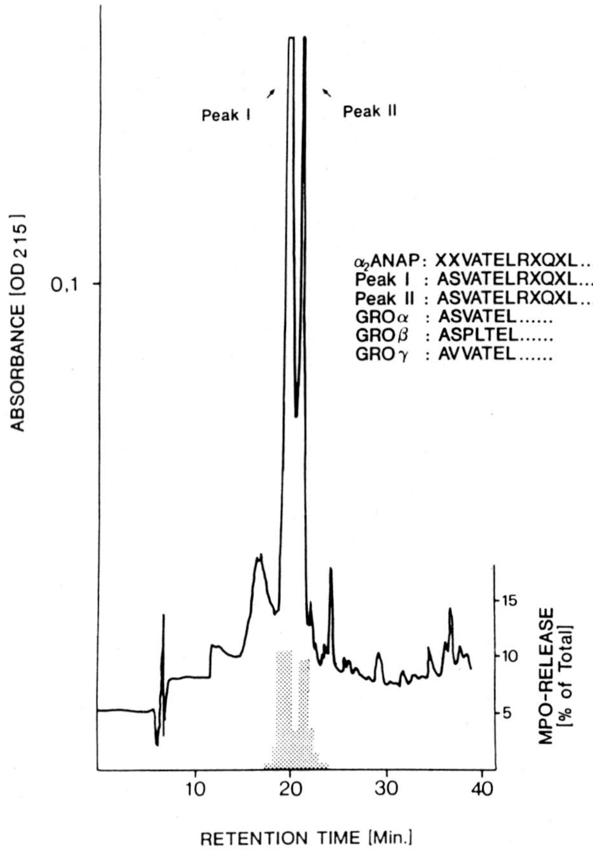

Figure 3 Identification of two additional neutrophil attractants in psoriatic scale extracts. Chemotactic activity in α-ANAP fractions of cation-exchange HPLC was finally purified by RP-4-reversed phase HPLC. Chemotactic activity is shown in the shaded area. Note the presence of two biochemically distinct peaks, which show the same N-terminal sequence (inset).

ROLE OF OTHER α-CHEMOKINES IN PSORIASIS

Neutrophil-activating chemokines are known to contain the Glu-Leu-Arg (ELR) motif, which is absent in the C–X–C chemokines platelet factor 4 (PF-4), γ-interferon-inducible protein 10 (IP-10), and a monokine induced by γ-interferon (MIG) (Fig. 2).

Whereas PF-4 is absent in lesional scale material containing no serum components, there is strong evidence that IP-10 plays a role in psoriasis: the IP-10 gene originally was discovered as a gene transcriptionally regulated by γ-interferon (45). Major IP-10-producing cells appeared to be keratinocytes and macrophages (46). In delayed immune responses in human skin, staining for IP-10 immunoreactivity was seen in endothelial cells, in macrophages, and to a strong extent in basal keratinocytes. It is believed that the dermal T-lymphocyte infiltrate is responsible for the expression of IP-10.

In psoriatic plaques, similarly strong expression of IP-10 in the basal layer is visible (46). Also in that case the lymphocyte tissue infiltrate seems to be the inducer of IP-10 production by release of γ-interferon.

Previous studies have shown that recombinant IP-10 is a potent chemotactic factor preferentially for CD4+ T lymphocytes (47). Thus it could be important in explaining at least part of the dermal CD4+–T-lymphocyte infiltrate. More recently it has been hypothesized that IP-10 explains the epidermotropism of cutaneous T-cell lymphoma (48). This idea came from the observation that IP-10 overexpression was seen in epidermal keratinocytes overlying the lymphomatous infiltrates. Apart from its possible role in regulation of CD4+–T-lymphocyte migration into skin, IP-10 may play a role in regulating angiogenesis: It was shown that ELR-motif-containing C–X–C chemokines like IL-8, Gro, and ENA-78 have angiogenic properties (49). Wound-associated angiogenesis is locally transient and tightly controlled. This observation led to the detection of a proteinaceous inhibitor of IL-8- and b-FGF-induced angiogenesis, which was found to be identical with IP-10 (50).

Human MIG represents a more recently described C–X–C chemokine, originally discovered by differential screening of a cDNA library prepared from lymphokine-activated macrophages (51). rMIG is able to activate Ca^{2+} fluxes in T lymphocytes and seems to be an attractant for activated T lymphocytes (52). Thus this chemokine could also play a role in T-cell trafficking into skin. So far no data are available on whether MIG is generated in the skin.

ROLE OF β-CHEMOKINES IN PSORIASIS

β-Chemokines (Fig. 2) have been reported to show selective or preferential chemotactic properties for monocytes, T lymphocytes and subsets, eosinophils, and basophils (Table 2, for review see 53–55), but not for neutrophils. Therefore, members of this chemokine subfamily are attractive candidates for explaining disease-specific mononuclear cell and/or eosinophil infiltrates. Depending on the disease stage, psoriatic lesions show apart from the characteristic neutrophil

Table 2 Chemotactic Properties of Chemokines

Chemokine	Major chemotactic activities	Minor chemotactic activities	Not active
IL-8	PMN	T-Ly, Bas	MØ, Eo
Gro_{α}	PMN	T-Ly	MØ, Eo
Gro_{β}	PMN	T-Ly	MØ, Eo
Gro_{γ}	PMN	T-Ly	MØ, Eo
NAP-2	PMN	T-Ly?	MØ, Eo
ENA-78	PMN	T-Ly	MØ, Eo
GCP-2	PMN	?	?
PF-4	—	PMN	MØ, Eo
IP-10	T-Ly	MØ	PMN
MIG	T-Ly	?	PMN
MIP-1a	CD-8-T-Ly	MØ	PMN, Eo
MIP-1β	CD-4-T-Ly	MØ	PMN, Eo
MCP-1	MØ, T-Ly, Bas		PMN
MCP-2	MØ, T-Ly, Bas	Eo	PMN
MCP-3	MØ, Eo, Bas	T-Ly	PMN
RANTES	memory-T-Ly, MØ		PMN
Eotaxin	Eo	?	PMN, MØ, T-Ly
Lymphotactin	T-Ly	?	PMN, MØ

infiltrate also an epidermal infiltration by CD8+ T lymphocytes and dermal infiltration by CD4+ T lymphocytes (56). Therefore, one could speculate whether β-chemokines are involved in T-lymphocyte tissue migration.

MIP-1α has been reported to preferentially attract CD8+ T lymphocytes. So far there is no evidence that MIP-1α is released within psoriatic lesions. This was proven by investigating crude psoriatic scale extracts as well as RP-HPLC-fractions for MIP-1α-immunoreactivity using a specific MIP-1α ELISA, where we did not detect any activity (our unpublished results). We obtained similar findings for MIP-1β. In support of these observations, in situ hybridization experiments using antisense MIP-1α- and MIP-1β-riboprobes so far have not shown any expression of its mRNA (R. Kulke, unpublished results).

Macrophages are known to accumulate near the basal cell layer of the epidermis in psoriasis. These lining cells could be attracted by selective monocyte/macrophage chemotaxins. In a recent study Gillitzer and co-workers (57) were able to show that in active psoriasis MCP-1 mRNA is expressed in basal keratinocytes, exactly close to the macrophages, thus making it attractive to speculate that MCP-1 is indeed released from basal keratinocytes and possibly is responsible for monocyte attraction. So far we have no evidence that biologically active MCP-1 is indeed released within the psoriatic lesion.

When we analyzed psoriatic scale extracts for the presence of monocyte attractants, we found that in the heparin-binding protein fraction after RP-HPLC only $C5a_{des\ arg}$ could be identified as a monocyte attractant (58). Although there seems to be some immunoreactive MCP-1 present in HPLC fractions, there is no evidence for biologically active MCP-1 (59).

A number of C–C chemokines are known to be preferential or selective attractants for eosinophils. The most prominent factors are RANTES (60), monocyte-chemotactic protein 3 (MCP-3) (61) as well as eotaxin (62,63). In psoriasis there is no evidence for a prominent eosinophil infiltrate in the epidermis. Thus it would be interesting to know whether or not eosinophil-attracting chemokines are present in psoriasis. We therefore have investigated lesional psoriatic scale extracts for the presence of both eosinophil-chemotactic activity and immunoreactive RANTES (detectable by an ELISA).

In numerous investigations where we tested extracts obtained from 50-g amounts each after heparin-sepharose chromatography and separation of bound proteins by RP-HPLC, we were not able to see any-eosinophil-chemotactic activity as well as iRANTES in HPLC fractions (Fig. 4).

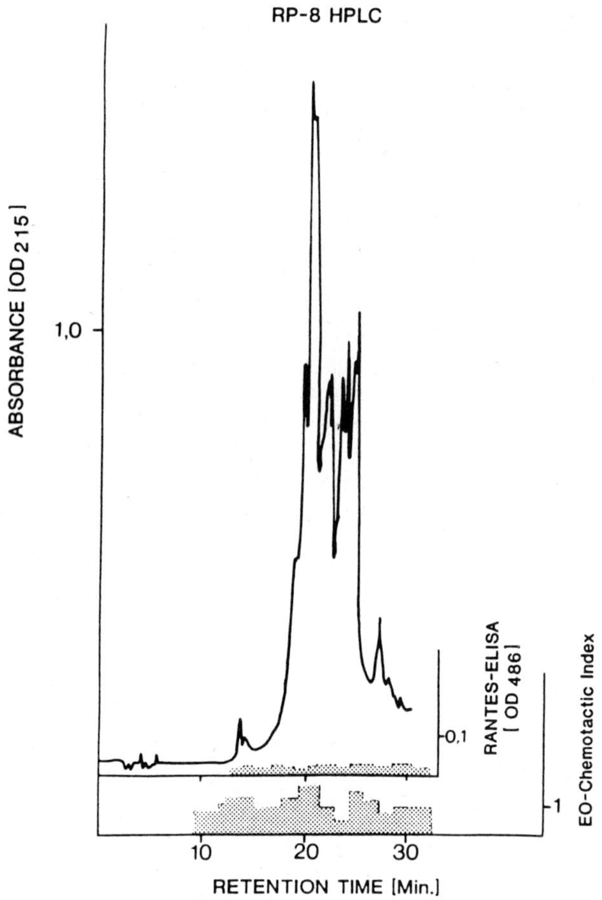

Figure 4 Absence of eosinophil-chemotactic activity and immunoreactive RANTES in heparin-bound psoriasis-derived proteins. Lower panel, eosinophil chemotactic activity (shaded area); upper panel, results of a specific RANTES ELISA.

Thus, eosinophil-chemotactic chemokines are absent in psoriatic lesions. In contrast, we were able to find eosinophil chemotactic activity in extracts of scales obtained from skin diseases with known tissue eosinophilia such as drug reaction and atopic dermatitis (64). This activity could be identified as chemokine RANTES (64).

SUMMARY

Chemokines represent a novel family of leukocyte-selective or specific chemotactic cytokines. Among the two branches of this family (α- or C–X–C chemokines, β- or C–C chemokines) members of the α-chemokine family are neutrophil-selective attractants without having activity for monocytes or eosinophils. In contrast, β-chemokines mainly act on monocytes, T lymphocytes, basophils, and eosinophils, but not neutrophils. Thus α-chemokines rather than β-chemokines are attractive candidate mediators explaining neutrophil accumulation in active psoriatic lesions. There is strong biochemical evidence that indeed α-chemokines IL-8 and Gro_α represent the predominant neutrophil-selective proteinaceous attractants in psoriatic lesions. On the other hand, monocyte-chemotactic β-chemokines appear to be of less importance in the upper part of affected skin.

Eosinophil chemotactic chemokines are absent in lesional skin material thus supporting the finding that eosinophils are also absent in lesional psoriatic skin.

The presence of high amounts of the α-chemokines IL-8 and Gro_α led us to speculate about a significant contribution of both chemokines to the inflammatory response in active psoriatic lesions.

REFERENCES

1. Rot, A (1992). The role of leukocyte chemotaxis in inflammation. In *Biochemistry of Inflammation.* J.T. Whicher and S.W. Evans (Eds.). Kluver Academic Publisher, Dordrecht, Netherlands, pp. 271–304.
2. Langhof, H., and Müller, H. (1966). Eigenschaften von Psoriasisschuppen. *Hautarzt* 3:101–104.
3. Tagami, H., and Ofuji, S. (1977). Characterization of a leukotactic factor derived from psoriatic scale. *Br. J. Dermatol.* 97:509–518.
4. Schröder, J.-M., and Christophers, E. (1986). Identification of $C5a_{des\ arg}$ and an anionic neutrophil-activating peptide (ANAP) in psoriatic scales. *J. Invest. Dermatol.* 87:53–58.
5. Hammarström, S., Hamberg, M., Samuelsson, B., et al. (1975). Increased concentrations of nonesterified arachidonic acid, 12-L-hydroxy-5,8,10,14-eicosatetraenoic acid, prostaglandin E_2 and prostaglandin F_2 in epidermis of psoriasis. *Proc. Natl. Acad. Sci. U.S.A.* 72:5130–5134.
6. Woollard, P.M. (1986). Stereochemical difference between 12-hydroxy-5,8,10,14-eicosatetraenoic acid (12 HETE) in platelets and psoriatic lesions. *Biochem. Biophys. Res. Commun.* 136:169–173.
7. Brain, S., Camp, R., Dowd, P., et al. (1984). The release of leukotriene B_4-like material in biologically active amounts from the lesional skin of patients with psoriasis. *J. Invest. Dermatol.* 83:70–73.
8. Fogh, K., Herlin, T., and Kragballe, K. (1989). Eicosanoids in acute and chronic psoriatic lesion. Leukotriene B_4 but not 12-hydroxy-eicosatetraenoic acid is present in biologically active concentrations in acute guttate lesion. *J. Invest. Dermatol.* 92:837–841.

9. Camp, R.D.R., Cunningham, F.M., Fincham, N.J., et al. (1988). Psoriatic skin lesions contain a novel lipid neutrophil chemokinetic eicosanoids. *Br. J. Pharmacol.* 94:1043–1050.
10. Sauder, D.N., Mounessa, N.L., Katz, S.I., et al. (1984). Chemotactic cytokines: The role of leukotactic pyrogen and epidermal cell thymocyte activating factor in neutrophil chemotaxis. *J. Immunol.* 132:828–832.
11. Luger, T.A., Charon, J.A., Colot, M., et al. (1983). Chemotactic properties of partially purified human epidermal cell-derived thymocyte-activating factor (ETAF) for polymorphonuclear and mononuclear cells. *J. Immunol.* 131:816–820.
12. Georgilis K., Schäfer, C., Dinarello, C.A., and Klempner, M.S. (1987). Human recombinant interleukin 1β has no effect of intracellular calcium or on functional responses of human neutrophils. *J. Immunol.* 139: 3403–3407.
13. Fincham, N.J., Camp, R.D.R., Gearing, A.J.H., et al. (1988). Neutrophil chemoattractant and Il-1-like activity in samples from psoriatic lesions: further characterization. *J. Immunol.* 140:4294–4299.
14. Schröder, J.-M., Mrowietz, U., Morita, E., and Christophers, E. (1987). Purification and partial biochemical characterization of a human monocyte-derived neutrophil-activating peptide that lacks interleukin 1 activity. *J. Immunol.* 139:3474–3483.
15. Yoshimura, T., Matsushima, K., Tanake, S., et al. (1987). Purification of a human monocyte-derived neutrophil chemotactic factor that shares sequence homology with other host defense cytokines. *Proc. Natl. Acad. Sci. U.S.A.* 84:9233–9237.
16. Walz, A., Peveri, P., Aschauer, H., and Baggiolini, M. (1987). Purification and amino acid sequencing of NAF, a novel neutrophil activating factor produced by monocytes. *Biochem. Biophys. Res. Commun.* 149: 755–761.
17. Gronhoj-Larsen, C. Anderson, A.O., Apella, E., Oppenheim, J.J., and Matsushima, K. (1989). The neutrophil-activating protein (NAP-1) is also chemotactic for T lymphocytes. *Science* 243:1464–1467.
18. Schröder, J.M. (1991). Biochemical and biological characterization of NAP-1/IL-8 related cytokines in lesional Psoriatic scale. In *Chemotactic Cytokines.* J. Westwick, S. Kunkel, and R.D.R. Camp (Eds.). Plenum Press, New York, pp. 97–107.
19. Schröder, J.M. (1992). Generation of NAP-1 and related peptides in psoriasis and other inflammatory skin diseases. In *Cytokines: Neutrophil-Activating Peptides and Other Chemotactic Cytokines.* M. Baggiolini, and C. Sorg (Eds.). Karger, Basel, pp. 54–76.
20. Schröder, J.-M., Gregory, H., Young, J., and Christophers, E. (1992). Neutrophil activating proteins in psoriasis. *J. Invest. Dermatol.* 98:241–247.
21. Hebert, C.A., Vitangcol, R.V., and Baker, J.B. (1991). Scanning mutagenesis of interleukin-8 identifies a cluster of residues required for receptor binding. *J. Biol. Chem.* 266:18989–18994.
22. Baggiolini, M., Dewald, B., and Walz, A. (1992). Interleukin-8 and related chemotactic cytokines. In *Inflammation: Basic Principles and Clinical Correlates*, 2nd ed. J.I. Gallin, I.M. Goldstein, and R. Synderman (Eds.). Raven Press, New York, pp. 247–262.
23. Ayesh, S.K., Azar, Y., Babior, B.M., and Matzner, Y. (1993). Inactivation of interleukin-8 by the C5a-inactivating protease from serosal fluid. *Blood* 81: 1424–1427.
24. Richmond, A., Balentien, E., Thomas, H.G., et al. (1988). Molecular characterization and chromosomal mapping of melanoma growth stimulatory activity, a growth factor structurally related to β-thromboglobulin. *EMBO J.* 7:2025–2033.
25. Anisowicz, A., Bardwell, L., and Sager, R. (1987). Constitutive overexpression of a growth-regulated gene in transformed Chinese hamster and human cells. *Proc. Natl. Acad. Sci. U.S.A.* 84:7188–7192.
26. Schröder, J.-M., Persoon, N., and Christophers, E. (1990). Lipopolysacchardie-stimulated human monocytes secrete apart from NAP-1/IL-8 a second neutrophil-activating protein: NH2-terminal amino acid sequence—identity with melanoma growth stimulatory activity (MGSA/gro). *J. Exp. Med.* 171: 1091–1100.
27. Richmond, A., and Thomas, H.G. (1988). Melanoma growth stimulatory activity: Isolation from human melanoma tumors and characterization of tissue distribution. *J. Cell Biochem.* 36:185–198.
28. Schägger, H., and von Jagow, G.V. (1987). Tricine-sodium dodecylsulfate-polyacrylamide gel electrophoresis for the separation of proteins in the range from 1 to 100 kD. *Anal. Biochem.* 166:368–379.
29. Witt, D.P., and Lander, A.D. (1994). Differential binding of chemokines to glycosaminoglycan subpopulations. *Curr. Biol.* 4:394–400.
30. Kojima, T., Cromie, M.A., Fisher, G.J., et al. (1993). Gro-α mRNA is selectively overexpressed in psoriatic epidermis and is reduced by cyclosporin A in vivo, but not in cultured keratinocytes. *J. Invest. Dermatol.* 101: 757–772.
31. Walz, A., Burgener, R., Car, B., Baggiolini,M., Kunkel, S.L., and Strieter, R.M. (1991). Structure and neutrophil-activating properties of a novel inflammatory peptide (ENA-78) with homology to interleukin 8. *J. Exp. Med.* 174:1355–1362.
32. Walz, A., Strieter, M., and Schnyder, S. (1993). Neutrophil-activating peptide ENA-78. In *The Chemokines.* I.J.D. Lindley et al. (Eds.). Plenum Press, New York, pp. 129–137.
33. Walz, A., and Baggiolini, M. (1989). A novel cleavage product of β-thromboglobulin formed in cultures of stimulated mononuclear cells activates human neutrophils. *Biochem. Biophys. Res. Commun.* 159:969–975.

34. Proost, P., De Wolf-Peeters, C., Conings, R., Opdenakker, G., Billiau, A., and Van Damme, J. (1993). Identification of a novel granulocyte chemotactic protein (GCP-2) from human tumor cells: In vitro and in vivo comparison with natural forms of GRO, IP-10, and IL-8. *J. Immunol.* 150:1000–1010.
35. Gillitzer, R., Berger, R., Mielke, V., et al. (1991). Upper keratinocytes of psoriatic skin lesions express high levels of NAP-1/IL-8 mRNA in situ. *J. Invest. Dermatol.* 97:73–79.
36. Bazzoni, F., Cassatella, M.A., Rossi, F., Ceska, M., Dewald, B., and Baggiolini, M. (1991). Phagocytosing neutrophils produce and release high amounts of the neutrophil-activating peptide 1/interleukin 8. *J. Exp. Med.* 173:771–774.
37. Sticherling, M., Bornscheuer, E., Schröder, J.-M., and Christophers, E. (1991). Localization of neutrophil-activating peptide-1/interleukin-8-immunoreactivity in normal and psoriatic skin. *J. Invest. Dermatol.* 96:1–5.
38. Kulke, R., Tödt-Pingel, I., Rademacher, D., Röwert, J., Schröder, J.-M., and Christophers, E. (1996). Co-localized overexpression of GRO-α and IL-8 mRNA is restricted to the suprapapillary layers of psoriatic lesions. *J. Invest. Dermatol.* 526–530.
39. Richmond, A., Mueller, S., Bueno, R., and Nanney, L.B. (1995). Localization of MGSA/GRO protein and its receptor in human burn wounds. *J. Invest. Dermatol.* 104:650 (abstract).
40. Schröder, J.-M., and Christophers, E. (1989). Secretion of novel and homologous neutrophil activating peptides by LPS-stimulated human endothelial cells. *J. Immunol.* 142:244–251.
41. Schröder, J.-M., Sticherling, M., Henneicke, H.-H., Preissner, W.C., and Christophers, E. (1990). IL-1α or tumor necrosis factor-α stimulate release of three NAP-1/IL-8-related neutrophil chemotactic proteins in human dermal fibroblasts. *J. Immunol.* 144:2223–2332.
42. Schröder, J.-M., Sticherling, M., Smid, P., and Christophers, E. (1994). Interleukin 8 and other structurally related cytokines. In *Epidermal Cytokines.* T.A. Luger, and T. Schwarz (Eds.). CRC Press, Boca Raton, FL, pp. 89–112.
43. Barker, J.N.W.N., Sama, V., Mitra, R.S., et al. (1990). Marked synergism between tumor necrosis factor α and inteferon-γ in regulation of keratinocytes of psoriatic lesions. *J. Invest. Dermatol.* 101:127–131.
44. Bartels, J., Sticherling, M., Kulke, R., et al. (1994). The regulation of IL-8 mRNA expression in human keratinocytes after stimulation with a combination of interferon-γ and tumor necrosis factor-α involves interleukin-8 mRNA length polymorphism. *Eur. J. Cell Biol.* 63(Suppl. 40):1 (abstract).
45. Luster, A.D., and Raveteh, J.V. (1987). Biochemical characterisation of a γ-interferon-inducible cytokine (IP-10). *J. Exp. Med.* 166:1084–1097.
46. Gottlieb, A.B., Luster, A.D., Posnett, D.N., and Carter, D.M. (1988). Detection of a γ interferon-induced protein IP-10 in psoriatic plaques. *J. Exp. Med.* 168: 941–948.
47. Taub, D.D., Lloyd, A.R., Conlon, K., Wang, J.M., Ortaldo, J.R., Harada, A., Matsushima, K., Kelvin, D.J., and Oppenheim, J.J. (1993). Recombinant human interferon-inducible protein 10 is a chemosttractant for human monocytes and T lymphocytes and promotes T cell adhesion to endothelial cells. *J. Exp. Med.* 177: 1809–1814.
48. Sarris, A.H., Esgleyes-Ribot, T., Crow, M., Broxmeyer, H.E., Karasavvas, N., Pugh, W., Grossman, D., Deisseroth, A., and Duvic, M. (1995). Cytokine loops involving interferon-γ and IP-10, a cytokine chemotactic for CD4+ lymphocytes: an explanation for the epidermatropism of cutaneous T-cell lymphoma? *Blood* 86: 651–658.
49. Koch, A.E., Polverini, P.J., Kunkel, S.L., Harlow, L.A., Di Pietro, L.A., Elner, V.M., Elner, S.G., and Strieter, R.M. (1992). Interleukin-8 as a macrophage-derived mediator of angiogenesis. *Science* 258:1798–1801.
50. Strieter, R.M., Kunkel, S.L., Arenberg, D.A., Burdick, M.D., and Polverini, P.J. (1995). Interferon γ-inducible protein 10 (IP-10), a member of the C–X–C chemokine family is an inhibitor of angiogenesis. *Biochem. Biophys. Res. Commun.* 210:51–57.
51. Farber, J.M. (1993). HuMig: a new human member of the chemokine family of cytokines. *Biochem. Biophys. Res. Commun.* 192:223–230.
52. Liao, F., Rabin, R.L., Yannelli, J.R., Koniaris, L.G., Vanguri, P., and Farber, J.M. (1995). Human mig chemokine: biochemical and functional characterization. *J. Exp. Med.* 182:1301–1314.
53. Schall, T.J. (1991). Biology of the RANTES/SIS cytokine family. *Cytokine* 3:165–183.
54. Baggiolini, M., and Dahinden, C.A. (1994). CC chemokines in allergic inflammation. *Immunol. Today* 15: 127–133.
55. Bacon, K.B., and Schall, T.J. (1996). Chemokines as mediators of allergic inflammation. *Int. Arch. Allergy Immunol.* 109:97–109.
56. Hammar, H., Gu, S.-Q., Johannesson, A., Sundkvist, K.G., and Bieberfeld, P. (1984). Subpopulations of mononuclear cells in microscopic lesions of psoriatic patients. Selective accumulation of suppressor/cytotoxic T cells in epidermis during the evolution of the lesion. *J. Invest. Dermatol.* 83:416–420.
57. Gillitzer, R., Wolff, K., Tong, D., et al. (1993). MCP-1 mRNA expression in basal keratinocytes of psoriatic lesions. *J. Invest. Dermatol.* 101:127–131.
58. von der Lage, P., Mrowietz, U., Christophers, E., and Schröder, J.-M. (1994). Monocyte-chemotactic cytokines in psoriatic scales. *Arch. Dermatol. Res.* 286:228.
59. von der Lage, P., Mrowietz, U., Christophers, E., and Schröder, J.-M. (1995). Immunoreactivity of chemo-

tactic cytokines in psoriatic scales. *Arch. Dermatol. Res.* 287:395.

60. Kameyoshi, Y., Dörschner, A., Mallet, A.I., Christophers, E., and Schröder, J.-M. (1992). Cytokine RANTES released by thrombin-stimulated platelets is a potent attractant for human eosinophils. *J. Exp. Med.* 176:587–592.
61. Noso, N., Proost, P., Van Damme, J., and Schröder, J.-M. (1994). Human monocyte chemotactic proteins-2 and 3 (MCP-2 and MCP-3) attract human eosinophils and desensitize the chemotactic responses towards RANTES. *Biochem. Biophys. Res. Commun.* 200: 1470–1476.
62. Ponath, P.D., Qin, S., Ringler, D.J., Clark-Lewis, I., Wang, J., Kassam, N., Smith, H., Shi, X., Gonzalo, J.A., Newman, W., Gutierrez-Ramos, J.C., and Mackay, C.R. (1996). Cloning of the human eosinophil chemoattractant, ecotaxin. *J. Clin. Invest.* 97:604–612.
63. Noso, N., Bartels, J., Christophers, E., and Schröder, J.-M. (1996). Identification of a novel eosinophil-specific chemokine. *Arch. Dermatol. Res.*. 326 (abstract).
64. Schröder, J.-M., Noso, N., Sticherling, M., and Christophers, E. (1996). Role of eosinophil-chemotactic C–C–chemokines in cutaneous inflammation. *J. Leukocyte Biol.* 59:1–5.

21

Immunological Pathways in Psoriasis

Christopher E. M. Griffiths
University of Manchester, Manchester, England

Although psoriasis is one of the more common dermatoses, well known to dermatologist and internist alike, its underlying etiology and pathological mechanisms are still relatively poorly elucidated. That being said, it is remarkable how much progress has been made by cutaneous biologists in investigating the mysteries of this disease. Undoubtedly, the greatest influence on how we view the psoriatic process has come from recognition that cells of the immune system are more than innocent bystanders in this process and indeed are integral. This recognition develops from two lines of observation—laboratory studies and immunotherapy. Laboratory, basic-science investigation is the linchpin of clinical progress, and the skin with its inherent facilitation of direct observation of disease and tissue procurement may more readily yield its secrets than do other organs. Immunotherapy of inflammatory disease indirectly allows one to test suppositions regarding pathogenesis and pathways important to clinically apparent disease—psoriasis exemplifies this dictum.

Immunology, as a discipline, is ubiquitous to any disease pathway and immunological functions can be ascribed to almost any cell type. The ubiquity of immunology implies that one must take care in segregating primary from secondary events, i.e., look as far "upstream" as possible for initiating signals that may be specific to psoriasis rather than common to inflammatory dermatoses in general. Other authors in this book have concentrated on single cell types and single therapeutic interventions. I will attempt to provide an immunological overview of psoriasis, which by definition cannot be exhaustive, drawing from observations made in the laboratory and the clinic.

T CELLS

A histological study of skin involved by psoriasis reveals keratinocyte hyperproliferation and an inflammatory infiltrate. Work in the late 1970s (1) and early 1980s (2) established that the inflammatory infiltrate, in both the dermis and epidermis, is composed primarily of T cells. Established plaques of psoriasis often contain a dense T-cell infiltrate in the dermis composed mainly of CD4+ T cells and a relatively scanty but crucial infiltrate of T cells in the epidermis. The nature of these intraepidermal T cells has generated a good deal of debate—it appears that early, i.e., developing, psoriatic lesions contain predominantly activated (HLA-DR+) CD4+ T cells in the epidermis (2) whereas an established lesion contains relatively more CD8+ T cells (3). It is possible that induction of a plaque of psoriasis is mediated by activated (HLA-DR+, CD25-IL-2 receptor+) CD4+ T cells and maintenance is dependent on CD8+ T cells. Resolution of plaques correlates with reduced numbers of either intraepidermal DR+ CD4+ T cells (2) or CD8+ T cells (3). The presence of T cells within the epidermis appears to be a driving influence on the psoriasis phenotype as clearance of psoriasis plaques by cyclosporin is associated with a marked reduction in intraepidermal T cells but only a modest reduction in dermal T cells (4).

T cells in psoriatic plaques are activated in that they are HLA-DR+ (2) and express the interleukin-2 receptor CD25 (5). Activation implies functionality and ability to secrete cytokines that can influence the function of other cell types within the skin. As to whether the activation signal for T cells occurs within the skin or elsewhere is disputed. Morganroth et al. (6) demonstrated that proliferation, and possibly activation, of T cells occurred within the dermis of psoriatic plaques in that 37% of $CD45RO^+$ (memory) T cells at this site are actively proliferating (6). I believe it more likely that skin-homing T cells are activated elsewhere, maybe by superantigen (see below), and then migrate to the skin. Assuming that intracutaneous T cells are activated, what cytokines are they producing and how may these distinguish psoriasis from other inflammatory dermatoses?

CYTOKINES

A variety of techniques have enabled us to establish that interferon-γ (IFN-γ) is present within plaques of psoriasis at both the mRNA (7) and protein (8) levels. Anecdotally IFN-γ may be an important cytokine in the initiation of psoriasis in that subcutaneous injections of IFN-γ an induce psoriatic foci in patients with psoriasis, but not in normal individuals, whereas similar injections of normal saline do not produce this response (9). No cytokine in isolation can orchestrate the inflammatory cascade, and levels of other cytokines are elevated in psoriatic lesions. It is beyond the scope of this chapter to detail all growth factors and cytokines whose levels are elevated in plaques of psoriasis as compared to normal skin, although particular attention should be paid to IL-2 (10) and IL-8 (11), in addition to IFN-γ (7,8). Such a pattern, i.e., increased IL-2 and IFN-γ, is in keeping with the so-called Th1 cytokine profile as designated by Mossman et al. (12). They described two distinct cytokine profiles: Th1 and Th2 (12). Th1 cytokines are mainly represented by IFN-γ, IL-2, and IL-12 (12,13) whereas predominant Th2 cytokines are IL-4, IL-5, IL-6, and IL-10 (12,13). In essence Th1 and Th2 cytokines are opposing forces. Cutaneous diseases in which Th1 cytokines predominate are mycosis fungoides (14) and tuberculoid leprosy (13) whereas Th2 cytokines predominate in atopic dermatitis (15) and lepromatous leprosy (13). Psoriasis "fits" best with a Th1 profile disease and this is underscored by the relative rarity of concurrence of atopic dermatitis (Th2) and psoriasis (Th1) in the same individual (16).

IL-8 produced predominantly by keratinocytes is also overexpressed in psoriasis plaques (11,17) and appears to be pluripotential in that it can induce both keratinocyte proliferation and leukocyte chemotaxis (18).

SUPERANTIGENS

The precipitating or activation signal in psoriasis is unknown although there are various candidates for this role. The most likely are infectious agents and "stress." Most research has focused on the more tangible of these two precipitants, namely infectious agents, although the role of stress in induction and maintenance of psoriasis and other inflammatory dermatoses (19) must not be underestimated. Considerable interest has been shown in the ability of infection, in the form of superantigens, to precipitate psoriasis in genetically predisposed individuals. Genetic predisposition relates to the genotype of the individual in that he or she carries the gene or genes that predispose to development of psoriasis in response to certain environmental antigens (20). The genetic locus/loci for psoriasis are for the most part unknown although one kindred in Texas exhibits linkage to the end of chromosome 17q (21). But researchers elsewhere in the United States and Europe (22) have been unable to demonstrate the same or any linkage in families under their investigation. There is a strong association between the MHC-I molecule HLA CW6 and psoriasis in that 85% of people who present with psoriasis before 40 years of age are HLA-CW6+ (23). Indeed the concurrence of HLA-DQ9 and HLA-CW6 appears to be highly predictive of psoriasis susceptibility (24).

Streptococcus appears to be a firm candidate for a necessary environmental factor that may precipitate psoriasis in people who are genetically predisposed. For more than 200 years it has been known that guttate psoriasis can be preceded by a streptococcal pharyngitis or tonsillitis (25,26). The majority of patients with guttate psoriasis have both serological and microbiological evidence for recent infection with nonspecific, β-hemolytic *Streptococcus* (26). T-cell lines isolated from plaques of psoriasis proliferate in vitro in response to the M-protein component of *Streptococcus* (25). It is the M-protein portion of *Streptococcus* that confers on it the capacity to perform as a superantigen. Simplistically, superantigens are proteins that can be presented by antigen-presenting cells, such as Langerhans cells and dermal dendrocytes, without prior intracellular processing or the necessity of being presented within the peptide-binding groove of the antigen-presenting cell (27). Superantigens are presented to a particular portion of the T-cell receptor known as the Vβ region, such presentation eventuating in clonal expansion of T cells expressing that particular Vβ subtype (27). In the case of *Streptococcus* this Vβ subtype is usually Vβ13.1. Several research groups have demonstrated that Vβ-expressing T cells of various subtypes are preferentially overrepresented within skin lesions of chronic plaque and acute guttate psoriasis as compared to the peripheral blood of the same individuals (28–30). Whether the Vβ clonal expression occurs within the skin or elsewhere is currently under investigation. It is possible that superantigen-induced activation and expression of Vβ-expressing T cells occurs extracutaneously and this imbues such cells with preferential skin homing. Evidence for this hypothesis is the observation that streptococcal toxin can induce HECA-452 on T cells (31). HECA-452 is a marker for cutaneous lymphocyte–associated antigen (CLA), a ligand for the adhesion molecule, E-selectin, expressed on endothelium, and a designated addressin for T cells that home to the skin (32). CLA^+ T cells constitute approximately 15% of circulating peripheral blood T cells but more than 85% of T cells within skin of inflammatory dermatoses (32).

Superantigen-induced activation and proliferation of T cells may be the initiating event but it is probable that maintenance of the psoriatic process is dependent on recognition of other, possibly "self"-antigens. The identity of self-antigens is a crucial component to understanding of the pathogenesis and perhaps treatment of this disease. As the immune process appears directed at the epidermis, the most likely candidate for a self-antigen is keratin or some component of keratin. Cross-reactivity exists between keratin and streptococci (33,34) in that there is sequence homology between streptococcal protein M6 and a type I keratin (keratin 14) (33).

Antigen presentation, whether of self or foreign antigen, to T cells occurs in epidermis and probably dermis and is performed by a variety of antigen-presenting cells. Within psoriatic epidermis are a population of antigen-presenting cells distinct from classical Langerhans cells in that they lack expression of CD1a but are still HLA-DR+ (35,36). These antigen-presenting cells express macrophage markers including Mo-1, CD11b, and Mac387 and may be responsible for self-antigen presentation to T cells. The ability of psoriatic epidermal cell suspensions to stimulate autologous T cells seems dependent on this CD1a−DR+ group (36). Langerhans cell numbers are variable in psoriatic epidermis although they are increased in the dermis. Also within the dermis are a resident population of antigen-presenting cells/macrophages that express macrophage markers and factor XIIIa—dermal dendrocytes (37). These cells are increased in number and appear to be activated in the dermis of plaques of psoriasis (38). It should not be forgotten that epidermal keratinocytes may function as nonprofessional antigen-presenting cells in certain circumstances, e.g., if HLA-DR+, as can occur in psoriasis.

The earliest microscopically identifiable changes within uninvolved skin of a patient prior to the skin developing clinically overt psoriasis are within the endothelium (39). The exact signals that induce these changes are unknown although cytokines such as tumor necrosis factor-α (TNF-α) produced by mast cells, keratinocytes, antigen-presenting cells, and leukocytes have profound effects on endothelial cells particularly on their ability to express adhesion molecules (40). Ordinarily leukocytes within peripheral blood are unable to gain access to extravascular sites without the ability to bind to endothelial cells. The earliest adhesion molecules to be expressed on the surface of endothelial cells are GMP-140 (41) and E-selectin induced by IL-1 and TNF-α (42). Receptors or ligands on the cell surface of leukocytes engage their cognate sites or selectins—such a leukocyte ligand for E-selectin is sialyl Lewis × (43) or CLA (32). E-selectin-mediated endothelial cell/leukocyte binding is relatively weak but strong enough to precipitate margination of lymphocytes to the edge of capillary flow, a process known as margination and "rolling" (40). Subsequently, intercellular adhesion molecule-1 (ICAM-1) and vascular cell adhesion molecule-1 (VCAM-1) are up-regulated on endothelial cells (40). CAMs are more rigorous binders of leukocytes and allow firm adherence of leukocytes to endothelial cells thus enabling diapedesis between endothelial cells and egress from the vascular component along chemotactic gradients (40).

Adhesion molecules also play a crucial role in enabling lymphocytes to bind to other cells of the cutaneous compartment, most particularly keratinocytes. ICAM-1 is not expressed by keratinocytes in normal epidermis but is strongly and focally expressed by epidermal keratinocytes in psoriasis plaques as a result of exposure to TNF-α and/or IFN-γ (44). Thus, wherever T cells are observed within psoriatic epidermis they are juxtaposed to ICAM-1-expressing keratinocytes, the binding occurring consequent on ICAM-1/lymphocyte function associated antigen-1 (LFA-1) interactions (45).

Thus, a considerable body of evidence points to the presence of activated T cells within psoriatic lesions and speculation as to how they were activated. Psoriasis is not primarily a dermatosis exemplified by a lymphocytic infiltrate but is more one of epidermal kertinocyte hyperproliferation (46). What is the evidence that T cells, or other cells of the immune system, can induce keratinocyte proliferation?

Work by Bata-Csorgo and colleagues (47,48) has provided some insight into this process. It is well established that human epidermis contains two types of proliferative keratinocytes both of which express the β_1 integrin CD29 (47). Basal keratinocytes contain a group of slow-cycling, undifferentiated, small cells identified as expressing CD29 but not the differentiation keratins K1 and K10 (47)—this phenotype fulfills acknowledged criteria for a stem cell. The other potentially proliferative population of keratinocytes expresses both CD29 and K1/K10 and as such is committed to differentiation—transit-amplifying cells (47). In psoriasis, as compared to normal skin, the CD29+ K1/K10− stem cell population is actively proliferative. It appears that cytokines derived from T cells isolated from plaques of psoriasis are able to stimulate proliferation of CD29+ K1/K10− stem cells isolated from uninvolved skin from patients with psoriasis but are relatively poor at stimulating proliferation of stem cells taken from normal skin (48). The range of cytokines/growth factors produced by T cells cloned from psoriasis plaques is immense. Although, granulocyte-macrophage colony-stimulating factor (GM-CSF) and IFN-γ are predominant within these T-cell supernatants, no cytokine/growth factor appears able to "singlehandedly" stimulate keratinocyte proliferation (49). However, IFN-γ acts as a vital enabler of other cytokines to move stem cells into the proliferative cell cycle (47).

Psoriasis research, as compared to research into rheumatoid arthritis, diabetes, and multiple sclerosis, is hindered greatly by the absence of an animal model for this disease. Psoriasis seemingly does not occur in animals other than humans, and experimental models of the disease are not completely representative, e.g., HLA-B27 transgenic rat (50), "flaky mouse" (51), and transplantation of involved and uninvolved skin from psoriatic patients onto a nude mouse (52). Thus, there is considerable promise in a new animal model for psoriasis: psoriatic skin transplanted onto severe combined immunodeficiency mice (SCID) (53,54) retains its pretransplantation immunophenotype and may well prove appropriate to enable investigation of pathological mechanisms and potential treatments in psoriasis. Until the SCID mouse model is fully validated, testing of hypotheses regarding immunological mechanisms can be validated only by immunotherapeutic approaches to psoriasis in humans. If the gene or genes for psoriasis are identified, then this knowledge could be used to produce mice transgenic for such genes, the ideal animal model for psoriasis research. Understandably such hypothesis testing is a by-product of clinical trials of various specific immunosuppressive agents for the treatment of psoriasis. Indeed much of our knowledge regarding the immunology of psoriasis has derived from data collected during clinical trials.

The first relatively specific immunosuppressive drug to be used for treating psoriasis was cyclosporin (55), and both the utility and the mechanism(s) of action of cyclosporin in the treatment of psoriasis are well established (56–58). Cyclosporin acts as a prodrug by binding to a cytoplasmic immunophilin receptor, cyclophilin (59). The consequent complex of cyclosporin and cyclophilin acts to inhibit a key cytoplasmic enzyme, calcineurin phosphatase. Calcineurin phosphatase dephosphorylates the cytoplasmic precursor of nuclear factor of activated T cells (NFAT) thereby facilitating the passage of NFAT into the T-cell nucleus and subsequent transcription of IL-2, an indicator of T-cell activation (59). Thus cyclosporin inhibits T-cell activation and all dependent processes such as cytokine production and T-cell proliferation. Although other immunological pathways are undoubtedly impaired by cyclosporin, there is little evidence that keratinocyte proliferation is directly affected by this drug in vivo. Elder and colleagues (60) analyzed skin biopsies from plaques of psoriasis during patients' first week of cyclosporin treatment and before any clinical improvement. This analysis showed that significant reductions in mRNA for IL-1β and IL-8 had already occurred—circumstantial evidence that T-cell function and cytokine production was already impaired by cyclosporin. Gerritsen et al. (61) also showed in vivo that cyclosporin indirectly inhibits keratinocyte proliferation (via its effects on T cells) and not directly. Before and during treatment with cyclosporin, patients with psoriasis had a small area of skin tape-stripped, a process that induces, in a non-lymphocyte-dependent manner, epidermal keratinocyte proliferation. There was no difference in rate of keratinocyte proliferation in tape-stripped skin before or during cyclosporin treatment. FK506 is a macrolide drug that is structurally and phylogenetically different from cyclosporin but also binds an immunophilin receptor (FK binding protein) in cytoplasm thereby inhibiting calcineurin phosphatase and consequently NFAT (62). Not surprisingly, systemic administration of FK506 is also a highly effective treatment for psoriasis (63,64).

More specific approaches to immunosuppression in psoriasis supply additional, corroborative evidence that T cells are important to the psoriatic process. Intravenously administered anti-CD3 (65) and anti-CD4 (66,67) monoclonal antibodies produce temporary but marked improvement in psoriasis although neither of these markers (CD3 and CD4) is unique to T cells. Strong expression of high-affinity IL-2 receptors is unique to T cells and targeting of such receptors would be highly T-cell-specific. A fusion protein, DAB_{389}IL-2, in which IL-2 replaces the receptor-binding domain of diphtheria toxin is specific and toxic for cells expressing the high-affinity IL-2 receptor. Gottlieb et al. (3) demonstrated that DAB_{389}IL-2 administered intravenously to patients with severe psoriasis does produce marked, but temporary, improvement in their psoriasis. The clinical improvement engendered by DAB_{389}IL-2 strongly correlates with reduction in intraepidermal T cells within psoriatic plaques.

Immune targeting is undoubtedly the way ahead for psoriasis treatment in the next millennium. In retrospect, even psoriasis treatments that were not initially believed to be immunosuppressive in their mechanism of action are now understood to work at least partially in this way. Such treatments are PUVA and methotrexate, the latter acting as an anti-inflammatory agent by virtue of inhibition of leukocyte accumulation (68). It is possible that retinoids, vitamin D, and glucocorticoids may produce at least some of their antipsoriatic effects by inhibiting the formation of complexes between the transcription factor, AP-1, and NFAT and consequent impairment of IL-2 production by T cells (69).

In summary, immunological pathways are crucial to the development and perpetuation of plaques of psoriasis although it must be appreciated that they are only one of many such conspiring mechanisms occurring amid a permissive genotype. Research is currently targeted at understanding the precipitating events and the identity of the autoantigens in this common, disabling disease.

REFERENCES

1. Bjerke, J.R., Krough, H.K., and Matre, R. (1978). Characterisation of mononuclear cell infiltrate in psoriatic lesions. *J. Invest. Dermatol.* 71:340.
2. Valdimarsson, H., Baker, B.S., Jonsdottir, I., and Fry, L. (1986). Psoriasis: a disease of abnormal keratinocyte proliferation induced by T lymphocytes. *Immunol. Today* 7:256–259.
3. Gottlieb, S.L., Gilleaudeau, P., Johnson, R., et al. (1995). Response of psoriasis to a lymphocyte-selective toxin (DAB_{389}IL-2) suggests a primary immune, but not keratinocyte, pathogenic basis. *Nature Med.* 1:442–447.
4. Baker, B.S., Griffiths, C.E.M., Lambert, S., et al., (1987). The effects of cyclosporin A on T lymphocyte and dendritic cell sub-populations in psoriasis. *Br. J. Dermatol.* 116:503–510.
5. de Boer, O.J., van der Loos, C.M., Hamerlinck, F., Bos, J.D., and Das, P.K. (1994). Reappraisal of in situ immunophenotypic analysis of psoriasis skin: interaction of activated HLA-DR^+ immunocompetent cells and endothelial cells is a major feature of psoriatic lesions. *Arch. Dermatol. Res.* 286:87–96.
6. Morganroth, G.S., Chan, L.S., Weinstein, G.D., Voorhees, J.J., and Cooper, K.D. (1991). Proliferating cells in psoriatic dermis are comprised primarily of T cells, endothelial cells, and factor $XIIIa^+$ perivascular dendritic cells. *J. Invest. Dermatol.* 96:333–340.
7. Barker, J.N.W.N., Karabin, G.D., Stoof, T.J., Sarma, V.J., Dixit, V.M., and Nickoloff, B.J. (1991). Detection of interferon-gamma mRNA in psoriatic epidermis by polymerase chain reaction. *J. Dermatol. Sci.* 2:106–111.
8. Takematsu, H., and Tagami, H. (1991). Interleukin-2, soluble interleukin-2 receptor and interferon gamma in the suction blister fluids from psoriatic skin. *Arch. Dermatol. Res.* 283:138–139.
9. Fierlbeck, G., Rasner, G., and Muler, G. (1990). Psoriasis induced at injection site by recombinant gamma interferon. *Arch. Dermatol.* 126:351–355.
10. Schlaak, J.F., Buslau, M., Jochum, W., et al. (1994). T cells involved in psoriasis vulgaris belong to the Th_1 subset. *J. Invest. Dermatol.* 102:145–149.
11. Christophers, E., Schroder, J.M., and Mrowietz, U. (1989). Identification of two endogenous neutrophil-activating peptides in psoriatic skin and inflammatory cells: CSa and NAP-1. *Dermatologica* 179(1)(Suppl.): 9–15.
12. Mossman, T.R., Cherwinski, H., Bond, M.W., Giedlin, M.A., and Coffman, R.L. (1986). Two types of murine

helper T cell clones. I. Definition according to profiles of lymphokine activites and secreted proteins. *J. Immunol.* 136:2348–2357.
13. Modlin, R.L. (1994). Th_1–Th_2 paradigm: insights from leprosy. *J. Invest. Dermatol.* 102:828–832.
14. Saed, G., Fivenson, D.P., Naidu, Y., and Nickoloff, B.J. (1994). Mycosis fungoides exhibits a TH1 cell-mediated cytokine profile whereas Sézary syndrome expresses a TH2-type profile. *J. Invest. Dermatol.* 103: 29–33.
15. Kay, A.B., Ying, S., Varney, V., et al. (1991). Messenger RNA expression of the cytokine gene cluster, interleukin 3 (IL-3), IL-4, IL-5, and granulocyte/macrophage colony stimulating factor, in allergen-induced late-phase cutaneous reactions in atopic subjects. *J. Exp. Med.* 173:775–778.
16. Henseler, T., and Christophers, E. (1995). Disease concomitance in psoriasis. *J. Am. Acad. Dermatol.* 32: 982–986.
17. Nickoloff, B.J., Karabin, G.D., Barker, J.N.W.W., et al. (1991). Cellular localization of interleukin-γ and its inducer tumor necrosis factor alpha in psoriasis. *Am. J. Pathol.* 138:129–140.
18. Larsen, C.G., Anderson, A., Appella, E., Oppenheim, J.J., and Matsushima, K. (1989). The neutrophil-activating protein (NAP-1) is also chemotactic for T lymphocytes. *Science* 243:1464–1466.
19. Gupta, M.A., and Gupta, A.K. (1996). Psychodermatology: an update. *J. Am. Acad. Dermatol.* 1030–1046.
20. Elder, J.T., Nair, R.P., Guo, S.-W., Henseler, T., Christophers, E., and Voorhees, J.J. (1994). The genetics of psoriasis. *Arch. Dermatol.* 130:216–224.
21. Tomfohrde, J., Silverman, A., Barnes, R., et al. (1994). Gene for familial psoriasis susceptibility mapped to the distal end of human chromosome 17q. *Science* 264: 1141–1145.
22. Nair, R.P., Guo, S.W., Janish, S., et al. (1995). Scanning chromosome 17 for psoriasis susceptibility: lack of evidence for a distal 17q locus. *Hum. Hered.* 45: 219–230.
23. Henseler, T., and Christophers, E. (1985). Psoriasis of early and late onset: characterization of two types of psoriasis vulgaris. *J. Am. Acad. Dermatol.* 13:450–456.
24. Jenisch, S., Henseler, T., Westphal, E., et al. (1995). HLA-DQ9 (9DQB1*0303) increases susceptibility to type 1 psoriasis in multiplex families but only in the presence of HLA-Cw6. *J. Invest. Dermatol.* 104:629.
25. Valdimarsson, H., Baker, B.S., Jonsdottir, I., Powles, A., and Fry, L. (1995). Psoriasis: a T-cell-mediated autoimmune disease induced by streptococcal superantigens? *Immunol. Today* 16:145–149.
26. Telfer, N.R., Chalmers, R.J.C., Whale, K., and Colman, G. (1992). The role of streptococcal infection in the initiation of guttate psoriasis. *Arch. Dermatol.* 126: 39–42.
27. Drake, C.G., and Kotzin, B.L. (1992). Superantigens: biology, immunology, and potential role in disease. *J. Clin. Immunol.* 12:149–162.
28. Leung, D.Y.M., Walsh, P., Giorno, R., and Norris, D.A. (1993). A potential role for superantigens in the pathogenesis of psoriasis. *J. Invest. Dermatol.* 100: 225–228.
29. Lewis, H.M., Baker, B.S., Bokth, S., et al. (1993). Restricted T-cell receptor Vβ gene usage in the skin of patients with guttate and chronic plaque psoriasis. *Br. J. Dermatol.* 129:514–520.
30. Chang, J.C.C., Smith, L.R., Froning, K., et al. (1994). $CD8^+$ T cells in psoriatic lesions preferentially use T-cell receptor $V_\beta 3$ and/or $V_\beta 13.1$ genes. *Proc. Natl. Acad. Sci. U.S.A.* 91:9282–9286.
31. Baker, B.S., Powles, A.V., and Fry, L. (1996). Induction of CLA antigen expression by group A streptococcal antigens in psoriasis. *Br. J. Dermatol.* (in press).
32. Picker, L.J., Treer, J.R., Ferguson-Darnell, B., Collins, P.A., Bergstresser, P.R., and Terstappen, L.W.M.M. (1993). Control of lymphocyte recirculation in man. II. Differential regulation of the cutaneous lymphocyte associated antigen, a tissue-selective homing receptor for skin-homing T cells. *J. Immunol.* 150:1122–1136.
33. McFadden, J., Valdimarsson, H., and Fry, L. (1991). Cross-reactivity between streptococcal M surface antigen and human skin. *Br. J. Dermatol.* 125:343–347.
34. Swerlick, R.A., Cunningham, M.W., and Hall, N.K. (1986). Monoclonal antibodies cross-reactive with group A streptococci and normal and psoriatic human skin. *J. Invest. Dermatol.* 87:367–371.
35. Baker, B.S., Lambert, S., Powles, A.V., Valdimarsson, H., and Fry, L. (1988). Epidermal DR^+T6^- dendritic cells in inflammatory skin diseases. *Acta Derm. Venereol.* 68:209–217.
36. Baadsgaard, O., Gupta, A.K., Taylor, R.S., Ellis, C.N., Voorhees, J.J., and Cooper, K.D. (1989). Psoriatic epidermal cells demonstrate increased numbers and function of non-Langerhans antigen-presenting cells. *J. Invest. Dermatol.* 92:190–195.
37. Cerio, R., Griffiths, C.E.M., Cooper, K.D., Headington, J.T., and Nickoloff, B.J. (1989). Characterization of factor XIII—positive dermal dendritic cells in normal and inflamed skin. *Br. J. Dermatol.* 121:421–431.
38. Nickoloff, B.J., and Griffiths, C.E.M. (1990). Lymphocyte trafficking in psoriasis: a new perspective emphasizing the dermal dendrocyte with active dermal recruitment mediated via endothelial cells followed by intra-epidermal T cell activation. *J. Invest. Dermatol.* 95:35s–37s.
39. Braverman, I.M., and Yen, A. (1974). Role of the microcirculation in the treatment and pathogenesis of psoriasis. *J. Invest. Dermatol.* 78:12.

40. Barker, J.N.W.N., and Nickoloff, B.J. (1992). Cutaneous leukocyte–vascular endothelium interactions. *Spring Semin. Immunopathol.* 13:355–367.
41. Hattori, R., Hamilton, K.K., Fugate, R.D., McEver, R.D., and Sims, P.J. (1989). Stimulated secretion of endothelial von Willebrand factor is accompanied by rapid redistribution to the cell surface of the intracellular granule membrane protein GMP-140. *J. Biol. Chem.* 264:7768–7771.
42. Bevilacqua, M.P., Stengelin, S., Gimbrone, M.A., and Seed, B. (1989). Endothelial leukocyte adhesion molecule-1: an inducible receptor for neutrophils related to the complement regulatory proteins and lectins. *Science* 243:1160–1165.
43. Lowe, J.B., Stoolman, L.M., Nair, R.P., Larsen, R.D., Berhend, T.L., and Marks, R.M. (1990). ELAM-1 dependent cell adhesion to vascular endothelium determined by a transfected human fucosyl transtense DNA. *Cell* 63:475–484.
44. Griffiths, C.E.M., Voorhees, J.J., and Nickoloff, B.J. (1989). Gamma interferon induces different keratinocyte cellular patterns of expression of HLA-DR and D4 and intercellular adhesion molecule-1 (ICAM-1) antigens. *Br. J. Dermatol.* 120:1–7.
45. Griffiths, C.E.M., Voorhees, J.J., and Nickoloff, B.J. (1989). Characterization of intercellular adhesion molecule-1 and HLA-DR expression in normal and inflamed skin. Modulation by recombinant gamma interferon and tumor necrosis factor. *J. Am. Acad. Dermatol.* 20:617–629.
46. Barker, J.N.W.N. (1991). The pathophysiology of psoriasis. *Lancet* 338:227–230.
47. Bata-Csorgo, Z., Hammerberg, C., Voorhees, J.J., and Cooper, K.D. (1993). Flow cytometric identification of proliferative subpopulations within normal human epidermis and the localization of the primary hyperproliferative population in psoriasis. *J. Exp. Med.* 178: 1271–1281.
48. Bata-Csorgo, Z., Hammerberg, C., Voorhees, J.J., and Cooper, K.D. (1995). Kinetics and regulation of human keratinocyte stem cell growth in short-term primary ex vivo culture. *J. Clin. Invest.* 95:317–327.
49. Strange, P., Cooper, K.D., Hansen, E.R., et al. (1993). T-lymphocyte clones initiated from lesional psoriatic skin release growth factors that induce keratinocyte proliferation. *J. Invest. Dermatol.* 101:695–700.
50. Hammer, R.E., Maika, S.D., Richardson, J.A., Tang, T.P., and Tanroy, J.D. (1990). Spontaneous inflammatory disease in transgenic rats expressing HLA-B27 and human β-2M: animal model of HLA-B27-associated human disorders. *Cell* 63:1099–1105.
51. Sundberg, J.P., Dunstan, R.W., Roop, D.R., and Beamer, W.G. (1994). Full-thickness skin grafts from flaky skin mice to nude mice: maintenance of psoriasiform phenotype. *J. Invest. Dermatol.* 102:781–788.
52. Krueger, G.C. (1975). Long-term maintenance of psoriatic human skin on congenitally athymic (nude) mice. *J. Invest. Dermatol.* 64:307–312.
53. Nickoloff, B.J., Kunkel, S.L., Burdick, M., and Strieter, R.M. (1995). Severe combined immunodeficiency mouse and human psoriatic skin chimeras. *Am. J. Pathol.* 146:580–588.
54. Boehncke, W.H., Dressel, D., Zollner, T.M., and Haufmann, R. (1996). Pulling the trigger on psoriasis. *Nature* 379:777.
55. Mueller, W., and Herrmann, B. (1979). Cyclosporin A for psoriasis. *N. Engl. J. Med.* 301:555.
56. Griffiths, C.E.M., Powles, A.V., Leonard, J.N., Baker, B.S., Fry, L., and Valdimarsson, H. (1986). Clearance of psoriasis with low dose cyclosporin. *Br. Med. J.* 293: 731–732.
57. Ellis, C.N., Fradin, M.S., Messana, J.M., et al. (1991). Cyclosporine for plaque type psoriasis. Results of a multidose, double-blind trial. *N. Engl. J. Med.* 324: 277.
58. Cooper, K.D., Voorhees, J.J., Fisher, G.J., Chan, L.S., Gupta, A.K., and Baadsgaard, O. (1990). Effect of cyclosporine on immunologic mechanisms in psoriasis. *J. Am. Acad. Dermatol.* 23:1318–1328.
59. Emmel, E.A., Verweije, C.L., Durand, D.B., Higgins, K.M., Lacy, E., and Crabtree, G.R. (1989). Cyclosporin A specifically inhibits function of nuclear proteins involved in T cell activation. *Science* 246:1617.
60. Elder, J.T., Hammerberg, C., Cooper, K.D., et al. (1993). Cyclosporin A rapidly inhibits epidermal cytokine expression in psoriasis lesions, but not in cytokine-stimulated cultured keratinocytes. *J. Invest. Dermatol.* 101:761–766.
61. Gerritsen, M.J.P., Rulo, H.F.C., Arnold, W.P., Van de Kerkhof, P.C.M. (1994). Response of the clinically uninvolved skin of psoriatic patients to repeated tape stripping during cyclosporin A treatment. *Br. J. Dermatol.* 130:181–188.
62. Thomson, A.W. (1993). The new immunosuppressive macrolides—mechanisms of action. In M. Rose and M. Yacoub (Eds.). *Immunology of Heart-Lung Transplantation*, Edward Arnold, London.
63. Jegasothy, B.V., Ackerman, C.D., Todo, S., Fung, J.J., Abu-Elmayd, K., and Starzl, T.E. (1991). Tacrolimus (FK506)—a new therapeutic agent for severe recalcitrant psoriasis. *Arch. Dermatol.* 128:781–785.
64. The European FK506 Multicentre Psoriasis Study Group. (1996). Systemic tacrolimus (FK506) is effective for the treatment of psoriasis in a double-blind, placebo-controlled study. *Arch. Dermatol.* 132: 419–423.
65. Weinshenker, B.G., Bass, B.H., Ebers, G.C., and Rice, G.P.A. (1989). Remission of psoriatic lesions with muromonab-CD3 (orthoclone OKT3) treatment. *J. Am. Acad. Dermatol.* 20:1132–1133.

66. Poizot-Martin, I., Dhiver, C., Mawas, C., Olive, D., and Gastraut, J.A. (1991). Are CD4 antibodies and peptide T new treatments for psoriasis? *Lancet* 337: 1477.
67. Prinz, J., Braun Falco, O., Meurer, M., Daddona, P., Reiter, C., Rieber, P., and Riethmuller, G. (1991). Chimaeric CD4 monoclonal antibody in treatment of generalised pustular psoriasis. *Lancet* 338:320.
68. Cronstein, B.N., Naime, D., and Ostad, E. (1993). The antiinflammatory mechanism of methotrexate. *J. Clin. Invest.* 92;2675–2682.
69. Guyre, P.M., Girard, M.T., Morgarelli, P.M., et al. (1988). Glucocorticoid effects on the production and actions of immune cytokines. *J. Steroid Biochem.* 30: 89–93.

22

Molecular and Immunological Aspects of Psoriasis

Madeleine Duvic
M.D. Anderson Cancer Center, Houston, Texas

Noreen Lemak
University of Texas Medical School, Houston, Texas

The advent of molecular biology has resulted in the identification and sequencing of genes, DNA base pairs encoding proteins. It is estimated that approximately 100,000 genes exist in humans; the function of many genes already identified is unknown. Differences in genes or polymorphic markers have been used to assign phenotypic traits to specific regions of the chromosome by genetic linkage analysis and to locate disease-causing genes inherited in families.

Genetic analysis in psoriasis is complicated by the fact that we do not know if psoriasis is a single disease. Two possibilities are likely: (1) Psoriasis is a multigenetic disease; i.e., a number of different genes must all be present for the expression of a psoriatic phenotype, or (2) psoriasis can result from single mutations in several separate genes (1). Studies of psoriasis in a few large kindreds have supported an autosomal dominant inheritance with penetrance of approximately 60% (2). Genetic linkage studies to date have found evidence for linkage in one family with psoriatic arthritis to chromosome 17q (3). This has not been confirmed by other studies, supporting genetic heterogeneity (4,5).

PSORIASIS IS A T-CELL-MEDIATED HOST RESPONSE IN A GENETICALLY PROGRAMMED HOST

The T cell is thought to play an essential role for the development of psoriasis (6,7). The hypothesis currently in favor is that psoriasis is a host-determined autoimmune or immune reaction pattern, occurring in the setting of a skin programmed for accelerated wound healing. Juvenile-onset diabetes, another immune reaction, has been linked to as many as 11 different genetic loci, and there is no reason to suspect otherwise for psoriasis (8). Psoriasis is most likely initiated as a T-cell-mediated immune response against an endogenous or exogenous antigen, bacterial, viral, or superantigen (9,10). The immune reaction occurs in the epidermis and papillary dermis between antigen-presenting cells and T cells (11).

The central role of the T cell in the pathogenesis of psoriasis is supported by the observations that psoriasis will remit with the use of immunosuppressive therapy (cyclosporin, steroids, methotrexate), in end-stage AIDS (12), and following allogeneic bone marrow transplant from a donor without psoriasis (13). Gottlieb et al. have shown that IL-2 diphtheria conjugated fusion protein reverses psoriasis and is associated with a decrease in the CD8+ T cells within the epidermis (14). Krueger has shown that ultraviolet light administration will cause T-cell apoptosis with reduction of the psoriasis lesion inflammatory infiltrates (15).

Of interest, Chang et al. have recently shown that CD8+ cells isolated from psoriatic plaques over time may show mono- or oligoclonal T-cell Vβ gene rearrangements (16). Clonal expansion of T cells suggests that they are being stimulated by a specific antigen. However, it is not known for certain whether these are effector or disease-limiting (suppressor) lymphocytes. In patients with poststreptococcal psoriasis, T-cell clones responsive to strep toxins have been identified (17,18). However superantigen-stimulated Vβ clones are not found by some investigators (19).

When psoriasis-normal skin is transplanted onto nude mice, it may become psoriasiform (20). This model has been further developed using an immunocompromised SCID mouse that lacks both cellular and humoral immunity. On the SCID mouse, a psoriatic phenotype will result in the graft if superantigen is applied to the skin graft (21) or if T cells from a psoriatic patient stimulated with IL-2 are added to the animal (22).

PSORIASIS IS A CYTOKINE SYMPHONY

Damage of the epidermis, whether through trauma, infection, or immune reaction, has been hypothesized to set off a cascade of cytokines and chemokines that will amplify the reaction and result in local perturbations of gene expression. A variety of cytokines including IL-1, IL-6, IL-8, TNF-α, interferon-gamma, IP-10, and others are implicated in the pathogenesis of psoriasis, since their expression profoundly influences the pattern of epidermal gene expression (differentiation program) and the rate of cell division (23–25). IL-1 is key because it induces other cytokines, such as IL-6 and IL-8, that are capable of stimulating the rate of keratinocyte proliferation (23,26).

Psoriasis is characterized by a predominance of Th1 cytokines (IL-2 and IFN-γ) that can invoke expression of HLA-DR, I-CAM, and IP-10 (27). Psoriasis might be best envisioned as a "cytokine symphony" played by the orchestra composed of sections: the chemotaxis section, the epidermal proliferator section, the Th1 T-cell section, the dermal-angiogenesis section. Abnormalities or imbalances in any molecule, its receptor, or its antagonists might contribute to the inheritance of this and other similar disorders, as suggested by Cork et al. (28). A commonality in all psoriasis may involve altered signal transduction set off by pathways of cytokines or interleukins. Factors that limit the spread of a psoriatic lesion to the surrounding normal skin are completely unknown.

THE WOUND-HEALING PHENOTYPE

Since similar T-cell-mediated responses are also found in patients with eczema/dermatitis, psoriatic patients must also have an intrinsic responsiveness in their skin. This quality, called Koebner's phenomenon, was also described as "the wound healing phenotype" by Mansbridge and Knapp (29). The ability to heal quickly or better than others or to react to bacterial skin infections in a benign fashion would have certainly conferred a selective advantage to cave-dwelling ancestors.

Saiag et al. first showed that psoriatic fibroblasts would support an accelerated outgrowth of epidermal keratinocytes placed above them (30). Priestley has suggested that psoriatic fibroblasts are hyperproliferative and are stimulated by serum factors (31). We have recently reexamined the psoriasis fibroblast in a skin-equivalent model.

In our skin equivalent, the majority, but not all, fibroblast lines derived from psoriatic nonlesional or lesional skin will induce epidermal hyperproliferation, as defined by epidermal thickness, on overlying normal foreskin keratinocytes (32,33). In addition, we found that psoriatic fibroblasts when combined with normal keratinocytes, in the absence of any inflammatory cells, induce significantly higher levels of interleukin-8 (IL-8) over the course of 14 days of culture in comparison with fibroblast strains from controls without psoriasis (34). The IL-8 level is correlated with epidermal thickness at 14 days (34).

IL-8 levels have been shown to be increased within psoriatic lesions (35–38) in association with the IL-8 receptor (39,40). Kojima et al. suggested that the elevation in IL-8 was secondary to the effect of activated T cells (38), and Nickoloff et al. demonstrated that TNF-α expression was associated with the increased IL-8 (41). A critical role for IL-8 in psoriasis (42) is also suggested by the findings that it can increase keratinocyte proliferation (43), cause T-cell chemotaxis (44), and influence the migration of keratinocytes on collagen (45). Our work in the skin-equivalent model, which lacks T cells, supports the hypothesis that intrinsic IL-8 levels induced by psoriatic fibroblasts may be important in the wound-healing phenotype of psoriasis patients. Even in the SCID model, psoriatic-normal skin grafts are required and they contain a dermal component.

INHERITANCE

Psoriasis has been subclassified into two forms based on age of onset (46,47), but this may be an oversimplification of the genetic diversity of psoriasis. Early-onset psoriasis, before the age of 20, is more likely to be inherited (type 1) than onset in later life. About 58% of patients with early-onset psoriasis have a first-degree relative with psoriasis, while only about 2% of patients with late-onset psoriasis have known relatives with the disease (46). Studies of the age of onset show two peaks, one at 16 years (for females) or 22 years (for males) and a second peak at the age of 60 years (for females) or 57 years (for males) (46). In addition, onset before age 15 carries the prospects of severe disease, involvement of a high percentage of the body, and a poor response to therapy (47). The predisposition for psoriasis evidently represents a multifactorial inheritance, and HLA studies (below) support this conclusion. The reason for the affinity between the HLA system and psoriasis, however, has not been explained.

HOST PREDISPOSITION

HLA or the major histocompatibility complex (MHC), contains a large family of polymorphic genes on the short arm of human chromosome 6. HLA protein chains on the surface of cells are markers for self-recognition and are necessary to present antigens to T and B cells to stimulate an immune response. Class I loci limit antigen recognition by cytotoxic (CD8+) T lymphocytes, and their MHC products are found on nearly all cells of the body.

Specific amino acid sequences within the HLA chains determine which peptide antigens may be bound, and thus presented to a T cell. The HLA chain is critical in initiating an immune response and thus could play a critical role in disease susceptibility. HLA disease associations have been found in psoriasis, as well as other immune skin diseases. Russell et al. (48) first reported an increased frequency of HL-A13 in patients with psoriasis in 1972. The antigen was present in 12 of 44 unrelated patients and in three of 89 controls (a difference significant at $p \leq 0.0001$). There have been many subsequent reports (often conflicting); however, certain antigens appear to be significantly associated with psoriasis and its subsets. Cw6 seems to be firmly linked with type I, or early-onset, psoriasis (47), DR7 and B27 with the arthritic manifestations of psoriasis, and DR3 with erosive psoriatic arthropathy (49).

It is not known how HLA antigens are linked with diseases, and the antigens may be only genetic markers for the true disease genes, which are located near the HLA genes on chromosome 6. The relative risk for psoriasis with Cw6 is 13 in Caucasians and 25 in Japanese (50). This means that a person carrying the Cw6 antigen has 13 times more chance (if Caucasian) or 25 times more chance (if Japanese) of getting psoriasis than the person who does not carry the antigen.

AUTOANTIBODIES AND HLA

In 1993 Parker wrote, "The function of class II MHC is to induce help in the T cell, rather than to deliver help to the B cell" (51). In other autoimmune diseases such as lupus and scleroderma, the HLA associations have been shown to be more closely tied with the presence of specific autoantibodies (52,53). This is not the case for psoriasis, to date. However, antibodies to streptococcal M protein that are cross-reactive to the stratum cornium have been demonstrated (54,55). Interestingly, serum and salivary IgA concentrations are significantly higher in psoriatics than controls ($p \leq 0.00001$). An increase in serum IgG concentration was also statistically significant ($p \leq 0.001$), and in 18 of 40 patients with psoriasis, anti-IgG activity was present in the serum (56).

EPIDERMAL DIFFERENTIATION PATHWAY IN PSORIASIS: A PRIMARY OR SECONDARY ALTERATION?

One of the controversies in the pathogenesis of psoriasis is whether the psoriatic keratinocyte is intrinsically different or is the victim of its cytokine milieu (57–59). In vitro, lymphokines from T-cell clones apparently stimulate keratinocyte proliferation and change their function by bringing about intercellular adhesion molecule-1 (ICAM-1) and HLA-DR cell-surface expression (60). The cytokine cascade evoked by the release of IL-1 is clearly able to stimulate epidermal proliferation (24). TNF-α as well as TGF-α may similarly increase epidermal proliferation (61,62).

We have found that many psoriatic keratinocytes are more difficult to culture and when placed in a skin equivalent have marked abnormalities in their ability to correctly differentiate (32,33). Nickoloff and associates have suggested that psoriatic keratinocytes may be abnormal in their ability to respond to the growth inhibition of IFN-γ (63–66). IFN-γ induces a cascade of genes through the STAT-1 pathway (67). These include the hyperproliferative keratins, K17, K6, and K16, and chemokines, including IP-10, that may inhibit keratinocyte growth and be chemotactic for T cells (68–70). The IFN-γ pathway may be susceptible to blockade by RAR-specific retinoid therapy (71), and the actions of retinoids in psoriasis may be anti-inflammatory, as well as effecting epidermal differentiation (72).

Bernard and associates noted that the differentiation program in psoriatic epidermis is abnormal in that there is precocious expression of both involucrin and keratinocyte transglutaminase, normally expressed in the upper stratum granulosum (73,74). We have shown that keratinocyte transglutaminase, the enzyme that forms crosslinking bonds to create the cornified layer, is overexpressed at the RNA level in psoriatic lesions and suggested that this in part explains the hyperkeratosis feature of psoriasis (75). Involucrin is one of a cluster of epidermal differentiation genes, also including psoriasin, CRABP-2, and MRP-8, that are overexpressed in the psoriasis lesion and may be coordinately regulated (76). Retinoids may be effective in psoriasis therapy by their action in down-regulating the expression of abnormally expressed epidermal genes, including but not limited to hyperproliferative keratins, epidermal growth factor receptor, keratinocyte transglutaminase, MRP-8, and SKALP (67, 77–80). Retinoids with specificity for receptors may be useful as tools for studying psoriatic gene regulation. Tazarotene, a new topical retinoid with selectivity for RAR $\beta\gamma$ receptors, has been found to upregulate the expression of several novel genes (tazarotene-inducible genes, TIG), which are induced in psoriatic plaques by the drug (71,81). TIG-1 is selective for the RAR class of receptors (81) and appears to be a cell surface molecule.

ANGIOGENESIS—PRIMARY OR SECONDARY?

The capillaries are known to be abnormal in psoriatic lesions with fenestrations present (82). Psoriatic capillaries become elongated as they orient themselves parallel with the acanthosis of the epidermal rete ridges. Alterations in epidermal differentiation have been shown to precede the abnormalities of angiogenesis within the psoriatic plaque (83). This suggests that IL-8 or other epidermal cytokines may invoke neovascularization as a secondary feature. Interferon-inducible protein 10 (IP-10), over expressed in psoriatic epidermis (68), has been shown to inhibit angiogenesis (84). Moreover, the inhibitory effects of IL-12 on IFN-γ may be effected by IP-10 (84).

CONCLUSIONS

The central role of the T cell (85) is supported by the recent finding of CD8+ T-cell clones within psoriasis lesions (16) and by observing the effect of therapy on psoriasis, especially relating to the use of cyclosporin A DAB-IL2 fusion toxin and ultraviolet light (15, 23,38,86). Krueger et al. found that most of the cellular and molecular changes that occur in the psoriatic epidermis are restored to normal following repeated ultraviolet B (UVB) irradiation. Epidermal thickening was reduced by 60%, keratinocyte pathology was reversed, and activated intraepidermal T cells were markedly decreased. Also, UVB depleted ≥90% of the CD3+, CD8+, and CD25+ T cells from the epidermis but not from the dermis (15). Translational research using new agents such as retinoids with selectivity for specific receptor classes may also result in the discovery of new genes with abnormal expression in psoriasis; retinoids can interfere with transcription factors necessary for cell signaling (71,81,87,88).

The "framework hypothesis" for the pathogenesis of psoriasis suggests that the entire skin of a patient with psoriasis is genetically programmed with the ability to express the disease (89); however, active manifestations of psoriasis require additional stimuli (environmental factors) (90). Common factors that may bring about an outbreak of lesions include skin injury, drugs, infections especially with bacterial superantigens, and stress (90). Although the skin is the principal organ affected in psoriasis, it is not entirely a skin disease because nails or joints may be involved, and disorders of various internal tissues have been associated. The keratinization of the psoriatic epidermis, the increased utilization of glucose and oxygen in the lesions, the possibility of an enzyme deletion, and the plausibility of a defect in the cyclic AMP cascade have all been thoroughly investigated. Recently, molecular biologists have seen psoriasis as an error of communication, a disorganization of the normal pathway of information. A pathway associated with the inflammatory response has been suggested (91).

REFERENCES

1. Meyer, L.J. (1990). Psoriasis: the application of genetic technology and mapping. *J. Invest. Dermatol.* 95: 5S–6S.
2. Wuepper, K.D., Coulter, S.N., and Haberman, A. (1990). Psoriasis vulgaris: a genetic approach. *J. Invest. Dermatol.* 95:2S–4S.
3. Tomfohrde, J., Silverman, A., Barnes, R., et al. (1994). Gene for familial psoriasis susceptibility mapped to the distal end of human chromosome 17q. *Science* 264: 1141–1145.
4. Theeuwes, M., and Leder, R.O. (1993). Hereditary insights in psoriasis. *Eur. J. Dermatol.* 3:335–341.
5. Nair, R.P., Sun-Wei, G., Jenisch, S., et al. (1995). Scanning chromosome 17 for psoriasis susceptibility; lack of evidence for a distal 17q locus. *Hum. Hered.* 45: 219–230.
6. Baadsgaard, O., Tong, P., Elder, J.T., et al. (1990). UM4D4+ (CDw60) T cells are compartmentalized into psoriatic skin and release lymphokines that induce a keratinocyte phenotype expressed in psoriatic skin lesions. *J. Invest. Dermatol.* 95:275–282.
7. Baker, B.S., and Fry, L. (1992). The immunology of psoriasis. *Br. J. Dermatol.* 126:1–9.
8. Davies, J.L., Kawaguchi, Y., Bennett, S.T., et al. (1994). A genome-wide search for human type 1 diabetes susceptibility genes. *Nature* 371:130–135.
9. Asselineau, D., and Prunieras, M. (1984). Reconstruction of "simplified" skin: control of fabrication. *Br. J. Dermatol.* 111:219–222.
10. Breathnach, S.M. (1993). The skin immune system and psoriasis. *Clin. Exp. Immunol.* 91:343–345.
11. Baadsgaard, O., Gupta, A.K., Taylor, R.S., et al. (1989). Psoriatic epidermal cells demonstrate increased numbers and function of non-Langerhans antigen-presenting cells. *J. Invest. Dermatol.* 92:190–195.
12. Johnson, T.M., Duvic, M., Rapini, R.P., et al. (1985). AIDS exacerbates psoriasis. *N. Engl. J. Med.* 313:1415 (letter).
13. Eedy, D.J., Burrows, J.M., Bridges, J.M., et al. (1990). Clearance of severe psoriasis after allogeneic bone marrow transplantation. *Br. Med. J.* 300:908–909.
14. Gottlieb, S.L., Gilleaudeau, P., Johnson, R., et al. (1995). Response of psoriasis to a lymphocyte-selective toxin (DAB-IL2) suggests a primary immune, but not keratinocyte pathogeneic basis. *Nature Med.* 1: 442–447.
15. Krueger, J.G., Wolfe, J.T., Nabeya, R.T., et al. (1995). Successful ultraviolet B treatment of psoriasis is accompanied by a reversal of keratinocyte pathology and by selective depletion of intraepidermal T cells. *J. Exp. Med.* 182:2057–2068.
16. Chang, J.C.C., Smith, L.R., Froning, K.J., et al. (1994). CD8+ T cells in psoriatic lesions preferentially use T-cell receptor Vβ3 and/or Wβ13.1 genes. *Proc. Natl. Acad. Sci. U.S.A.* 91:9282–9286.
17. Baker, B.S., Bokth, S., Powles, A., et al. (1993). Group A streptococcal antigen-specific T lymphocytes in guttate psoriatic lesions. *Br. J. Dermatol.* 128:493–499.
18. Yokote, R., Tokura, Y., Furukawa, F., et al. (1995). Susceptible responsiveness to bacterial superantigens in peripheral blood mononuclear cells from patients with psoriasis. *Arch. Dermatol. Res.* 287:443–447.
19. Boehncke, W.H., Dressel, D., Manfras, B., et al. (1995). T-cell-receptor repertoire in chronic plaque-stage psoriasis is restricted and lacks enrichment of superantigen-associated Vβ regions. *J. Invest. Dermatol.* 104:725–728.
20. Fraki, J., Briggaman, R., and Lazarus, G. (1982). Uninvolved skin from psoriatic patients develops signs of involved psoriatic skin after being grafted onto nude mice. *Science* 215:685–687.
21. Boehncke, W.H., Zollner, T.M., Dressel, D., et al. (1996). Induction of psoriasiform inflammation by a bacterial superantigen in human skin grafts transplanted onto SCID mice. *J. Invest. Dermatol.* 106:833.
22. Wrone-Smith, T., and Nickoloff, B.J. (1996). Dermal injection of immunocytes induces psoriasis. *J. Clin. Invest.* 98:1878–1887.
23. Krueger, J.G., Krane, J.F., Carter, M., et al. (1990). Role of growth factors, cytokines, and their receptors in the pathogenesis of psoriasis. *J. Invest. Dermatol.* 94:135S–140S.
24. Kupper, T.S. (1993). Cytokines in pathophysiologic responses in skin: recruitment of inflammatory infiltrates to cutaneous tissues. In *Clinical Applications of Cytokines: Role in Pathogenesis, Diagnosis, and Therapy.* J.J. Oppenheim, J.L. Rossio, and A.S.H. Gearings (Eds.). Oxford University Press, Oxford, pp. 251–255.
25. Elder, J.T. (1995). Cytokine and genetic regulation of psoriasis. *Adv. Dermatol.* 10:99–133.
26. Grossman, R.M., Krueger, J., Yourish, D., et al. (1989). Interleukin 6 is expressed in high levels in psoriatic skin and stimulates proliferation of cultured human keratinocytes. *Proc. Natl. Acad. Sci. U.S.A.* 86: 6367–6371.
27. Uyemura, K., Yamamura, M., Fivenson, D.F., et al. (1993). The cytokine network in lesional and lesion-free psoriatic skin is characterized by a T-helper type 1 cell-mediated response. *J. Invest. Dermatol.* 101: 701–705.

28. Cork, M.J., Tarlow, J.K., Blakemore, A.I.F., et al. (1993). Genetics of interleukin 1 receptor antagonist Cr2 q14 in inflammatory skin diseases. *Clin. Res.* 41: 179A.
29. Mansbridge, J.N., and Knapp, A.M. (1987). Changes in keratinocyte maturation during wound healing. *J. Invest. Dermatol.* 89:253–263.
30. Saiag, P., Coulomb, B., Lebreton, C., et al. (1985). Psoriatic fibroblasts induce hyperproliferation of normal keratinocytes in a skin equivalent model in vitro. *Science* 230:669–672.
31. Priestley, G., and Adams, L. (1985). Mitogenic effects of sera from normal and psoriatic subjects on human skin fibroblasts. *Arch. Dermatol. Res.* 227:13–15.
32. Remenyik, E., Ellard, J., Cho, J., et al. (1994). Psoriatic raft model: effect of fibroblasts. *Clin. Res.* 42: 230A.
33. Remenyik, E., Davies, P.J.A., and Duvic, M. (1995). Skin-equivalent model. *Borgyogyaszati Venerol. Szemle* 71:19–24.
34. Konstantinova, N.V., Duong, D.-M.T., Remenyik, E., et al. (1996). IL-8 is induced in skin equivalents and is highest in those derived from psoriatic fibroblasts. *J. Invest. Dermatol.* 107:615–621.
35. Sticherling, M., Bornscheuer, E., Schroder, J.-M., et al. (1991). Localization of neutrophil-activating peptide-1/interleukin-8-immunoreactivity in normal and psoriatic skin. *J. Invest. Dermatol.* 96:26–30.
36. Schroder, J.-M., and Enno, C. (1986). Identification of C5a Des Arg and an anionic neutrophil-activating peptide (ANAP) in psoriatic scales. *J. Invest. Dermatol.* 87:53–58.
37. Gillitzer, R., Berger, R., Mielke, V., et al. (1991). Upper keratinocytes of psoriatic skin lesions express high levels of NAP-1/IL-8 mRNA in situ. *J. Invest. Dermatol.* 97:73–79.
38. Kojima, T., Cromie, M.A., Fisher, G.J., et al. (1993). GRO-A mRNA is selectively overexpressed in psoriatic epidermis and is reduced by cyclosporin A in vivo, but not in cultured keratinocytes. *J. Invest. Dermatol.* 101:767–772.
39. Schulz, B.S., Michel, G., Wagner, S., et al. (1993). Increased expression of epidermal IL-8 receptor in psoriasis. *J. Immunol.* 151:4399–4406.
40. Arenberger, P., Kemeny, L., Suss, R., et al. (1992). Interleukin-8 receptors in normal and psoriatic polymorphonuclear leukocytes. *Acta Derm. Venereol. (Stockh.)* 72:334–336.
41. Nickoloff, B.J., Karabin, G.D., Barker, J.N.W.N., et al. (1990). Cellular localization of IL-8 and its inducer, tumor necrosis factor alpha in psoriasis. *Am. J. Pathol.* 138:129–140.
42. Schroder, J.-M. (1995). Cytokine networks in the skin. *J. Invest. Dermatol.* 105:20S–24S.
43. Tuschil, A., Lam, C., Halsberger, A., et al. (1992). Interleukin-8 stimulates calcium transients and promotes epidermal cell proliferation. *J. Invest. Dermatol.* 99:294–298.
44. Larsen, C.G., Anderson, A.O., Appella, E., et al. (1989). The neutrophil-activating protein (NAP-1) is also chemotactic for T lymphocytes. *Science* 243: 1464–1466.
45. Michel, G., Kemeny, L., Peter, R.U., et al. (1992). Interleukin-8 receptor-mediated chemotaxis of normal human epidermal cells. *FEBS Lett* 305:241–243.
46. Henseler, T., and Christophers, E. (1985). Psoriasis of early and late onset: characterization of two types of psoriasis vulgaris. *J. Am. Acad. Dermatol.* 13:450–456.
47. Elder, J.T., Nair, R.P., Guo, S.-W., et al. (1994). The genetics of psoriasis. *Arch. Dermatol.* 130:216–224.
48. Russell, T.J., Schultes, L.M., and Kuban, D.J. (1972). Histocompatibility (HL-A) antigens associated with psoriasis. *N. Engl. J. Med.* 287:738–740.
49. Moll, J.M.H. (1986). Psoriatic arthropathy. In *Textbook of Psoriasis.* P.D. Mier and P.C.M. van de Kerkhof (Eds.). Churchill Livingstone, London, pp. 55–83.
50. Zachariae, H. (1986). Epidemiology and genetics. In *Textbook of Psoriasis.* P.D. Mier and P.C.M. van de Kerkhof (Eds.). Churchill Livingstone, London, pp. 4–12.
51. Parker, D.C. (1993). The functions of antigen recognition in T cell-dependent B cell activation. *Semin. Immunol.* 5:413–420.
52. Arnett, F.C., Bias, W.B., and Reveille, J.D. (1989). Genetic studies in Sjögren's syndrome and systemic lupus erythematosus. *Autoimmunity* 2:404–413.
53. Reveille, J.D., Durban, E., MacLeod-St. Clair, M.J., et al. (1992). Association of amino acid sequences in the HLA-DQB1 first domain with the anti-topoisomerase antibody response in scleroderma (progressive systemic sclerosis). *J. Clin. Invest.* 90:973–980.
54. Swerlick, R.A., Cunningham, M.W., and Hall, N.K. (1986). Monoclonal antibodies cross-reactive with group A streptococci and normal and psoriatic human skin. *J. Invest. Dermatol.* 87:367–371.
55. Shikman, A.R., and Cunningham, M. (1994). Immunological mimicry between *N*-acetyl-B-D-glucosamine and cytokeratin peptides. *J. Immunol.* 152:4375–4387.
56. Guilhou, J.J., Clot, J., Meynadier, J., et al. (1976). Immunologic aspects of psoriasis. *Br. J. Dermatol.* 94: 501–507.
57. Lui, S.C.C., and Parsons, C.S. (1983). Serial cultivation of epidermal keratinocytes from psoriatic plaques. *J. Invest. Dermatol.* 81:54–61.
58. West, M., Kernicer,K., and Faed, M. (1983). In vitro growth rates of epidermal cells derived from the skin of psoriatic patients and nonpsoriatic controls. *Br. J. Dermatol.* 108:533–540.
59. Krabelle, K., Desjarlais, L., and Marcelo, C. (1985). Increased DNA synthesis of uninvolved psoriatic epidermis is maintained in vitro. *Br. J. Dermatol.* 112: 263–270.

60. Baadsgaard, O., Fisher, G., Voorhees, J.J., et al. (1990). The role of the immune system in the pathogenesis of psoriasis. *J. Invest. Dermatol.* 95:32S–34S.
61. Christophers, E., and Krueger, G.G. (1987). Psoriasis. In *Dermatology in General Medicine*, 3rd ed., Vol. I. T.B. Fitzpatrick, A.Z. Eisen, K. Wolff, et al. (Eds.). McGraw-Hill, New York, Chapter 42, pp. 461–491.
62. Elder, J.T., Fisher, G.J., Lindquiest, P.B. et al. (1989). Overexpression of transforming growth factor alpha in psoriatic epidermis. *Science* 243:811–814.
63. Nickholoff, B.J., Mitra, R.S., Elder, J.T., et al. (1989). Decreased growth inhibition by recombinant gamma interferon is associated with increased transforming growth factor-alpha production in keratinocytes cultured from psoriatic lesions. *Br. J. Dermatol.* 121: 161–174.
64. Nickoloff, B.J., Fisher, G.J., Mitra, R.S., et al. (1988). Additive and synergistic antiproliferative effect of cyclosporin A and gamma interferon on cultured human keratinocytes. *Am. J. Pathol.* 131:12–18.
65. Nickoloff, B.J., and Mitra, R.S. (1989). Inhibition of ^{125}I-epidermal growth factor binding to cultured keratinocytes by antiproliferative molecules gamma interferon, cyclosporin A, and transforming growth factor-beta. *J. Invest. Dermatol.* 39:799–803.
66. Nickoloff, B.J. (1991). The cytokine network in psoriasis. *Arch. Dermatol.* 127:871–874 (editorial).
67. Komine, M., Freedberg, I.M., and Blumenberg, M. (1996). Regulation of epidermal expression of keratin K17 in inflammatory skin diseases. *J. Invest. Dermatol.* 107:569–575.
68. Gottlieb, A.B., Luster, A.D., Postnett, D.N., et al. (1988). Detection of a gamma interferon induced protein IP-10 in psoriatic plaques. *J. Exp. Med.* 168: 941–948.
69. Sarris, A.H., Esgleyes-Ribot, T., Crow, M., et al. (1995). Cytokine loops involving interferon-gamma and IP-10, a cytokine chemotactic for CD4-positive lymphocytes: an explanation for the epidermotropism of cutaneous T cell lymphoma. *Blood* 86:651–658.
70. Luster, A.D., and Leder, P. (1993). IP-10, a C-X-C chemokine, elicits a potent thymus-dependent antitumor response in vitro. *J. Exp. Med.* 178:1057–1065.
71. Duvic, M., Nagpal, S., Asano, A., et al. (1997). Molecular mechanisms of tazarotene action. *J. Am. Acad. Dermatol.* (in press).
72. Esgleyes-Ribot, T., Chandraratna, R.A., Lew-Kaya, D.A., et al. (1994). Response of psoriasis to a new topical retinoid, AGN 190168. *J. Am. Acad. Dermatol.* 30:581–590.
73. Bernard, B.A., Reano, A., Darmon, Y.M., et al. (1986). Precocious appearance of involucrin and epidermal transglutaminase during differentiation of psoriatic skin. *Br. J. Dermatol.* 114:279–283.
74. Bernard, B.A., Magnaldo, T., and Darmon, Y.M. (1992). Delayed onset of epidermal differentiation in psoriasis. *J. Invest. Dermatol.* 98:902–910.
75. Schroeder, W.T., Thacher, S.M., Stewart-Galetka, S., et al. (1992). Type I human keratinocyte transglutaminase: expression in normal skin and psoriasis. *J. Invest. Dermatol.* 99:27–34.
76. Gillitizer, R., Wolff, K., Tong, D., et al. (1993). MCP-1 mRNA expression in basal keratinocytes of psoriatic lesions. *J. Invest. Dermatol.*101:127–131.
77. Esgleyes, T., Annarella, M., Chandraratna, R., et al. (1993). Effect of topically applied retinoid, AGN 190168, on epidermal gene expression psoriasis. *Clin. Res.* 41(2):491A.
78. Nagpal, S., Thacher, S.M., Patel, S., et al. (1996). Negative regulation of two hyperproliferative keratinocyte differentiation markers by a retinoic acid receptor-specific retinoid: insight into the mechanism of retinoid action in psoriasis. *Cell Growth Differ.* 7:1783–1791.
79. Griffiths, C.E.M., Rosenthal, D.S., Reddy, A.P., et al. (1992). Short-term retinoic acid treatment increases in vivo, but decreases in vitro, epidermal transglutaminase-K enzyme activity and immunoreactivity. *J. Invest. Dermatol.* 99:283–288.
80. Alkemade, H.A.C., de Jongh, G.J., Arnold, W.P., et al. (1995). Levels of skin-derived antileukoprotease (SKALP)/elafin in serum correlate with disease activity during treatment of severe psoriasis with cyclosporin A. *J. Invest. Dermatol.* 104:189–193.
81. Nagpal, S., Patel, S., Asano, A.T., et al. (1996). Tazarotene-induced gene 1, (TIG1), a novel retinoic acid receptor-responsive gene in skin. *J. Invest. Dermatol.* 106:269–274.
82. Braverman, I.M., and Yen, A. (1977). Ultrastructure of the capillary loops in the dermal papillae of psoriasis. *J. Invest. Dermatol.* 68:53–60.
83. Parent, D., Bernard, B.A., Desbas, C., et al. (1990). Spreading of psoriatic plaques: alteration of epidermal differentiation precedes capillary leakiness and anomalies in vascular morphology. *J. Invest. Dermatol.* 95: 333–340.
84. Sgadari, C., Angiolillo, A.L., and Tosato, G. (1996). Inhibition of angiogenesis by interleukin-12 is mediated by the interferon-inducible protein 10. *Blood* 87: 3877–3882.
85. Valdimarsson, H., Baker, B.S., Jónsdóttir, I., et al., (1987). Psoriasis: a disease of abnormal keratinocyte proliferation induced by T lymphocytes. *Immunol. Today* 7:256–259.
86. Elder, J.T., Hammerberg, C., Cooper, K.D., et al. (1993). Cyclosporin A rapidly inhibits epidermal cytokine expression in psoriasis lesions, but not in cytokine stimulated keratinocytes. *J. Invest. Dermatol.* 101:761–766.

87. Chandraratna, R., Patel, S., Duvic, M., et al. (1994). Subtractive hybridization cloning of a candidate marker gene from skin raft cultures reveals the anti-inflammatory action of retinoids. *J. Invest. Dermatol.* 102:625.
88. Nagpal, S., Athanikar, J., and Chandraratna, R.A.S. (1995). Separation of transactivation and AP1 antagonism functions of retinoic acid receptor alpha. *J. Biol. Chem.* 270:923–927.
89. Krueger, G., Chambers, D., and Shelby, J. (1981). Involved and uninvolved skin from psoriatic patients: are they equally diseased? *J. Clin. Invest.* 68:1548–1557.
90. Krueger, G.G., and Duvic, M. (1994). Epidemiology of psoriasis: clinical issues. *J. Invest. Dermatol.* 102: 14s–18s.
91. Van Erp, P.E.J., and Mier, P.D. (1986). Molecular biology. In *Textbook of Psoriasis.* P.D. Mier and P.C.M. van de Kerkhof (Eds.). Churchill Livingstone, London, pp. 125–149.

23

Cytokine Abnormalities in the Epidermis

Lloyd E. King, Jr.
Vanderbilt University School of Medicine and Department of Veterans Affairs Medical Center, Nashville, Tennessee

Lillian B. Nanney
Vanderbilt University School of Medicine, Nashville, Tennessee

John Paul Sundberg
The Jackson Laboratory, Bar Harbor, Maine

Many hypotheses have been postulated to explain the cause of or propose a cure for psoriasis. The current prevailing hypothesis is that the epidermal proliferation and skin inflammation, hallmarks of psoriasis, are either primarily or secondarily due to aberrant T-lymphocyte dysfunction (1,2). An alternative yet viable hypothesis is that epidermal keratinocytes may be genetically abnormal. This view is supported by studies showing that affected psoriatic skin grafted onto immunodeficient mice maintains a psoriatic phenotype for months (3–5) and that transgenic mice overexpressing certain integrins develop a psoriatic phenotype (6) (see below). It is entirely possible that these two hypotheses, aberrant T-cell activation and intrinsically defective keratinocytes, may not be mutually exclusive. Abnormal growth factor and cytokine regulation exhibited by psoriatic keratinocytes may be due to their genetically defective interactions with dermal cells, endothelial cells, or immunocytes (7,8).

The seminal paper reporting cytokine receptor alterations in psoriasis first appeared approximately 10 years ago (9). This report showed that the epidermal growth factor receptor tyrosine kinases (EGF-R) were markedly increased in active psoriatic lesions owing to their persistence into the suprabasal epidermal compartment (Fig. 1). This observation contrasted sharply with a previous report describing the primary localization of EGF-R to the basal compartment in normal human epidermis (10) (Fig. 2). The potential clinical relevance of EGF-R was initially indicated by the observation that the altered EGF-R distribution pattern in psoriasis resumed its normal basal epidermal layer distribution in regressing or healing lesions (9). Subsequent studies by many other groups now strongly support the relevance of the EGF-R pathway in psoriasis (see below) and are the foundation for the now popular hypotheses that (1) EGF-R serve a functional role in normal epidermis and (2) EGF-R play a causal role in the pathophysiology of hyperproliferative skin diseases. This chapter focuses on the role(s) of the EGF receptor family signaling pathways in the proliferative epidermis present in psoriasis and other hyperproliferative skin conditions and provides an overview of this receptor and its interactions with numerous related ligands and signaling molecules that regulate epidermal proliferation. The EGF-R research area is very active and insights into the mechanisms along its signaling pathway in normal and pathological states continue to increase. Thus, it is appropriate to review recent data pertaining to EGF-R and related cytokines before discussing what is already known about the specific roles of EGF-R in the pathogenesis and treatment of psoriasis.

EGF RECEPTOR SUPERFAMILY, THEIR LIGANDS AND MOLECULES WITH EGF-LIKE MOTIFS

EGF and Molecules with EGF-like Motifs

Over the past 10 years, it has become apparent that a number of molecules exhibit strong homologies with EGF. To date, those with the closest similarity include TGF-α, amphiregulin (AR), heparin-binding EGF-like molecule (HB-EGF), *neu* differentiation factor (NDF), and betacellulin (Table 1). Currently, the presence and/or expression of these ligands in normal epidermis has been confirmed for TGF-α (11), amphiregulin (12,13), and NDF (14). The existence of multiple EGF-R ligands is both puzzling and challenging. These ligands appear to have equal binding affinities, stimulate mitogenesis, and induce mRNA expression of other EGF family members (15). However, reports are just beginning to document that EGF ligands also exhibit subtly different effects in their regulatory mechanisms. For example, EGF and TGF-α both bind in subdomain IV of the extracellular portion of the EGF-R; however, subdomain IV of the receptor regulates only TGF-α-mediated signal transduction across the membrane (16). A recent study reported that keratinocyte motility was enhanced more effectively by TGF-α than EGF; however, mitogenic responses were equally matched (17). Amphiregulin and HB-EGF, both present in human keratinocytes, have, in addition to their binding affinities for the EGF-R, a marked binding affinity for heparin. As a result, both are subject to additional regulatory variables determined by the glycosaminoglycan composition within the extracellular matrix (18).

Tenascin, a large glycoprotein of the extracellular matrix, is another molecule with numerous EGF-like motifs in its structure and is reportedly increased in hyperproliferative skin disease such as psoriasis (19). Laminin, a prominent molecule of the extracellular matrix, also reportedly has multiple EGF-like repeats in its structure, but it is unclear how this finding fits into the regulatory pathway (20). NDF (or heregulin), another structurally related EGF-like molecule, can also bind to a variant within the EGF-R family known as *erb*B2 or HER-2 (21). The *neu* ligand is expressed by proliferating keratinocytes in culture but has not been detected in normal skin to date (22). Additional EGF-like molecules such as betacellulin have been identified and characterized but their presence in cutaneous structures has not yet been confirmed. The mechanistic reasons for the redundancy of EGF-like molecules potentially capable of regulating keratinocyte growth through EGF-R activation are not yet clearly identified.

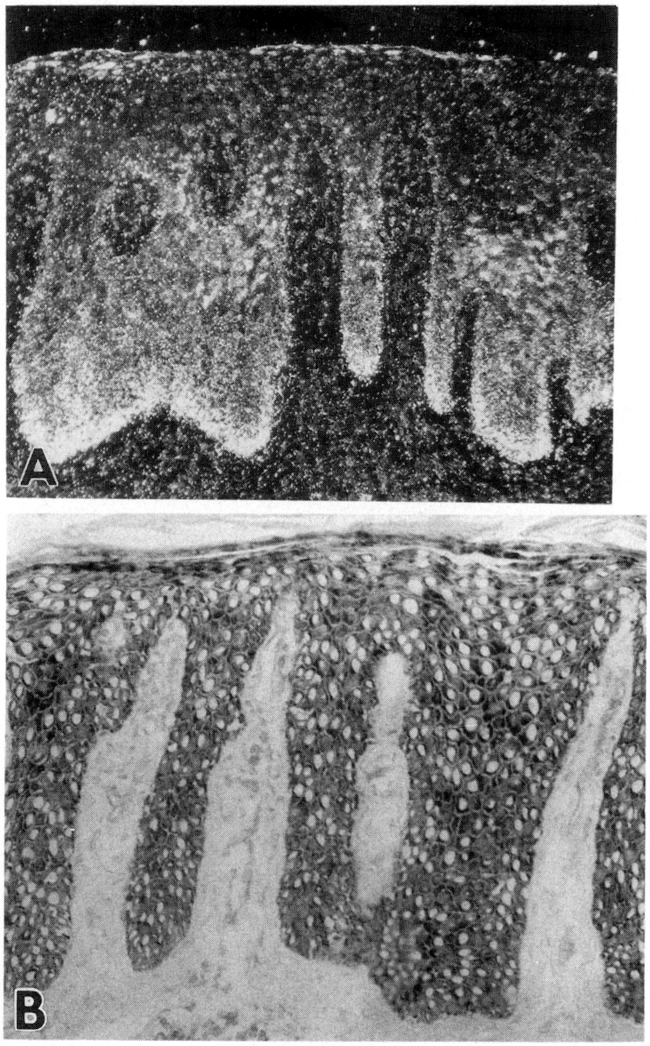

Figure 1 (A) Dark-field micrograph showing the localization of ^{125}I-EGF binding to the EGF-R in psoriatic epidermis. Silver grains are greatest in the basal compartment, yet persist into the outer layers. (B) Immunostaining for EGF-R in a psoriatic lesion shows receptors throughout all layers of the epidermis.

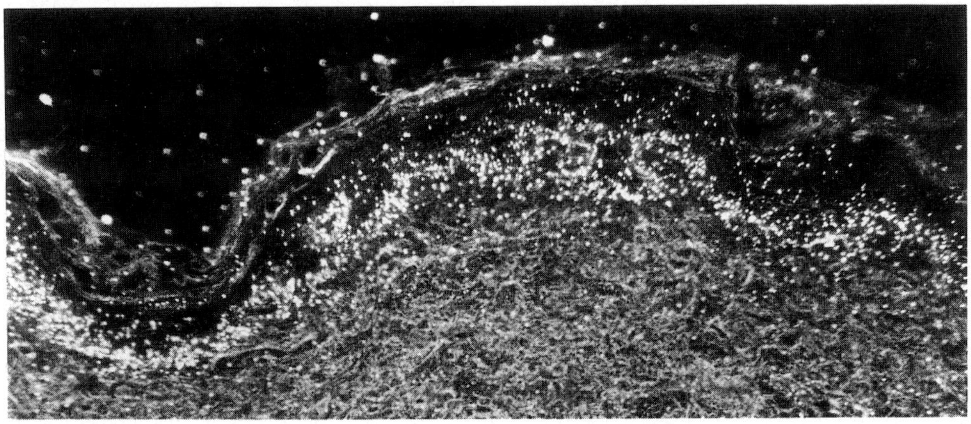

Figure 2 Dark-field micrograph showing the localization of ^{125}I-EGF binding to the EGF-R in normal epidermis. Binding is greatest in the stratum basalis.

EGF Receptor Superfamily

Diversity in the signal transduction pathway also exists at the receptor level (Table 1). Currently, four members of the EGF-R family have been identified (Table 1). Both EGF-R and *erb*B2 (HER-2) have been localized in normal human skin (10,14) but only EGF-R has been reported in psoriasis (9). The characterization of other receptor forms in normal skin is just beginning. A preliminary report suggested that transcripts for HER-3 were most strongly expressed in the differentiated layers of the normal epidermis and that HER-4 was not present in normal epidermis (22). The HER-2 receptor, which preferentially binds the *neu* ligand, has been previously reported in normal skin; the *neu* ligand itself was not detected in normal epidermis, according to a recent study (22). While the *neu* (*erb*B2) receptor has been reported in normal skin (14), it has most recently been reported in another very important keratinocyte population—metastatic keratinocytes (23–25). In cultured cells it is known that the *neu* ligand binds to either HER-3 or HER-4 receptor forms and can indirectly induce tyrosine phosphorylation of HER-2 through heterodimerization (26–28).

EGF-R MEDIATED SIGNAL TRANSDUCTION PATHWAYS TO THE NUCLEUS

Ultimately mitogenic signals must be delivered to the nucleus to trigger mitogenesis either directly or indirectly or regulated gene expression. Motifs in the membrane distal intracellular domain of the EGF-R tyrosine kinases mediate signaling by regulating the association of signaling molecules with the activated EGF-R (Fig. 3). More recently, another pathway has been identified that transduces signals from the membrane proximal region of the EGF-R and other cytokine receptors to the nucleus (STAT pathway, Fig. 4).

Regulation of Membrane Receptor Tyrosine Kinases by Dimerization

EGF receptor responses are triggered by ligands interacting with the extracellular domain of this trans-

Table 1 Molecules with Strong Homologies with EGF

Possible ligands for the EGF receptor
Epidermal growth factor (EGF)
Transforming growth factor-alpha (TGFα)
neu differentiation factor/heregulin (*neu*)
Amphiregulin (AR)
Heparin-binding epidermal growth factor like molecule (HB-EGF)
Betacellulin
Tenascin
Laminin
Tyrosine kinase receptor molecules in the EGF-R series
Epidermal growth factor receptor (EGF-R)
Heregulin receptor 2 (*erb*-B2, HER2)
Heregulin receptor 3 (*erb*-B3, HER3)
Heregulin receptor 4 (*erb*-B4, HER 4)

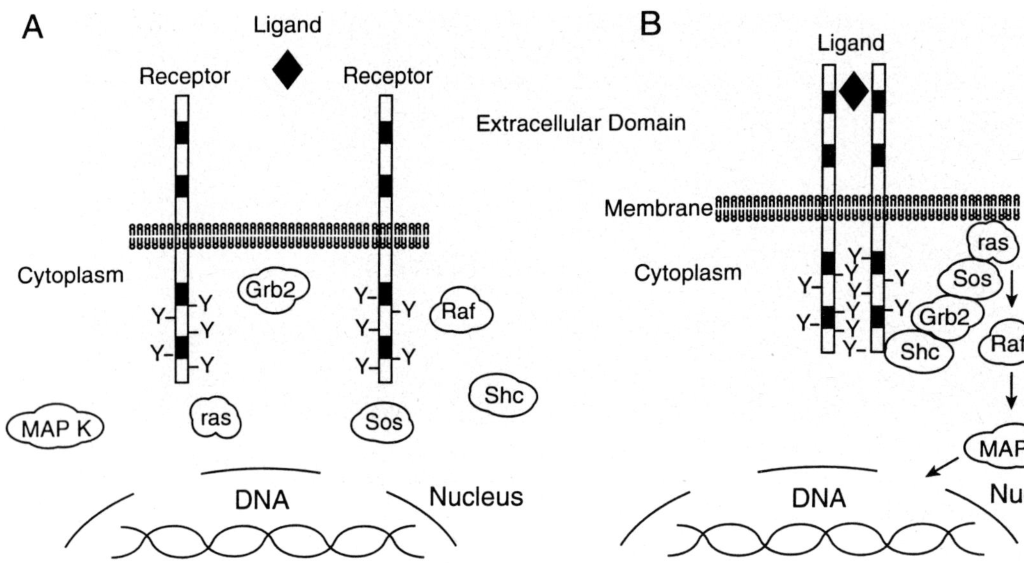

Figure 3 Molecules along the *ras* signal transduction pathway for EGF-R. (A) Molecules before ligand binding. (B) Molecules following receptor activation.

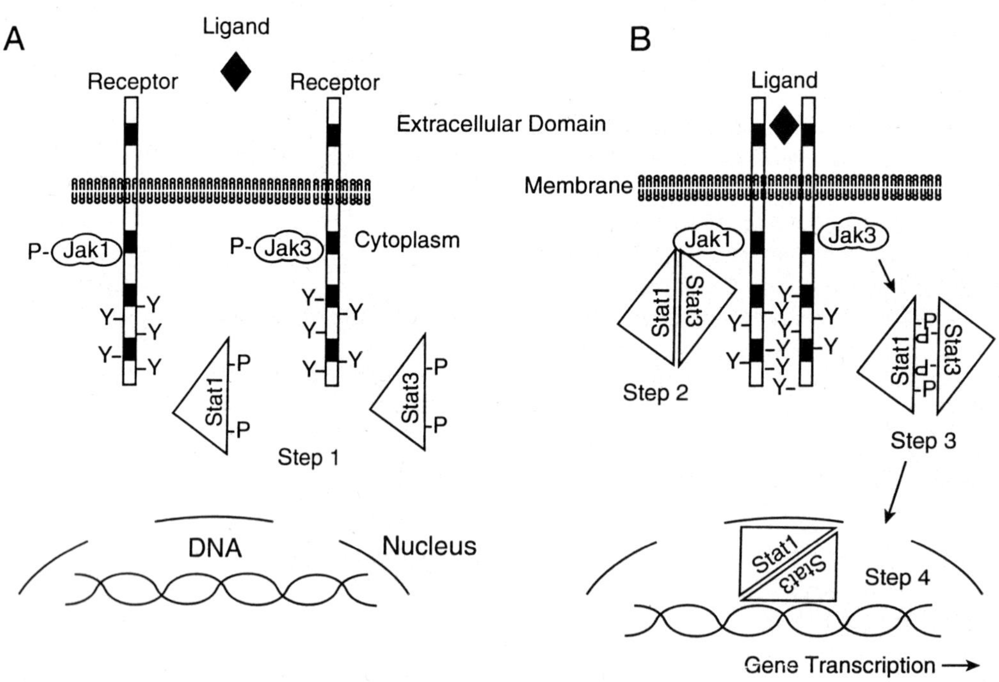

Figure 4 Molecules along the Jak-STAT signal transduction pathway for EGF-R. (A) Molecules before ligand binding. (B) Molecules after activation.

membrane receptor leading to dimerization and activation of intrinsic tyrosine kinase activity (29) (Fig. 3). By analogy, other cytokines acting through their tyrosine kinase receptors are thought to have a similar final common pathway to trigger their effects such as migration or mitogenesis. Receptor dimerization is but one potential point along the EGF-R cascade where selective signaling can lead to divergent cellular consequences (16,30). Although precise mechanisms of EGF-R dimerization are unclear (31), an intracellular dimerization domain in EGF-R was recently identified using deletion analysis (32). Heterodimerization studies between EGF-R and another receptor form p185, *erb*B2 (HER-2) suggest that simultaneous activation of two types of receptor kinases may result in more efficient (transforming) or distinct signal transduction pathways (30,31,33,34). Conversely, *neu* (heregulin), an EGF-like molecule, was recently shown to *trans*-regulate or negatively impact the dimerization of EGF-R forms (21,35). Thus, many more regulatory points along the EGF-R signaling cascade are being identified (17). Each addition along the signaling pathway marks yet another potential point where misregulation can either block or amplify the pathway. How these homeostatic mechanisms involving EGF-like ligands, EGF-R family members, and other cytokine receptors are persistently disrupted in psoriasis is uncertain, but clearly the EGF-R-related pathways that control normal epidermal proliferation and differentiation are markedly affected in this patient population.

Ligand-Binding-Induced Phosphorylation of Adaptor Molecules Binding to EGF-R

The various domains within this receptor tyrosine kinase govern the downstream signals that are generated following interaction with appropriate ligands (39,40,52,53,54). Five phosphorylation sites are clustered in the carboxy-terminus of the native form of EGF-R. These can become autophosphorylated or can be *trans*-phosphorylated when two receptor molecules form a dimer. Three of these autophosphorylation sites and the SH2-binding sites are removed by calcium-activated proteolysis that occurs in vivo or in vitro in response to cell lysis (36). These phosphotyrosine residues serve as recognition sites for intracellular proteins that contain *src*-homology 2 (SH2) motifs (29). A few of the growing list of SH2 proteins that have been implicated in the EGF-R-mediated signal transduction pathways are depicted in Figure 3A. Although details are still emerging, it appears that following receptor activation, the Shc adaptor protein molecule becomes associated with the carboxy-terminal region of the EGF-R (Fig. 3B). This phosphorylation and molecular association elicits movement of two other SH2-containing molecules known as Grb2 and Sos (son of sevenless, a guanine nucleotide exchange factor) to associate with each other (39,54). This complex, Gbr2:Sos, rapidly moves to the membrane where it catalyzes the conversion of inactive GDP-bound *ras* to the activated GTP *ras* form (Fig. 3B). At this point, yet another cascade of protein molecules become phosphorylated along the mitogen-activated protein (MAP) kinase pathway (59). Although the details of this pathway are still emerging, it is clear that the signal transduction pathway from the EGF-R into the nucleus involves both the movements and the associations between a host of adaptor and regulatory molecules. The existence of the *ras* pathway has been confirmed in cultured keratinocytes but to date has not been directly implicated in benign hyperproliferative skin diseases. Preliminary data have shown that activation of the *ras* signaling pathway leads to gene expression for the proliferation-associated keratins, K6 and K16, that are characteristically expressed in involved psoriatic epidermis (37). It is also quite likely that additional genes are also regulated by this signaling pathway.

Many of these EGF-R substrates interact with a variety of other receptors in the tyrosine kinase receptor family, but the EGF-R appears unique in that its autophosphorylation sites seem to be more flexible or not as stringent as others, allowing it to interact with a wider range of adaptor molecules (38–40). This rapidly growing group of adaptor molecules include enzymes such as PLCγ1, syp-phosphatase, and nonenzymatic adapter molecules such as the p85 subunit of phosphatidylinositol 3-kinase (41). Most of these molecules either recognize phosphotyrosine or contain SH2 domains. Exposure of keratinocytes to either ultraviolet A or B irradiation results in increased phosphorylation of the EGF-R which is also independent of the PLCγ1 or *ras* signaling molecules (42,43). Although the interplay between these additional SH2 molecules and the *ras* signaling pathway has not been fully worked out, it seems likely that these molecules represent potential spots along the EGF-R signaling cascade where selective signaling could lead to divergent outcomes or be aberrantly regulated in disease states (16,31,44,45).

Interplay and Transmodulation of EGF-R and Other Receptor Tyrosine Kinases

Interplay and transmodulation exist between the TGF-α/EGF-R pathway and other receptor tyrosine kinases. Another tyrosine kinase receptor, IGF-R, is also overexpressed in psoriatic epidermis (5–20-fold) but is differentially regulated from EGF-R (46). In vitro, an increase in EGF-R can be rapidly induced by an IGF-R-mediated transmodulation (47), but it remains unproved whether activation of increased IGF-R that are present in lesional psoriatic skin might increase EGF-R expression. A reciprocal relationship also exists between TGF-α and IFN-γ and their receptors (48). If TGF-α/EGF are increased, IFN-γ receptors are decreased, and vice versa (49). Additional tyrosine kinase family members such as TNF-α and TGF-β are also known to *trans*-activate the EGF-R (50). An EGF-like molecule, *neu* (heregulin), was recently shown to *trans*-regulate or negatively impact the dimerization of EGF-R forms (21). Clearly tyrosine kinase receptors by either dimerization or transactivation can form complexes that can differentially modify signal transmission (51,52).

EGF-R and JAK/STAT Pathway (Fig. 4)

Six different members of the STAT family (Signal Transducers and Activators of Transcription) have been identified that appear to form dimers and *trans*-locate to the nucleus to direct gene transcription (55–59). These regulatory factors appear to be preformed proteins that become immediately phosphorylated following receptor activation. At present it appears that inactivated Janus kinase molecules (Jaks) are constitutively associated with cytoplasmic portions of receptors (Fig. 4A). Upon stimulation by ligand binding to a tyrosine kinase receptor such as the EGF-R and subsequent receptor dimerization, select STATs become phosphorylated on tyrosine by Jak protein kinases. These STAT complexes rapidly translocate to the nucleus (Fig. 4B). Activation of the same Jaks by multiple cytokines raises the question of how these cytokines utilize distinct intracellular signaling pathways, an area under extensive scrutiny (56–60). Although stimulation of the Jak/STAT pathway in response to EGF binding has been reported from in vivo liver studies (61), to date this pathway has not been identified in cultured keratinocytes but has been explored for numerous other tyrosine kinase receptor motifs in the interferon family (57,59). Very little is known of whether and how specific EGF-activated STATs function in normal keratinocytes and which ones are possibly altered in psoriasis. These pathways have been implicated in the regulation of keratin profiles in keratinocytes. Keratin genes (K6 and K16), which are present as part of the hyperproliferative phenotype in psoriatic epidermis, contain upstream regulatory response elements that are activated following ligand stimulation of EGF-R (62).

MISREGULATION OF EGF-R PATHWAYS IN PSORIASIS

Review of EGF-R-Associated Abnormalities in Lesions of Psoriasis

A number of abnormalities in the EGF-R signal transduction pathway have been detected and confirmed in psoriasis from both in vitro and in vivo experiments. Multiple EGF-R ligands are overexpressed in psoriatic lesions including TGF-α (14,63–66) and, most recently, amphiregulin mRNA (67). In vitro, psoriatic keratinocytes produce twice as much TGF-α as normal keratinocytes (48). Higashiyama and colleagues (68) performed studies that confirmed the earlier increased expression of EGF-R (9) and TGF-α in active lesions (63). They reported differential expression of TGF-α and EGF-R in the transitional area between lesional and perilesional psoriatic epidermis. Their study also reported that increased levels of immunoreactive EGF-R precede an increase for TGF-α in psoriatic plaque formation (68). TGF-α expression also decreases in regressing lesions but remains elevated in lesions not responding to treatment (70). The sequence leading to gene expression is still sketchy. The increased EGF-R present in psoriatic skin was shown to be biologically responsive when tested after grafting onto immunodeficient mice (4). The concomitant modulation of increased levels of immunoreactive EGF-R and its substrate, phospholipase Cγ1 (PLCγ1), in active lesions as well as a simultaneous decrease in both EGF-R and PLCγ1 in regressing lesions provided additional evidence that the pathway was biologically active and possibly relevant to the disease state (4,69).

Review of the Effects of Potential Therapeutic Agents on EGF-R Pathways

To determine if the regulation of EGF-R expression in psoriatic lesions is clinically significant, numerous evaluations of the impact of standard psoriatic therapies on the EGF-R signaling cascade have been made.

Most studies with potential or commonly used psoriatic pharmaceutical agents have been conducted on cultured human normal and psoriatic keratinocytes. Not surprisingly, nearly all studies to date have clearly shown that down-regulation of EGF-R or internalization of active EGF-R in both normal and psoriatic keratinocytes can be induced by standard antipsoriatic treatments such as dithranol (71), ultraviolet B (43, 72), or IFN-γ (48). Anthralin decreased both TGF-α expression and EGF binding (73) in psoriatic keratinocytes. Inhibitors of EGF-R kinase activity termed tyrophostins suppressed the growth of psoriatic keratinocytes in culture (74).

Examinations of human psoriatic lesions have produced hints of still more disturbances along the EGF-R signaling pathway. EGF-R substrates such as PLCγl were concomitantly elevated with EGF-R in psoriasis and other hyperproliferative skin lesions. When grafted human psoriatic lesions on nude mice were treated and began to resolve, PLCγl and EGF-R simultaneously decreased (4), suggesting that the EGF-R signaling pathway was biologically active and responsive in this disease state. High doses of topically delivered EGF induced remission of active lesions and decreased levels of immunoreactive EGF-R and its substrates in this in vivo model (4). In human patients, TGF-α mRNA levels were down-regulated during successful treatment of psoriatic plaques but no TGF-α changes were detected in lesions unresponsive to standard psoriatic treatments (70).

Annexin-1 (lipocortin), another of the potential EGF-R substrates, is likewise elevated in psoriatic lesions but its significance is not yet obvious (75). Another key enzyme regulating Ca^{2+}-dependent phosphorylation events was found to be abnormal in human psoriatic lesions. A calmodulin-containing enzyme, phosphorylase kinase, is elevated in active lesions but decreased in resolving lesions (76) and could increase ATP availability for phosphorylation reactions such as those necessary for signal transduction.

EGF-R, OTHER CYTOKINES, IMMUNOCYTES IN THE PATHOGENESIS OF PSORIASIS

Interplay Between Psoriasis and the Immunomediators in the Dermis

The evidence that many features of psoriasis are due to the effects of the immune system is overwhelming, continues to grow, and is reviewed in many other chapters in this book. The evidence of skin-associated lymphoid tissue (SALT, 77) and an epidermal-dermal cytokine network produced by CD4+, CD8+ lymphocytes, macrophages, dermal dendrocytes, and keratinocytes similarly has been reviewed (78,79). The challenge has been to identify and distinguish those features associated exclusively with psoriasis and those features that are also commonly found in other benign proliferative skin diseases, wound healing, and carcinomas.

EGF-R, Psoriasis, and Other Hyperproliferative Skin Conditions

Although gene linkage studies are well on their way toward proving that psoriasis is a polygenic disease (80–83), many similarities have been reported between psoriasis and other hyperproliferative epidermal diseases. Altered EGF-R expression patterns were detected in growing seborrheic keratoses, acrochordons, acanthosis nigricans, molluscum contagiosum, and several forms of ichthyoses (84–86). However, EGF-R expression was not constitutively increased in all presumptively hyperproliferative epidermal disorders as evidenced by the absence of EGF-R in lesions of verruca vulgaris and mild ichthyoses (84). In a case report of a unique melanoma patient who produced excessive TGF-α, EGF-R levels were elevated in hyperproliferative skin lesions as long as TGF-α levels were high (87). In contrast, transgenic mice overexpressing TGF-α exhibited little or no detectable EGF-R within the papillomas that developed in these mice (88).

EGF-R, Psoriasis, Wound Healing, and the Regenerative Phenotype

Similarities abound between the regenerative phenotype seen in wound healing and the psoriasiform phenotype. The connection between cytokines and the psoriasiform hyperplasia of wound repair and psoriasis grows stronger every day. Although EGF-R have long been known to be increased in the hyperproliferative epidermis of psoriasis (9), later studies reported an increase in receptors during the initial phases of wound repair (89–91) where they are closely correlated with cellular proliferation. Another example of similarities between the regenerative phenotype and psoriasis was recently reported. Application of keratinocyte growth factor (KGF), a member of the fibroblast growth family (FGF-7), induced a psoriasiform hyperplasia in the resurfacing of the epidermis following a burn injury (92). In both psoriasis and wound repair, the hyperproliferative keratins K6 and 16 are detected in the epidermis. Similarities have also been detected between cytokine profiles that are known to regulate capillary proliferation. In psoriatic lesions, the capillary overgrowth in the papillary dermis may well be explained by an overexpression of vascular endothelial growth factor (VEGF), which is likely regulated by the excessive TGF-α expression derived from the epidermis (93,94). Preliminary wound-healing data suggest that HB-EGF induce vascular permeability factor, thereby regulating the capillary proliferation, a hallmark of the hyperproliferative phenotype (93).

Studies on integrins in both psoriasis and wound repair have led some investigators to suggest that epidermal hyperplasia within psoriatic lesions is secondary to primary immunological events (6,95). Integrin patterns are similar in both the psoriasiform phenotype and the hyperproliferative epidermis following wounding (95). Recent overexpression of β integrin in the suprabasal epidermis in transgenic mice produced a phenotype that closely resembled psoriasis and was secondarily associated with immunological responses (95). These data suggest that it is also plausible that genetic abnormalities are present within psoriatic keratinocytes that permit a chronic cytokine-driven benign hyperproliferation that is distinct from both malignant growth of the epidermis in squamous cell carcinoma and the transient proliferative state observed during wound healing.

Malignant Skin Disease

Overexpression of EGF and its ligands has been detected in a variety of epithelial carcinomas, especially squamous cell carcinomas (96,97). Levels of EGF-R and its forms are currently being advocated as a prognostic tool for various neoplasms arising from keratinocytes in breast cancer (23,24). Studies with squamous cell carcinoma cell lines have shown that inhibitors of EGF-R tyrosine kinase can block mitogenesis and phosphorylation (25,98). Thus, therapeutic modulation of the EGF-R signaling pathway for the purposes of inhibiting keratinocyte proliferation is both theoretically and practically feasible (99).

SPONTANEOUS AND INDUCED MOUSE MUTATION MODELS OF PSORIASIS

Identification of spontaneous and induced transgenic mouse mutations that have a psoriasiform phenotype has begun and continues to provide exciting new opportunities to examine the molecular bases of epidermal proliferation and differentiation (100). Figure 5 shows the gross appearance of the flaky skin mutation known as *fsn/fsn*. In addition, the use of immunodeficient mice (nude, $Hfh11^{nu}$, severe combined immunodeficiency, and others) that do not reject human psoriatic skin grafts has greatly facilitated in vivo analysis of psoriasis not possible in humans as well as testing of potentially toxic therapeutic agents (4,5).

Flaky Skin Mice (*fsn/fsn*): Chromosome 17

An inbred mouse strain, flaky skin (*fsn/fsn*) was identified in 1986 at the Jackson Laboratory (101) and found to have a highly proliferative epidermis, neutrophils within the epidermis, and other features of one form of psoriasis (Fig. 6). These mice have dendritic cell abnormalities (102) suggesting that *fsn/fsn* mice have inherent abnormalities in the immune system. This mutation is also characterized by ultrastructural features typical of human psoriasis including basal cell edema and herniations, intraepidermal neutrophils, and excessive epidermal scaling (103,104) (Fig. 7). *Fsn/fsn* skin maintains this psoriatic phenotype when grafted on nude mice (105). We recently reported increased EGF-R in *fsn/fsn* epidermis (106) in a cytokine profile that closely mimics the data in our earlier report from human psoriasis (9). This *fsn/fsn* epidermis exhibited the Koebner reaction in response to mild trauma and regressed in response to standard psoriatic treatments. This constellation of features suggests a high degree of correlation between *fsn/fsn*

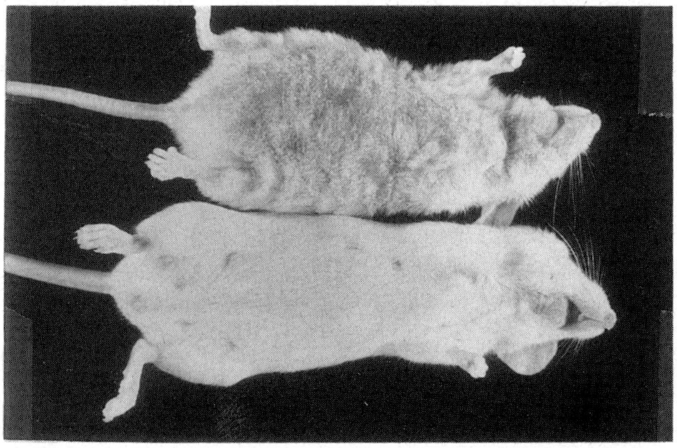

Figure 5 Gross appearance of (top) normal littermate and (bottom) *fsn/fsn* mice. The affected *fsn/fsn* mouse has relative alopecia and noticeable scaling.

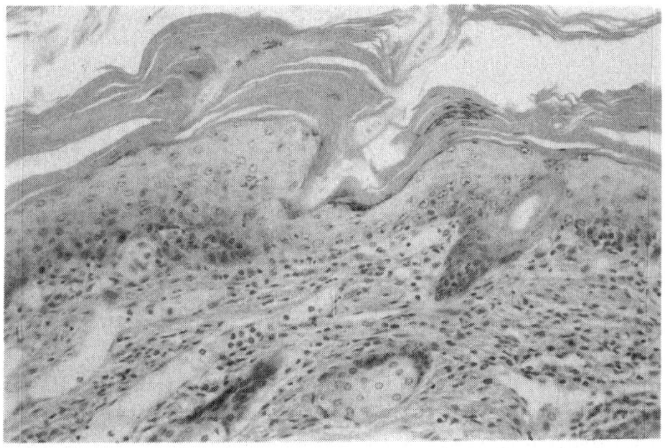

Figure 6 Histological appearance of *fsn/fsn* skin. Note the increased thickness and presence of neutrophils in the epidermis.

skin pathology and human psoriasis. It further suggests that alteration in cytokine profiles is a constant feature of psoriatic lesions in both animals and humans. Characterization of additional mouse mutations such as chronic proliferative dermatitis mice (*cpdm*) (107), flaky tail (*ft*), ichthyosis (*ic*), and others is undoubtedly offering new avenues for the study of psoriasis and hyperproliferative skin diseases within its systemic context (100,108).

Transgenic Mice with Mutations Affecting EGF-R and Its Ligands

The epidermal targeting of transgenes using keratin or involucrin promoters has produced transgenic mice that overexpress cytokines and often exhibit psoriatic or hyperproliferative phenotypes (Table 2). Cytokines such as TGF-α (109), IL-1, TGF-β superfamily members (bone morphogenetic proteins BMP2,4) (110,111), and adhesion molecules such as integrins (6), which may be relevant to the pathogenesis of human psoriasis, have been overexpressed or eliminated in these innovative in vivo models.

Transgenic Mice Overexpressing TGF-α

Transgenic mice overexpressing TGF-α developed a hyperproliferative epidermal phenotype with a tendency to form papillomas (88,109,112) whereas the epidermis and hair follicles in the BMP-4 mice were hypoproliferative and did not produce papillomas even using the standard two-stage carcinogenesis protocol of applying an initiator (TPA) followed by a promoter (DMBA) to induce papillomas (110,111).

Transgenic Mice with TGF-α Deficiency

Generation of TGF-α null mice (112), an allele of the waved-1 mouse mutation (113), produced mice whose only obvious phenotype were wavy vibrissae and hair and problems with eyelid opening with corneal abnormalities (112). The genetic mimic, waved-2 (wa2), was subsequently determined to be a point mutation in the tyrosine kinase domain of the EGF-R gene (114). Additional mimics, mapping to other chromosomes, have recently been found that will expand our knowledge of those complex cycles. Redundancies in cytokine signaling cascades are fairly common. Seemingly critical molecules may be deleted with minor biological damage in vivo. The mild phenotype in the case of the TGF-α null mice is likely the result of compensation by the presence of other EGF ligands such as EGF, HB-EGF, betacellulin, or amphiregulin.

Transgenic Mice with Defective EGF-R

In mice, targeted disruption of the mouse EGF-R produced a phenotype with deformities of hair follicle orientation and maturation with a decrease in epidermal proliferation (115,116). When a dominant negative mutation of EGF-R was expressed in transgenic mice, the predominant feature was an inexplicable perpetuation of the growing phase of hair follicle growth (117). The obvious phenotype on this mouse was the short and waved hair, which culminated in severe alopecia and inflammation related to the follicular dystrophy. These unexpected phenotypes have produced undeniable evidence that the EGF-R pathways plays a pivotal role in epidermal growth and differentiation. These emerging new mouse models can facilitate testing of new hypotheses of cell growth and new treatments aimed at better regulation of cell proliferation. Most recently the targeted disruption of EGF-R in these mouse keratinocytes has been used to prove that loss of the EGF-R impairs the growth of v-*ras*-induced epidermal tumors (118).

Transgenic Mice Overexpressing Integrins in Epidermis

When specific adhesion molecules were targeted for expression in the suprabasal layer of the epidermis using an involucrin promoter, transgenic mice were generated that had developmental defects and a phe-

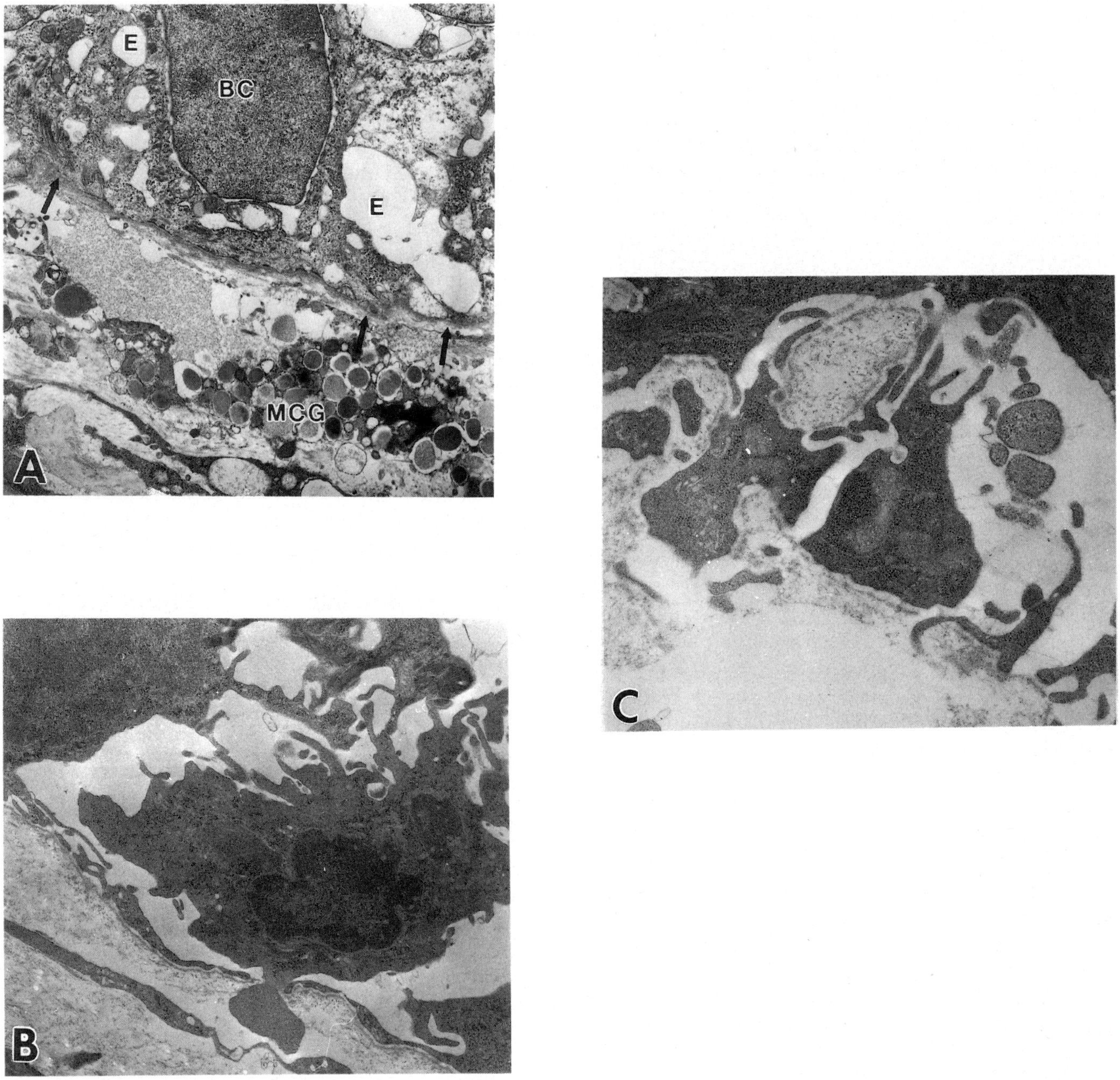

Figure 7 Ultrastructural features of *fsn/fsn* epidermis that resemble those characteristics of human psoriasis. (A) Dissolution of the basal lamina at the dermal-epidermal junction in the vicinity of degranulating mast cells (MCG). (B,C) Passage of a neutrophil (N) into the epidermis through a gap in the basal lamina with edema between the basal keratinocytes.

Table 2 Functions of Transgenic, and Spontaneous Knockout Mutations In Vivo

Mutation	Regulation	Effect
TGFαTg	Up	Psoriasiform skin
TGFα -/-(wa-1)	None	Curly hair, skin normal
EGFR -/-(wa-2)	None	Curly hair, juvenile lethal
wa-3	?	Curly hair
EGF -/- mild	Down(?)	Curly hair
EGF -/-	Down	Misdirected hair, alopecia

notype resembling psoriasis (6). Transgenic mice expressing integrin $\beta 1$ alone or in combination with $\alpha 2$ or $\alpha 5$ had epidermal hyperproliferation, abnormal keratinocyte differentiation, and inflammation that included subcorneal pustules and exocytosis of T lymphocytes. These authors conclude that the phenotypic features induced by overexpressing integrins in these transgenic mice strongly support the view that the defect responsible for psoriasis is present in the keratinocytes as opposed to psoriasis being primarily a disorder of the immune system. Since the mice were not strictly in a barrier-pathogen-free environment, it is possible to conclude that the waxing and waning of the psoriasiform phenotype may be due to environmental factors such as trauma, barbering, and infection that unmasked the genotypic predisposition to increased proliferation and inflammation in response to trauma.

CONCLUSIONS

There is growing evidence that genetic abnormalities are present within psoriatic keratinocytes that permit a chronic, cytokine-driven benign hyperproliferation distinct from both malignant hyperproliferation and the transient proliferative state observed during wound healing. EGF-R expression, its ligands, and related signaling molecules appear to be important targets in the induction, persistence, and therapy of psoriasis. At present, a multitude of standard psoriatic treatments may cause temporary or prolonged regression in skin lesions, but research has yielded only a few clues as to how cytokine pathways induce or are affected by remission. New compounds such as tryphostins inhibit EGF-R kinase activity and represent novel leads for the therapy of psoriasis (74). Therapy that specifically targets or depletes T cells is likely to reduce the severity and chronicity of psoriasis (2). Continued in vitro and in vivo work is important to gain an understanding of how the EGF-R-associated signal pathways regulate the pathophysiology and therapeutic response in psoriasis and quite possibly other hyperproliferative skin diseases.

ACKNOWLEDGMENTS

This work was supported by P30 AR41943 (LEK, LBN), GM40437 (LBN), and the Department of Veterans Affairs (LEK, LBN), RR8911 (JPS), and a grant from the Center for Innovative Biotechnology (JPS).

REFERENCES

1. Gottlieb, A.B., Krueger, J.G., Khandke, L., Grossman, R.M., Krane, J., and Carter, D.M. (1991). Role of T-cell activation in the pathogenesis of psoriasis. *Ann. N.Y. Acad. Sci.* 636:377–379.
2. Gottlieb, J.L., Gilleaudeau, P., Johnson, R., Estes, L., Woodworth, T.G., Gottlieb, A.B., and Krueger, J.G. (1995). Response of psoriasis to a lymphocyte-selective toxin (DAB389IL-2) suggests a primary immune, but not keratinocyte, pathogenic basis. *Nature Med.* 1:442–447.
3. Krueger, G.G., Manning, D.D., Malouf, J., and Ogden, B. (1975). Long-term maintenance of psoriatic human skin on congenitally athymic (nude) mice. *J. Invest. Dermatol.* 64:307–312.
4. Nanney, L.B., Yates, R.A., and King, L.E., Jr. (1992). Modulation of epidermal growth factor receptors in psoriatic lesions during treatment with topical EGF. *J. Invest. Dermatol.* 98(3):296–301.
5. Nickoloff, B.R., Kunkel, S.L., Burdick, M., and Strieter, R.M. (1995). Severe combined immunodeficiency mouse and human psoriatic skin chimeras. *Am. J. Pathol.* 146:580–588.
6. Carroll, J.M., Romero, M.R., and Watt, F.M. (1995). Suprabasal integrin expression in the epidermis of transgenic mice results in developmental defects and a phenotype resembling psoriasis. *Cell* 83:957–968.
7. Nickoloff, B.J. (1991). Cytokine network in psoriasis. *Arch. Dermatol.* 127:871–84.
8. Nickoloff, B.J., Karabin, G.D., Barker, J.N., Griffiths, C.E.M., Sarma, V., Mitra, R.S., Elder, J.T., Kunkel, S.L., and Dixit, V.M. (1991). Cellular localization of interleukin-8 and its inducer tumor necrosis factor-alpha in psoriasis. *Am. J. Pathol.* 138:129–140.
9. Nanney, L.B., Stoscheck, C.M., Magid, M., and King, L.E. (1986). Altered ^{125}I-EGF binding and receptor distribution in psoriasis. *J. Invest. Dermatol.* 86: 260–265.
10. Nanney, L.B., Magid, M., Stoscheck, C.M., and King, L.E. (1984). Comparison of epidermal growth factor

binding and receptor distribution in normal human epidermis and epidermal appendages. *J. Invest. Dermatol.* 83:385–93.

11. Coffey, R.J., Derynck, R., Wilcox, J.N., Bringman, T.S., Goustin, A.S., Moses, H.L., and Pittelkow, M.R. (1987). Production and autoinduction of transforming growth factor-α in human keratinocytes. *Nature* 328: 817–820.
12. Cook, P.W., Pittelkow, M.R., and Shipley, G.D. (1991). Growth factor-independent proliferation of normal human neonatal keratinocytes: production of autocrine and paracrine acting mitogenic factors. *J. Cell Physiol.* 146:277–289.
13. Piepkorn, M., Underwood, R.A., Henneman, C., and Smith, L.T. (1995). Expression of amphiregulin is regulated in cultured human keratinocytes and in developing fetal skin. *J. Invest. Dermatol.* 105:802–809.
14. Maguire, H.D., Jaworsky, C., Cohen, J.A., Hellman, M., Weiner, D.B., and Greene, M.I. (1989). Distribution of *neu* (c-*erb*B2) protein in human skin. *J. Invest. Dermatol.* 92:786–90.
15. Barnard, J.A., Graves-Deal, R., Pittelkow, M.R., DuBois, R., Cook, P., Ransey, G.W., Bishop, P.R., Damstrup, L., and Coffey, R.J. (1994). Auto-and cross-induction within the mammalian epidermal growth factor-related peptide family. *J. Biol. Chem.* 269:22817–22.
16. Moriai, T., Kobrin, M.S., Hope, C.H., Speck, L., and Korc, M. (1994). A variant epidermal growth factor receptor exhibits altered TGFα binding and transmembrane signaling. *Proc. Natl. Acad. Sci. U.S.A.* 91: 10217–10221.
17. Cha, D., O'Brien, P., O'Toole, E.A., Woodley, D.T., and Hudson, L.G. (1996). Enhanced modulation of keratinocyte motility by transforming growth factor-α (TGFα) relative to epidermal growth factor (EGF). *J. Invest. Dermatol.* 106:590–597.
18. Hashimoto, K., Higashiyama, S., Asada, H., Hashimura, E., Kobayashi, T., Sudo, K., Nakagawa, T., Damm, D., and Yoshikaw, K. (1994). Heparin binding epidermal growth factor like growth factor is an autocrine growth factor for human keratinocytes. *J. Biol. Chem.* 269:20060–20066.
19. Schalkwijk, J., VanVlijmen, I., Oosterling, B., Perrit, C., Koopman, R., VandenBorn, J., and Mackie, E.J. (1991). Tenascin expression in hyperproliferative skin diseases. *Br. J. Dermatol.* 124:13–20.
20. Aumailley, M., and Krieg, T. (1996). Laminins: A family of diverse multifunctional molecules of basement membranes. *J. Invest. Dermatol.* 106:209–214.
21. Karunagaran, D., Tzahar, E., Liu, N., Wen, D., and Yarden, Y. (1995). *Neu* differentiation factor inhibits EGF binding: a model for trans-regulation within the *Erb*B family of receptor tyrosine kinases. *J. Biol. Chem.* 270:9982–9990.
22. Poumay, Y., Leclercq-Smekens, M., Deom, R., and Pittelkow, M.R. (1996). Expression of receptors of the human epidermal growth factor receptor (HER) family and NDF/Heregulin in normal skin. *J. Invest. Dermatol.* 106:820.
23. Katsumata, M., Okudaira, T., Samanta, A., Clark, D.P., Drebin, J.A., Jolicoeur, P., and Greene, M.I. (1995). Prevention of breast tumor development in vivo by downregulation of the p185 neu receptor. *Nature Med.* 1:644–648.
24. LeMaistre, C.H., Meneghetti, C., Howes, L., and Osborne, C.K. (1994). Targeting the EGF receptor in breast cancer treatment—a review. *Breast Cancer Res. Treat.* 32:97–103.
25. Modjtahedi, H., Eccles, S., Sandle, J., Box, G., Titley, J., and Dean, C. (1994). Differentiation or immune destruction: two pathway for therapy of squamous cell carcinomas with antibodies to the epidermal growth factor receptor. *Cancer Res.* 54:1695–1701.
26. Plowman, G.D., Culouscou, J.M., Whitney, G.S., Green, J.M., Cariton, G.W., Foy, L., Neubauer, M.G., and Shoyab, M. (1993). Ligand-specific activation of HER4/p180^{erbB4}, a fourth member of the epidermal growth factor receptor family. *Proc. Natl. Acad. Sci. U.S.A.* 90:1746–1750.
27. Plowman, G.D., Green, J.M., Culouscou, J-M., Cariton, G.W., Rothwell, V.M., and Buckley, S. (1993). Heregulin induces tyrosine phosphorylation of HER4/p180^{erbB4}. *Nature* 366:473–475.
28. Carraway, K.L., Sliwkowski, M.X., Akita, R., Platko, J.V., Guy, P.M., Nuijens, A., Diamonti, A.J., Vandlen, R.L., Cantley, L.C., and Cerione, R.A. (1994). The erbB3 gene product is a receptor for heregulin. *J. Biol. Chem.* 269:14303–14306.
29. Carpenter, G. (1992). Receptor tyrosine kinase substrates: *src* homology domains and signal transduction. *FASEB J.* 6:3283–89.
30. Wada, T., Qian, W., Greene, M. (1990). Intermolecular association of the p185 *neu* protein and EGF receptor modulates EGF receptor function. *Cell* 61: 1339–47.
31. Qian, X., LeVea, C.H., Freeman, J.K., Dougall, W.E., and Greene, J.I. (1994). Heterodimerization of epidermal growth factor receptor and wild-type or kinase-deficient *Neu*: A mechanism of interreceptor kinase activation and transphosphorylation. *Proc. Natl. Acad. Sci. U.S.A.* 91:1500–04.
32. Chantry, A. (1995). The kinase domain and membrane localization determine intracellular interactions between EGF receptor. *J. Biol. Chem.* 270: 3068–73.
33. Weernink, O., Ottenhoff-Kalff, A.E., Vendrig, M.P., Beurden, E.A., Staal, G.E., and Rijken, G. (1994). Functional interaction between the EGF receptor and c-Src kinase activity. *FEBS Lett.* 352:296–300.

34. Kashles, L., Yarden, Y., Fisher, R., Ullrich, A., and Schlessinger, J. (1991). A dominant negative mutation suppresses the function of normal EGF receptors by heterodimerization. *Mol. Cell. Biol.* 11: 1453–1463.
35. Qian, X., Decker, S.J., and Greene, M.I. (1992). p185c-*neu* and epidermal growth factor receptor associate into a structure composed of activated kinases. *Proc. Natl. Acad. Sci. U.S.A.* 89:1330–1334.
36. Gates, R.E., King, L.E. (1982). Calcium facilitates endogenous proteolysis of the EGF receptor-kinase. *Mol. Cell. Endocrinol.* 27:263–276.
37. Blumenberg, J., Komine, M., Gorelick, S., and Freedberg, I.M. (1995). Signal transduction in epidermal keratinocytes: two independent cascades. *J. Invest. Dermatol.* 104:591.
38. Soler, C., Beguinot, L., and Carpenter, G. (1994). Individual EGF receptor autophosphorylation sites do not stringently define association motifs for SH2-containing proteins. *J. Biol. Chem.* 269: 12320–12324.
39. Batzer, A.G., Rotin, D., Uren, J.M., Skolnik, E.Y., and Schlessinger, J. (1994). Hierarchy of binding sites for Grb2 and Shc on the epidermal growth factor receptor. *Mol. Cell. Biol.* 14:5192–5201.
40. Li, N., Schlessinger, J., and Margolis, B. (1994). Autophosphorylation mutants of the EGF receptor signal through auxiliary mechanisms involving SH2 domain proteins. *Oncogene* 9:3457–3465.
41. Okabayashi, Y., Kido, Y., Okutani, T., Sugimoto, Y., Sakagucki, K., and Kasuga, M. (1994). Tyrosines 1148 and 1173 of activated human EGF receptors are binding sites of Shc in intact cells. *J. Biol. Chem.* 269:18674–1868.
42. Schindler, C., and Darnell, J.E. (1995). Transcriptional responses to polypeptide ligands the Jak-STAT pathway. *Annu. Rev. Biochem.* 64:621–651.
43. Y, E., Morraro, R., Levit, E., Zhu, H., and DeLeo, V. (1996). Ultraviolet radiation induced phosphorylation of the EGF receptor in keratinocytes by a novel mechanism. *J. Invest. Dermatol.* 106:821.
44. Qian, X., Dougall, W.C., Hellman, M.E., and Greene, M.I. (1994). Kinase-deficient *neu* proteins suppress epidermal growth factor receptor function and abolish cell transformation. *Oncogene* 9:1507–1514.
45. Griswold-Penner, I., Carlin, C.R., and Rosner, M.R. (1993). Mitogen-activated protein kinase regulates the epidermal growth factor receptor through activation of a tyrosine phosphatase. *J. Biol. Chem.* 268: 13050–13054.
46. Krane, J.F., Gottlieb, A.B., Carter, D.M., and Krueger, J.G. (1992). Insulin-like growth factor I receptor is overexpressed in psoriatic epidermis, but is differentially regulated from the epidermal growth factor receptor. *J. Exp. Med.* 175:1081–1090.
47. Krane, J.F., Murphy, D.P., Carter, D.M., and Krueger, J.G. (1991). Synergistic effects of EGF and insulin-like growth factor I/somatomedin C (IGFI) on keratinocyte proliferation may be mediated by IGF-I transmodulation of the EGF receptor. *J. Invest. Dermatol.* 96:419–424.
48. Nickoloff, B.J., Mitra, R.S., Elder, J.T., Fisher, G.J., and Voorhees, J.J. (1989). Decreased growth inhibition by recombinant gamma interferon is associated with increased transforming growth factor-alpha production in keratinocytes cultured from psoriatic lesions. *Br. J. Dermatol.* 121:161–174.
49. Mitra, R.S., and Nickoloff, B.J. (1992). Epidermal growth factor and TGFα decrease gamma interferon receptor and induction of intercellular adhesion molecule-1 (ICAM-1). *J. Cell. Physiol.* 150:264–268.
50. Izumi, H., Ono, M., Ushiro, S., Kohno, K., Kung, H., and Kuwano, M. (1994). Cross talk of tumor necrosis factor-α and epidermal growth factor in human microvascular endothelial cells. *Exp. Cell Res.* 214: 654–662.
51. Dougall, W.C., Qian, X., Peterson, N.C., Miller, M.J., Samanta, A., and Greene, M.I. (1994). The *neu*-oncogene signal transduction pathways, mechanisms and evolving therapies. *Oncogene* 9:2109–2123.
52. Qian, X., Dougall, W.C., Fei, Z., and Greene, M.I. (1995). Intermolecular association and *trans*-phosphorylation of different *neu*-kinase forms permit SH2-dependent signaling and oncogenic transformation. *Oncogene* 10:211–219.
53. Hall, A. (1994). A biochemical function for *ras*—at last. *Science* 264:1413–1416.
54. Sasaoka, T., Langlois, W.J., Leitner, J.W., Draznin, B., and Olefsky, J.M. (1994). The signaling pathway coupling epidermal growth factor receptors to activation of $p21^{ras}$. *J. Biol. Chem.* 269:32621–32625.
55. Wen, Z., Zhong, Z., and Darnell, J.E. (1995). Maximal activation of transcription by STAT1 and STAT3 requires both tyrosine and serine phosphorylation. *Cell* 82:241–250.
56. Heim, M.H., Kerr, I.M., Stark, G.R., and Darnell, J.E. (1995). Contribution of Stat SH2 groups to specific interferon signaling by the Jak-STAT pathway. *Science* 267:1347–49.
57. Darnell, J.E., Kerr, I.M., and Stark, G.R. (1994). Jak-STAT pathways and transcriptional activation in response to IFNs and other extracellular signaling proteins. *Science* 264:1415–1420.
58. Fu, X.Y., and Zhang, J.J. (1993). Transcription factor p91 interacts with the epidermal growth factor receptor and mediates activation of the c-*fos* gene promoter. *Cell* 74:1135–1143.
59. Ihle, J.N. (1995). Cytokine receptor signalling. *Nature* 377:591–594.
60. Stahl, J., Farruggella, T.J., Boulton, T.G., Zhong, Z., Darnell, J.E., and Yancopoulos, G.D. (1995). Choice

of STATs and other substrates specified by modular tyrosine-based motifs in receptors. *Science* 267: 1349–1353.

61. Jamison-Ruff, S., Zhong, Z., Wen, Z., Chen, K., Darnell, J.E., and Cohen, S. (1994). Epidermal growth factor and lipopolysaccharide activate STAT3 transcription factor in mouse liver. *J. Biol. Chem.* 269: 21933–21935.
62. Jiang, C.K., Magnaldo, T., Ohtsuki, M., Freedberg, I.M., Bernerd, F., and Blumenberg, M. (1993). EGF and TGFα specifically induce the activation and hyperproliferation-associated keratins 6 and 16. *Proc. Natl. Acad. Sci. U.S.A.* 90:6786–6790.
63. Gottlieb, A.B., Chang, C.K., Posnett, D.N., Fanelli, B., and Tam, J.P. (1988). Detection of transforming growth factorα in normal, malignant, and hyperproliferative human keratinocytes. *J. Exp. Med.* 167: 670–675.
64. Elder, J.T., Fisher, G.J., Lindquist, P.B., Bennett, G.L., Pittelkow, M.R., Coffey, R.J., Ellingsworth, L., Derynck, R., and Voorhees, J.J. (1989). Overexpression of TGFα in psoriatic epidermis. *Science* 243: 811–814.
65. Turbitt, M., Akhur, R.J., White, S.I., and Mackie, R.M. (1990). Localization of elevated TGFα in psoriatic epidermis. *J. Invest. Dermatol.* 95:229–232.
66. Schmid, P., Cox, D., McMaster, G.K., and Itin, P. (1993). In situ hybridization analysis of cytokine, proto-oncogene and tumour suppressor gene expression in psoriasis. *Arch. Dermatol. Res.* 285:334–340.
67. Cook, P.W., Pittelkow, M.R., Keeble, W.N., et al. (1992). Amphiregulin mRNA is elevated in psoriatic epidermis and gastrointestinal carcinomas. *Cancer Res.* 52:3224–3227.
68. Higashiyama, M., Hashimoto, K., Matsumoto, K., and Yoshikawa, K. (1994). Differential expression of TGFα and EGF receptor in the transitional area of psoriatic epidermis. *J. Dermatol. Sci.* 7:45–53.
69. Nanney, L.B., Gates, R.E., Todderud, G., King, L.E., Jr., and Carpenter, G. (1992). Altered distribution of phospholipase Cγ1 in benign hyperproliferative epidermal diseases. *Cell Growth Differ.* 3:233–239.
70. Watts, P., Stables, G.S., Akhurst, R.J., and Mackie, R.M. (1994). Localization of transforming growth factor-alpha RNA and protein in the skin of psoriatic patients receiving therapy. *Br. J. Dermatol.* 131: 64–71.
71. Kemeny, L., Michel, G., Arenberger, P., and Ruzicka, T. (1993). Down-regulation of epidermal growth factor receptors by dithranol. *Acta Derm. Venereol.* 73: 37–40.
72. Matsui, M.S., Laufer, L., Scheide, S., and DeLeo, V. (1989). Ultraviolet-B (290–320 nm)-irradiation inhibits epidermal growth-factor binding to mammalian cells. *J. Invest. Dermatol.* 92:617–622.
73. Gottlieb, A.B., Khandke, L., Krane, J.F., Staiano-Coico, L., Ashinoff, R., and Krueger, J.G. (1992). Anthralin decreases keratinocyte TGFα expression and EGF receptor binding in vitro. *J. Invest. Dermatol.* 98:680–685.
74. BenBassat, H., Vardi, D.V., Gazit, A., Klaus, S.N., Chaouat, M., Hartzstark, Z., and Levitzki, A. (1995). Tryphostins suppress the growth of psoriatic keratinocytes. *Exp. Dermatol.* 4:82–88.
75. Fava, R., Nanney, L.B., Wilson, D., and King, L.E. (1993). Annexin-1 (p35/lipocortin-1) localization in adult, embryonic and diseased human skin: possible association with cytoskeletal elements in keratinocytes of the stratum spinosum. *J. Invest. Dermatol.* 101(5):732–737.
76. Heng, M.C.Y., Song, M.K., and Heng, M.K. (1994). Elevated phosphorylase kinase activity in psoriatic epidermis correlation with increased phosphorylation and psoriatic activity. *Br. J. Dermatol.* 130:298–306.
77. Streilein, J.W. (1983). Skin-associated lymphoid tissues (SALT): origins and functions. *J. Invest. Dermatol.* 80:12S–16S.
78. Nestle, F.O., Turka, L.A., and Nickoloff, B.J. (1994). Characterization of dermal dentritic cells in psoriasis. Auto stimulation of T lymphocytes and induction of Th1 type cytokines. *J. Clin. Invest.* 94:202–209.
79. Prens, E., Debets, R., and Hegmans, J. (1995). T lymphocytes in psoriasis. *Clin. Dermatol.* 13:115–129.
80. Tomfohrde, J., Silverman, A., Barnes, R., Fernandez-Vina, M.A., Young, M., Lory, D., Morris, L., Wuepper, K.D., Stastny, P., Neter, A., and Bowcock, A. (1994). Gene for familial psoriasis susceptibility mapped to the distal end of chromosome 17q. *Science* 264:1141–1144.
81. Hensler, T., and Christophers, E. (1995). Disease concomitance in psoriasis. *J. Am. Acad. Dermatol.* 32: 982–986.
82. Nair, R.P., Jenisch, S., Guo, S.W., Henseler, T., Kokx, S., Terhunc, M., Woodburn, M., Westphal, E., Christophers, E., Voorhees, J.J., and Elder, J.T. (1995). Evidence for psoriasis susceptibility gene(s) on human chromosome 6p. *J. Invest. Dermatol.* 104:598.
83. Nair, R.P., Henseler, T., Jenisch, S., Stuart, P., Rasmussen, B., Bichakjian, C., Guo, S.W., Westphal, E., Christophers, E., Voorhees, J.J., and Elder, J.T. (1996). A recombination based genome-wide scan for psoriasis genes: the hunt continues. *J. Invest. Dermatol.* 106:985.
84. Nanney, L.B., Ellis, D.L., Levine, J., and King, L.E. (1992). EGF-R in idiopathic and virally induced skin diseases. *Am. J. Pathol.* 140(4):915–925.
85. Ellis, D.L., Nanney, L.B., and King, L.E. (1990). Increased EGF receptors in seborrheic keratoses and acrochordons of dysplastic nevus syndrome patients. *J. Am. Acad. Dermatol.* 23:1070–1077.

86. Nanney, L.B., King, L.E., and Dale, B.A. (1991). Epidermal growth factor receptor in genetically induced hyperproliferative skin disorders. *Pediatr. Dermatol.* 7:265–272.
87. Ellis, D.L., Kafka, S., Chow, J., Nanney, L.B., Inman, W., McCadden, M., and King, L.E. (1987). Melanoma, growth factors, acanthosis nigricans, the sign of Leser-Trelat and multiple acrochordons: a role for TGFα in cutaneous paraneoplastic syndromes. *N. Engl. J. Med.* 317:1582–1587.
88. Dominey, A.M., Wang, X-J., King, L.E., Jr., Nanney, L.B., Gagne, T.A., Sellheyer, C., Bundman, D.S., Longley, M.A., Rothnagel, J.A., Greenhalgh, D.A., and Roop, D.R. (1993). Targeted over-expression of transforming growth factors-α in the epidermis of transgenic mice elicits anomalous proliferation and differentiation and spontaneous squamous papillomas. *Cell Growth Differen.* 4:1071–1082.
89. Wenczak, B.A., Lynch, J.B., and Nanney, L.B. (1992). Epidermal growth factor distribution in burn wounds: implications for growth factor mediated repair. *J. Clin. Invest.* 90:2392–2401.
90. Wenczak, B.A., and Nanney, L.B. (1993). Correlation of TGFα and EGF-R with proliferating cell nuclear antigen in human burn wounds. *J Wound Repair Regen.* 1:41–46.
91. Stoscheck, C.M., Nanney, L.B., and King, L.E. (1992). Quantitative determination of EGF-R during epidermal wound healing. *J. Invest. Dermatol.* 99(5): 645–649.
92. Danielenko, D.M., Ring, B.D., Tarpley, J.E., Morris, B., Van, G.Y., Morawiecki, A., Callahan, W., Goldenberg, M., Hershenson, S., and Pierce, G.F. (1995). Growth factors in porcine full and partial thickness burn repair: differing targets and effects of keratinocyte growth factor, platelet-derived growth factor-BB, epidermal growth factor, and *neu* differentiation factor. *Am. J. Pathol.* 147:1261–1277.
93. Stoll, S.W., and Elder, J.T. (1995). Heparin-binding EGF-like growth factors induce vascular permeability factor via autocrine EGF receptor activation: Early events in wound healing. *J. Invest. Dermatol.* 104: 678.
94. Detmar, M., Brown, L.F., Claffey, K.P., Yeo, K-T., Kocher, O., Jackman, R.W., Berse, B., and Dvorak, H.F. (1994). Overexpression of vascular permeability factor/vascular endothelial growth factor and its receptors in psoriasis. *J. Exp. Med.* 180:1141–46.
95. Hertie, M.D., Kubler, M-D., Leigh, I.M., and Watt, F.M. (1992). Aberrant integrin expression during epidermal wound healing and in psoriatic epidermis. *J. Clin. Invest.* 89:1892–901.
96. Yamamoto, T., Kamata, N., Kawano, H., Shimizu, S., Kuroki, T., and Shimizu, N. (1986). High incidence of amplification of the epidermal growth factor receptor gene in human squamous carcinoma cell lines. *Cancer Res.* 46:414–416.
97. Derynck, R., Goeddel, D.V., Ullrich, A., Gutterman, J.U., Williams, R.D., Bringman, T.S., and Berger, W. (1987). Synthesis of messenger RNAs for transforming growth factors α and β and the epidermal growth factor receptor by human tumors. *Cancer Res.* 47: 707–712.
98. Fry, D.W., Kraker, A.J., McMichael, A., Ambroso, L.A., Nelson, J.M., Leopold, W.R., Connors, R.W., and Bridges, A.J. (1994). A specific inhibitor of the epidermal growth factor receptor tyrosine kinase. *Science* 265:1093–1095.
99. Le Maistra, C.H., Meneghetti, C., Howes, L., and Osborne, C.K. (1994). Targeting the EGF receptor in breast cancer treatment—review. *Breast Cancer Res. Treat.* 32:97–103, 1994.
100. Sundberg, J.P., and King, L.E. (1996). Mouse mutations as animal models and biomedical tools for dermatological research. *J. Invest. Dermatol.* 106: 368–376.
101. Compton, J.G., Dunstan, R.W., Beamer, W.G., Roop, D.R., and Sundberg, J.P. (1989). Flaky skin: a new mutant mouse developing a heritable papulosquamous disease. *J. Invest. Dermatol.* 92:414.
102. Sundberg, J.P., Boggess, D., Sundberg, B.A., Beamer, W.G., and Shultz, L.D. (1993). Epidermal dendritic cell populations in the flaky skin mutant mouse. *Immunol. Invest.* 22:389–401.
103. Morita, K., Hogan, M.E., Nanney, L.B., King, L.E., Monabe, M., Sun, T.-T., and Sundberg, J.P. (1995). Cutaneous ultrastructural features of the flaky skin (*fsn/fsn*) mouse mutation. *J. Dermatol.* 22:385–395.
104. Sundberg, J.P., Boggess, D., Shultz, L.D., and Beamer, W.G. (1994). The flaky skin (*fsn*) mutation, Chromosome? In *Handbook of Mouse Mutations with Skin and Hair Abnormalities: Animal Models and Biomedical Tools.* J.P. Sundberg (Ed.), CRC Press, Boca Raton, FL.
105. Sundberg, J.P., Dunstan, R.W., Roop, D.R., and Beamer, W.G. (1994). Full-thickness skin grafts from flaky skin mice to nude mice: maintenance of the psoriasiform phenotype. *J. Invest. Dermatol.* 102: 781–788.
106. Nanney, L.B., Sundberg, J.P., and King, L.E. (1996). Increased epidermal growth factor receptor in *fsn/fsn* mice. *J. Invest. Dermatol.* 106:1169–1176.
107. HoganEsch, H., Gijebeis, M.J.J., Offerman, E., van Hooft, J., van Bekkum, D.W., and Zurcher, C. (1993). A spontaneous mutation characterized by chronic proliferative dermatitis in C57BL mice. *Am. J. Pathol.* 143:972–982.
108. Sundberg, J.P., HogenEsch, J., and King, L.E. (1995). Mouse models for scaly skin diseases. In *Models for Dermatology Research.* H. Maibach (Ed.). CRC Press, Boca Raton, FL.

109. Sandgren, E.P., Luetteke, N.C., Palmiter, R.D., Brinster, R.L., and Lee, D.C. (1990). Overexpression of TGFα in transgenic mice induction of epithelial hyperplasia, pancreatic metaplasia, and carcinoma of the breast. *Cell* 61:1121–1130.
110. Blessings, M., Nanney, L.B., King, L.E., Jones, C.M., and Hogan, B.I.M. (1993). Transgenic mice as a model to study the role of TGFβ related molecules in hair follicles. *Genes Dev.* 7:204–215.
111. Blessing, M., Nanney, L.B., King, L.E., and Hogan, B.L.M. (1995). Chemical skin carcinogenesis is prevented in mice by induced expression of a TGF-β related transgene. *Teratogen. Carcinogen. Mutagen.* 15:11–21.
112. Luetteke, N.C., Qiu, T.H., Peiffer, R.L., Oliver, P., Smithies, O., and Lee, D.C. (1993). TGFα deficiency results in hair follicle and eye abnormalities in targeted and waved-1 mice. *Cell* 73:263–278.
113. Mann, G.B., Fowler, K.J., Gabriel, A., Nice, E.C., Williams, R.L., and Dunn, A.R. (1993). Mice with a null mutation of the TGFα gene have abnormal skin architecture, wavy hair, and curly whiskers and often develop corneal inflammation. *Cell* 73:248–261.
114. Luetteke, N.C., Phillps, H.K., Qiu, T.H., Copeland, N.G., Earp, H.S., Jenkins, N.A., and Lee, D.C. (1994). The mouse waved-2 phenotype results from a point mutation in the EGF receptor tyrosine kinase. *Genes Dev.* 8:399–413.
115. Threadgill, D.W., Dlugosz, A.A., Hansen, L.A., Tennenbaum, T., Lichti, U., Yee, D., LaMantia, C., Mourton, T., Herrup, K., Harris, R.C., Barnard, J.A., Yaspa, S.H., Coffey, R.J., and Magnuson, T. (1995). Targeted disruption of mouse EGF receptor: effects of genetic background on mutant phenotype. *Science* 269: 230–234.
116. Sibilia, M., and Wagner, E.F. (1995). Strain-dependent epithelial defects in mice lacking the EGF receptor. *Science* 269:234–238.
117. Murillas, R., Larcher, F., Conti, C.J., Santos, M., Ullrich, A., and Jorcano, J.L. (1995). Expression of a dominant negative mutant of epidermal growth factor receptor in the epidermis of transgenic mice elicits striking alterations in hair follicle development and skin structure. *EMBO J.* 14:5216–5223.
118. Dlugosz, A.A., Hensen, L., Cheng, C., Denning, M.F., Threadgill, D.W., Magnuson, T., Coffey, R.J., and Yuspa, S.H. (1996). Targeted disruption of EGFR impairs keratinocyte responses to the v-*ras* oncogene in vitro and in vivo. *J. Invest. Dermatol.* 106:811.

24

Anti-Infectious Therapy of Psoriasis

E. William Rosenberg, Robert B. Skinner, Jr., and Patricia W. Noah
University of Tennessee, Memphis, Tennessee

Create a concept, and reality leaves the room
—Ortega y Gasset

The past 40 years have seen a succession of concepts advanced to explain the various, and often changing, manifestations of psoriasis. These (real) phenomena include redness, thickness, and scaling of the skin, a proclivity to localize on the knees, elbows, shins, scalp, or skinfolds, an associated, often mutilating arthritis, and a rarer, but devastating, appearance of thin, moist, often pustular, red skin. Add to that some indisputable associations with HLA haplotypes, HIV-induced immunodeficiency, preceding sore throat, seborrheic dermatitis, and Reiter's disease and it becomes understandable how one could find plausible support in this rich mix of pathological events for any number of theories of pathogenesis.

One can recall, for instance, the thought that psoriasis must represent a defect in the G-phase, S-phase aspects of mitotic regulation (the thickness and scaliness and response to aminopterin), or, perhaps, a defect in the cyclic-AMP, cyclic-GMP influence on cell division. Later theories focused on disorders of arachidonic acid derivatives (the redness, and associated joint disease that responded to treatment with nonsteroidal anti-inflammatory drugs).

ROLE OF THE IMMUNE SYSTEM IN PSORIASIS

More recently it has been possible to demonstrate a multiplicity of signs of increases in number and amount of cytokines present in psoriatic skin and in the blood vessels that support it. The presence of those cytokines, among other, supporting findings, has helped to focus most present-day attention on the cells of the immune system and their possible role in psoriasis. Cytokines, of course, are the chemical messengers by which the immune system, second in complexity of its function only to the nervous system, coordinates and regulates its activities.

Further reasons to pay attention to immune function as the possible critical event in the appearance of psoriasis include the effect of immunosuppressive drugs like cyclosporin and methotrexate on the disease, and the association of psoriasis with HLA types, HLA now recognized as an essential part of the immune cells' recognition system.

A number of loose ends remain to be dealt with before we can decide that the mysteries of psoriasis have been solved and that we can now, confidently, sit back and precisely dissect the immune derangements responsible for the disease. For one thing, there is still the often overwhelming *scaliness* of psoriasis. Sunburns scale, scarlet fever scales, eczema scales but nothing quite scales the way that psoriasis does. In addition is the old clinical observation that "psoriasis is a disease of healthy people," something that does not quite jibe with a profound systemic defect in immune function. Nor is it clear why a systemic disorder of lymphocytes should show itself preferentially on places like knees, elbows, shins, and gluteal folds. And, because whatever the correct understanding of what psoriasis' pathogenesis is will have to explain all of its varied manifestations, it seems likely that however promising the immunological theory of psoriasis is, it requires considerably more insights than are now available.

By far the most pressing of those needs is to try to determine to what it is that the body's immune system is reacting. At present three such explanations are being proffered.

The first is that the body's immune system is reacting inappropriately against some part of its own skin or joints in the mistaken recognition of self-tissue as foreign pathogen. This concept of autoimmunity is now widely accepted and was asserted as fact in an editorial in the *New England Journal of Medicine* (1).

The second, based on some evidence in patients with streptococcal guttate psoriasis, is that some microbial "superantigen," in this case of streptococcal origin, has, by virtue of its ability to interfere with T-cells' usual antigen recognition system, been able to set off an indiscriminate, self-perpetuating T-cell reaction (2).

A third explanation of the immunological reactivity seen in psoriasis and psoriatic arthritis is that it represents a coordinated and complex response to microbial antigen present in the skin or joints (13). This is a concept we have accepted after more than 25 years of pursuing possible associations of microbial factors in both seborrheic dermatitis and psoriasis.

The rest of this chapter will be a further exposition of that proposition.

THE INFLAMMATORY REACTION

But first it is necessary to argue *why* it is so important to try to discover if the special kind of inflammatory reaction we call psoriasis is due to persisting microbial antigen or to inappropriate T-cell reactivity.

Forty or 50 years ago psoriasis and psoriatic arthritis were treated mostly with the judicious use of tars, baths, sunshine, artificial light, and aspirin. Most patients did reasonably well, although for many at great cost in time and inconvenience. Although it was known that psoriasis could usually be controlled by the use of Fowler's solution (arsenic), knowledge of Fowler's solution's tendency to promote cancer at some later date limited its attractiveness as an option.

If Fowler's solution constituted the preaminopterin armamentarium against the white blood cell, tonsillectomy was almost the only option for ending chronic streptococcal carrier state. Today, we have far more potent agents for moving in either direction. It is a matter of which we choose, and ultimately that choice will depend on individual preference. (An exception is the use of antibiotics for their anti-inflammatory side effects. The antibacterial sulfasalazine is an important agent, among others.)

Before we try to present the case for antibiotics as the preferred treatment for psoriasis, further brief comments seem in order about both autoimmunity and superantigen.

The concept that psoriasis is a disease of autoimmunity has been based on evidence that seems to us far too flimsy to support the kinds of powerful attacks on the immune system that are now being suggested as following from that assumption. Reeves, whose special field of interest is autoimmunity, concluded that maybe psoriasis was not, after all, an autoimmune disease (3). More recently, Burmester called autoimmunity in the reactive arthritides "not proven" (4). And in Taurog's important study of rats with a human B27 gene raised in a germ-free state he ascribes the psoriasis-like scaling on their tails to microbial antigen still present in the autoclaved sawdust, and not to autoimmunity (5).

ROLE OF MICROBIAL SUPERANTIGEN

There is now considerable interest in the possibility that microbial superantigen may play an important role in the pathogenesis of psoriasis. Evidence for this has come from findings of Vβ regions on T-cell receptors in psoriatic lesions (6) and from the actual demonstration of superantigen in some patients with guttate psoriasis (7). Even more impressive has been the demonstration that streptococcal superantigen is capable of inducing a psoriasis-like response on previously uninvolved skin that had been grafted onto immunocompromised mice. Comparable grafts from patients with no history of psoriasis did not develop psoriasis under the same experimental conditions (8).

The therapeutic implications of microbial superantigens, however, are less clear. While there are those who see superantigens as having unsettled the T-cell community sufficiently to want to treat patients with methotrexate and beyond, our reaction would be to first try antibiotics. Penicillin, after all, is the first treatment for toxic shock, and dicloxacillin for scalded skin, diseases associated with streptococcal and staphylococcal superantigens, respectively.

Our argument that psoriasis is a result of persisting stimulation of the alternative complement pathway (9) by actual microbial antigen seems strengthened by Basset-Séguin et al's demonstration that the keratinocyte makes and deploys constituents of the alternative complement pathway cascade in psoriasis (10). This, along with the insights of Kirkpatrick (11), Sohnle (12) and their collaborators on the role of the alternative complement pathway in chronic mucocutaneous candidiasis, is discussed at length by us elsewhere (13).

Recent studies by Talanin et al. (14) and us (15) point to the presence of microbial antigen and not cross-reacting skin epitope in psoriasis.

Talanin used confocal laser immunofluorescence to demonstrate reactive particles clustered around the dilated capillaries of the psoriatic plaque. Belew-Noah, Handorf, et al. (16) used an amplified avidin-biotin alkaline phosphatase system to test anti-*Candida* antibody on biopsy specimens of patients whose psoriasis had been characterized by previous workup and treatment as being related to streptococcal, candidal, or gram-negative rod colonization. The only positive reactions to the anti-*Candida* antibody occurred in those patients whose disease had been characterized previously as candidal. Of even more interest were the positive findings of a bandlike amorphous staining pattern high in the dermis just below the basement membrane in the biopsies from unaffected, normal-looking skin of those same patients. Again, there were no positive reactions to the anti-*Candida* reagent in either the characterized streptococcal or gram-negative-rod-related specimens. This suggests that the skin may play a much larger role than has been previously thought in the body's overall response to circulating microbial antigen.

Noah has reviewed the commonest microbial findings from the customary laboratory workup given to patients seen at our Problem Psoriasis Clinic (17). Interestingly, the discovered organisms correspond quite closely to those that Juhlin and Shelley found produced star-shaped microclots when added to the plasma of psoriasis patients (18).

ANTIMICROBIAL THERAPY

For the past 5 years we have been conducting a Problem Psoriasis Clinic at the University of Tennessee, Memphis. Approximately 3000 patients have been examined, subjected to a microbiological laboratory workup, and treated with antimicrobial agents or surgery. Skinner et al. have recently described these workups and treatments in detail (19).

Takegami et al. (20) assessed the effectiveness of our treatment by reviewing 59 charts and then sending follow-up questionnaires that asked patients how they thought antibiotic treatment of their psoriasis compared with conventional treatments they had received previously. Based on separate assessments of our medical records and the patients' replies to the questionnaires, Takegami et al. concluded that about 50% of our patients cleared totally or almost so, and another one-third improved substantially. Twenty percent were not helped. We are impressed enough by our results to urge others who treat psoriasis to try this approach before considering PUVA, clobetasol, methotrexate, cyclosporin, or any of the other newer systemic treatments.

Following is an outline of our protocol.

1. Usually a 4-month course of ketoconazole 200–400 mg/day will clear seborrheic-distribution psoriasis. Often these patients can be kept well by frequent or daily shampoos with 2% ketoconazole shampoo or 2.5% selenium sulfide lotion. Patients taking oral ketoconazole receive monthly liver function profile tests.
2. Patients younger than 30 with almost any pattern of psoriasis on their limbs or trunk, especially if the appearance is of thin, light-pink plaques, often turn out to be carriers of beta-hemolytic streptococci (21). To search for evidence of the *Streptococcus*, their workup must include a throat culture on blood agar (not a latex screen) with report of any beta-hemolytic streptococci, including not only group A, but also groups B, C, D, or G. Serological evidence of carrier state can be gained from a combination of anti-DNAse-B, antihyaluronidase, Streptozyme® (Wampole), and anti-streptolysin-O (ASO). The last by itself is not adequate; the ASO test is better for acute streptococcal infection than for the chronic carrier state.

Table 1 Positive Bacteriological Tests

	Face/scalp, ear	Throat	Dental plate	Nail fold	Glut fold	Groin/penis	Urine
Beta-hemolytic streptococci							
Group A		1					
Group B		1	1		4	1	3
Group C		2					
Enterococcus Group D					2		2
Group G		1				1	1
Misc: *Sanguis/Mitis/Morbillorum*				2			1
Haemophilus-Moraxella		9				1	
Klebsiella		4	2	1			
Enterobacter/Proteus	2	4	1	1			
Escherichia coli		2		1			2
Pseudomonas-Flavimonas-Acetinobacter	4	1	1	2			
Bacillus	1			1			

Patients who have either a positive throat culture or any of the serological tests above normal are treated vigorously in an attempt to clear the carrier state with clindamycin 300 mg qid for 10 days. Patients receive a diarrhea warning (30). We have foiund this superior to our previous experience with penicillin and rifampin, and erythromycin (22).

3. Patients with red, scaly or thick, scaly psoriasis of the palms and/or soles are studied for oropharyngeal candidiasis.

Both throat and dental plates (if present) are cultured for the presence of *Candida*. Dental plates are best cultured by first removing them from the patient's mouth and then swabbing the surface that touches the hard palate. Treatment is with fluconazole 200 mg/day for 2–4 weeks if the patients can afford it, and nystatin 500,000 units qid for 30–90 days if they cannot. If the dental plate culture is positive for *Candida*, patients are urged to purchase an ultrasonic cleaning device for dental plates and to be sure to take their plates out while they sleep. Such a machine is available from the Sharper Image catalog (1-800-344-4444) for about $100.

Most of our patients manage very well with what can often be an extremely troublesome or even disabling form of psoriasis (23).

4. Look for acute, but clinically inapparent urinary tract infection with the usual gram-negative rods or group D (*Enterococcus*), or group B beta-hemolytic streptococci in middle-aged or older patients with sudden flares of florid, widely scattered lesions. Try to find a microbiology laboratory that will identify all discovered pathogens, even if more than three, instead of considering them to be skin contaminants.* Treat according to reported sensitivities.

5. We have come to think that the frequently present large patch of psoriasis over the sacrum relates to the microflora of the colon, perhaps modified by diverticulosis. Patients with axial psoriatic arthritis were more likely than those with acral arthritis to have demonstrable bowel pathology on colonoscopy, and there is a literature on "translocation" of colon microflora to the regional lymphatics (24,25).

Such patients should have a trial of at least 3 months with sulfasalazine at doses of 500 mg or more qid, or a comparable course of metronidazole, usually at a somewhat lower dose.

6. In patients with either throat culture or antistreptococcal antibody evidence of streptococcal carrier state who do not clear with clindamycin treatment or who clear and then relapse, we have been impressed with the efficacy of tonsillectomy as definitive treatment for their psoriasis. In nine of 14 such patients, tonsillectomy was followed by complete clear-

*We often use North Coast Clinical Labs, Inc., 2215 Cleveland Road, Sandusky, OH 44870.

Table 2 Positive Mycological Tests

	Face	Back	Scalp	Ear	Nailfold	Throat	Dental plate	Feet/legs
Candida albicans			4	1	2	11	5	
Malassezia (pityrosporum)	2	2	11					
(KOH+) dermatophyte								5

ing. Tonsillectomy was of no help, however, in any of our patients from whom *Enterococcus faecalis* was grown on culture from any site including throat, urine, or skin (26).

7. Chronic leg psoriasis cleared in a few patients after they were treated with itraconazole for toenail onychomycosis.

8. We do not find culture of skin lesions themselves very helpful except in skinfolds (red fingernail folds, inguinal folds, inframammary folds, postauricular and axillary folds, the umbilicus). Most positive skinfold cultures grow group B beta-hemolytic streptococci, but some grow group G beta-hemolytic streptococci which are particularly difficult to treat, *Pseudomonas, Enterococcus*, or *Klebsiella* folds can be difficult to treat but sometimes respond to combinations of systemic and topical antibiotic. Upjohn's 1% clindamycin lotion (not the solution or gel) seems useful often.

Most of the time we think the microbial stimuli to psoriatic plaques comes from circulating microbial antigen, the identification of which becomes a challenging and difficult task.

9. Patients with rosacea or a history of upper gastrointestinal disease are studied and treated for the presence of *Helicobacter pylori.* At present we use what has been called "quadruple therapy" with (a) tetracycline 500 mg qid, (b) metronidazole 500 mg tid (antabuse warning), (c) Pepto-Bismol 1/2 oz qid (may darken stool and constipate), and (d) omperazole 20 mg bid. All are taken for 7 days.

There are other patterns and other histories. Often our laboratory survey shows unexpected pathogens. The *Enterococcus* when found is always difficult to treat (27,28).

Our initial treatments are always based on either the history/physical examination or the laboratory reports. We are encouraged when the laboratory reports appear to corroborate suspicions from the history/physical examination. In perhaps one-third to one-half of our patients these initial treatments do not seem to work. At that point we sometimes try alternative treatments directed at the same organisms or fall back on empirical, wider-spectrum antimicrobial agents.

Most recently we have been using levofloxacin and loracarbef as empirical antibacterials and fluconazole as an empirical anticandidal.

Belew-Noah (29) recently reviewed the laboratory findings, antimicrobial treatments, and response to therapy of 77 randomly selected patients being cared for in our Problem Psoriasis Clinic. These were not all new patients; some were those who had not improved after initial treatment and who were returning for trials of different or additional agents. Tables 1, 2, 3, and 4 summarize her findings.

Table 1 shows the number of positive bacterial recoveries from this group of patients and the sites from which the specimens were obtained.

Table 2 shows results of tests for *Candida* and *Malassezia ovalis,* and also for dermatophytes using the KOH preparation. The *Candida* reports are of growth on culture; the *Malassezia* reports are a numerical assessment of Giemsa-stained smears of wet cotton swabs rubbed over the face, back, or scalp.

Table 3 shows the positive serological test for organisms that we thought might be relevant.

Table 3 Positive Serological Tests

Anti-Group A streptococcal				Anti-*Helicobacter pylori*	Anti-CMV IgG
ASO	Streptozyme	DNase B	Hyaluronidase		
5	6	16	11	10	3

Table 4 Response to Antimicrobial Therapy in 77 Psoriasis Patients During 1995—207 Treatment Episodes of 1–4 Months

	Postive response	Negative response		Positive response	Negative response
Oral ketoconazole	24	13	Penicillin G benzathine	4	5
Oral ketoconazole plus additional oral antibiotic	6	5	Penicillin G benzathine plus additional oral antibiotic	9	4
Oral fluconazole	7	7	Amoxicillin	4	1
Oral fluconazole plus additional oral antibiotic	2	2	Amoxicillin plus additional oral antibiotic	4	4
Oral itraconazole	6	6	TMP/SMX plus 2nd antibiotic	2	5
Oral itraconazole plus additional oral antibiotic	1	0	Loracarbef	4	4
Oral nystatin	7	5	Loracarbef plus additional oral antibiotic	13	3
Terbinafine cream	0	1	Triple or quadruple therapy for *H. pylori*	2	3
Tonsillectomy plus additional oral antibiotic	2	0	Sulfasalazine	6	2
Pencillin/rifampin	8	3	Calcipotriene	2	3
Pencillin/rifampin plus additional oral antibiotic	7	0	Calcipotriene plus additional oral antibiotic	8	3

Table 4 summarizes the 207 different treatments prescribed for those 77 patients during a 4-month period and their responses. Of the 207 treatment episodes, 128 produced an apparent favorable effect.

These drugs are safer and no more expensive than methotrexate and cyclosporin. Patients who can be cleared or even controlled with antibiotics would be better off than those receiving "rotational therapy" with superpotent antisymptomatic agents.

REFERENCES

1. Krueger, G.G. (1991). Psoriasis therapy—observational or rational? *N. Engl. J. Med.* 328: 1845–1846.
2. Leung, D.Y.M., Walsh, P., Giorno, R., and Norris, D.A. (1993). A potential role for superantigens in the pathogenesis of psoriasis. *J. Invest. Dermatol.* 100: 225–228.
3. Reeves, W.H. (1991). Autoimmune mechanisms in psoriasis. *Semin. Dermatol.* 10:217–224.
4. Burmester, G.R. (1995). Immunology of reactive arthritides. *Annu. Rev. Immunol.* 13:229–250.
5. Taurog, J.D., Richardson, J.A., Croft, J.T., Simmons, W.A., Zhou, M., et al. (1994). The germfree state prevents development of gut and joint inflammatory disease in HLA-B27 transgenic rats. *J. Exp. Med.* 180: 2359–2364.
6. Lewis, H.M., Baker, B.S., Bokth, S., Powles, A.V., Garioch, J.J., et al. (1993). Restricted T-cell receptor Vβ gene usage in the skin of patients with guttate and chronic plaque psoriasis. *Br. J. Dermatol.* 129: 514–520.
7. Leung, D.Y.M., Travers, J.B., Giorno, R., Norris, D.A., Skinner, R., et al. (1995). Evidence for a streptococcal superantigen-driven process in acute guttate psoriasis. *J. Clin. Invest.* 96:2106–2112.
8. Boehncke, W.H., Dressel, D., Zollner, T.M., and Kaufmann, R. (1996). Pulling the trigger on psoriasis. *Nature* 379:777.
9. Rosenberg, E.W., Noah, P.W., Wyatt, R.M., Jones, R.M., and Kolb, W.P. (1990). Complement activation in psoriasis. *Clin. Exp. Dermatol.* 15:16–20.
10. Basset-Séguin, N., Porneuf, M., Dereure, O., et al. (1993). C3d,g deposits in inflammatory skin diseases: use of psoriatic skin as a model of cutaneous inflammation. *J. Invest. Dermatol.* 101:827–831.
11. Kirkpatrick, C.H. (1989). Chronic mucocutaneous candidiasis. *Eur. J. Clin. Microbiol. Infect. Dis.* 8: 448–456.
12. Sohnle, P.G., and Hahn, B.L. (1989). Epidermal proliferation and the neutrophilic infiltrates of experimental cutaneous candidiasis in mice. *Arch. Dermatol. Res.* 281:279–283.

13. Rosenberg, E.W., Noah, P.W., and Skinner, R.B., Jr. (1994). Psoriasis is a visible manifestation of the skin's defense against micro-organisms. *J. Dermatol.* 21: 375–381.
14. Talanin, N.Y., Shelley, V.B., Raeder, R., et al. (1997). Detection of streptococcal class I M protein in psoriasis by confocal immunofluorescent microscopy. *Acta Derm. Venereol. (Stockh)*, 77:175–180.
15. Noah, P.W., Bale, G., Eilert, V., et al. (1986). Streptococcal products in the epidermis of patients with streptococcal associated psoriasis: detection by immunofluorescence with monoclonal and polyclonal antistreptococcal antibodies. *J. Invest. Dermatol.* 86:497. (abstract).
16. Belew-Noah, P.W., Handorf, C.R., Rosenberg, E.W., Skinner, R.B., Jr., and Murphy, M. (1995). The psoriasis band test: detection of microbial antigen deposited in the skin of psoriasis patients using amplification staining with streptavidin-biotin alkaline phosphatase, DAKO, LSAB Kit. *J. Invest. Dermatol.* 43:2A (abstract).
17. Noah, P.W. (1990). The role of microorganisms in psoriasis. *Semin. Dermatol.* 9:269–276.
18. Juhlin, L., and Shelley, W.B. (1977). Oriented fibrin crystallization: a phenomenon of hypersensitivity to bacteria in psoriasis, vasculitis and other dermatoses. *Br. J. Dermatol.* 96:577–585.
19. Skinner, R.B., Jr., Rosenberg, E.W., and Noah, P.W. (1995). Antimicrobial treatment of psoriasis. *Dermatol. Clin.* 13:909–913.
20. Takegami, K.T., Ross, S.O., Rosenberg, E.W., et al. (1991). Antimicrobial treatment of psoriasis. *J. Invest. Dermatol.* 98:607 (abstract).
21. Rosenberg, E.W., Noah, P.W., Skinner, R.B., Jr. et al. (1989). Microbial associations of 167 patients with psoriasis. *Acta Derm. Venereol. (Stockh.)* 146:72–75.
22. Rosenberg, E.W., Noah, P.W., Zanolli, M.D., et al. (1986). Use of rifampin with penicillin and erythromycin in the treatment of psoriasis. *J. Am. Acad. Dermatol.* 14:761–764.
23. Skinner, R.B., Jr., Rosenberg, E.W., and Noah, P.W. (1994). Psoriasis of the palms and soles is frequently associated with oropharyngeal *Candida albicans. Acta Derm. Venereol. (Stockh.)* (Suppl.) 186:149–150.
24. Schatteman, L., Mielants, H., Veys, E.M., Cuvelier, C., De Vos, M., et al. (1995). Gut inflammation in psoriatic arthritis: a prospective ileocolonoscopic study. *J. Rheumatol.* 22:680–685.
25. Van Leeuwen, P.A.M., Boermeester, M.A., Houdijk, A.P.J., Ferwerda, C.C., Cuesta, M.A., et al. (1994). Clinical significance of translocation. *Gut* 1:S28–S34.
26. Rosenberg, E.W., Duberstein, L.E., Duberstein, A.J., Skinner, R.B., Jr., Noah, P.W., et al. (1994). Effect of tonsillectomy and other otorhinolaryngologic surgery on psoriasis. Poster. Presented at The Society of Investigative Dermatology annual meeting. Baltimore, Maryland, April 27–30.
27. Swartz, J.H. (1945). The possible inter-relation of psoriasis and streptococcus faecalis. *N. Engl. J. Med.* 233: 296–297.
28. Robinson, M.M. (1953). The relationship of streptococcus faecalis to psoriasis. *J. Invest. Dermatol.* 20: 455–459.
29. Belew-Noah, P.W. (1996). Antimicrobial treatment of psoriasis. Forum. Presented at the 54th Annual Meeting of the American Academy of Dermatology. Washington, DC, February 10–15.
30. St. Jennquist-Desatnik, A., Orrling, A., Schalén, C., and Kamme, C. (1997). Clindamycin in recurrent group A streptococcal pharyngotonsillitis—an alternative to tonsillectomy. In Horaud, T., Bouvet, A., Leclerq, R., de Montclos, H., and Sicard, M., (eds.) Advances in Experimental Medicine and Biology: Streptococci and the Host. Plenum, New York, pp. 435–437.

Part IV

HISTOLOGY

25

Neuropeptides and Neurogenic Inflammation in Psoriasis

Siba Prasad Raychaudhuri and Eugene M. Farber
Psoriasis Research Institute, Palo Alto, California

Psoriasis is a complex, mulifactorial, lifelong disease of unknown etiology. The concept of cutaneous neuroimmunology as it relates to psoriasis is relatively new. Farber et al. in 1986 first proposed a possible role for neuropeptides in the pathogenesis of psoriasis (1). Subsequently other investigators have observed upregulation of various neuropeptides in the psoriatic lesions (2–4). In this chapter we will discuss the role of neuropeptides in the inflammatory and vascular changes associated with psoriasis and will review the pharmacological agents that modulate the local actions of neuropeptides in the skin.

STRESS, PSORIASIS, AND PSYCHONEUROIMMUNOLOGY

In several studies of large groups of patients, it has been observed that stress plays an important role in the onset and course of psoriasis. In a questionnaire survey Farber and Nall reported that 33% of 5600 patients noticed appearance of new lesions at the time of worry (5). In a similar series of 536 patients, Braun-Falco et al. reported that in 42% of patients worry precipitates an exacerbation of psoriasis (6). Fava et al. correlated the appearance or exacerbation of psoriasis in 80% of patients (7). Seville followed 132 patients for 3 years and observed that a specific stress occurred within a month before the appearance of psoriasis in 39% of subjects (8). Our recent data from the Psoriasis Research Institute reveal that in 607 patients with psoriasis 31.8% mentioned stress as an initiating event and in 46.3% stress caused exacerbation of psoriasis (9).

How stress influences the inflammatory and the proliferative processes of psoriasis is not clearly understood. Current evidence suggests an existence of complex bidirectional interactions between the nervous system, the endocrine system, and the immune system (10,11). This new field of study is known as psychoneuroimmunology. The bidirectional communication between the nervous system and the immune system is mediated by the endocrine system. Both the nervous system and the immune system have been found to share recognition molecules originating from both systems. There is now ample evidence that immunocompetent cells express receptors for neurohoromones, neurotransmitters, and neuropeptides. Receptors for neuropeptides like vasoactive intestinal peptide (VIP) and somatostatin have been found on lymphocytes (12). Receptors for glucocorticoids, estrogens, androgens, β-adrenergic catecholamines, and neurotensin have been found on T cells (13,14). Receptors for the cytokines IL-1 and IL-3 have been demonstrated in the brain (15).

Stressful events can alter substance P level in the CNS and in the periphery. In an animal model it has been reported that stress can increase levels of substance P in the adrenal glands by activating the descending autonomic fibers (16). Local release of neuropeptides from sensory nerves in the skin, however, has not been measured after stressful stimuli in either animals or humans. Some of the descending autonomic fibers innervate opioid interneurons in the dorsal horn, and as interneurons exist in the spinal cord for the substance P–containing nerves, it is possible that descending autonomic paths can cause release of cutaneous neuropeptides (17).

Correlating the concepts of psychoneuroimmunology and clinical observations that stress exacerbates psoriasis and psoriasis is distributed symmetrically in the skin, Farber et al. proposed a role for neuropeptides in the pathogenesis of psoriasis. The authors suggested that release of SP and other neuropeptides from sensory cutaneous nerves in response to stress causes local inflammatory response that triggers psoriasis in a genetically predisposed individual (1).

NEUROGENIC INFLAMMATION AND THE SKIN

Activation of unmyelinated capsaicin-sensitive fibers can cause vasodilation and plasma extravasation. Antidromic stimulation of dorsal roots causes not only vasodilatation, it also evokes characteristic inflammatory response in the skin and in various internal organs. This process is called neurogenic inflammation.

Goltz and Stricker in the late 1880s were the first to observe that the nerves of the dorsal root ganglia can cause peripheral vasodilatation. Bayliss in the early part of this century demonstrated that antidromic stimulation of peripheral sensory nerves results in cutaneous vasodilatation (18). Thomas Lewis established the concept of the "triple response" that is observed in human skin in response to a pinpoint injury (19). Triple response relates to the morphological changes manifested as wheal, local erythema, and flare in response to an external stimulus. Lewis suggested that injury to the skin leads to stimulation of sensory nerves, resulting in transmission of impulses to the spinal cord, as well as antidromic stimulation of connecting fibers that innervate the adjacent skin. Jancsó et al. in the 1960s showed that the inflammatory response in the skin secondary to stimulation of sensory nerves could be abolished by denervation and they postulated that the inflammatory response was due to release of neurohormones (20). In last 30 years extensive research has been carried out to elucidate these neurohormones. Now we know that the neurogenic inflammation results from the release of neuropeptides from the nerve endings, and this can affect a variety of immune cells through specific neuropeptide receptors (21,22). These observations suggest that the cutaneous sensory nervous system in addition to conduction of sensory impulses has an effector role in producing an inflammatory response.

A large number of neuropeptides have been identified in the skin by immunohistochemical staining and/or radioimmunoassay. Table 1 lists the neuropeptides in the human skin. We will discuss in detail some of the neuropeptides that have potent effects on various components of the cutaneous tissue.

The neurokinins (NKs) are substance P, neurokinin A, and neurokinin B. They share the same C-terminal amino acid sequences. NK-A and substance P are encoded by the same gene and their distributions are similar (23). In normal human skin substance P nerve fibers are present in the dermis, epidermis, Meissner's corpuscles, and around the sweat glands (24,25). Neurokinin B is not found in the skin. Intradermal injection of substance P induces a triple response. The flare component of the triple response can be inhibited by H-1 receptor antagonist (26). This indicates that the flare response is due to the actions of histamine released by the mast cells. Substance P increases permeability of the vessels by activation of the NK-1 receptors on postcapillary venules and by releasing histamine from the mast cells (27).

CGRP is widely distributed in the skin and is one of the most abundant neuropeptides. It is commonly colocalized with substance P (28). Distribution of CGRP-positive nerve fibers in the skin is similar to that of substance P nerve fibers. Intradermal injection of CGRP induces a local erythema, which can be observed for several hours.

VIP is mainly found in nerve fibers around the arterial walls and acini of sweat glands (24). Intradermal injection of VIP causes a wheal-and-flare response. As

Table 1 Neuropeptide-Positive Fibers Identified in Human Skin

Substance P
Vasoactive intestinal polypeptide
Calcitonin-gene-related peptide
Neuropeptide Y
Neurokinin A
Somatostatin
Neurotensin
Galanin
Atrial natriuretic peptide
Peptide histidine methionine
γ-Melanocyte-stimulating hormone

the axon-reflex flare response fades, a local area of erythema appears due to increased blood flow (29).

In addition to the vasoactive activities, substance P, VIP, and CGRP have extremely potent effects on various cellular components of an inflammatory response. Various biological effects of these neuropeptides are listed in Tables 2–4.

EVIDENCE FOR THE INVOLVEMENT OF NEUROPEPTIDE IN THE PATHOGENESIS OF PSORIASIS

The actions of neuropeptides like SP, VIP, and CGRP can be of great significance in the inflammatory and proliferative process in psoriasis. Keratinocyte hyperproliferation, the hallmark of psoriasis, can be triggered by VIP (30), CGRP acts synergistically with SP to stimulate keratinocyte proliferation (31), and both SP and VIP can enhance the mitogenic effect of leukotrine B4 on human keratinocyte (32). Degranulation (33) and increased number of mast cells (34) seen in early lesions of psoriasis can both be induced by substance P (35). CGRP, a potent mitogenic factor for endothelial cells (36), can explain angiogenesis observed in the developing lesions of psoriasis (37). One of the earliest histological changes occurring in the psoriatic lesions is infiltration by leukocytes (38). Increased adhesion of peripheral blood lymphocytes to endothelium has been observed in psoriasis (39,40). Both SP and CGRP have been reported to enhance adhesion of lymphomononuclear cells (41,42). Further, it has been shown that substance P can induce the expression of endothelial leukocyte adhesion molecules (ELAM-1) on postcapillary dermal vessels (43). Substance P can cause chemotaxis of neutrophils (44), stimulates IL-2 synthesis (45) in T cells, and can induce IL-1 secretion from keratinocytes (46). All of these functions can contribute significantly to the pathogenesis of psoriasis. Intradermal injection of SP, VIP, and CGRP in normal human skin has been reported to induce rapid time-dependent neutrophil infiltration (47). The same authors also observed that SP induced marked up-regulation of E-selectin expression in the vessels together with increased accumulation of eosinophils in the dermis.

Table 2 Biological Actions of Substance P

Keratinocyte	Stimulation of IL-1, GM-CSF Synthesis and Secretion, Comitogen with CGRP, LTB 4.
Fibroblasts	Stimulates proliferation
Endothelial cells	Stimulates proliferation, increases permeability, up-regulation of ELAM-1
Neutrophil	Stimulates chemotaxis, phagocytosis
Mast cell	Degranulation, stimulates proliferation and survival in culture
Lymphocytes	Stimulates proliferation and IL-2 synthesis, increases IgA, IgM, and heavy-chain mRNA production
Macrophage/monocyte	Increases chemotaxis, phagocytosis, and arachadonic acid synthesis

Table 3 Biological Actions of Calcitonin Gene-Related Peptide

Keratinocyte	Proliferation in association with substance P
Endothelial cell	Proliferation, up-regulation of ELAM-1
Mast cell	Degranulation
Langerhans cell	Inhibits antigen presentation
T lymphocytes	Chemotactic, inhibits mitogen-induced T-cell proliferation

A functional role for cutaneous nerves with their neuropeptides in the pathogenesis of psoriasis is supported by increasing numbers of biochemical and clinical studies. An increased number of neural filaments in both lesional and symptomless psoriatic skin have been reported much earlier by Weddell et al. in 1965 (48). By using immunohistochemical staining, we have demonstrated an increased number of substance P–containing nerves in psoriatic epidermis (2). Subsequent study has confirmed these findings and also demonstrated VIP-containing nerves in psoriatic plaques (4). Direct measurement of neuropeptides by radioimmunoassay from the lesional psoriatic biopsies in a majority of studies have shown increased levels of substance P and/or VIP (49–51). However, there are some differences in their results. Wallengren et al. reported reduced VIP level in suction blisters raised from psoriatic plaques (49), Pincelli et al. reported reduced levels of substance P in chronic psoriatic plaques (50), Anand et al. found no difference in SP levels in the psoriatic plaques compared to normal skin (52). The conflicting results obtained in these studies may be due to several factors. It is unknown when SP and VIP appear and where they are located in the developing lesion. In addition, neuropeptide lev-

Table 4 Biological Actions of Vasoactive Intestinal Polypeptide

Keratinocytes	Proliferation, increased adenylate cyclase activity
Mast cell	Degranulation
Endothelial cell	Proliferation
Neutrophil	Chemotaxis
Lymphocyte	Inhibits proliferation, inhibits NK cell activity

els are difficult to measure because they are readily metabolized. In a relatively new study Naukkarinen et al. studied the dynamics of neuropeptides in tape-strip-induced evolving psoriatic lesions and mature psoriatic plaques. The authors observed very few nerves to contain SP, VIP, or CGRP in control skin, nonlesional skin, and Koebner-negative psoriatic skin. In the evolving Koebner-positive lesions, at the end of a week SP-positive fibers were found in the papillary dermis in all the lesions and VIP-positive fibers were observed around the capillaries in 66% of the lesions (53). SP fibers were most abundant in mature psoriatic plaques. We conducted a study in 28 patients with psoriasis to identify SP, VIP, and CGRP in the skin biopsies and observed an increase in the number of SP-positive intraepidermal nerve fibers in lesional psoriatic skin specimens (2.8 nerves/mm biopsy) compared with nonlesional psoriatic skin (0.01 nerves/mm biopsy) and normal skin (0.04 nerves/mm biopsy). Increased intraepidermal VIP- and CGRP-positive fibers were also observed in the psoriatic lesions (54).

In addition to SP, VIP, and CGRP, other neuropeptides may be involved in the pathogenesis of psoriasis. Proliferating keratinocytes can synthesize and release nerve growth factor (55). NGF exerts a number of effects like degranulation of mast cells (56), regulation of the synthesis and expression of neuropeptides (57), and proliferation of keratinocytes (58). Recently it was reported that NGF is increased in psoriatic skin (59).

Krogstad et al. observed that local infiltration of the psoriatic plaques with mepivacaine caused 40% reduction of blood flow in the lesions, whereas surface anesthesia of UVB-induced erythema did not affect the regional blood flow (60). It is known that cutaneous anesthesia can prevent vasodilatation induced by axon reflex (61). This observation supports the idea that a local neurogenic mechanism is active in the psoriatic plaques. The most striking evidence for the role of neurogenic inflammation in psoriasis comes from studies where peripheral nerve sectioning resulted in clearing of psoriatic plaques. We have reported a number of cases where psoriatic lesions resolved at the site of anesthesia subsequent to damage of sensory nerves (62,63). In one patient it was interesting that psoriasis resolved at the anesthetic area over the knee, and with the return of sensation, psoriasis reappeared at the same site (62).

THE APPLICATION OF PSYCHONEUROIMMUNOLOGY TO THE TREATMENT OF PSORIASIS

There is unequivocal evidence that stress is a triggering factor for the appearance or exacerbation of psoriasis (5–8). This indicates that, in addition to the standard therapies available to dermatologists, it is advisable to consider stress reduction measures. Psychological evaluation should be an integral part of the management of psoriasis. It is helpful to know whether a patient has a primary emotional disorder or an emotional instability secondary to the psychosocial impact of psoriasis. In patients with anxiety or depression, psychopharmacological medications like antidepressants or anxiolytics may be appropriate. The other aspect of psychological evaluation is to find out the various underlying factors, the patient's personality, and the way the patient reacts to a stressful situation. Analysis of these factors will indicate desirability of stress reduction modalities like hypnosis (64–66), biofeedback (67,68), meditation (69), and visual imagery and cognitive organization (70).

A direct pharmacological approach is to develop drugs that can deplete or block the release of neuropeptides, block the receptor sites of neuropeptides, or activate the enzyme neutral endopeptidase (NEP). Until now only a few neuropeptide-modulating agents have been evaluated.

Capsaicin (trans-8-methyl-*N*-vanillyl-G-nonenamide), the extract of the hot pepper, depletes the neuropeptides from the sensory C nerve fibers (71). Topical use of capsaicin has been reported to be effective in psoriasis (72), but it is unsuitable because it causes significant burning of the skin.

Neuropeptide receptor analogs have been reported to block inflammatory effects of neuropeptides such as plasma extravasation (73), nociceptor flexor reflexes (74), and erythematous responses (75). In vitro effects of neuropeptides on lymphocytes (76), keratinocytes (32), and mast cells (77) can be modulated by neuropeptide receptor antagonists as well. These results indicate that neuropeptide analogs can be applied to inhibit the inflammatory and vascular changes associated with psoriasis.

Peptide T, a synthetic octapeptide, is a protease-resistant analog of VIP (87). The first report of efficacy of peptide T in psoriasis came from an anecdotal case report where psoriasis in an AIDS patient significantly improved following the intravenous infusion of peptide T (79). Subsequently IV use of peptide T has been reported to improve psoriasis (80,81). Farber et al. evaluated the efficacy of peptide by direct administration into psoriatic lesion by miniosmotic pump (82). In this double-blind, placebo-controlled study authors observed that infusion of peptide T in nanogram amounts improved psoriatic lesions both clinically and histopathologically. The mechanism of action of peptide T in psoriasis is not clear; possibilities suggested are antagonizing the action of VIP, upregulation of somatostatin in the psoriatic lesion, and immunomodulation (82–84).

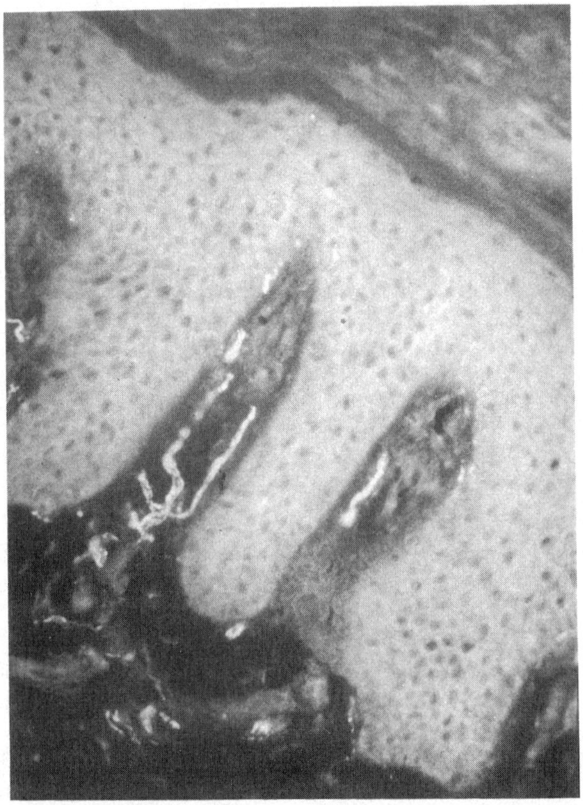

Figure 1 Psoriasis biopsy stained with general neuronal marker (PGP 9.5). Note nerve fibers in the papillary dermis. (Courtesy of J. Wallengren.)

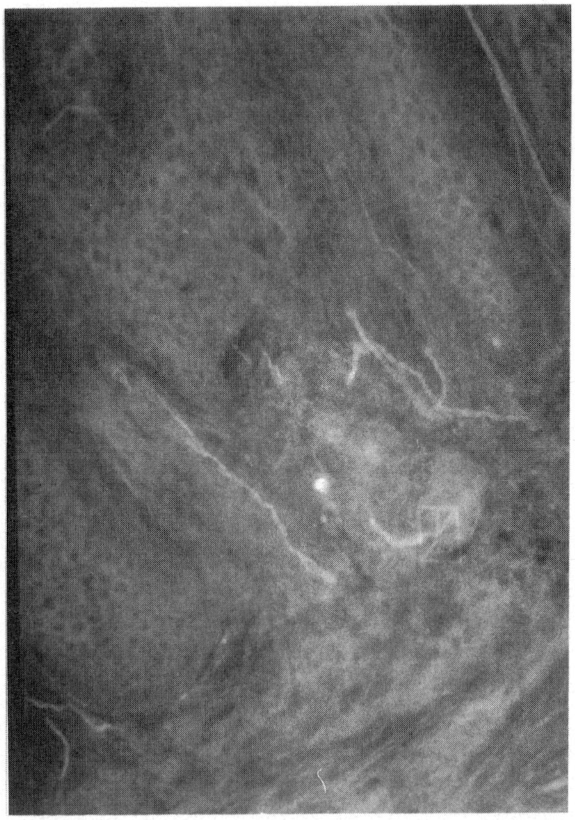

Figure 2 NGF receptor antibody reveals multiple nerve fibers in epidermis and upper dermis. Magnification ×200.

Somatostatin analog (Sandostatin) is the other neuropeptide analog that has been found to be efficacious in psoriasis (85). Six of nine patients treated with Sandostatin showed minimal to marked improvement. However, a high frequency of gallstones was noted among these patients. Somatostatin is a well-known SP inhibitor (86).

Substance P antagonists may also be useful therapeutic agents for psoriasis. Spantide, a structural analog of SP, has been reported to cause inhibition of delayed-type cutaneous hypersensitivity reactions in healthy human volunteers (87). Spantide can also inhibit SP-induced keratinocyte proliferation in vitro (32). Peptide antagonists are metabolically unstable and can cause hypersensitivity reaction. The discovery of CP-96,345, a synthetic, nonpeptide SP receptor

(NK-1 receptor) antagonist, has made it possible to evaluate the effects of NK-1 receptor antagonism in humans (88). In animal models CP-96,345 has been found to inhibit plasma exudation induced by SP and can block nociceptor responses to noxious cutaneous stimuli (89,90). These results indicate the applicability of SP antagonists in various inflammatory conditions, including psoriasis. Currently various synthetic substance P antagonists are in phase II trial for evaluation of its efficacy and safety in psoriasis.

Activating the enzyme neutral endopeptidase (NEP), which degrades the neuropeptides, would be an alternative way to counter the actions of neuropeptides (91). It has been reported that glucocorticoids can induce NEP (92). This provides another explanation for the efficacy of glucocorticoids in the treatment of psoriasis. Neurogenic inflammation induced by substance P can be suppressed with exogenous human recombinant NEP (93).

In conclusion, we want to emphasize that psoriatic lesions have a significantly larger number of nerves (Figs. 1 and 2) with increased content of neuropeptides. It has been documented that the damage to sensory nerves results in clearance of psoriatic lesions in the anesthetic areas and neuropeptide-modulating drugs have been found to be efficacious in psoriasis. All these observations substantiate that neuropeptides play a significant role in the pathogenesis of psoriasis.

REFERENCES

1. Farber, E.M., Nickoloff, B.J., Recht, B., et al. (1986). Stress, symmetry, and psoriasis: possible role of neuropeptides. *J. Am. Acad. Dermatol.* 14:305–311.
2. Naukkarinen, A., Nickoloff, B.J., and Farber, E.M. (1989). Quantification of cutaneous sensory nerves and their substance P content in psoriasis. *J. Invest. Dermatol.* 92:126–129.
3. Naukkarinen, A., Harvima, I.T., Paukkonen, K., et al. (1991). Quantitative analysis of contact sites between mast cells and sensory nerves in cutaneous psoriasis and lichen planus based on histochemical double staining technique. *Arch. Dermatol. Res.* 283:433–437.
4. Al-Abadie, M.S.K., Senior, H. J., Bleehen, S.S., et al. (1992). Neurogenic changes in psoriasis. An immunohistochemical study. *J. Invest. Dermatol.* 98:535.
5. Farber, E.M., and Nall, M.L. (1974). The national history of psoriasis in 5,600 patients. *Dermatologica* 148: 1–18.
6. Braun-Falco, O., Burg, G., and Farber, G.M. (1972). Psoriasis: eine Fragebogen—studie bei 536 Patienten. *Munch–Med. Wochenschr.* 114:1–15.
7. Fava, G.A., Perini, G.I., Santonastaso, P., et al. (1980). Life events and psychological distress in dermatological disorders: psoriasis, chronic urticaria, and fungal infections. *Br. J. Med. Psychol.* 53:277–282.
8. Seville, R.H. (1977). Psoriasis and stress I. *Br. J. Dermatol.* 97:297–302.
9. Farber, E.M., and Nall, L. (1993). Psoriasis: a stress-related disease. *Cutis* 51:322–326.
10. Ader, R., ed. (1981). *Psychoneuroimmunology.* Academic Press, New York, 1981, pp. 230–257.
11. Jankovic, B.D., Markovic, B.M., and Spector, N.H. (1987). Neuroendocrine correlates of neuroimmunomodulation. *Ann. N. Y. Acad. Sci.* 496:3–107.
12. Goetzl, E.J., Turck, C.W., and Sreedharan, S.P. (1991). Production and recognition of neuropeptides by cells of the immune system. *Psychoneuroimmunology (II).* Academic Press, New York, pp. 263–282.
13. Motulsky, H.J., and Insel, P.A. (1982). Adrenergic receptors in man: direct identification, physiological regulation, and clinical alterations. *N. Engl. J. Med.* 307: 18–29.
14. Gorman, J.R., and Locke, S.E. (1989). Neural, endocrine and immune interactions. In *The Comprehensive Textbook of Psychiatry*, H.I. Kapland and B.J. Sadock (Eds.). Williams & Wilkinson, Baltimore, pp. 111–125.
15. Farrar, W.I., Hill, J.M., Hard-Bellam, A., et al. (1987). The immunological brain. *Immunol. Rev.* 100: 361–378.
16. Vaupel, R., Jarry, H., Schlomer, H.T., et al. (1988). Differential response of substance P containing subtypes of adrenomedullary cells to different stressors. *Endocrinology* 123:2140–2145.
17. Farber, E.M., Rein, G., and Lanigan, S.W. (1991). Stress and psoriasis—psychoneuroimmunologic mechanisms. *Int. J. Dermatol.* 30:8–12.
18. Bayliss, W.M. (1901). On the origin from the spinal cord of the vasodilator fibres of the hind limb, and on the nature of these fibres. *J. Physiol.* 26:173.
19. Lewis, T. (1930). Observation upon reaction of vessels in human skin to cold. *Heart* 15:177.
20. Jancsó, N., Janscó-Gábor, A., and Szolcsányi, J. (1967). Direct evidence for neurogenic inflammation and its prevention by denervation and by pretreatment with capsaicin. *Br. J. Pharmacol.* 31:138–151.
21. Blalock, J.E., Bost, K.L., and Smith, M.E. (1985). Neuroendrocine peptide hormones and their receptors in the immune system production, processing and action. *J. Neuroimmunol.* 10:31–40.
22. Widermann, C.J. (1987). Shared recognition molecules in the brain and lymphoid tissues: the polypeptide mediator network of psychoneuroimmunology. *Immunol. Lett.* 16:371–378.
23. Weihe, E., and Hartschuh, W. (1988). Multiple peptides in cutaneous nerves: regulator under physiologi-

cal conditions and a pathogenetic role in skin disease? *Semin. Dermatol.* 7:284.
24. Bloom, S.R., and Polak, J.M. (1983). Regulatory peptides and the skin. *Clin. Exp. Dermatol.* 8:3.
25. Tanio, H., Vaalastic, A., and Rechardt, L. (1983). The distribution of substance P, CGRP, galanin and ANP like immunoreactive nerves in human sweat glands. *Histochem. J.* 39:1018.
26. Hagermark, O., Hokfelt, T., and Pernow, B. (1980). Flare and itch induced by substance P in human skin. *J. Invest. Dermatol.* 71:233.
27. Deviller, P., Regoli, D., Asseraf, A., et al. (1986). Histamine release and local response of rat and human skin to substance P and other mammalian tachykinins. *Pharmacology* 32:340.
28. Gibbins, I.L., Wattchow, D., and Conventry, G. (1987). Two immunohistochemically identified populations of calcitonin gene-related peptide (CGRP)-immunoreactive axons in human skin. *Brain Res.* 414: 143.
29. Anand, A., Bloom, S.R., and McGregor, G.P. (1983). Topical capsaicin pretreatment inhibits axon reflex vasodilation caused by somatostatin and vasoactive intestinal polypeptide in human skin. *Br. J. Pharmacol.* 78:665.
30. Haegerstrand, A., Jonzon, B., Dalsgaard, C.J., et al. (1989). Vasoactive intestinal polypeptide stimulates cell proliferation and adenylate cyclase activity of cultured human keratinocytes. *Proc. Natl. Acad. Sci. U.S.A.* 86:5993–5996.
31. Wilkinson, D.I. (1989). Mitogenic effect of substance P and CGRP on keratinocytes. *J. Cell Biol.* 107:509a.
32. Rabier, M., and Wilkinson, D.I. (1991). Neuropeptides modulate leukotrine B 4 mitogenicity toward cultured keratinocytes. *Clin. Res.* 39:536a.
33. Brody, I. (1984). Mast cell degranulation in the evolution of acute eruptive guttate psoriasis vulgaris. *J. Invest. Dermatol.* 82:460–464.
34. Cox, A.J. (1976). Mast cells in psoriasis. In *Psoriasis. Proceedings of the Second International Symposium*, E.M. Farber and A.J. Cox (Eds.). York Medical Books, New York, pp. 36–37.
35. Erjavec, F., Lembeck, F., Irman, I.F., et al. (1981). Release of histamine by substance *P. Naunyn Schmiedebergs Arch. Pharmacol.* 317:67–70.
36. Haegerstrand, A., Dalsgaard, C.J., Jonzon, B., et al. (1990). Calcitonin gene-related peptide stimulates proliferation of human endothelial cells. *Proc. Natl. Acad. Sci. U.S.A.* 87:3299–3303.
37. Pinkus, H., and Mehregan, A.M. (1966) The primary histologic lesion of seborrheic dermatitis and psoriasis. *J. Invest. Dermatol.* 46:109–116.
38. Ragaz, A., and Ackerman, B. (1979). Evolution, motivation and regression of lesions of psoriasis. *Am. J. Dermatopathol.* 1:199–214.
39. Le Roy, F., Brown, K.A., and Graes, M.W. (1991). Blood mononuclear cells from patients with psoriasis exhibit an enhanced adherence to cultured vascular endothelium. *J. Invest. Dermatol.* 97:511–516.
40. Sackstein, R., Falnga, V., Streilein, J.W., et al. (1988). Lymphocyte adhesion to psoriatic dermal endothelium is medicated by a tissue-specific receptor/ligand interaction. *J. Invest. Dermatol.* 91:423–428.
41. Rein, G., and Karasek, M. (1992). Effect of substance P on adhesion of a human monocyte cell line to fibronectin. *Clin. Res.* 40:45a.
42. Sung, C.P., Arleth, A.J., Aiyar, N., et al. (1992). CGRP stimulates the adhesion of leukocytes to vascular endothelial cells. *Peptides* 13:429–434.
43. Matis, W.L., Lavker, R.M., and Murphy, G.F. (1990). Substance P induces the expression of an endothelial-leukocyte adhesion molecule by microvascular endothelium. *J. Invest. Dermatol.* 94:492–495.
44. Tomoe, S., Iwamoto, I., Tomioka, H., et al. (1992). Comparison of substance P–induced and compound 48/80 induced neutrophil infiltrations in mouse skin. *Int. Arch. Allergy Appl. Immunol.* 97:237–242.
45. Calvo, C.F., Chavanel, G., and Senica, A. (1992). Substance P enhances interleukin-2 expression in activated human T cells. *J. Immunol.* 148:3498–3504.
46. Ansel, J., Perry, P., Brown, J., et al. (1990). Cytokine modulation of keratinocyte cytokines. *J. Invest. Dermatol.* 94:101S–107S.
47. Smith, C.H., Barker, J., Morris, R.W., et al. (1993). Neuropeptides induce rapid expression of endothelial cell adhesion molecules and elicit granulocytic infiltration in human skin. *J. Immunol.* 151:3274–3282.
48. Weddell, G., Cowan, M.A., Palmer, E., et al. (1965). Psoriatic skin. *Arch. Dermatol.* 91:252–266.
49. Wallengren, J., Ekman, R., and Sunder, F. (1987). Occurrence and distribution of neuropeptides in human skin. An immunochemical study of normal skin and blister fluid from inflamed skin. *Acta Derm. Venerol. (Stockh.)* 67:185–192.
50. Pincelli, C., Fantini, F., Romualdi, P., et al. (1992). Substance P is diminished and VIP is augmented in psoriatic lesions and these peptides exert diparate effects on the proliferation of cultured human keratinocytes. *J. Invest. Dermatol.* 98:421–427.
51. Eedy, D.J., Johnson, C.F., Shaw, C., et al. (1991). Neuropeptides in psoriasis: an immunocytochemical and radioimmunoassay study. *J. Invest. Dermatol.* 96: 434–438.
52. Anand, P., Springail, D.R., Blank, K., et al. (1991). Neuropeptides in skin disease: increased VIP in eczema and psoriasis but not axillary hyperhidrosis. *Br. J. Dermatol.* 124:547–549.
53. Naukkarinen, A., Harvima, I., Paukkonen, et al. (1993). Immunohistochemical analysis of sensory nerves and neuropeptides and their contacts with mast

cells in developing and mature psoriatic lesions. *Arch. Dermatol. Res.* 285:341–346.
54. Chan, J., Smoller, B., Raychaudhuri, S.P., et al. (1997). Interaepidermal nerve fibre expression of calcitonin gene related peptide, vasoactive intermittent peptide and substance P confirms the role of neuropeptides in pathogens of psoriasis. *J. Arch. Dermatol. Res.* (in press).
55. Pincelli, C., Sevignanic, C., Mantredini, R., et al. (1994). Expression and function of nerve growth factor receptor on cultured keratinocytes. *J. Invest. Dermatol.* 103:13–18.
56. Pearce, F.L., and Thompson, H.L. (1986). Some characteristics of histamine secretion from rat peritoneal mast cells stimulated with nerve growth factors. *J. Physiol.* 372:379–393.
57. Lindsay, R., and Harmar, A. (1989). Nerve growth factor regulates expression of neuropeptide genes in adult sensory neurons. *Nature* 337:362–364.
58. Wilkinson, D.I., Theeuwes, M.J., and Farber, E.M. (1994). Nerve growth factor increases the mitogenicity of certain growth factors for cultured human keratinocytes: a comparison with epidermal growth factor. *Exp. Dermatol.* 3:239–245.
59. Fantini, F., Magnoni, C., Bracci-Laudierol, L., et al. (1995). Nerve growth factor is increased in psoriatic skin. *J. Invest. Dermatol.* 104:854–855.
60. Krogstad, A.L., Swanbeck, G., and Wallin, G. (1995). Axon-reflex mediated vasodilatation in the psoriatic plaque? *J. Invest. Dermatol.* 104:872–876.
61. Wardell, K., Naver, H.K., Nilsson, G.E., et al. (1993). The cutaneous vascular axon reflex in humans characterized by laser doppler perfusion imaging. *J. Physiol. (Lond.)* 460:185–190.
62. Farber, E.M., Lanigan, S.W., and Boer, J. (1990). The role of cutaneous sensory nerves in the maintenance of psoriasis. *Int. J. Dermatol.* 29:418–420.
63. Raychaudhuri, S.P. and Farber, E.M. (1993). Are sensory nerves essential for the pathogenesis of psoriasis? *J. Am. Acad. Dermatol.* 28:488–489.
64. Zachariae, R., and Bjerring, P. (1993). Increase and decrease of cutaneous reaction obtained by hypnotic suggestion during sensitization—studies on dinitrochlorobenzene (DNCB) and diphenylcyclopropenone (DCP). *Allergy* 48:6–11.
65. Zachariae, R., and Bjerring, P. (1990). The effect of hypnotically induced analgesia on flare reaction of cutaneous histamine prick test. *Arch. Dermatol. Res.* 282: 539–543.
66. Waxman, D. (1973). Behavior therapy of psoriasis—a hypnoanalytic and counter conditioning technique. *Postgrad. Med. J.* 49:591–585.
67. Hughes, H.H., England, R., and Goldsmith, D.A. (1981). Biofeedback and psychotherapeutic treatment of psoriasis: a brief report. *Psycho. Rep.* 48:99–102.
68. Basmajian, J.V. (Ed.) (1989). *Biofeedback. Principles and Practice for Clinicians*, 3rd ed. Williams & Wilkins, Baltimore, 1989.
69. Marcer, D. (1986). *Biofeedback and Related Therapies in Clinical Practice.* Aspen Publishers, Rockville, MD, 1986.
70. Horowitz, M.J. (1972) Visual imagery and cognitive organization. *Am. J. Psychiatry* 123:938–946.
71. Fitzgerald, M. (1983). Capsaicin and sensory neurons: a review. *Pain* 15:109–130.
72. Brenstein, J.E., Parish, L.C., Rappaport, M., et al. (1986). Effects of topically applied capsaicin on moderate and severe psoriasis vulgaris. *J. Am. Acad. Dermatol.* 15:504–507.
73. Xu, Xj, Hao, J.X., Wiesenfeld-Hallin, Z., et al. (1991). Spantide II, a novel tachykinin antagonist inhibits plasma extravasation induced by antidromic C-fiber stimulation in rat hind paw. *Neuroscience* 42:731–737.
74. Wiesenfeld-Hallin, Z., Xu, X.J., Hakanson, R., et al. (1990). The specific antagonistic effect of intrathecal spantide II on substance P stimulation-induced facilitation of the nociceptive flexor reflex in rat. *Brain Res.* 526:284–290.
75. Wallengren, J., and Moller, H. (1988). Some neuropeptides as modulators of experimental contact allergy. *Contact Derm.* 19:351–354.
76. Gozes, Y., Brenneman, D.E., Friedkin, M., et al. (1991). A VIP antagonist distinguishes spinal cord receptors on spinal cord cells and lymphocytes. *Brain Res.* 540:319–320.
77. Krumin, S.A., and Broomfield, C. (1992). Evidence of NK 1 and NK 2 tachykinin receptors and their involvement in histamine release in a murine mast cell line. *Neuropeptides* 21:65–72.
78. Ruff, M.R. (1989). Peptide T. *Drugs Future.* 14: 1049–1051.
79. Wetterberg, L., Alexius, B., Saaf, J., et al. (1987). Peptide T in treatment of AIDS. *Lancet* 1:159 (letter).
80. Marcusson, J.A., Lazega, D., Pert, C.B., et al. (1989). Peptide T and psoriasis. *Acta Derm. Venereol. (Stockh.)* 146:117–121.
81. Talme, T., and Lund-Rosell, B., Sundquist, K.G., et al. (1994). Peptide T: a new treatment for psoriasis? *Acta Derm. Venereol. (Stockh.)* (Suppl 186):76–78.
82. Farber, E.M., Cohen, E.N., Trozak, D.J., et al. (1991). Peptide T improves psoriasis when infused into lesions in nanogram amounts. *J. Am. Acad. Dermatol.* 25: 658–664.
83. Johansson, O., Hilliges, M., Talme, T., et al. (1994). Somatostatin immunoreactive cells in lesional psoriatic human skin during peptide T treatment. *Acta Derm. Venereol. (Stockh.)* 74:106–109.
84. Johansson, O., Hilliges, M., Talme, T., et al. (1993). Speculation around the mechanism behind the action of peptide T in the healing of psoriasis. *Acta Dermatol. Venereol. (Stockh.)* 73:401–403.

85. Camisa, C., O'Dorisio, T.M., Maceyko, R.F., et al. (1990). Treatment of psoriasis with chronic subcutaneous administration of somatostatin analog 201-295 (Sandostatin). An open-label pilot study. *Clev. Clin. J. Med.* 57:71–76.
86. Leeman, S.E., Krause, J.E., and Lembeck, F. (Eds.) (1991). Substance P and related peptides: cellular and molecular physiology. *Ann. N.Y. Acad. Sci.* 632:1–58, 263–271.
87. Wallengren, J. (1991). Substance P antagonist inhibits immediate and delayed type cutaneous hypersensitivity reactions. *Br. J. Dermatol.* 124:324–328.
88. Snider, R.M., Constantine, J.W., Lowe, J.A., et al. (1991). A potent nonpeptide antagonist of the substance P (NK1) receptor. *Science* 251(4992):435–437.
89. Lei, Y.H., Barnes, P.J., and Rogers, D.F. (1992). Inhibition of neurogenic plasma exudation in guinea-pig airways by CP-96,345, a new nonpeptide NK1 receptor antagonist. *Br. J. Pharmacol.* 105:261–262.
90. Radhakrishna, V., and Henry, J.L. (1991). Novel substance P antagonist, CP-96,345, blocks responses of cat spinal dorsal horn neurons to noxious cutaneous stimulation and substance P. *Neurosci. Lett.* 132: 39–43.
91. Erdos, E.G., and Skidgel, R.A. (1989). Neutral endopeptidase and related regulators of peptide hormones. FASEB J. 3:145–151.
92. Borson, D.B., and Gruenert, D.C. (1991). Glucocorticoids induce neutral endopeptidase in transformed human tracheal epithelial cells. *Am. J. Physiol.* 260: L83–L89.
93. Nadel, J.A. (1991). Neutral endopeptide modulates neurogenic inflammation. *Eur. Respir. J.* 4:745–754.

26

Neuropeptides and Psoriasis

Carlo Pincelli
University of Modena, Modena, Italy

Psoriasis is a skin disorder that can be provoked or exacerbated by both endogenous and exogenous factors. Among others, various forms of stress can influence its natural course. There is a large body of literature on this concept (1–3), although most reports of a psoriatic rash being triggered by emotional stress are based on anecdotal observations, which every physician has made in daily clinical practice. This has led many authors in recent years to erroneously think in terms of a direct connection between psyche and neural factor release in skin. Farber et al. have hypothesized that, during stress, descending autonomic nerves can trigger antidromic release of neuropeptides (NP) in the skin (4). Although intriguing, this idea is still vague and needs further investigation. So far, there are no studies demonstrating local release and alterations of NP in normal as well as pathological skin in response to stress in humans. In addition, we feel that the concept of "stress" as related to clinical conditions is undefined. At present, in our view, the clinical finding of certain dermatoses, and in particular psoriasis, being exacerbated by psychological factors cannot be satisfactorily explained with alterations of NP release in the skin. After these preliminary remarks, which are necessary to avoid possible misunderstanding by the reader, I would like to point out that this chapter will deal with the correlations among peripheral nerves, neural factors, and the mechanisms underlying the development of the psoriatic lesion.

NERVES, NEUROPEPTIDES, AND PSORIASIS

A role for peripheral nerves releasing NP in the etiopathogenesis of psoriasis was first proposed by Farber et al., who suggested that these substances, which mediate neurogenic inflammation, could be an important mechanism associated with the psoriatic lesion (5). NP are protein compounds contained in the central and peripheral nervous system. In skin, they can be antidromically released by sensory fibers and cause local inflammatory reactions (6). NP possess numerous functions within both the inflammatory and the immune system and exert trophic and growth stimulatory actions (7). There are pathogenetic mechanisms in psoriasis that suggest an influence of NP in this disease. Thus, for example, most NP exert major effects on blood vessels (8), which are characteristically altered in psoriasis (9). In this respect, it has recently been demonstrated by Doppler laser analysis that skin blood flow in psoriatic plaque is significantly higher than in normal skin. In addition, this study has shown that, after surface anesthesia, there is considerable reduction of blood perfusion in psoriatic plaque, suggesting that a local neurogenic mechanism contributes to the high blood flow in the psoriatic lesion (10). Furthermore, NP such as vasoactive intestinal peptide (VIP) and substance P (SP) degranulate mast cells (11), which have been shown to appear early in the development of psoriatic lesions (12). Naukkarinen et al. have shown that in psoriatic plaques, nerve–mast cell contacts are significantly increased as compared with nonlesional skin (13). Moreover, immunohistochemical studies have revealed that the activity of mast cell tryptase, an enzyme that degrades certain NP, is increased in psoriatic lesions (14). Keratinocyte hyperproliferation is the hallmark of psoriasis, and SP and VIP exert different effects on the proliferation of cultured human keratinocytes (15). VIP, and in particular the VIP carboxyterminal fragment, exerts mitogenic activity on keratinocytes in vitro (16), acting through a specific receptor (15). By contrast, SP not only fails to stimulate keratinocyte growth, but is also capable of inhibiting the VIP-induced keratinocyte proliferation (16). These different modulating effects of NP on human keratinocytes support the idea first proposed by Hanley that these substances may exert a tonic control over normal basal layer cell division and that in psoriasis there appears to be an alteration of such a regulation (17). Finally, several NP affect the function of various immunocompetent cells involved in the psoriatic lesion (18), such as lymphocytes, neutrophils, and mast cells.

There are clinical observations that support the idea of NP being involved in the mechanisms associated with psoriasis. For instance, the neurotoxin capsaicin, which is able to deplete sensory nerves from their NP content (19), can clear psoriatic lesions when applied topically (20). Interestingly, in a number of patients, psoriasis clears after surgical operations in that area of the skin or even when treated with dermabrasion (21,22). A "reverse Koebner phenomenon" has been used to describe the clearance of a psoriatic lesion that had been injured (23). It has been hypothesized that this phenomenon can be caused either by humoral factors or by destruction of cutaneous microvasculature (24). Farber et al. suggest that, alternatively, this phenomenon could be consistent with ablation of epidermal and superficial dermal nerves and, possibly, by consequent NP release (25).

Besides these clinical observations, histological and electron microscopic studies have shown an accelerated turnover of neural elements (26) and a more dense innervation in psoriatic lesions (27). Immunohistochemical studies have been numerous, although they have led to rather conflicting and disappointing results. No defined alterations of specific subsets of peptidergic fibers have been found (28–30). The increased number of SP-containing fibers first reported by Naukkarinen et al. (31) has never been confirmed by other authors (32,33). These discrepancies are not surprising. It should be considered that immunocytochemistry of nerve fibers needs a rigorous sampling and counting method, and that results can hardly be correlated to functional activity. Pincelli and coworkers have reported no differences in the distribution and expression of SP and VIP in psoriatic lesions, but, interestingly, they have shown that neutrophils from lesional psoriatic skin express both SP and VIP immunoreactivity (16). Strong evidence of the important role played by a mediator in a given tissue is the demonstration of the expression of its receptor. SP receptors have been detected in both normal and psoriatic skin, indicating the existence of SP cutaneous target structures (34).

The findings mentioned above strongly suggest a role for NP in the mechanisms associated with psoriatic lesions. To confirm this hypothesis, Pincelli et al. have directly measured SP and VIP levels in whole skin homogenates from psoriatic lesions using a radioimmunoassay technique. Radioimmunological evaluations on tissue specimens from lesional skin have resulted in more homogeneous results. VIP was found in significantly increased amounts in lesional psoriatic skin as compared to skin from healthy subjects, whereas SP concentrations were decreased in psoriatic skin as compared to controls (16). Although others have obtained conflicting results (35,36), a fourfold amount of capsaicin was needed to induce neurogenic inflammation in psoriatic as compared to control skin, possibly due to a lower content of SP in psoriatic nerve fibers (37). The imbalance of SP and VIP in psoriatic lesions does not appear to be specific, since similar data have been obtained in other inflammatory dermatoses, such as atopic dermatitis (38). A reduction in cutaneous SP levels has also been documented in the course of allergic contact dermatitis in mice (39), and other types of chronic peripheral inflammation, such as arthritis and inflammatory bowel disease, show similar NP alterations (40,41). Experimental evidence suggests these alterations are reactive phenomena of neurogenic origin. In fact, stereotyped changes in NP pattern in sensory ganglia and spinal cord similar to those found in inflammatory dermatoses (in particular, up-regulation of VIP and down-regulation of SP levels) can be evoked by peripheral nerve damage (42). Therefore, we hypothesize that cutaneous inflammation could represent a mechanism analogous to nerve injury, inducing changes in the neuronal NP content. It should be noticed that modifications of the NP content at the neuronal level may not parallel the peripheral changes in inflamed tissues, probably depending on an increased rate of peripheral release that reduces the nerve stores of NP (43). Furthermore, the imbalance of SP and VIP in psoriatic skin seems to parallel a similar alteration in the synthesis of these NP, which takes place in both dorsal root ganglia and spinal cord after peripheral nerve injury in rats (44). This finding may lead to the hypothesis that a similar imbalance in the synthesis of SP and VIP in the central nervous system may occur during peripheral inflammatory processes in the skin.

NERVE GROWTH FACTOR AND PSORIASIS

The mechanisms leading to biochemical alterations in the peptidergic neurons during peripheral inflammation remain largely speculative. It is known that a sustained electrical activity in afferent terminals is able to induce changes in the NP content of the corresponding neurons (45). Several inflammatory mediators, locally released in the course of inflammatory reactions, are able to sensitize (prostaglandins) and/or activate (potassium ions, ATP, histamine, bradykinin, serotonin) unmyelinated sensory terminals, inducing an increased neural discharge (46). Alternatively, a chemical mediation exerted by neurotrophic molecules released by peripheral tissues could be operating. Recent experimental evidence suggests a role for the neurotrophin nerve growth factor (NGF) in the neuropeptidergic alterations during peripheral inflammation. It is known that NGF exert a continuous control over NP synthesis in primary sensory neurons (47). NGF is produced in the skin by proliferating keratinocytes (48), and NGF receptors are present in cutaneous nerve terminals (49). It has been shown that in rat adjuvant arthritis NGF levels are rapidly increased in the nerves supplying the inflamed area, and that pretreatment with an anti-NGF serum prevents the NP changes (43). Moreover, local treatment with exogenous NGF induces changes in the neuronal NP content similar to those observed during the course of inflammatory dermatoses, i.e., decreased cutaneous SP levels (43). NGF is thought to be taken and retrogradely transported by receptor-bearing nerve terminals from inflamed tissues to the neuronal body (50), where it stimulates NP production. According to this hypothesis, NGF, locally produced in increased amounts during inflammation, would represent the chemical mediator of the NP changes.

CONCLUSION

In psoriasis, hyperproliferating keratinocytes could be responsible for the increased local NGF synthesis, which in turn could contribute to the maintenance of the psoriatic lesion through both the induction of NP synthesis and the stimulation of keratinocyte proliferation (48,51). In addition, both NGF (52–54) and NP (8,11,55) possess a number of proinflammatory activities that could be relevant in amplifying the pathogenetic events leading to the formation of the psoriatic lesion. Finally, of great interest is our recent observation of increased NGF levels in chronic plaques of psoriasis (56).

REFERENCES

1. Seville, R.H. (1989). Stress and psoriasis: the importance of insight and empathy in prognosis. *J. Am. Acad. Dermatol.* 20:97–100.
2. Farber, E.M. (1993). Psychoneuroimmunology and dermatology. *Int. J. Dermatol.* 32 (2):93–94.
3. Polenghi, M.M., Gala, C., Citeri, A., Manca, G., Guzzi, R., Barcella, M., and Finzi, A. (1989). Psychoneurophysiological implications in the pathogenesis and treatment of psoriasis. *Acta Derm. Vernereol.* 146(Suppl):84–86.
4. Farber, E.M., Rein, G., and Lanigan, S.W. (1991). Stress and psoriasis: psychoneuroimmunologic mechanisms. *Int. J. Dermatol.* 30:8–11.
5. Farber, E.M., Nicoloff, B.J., Recht, B., and Fraki, J.E. (1986). Stress, symmetry and psoriasis: possible role of neuropeptides. *J. Am. Acad. Dermatol.* 14:305–311.
6. Maggi, C.A., and Meli, A. (1988). The sensory-efferent function of capsaicin-sensitive sensory neurons. *Gen. Pharmacol.* 19:1–43.
7. Holzer, P. (1988). Local effector functions of capsaicin-sensitive sensory nerve endings: involvement of tachikinins, calcitonin gene-related peptide and other neuropeptides. *Neuroscience* 24:739–768.
8. Wallengren, J., and Hakanson, R. (1987). Effects of substance P, neurokinin A and calcitonin gene-related peptide in human skin and their involvement in sensory nerve-mediated responses. *Eur. J. Pharmacol.* 143: 267–273.
9. Pinkus, H., and Mehregan, A.H. (1966). The primary histologic lesion in seborrheic dermatitis and psoriasis. *J. Invest. Dermatol.* 46:109–116.
10. Krogstad, A.L., Swanbeck, G., and Wallin, B.G. (1995). Axon-reflex-mediated vasodilation in the psoriatic plaque? *J. Invest. Dermatol.* 104:872–876.
11. Piotrowsky, W., and Foreman, J.C. (1985). On the actions of substance P, somatostatin, and vasoactive in-

testinal polypeptide on rat peritoneal mast cells and in human skin. *Naunyn Schmiedeberg's Arch. Pharmacol.* 331:364–368.

12. Schuber, C. and Chrostopers, E. (1985). Mast cells and macrophages in early relapsing psoriasis. *Arch. Dermatol. Res.* 277:352–358.
13. Naukkarinen, A., Harvima, I., Paukkonen, K., Aalto, M.L., and Horsmanheimo, M. (1993). Immunohistochemical analysis of sensory nerves and neuropeptides, and their contacts with mast cells in developing and mature psoriatic lesions. *Arch. Dermatol. Res.* 285: 341–346.
14. Naukkarinen, A., Harvima, I., Aalto, M.L. and Horsmanheimo, M. (1994). Mast cell tryptase and chimase are potential regulators of neurogenic inflammation in psoriatic skin. *Int. J. Dermatol.* 33(5):361–366.
15. Haegerstrand, A., Jonzon, B., Dalsgaard, C.J., and Nilsson, J. (1989). Vasoactive intestinal polypeptide stimulates cell proliferation and adenylate cyclase activity of cultured human keratinocytes. *Proc. Natl. Acad. Sci. U.S.A.* 86:5993–5996.
16. Pincelli, C., Fantini, F., Romualdi, P., Sevignani, C., Lesa, G., Benassi, L., and Giannetti, A. (1992). Substance P is diminished and vasoactive intestinal peptide is augmented in psoriatic lesions and these peptides exert disparate effects on the proliferation of cultured human keratinocytes. *J. Invest. Dermatol.* 98:421–427.
17. Hanley, M.R. (1985). Neuropeptides as mitogens. *Nature* 315:14–15.
18. O' Dorisio, M.S. (1988). Neuropeptide modulation of the immune response in gut associated lymphoid tissue. *Int. J. Neurosci.* 38:189–198.
19. Buck, S.H., and Burks, T.F. (1983). Capsaicin: hot new pharmacological tool. *Trends Pharmacol. Sci.* 4:84–87.
20. Bernstein, J.E., Parish, L.C., Rapaport, M., Rosenbaum, M.M. and Roengigk, H.H. (1986). Effects of topically applied capsaicin on moderate and severe psoriasis vulgaris. *J. Am. Acad. Dermatol.* 15:504–507.
21. Farber, E.M., Lanigan, S.W., and Boer, J. (1990). The role of cutaneous sensory nerves in the maintenance of psoriasis. *Int. J. Dermatol.* 29:418–420.
22. Gold, M.H. and Roenigk, H.H. (1987). Surgical treatment of psoriasis: a review including a case of dermabrasion of hypertrophic psoriatic plaque. *J. Dermatol. Surg. Oncol.* 13:1326–1331.
23. Eyre, R.W., and Krueger, G.G. (1982). Response to injury of skin involved and uninvolved with psoriasis, and its relation to disease activity: Koebner and "reverse" Koebner reactions. *Br. J. Dermatol.* 106: 153–159.
24. Bekassy, Z., and Astedt, B. (1986). Carbon dioxide laser vaporization of plaque psoriasis. *Br. J. Dermatol.* 114:489–492.
25. Farber, E.M., Rein, G., and Lanigan, S.W. (1991). Stress and psoriasis. Psychoneuroimmunologic mechanisms. *Int. J. Dermatol.* 30:8–12, 1991.
26. Weddel, G., Cowan, M.A., Palmer, E., and Ramaswamy, S. (1965). Psoriatic skin. *Arch. Dermatol.* 91: 252–266.
27. Armagni, C., Di Francesco, C., and Schaltegger, H. (1979). Electron microscopy studies on dermal nerves in psoriasis. *Acta Derm. Venereol. (Stockh.)* (Suppl.) 87:68–70.
28. Wallengren, J., Ekman, R., and Möller, H. (1986). Substance P and vasoactive intestinal peptide in bullous and inflammatory skin disease. *Acta Derm. Venereol.* 66:23–28.
29. Pincelli, C., Fantini, F., Massimi, P., Girolomoni, G., Seidenari, S., and Giannetti, A. (1990). Neuropeptides in skin from patients with atopic dermatitis: an immunohistochemical study. *Br. J. Dermatol.* 122: 745–750.
30. Anand, P., Springall, D., Blank, M., Sellu, D., Polak, J., and Bloom, S. (1991). Neuropeptides in skin diseases: increased VIP in eczema and psoriasis but not axillary hyperhidrosis. *Br. J. Dermatol.* 124:547–549.
31. Naukkarinen, A., Nickoloff, B.J., and Farber, E.M. (1989). Quantification of cutaneous sensory nerves and their substance P content in psoriasis. *J. Invest. Dermatol.* 92:126–129.
32. Fantini, F., Pincelli, C., Massimi, P., and Giannetti, A. (1990). Neuropeptide-like immunoreactivity in skin lesions of atopic dermatitis and psoriasis. *Br. J. Dermatol.* 122:838–839.
33. Johansson, O., Olsson, A., Enhamre, A., Hammar, H., and Goldstein, M. (1987). Phenylethanolamine *N*-methyl-transferase-like immunoreactivity in psoriasis. An immunohistochemcial study on catecholamine synthesizing enzymes and neuropeptides of the skin. *Acta Derm. Venereol. (Stockh.)* 67:1–7.
34. Pincelli, C., Fantini, F., Giardino, L., Zanni, M., Calzá, L., and Giannetti, A. (1993). Autoradiographic detection of substance P receptors in normal and psoriatic skin. *J. Invest. Dermatol.* 101:301–304.
35. Eedy, D.J., Johnston, C.F., Shaw, C., and Buchanan, K.D. (1991). Neuropeptides in psoriasis: an immunocytochemical and radioimmunoassay study. *J. Invest. Dermatol.* 96:434–438.
36. Anand, P., Springall, D.R., Blank, M.A., Sellu, D., Polak, J.M., and Bloom, S.R. (1991). Neuropeptides in skin diseases: increased VIP in eczema and psoriasis but not axillary hyperhidrosis. *Br. J. Dermatol.* 124: 547–549.
37. Glinski, W., Glinska-Ferenz, M., and Pierozynska-Dubowska, M. (1991). Neurogenic inflammation induced by capsaicin in patients with psoriasis. *Acta Derm. Venereol. (Stockh.)* 71:51–54.
38. Giannetti, A., Gantini, F., Cimitan, A., and Pincelli, C. (1992). Vasoactive intestinal polypeptide and substance P in the pathogenesis of atopic dermatitis. *Acta Derm. Venereol. (Stockh.)* (Suppl.) 176:90–92.

39. Ek, L., and Theodorsson, E. (1990). Tachykinins and calcitonin gene-related peptide in oxazolone-induced allergic contact dermatitis in mice. *J. Invest. Dermatol.* 94:761–763.
40. Bishop, A., Polak, J., Bryant, M., Bloom, S., and Hamilton, S. (1980). Abnormalities of vasoactive intestinal polypeptide-containing nerves in Crohn's disease. *Gastroenterology* 79:853–860.
41. Hernanz, A., De Miguel, E., Romera, N., Perez-Ayala, C., Gijon, J., and Arnalich, F. (1993). Calcitonin gene-related peptide II, substance P and vasoactive intestinal peptide in plasma and synovial fluid from patients with inflammatory joint disease. *Br. J. Rhuematol.* 32: 31–35.
42. Villar, M., Cortes, R., Theodorsson, E., Wiesenfeld-Hallin, Z., Schalling, M., Fahrenkrug, J., Emson, P., and Hökfelt, T. (1989). Neuropeptide expression in rat dorsal root ganglion cells and spinal cord after peripheral nerve injury with special reference to galanin. *Neuroscience* 33:587–604.
43. Donnerer, J., Schuligoi, R., and Stein, C. (1992). Increased content and transport of substance P and calcitonin gene-related peptide in sensory nerves innervating inflamed tissue: evidence for a regulatory function of nerve growth factor *in vivo. Neuroscience* 49:693–698.
44. Nielsch, U., and Keen, P. (1989). Reciprocal regulation of tachykinin- and vasoactive intestinal peptide-gene expression in rat sensory neurons following cut and crush injury. *Brain Res.* 481:25–30.
45. Donaldson, L., McQueen, D., and Seckl, J. (1994). Local anaesthesia prevents acute inflammatory changes in neuropeptide messenger RNA expression in rat dorsal root ganglia neurons. *Neurosci. Lett.* 175:111-113.
46. Rang, H., Bevan, S., and Dray, A. (1991). Chemical activation of nociceptive peripheral neurons. *Br. Med. Bull.* 47:534–548.
47. Lindsay, R., and Harmar, A. (1989). Nerve growth factor regulates expression of neuropeptide genes in adult sensory neurons. *Nature* 337:362–364.
48. Pincelli, C., Sevignani, C., Manfredini, R., Grande, A., Fantin, F., Bracci-Laudiero, L., Aloe, L., Ferrari, S., Cossarizza, A., and Giannetti, A. (1994). Expression and function of nerve growth factor and nerve growth factor receptor on cultured keratinocytes. *J. Invest. Dermatol.* 103:13–18.
49. Fantini, F., and Johansson, O. (1992). Expression of growth-associated protein 43 and nerve growth factor receptor in human skin: a comparative immunohistochemical investigation. *J. Invest. Dermatol.* 99: 734–742.
50. Raivich, G., Hellweg, R., and Kreutzberg, G. (1991). NGF receptor-mediated reduction in axonal NGF uptake and retrograde transport following sciatic nerve injury and during regeneration. *Neuron* 7:151–164.
51. Di Marco, E., Mathor, M., Bondanza, S., Cutuli, N., Marchisio, P.C., Cancedda, R., and De Luca M. (1993). Nerve growth factor binds to normal human keratinocytes through high and low affinity receptors and stimulates their growth by a novel autocrine loop. *J. Biol. Chem.* 268:22838–22846.
52. Bischoff, S.C., and Dahinden, C.A. (1992). Effect of nerve growth factor on the release of inflammatory mediators by mature human basophils. *Blood* 79: 2662–2669.
53. Pearce, F.L., and Thompson, H.L. (1986). Some characterisitcs of histamine secretion from rat peritoneal mast cells stimulated with nerve growth factor. *J. Physiol.* 372:379–393.
54. Alehim, K., Andersson, C., Tingsborg, S., Ziolkowska, M., Schultzberg, M., and Bartfai, T. (1991). Interleukin 1 expression is inducible by nerve growth factor in PC12 pheochromocytoma cells. *Proc. Natl. Acad. Sci. U.S.A.* 88:9302–9306.
55. Smith, C., Barker, J., Morris, R., MacDonald, D., and Lee, T. (1993). Neuropeptides induce rapid expression of endothelial cell adhesion molecules and elicit granulocytic infiltration in human skin. *J. Immuol.* 151: 3274–3282.
56. Fantini, F., Magnoni, C., Bracci-Laudiero, L., and Pincelli, C. (1995). Nerve growth factor is increased in psoriatic skin. *J. Invest Dermatol.* 105:854–855.

27

Microcirculation

Irwin M. Braverman
Yale University School of Medicine, New Haven, Connecticut

The microcirculatory vessels in the horizontal plexus of the dermis and in the capillary loops are an integral component of the lesions in psoriasis vulgaris and pustular psoriasis of von Zumbusch. Two types of alterations have been found. The first is the ultrastructural configuration of the capillary loops in the dermal papillae of psoriatic plaques and how they respond sequentially during successful phototherapy. The second, a structural abnormality in the vessels themselves, is unaffected by phototherapy. Both types are discussed.

The major emphasis in psoriatic research has been on epidermal hyperplasia. Whether the accelerated epidermal cell turnover is a primary defect or a secondary response to an unidentified stimulus is unresolved. The possibility that a vascular defect plays a major role in the pathogenesis of psoriasis has been long debated. Morphological studies employing capillary microscopy and cleared whole mounts of skin support this notion with the following observations. The capillary loops in the dermal papillae of psoriatic lesions become dilated and tortuous, before epidermal hyperplasia has been detected morphologically (Telner and Fekete, 1961; Kulka, 1964). Abnormally dilated capillary loops have frequently been found in the normal-appearing skin of psoriatic patients (Kulka, 1964). Convoluted capillaries may persist for 1–9 months after the skin has returned to normal (Lawler and Vineyard, 1960; Gordon et al., 1967). Based upon light microscopic studies of developing psoriatic lesions, Pinkus and Mehregan (1966) concluded that initial vasodilatation accompanied by an exudate of inflammatory cells and serum in the papilla was the initiating event in psoriasis. Several investigators, who studied developing 1-mm psoriatic lesions, found an upward proliferation of the dermal papillae at the edges of psoriatic lesions. They believed this enlargement was one of the initiating events, although the stimulus was unknown (Van Scott and Ekel, 1963; Braun-Falco and Christophers, 1974).

In chronic psoriatic plaques, several studies have shown marked vascular and lymphatic dilatation, with a blood flow twice normal (Nyfors and Rothenberg, 1970; DiLorenzo et al., 1971; Braverman, 1972; Braverman and Yen, 1974). Endothelial cell gaps, present in the venous capillaries of the capillary loops and postcapillary venules of the superficial horizontal plexus (Braverman et al., 1972; Mottaz et al., 1973; Braverman, 1974) provide a morphological basis for the proposal that capillary loop dilatation with a presumed protein-rich exudate is responsible for initiating epidermal hyperplasia (Kulka, 1964; Pinkus and Mehregan, 1966).

Our previous studies on the normal dermal microcirculation (Yen and Braverman, 1976; Braverman and Yen, 1977) confirmed by others (Higgins and Eady, 1979), showed that it is possible to differentiate arterioles, arterial capillaries, venous capillaries, and postcapillary venules by their ultrastructural features. Reconstruction of the capillary loops within the dermal papillae of normal skin showed them to have the fine structure of arterial capillaries: homogeneous-appearing basement membrane material in the wall and an absence of bridged fenestrations in the endothelial layer. The efferent limb develops a multilayered basement membrane (venous capillary characteristic) after it has left the papilla on its way to its venous connection in the horizontal plexus of the papillary dermis (Fig. 1). In psoriasis, the capillary loops within the dermal papillae display the characteristics of venous capillaries: single or multilayered basement membrane material in the wall and the presence of bridged fenestrations of the endothelial cell layer. It is possible to describe each loop in a psoriatic lesion by the extent of its venous capillary component (Fig. 2) (Braverman and Yen, 1977). We noted that the venous capillary loops in psoriatic plaques were replaced by arterial capillaries after the skin had returned to normal following Goeckerman therapy, and that the capillary loops had begun to revert toward a normal pattern within 24–72 hr after the initiations of Goeckerman therapy; biopsy specimens were taken at 24-hr intervals for the first 96 hr only.

To extend these observations, we combined autoradiography, histological evaluation by light microscopy, and ultrastructural reconstruction of capillary loops in sequential biopsy specimens from psoriatic plaques over a longer period to determine whether the histological features of psoriasis and epidermal hyperplasia as measured by the basal cell labeling index precede or follow the return of venous capillary loops toward normal during Goeckerman and psoralen/ultraviolet A (PUVA) therapy. We studied the normal-appearing buttock skin of untreated psoriatic patients by this combined approach to relate the ultrastructural pattern of the capillary loops to the labeling index and the histological appearance of the epidermis. We applied these techniques to the acute lesions of pustular psoriasis of von Zumbusch to identify the segments of the microvasculature responsible for capillary elongation in the enlarging dermal papillae of developing psoriatic lesions (Braverman and Sibley, 1982).

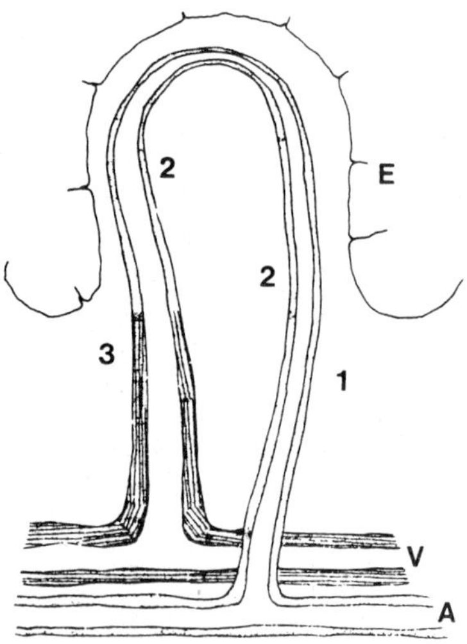

Figure 1 Anatomy of normal capillary loop. A, terminal arteriole; V, postcapillary venule in upper horizontal plexus; 1, extrapapillary ascending arterial limb; 2, intrapapillary loop; 3, extrapapillary descending venous limb; *stippled wall*, homogeneous basement membrane material; *striped wall*, multilaminated basement membrane material; E, epidermis. (From Braverman and Yen, 1977.)

The experimental design was as follows. Six patients treated by inpatient Goeckerman therapy with coal tar and UVB irradiation or photochemotherapy with 8-methoxypsoralen and UVA (PUVA) volunteered for these studies. In each patient, biopsy specimens were taken just inside the edge of a plaque the day before therapy was begun and, subsequently, at similar sites along the edge of the same plaque at intervals during therapy. The sampled plaques were on the buttock or trunk. In the Goeckerman-treated patients, specimens were obtained daily for the first 2 or 3 days and at intervals of 3–4 days thereafter. In the PUVA-treated patients, treated twice a week, biopsy specimens were obtained at 3- or 4-day intervals just before patients' next scheduled treatment. Three percent coal tar in Plastibase was the only topical treatment used in the Goeckerman-treated patients. No topical preparations were applied by the PUVA-treated patients to their plaques. These experiments continued for 6–29 days until the plaques almost disappeared or showed marked improvement characterized by flattening, loss of scale, and decreased erythema. Anesthesia using 1% lidocaine without epinephrine was injected as an intradermal ring around the site to be biopsied and the center was removed with a 3-mm skin trephine. The plaques selected for study were large enough that the subsequent areas to be biopsied were not infiltrated by the previous rings of anesthesia.

Each biopsy specimen was split in half. One piece was processed for electron microscopic examination by procedures described previously (Braverman and Yen, 1974). The ultrastructural patterns of four or five capillary loops were reconstructed by correlating 1-mm sections studied by light microscopy with the corresponding ultrathin sections used for electron microscopy. Our previous studies have shown that all the

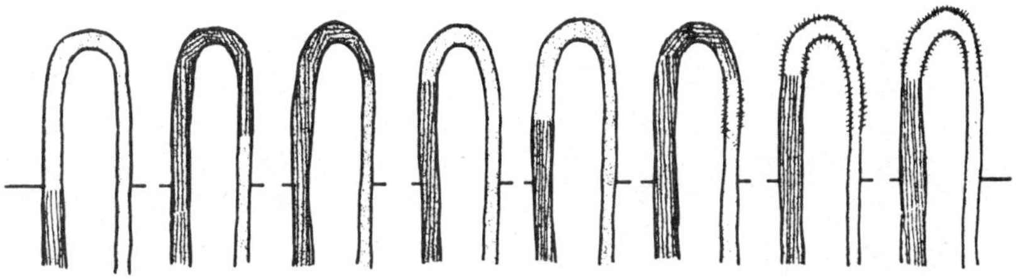

Figure 2 Capillary loop patterns in normal and psoriatic skin. NL, normal loop; 1–4c, psoriatic patterns; *horizontal line* delimits the intrapapillary portion from the extrapapillary portion of the loop; *striped areas*, venous ultrastructure; *stippled areas*, arterial ultrastructure; *clear area with slashes*, transitional zone vessel in which the basement membrane has both homogeneous and multilaminated features and bridged fenestrations and is probably equivalent to a venous capillary in physiological function. (From Braverman and Sibley, 1982.)

capillary loops in a given area of psoriasis (1–2 mm diameter) have the same ultrastructural characteristics. The other half of the specimen was processed for autoradiography by the in vitro technique of Lachapelle and Gillman (1969) to determine the labeling index of the basal (germinative) cell layers. Only the basal cells between appendages were scored. The labeling index (LI) was calculated as follows:

$$\mathrm{LI} = \frac{\text{Number of labeled basal cell nuclei}}{\text{Number of counted basal cell nuclei}} \times 100$$
$$= \begin{array}{l}\text{Mean percentage of labeled}\\ \quad\text{basal cells in epidermis}\end{array}$$

The LI for normal skin by the in vitro method ranges from 2 to 5% (Lachapelle, 1969; Lachapelle and Gillman, 1969). In our own controls, the LI of skin from the buttocks and forearms of six healthy adult men and women ranged from 2.4 to 3.9%.

The autoradiographs (see Figs. 1 and 2) were scored for the presence of histological abnormalities using the following notations. PS indicates the presence of parakeratosis, loss of the granular layer, acanthosis, and in most instances the presence of Munro's microabscesses. N1 indicates the presence of orthokeratosis and the presence of a granular layer. The epidermis was either slightly to moderately acanthotic or of normal thickness.

Biopsy specimens were obtained from normal-appearing buttock skin of eight men and three women being evaluated for PUVA or Goeckerman therapy. These individuals had been applying only lubricants to their skin for the preceding 2–3 weeks. The LI, capillary loops, and histological findings were evaluated in these biopsy sections.

We studied an early pustule and an erythematous macule in a man with pustular psoriasis (von Zumbusch) to determine the LI of the epidermal cells and the pattern of endothelial cell labeling in the microvasculature. Capillary loops were reconstructed from serial 5-μm autoradiographic sections to determine the localization pattern of endothelial cell labeling.

The results can be summarized as follows (Braverman and Sibley, 1982). In all instances, the return of the capillary loops toward normal proceeded in a uniform, orderly, and identical way. The arterial characteristics of the ascending limb increased progressively in length with a reciprocal decrease in the venous features of the rest of the loop. By the end of these studies, the intrapapillary portion of the capillary loop was almost completely arterial except for the short terminal segment of the intrapapillary descending limb which still showed venous characteristics. At no time did arterial features develop as isolated segments within the venous portions of the loops. In all six patients, only an occasional endothelial cell was labeled by autoradiography, even though the epidermis of these chronic psoriatic plaques was heavily labeled.

Figure 3 shows the correlation between LI, histological appearance of the biopsy, and ultrastructural configuration of the capillary loops. For the sake of conciseness, the data for days 3 and 7 in PUVA-1, day 4 in PUVA-2, and days 4 and 8 in UV-tar-1 have not been included. There were no signs of improvement in the LI or loop configurations at these times. In the successfully treated patients, the capillary loops began to return toward normal 3–8 days before the LI did. The histological features of psoriasis in the biopsy specimens began to show signs of improvement concomitant with the return of the capillary loops toward normal. The first change was a spotty and focal return of the granular cell layer with overlying orthokerato-

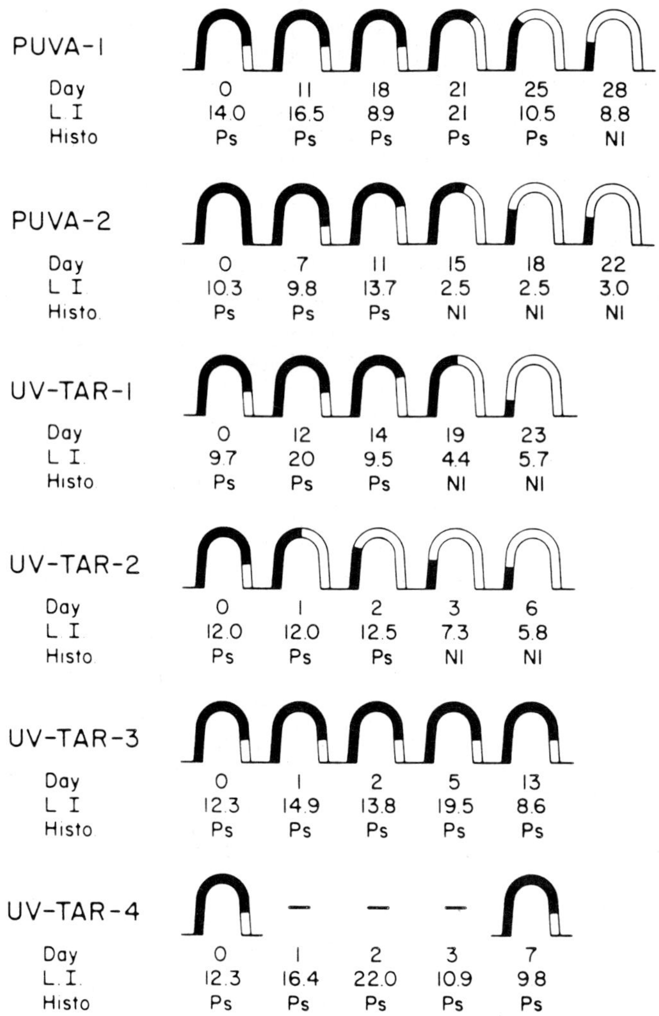

Figure 3 Correlation of capillary loop configuration, labeling index (LI), and histological findings in serial sections. Only the intrapapillary portions of the loops are shown. *Black area*, venous component; *clear area*, arterial component; *Ps*, psoriatic features present; *NL*, normal epidermis; LI expressed in percent; —, not determined. (From Braverman and Sibley, 1982.)

sis. Complete restoration of the granular layer with orthokeratosis in the entire biopsy specimen took 3–8 days. At this point (NL in Fig. 3), the epidermis was still slightly to moderately acanthotic. In patients UV-tar-3 and 4, none of the three parameters showed any change toward normal even though the plaque was thinner and less scaly when the experiment was ended.

In four of the six subjects, the LI in the serial biopsy specimens fluctuated over a twofold range in the early and midportions of the experiments.

In 11 patients with extensive psoriasis who had not yet begun treatment with either PUVA or Goeckerman therapy, the same three parameters were evaluated in biopsy specimens from their normal-appearing uninvolved buttock skin. Figure 4 shows these data. In six normal controls, the LI of buttock and flexor forearm skin ranged from 2.4 to 3.9%, and the capillary loops in the papillae were arterial in configuration. In five of the 11 psoriatic patients, the LI (1.8–3.4%) and capillary loops were normal. In six of the 11, the LI (5.1–8.6%) was abnormally elevated, but in only two of these individuals (LI 5.9 and 7.4%) did the capillary loops have venous features. The other four had arterial loops.

The histological appearance of the skin in both the controls and in eight of the 11 psoriatic patients was normal. In the two psoriatic patients who had both an elevated LI and venous capillary loops, the epidermis was normal except for a few small foci of basal cell hyperplasia. In both individuals, a granular cell layer and orthokeratosis were present. In one psoriatic patient with an elevated LI (7.3%) and arterial loops, the epidermis showed a few small foci of basal cell hyperplasia as the only histological abnormality. Thus,

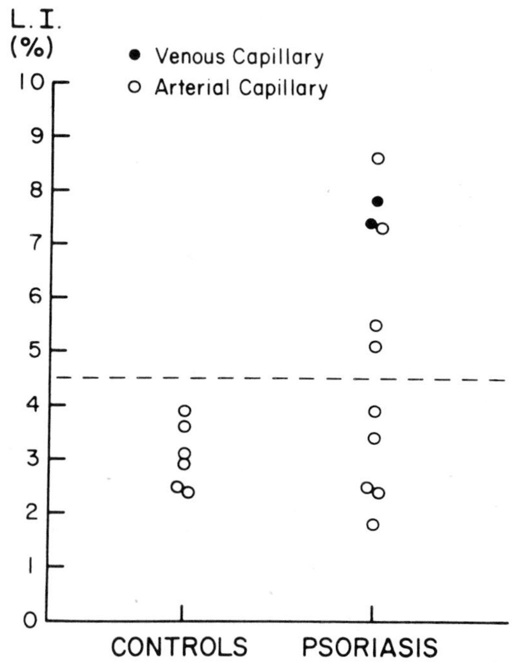

Figure 4 Correlation between labeling index and capillary loop configuration in normal-appearing buttock skin of 11 psoriatic patients and 6 controls. (From Braverman and Sibley, 1982.)

we found an elevated LI in association with normal capillary loops and normal epidermal histological findings in the clinically uninvolved buttock skin of three psoriatic patients. In a fourth psoriatic patient, a few foci of basal cell hyperplasia were present in association with an elevated LI and arterial loops.

In the pustular and macular lesions of von Zumbusch disease, there was extensive labeling of the endothelial cells by tritiated thymidine in the superficial horizontal plexus and the vessels passing from the dermal papillae to this layer. Three well-labeled capillary loops were reconstructed in three dimensions from the 5-μm autoradiographic sections. Identical findings were present in all three loops. The labeled or dividing endothelial cells (asterisks) were limited to the extrapapillary portion of the descending venous limb of the capillary loop (Fig. 5) and to the vessels in the superficial horizontal plexus (not shown). Labeled endothelial cells were never found in the intrapapillary portion of the loop.

From these observations we have drawn the following conclusions. The infrequent labeling of endothelial cells in the psoriatic plaques probably reflects the chronicity and stability of such lesions. In contrast, the pustules and red macules of von Zumbusch disease which are active and rapidly evolving lesions, displayed marked vascular labeling. de la Brassinne and Lachapelle (1977) reported that labeling of endothelial cells by tritiated thymidine can be seen in all forms of psoriasis (vulgaris, erythroderma, and von Zumbusch disease), but they did not state whether the extent of labeling differed among these three varieties.

Based upon the pattern by which the loops in psoriasis vulgaris return to normal, and the pattern of vascular labeling in von Zumbusch disease, the mechanism illustrated in Figure 6 is offered as an explanation of the process of elongation of the capillary loops in psoriasis. The endothelial cells in the extrapapillary portion of the venous divide to supply the cells required for the lengthening of the loop within the enlarging dermal papilla. Since the venous limb is the source of the endothelial cells, the intrapapillary venous limb enlarges and the arterial limb becomes proportionally shorter. Eventually, almost the entire intrapapillary loop has the ultrastructural features of a venous capillary. The white dots indicate the region of the bridged fenestrations. Successful antipsoriatic therapy is associated with a decrease in the volume of the dermal papillae and a concomitant shortening of the capillary loops. As the extraendothelial cells in the venous limb are resorbed, the venous limb shortens and the arterial limb becomes proportionally longer. The bridged fenestrations decrease in number until they are no longer present in the normal arterial loop. We never observed necrosis of endothelial cells in the intrapapillary loops or a spotty return to normal within these loops. The loss of endothelial cells could occur from the segment that was the site of proliferation, or from the intrapapillary portion. However, it seems more likely that the segment responsible for hyperplasia would also be the site from

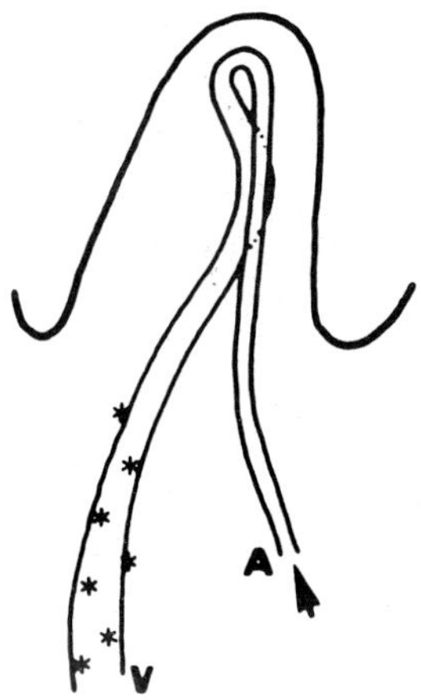

Figure 5 Reconstruction of loop showing arterial limb (A), direction of flow (arrow), and localization of labeled endothelial cells (asterisks) to extrapapillary portion of descending venous limb (V). (From Braverman and Sibley, 1982.)

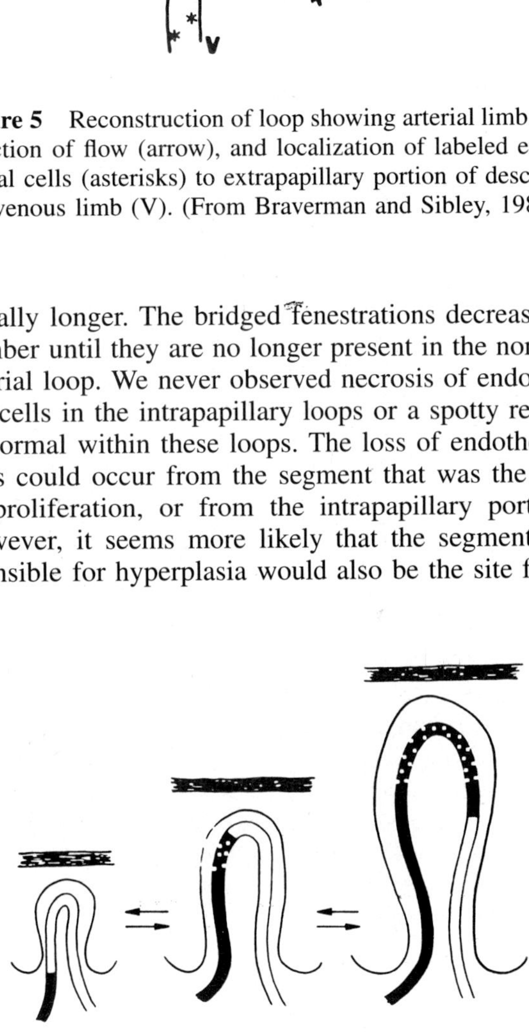

Figure 6 Proposed mechanism for shortening and elongation of capillary loops in psoriasis: (a) normal loop; (b) partial elongation or shortening depending upon direction; (c) maximal elongation. *White dots* indicate area of bridged fenestrations; *black zone*, venous component; *clear zone*, arterial component. (From Braverman and Sibley, 1982.)

which endothelial cells would be lost. An analogous phenomenon develops in the microvasculature of rat skin during the hair growth cycle (Sholley and Cotran, 1976). The capillary network around actively growing follicles increases in size by endothelial cell proliferation. Virtually all the endothelial cells are supplied by the capillaries. (In human skin, both glabrous [Braverman, I.M., unpublished data] and scalp [McLeod, 1970], the capillary network around the hair follicles has a venous ultrastructure: bridged fenestrations and a laminated basement membrane.) When the rat hair follicle enters catagen, the vascular network is greatly reduced in size, partly through loss and partly through collapse.

Morphologically, the return of the capillary loops toward normal preceded improvement in the LI by 3–8 days. In two patients, there was neither significant healing of the plaques nor improvement in the three parameters during the experimental period. Of the four patients who did show improvement, three still had an elevated LI (8.8, 5.8, and 5.7%) even though the loops had returned almost to normal and the histological features of psoriasis were no longer present. Similarly, the studies of normal-appearing buttock skin in psoriatic patients showed that an elevated LI may exist in the presence of both normal epidermal histological characteristics and a normal capillary loop configuration. In one of these subjects, an elevated LI was associated with normal arterial loops and a few foci of basal cell hyperplasia in an otherwise histologically normal epidermis.

These two complementary studies support the concept that the initial stimulus for epidermal hyperplasia in psoriasis resides in the epidermis and not in the microvasculature. We never observed venous capillaries in the papillae of clinically uninvolved psoriatic skin that had a normal LI and was also histologically normal. These studies do not support previous proposals that epidermal hyperplasia may be initiated by a protein-rich exudate in underlying papillae resulting from venous capillaries made more permeable by endothelial cell gaps and bridged fenestrations (Kulka, 1964; Pinkus and Mehregan, 1966).

Instead, our studies suggest that the microvasculature plays a modulating role in psoriasis. Morphologically, the response to PUVA and Goeckerman therapies appears to be mediated through the microvasculature rather than through any observable antiproliferative effect on the basal cells. In the normal-appearing buttock skin of psoriatic patients, the combination of normal capillary loops was a histologically normal epidermis that has an elevated LI suggests a possible inhibition of endothelial cell proliferation. Such inhibition would prevent basal cells from multiplying to produce a psoriatic lesion by failing to generate an adequate blood supply.

PUVA and Goeckerman therapies are believed to produce beneficial effects in psoriasis through mechanisms related to phototoxicity, but which have never been clearly defined. Although the inhibition of deoxyribonucleic acid (DNA) synthesis in epidermal cells has been shown to occur in vivo following phototherapy (Walter et al., 1973, 1978), this may not be the major or only mechanism by which these modalities are effective. In our studies, psoriasis began to improve before the LI showed a return toward normal as measured by autoradiographic techniques. Concomitant with the return of the capillary loops toward normal and before the LI began to decrease, the granular layer began to reform in a spotty fashion. Fry and McMinn (1968) made the same observation in their studies, in which serial biopsy specimens were taken from psoriatic plaques treated topically with coal tar coupled with UVB. The earliest morphological change was a return of the granular layer before the elevated mitotic count showed a significant fall. Goldberg et al. (1980) made similar observations in their study of the mitotic index in psoriatic plaques treated by PUVA therapy. The vessels were not studied in these two experiments. Since both UVA and UVB penetrate the dermis to the level of the capillary loops, UV irradiation may be exerting its beneficial effects by inducing endothelial cells in the venous limbs to be resorbed, thereby shortening the loops. In effect, this would increase the length of the arterial limbs which lack the bridged fenestrations believed to represent the large-pore system of the capillaries responsible for facilitating the transport of nutrients (Simionescu et al., 1972). Such a change in the morphology of the capillary loop would result in less nutrient support for the continuing epidermal hyperplasia, and the epidermal proliferation might thus be damped by a restriction of its energy sources. The mechanism by which UV irradiation exerts these effects is unknown. Both PUVA and Goeckerman therapy require an average of 23 treatments to produce healing of psoriasis. The number of UV interactions with the skin, not the total duration of therapy, appears to be the significant feature of these two forms of phototherapy.

An alternative hypothesis for the beneficial effects of UV irradiation is that it produces an epidermal signal that causes the microvasculature to regress, which in turn results in normalization of the epidermis. Our data do not exclude such a possibility.

The microvasculature has been implicated in the pathogenesis of psoriasis by previous studies employing light and capillary microscopy in which the capillary loops remained dilated for months after the skin lesions had healed (Lawler and Vineyard, 1960; Gordon et al., 1967). Our electron microscopy studies of healed lesions indicate that although dilatation is present, the loops are arterial rather than venous (Braverman and Yen, 1977). A relationship between the persistent vasodilatation and possible inhibitory processes on the microvasculature remains to be determined.

The epidermis and microvasculature act as a unit once the epidermal hyperplasia of psoriasis begins. Understanding the factors responsible for the shortening of the capillary loops that leads to epidermal normalization and for the inhibition of capillary growth in the presence of an increased LI could lead to other methods of controlling psoriasis.

A second vascular abnormality exists in psoriasis. Endothelial cell gaps are present in the postcapillary venules of the upper horizontal plexus and less frequently in the venous capillaries of the dermal papillae in psoriatic lesions. They were also found, but less often, in the normal-appearing skin of patients with psoriasis. We have not observed them in normal skin or in other inflammatory skin diseases we have studied.

The endothelial cell gaps ranged from 0.03 to 1.9 μm in width and had a characteristic appearance (Fig. 7). One edge of the gap usually had a fragment of one or more endothelial cells still attached to each other by intercellular junctions. These endothelial cell gaps were found in the absence of inflammatory cells. Their prevalence did not appear to change following complete clearing of psoriatic plaques after Goeckerman therapy. Mottaz et al. (1973) have confirmed the presence of these gaps and found that they were still present after topical corticosteroid therapy.

These endothelial cell gaps are identical to the gaps produced in postcapillary venules of animals by local injection of histamine in human skin (Majno et al., 1969). Two possible explanations for the gaps in psoriasis include an inherent weakness of the intercellular junctions of the endothelial cells and a histaminelike response of endothelial cells to as yet unidentified stimuli. The former hypothesis suggests that the gaps may be useful as genetic markers for latent psoriasis in as yet unaffected patients. The latter hypothesis suggests that low-grade inflammatory mechanisms may be constantly present in psoriatic skin.

A role for the endothelial cell gaps in the pathogenesis of psoriasis has not yet been found. However these gaps may be responsible in part for the known increased transcapillary loss of albumin and other plasma proteins in extensive psoriasis (Worm, 1981). These physiological studies are supported by morphological studies which have demonstrated abundant dilated lymphatics, some of which contain erythrocytes, in lesional and normal-appearing psoriatic skin (Braverman, 1972; Braverman and Yen, 1974).

Precise ultrastructural criteria are now available for delineating the different segments of the microcirculatory bed (Yen and Braverman, 1976; Braverman and Yen, 1977b). By studying the ultrastructural characteristics and sequential changes of the capillary loops in the advancing edges of psoriatic plaques, in the Koebner phenomenon, and in trials with different therapeutic modalities it should be possible to further our understanding of the role of the microcirculation in the pathogenesis of psoriasis. The accumulated evidence suggests that the vasculature is a modulator rather than an initiator of the psoriatic process, but therapy directed against its role as a modulator may provide an additional approach to treatment.

The recent advances in angiogenesis research allow one to consider several molecules as potential angiogenic factors responsible for the elongation and shrinkage of the dermal capillary loops during exacerbation and resolution respectively of the disease process. Classic angiogenesis in wound healing and tumor growth involves three phases: sprouting of endothelial cells, locomotion of endothelial cells to form solid sprouts that undergo lumen formation, and proliferation of endothelial cells to produce vessel elongation. In these situations many vessels are produced, but they grow in a random pattern (Folkman and Klagsbrun, 1987). In psoriasis, however, angiogenesis takes a different form. The capillary loop elongates in association with epidermal hyperplasia during disease activity and shortens with loss of endothelial cells during disease remission. The endothelial cells in the venous limb of the capillary loop are the cells responsible for this elongation and subsequent dropout (Braverman and Sibley, 1982). Therefore, in psoriasis one needs to look for factors that will not only induce a directed capillary loop elongation by endothelial cell proliferation and will also cause a directed capillary loop shortening by endothelial cell reabsorption.

Wolf and Harrison (1973) have shown that psoriatic epidermis contains a potent angiogenic factor, as measured by the hamster cheek pouch assay, which was

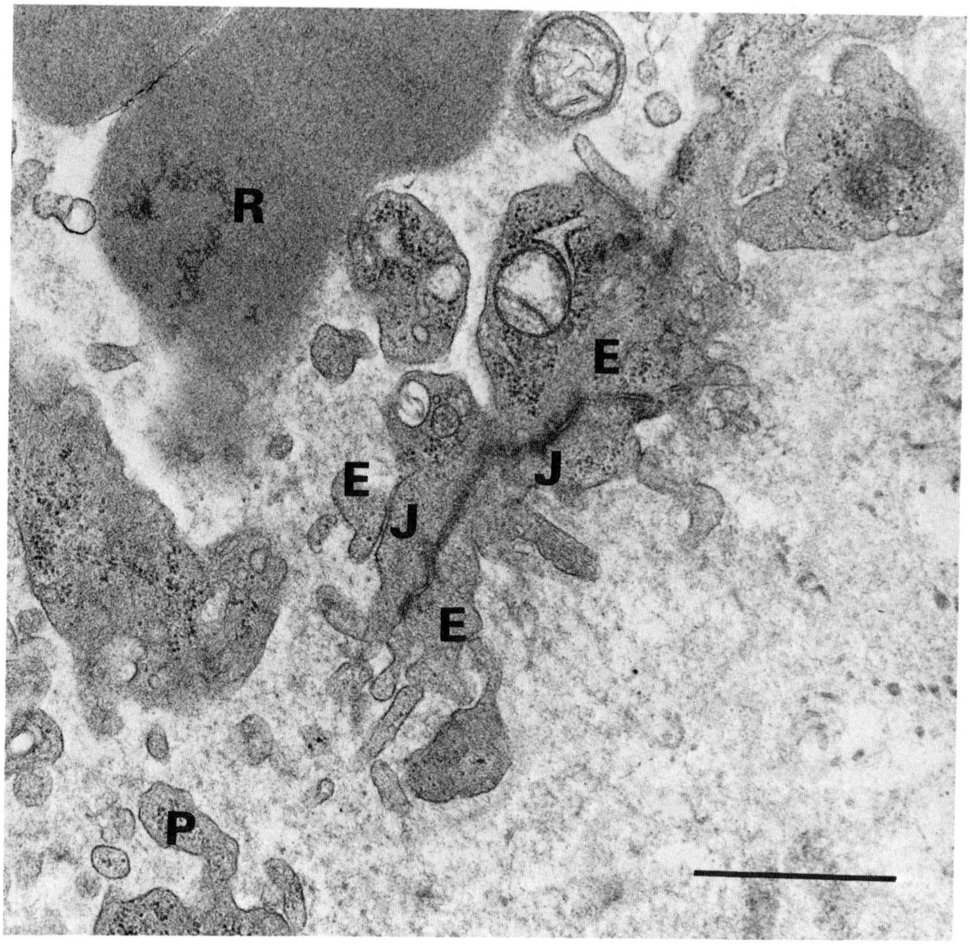

Figure 7 Endothelial gap in postcapillary venule of psoriatic lesion. One lip has portions of at least three endothelial cells (E) attached by intercellular junctions (J). R, erythrocyte; P, pericyte; bar, 1 μm (×27,160). (From Braverman and Yen, 1974.)

stable at 4°C and was heat labile. The activity from psoriatic skin was greater than that from treated psoriatic skin, the normal skin of psoriatics and normal patients, but was not as potent as that derived from tumors. Malhotra et al. (1989) showed that the epidermis from psoriatic lesions, the normal-appearing skin of psoriatics, and normal skin, but not the dermis, contains a potent angiogenic factor when tested in the rabbit corneal pocket assay. The factor in this latter study was stable to both heat (100°C) and freezing (−75°C), suggesting that most likely there is more than one angiogenic factor present in epidermis.

Currently, there are two angiogenic molecules produced in epidermis that directly cause endothelial cells to proliferate: basic fibroblast growth factor and transforming growth factor α (TGF-α) (Kupper, 1988). Elder et al. (1989) have demonstrated that TGF-α is overexpressed in psoriatic epidermis compared to both the clinically normal-appearing epidermis of psoriatics and normal epidermis. Which of these components or other as yet to be discovered factors potentially plays a central role in the angiogenesis of psoriasis awaits further experiments.

ACKNOWLEDGMENT

This work was supported by NIH Grant AM 15739.

REFERENCES

Braun-Falco, O., and Christophers, E. (1974). Structural aspects of initial psoriatic lesions. *Arch. Dermatol Forsch.* 251:95–110.

Braverman, I.M. (1972). Electron microscopic studies of the microcirculation in psoriasis. *J. Invest. Dermatol.* 59: 91–98.

Braverman, I.M., Cohen, I., and O'Keefe, E. (1972). Metabolic and ultrastructural studies in a patient with pustular psoriasis (von Zumbusch). *Arch. Dermatol.* 105:189–196.

Braverman, I.M., and Sibley, J. (1982). Role of the microcirculation in the treatment and pathogenesis of psoriasis. *J. Invest. Dermatol.* 78:12–17.

Braverman, I.M., and Yen, A. (1974). Microcirculation in psoriatic skin. *J. Invest. Dermatol.* 62:493–502.

Braverman, I.M., and Yen, A. (1977a). Ultrastructural study of the capillary loops in the dermal papillae of psoriasis. *J. Invest. Dermatol.* 68:53–60.

Braverman, I.M., and Yen, A. (1977b). Ultrastructural study of the human dermal microcirculation. II. The capillary loops of the dermal papillae. *J. Invest. Dermatol.* 68: 44–52.

de la Brassinne, M., and Lachapelle, J.M. (1977). Epidermal and dermal cell renewal in pustular psoriatic erythroderma. In *Psoriasis, Proceedings of the 2nd International Symposium.* E.M. Farber and A.J. Cox (Eds.). Yorke Medical Books, New York, pp. 368–370.

DiLorenzo, P.A., Brown, D.M., Walker, S.H., Deern, P.L., and Goltz, R.W. (1971). Technetium 99m pertechnetate disappearance studies in normal and psoriatic skin. *J. Invest. Dermatol.* 56:39–43.

Elder, J.T., Fisher, G.J., Lindquist, P.B., Bennett, G.L., Pittelkow, M.R., Coffey, R.J., Jr., Ellingsworth, L., Derynck, R., and Voorhees, J.J. (1989). Overexpression of transforming growth factor alpha in psoriatic epidermis. *Science* 243:811–814.

Folkman, J., and Klagsburn, M. (1987). Angiogenic factors. *Science* 235:442–447.

Fry, L., and McMinn, R.M.H. (1968). The action of chemotherapeutic agents on psoriatic epidermis. *Br. J. Dermatol.* 80;373–383.

Goldberg, L.H., Cox, A.J., and Abel, E.A. (1980). The mitotic index in psoriatic plaques and their response to PUVA therapy. *Br. J. Dermatol.* 102:401–405.

Gordon, M., Johnson, W.C., and Burgoon, C.F., Jr. (1967). Histopathology and histochemistry of psoriasis. II. Dynamics of lesion during treatment. *Arch. Pathol.* 84: 443–450.

Higgins, J.C., and Eady, R.A.J. (1981). Human dermal microvasculature: a morphological and enzyme histochemical investigation at the light and electron microscope levels. *Br. J. Dermatol.* 104:117–129.

Kulka, J.P. (1964). Microcirculatory impairments as a factor in inflammatory tissue damage. *Ann. N.Y. Acad. Sci.* 116: 1018–1044.

Kupper, T.S. (1988). Interleukin-1 and other human keratinocyte cytokines: molecular and functional characterization. *Adv. Dermatol.* 3:293–308.

Lachapelle, J.M. (1969). Isotopic labelling of cutaneous structures. *Br. J. Dermatol.* 81:299–305.

Lachapelle, J.M., and Gillman, T. (1969). Tritiated thymidine labelling of normal human epidermal cell nuclei. *Br. J. Dermatol.* 81:603–616.

Lawler, J.C., and Vineyard, W.R. (1960). The effect of treatment on the vascular component of the psoriatic lesion. *Arch. Dermatol.* 82:190–193.

Majno, G., Shea, S.M., and Leventhal, M. (1969). Endothelial contraction induced by histamine-type mediators. *J. Cell Biol.* 42:647–672.

Malhotra, R., Stenn, K.S., Fernandez, L.A., and Braverman, I.M. (1989). *Lab. Invest.* 61:162–165.

McLeod, W.A. (1970). Observations of fenestrated capillaries in the human scalp. *J. Invest. Dermatol.* 55:354–357.

Mottaz, J., Zelickson, A.S., Thorne, E.G., and Wachs, G. (1973). Blood vessel changes in psoriatic skin. *Acta Derm. Venereol. (Stockh.)* 53:195–198.

Nyfors, A., and Rothenborg, H.W. (1970). Cutaneous blood flow in psoriasis measured by ^{133}Xenon clearance. *J. Invest. Dermatol.* 54:381–385.

Pinkus, H., and Mehregan, A.H. (1966). The primary histologic lesion of seborrheic dermatitis and psoriasis. *J. Invest. Dermatol.* 46:109–116.

Simionescu, N., Simionescu, M., and Palade, G.E. (1972). Permeability of intestinal capillaries. Pathway followed by dextrous and glycogens. *J. Cell Biol.* 53:365–392.

Sholley, M.M., and Cotran, R.S. (1976). Endothelial DNA synthesis in the microvasculature of rat skin during the hair growth cycle. *Am. J. Anat.* 147:243–254.

Telner, P., and Fekete, Z. (1961). The capillary responses in psoriatic skin. *J. Invest. Dermatol.* 36:225–230.

Van Scott, E.F., and Ekel, T.M. (1963). Kinetics of hyperplasia in psoriasis. *Arch. Dermatol.* 88:373–381.

Walter, J.F., Voorhees, J.J., Kelsey, W.H., and Duell, E.A. (1973). Psoralen plus black light inhibits epidermal DNA synthesis. *Arch. Dermatol.* 107:861–865.

Walter, J.F., Stoughton, R.B., and DeQuoy, P.R. (1978). Suppression of epidermal proliferation by ultraviolet light, coal tar and anthralin. *Br. J. Dermatol.* 99:89–96.

Wolf, J.E., Jr., and Harrison, R.G. (1973). Demonstration and characterization of an epidermal angiogenic factor. *J. Invest. Dermatol.* 59:40–43.

Worm, A.-M. (1981). Exchange of macromolecules between plasma and skin interstitium in extensive skin disease. *J. Invest. Dermatol.* 76:489–492.

Yen, A., and Braverman, I.M. (1976). Ultrastructure of the human dermal microcirculation: the horizontal plexus of the papillary dermis. *J. Invest. Dermatol.* 66:131–142.

28

Histopathology and Electron Microscopy of Psoriasis

Sven Krengel, Christoph C. Geilen, and Constantin E. Orfanos
Free University, Berlin, Germany

Gundula M. Schaumburg-Lever
Eberhard Karls University, Tübingen, Germany

HISTOPATHOLOGICAL CHANGES

The histological picture of psoriasis varies considerably depending on the stage and the clinical characteristics of each lesion. The sequence of events in acute eruptive guttate psoriasis has been studied (1) in *early pinpoint lesions*, consisting of a 1-mm macule or smooth-surfaced papule, and (2) in *fully developed guttate lesions*. There are further differences to the histopathological changes characteristic for (3) *chronic psoriatic plaques* and (4) *pustular lesions* as seen in pustular types of psoriasis, respectively.

Early Smooth-Surfaced Papules

In very early psoriatic lesions the histological picture is not diagnostic. Epidermal changes may include a bandlike epidermal hyperplasia and small foci of parakeratosis with absence of the granular layer (1,2). In the stratum basale and stratum spinosum there are areas of focal spongiosis, with dilatation of the intercellular spaces between the keratinocytes, especially at sites of some initial invasion of mononuclear cells. The epidermal cells show an increase in volume with enlarged nuclei and nucleoli (1). The presence of increased numbers of HLA-DR+/CD1a- dendritic cells and neighboring HLA-DR+ T-helper lymphocytes has been demonstrated in the basal epidermal layer of such lesions, whereas the number of HLA-DR+/CD1a+ Langerhans cells is slightly decreased (3–5). A few polymorphonuclear leukocytes (PMNL) may be found at all levels of the psoriatic epidermis (2).

At this early stage, dermal changes are often more pronounced than epidermal alterations. The dermal papillae regularly show capillary dilatation and also edema to a certain degree (6). An inflammatory infiltrate consisting of lymphocytes and macrophages is seen in the upper dermis and is most pronounced in the center of initial psoriatic lesions, sometimes involving only two or three papillae (1,2,7). There are a few reports describing a significant role of PMNL in the early dermal infiltrate of psoriatic lesions (8,9).

The light microscopic examination of clinically uninvolved skin of patients with eruptive psoriasis has revealed an increase in the number of both T-helper and T-suppressor lymphocytes in the dermis (3) and punctiform spongiotic areas in the overlying epidermis (2). Vascular changes have been observed at this stage by electron microscopy and will be discussed below. Further changes in clinically uninvolved psoriatic skin include marked increase of the expression of $\alpha 1\beta 5$-integrin (fibronectin-receptor) on keratinocytes (10), cytoplasmic retinoic acid–binding protein type 2 (11), and up-regulation of HLA-DR on endothelial cells and in mononuclear infiltrates (12).

Fully Developed Guttate Lesions

In fully developed guttate lesions the epidermal and dermal changes are usually sufficiently pronounced to make it possible to recognize the typical features of psoriasis and make the diagnosis. In the granular layer, the keratinocytes become vacuolated and finally disappear, resulting in areas of agranulosis with overlying parakeratosis (13). Also, the phenomenon of "squirting papillae" becomes visible (14): PMNL are discharged intermittently from dilated papillary capillaries and migrate into the epidermis to the areas of parakeratosis. These areas then move together with the migrating PMNL into the stratum corneum. Since the areas of parakeratosis may be formed at different times, they appear scattered through an otherwise orthokeratotic stratum corneum as parakeratotic mounds (Fig. 1), containing some degenerated PMNL (15). These areas obviously represent the earliest manifestation of Munro microabscesses (6). In some cases, marked exudation of PMNL occurs into the epidermis, where the cells aggregate in the upper portion of the stratum spinosum to form the small spongiform pustules described by Kogoj (Fig. 2).

An increase in the number of HLA-DR+ T-suppressor lymphocytes has been observed in the upper epidermis (3) and has been interpreted as a feature of initial resolution of eruptive guttate lesions. The epidermal changes are initially restricted to microscopic focal areas, but later they become confluent, thus leading to the formation of clinically visible lesions.

Psoriatic Plaques of Vulgar Psoriasis

In fully developed psoriatic plaques, as best seen at the marginal areas of enlarging lesions, the histological picture is characterized by: (1) regular elongation of the rete ridges with thickening in their lower portions; (2) elongation and edema of the dermal papillae; (3) thinning of the suprapapillary portions of the malpighian layer; (4) absence of a granular layer; (5) parakeratosis and, finally, (6) the presence of microabscesses here and there (13).

The rete ridges are elongated and extend downward to a uniform level, resulting in regular acanthosis (13) (Fig. 3). They are usually club-shaped: slender in the upper portion but thickened in the lower portion. At

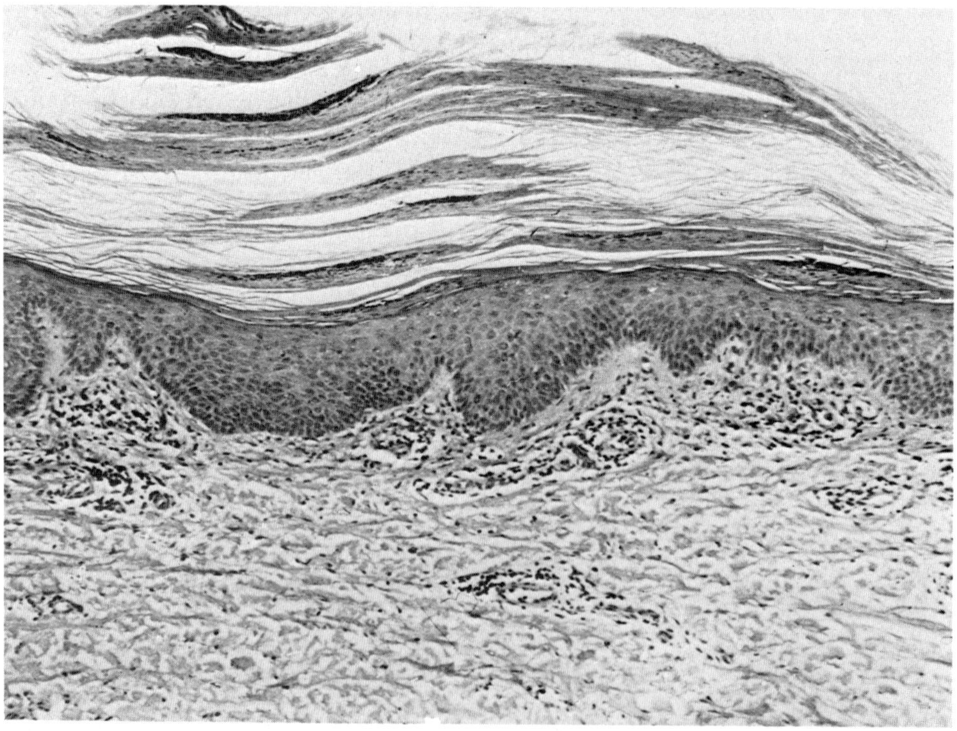

Figure 1 Earliest diagnostic lesion: scattered parakeratotic mounds within an orthokeratotic stratum corneum (×50).

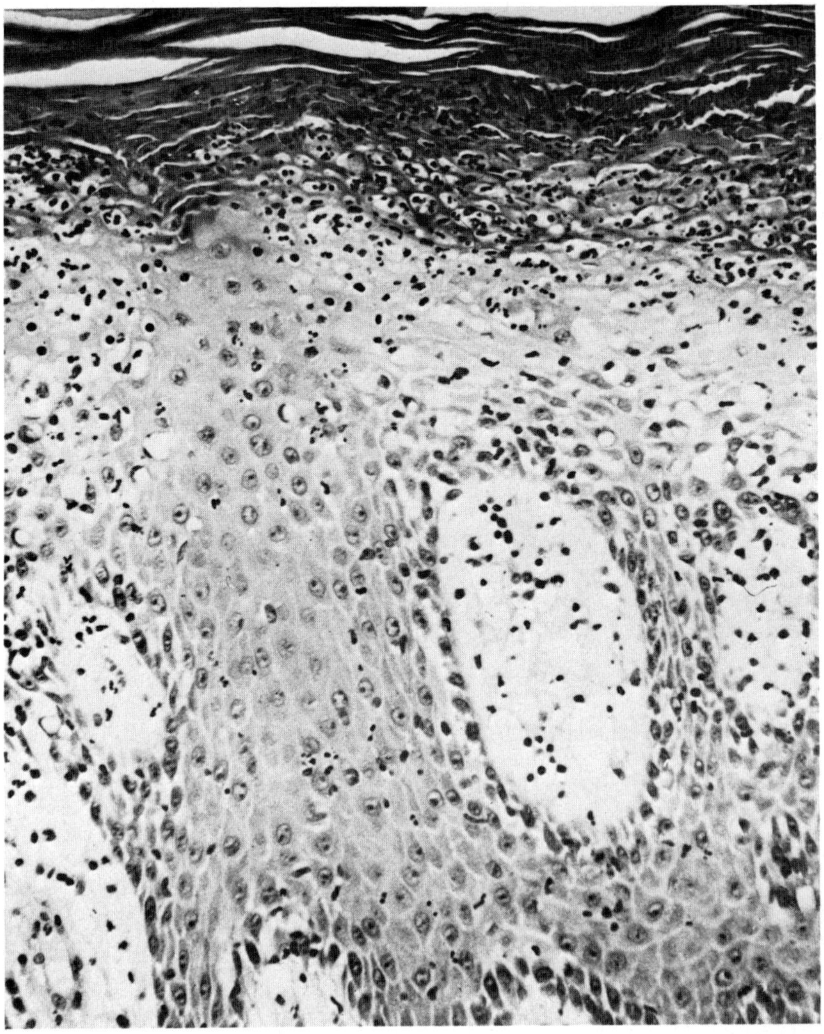

Figure 2 In the uppermost stratum malpighii, small aggregates of neutrophils result in spongiform pustules of Kogoj, which are highly diagnostic for psoriasis (×125).

times, neighboring rete ridges coalesce at their bases. There is an increase in the number of mitoses (15), not limited to the basal layer as in normal skin, but also extending to two rows of the cells above.

The papillae, in accordance with the elongation and basal thickening of the rete ridges, are elongated and club-shaped (13). The capillaries are dilated and tortuous (15). The inflammatory infiltrate around the blood vessels is sparse and consists usually only of mononuclear cells, but shows an admixture of neutrophils during periods of exacerbation. The number of mast cells has been shown to be elevated in the center of a psoriatic plaque, as compared to the adjacent uninvolved skin (16). Recently, a special subset of flat-shaped macrophages, called "epithelium-lining macrophages" has been described to form an almost continuous single-cell row at the dermoepidermal junction in many cases of psoriatic plaques (17).

The stratum malpighii overlying the papillae appears thin (13) and exerts significantly different characteristics compared to the stratum malpighii overlying the rete ridges. Because of intracellular edema, the cells of the upper malpighian layer appear pale-stained. The epidermal cells located beneath the parakeratotic stratum corneum may be intermingled with neutrophils, forming a small spongiform pustule (Kogoj) that is diagnostic for psoriasis (13). The pustule is formed by aggregates of neutrophils within the in-

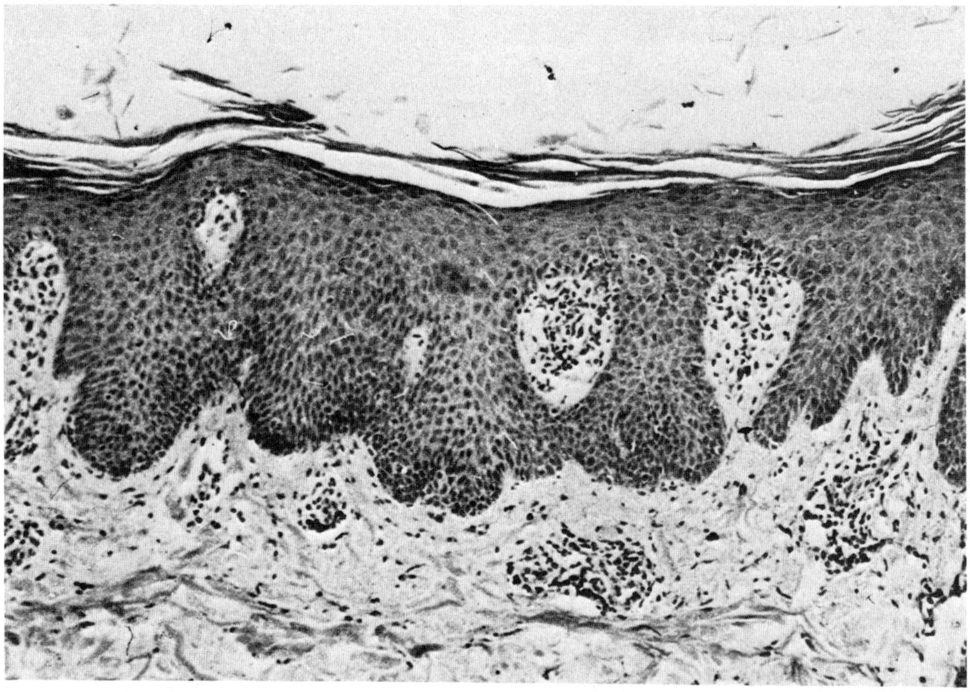

Figure 3 The epidermis shows regular acanthosis. The rete ridges are elongated and club-shaped. Neighboring rete ridges are seen to coalesce at their bases (×70).

terstices of a spongelike network formed by degenerated and thinned epidermal cells (18).

The cornified layers of psoriatic plaques usually show confluent parakeratosis with only small foci of orthokeratosis (15). Since a direct relationship exists between the absence of keratohyaline granules and the development of parakeratosis in psoriatic epidermis, widespread absence of stratum granulosum is a characteristic feature. However, fluctuations in the activity of the psoriatic processes may result in layers of parakeratosis intermingled with layers of orthokeratosis and with well-developed stratum granulosum underneath. Munro microabscesses, located within paraeratotic areas, show accumulations of pyknotic nuclei of neutrophils migrated from the dilated capillaries of the dermal papillae (13). With increasing age of the psoriatic lesion, fewer Munro microabscesses and less parakeratosis are usually found.

Pustular Psoriatic Lesions

The spongiform pustule of Kogoj remains, among all other features, the most prominent diagnostic feature of psoriasis. It starts as a micropustule located in the upper malpighian layer, with neutrophils aggregating within the interstices of a spongelike network formed by degenerated and thinned epidermal cells. It is seen mainly in early, active lesions. This type of pustule also occurs as a micropustule in both generalized and localized pustular psoriasis and represents the characteristic lesion of pustular psoriasis. As the pustule grows, the epidermal cells in the center of the lesion dissolve, so that a large cavity forms, filled with neutrophils. (13). At the periphery of the large cavity, the network of thinned epidermal cells persists over a longer period of time, thus allowing one to recognize that the cavity has been derived from a spongiform pustule. As the neutrophils of the spongiform pustule move up into the horny layer, they become pyknotic and assume the appearance of a large Munro microabscess.

IMMUNOHISTOLOGY

During the last decade, immunohistological examinations have provided some further insights into the pathophysiological aspects of psoriatic transformation.

Keratins 5 and 14 are equally expressed by basal keratinocytes in both normal and psoriatic epidermis; however, in the suprabasal layer, the normal expression of keratins 1 and 10 seems to be replaced by keratins 6, 16, and 17 in manifested psoriatic lesions (19). In the malpighian area, TGF-α is overexpressed and could be responsible for the concomitant suppression of the anti-proliferative IFN-γ receptor (20,21). Involved psoriatic skin revealed marked reduction of filaggrin in the stratum granulosum and stratum corneum (22), and psoriatic keratinocytes showed a loss of the normally polarized expression of certain integrins (10). Expression of ICAM-1 may be detected on epidermal keratinocytes early, during the appearance of initial pinpoint lesions, being possibly important for the recruitment of inflammatory cells and for controlling effector cell functions in psoriatic epidermis (23,24). In contrast to normal epidermis, which releases a balance of cytokines that is neither immunostimulatory nor inhibitory, the cytokines released in psoriatic epidermis (i.e., IL-1, IL-6, IL-8, GRO-α, MCP-1) strongly potentiate T-cell activation in the dermis in response to a suboptimal T-cell-receptor-mediated signal (25–27).

The T-cell population invading the epidemis consists primarily of activated T-helper lymphocytes, whose production of mRNAs for lymphokines such as IL-2, IFN-γ, and TNF-α is elevated (28). TNF-α was also shown to be expressed by psoriatic dermal dendrocytes (macrophages) (26). Activated (CD45 RO+) T lymphocytes as well as perivascular dendritic cells and endothelial cells represent the majority of proliferating cells in the dermis of psoriatic lesions (29). In addition, flow cytometric analyses suggest certain basal cells of stem cell phenotype to be the most likely target population for the lymphokines released by activated T lymphocytes resulting in keratinocyte hyperproliferation (30).

ULTRASTRUCTURE

Ultrastructural investigations have shown mild abnormalities of psoriatic keratinocytes in all epidermal layers, whereas differences between normal and unaffected psoriatic epidermis were not observed (31,32). *In vitro*, it was demonstrated that he characteristic hyperproliferation of psoriatic keratinocytes and the defective terminal differentiation could only be maintained over a short period in primary culture (33). However, skin specimen of psoriatic lesions transplanted into nude mice showed the same ultrastructural morphology as biopsies from untransplanted psoriatic lesions (34) and provided a valuable model system.

In psoriasis, the stratum corneum is formed by up to 40–50 cell layers. Most of its cells contain remnants of nuclei (Fig. 4) and other cytoplasmic organelles. Also, lipid droplets were found within the cytoplasm of horny cells (1). In some psoriatic horny cells the trilaminar plasma membrane is preserved and prominent cornified envelopes, as seen in normal stratum corneum, are rare (35). The keratinocytes of the stratum corneum contain a large number of vesicles that are rarely seen in unaffected psoriatic or in normal keratinocytes (32,36,37). These so-called parakeratotic granules are not sufficiently characterized yet (36,38). Involucrin, the major protein precursor of the cornified envelope, proved by immunoelectron microscopy to be present throughout the parakeratotic stratum corneum (40). The keratin pattern differs from that of normal keratinocytes. This is in agreement with biochemical findings, but seems to be a secondary effect of hyperproliferation (41,42) and could be normalized by retinoids (43).

The keratinocytes in the stratum malpighii have enlarged nuclei, an edematous cytoplasm with abundant ribosomes, and increased numbers of mitochondria (39). It has been shown that in skin biopsies from psoriatic lesions after dithranol therapy an unusual perinuclear arrangement of these mitochondria occurs in keratinocytes and also Langerhans cells exhibit remarkable changes of their cell organelles (44,45). Keratohyalin granules are reduced in number and are smaller than in normal epidermis (1) (Fig. 5); occasionally, they are absent. The tonofilaments are decreased in number and in diameter and lack their normal aggregation (13,32). Particularly in the upper layers of the stratum malpighii, microvillous transformation of the plasma membranes occurs. The microvilli often appear intertwined (35). No tight junctions are observed in the psoriatic epidermis (35). In electron microscopic histochemistry and immunolabeling a reduced occurrence or almost complete absence of glycoconjugates has been detected, which results in decreased adhesiveness (35,46).

The basal cells show a large number of pinocytotic vesicles in their basal portions (1). The intercellular spaces are considerably widened between desmosomes (47,35). Mitoses occur frequently (Fig. 5). Although basal keratinocyte herniations through the lamina basalis into the dermis are demonstrable in

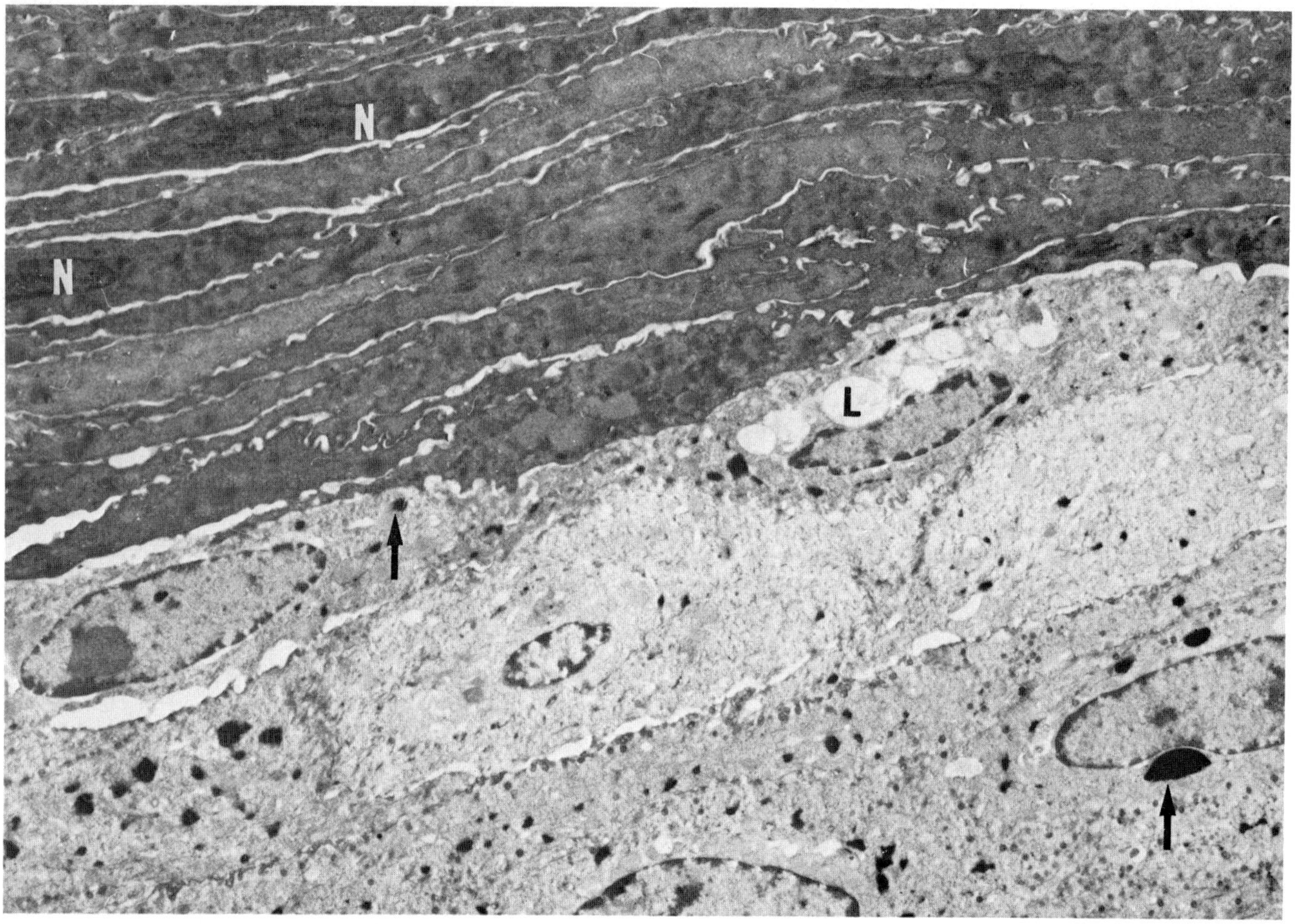

Figure 4 The keratohyalin granules (arrows) are reduced in number and smaller thanin the normal epidermis. The horny cells contain remnants of nuclei (N). L,lipid droplets in the cytoplasmof a granular cell (×520).

psoriatic lesions and appear to correlate with disease activity, the attachment of hemidesmosomes to the lamina basalis seems to be unaffected (48).

In the dermis, an increased number of capillaries are seen, dilated and with thinned and fenestrated endothelium (1,49), indicating increased capillary permeability. The coiled and twisted psoriatic capillaries also differ from the capillary loops in normal skin by an earlier change from the homogeneous (arterial) basement membrane to the multilaminated (venous) basement membrane (50). In addition, immunoelectronmicroscopic studies revealed differences in the expression of microvascular endothelial adhesion molecules (49).

The dermal infiltrate in psoriatic lesions is composed of macrophage-like cells, lymphocytes, and neutrophis (39,51). Using immunoelectronmicroscopy, it could be found that approximately 60% of the infiltrating cells are lymphocytes and another 30% macrophage-like cells. The T4/T8 lymphocyte ratio in tissue has been determined as 3.7 (52). Mast cell degranulation has been suggested to be a prerequisite for the development of psoriatic lesions (2). The basement membrane at the dermoepidermal junction shows large gaps (46) through which inflammatory cells enter the epidermis. Heng et al. (53) described cellular interactions between predominantly CD8+ T lymphocytes and keratinocytes via microvillous cytoplasmic processes in the epidermis of Koebner-positive psoriatic patients. Furthermore, they observed interactions between Langerhans cells and keratinocytes and, in older lesions, between macrophages and lympocytes. Under oral retinoid treatment mucous degeneration phenomena occur in the psoriatic epider-

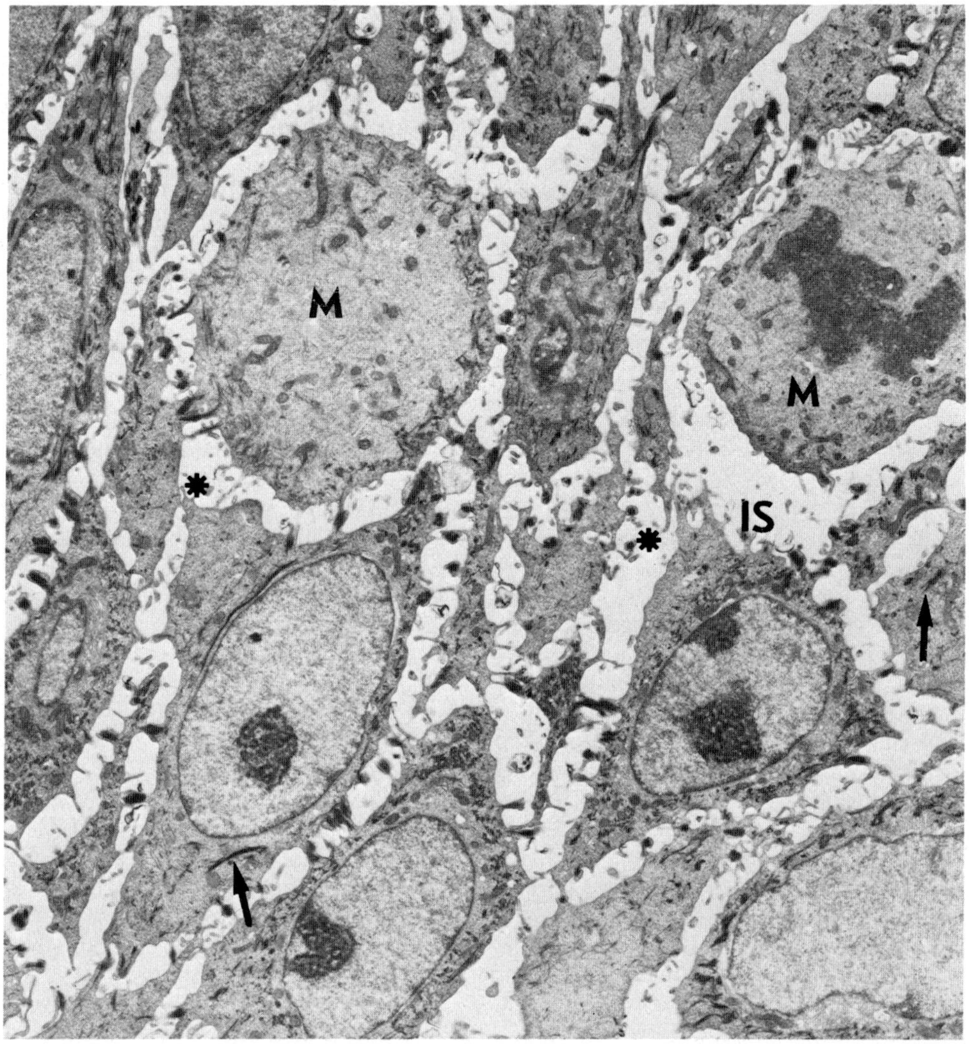

Figure 5 The intracellular spaces (IS) are considerably widened. Two cells are undergoing mitosis (M). The tonofilaments (arrows) are decreased in number and diameter. The plasma membrane shows microvillous transformation (asterisks) (× 6500).

mis (54), together with stimulation of dermal cells including Langerhans cells and macrophages (55), indicating immunomodulation.

REFERENCES

1. Stadler, R., Schaumburg-Lever, G., and Orfanos, C.E., (1986). Histology of psoriatic lesions. In *Textbook of Psoriais.* P.D. Mier and P.C.M. Van de Kerkhof. (Eds.). Churchill Livingstone, Edinburgh, pp. 40–54.
2. Brody, I. (1984). Dermal and epidermal involvement in the evolution of acute eruptive guttate psoriasis vulgaris. *J. Invest. Dermatol.* 82:465–470.
3. Baker, B.S., Swain, A.F., Fry, L., and Valdimarsson, H. (1984). Epidermal T lymphocytes and HLA-DR expression in psoriasis. *Br. J. Dermatol.* 110:555–564.
4. Placek, W., Haftek, M., and Thivolet, J. (1988). Sequence of changes in psoriatic epidermis. *Acta Derm. Venereol. (Stockh.)* 68:369–377.
5. Prens, E.P., Benne, K., Van Joost, T., and Benner, R. (1991). The autologous mixed epidermal cell–T lymphocyte reaction is elevated inpsoriasis: a crucial role for HLA-DE+/CD 1a- antigen presenting cells. *J. Invest. Dermatol* 96:880–887.
6. Ragaz, A., and Ackerman, A.B. (1979). Evolution, maturation, and regression of lesions of psoriasis. *Am. J. Dermatopathol.* 1:199–214.

7. Braun-Falco, O. (1977). The initial psoriatic lesion. In *Psoriasis: Proceedings of the Second International Symposium.* E.M. Farber and A.J. Cox (Eds.). Yorke Medical Books, New York, pp. 1–11.
8. Chowaniec, O., Jablonska, S., Beutner, E.H. Proniewska, M., Jarzabek-Chorzrelaska, M., and Rzesa, G. (1981). Earliest clinical and histological changes in psoriasis. *Dermatologica* 163:42–51.
9. Schubert, Ch., Schlaak, H.E., Schröder, J.M., and Christophers, E. (1984). Ultrastructural sequences of papillary body changes in incipient psoriasis. *J. Invest. Dermatol.* 82:555.
10. De Luca, M., Pellegrini, G., Zambruno, G., and Marchisio, P.C. (1994). Role of integrins in cell adhesion and polarity in normal keratinocytes and human skin pathologies. *J. Dermatol.* 21:821–828.
11. Didierjean, L., Durand, B., and Saurat, J.-H. (1991). Cellular retinoic acid-binding protein type 2 mRNA is overexpressed in human psoriatic skin as shown by in situ hybridization. *Biochem. Biophys. Res. Commun.* 180:204–208.
12. De Boer, O.J., van der Loos, C.M. Hamerlinck, F., Bos, J.D., and Das, P.K. (1994). Reappraisal of in situ immunophenotypic analysis of psoriasis skin: interaction of activated HLA-DR+ immunocompetent cells and endothelial cells is a major feature of psoriatic lesions. *Arch. Dermatol. Res.* 286:87—96.
13. Lever, W.F., and Schaumburg-Lever, G. (1990). Psoriasis. In *Histopathology of the Skin*, 7th ed. J.B. Lippincott, Philadelphia, pp. 156–164.
14. Pinkus, H., and Mehregan, A.H. (1981). Psoriasis. In *A Guide to Dermatohistopathology*, 3rd ed. Appleton-Century-Crofts, New York, pp. 101–104.
15. Ackerman, B. (1978). Psoriasiform dermatitits. In *Histologic Diagnosis of Inflammatory Skin Diseases.* Lea & Febiger, Philadelphia, pp. 250–256.
16. Goodfield, M., MacDonald Hull, S., Holland, D., Roberts, G., Wood, E., Reid, S., and Cunliffe, W. (1994). Investigations of the 'active' edge of plaque psoriasis: vascular proliferation precedes changes in epidermal keratin. *Br. J. Dermatol.* 131:808–813.
17. Van Den Oord, J.J., and de Wolf-Peeters, C. (1994). Epithelium-lining macrophages in psoriasis. *Br. J. Dermatol.* 130:589–594.
18. Rupec, M. (1970). Zur Ultrastruktur der spongiformen Pustel. *Arch. Klin. Exp. Dermatol.* 239:30–49.
19. McKay, I.A., and Leigh, I.M. (1995). Altered keratinocyte growth and differentiation in psoriasis. *Clin. Dermatol.* 13:105–114.
20. Turbitt, M., Akhurt, R.J., White, S.I., and Mackie, R.M. (1990). Localization of elevates transforming growth factor alpha in psoriatic epidermis. *J. Invest. Dermatol.* 95:229–232.
21. Scheynius, A., Fransson, J., Johansson, C., Hammar, H., Baker, B., Fry, L., and Valdimarsson, H. (1992). Expression of interferon-gamma receptors in normal and psoriatic skin. *J. Invest. Dermatol.* 98:255–258.
22. Watanabe, S., Wagatsuma, K., Ichikawa, E., and Takahashi, H. (1991). Abnormal distribution of epidermal protein antigens in psoriatic epidermis. *J. Dermatol.* 18:143–151.
23. DEtmar, M. (1992). Mechanismen der Interaktion von Leukozyten und dermalen Endothelzellen in der kutanen Entzündung. *Hautarzt* 43:679–686.
24. Paukkonen, K., Naukkarinen, A., and Horsmanheimo, M. (1995). The development of manifest psoriatic lesions is linked with the appearance of ICAM-1 positivity on keratinocytes. *Arch. Dermatol. Res.* 287: 165–170.
25. Baker, B.S., Powles, A.V., Valdimaresson, H., and Fry, L. (1988). An altered response by psoriatic keratinocytes to gamma interferon. *Scand. J. Immunol.* 28: 735–740.
26. Nickoloff, B.J., Krabin, G.D, Barker, J.N.W.N., Griffiths, C.E.M., Sarma, V., Mitra, R.S., Elder, J.T., Kunkel, S.L. and Dixit, V.M. (1991). Cellular localization of interleukin-8 and its inducer, tumor necrosis factor-alpha in psoriasis. *Am. J. Pathol.* 138:129–140.
27. Tettelbach, W., Nanney, L., Ellis, D., King, L., and Richmond, A. (1993). Localization of MGSA/GRO protein in cutaneous lesions. *J. Cutan. Pathol.* 20: 259–266.
28. Uyemura, K., Yamamura, M., Fivenson, D.F., Modlin, R.L., and Nickoloff, B.J. (1993). The cytokine network in lesional and lesion-free psoriatic skin is characterized by a T-helper type 1 cell mediated response. *J. Invest. Dermatol.* 101:701–705.
29. Morganroth, G.S., Chan, L.S., Weinstein, G.D., Voorhees, J.J., and Cooper, K.D. (1991). Proliferating cells in psoriatic epidermis are comprised primarily of T cells, endothelial cells, and factor VIIIa+ perivascular dendritic cells. *J. Invest. Dermatol.* 96:333–340.
30. Bata-Csorgo, Z.S., Hammerbert, C., Voorhees, J.J., and Cooper, K.D. (1993). Flow cytometric identification of proliferative subpopulations within normal human epidermis and the localization of the primary hyperproliferative population in psoriasis. *J. Exp. Med.* 178: 1271–1281.
31. Hashimoto, K., and Lever, W.F. (1966). Elektronenmikroskopische Untersuchungen der Hautveränderungen bei Psoriasis. *Dermatol. Wochenschr.* 152: 713–722.
32. Jahn H., Nielsen, E.H. Elberg, J.J., Bierring, F., Ronne, M., and Brandrup, F. (1988). Ultrastructure of psoriatic epidermis. *APMIS* 96:723–731.
33. Detmar, M., Mayer da Silva, A., Stadler, R., and Orfanos, C.E. (1990). Initial hyperproliferation and incomplete terminal differentiation of cultured human keratinocytes from lesional and uninvolved psoriatic skin. *Acta Derm. Venereol. (Stockh.)* 70:295–299.

34. Ueda, K., Yanagihara, M., Nakagawa, S., and Fujita, T. (1994). Functional morphology of lesions of psoriasis vulgaris transplanted into nude mice at an early stage. *J. Dermatol.* 21:940–946.
35. Orfanos, C.E., Schaumburg-Lever, G., Mahrle, G., and Lever, W.F. (1973). Alterations of cell surfaces as a pathogenetic factor in psoriasis. *Arch. Dermatol* 107: 38–46.
36. Brody, I., Mishima, Y., and Masahiro, M. (1974). Stratum corneum in psoriasis vulgaris. A transmission and scanning electron microscopic study. *J. Cutan. Pathol.* 1:33–46.
37. Barbareschi, M., Colzani, G., Motta, S., Angius, A., Sesana, S., and Monti, M. (1994). Psoriatic scales: an ultrastructural study. *Acta Derm. Venerol. (Stockh.)* (Suppl) 186:35–36.
38. Steigleder, G.K., and Jorda, V. (1971). Parakeratosegranula. *Arch. Klin. Exp. Derm.* 239:414–425.
39. Lupulescu, A.P., Chadwick, J.M., and Downham, T.F. II (1979). Ultrastructural and cell surface changes of human psoriatic skin following Goeckerman therapy. *J. Cutan. Pathol.* 6:347–363.
40. Ishida-Yamamoto, A., and Iizuka, H. (1995) Differences in involucrin immunolabeling within cornified cell envelopes in normal and psoriatic epidermis. *J. Invest. Dermatol.* 104:391–395.
41. Baden, H.P., McGilvray, N., Ching, C.K., Lee, L.D., and Kubilus, F. (1978). The keratin polypeptides of psoriatic epidermis. *J. Invest. Dermatol.* 70:294–297.
42. Bowden, P.E., Wood, E.J., and Cunlife, J.W. (1983). Comparation of prekeratin and keratin polypeptides in normal and psoriatic human epidermis. *Biochim. Biophys. Acta* 743:172–179.
43. Staquet, M.J., Faure, M.R., Reano, A., Viac, J., and Thivolet, J. (1983). Keratin polypetide profile in psoriatic epidermis normalized by treatment with etretinate (aromatic retinoid Ro 10-9359). *Arch. Dermatol. Res.* 275:124–129.
44. Klug, H., and Schulze, P. (1988). Unusual mitochondrial reaction in psoriatic keratinocytes. *Virchows Arch. B Cell Pathol.* 56:201–203.
45. Kanerava, L. (1990). Electron microscopy of the effects of dithranol on healthy and on psoriatic skin. *Am. J. Dermatopathol.* 12:51–62.
46. Paller, A.S., Siegel, J. N., Spalding, D.E., and Bremer, E.G. (1989). Absence of a stratum corneum antigen in disorders of epidermal cell proliferation: detection with an antiganglioside GM3 antibody. *J. Invest. Dermatol.* 92:240–246.
47. Brody, I. (1978). Alterations of clincially normal skin in early eruptive guttate psoriasis. *J. Cutan. Pathol.* 5: 219–233.
48. Heng, M.C.Y., Kloss, S.G., Kuehn, C.S., and Chase, D.G. (1986). Significance and pathogenesis of basal keratinocyte herniations in psoriasis. *J. Invest. Dermatol.* 87:362–366.
49. Patzelbauer, P., Pober, J.S., Keh, A., and Braverman, I.M. (1994). Inducibility and expression of microvascular endothelial adhesion molecules in lesional, perilesional, and uninvolved skin of psoriatic patients. *J. Invest. Dermato.* 103:300–305.
50. Braverman, I.M., and Yen, A. (1977). Ultrastructure of the human dermal microcirculation. II. The capillary loops of dermal papillae. *J. Invest. Dermatol.* 68: 44–52.
51. Bos, J.D., Hulsebosch, H.J., Krieg, S.R., et al. (1983). Immunocompetent cells in psoriasis. In situ immunophenotyping by monoclonal antibodies. *Arch. Dermatol. Res.* 275:181–189.
52. De Peanfilis, G., Manara, G.C., Ferrari, C., Torresani, C., Zucchi, A., and Devoto, R.M. (1989). Further characterization of the incipient lesion of chronic stationary type psoriasis vulgaris in exacerbation. *Acta Derm. Venereol. (Stockh.)* (Suppl) 146:26–30.
53. Heng, M.C.Y., Allen, S.G., Haberfelde, G., and Song, M.K. (1991). Electronmicroscopic and immunocytochemical studies of th sequence of events in psoriatic plaque formation after tape-stripping, *Br. J. Dermatol.* 125:548–556.
54. Schultz-Ehrenburg, U., and Orfanos, C.E., (1981). Light- and electron-microscopic changes of human epidermis under oral retinoid treatment. In *Retinoids: Advances in Basic Research and Therapy*, Springer verlag, Berlin, pp. 99–108.
55. Tsambaos, D., Orfanos, C.E. (1981). Ultrastructural evidence suggesting an immunomodulatory activity of oral retinoid. Its effect on dermal components in psoriasis. *Br. J. Dermatol.* 104:37–45.

Part V

TOPICAL THERAPY

29

Product Development for Psoriasis: Clinical Challenges and Opportunities

Alice Bendix Gottlieb
University of Medicine and Dentistry of New Jersey–Robert Wood Johnson Medical School, New Brunswick, New Jersey

The patient with psoriasis represents both a challenge and an opportunity for drug treatment. Although we have a number of treatments that can induce remission in a high percentage of psoriasis patients, in the absence of a cure, we do not have both safe and effective drugs to maintain patients in remission.

PROBLEMS WITH CURRENT THERAPY

For patients with mild to moderate psoriasis, topical therapies are generally used. This therapeutic repertoire includes emollients and moisturizers, tars, anthralins, topical corticosteroids, and vitamin D analogs. However, for approximately 30% of patients seeking physicians care, these treatments are insufficient and systemic therapies are required (Table 1) (1). Although definitions vary in their details, patients with moderate to severe psoriasis requiring systemic treatment (including phototherapy) include those with 10% or more of body surface area covered with psoriatic lesions, psoriasis not responsive to topical therapy or so extensive that it becomes economically impractical to treat topically. Additional criteria include patients who are either psychologically or physically handicapped by their psoriasis or who cannot work because of their disease. Patients with pustular or erythrodermic psoriasis, and with psoriatic arthritis unresponsive to nonsteroidal anti-inflammatory therapy, should be treated with systemic agents. Currently the systemic repertoire for treatment of moderate to severe psoriasis includes ultraviolet B (UVB) alone or in combination with topical tars, anthralin, emollients, and moisturizers, topical corticosteroids, and topical vitamin D analogs, in either an outpatient or day hospital setting. Unfortunately, hospital admission for topical tar and UVB treatment (Goeckerman protocol) is difficult in the United States owing to insurance reimbursement constraints. Psoralen and UVA irradiation (PUVA) is highly clinical and cost-effective; however, the long-term risks of increased skin cancer incidence and of extensive photodamage limit treat-

Table 1 Working Definitions of Moderate-to-Severe Psoriasis

10% or more body surface area involved
Psoriasis not responsive to topical therapy
Extensive disease not economically feasible to treat topically
Psychologically distressful disease
Gainful employment prevented
Pustular or erythrodermic psoriasis
Psoriatic arthritis unresponsive to nonsteroidal anti-inflammatory therapy

Source: Reproduced from Ref. 1 by permission from the National Psoriasis Foundation.

ment. Methotrexate, etretinate and its active metabolite acitretin, cyclosporin, and sulfasalazine remain the oral drugs used in varying degrees throughout the world for treatment of moderate to severe psoriasis. Each oral agent is associated with potentially severe toxicity and, in some cases, extensive monitoring requirements.

The multiplicity of current treatments for psoriasis suggests that none is a definitive treatment for the disease. In a patient survey performed by the National Psoriasis Foundation, the major patient support group for psoriasis in the United States, 70% of patients felt that their treatments were ineffective because of either lack of efficacy, toxicity, or rapid relapse after cessation of therapy (2). Additionally, many psoriasis treatments are expensive.

Governmental and pharmaceutical support for psoriasis research is relatively low considering the high incidence of psoriasis in the United States and in Europe. Of late, access to adequate care is challenged in the managed health care environment. Despite these challenges, the opportunity in psoriasis lies in the realization that the psoriatic plaque is "driven" by the activated T lymphocyte in situ (3,4). This observation plus the accessibility of skin and availability of validated pharmacodynamic markers has led to a renaissance in pharmaceutical industry-led, innovative treatments for psoriasis, which make use of agents developed for treatments in the transplantation, oncology, and autoimmunity therapeutic areas.

Table 2 Factors That Can Induce or Exacerbate Psoriasis in Susceptible Individuals

Physical trauma to skin
Superficial abrasion
Blister
Laceration/incision
Thermal burn
Photoxic reactions
Solar
Ultraviolet B
PUVA-induced
Activation of local cellular immunity
Contact allergens
Immunizations in skin
Infections in skin (bacterial or viral)
Systemic immunological activation or alteration
Hypersensitivity to drug or other antigen
Group A streptococcal infections
HIV infection
Systemic drugs
Corticosteroids
Interferons
Lithium
Antimalarials
Beta-blockers
Angiotensin-converting enzyme inhibitors
Gemfibrozil and a number of other drugs in case reports
?Nonsteroidal anti-inflammatory drugs
Emotional stress

Source: Reproduced from Ref. 1 by permission of the National Psoriasis Foundation.

EVIDENCE THAT THE EPIDERMAL CHANGES IN PSORIATIC PLAQUES ARE REVERSIBLE AND SECONDARY TO T-LYMPHOCYTE ACTIVATION: CLINICAL, LABORATORY, AND THERAPEUTIC RESPONSE AS CLUES

Clinically, a number of factors flare psoriasis (Table 2) and these observations provided early clues to the immune basis of its pathogenesis. The Koebner phenomenon with its associated increase in keratinocyte-derived lymphokines suggested that the keratinocyte could play an active role in sustaining localized cellular immune activation (1,4). Pertubation of cellular immune function by infection [e.g., role of streptococcal infection and superantigen-mediated T-cell activation in guttate psoriasis (5)], drug reactions, or HIV infection provided additional clinical support (1). The observations that treatment with a variety of interferons flared psoriasis (6), and that injection of interferon-gamma into nonlesional skin in a psoriasis patient induced new lesions (7), provided more support for the role of interferon-gamma and activated T cells in the pathogenesis of the psoriatic plaque. Conversely, treatment with immunomodulators such as cyclosporin, FK 506, methotrexate, anti-CD3 monoclonal antibodies, and an IL-2 diphtheria toxin fusion protein greatly improved psoriasis (3,8–14). Genetic data suggested an association with certain class I and class II MHC haplotypes, the strongest being with HLA-Cw6 (15).

Laboratory studies of psoriatic plaques provided further pathogenic clues and also led to the validation of pharmacodynamic markers for psoriasis. Psoriatic epidermis demonstrates abnormal proliferation and differentiation similar to that seen in acute and chronic wounds [regenerative maturation (16)]. As will be described later, this abnormal phenotype is reversible and is the result of localized immune activation of T cells, possibly epidermal CD8+ T cells (3). However, since the clinical phenotype of psoriasis, i.e., the scaling and thickness, is largely a manifestation of the epidermal changes, let us focus first on the psoriatic epidermal phenotype (Table 3). This regenerative maturation phenotype is characterized by increased keratinocyte proliferation as measured by either immunostaining with Ki67 monoclonal antibody, which detects a cyclin protein expressed in the S, G_2, and M phases of the cell cycle and which is turned off in G_1, or by autoradiography using radioactive nucleotides (3,8,9,16). Abnormal differentiation is easily detected by immunostaining of plaques with antibodies directed against hyperproliferative keratin, K-16, filaggrin, and alpha-3 integrin (3,8,9,17,18). The lipid barrier is abnormal with decreased deposition of interlamellar lipids in the stratum corneum within psoriatic plaques (19). These abnormalities are completely normalized by psoriatic treatments that do not require continuous administration to maintain remission (remittive agents), such as PUVA, UVB plus tar, and possibly the interleukin-2 (IL-2)-diphtheria toxin fusion protein (3,8,9). In contrast, K-16, filaggrin, and alpha-3 integrin expression are not consistently normalized after treatment with agents requiring continuous treatment to maintain remission (suppressive agents), such as cyclosporin, etretinate, and topical calcitriol (18–20).

A number of cytokines and/or their receptors are abnormally expressed in psoriatic plaques (Table 3) (21). The most interesting potential pharmacological target is the insulin-like growth factor-1 (IGF-1) receptor. The IGF-1 receptor is a tyrosine kinase receptor. Its ligand, IGF-1, or high doses of insulin are absolutely required in vitro for epidermal growth factor (EGF)-, transforming growth factor (TGF)-alpha-, keratinocyte growth factor (KGF)-, and IL-6-mediated keratinocyte mitogenesis (22). The IGF-1 receptor is both overexpressed and overactivated in psoriatic plaques, and its expression normalizes with treatment with remittive therapies such as PUVA (9,23). Both IGF-1 receptor and ligand (IGF-1 and IGF-2) knockout mice show profound epidermal keratinocyte abnormalities in vivo and in vitro (24) (J.G. Krueger, personal communication). In contrast, psoriasis is not a primary disorder of the TGF-α/EGF-receptor pathway for the following reasons: Although TGF-α and its receptor the EGF receptor are overexpressed in psoriatic plaques (25–27), TGF-α transgenic mice, in which TGF-α is overexpressed, do not have psoriasis (28). Knockout mice for TGF-α do not show epidermal atrophy; they exhibit wavy hair (29,30). Treatment of severe psoriasis with cyclosporin clears plaques without decreasing either TGF-α or EGF-receptor expression (20). EGF receptors are not overactivated in psoriatic plaques despite their increased immunostaining (23,27). High doses of EGF have been used to clear psoriasis-like lesions in a nude mouse model (31). Finally, the original experiments by Carpenter and Cohen with EGF showed much more effect on epidermal differentiation (hyperkeratosis) than on thickening of the epidermis (32). Platelet-derived growth factor (PDGF) receptors are over-

Table 3 Histological Epidermal Phenotype and Growth Factor Expression in Psoriatic Plaques, Nonlesional and Normal Skin

Marker	Psoriatic plaque	Nonlesional skin from psoriasis patients	Normal skin
Regenerative maturation marker			
Ki67	Increased numbers and suprabasal expression	Normal	Normal
K-16 keratin	Positive	Negative	Negative
Filaggrin	Patchy or absent	Confluent	Confluent
Alpha-3 integrin	Suprabasal	Basal	Basal
Growth factors			
IGF-1 receptor	Overactivated and overexpressed, in suprabasal distribution	Basal only	Basal only
TGF-alpha	Increased	Normal	Normal
EGF-receptor	Overexpressed, in suprabasal distribution	Basal	Basal
IL-6	Overexpressed	Normal	Normal

expressed in the dermis of active plaques. Keratinocytes do not have PDGF- receptors. IL-6 and its receptor are both overexpressed in psoriatic plaques (33–35). There are increased circulating levels of IL-6 in psoriasis patients and IL-6 is mitogenic for keratinocytes in vitro (34). However, the variable response to therapy, i.e., decreased with UVB and vitamin D therapy but not with cyclosporin or PUVA, implies that IL-6 may play a supportive role in maintaining the plaque, but is probably not primary in the pathogenesis of the plaque (9,20,36). Supportive roles for IL-6 in psoriasis may be in maintaining keratinocyte hyperproliferation, serving as a local T-cell growth factor in situ, or supporting joint inflammation and destruction in psoriatic arthritis (34).

Evidence for the key role of T-cell activation in the pathogenesis of psoriasis has accumulated especially over the past 10 years (Table 4). There is a significant genetic association of psoriasis with certain HLA haplotypes, especially HLA-Cw6 (15). Increased numbers of IL-2 receptor+, presumably activated, T lymphocytes are present in both the epidermis and dermis of psoriatic plaques (4,37). There is an inversion of the normal CD4/CD8 ratio in psoriatic epidermis, but not in psoriatic dermis (3,8,9,18,19,38,39). There is oligoclonal expression of certain T-cell receptor Vβ genes in activated T cells in psoriatic epidermis, but not in psoriatic dermis or in lesions from patients with atopic dermatitis (40,41). Decreases in epidermal thickness with therapy correlate much better with decreases in numbers of epidermal CD8+ T cells than with decreases in numbers of CD4+ T cells for treatment with PUVA, UVB plus tar, an IL-2 diphtheria toxin fusion protein, topical calcitriol, and etretinate (3,8,9,18,19,38). These observations are consistent with the clinical findings that the AIDS condition flares psoriasis and is remarkable for CD8+ T-cell infiltration into the epidermis (42). Additionally, the strongest HLA associations are with class I MHC antigens (15). Interferon-gamma is synthesized exclusiely by activated T lymphocytes. Increased interferon-gamma in psoriatic plaques is demonstrated directly and also evidenced by keratinocyte expression of the interferon-gamma-induced proteins HLA-DR, IP-10, and I-CAM-1 only in active psoriatic plaques but not in uninvolved skin (4,37,43–46). Additionally, there is increased expression of other lymphokines such as IL-6 and IL-8 in psoriatic plaques (34,47).

Table 4 Evidence for Immune Pathogenesis of Psoriasis

HLA associations
Increased numbers of activated T lymphocytes in psoriatic plaques
Inversion of CD4/CD8 ratio of T lymphocytes in psoriatic epidermis
Oligoclonal expression of T cell receptor Vβ genes in activated CD8+ T cells isolated from psoriatic plaques
Correlation of epidermal thickness with epidermal CD8+ T-cell numbers
Presence of interferon-gamma-induced proteins on keratinocytes (HLA-DR, ICAM-1, IP-10)
Increased expression of lymphokines
Interferon-gamma
IL-6
IL-8
Immunosuppressives improve psoriasis
IL-2 diphtheria toxin fusion protein
Cyclosporin
FK 506
Anti-CD3 monoclonal antibodies
Interferons flare psoriasis

The demonstration that treatment with an IL-2 diphtheria toxin fusion protein as a single agent clears, both clinically and histopathologically, psoriatic plaques provides definitive evidence that the activated T lymphocyte "drives" the psoriatic plaque and that the epidermal abnormalities of hyperproliferation and abnormal differentiation are secondary and reversible with elimination of T-cell activation (3). The details of this study are discussed in detail elsewhere in this volume, but suffice it to say that this study demonstrated the power (and economy) of well-designed clinical studies in making basic discoveries in disease pathogenesis. This is especially true in diseases such as psoriasis in which good animal models do not exist.

In summary, understanding of pathogenesis leads to improved drug development for psoriasis (Table 5): Activated T lymphocytes (antigen-specific and nonspecifically activated T cells), or other leukocytes directly, or via cytokine elaboration, cause increased keratinocyte proliferation and altered differentiation (regenerative maturation). This is recognized clinically as scale and thickness. CD8+ T cells might possibly cause direct sublethal keratinocyte injury, which could also turn on the wound healing (regenerative maturation) phenotype. Removal of activated T cells eliminates the regenerative maturation phenotype and thus normalizes both keratinocyte proliferation and differentiation. Once it is accepted that psoriasis is an immune-mediated disorder, the gate is opened for novel therapeutic agents that interfere with a number of steps in the T-cell activation pathway. These include

Table 5 Immunopathogenesis of Epidermal Activation (Regenerative Maturation) in Psoriasis

Initiator	Mediator	Epidermal effect
Antigen presentation with subsequent antigen-specific T-cell activation —?CD8+ T cells	Cytokines	Increased keratinocyte proliferation and induction of regenerative maturation phenotype
		Induction of interferon-gamma-induced proteins on keratinocytes (HLA-DR, ICAM-1, IP-10)
Non-antigen-specific T-cell activation —?CD4+ T cells	Cytokines	Increased keratinocyte proliferation and induction of regenerative maturation phenotype
		Induction of interferon-gamma-induced proteins on keratinocytes (HLA-DR, ICAM-1, IP-10)
CD8+ T-lymphocyte-mediated keratinocyte injury	Direct effect	Increased keratinocyte proliferation and induction of regenerative maturation phenotype

agents that interrupt antigen presentation and activation (e.g., superantigen approaches, therapeutic peptide vaccines of Vβ3 and Vβ13.1 peptides, antagonists of T-cell costimulatory receptor/ligand pathways, IL-2 diphtheria toxin fusion protein), inhibit T-cell cytokine synthesis (e.g., cyclosporin, FK 506, topical ascomycins, anti-tumor-necrosis factor agents, vitamin D analogs), decrease T-cell recruitment and trafficking (e.g., antisense therapy with I-CAM-1 antisense oligonucleotides, monoclonal antibodies to various adhesion proteins), and decrease the keratinocyte response to T-cell immune activation (e.g., retinoids and vitamin D analogs, photodynamic therapy using topical 5-aminolevulinic acid) (3,5,18,40,48–52).

Table 6 Psoriasis Is the First Disease to Study with Therapeutic Agents that Modulate Th1-Type Cellular Immunity: Comparison Between Psoriasis and Rheumatoid Arthritis

	Psoriasis	Rheumatoid arthritis
Similarities		
Key role of activated T lymphocytes	Yes	Yes
Proliferative "nonimmune" endorgan leads to many phenotypic manifestations	Epidermis	Pannus
Increased inflammatory cytokines	IL-6, IL-8, interferon-gamma in plaques	TNF-alpha, IL-6 in synovial fluid
Increased adhesion molecules	I-CAM-1	I-CAM-1
Incidence	2–4%	1%
Unsatisfactory therapies	Yes	Yes
Differences		
MHC association	Class I	Class II
Placebo effect	Low	High
Tissue accessibility	Easy	Difficult
Pharmacodynamic markers	Validated	Not validated, rudimentary knowledge
Patient population	Generally healthy	Multisystem disease
In-life study duration	3 months	1–2 years (for disease control indication)
Drug formulation	Topical, bath, intralesional, oral, parenteral	Oral, intralesional, and parenteral

PSORIASIS AS *THE* MODEL DISEASE FOR PROOF-OF-CONCEPT FOR NEW DRUGS THAT INTERFERE WITH Th1 T-CELL IMMUNE ACTIVATION

In the past, rheumatoid arthritis has served as the first disease studied when a new drug that interferes with Th1 T-cell immune activation became available for testing in humans. Psoriasis and rheumatoid arthritis share many similarities in pathogenesis and epidemiology; however, it is in the differences between the two diseases that psoriasis pulls far ahead of rheumatoid arthritis for proof-of-concept studies and for pivotal trials for NDA registration (Table 6). In both psoriasis and rheumatoid arthritis, a key role for activated T lymphocytes in their pathogenesis has been demonstrated (3,4,37,38,53). In both diseases, there is a proliferative "nonimmune" endorgan whose involvement leads to most of the phenotypic manifestations of the disease. For psoriasis it is the epidermis and for rheumatoid arthritis it is the pannus of the joint. In both diseases, increased inflammatory cytokines and increased expression of various adhesion molecules have been described (21,34,38, 44–47,54–73). Clinically, the incidence of psoriasis is at least as high as rheumatoid arthritis and the medical need and unsatisfied market are comparable and large in both diseases. However, drug development is much more convenient to study in psoriasis than in rheumatoid arthritis. The placebo effect in chronic plaque-type psoriasis is less than 10%. In contrast, the placebo effect in rheumatoid arthritis is at least 40%. The in-life portion of a clinical trial in psoriasis is no more than 3 months, whereas for a disease-controlling indication of rheumatoid arthritis, it is 1–2 years. Patient study populations are generally healthy in psoriasis, but in rheumatoid arthritis, patients have multisystem disease and limited mobility. Tissue accessibility is easy in psoriasis and difficult in rheumatoid arthritis. There are markers of both immune activation and keratinocyte proliferation and differentiation for psoriasis that have been validated for six anti-psoriasis therapies (3,8,9,18,20,21,38,74,75). There are no validated pharmacodynamic markers for rheumatoid arthritis. Finally, drug formulations for psoriasis can be topical, via bath or soaks, intralesional, oral, or parenteral. In contrast, for rheumatoid arthritis, only intralesional, oral, or parenteral routes of administration are feasible at this time.

Table 7 Pharmacodynamic Markers of Therapeutic Response in Psoriasis

Keratinocyte activation
Proliferation
Ki-67
Differentiation
K-16
Filaggrin
Alpha 3 integrin
Epidermal thickness
Immune activation
T lymphocytes (CD3, CD8, CD4, IL-2 receptor)
Interferon-gamma-induced keratinocyte proteins
HLA-DR
ICAM-1
IP-10

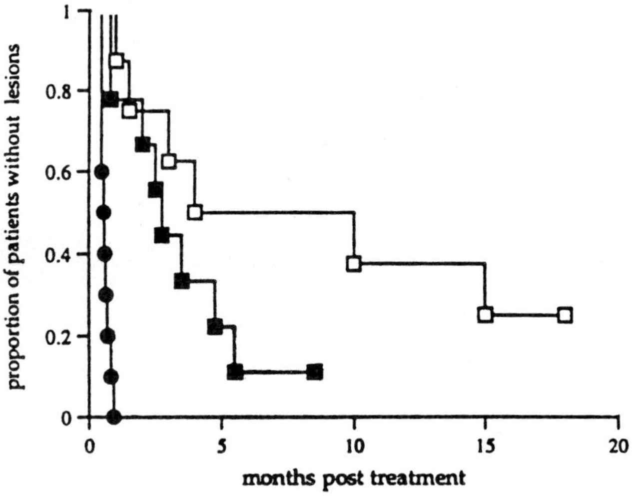

Figure 1 Recurrence of psoriasis after PUVA treatment in comparison with other therapies. Psoriasis was cleared in patients with comparable disease activity by cyclosporin treatment for at least 8 weeks (●), by treatment with bath PUVA (□), or by inpatient Goeckerman treatment with UVB light and topical tar treatment (■). All patients began follow-up with visually resolved psoriatic lesions. For each treatment, the time interval to relapse of clinically significant psoriatic plaques is shown. Cyclosporin provides a transient benefit upon discontinuation, whereas weeks to months of clear skin is produced by bath PUVA treatment. (Reproduced from Ref. 9 by copyright permission of The Rockefeller University Press.)

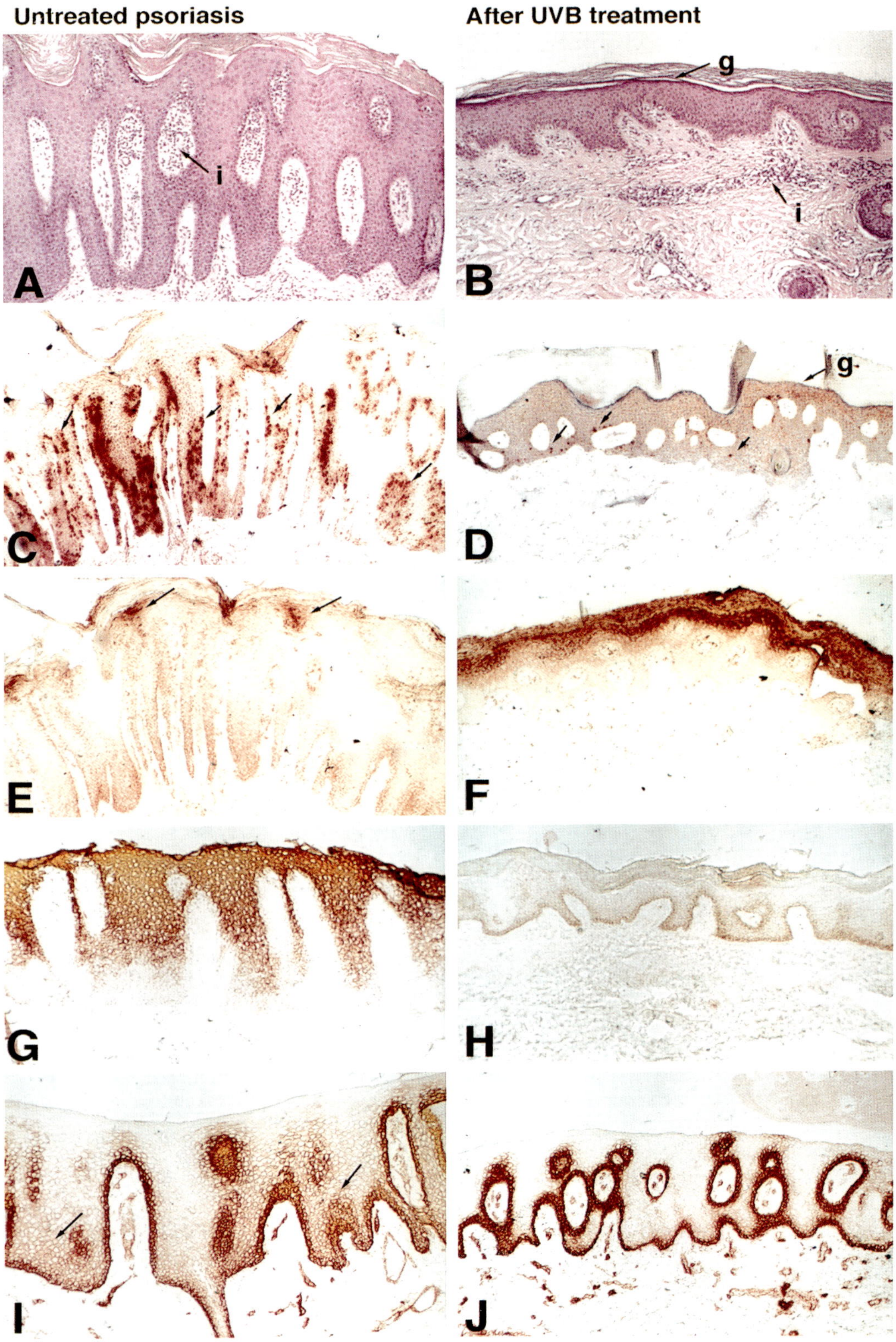

A/B- H&E (i= chronic inflam infiltrate, g= granular layer); C/D- Ki67
E/F- filaggrin; G/H- keratin 16; I/J- integrin alpha 3

Figure 3

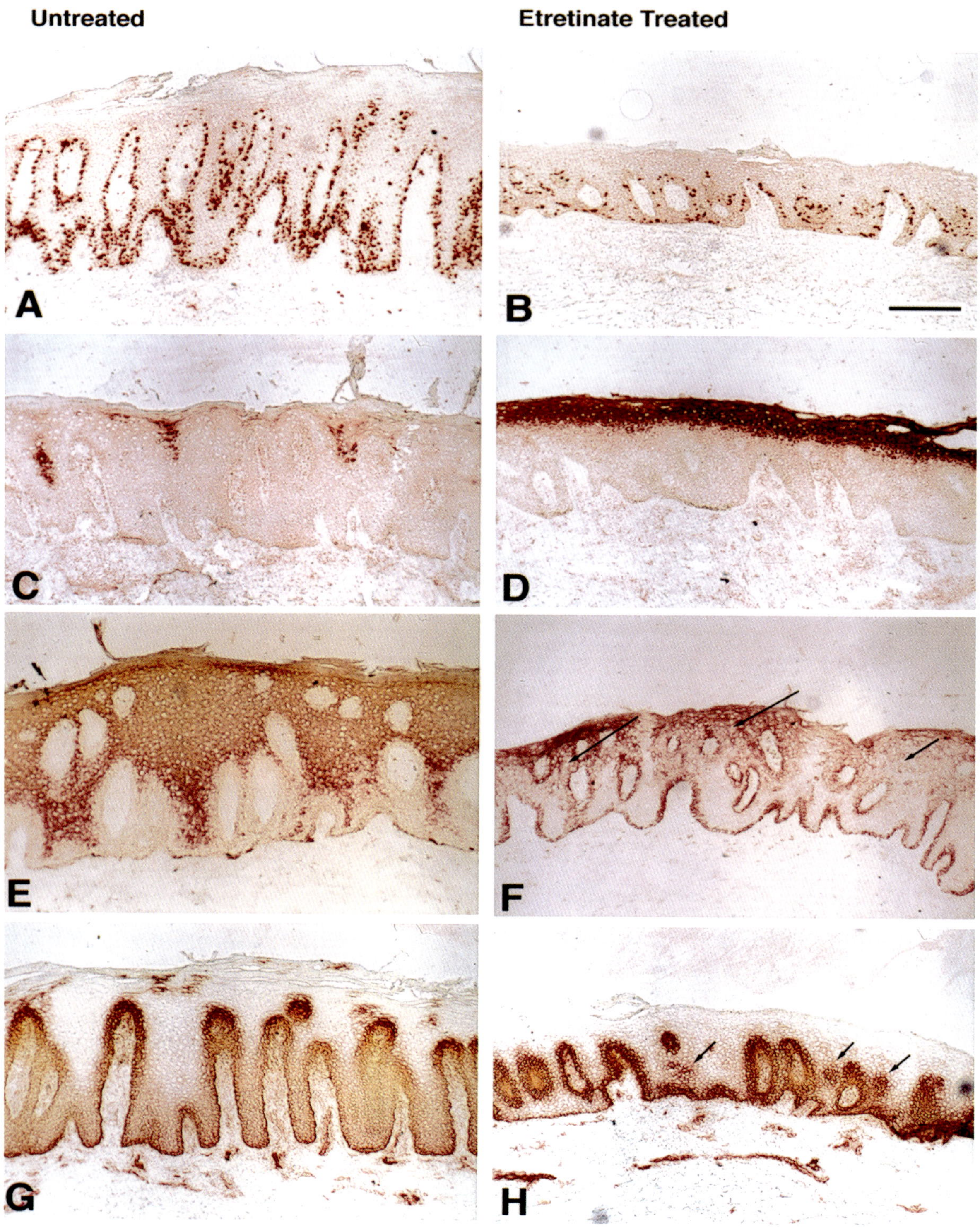

Expression of proteins marking keratinocyte proliferation, differentiation, and epidermal regenerative maturation

A,B = Ki67 E,F = keratin 16
C,D = filaggrin G,H = integrin alpha 3

Bar is 200 microns

Figure 3

Figure 2 Pathological and immunohistochemical assessment of psoriatic epidermis before and after UVB treatment. The left column displays micrographs from untreated psoriasis; the right column shows paired micrographs from UVB-treated psoriasis. Sections have been H&E stained (A,B) or reacted with antibodies to the Ki67 nuclear protein (C,D), to filaggrin (E,F), to keratin 16 (G,H) or to integrin-alpha$_3$ (I,J). In (A,B) "I" indicates chronic inflammatory dermal cells and "g" indicates a granular layer; in (C,D) arrows indicate some Ki67-positive nuclei; in (E) arrows indicate focal areas of epidermis expressing filaggrin; in (I) arrows indicate suprabasal keratinocytes expressing cell surface integrin-alpha$_3$. All micrographs are shown at the same magnification. (From Ref. 8.)

Figure 3 Expression of proteins marking proliferation, differentiation, or regenerative epidermal growth. Sections obtained from untreated (A,C,E,G) or etretinate-treated (B,D,F,H) lesions. Psoriatic lesions were reacted with antibodies to Ki67 (A,B), filaggrin (C,D), keratin 16 (E,F), or integrin-alpha$_3$ (G,H). Bar is 200 microns (shown in B). Arrows in F, H point to suprabasal keratinocytes showing residual staining for keratin 16 or integrin alpha$_3$. (Reproduced from Ref. 19 by permission from the Editor.)

PRACTICAL APPLICATIONS FOR DRUG DEVELOPMENT

Remittive Versus Suppressive Treatments

In Figure 1, we return to the major problem with current treatments for psoriasis, that is, the failure to obtain *both* safe and effective drugs for *maintenance* of remission. At one large psoriasis treatment center, all patients who cleared with cyclosporin therapy relapsed within 1 month after cessation of treatment. Cyclosporin is an example of a suppressive therapy. A *suppressive* therapy required continuous administration to maintain remission. In contrast, PUVA treatment led to approximately 6 months of clear skin after cessation of treatment in approximately 50% of patients. PUVA is an example of a remittive therapy. A *remittive* therapy does not require continuous administration to achieve long-lived remission. Inpatient UVB plus tar treatment is an example of another remittive therapy; however, the length of remission is somewhat less than that of PUVA (8,9).

Pharmacodynamic Markers for Psoriasis

Pharmacodynamic markers of immune activation and keratinocyte proliferation and differentiation can be carried out using simple immunostaining techniques on only one 6-mm punch biopsy before and after treatment (Table 7). These markers have been validated for treatment with PUVA, UVB plus tar, IL-2 diphtheria toxin fusion protein (remittive therapies), etretinate, cyclosporin, and topical calcitriol (suppressive therapies) (3,8,9,18,20,21,38,74,75). The value added by the use of these pharmacodynamic markers in addition to traditional clinical assessments [Psoriasis Activity and Severity Index (PASI), or other severity scores (20,76)] is that two therapies such as cyclosporin and PUVA clinically clear psoriatic plaques to a comparable degree; however, in one case, PUVA, potent decreases in T-cell numbers and activation and normalization of keratinocyte proliferation and differentiation are observed. In contrast, for cyclosporin, only moderate decreases in T-cell numbers are observed and normalization of epidermal keratinocyte proliferation and differentiation are not consistently achieved. This is despite the fact that the clinical response to these two agents looks identical. In addition, histological assessments are quantitative and more uniform (precise) than clinical assessments such as PASI or severity scores (20,76). This is especially true for treatments such as topical calcitriol, which often do not

Table 8 Histopathological Response Predicts Clinical Course in Psoriasis

Therapy	Decreased immune activation	Normalized keratinocyte differentiation and proliferation
Remittive		
PUVA	++++	++++
UVB/tar	++++ (epidermis)	++++
IL-2, diphtheria toxin fusion protein	+++	+++
Suppressive		
Etretinate	++	++
Cyclosporin	++	+−++
Vitamin D	++	++

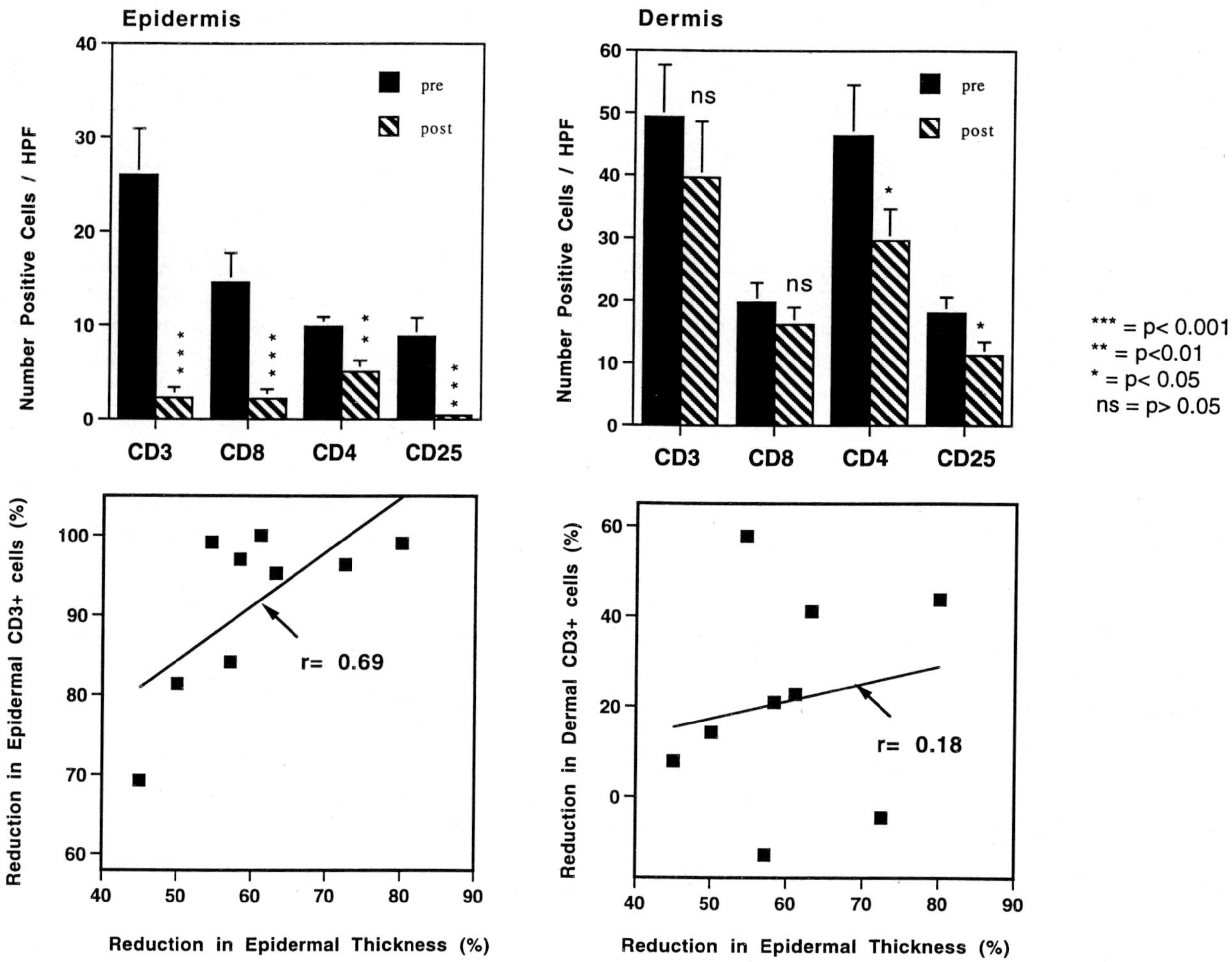

Figure 4 Quantitative analysis of T-cell infiltration in psoriatic lesional tissue before and after UVB treatment. (Top) Mean numbers of CD3+, CD8+, CD4+, or CD25+ cells in the epidermis or dermis of psoriatic lesional tissue before treatment (solid bars) or after UVB treatment (hatched bars); standard error is shown for each mean value. *p* values for differences between untreated and UVB treated tissue were $p < 0.001$ (***), $p < 0.01$ (**), $p < 0.05$ (*), or $p > 0.05$ (ns). (Bottom) The relationship between reduction in epidermal acanthosis (thickness) and reduction in the number of total T lymphocytes (CD3+) in either the epidermis or dermis of biopsies analyzed for individual patients. (Reproduced from Ref. 8 by copyright permission of The Rockefeller University Press.)

clear psoriatic plaques uniformly (18). Epidermal thickness can be quantitated on either frozen or routine paraffin-embedded skin sections. Keratinocyte proliferation can be measured by immunoperoxidase staining with a monoclonal anti-Ki 67 antibody. This technique is as quantitative and precise as in vivo studies with radioactive nucleotides (3,8,9,18,19). Normalization of keratinocyte differentiation can be assessed by looking for disappearance of keratin K-16, return of continuous expression of filaggrin in the granular layer, and return of alpha 3 integrin immunostaining to only the basal layer. Filaggrin has been demonstrated to normalize early in drug treatment (77); therefore, if filaggrin immunostaining is unaffected after 4 weeks of treatment, either the therapy is not effective or pharmaokinetic problems exist. Normalization of stratum corneum intercellular lipid depostion can be easily assessed with Nile Red staining and fluorescence microscopy (19).

Remittive treatments, such as PUVA, an IL-2 diphtheria toxin fusion protein, and UVB plus tar, completely normalize these parameters (3,8,9) (Fig. 2 and Table 8). Suppressive treatments, such as cyclosporin, topical calcitriol, and etretinate, do not consistently do

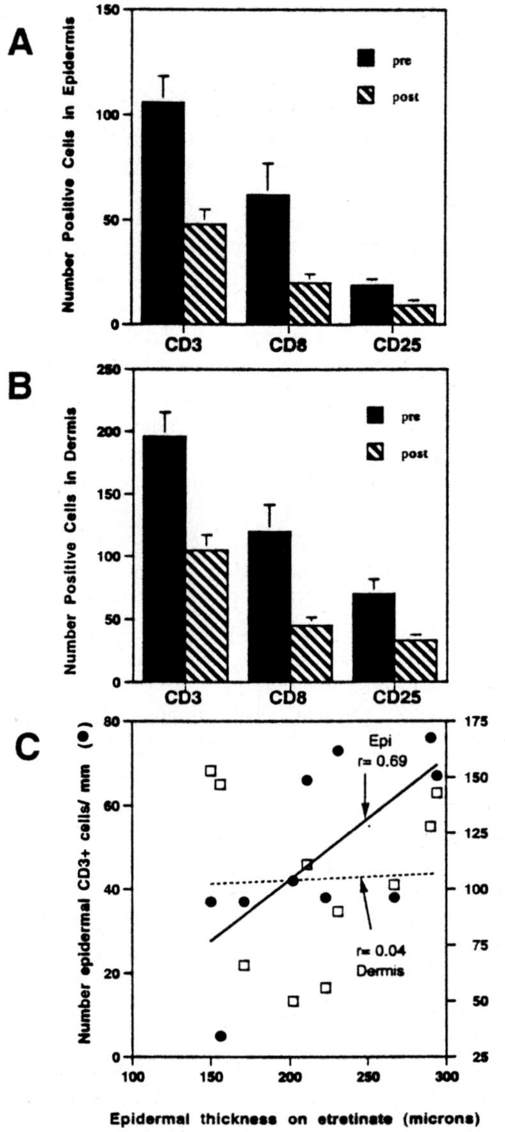

Figure 5 Quantitative analysis of T lymphocytes infiltrating untreated or etretinate-treated lesional psoriatic tissue. The number of cells reacting with antibodies to CD3, CD8, or CD25 has been measured separately for the epidermis (A) and the dermis (B). Bars are mean values for each cell type in all patients ± standard error. Cell numbers are expressed per image analysis field (1 mm of linear epidermal length). (C) Correlation for epidermal thickness versus the number of CD3+ T lymphocytes in the epidermis or in the dermis. Two correlation plots are superimposed. The solid circles show data points for epidermal CD3+ cell numbers and epidermal thickness measures, with the correlation plot illustrated by a solid line (r = 0.69). The open squares show data points for dermal CD3+ cell numbers and epidermal thickness measures, with the correlation plot illustrated by a dashed line (r = 0.04). (Reproduced from Ref. 19 by permission of the Editor.)

so (19) (Fig. 3 and Table 8). Immune activation can be simply assessed by looking for numbers of IL-2-receptor-positive (presumably activated) T lymphocytes and numbers of CD3+, CD4+, and CD8+ T cells. Interferon-gamma presence can be inferred by demonstration of keratinocyte HLA-DR or ICAM-1 expression. Cellular trafficking and endothelial cell proliferation can be assessed by ICAM-1 expression. Neutrophil microabcesses can be easily assessed using routine staining techniques. Remittive antipsoriasis therapies such as PUVA, UVB plus tar, and an IL-2 diphtheria toxin fusion protein potently decrease immune activation (Fig. 4 and Table 8) (3,9,19). Interestingly, the observed shorter length of remission seen in patients treated with UVB plus tar compared with those treated with PUVA (Fig. 1) may be due to the large decrease (approximately 95%) in T-cell numbers in the epidermis but not the dermis of UVB-plus-tar-treated patients. In contrast, large decreases in T-cell number were observed in both the epidermis and dermis of PUVA-treated patients (8,9). The differences in dermal T-cell response are due to the deeper penetration of UVA as compared with UVB irradiation. Suppressive treatments such as cyclosporin, etretinate, and topical calcitriol only mildly or moderately decrease immune activation (Fig. 5 and Table 8) (18–20). Thus one can refine the definition of a *remittive* treatment for psoriasis as one that results in complete histological normalization of immune activation, keratinocyte proliferation, and differentiation and is associated with a long-lived remission in the absence of continuous treatment. In contrast, a *suppressive* treatment for psoriasis is one that does *not consistently* normalize keratinocyte proliferation and differentiation, only moderately decreases immune activation, and requires continuous treatment to maintain clearing.

OPTIMISM FOR THE FUTURE

With the recognition of the immune basis of psoriasis, a potentially huge repertoire of therapeutic possibilities has become available for consideration, some of which are mentioned earlier in this article. Instead of being isolated in keratinocyte-based, dermatological therapies, psoriasis now can fully share immunomodulating drugs with transplantation, oncology, and autoimmunity. Additionally, vaccination-based treatments become therapeutic options to test. Because of the high incidence of moderate-to-severe disease, accessibility of skin, and the availability of validated pharmacodynamic markers, psoriasis becomes the *first* disease to investigate with drugs that interfere with Th1 cellular immunity. The recent scientific advances in understanding the pathogenesis of psoriasis and in biotechnology suggest an optimistic future in drug development for psoriasis.

REFERENCES

1. Weinstein, G.D., and Krueger, J.G. (1993). An overview of psoriasis. In *Therapy of Moderate-to-Severe Psoriasis*. G.D. Weinstein and A.B. Gottlieb (Eds.). National Psoriasis Foundation, Portland, OR, pp. 1–22.
2. *Dermatology Perspectives 6*. (1986). National Psoriasis Foundation, Portland, Oregon.
3. Gottlieb, S.L., Gilleaudeau, P., Johnson, R., Estes, L., Woodworth, T.G., Gottlieb, A.B., and Krueger, J.G. (1995). Response to psoriasis to a lymphocyte-selective toxin (DAB389IL-2) suggests a primary immune, but not keratinocyte, pathogenic basis. *Nature Med.* 1:442–447.
4. Gottlieb, A.B. (1988). Immunologic mechanisms in psoriasis. *J. Am. Acad. Dermatol.* 18:1376–1380.
5. Leung, D.Y., Walsh, P., Giorno, R., and Norris, D.A. (1993). A potential role for superantigens in the pathogenesis of psoriasis. *J. Invest. Dermatol.* 100: 225–228.
6. Funk, J., Langeland, T., Schrumpf, E., and Hanssen, L.E. (1991). Psoriasis induced by interferon-alpha. *Br. J. Dermatol.* 125:463–465.
7. Fierlbeck, G., Rassner, G., and Muller, C. (1990). Psoriasis induced at the injection site of recombinant interferon gamma. Results of immunohistologic investigations. *Arch. Dermatol.* 126:351–355.
8. Krueger, J.G., Wolfe, J.T., Nabeya, R.T., Vallat, V.P., Gilleaudeau, P., Heftler, N.S., Austin, L.M., and Gottlieb, A.B. (1995). Successful ultraviolet B treatment of psoriasis is accompanied by a reversal of keratinocyte pathology and by selective depletion of intraepidermal T cells. *J. Exp. Med.* 182:2057–2068.
9. Vallat, V.P., Gilleaudeau, P., Battat, L., Wolfe, J., Nabeya, R., Heftler, N., Hodak, E., Gottlieb, A.B., and Krueger, J.G. (1994). PUVA bath therapy strongly suppresses immunological and epidermal activation in psoriasis: a possible cellular basis for remittive therapy. *J. Exp. Med.* 180:283–296.
10. Thomson, A.W., Nalesnik, M., Abu-Elmagd, K., and Starzl, T.E. (1991). Influence of FK 506 on T lymphocytes, Langerhans cells and the expression of cytokine receptors and adhesion molecules in psoriatic skin lesions: a preliminary study. *Transplant. Proc.* 23: 3330–3331.
11. Weinshenker, B.G., Bass, B.H., Ebers, G.C., and Rice, G.P.A. (1989). Remission of psoriatic lesions with uromonab-CD3 (Orthoclone OKT3) treatment. *J. Am. Acad. Dermatol.* 20:1132–1133.
12. Ellis, C.N., Fradin, M.S., Messana, J.M., Brown, M.D., Siegel, M.T., Hartley, A.H., Rocher, L.L., Wheeler, S., Hamilton, T.A., Parish, T.G., Ellis-Madu, M., Duell, E., Annesley, T.M., Cooper, K.D., and Voorhees, J.J. (1991). Cyclosporine for plaque-type psoriasis. Results of a multidose, double-blind trial. *N. Engl. J. Med.* 324:277–284.
13. Bos, J.D., VanJoost, T., Powles, A.V., Meinardi, M.M.H.M., and Fry, L. (1989). Use of cyclosporin in psoriasis. *Lancet* 23:1500–1989.
14. Jeffes, W.M., III, McCullough, J.L., Pittelkow, M.R., McCormick, A., Almanzor, J., Liu, G., Dang, M., Voss, K., Voss, J., Schlotzhauer, A., and Weinstein, G.D. (1995). Methotrexate therapy of psoriasis: differential sensitivity of proliferating lymphoid and epithelial cells to the cytotoxic and growth-inhibitory effects of methotrexate. *J. Invest. Dermatol.* 104: 183–188.
15. Gottlieb, A.B., and Krueger, J.G. (1990). HLA region genes and immune activation in the pathogenesis of psoriasis. *Arch. Dermatol.* 126:1083–1086.
16. Mansbridge, J.N., and Knapp, A.M. (1987). Changes in keratinocyte maturation during wound healing. *J. Invest. Dermatol.* 89:253–263.
17. Kragballe, K., Gjertsen, B.T., de Hoop, D., Karlsmark, T., Van de Kerkhof, P.C.M., Larko, O., Nieboer, C., Roed-Petersen, J., Strand, A., and Tikjob, G. (1991). Double-blind, right/left comparison of calcipotriol and betamethasone valerate in treatment of psoriasis vulgaris. *Lancet* 337:193–196.
18. Lu, I., Gilleaudeau, P., McLane, J.A., Heftler, N., Kamber, M., Gottlieb, S., Krueger, J.G., and Gottlieb, A.B. (1996). Modulation of epidermal differentiation, tissue inflammation, and T-lymphocyte infiltration in psoriatic plaques by topical calcitriol. *J. Cutan. Pathol.* 23:419–434.
19. Gottlieb, S.L., Hayes, E., Gilleaudeau, P., Cardinale, I., Gottlieb, A.B., and Krueger, J.G. (1996). Etretinate promotes keratinocyte terminal differentiation and reduces T-cell infiltration in psoriatic epidermis. *J. Cutan. Pathol.* 23:404–418.
20. Gottlieb, A.B., Grossman, R.M., Khandke, L., Carter, D.M., Sehgal, P.B., Fu, S.M., Granelli-Piperno, A., Rivas, M., Barazani, L., and Krueger, J.G. (1992). Studies of the effect of cyclosporine in psoriasis in vivo: combined effects on activated T lymphocytes and epidermal regenerative maturation. *J. Invest. Dermatol.* 98:302–309.
21. Krueger, J.G., and Gottlieb, A.B. (1994). Cellular signalling in psoriasis: growth factors, cytokines and eicosanoids. In *Psoriasis*. L. Dubertret (Ed.). ISED Press, Brescie, Italy, pp. 18–28.
22. Krane, J.F., Murphy, D.P., Carter, D.M., and Krueger, J.G. (1991). Synergistic effects of epidermal growth factor (EGF) and insulin-like growth factor 1/somatomedin C (IGF-1) on keratinocyte proliferation may be

mediated by IGF-1 transmodulation of the EGF receptor. *J. Invest. Dermatol.* 96:419–424.
23. Krane, J.F., Gottlieb, A.B., Carter, D.M., and Krueger, J.G. (1992). The insulin-like growth factor 1 receptor is overexpressed in psoriatic epidermis, but is differentially regulated from the epidermal growth factor receptor. *J. Exp. Med.* 175:1081–1090.
24. Krueger, J.G., Liu, S., and Efatratiades, A. (1993). Targeted mutagenesis of the IGF-1 receptor suggests it is a critical pathway for normal epidermal differentiation and growth in vivo. *J. Invest. Dermatol.* 100:511 (abstract).
25. Gottlieb, A.B., Chang, C.K., Posnett, D.N., Fanelli, B., and Tam, J.P. (1988). Detection of transforming growth factor alpha in normal, malignant, and hyperproliferative human keratinocytes. *J. Exp. Med.* 167:670–675.
26. Elder, J.T., Fisher, G.J., Lindquist, P.B., Bennett, G.L., Pittelkow, M.R., Coffey, R.J., Ellingsworth, L., Derynck, R., and Voorhees, J.J. (1989) Overexpression of transforming growth factor alpha in psoriatic epidermis. *Science* 243:811–814.
27. Nanney, L.B., Stoscheck, C.M., Magid, M., and King, L.E., Jr. (1986). Altered ^{125}I epidermal growth factor binding and receptor distribution in psoriasis. *J. Invest. Dermatol.* 86:260–265.
28. Vassar, R., and Fuchs, E. (1991). Transgenic mice provide new insights into the role of TGF-alpha during epidermal development and differentiation. *Genes Dev.* 5:714–727.
29. Luettceke, N.C., Qiu, T.H., Peiffer, R.L., Oliver, P., Smithies, O., and Lee, D.C. (1993). TGF alpha deficiency results in hair follicle and eye abnormalities in targeted and waved-1 mice. *Cell* 73:263–278.
30. Mann, G.B., Fowler, K.J., Gabriel, A., Nice, E.C., Williams, R.L., and Dunn, A.R. (1993). Mice with a null mutation of the TGF-alpha gene have abnormal skin architecture, wavy hair, and curly whiskers and often develop corneal inflammation. *Cell* 73:249–261.
31. Nanney, L.B., Yates, R.A., and King, L.E., Jr. (1992). Modulation of epidermal growth factor receptors in psoriatic lesions during treatment with topical EGF. *J. Invest. Dermatol.* 98:296–301.
32. Carpenter, G., and Cohen, S. (1979). Epidermal growth factor. *Annu. Rev. Biochem.* 48:193–216.
33. Yoshizaki, K., Nishimoto, N., Matsumoto, K., Tagoh, H., Taga, T., Deguchi, Y., Kuritani, T., Hirano, T., Hashimoto, K., Okada, N., and Kishimoto, T. (1990). Interleukin 6 and expression of its receptor on epidermal keratinocytes. *Cytokine* 2:381–387.
34. Grossman, R.M., Krueger, J., Yourish, D., Granelli-Piperno, A., Murphy, D.P., May, L.T., Kupper, T.S., Sehgal, P.B., and Gottlieb, A.B. (1989). Interleukin-6 (IL-6) is expressed in high levels in psoriatic skin and stimulates proliferation of cultured human keratinocytes. *Proc. Natl. Acad. Sci. U.S.A.* 86:6367–6371.
35. Ohta, Y., Katayama, I., Funato, T., Yokozeki, H., Nishiyama, S., Hirano, T., Kishimoto, T., and Nishioka, K. (1991). In situ expression of messenger RNA of interleukin-1 and interleukin-6 in psoriasis: interleukin-6 involved in formation of psoriatic lesions. *Arch. Dermatol. Res.* 283:351–356.
36. Oxholm, A., Oxholm, P., Staberg, B., and Benditzen, K. (1989). Interleukin-6 in the epidermis of patients with psoriasis before and during PUVA treatment. *Acta Derm. Venereol. (Stockh.)* 69:195–199.
37. Gottlieb, A.B., Lifshitz, B., Fu, S.M., Staiano-Coico, L., Wang, C.Y., and Carter, D.M. (1986). Expression of HLA-DR molecules by keratinocytes and presence of Langerhans cells in the dermal infiltrate of active psoriatic plaques. *J. Exp. Med.* 164:1013–1028.
38. Gottlieb, A.B., and Krueger, J.G. (1994). The role of activated T lymphocytes in the pathogenesis of psoriasis, pp. 63–71. In *Psoriasis*, L. Dubertret (Ed.). ISED Press, Brescie, Italy.
39. Bos, J.D., and Krieg, S.R. (1985). Psoriasis infiltrating cell immunophenotype: changes induced by PUVA or corticosteroid treatment in T-cell subsets, Langerhans cells and interdigitating cells. *Acta Derm. Venereol.* 65: 390–397.
40. Chang, J.C., Smith, L.R., Froning, K.J., Schwabe, B.J., Laxer, J.A., Caralli, L.L., Kurland, H.H., Karasek, M.A., Wilkinson, D.I., Carlo, D.J., and Brostoff, S.W. (1995). CD8+ T cells in psoriatic lesions preferentially use T-cell receptor V beta 3 and/or V beta 13.1 genes. *Proc. Natl. Acad. Sci. U.S.A.* 91:9282–9286.
41. Menssen, A., Rommler, P., Vollmer, S., Schendel, D., Albert, E., Guertler, L., Riethmueller, G., and Prinz, J.C. (1995). Evidence for an antigen-specific cellular immune response in skin lesions of patients with psoriasis vulgaris. *J. Immunol.* 155:4078–4083.
42. McNutt, N.S., Hsu, A., Sadick, N.S., and Kaplan, M.H. (1989). Psoriasiform dermatitis of AIDS. *J. Cutan. Pathol.* 16:317 (abstract).
43. Gottlieb, A.B., Luster, A.D., Posnett, D.N., and Carter, D.M. (1988). Detection of a gamma-interferon-induced protein (IP-10) in psoriatic plaques. *J. Exp. Med.* 168: 941–948.
44. Livden, J.K., Nilsen, R., Bjerke, J.R., and Matre, R. (1989). In situ localization of interferons in psoriatic lesions. *Arch. Dermatol. Res.* 281:392–397.
45. Singer, K.H., Tuck, D.T., Sampson, H.A., and Hall, R.P. (1989). Epidermal keratinocytes express the adhesion molecule intercellular adhesion molecule-1 in inflammatory dermatoses. *J. Invest. Dermatol.* 92: 746–750.
46. Nickoloff, B.J. (1991). The cytokine network in psoriasis. *Arch. Dermatol.* 127:871–884.
47. Sticherling, M., Bornscheuer, E., Schroder, J.M., and Christophers, E. (1991). Localization of neutrophil-activating peptide-1/interleukin-8-immunoreactivity in

normal and psoriatic skin. *J. Invest. Dermatol.* 96: 26–30.

48. Rittenhouse-Diakun, K., vanLeengoed, H., Morgan, J., Hryhorenko, E., Paszkiewicz, G., Whitaker, J.E., and Oseroff, A.R. (1995). The role of transferrin receptor (CD71) in photodynamic therapy of activated and malignant lymphocytes using the heme precursor delta-aminolevulinic acid (ALA). *Photochem. Photobiol.* 61: 523–528.
49. Mak, V.H.W. (1995). Anti-TNF compounds as novel topical treatment for psoriasis. In *Psoriasis: Latest Advances in Understanding and Therapeutic Development.* C. Marie and K.L. Roderiques (Eds.). International Business Communications, Southborough, MA.
50. Robinson, M., and Rodriques, K.L. (1995). An engineered human antibody to E-selection for use in the treatment of psoriasis. In *Psoriasis: Latest Advances in Understanding and Therapeutic Development.* C. Marie and K.L. Rodrigues (Eds.). International Business Communications, Southborough, MA.
51. Bennett, C.F. (1995). Oligonucleotide-based therapeutics for the treatment of psoriasis. In *Psoriasis: Latest Advances in Understanding and Therapeutic Development.* C. Marie and K.L. Rodrigues (Eds.). International Business Communications, Southborough, MA.
52. Kragballe, K. (1989). Treatment of psoriasis by the topical application of the novel cholecalciferol analogue calcipotriol (MC 903). *Arch. Dermatol.* 125: 1647–1652.
53. Higgs, J.B., Zeldes, W., Kozarsky, K., Schteingart, M., Kan, L., Bohlke, P., Krieger, K., Davis, W., and Fox, D.A. (1988). A novel pathway of human T lymphocyte activation. Identification by monolonal antibody generated against a rheumatoid synovial T cell line. *J. Immunol.* 140:3758–3765.
54. Kaneko, F., Suzuki, M., Takiguchi, Y., Itoh, N., and Minagawa, T. (1990). Immunohistopathologic studies in the development of psoriatic lesion influenced by gamma-interferon and the producing cells. *J. Dermatol. Sci.* 1:425–434.
55. Baker, B.S., and Fry, L. (1992). The immunology of psoriasis. *Br. J. Dermatol.* 126:1–9.
56. Cooper, K.D. (1990). Psoriasis: leukocytes an cytokines. *Dermatol. Clini.* 8:737–745.
57. Oxholm, A., Oxholm, P., Staberg, B., and Bendtzen, K. (1989). Expression of interleukin-6-like molecules and tumour necrosis factor after topical treatment of psoriasis with a new vitamin D analogue (MC 903). *Acta Derm. Venereol.* 69:385–390.
58. Houssiau, F.A., Devogelaer, J., VanDamme, J., NagantdeDeuxchaisnes, C., and VanSnick, J. (1988). Interleukin-6 in synovial fluid and serum of patients with rheumatoid arthritis and other inflammatory arthridtides. *Arthritis Rheum.* 31:784–788.
59. Haynes, B.F., Grover, B.J., Whichard, L.P., Hale, L.P., Nunley, J.A., McCollum, D.E., and Singer, K.H. (1988). Synovial microenvironment T cell interactions. Human T cells bind to fibroblast-like synovial cells in vitro. *Arthritis Rheum.* 31:947–955.
60. Tugwell, P., Bombardier, C., Gent, M., Bennett, K., Ludwin, D., Grace, E., Buchanan, W.W., Gensen, W.G., Bellamy, N., Murphy, G.F., and vonGraffenried, B. (1987). Low dose cyclosporine in rheumatoid arthritis: a pilot study. *J. Rheumatol.* 14:1108–1114.
61. Miyasaka, N., Sato, K., Goto, M., Sasano, M., Natsuyama, M., Inoue, K., and Nishioka, K. (1988). Augmented interleukin-1 production and HLA-DR expression in the synovium of rheumatoid arthritis patients. Possible involvement in joint destruction. *Arthritis Rheum.* 31:480–486.
62. Holoshitz, J., Koning, F., Coligan, J.E., DeBruyn, J., and Strober, S. (1989). Isolation of CD4-CD8- mycobacteria-reactive T lymphocyte clones from rheumatoid arthritis synovial fluid. *Nature* 339:226–229.
63. Bucala, R., Richlin, C., Winchester, R., and Cerami, A. (1991). Constitutive production of inflammatory and mitogenic cytokines by rheumatoid synovial fibroblasts. *J. Exp. Med.* 173:569–574.
64. Holt, I., Cooper, R.G., and Hopkins, S.J. (1991). Relationships between local inflammation, interleukin-6 concentration and the acute phase protein response in arthritis patients. *Eur. J. Clin. Invest.* 21:479–484.
65. Guerne, P.A., Zuraw, B.L., Vaughan, J.H., Carson, D.A., and Lotz, M. (1989). Synovium as a source of interleukin 6 in vitro. Contribution to local and systemic manifestations of arthritis. *J. Clin. Invest.* 83: 585–592.
66. DeBenedetti, F., Massa, M., Robbioni, P., Ravelli, A., Burgio, G.R., and Martini, A. (1991). Correlation of serum interleukin-6 levels with joint involvement and thrombocytosis in systemic rheumatoid arthritis. *Arthritis Rheum.* 34:1158–1163.
67. Miyasaka, N., Sato, K., Hashimoto, J., Kohsaka, H., Yamamoto, K., Goto, M., Inoue, K., Matsuda, T., Kirano, T., and Kishimoto, T. (1989). Constitutive production of interleukin6/B cell stimulatory factor-2 from inflammatory synovium. *Clin. Immunol. Immunopathol.* 52:238–247.
68. Rosenbaum, J.T., Cugnini, R., Tara, D.C., Hefeneider, S., and Ansel, J.C. (1992). Production and modulation of interleukin 6 synthesis by synoviocytes derived from patients with arthritic disease. *Ann. Rheum. Dis.* 51: 198–202.
69. Wood, N.C., Symons, J.A., Dickens, E., and Duff, G.W. (1992). In situ hybridization of IL-6 in rheumatoid arthritis. *Clin. Exp. Immunol.* 87:183–189.
70. Field, M., Chu, C., Feldmann, M., and Maini, R.N. (1991). Interleukin-6 localization in the synovial membrane in rheumatoid arthritis. *Rheumtol. Int.* 11: 45–50.
71. Sawada, T., Hirohata, S., Inoue, T., and Ito, K. (1991). Correlation between rheumatoid factor and IL-6 activ-

ity in synovial fluids from patients with rheumatoid arthritis. *Clin. Exp. Rheumatol.* 9:363–368.

72. Tan, P.L., Farmiloe, S., Yeoman, S., and Watson, J.D. (1990). Expression of the interleukin 6 gene in rheumatoid synovial fibroblasts. *J. Rheumatol.* 17:1608–1612.
73. Hovdenes, J., Kvien, T.K., and Hovdenes, A.B. (1990). Il-6 in synovial fluids, plasma and supernatants from cultured cells of patients with rheumatoid arthritis and other inflammatory arthritides. *Scand. J. Rheumatol.* 19:177–182.
74. Gerritsen, M.J.P., Boezeman, J.B.M., Van Vlijmen-Willems, I.M.J.J., and Van de Kerkhof, P.C.M. (1994). The effect of tacalcitol (1,24(OH)2D3 on cutaneous inflammation, epidermal proliferation and keratinization in psoriasis: a placebo-controlled, double-blind study. *Br. J. Dermatol.* 131:57–63.
75. Baker, B.S., Griffiths, C.E.M., Lambert, S., Powles, A.V., Leonard, J.N., Valdimarsson, H., and Fry, L. (1987). The effects of cyclosporin A on T lymphocyte and dendritic cell sub-populations in psoriasis. *Br. J. Dermatol.* 116:503–510.
76. Frederiksson, T., and Pettersson, U. (1978). Severe psoriasis oral therapy with a new retinoid. *Dermatologica* 157:238–244.
77. Baker, B., Valdimarsson, H., Leonard, J.N., Griffiths, C.E.M., and Fry, L. (1984). The action of topical steroids, dithranol, and PUVA on T lymphocytes and dendritic cells in psoriasis. *Br. J. Dermatol.* 111:702.

30

Dithranol (Anthralin)

Stefan Kraft
Ludwig Maximilians University, Munich, Germany

Howard I. Maibach
University of California School of Medicine, San Francisco, California

Braham Shroot
Centre International de Recherches Dermatologiques, Sophia-Antipolis, France

Since Squire reported in 1877 (1) that the yellow powder extract from *Andera araroba*, formally used as a folk remedy for the treatment of mycoses of the skin, had a therapeutic effect in psoriasis, hydroxyanthracene derivatives have held an important place in the treatment of the disease. The active principle of Goa powder, as this extract was called, is chrysarobin, but during World War I, supply became scarce and a synthetic substitute, 1,8-dihydroxy-9-anthrone, anthralin or dithranol (see Fig. 1) was found. The substances differ by a methyl group located at C3 in chrysarobin and replaced by hydrogen in dithranol. Its biochemistry and pharmacology at the molecular, cellular, and clinical level are discussed here. The reader is referred to the *Proceedings of the Anthralin Symposium* for an earlier overview (2). The pivotal questions in dithranol research are: Is dithranol itself the active species, are the side effects of staining and irritation of uninvolved skin associated with this treatment essential for clinical efficacy, and what is its mode of action?

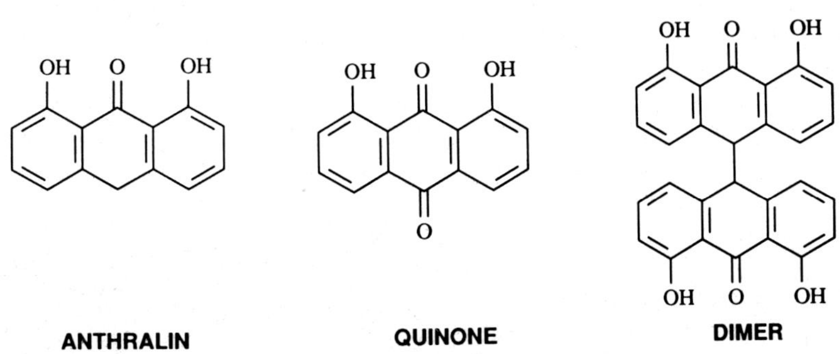

Figure 1 Chemical structures of dithranol, quinone, and dimer.

CHEMISTRY

The keynote of the chemical behavior of dithranol and related drugs is instability. That one of the major drawbacks of dithranol is shared by its forerunner, chrysarobin, is not surprising, since both molecules contain readily oxidizable centers at C10. Many chemical studies have been performed in this series, but the 1,8-dihydroxyanthraquinone (danthrone) and the dimeric 1,8,1′8′-tetrahydroxydianthrone (bianthrone) (see Fig. 1) are the only oxidation products that have been chemically characterized. Since dithranol, the quinone, and the dimer are, respectively, yellow, orange, and pale yellow, the violet brown staining of the skin and clothes associated with dithranol use is related to the uncharacterized products arising from extensive oxidation. These are referred to as dithranol-brown. As early as 1916, Unna (3) showed that oxidation of dithranol resulted in the production of hydrogen peroxide, which in turn oxidized unsaturated fatty acids in the skin. Muller and Kappus (4) pointed out the role of the hydroxyl radical OH as a secondary reaction product. This radical is generated from the iron-catalyzed degradation of hydrogen peroxide, which in turn is formed by interaction of the dithranol anion and oxygen (see Fig. 2). The therapeutic and/or toxic effects of dithranol are attributed to this sequence of redox reactions, and it is probable that the metabolic end products have little or no intrinsic biological action. The apparent pK of dithranol is 9.4: thus it is unlikely that the dithranol anion would be formed in vivo. Dithranol-containing radical species have been detected by electron spin resonance spectroscopy in pig skin (5,6). It is, however, conceivable that it is the unreactive and insoluble nature of these end products that explains the safe and effective topical use of the drug.

MODE OF ACTION

Extensive studies have been performed in this area. There is no single mode of action, but some of the major targets seen from different scientific viewpoints are the following:

1. Glucose-6-phosphate dehydrogenase
2. DNA synthesis, gene expression, cell growth and differentiation
3. Mitochondrial respiration
4. Molecules/cells involved in inflammatory processes

See Table 1 for a brief overview.

Glucose-6-Phosphate Dehydrogenase

Dithranol was originally thought to inhibit glucose-6-phosphate dehydrogenase (G6-PDH), an enzyme within the pentose phosphate shunt of the glycolytic pathway. The levels of this enzyme are elevated in psoriasis (7), and they return to baseline values following treatment of psoriatic lesions with dithranol (8). Raab and Gmeiner (9) indicated that ultraviolet (UV) irradiation of dithranol in dimethylformamide solution led to the production of highly potent inhibitors of G6-PDH, whose action was apparently modulated by the addition of proteins such as albumin (10). By careful selection of the experimental conditions, Cavey et al. (11) proved that dithranol itself as well as the quinone and the dimer are only weak inhibitors of the enzyme. Recent studies suggest that this inhibition is due to active oxygen species—especially the superoxide anion—resulting from dithranol oxidation (12).

Table 1 Selection of Dithranol Targets

Inflammation	1. Inhibition of 12-lipoxygenase (12-HETE synthesis) 2. Activation of transcription factor NF-kappa B 3. ROS release and chemotaxis of PMNL 4. Langerhans cells: ultrastructural changes, decreased ATPase activity and decreased density in treated skin
Mitochondrial respiration	1. Inhibition of glutamine metabolism 2. Inhibition of terminal reactions between ubiquinone pool and cytochrome oxidase 3. Ultrastructural changes
Keratinocyte proliferation	1. Down-regulation of TGF-alpha and EGF-receptor expression 2. Hyperproliferation of normal skin
Keratinocyte differentiation	1. Normalization of keratin expression
Other targets (biochemical level)	1. DNA synthesis (degradation of DNA sugar, modification of bases, enhancement of p53 expression) 2. Glucose-6-phosphate dehydrogenase 3. Tyrosine phosphorylation

DNA Synthesis, Gene Expression, Cell Growth, and Differentiation

Dithranol, its 10-acetyl analogue, as well as its dimer, completely inhibit cell growth and thymidine incorporation in cultured human fibroblasts at concentrations ranging from 0.1 to 1.0 μM. Except for the dimer, higher concentrations of these compounds (2–10 μM) cause cell destruction, suggesting a multiphasic cytotoxic process. The cytotoxic activity, as estimated by observing detachment of cultured fibroblasts, is reflected in the fact that dithranol treatment strongly decreased cell respiration, fermentation, and heat production as measured by Raab (13,14) and Pätel (15), respectively. Hsieh and Acosta (15a) demonstrated comparable effects in a model using primary cultures of rat epidermal keratinocytes. In contrast to the above-mentioned compounds, 1,8-dihydroxyanthraquinone had no effect at concentrations as high as 10 μM (16).

Recent experiments showed that dithranol reduced the expression of transforming growth factor-α and its receptor, the epidermal growth factor (EGF) receptor in cultured normal human keratinocytes, which are overexpressed in psoriasis (16a–e). In addition, dithranol also reduced the binding of EGF and insulin-like growth factor-I (IGF-1) to its receptors (see Fig. 2). The drug also acts at the level of tyrosine phosphorylation (16f).

Dithranol inhibits both DNA replication and repair synthesis, although it does not appear to form adducts with DNA in cultured human cells that can be repaired by an excision repair process (17). A direct interaction between dithranol and DNA as proposed initially by Swanbeck and Tyresson (18) was contested by both Caron et al. (19) and Sa e Melo et al. (20). Recently, Müller and Gürster (20a) demonstrated the ability of dithranol to degrade DNA sugar through the action of hydroxyl radicals. Treatment of DNA with dithranol resulted in a significant enhancement of DNA bases that were modified in a way that is typical for hydroxyl radicals (20b). Dithranol at concentrations of 1 μg/μl increases the levels of the tumor suppressor gene p53 as a marker for direct DNA damage at both the transcriptional and the translational level in human skin in vivo (20c).

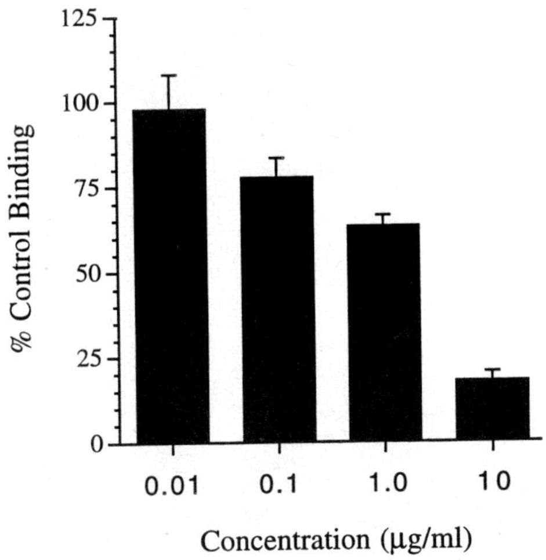

Figure 2 Route of dithranol auto-oxidation. (Adapted from Ref. 4.)

In the hairless mouse, topical application of a single dose of dithranol resulted in depression of the mitotic index and DNA synthesis (21). When 0.1% solutions of dithranol were repeatedly applied to the mouse tail over 10 days, a significant decrease in DNA synthesis was observed. In the same experiment a global reduction in protein synthesis was reported. Marked epidermal hyperplasia was noted from the third day of treatment. Importantly, by observing the presence of a continuous granular layer, these authors conclude that dithranol would induce orthokeratotic differentiation of the previously parakeratotic sections of the mouse tail epidermis (22).

This concept was undermined by newer data:

First, de Zwart et al. (22a) showed that dithranol applied to normal human skin induced epidermal hyperproliferation as measured in immunohistochemical studies with antibodies against proliferation markers. However, it remains unclear whether this effect is due to its mechanism of action or to irritation.

Second, Holland et al. (22b) demonstrated that dithranol applied to psoriatic plaques normalized levels of the differentiation markers keratin 1, 2, 16, and 18 in keratinocytes.

The skin tumor promotion caused by 12-*O*-tetradecanoylphorbol-13-acetate (TPA) was reduced by dithranol, as estimated by the reduction in the induction of ornithine decarboxylase (ODC), the [^{3}H]thymidine incorporation into DNA, and the incidence of tumors in mouse skin (23).

Mitochondrial Respiration

To determine the sensitivity of various cellular targets to dithranol, Reichert et al. (24) measured in the same experiment DNA synthesis (by thymidine incorporation), cytosolic enzyme activity, and mitochondrial respiration. These latter actions were estimated by monitoring $^{14}CO_2$ evolution from labeled glucose or glutamine, which reflect cytosolic oxidation processes and mitochondrial respiration, respectively. In cell culture, mitochondrial respiration was the most sensitive target (see Fig. 3). By electron microscopy it was revealed that after 15 min of contact with dithranol, the mitochondria of keratinocytes in culture increased in size and the cristae were less well defined. Fuchs et al. (24 a,b) and Salet et al. (24c) contributed to a better understanding of how dithranol affects mitochondrial respiration. In isolated mitochondria it inhibits ATP synthase activity, but not ATPase, stops the ADP/ATP translocation, and depletes mitochondria of ATP. Oxidative phosphorylation and uncoupler-induced respiratory stimulation is inhibited by dithranol in the presence of substrates, suggesting that it exerts its inhibitory action in the terminal reactions between the ubiquinone pool and cytochrome oxidase. They also observed a reduction of ubiquinones and cytochromes by dithranol, suggesting that it acts as an electron donor to the inner mitochondrial membrane in its oxidation process forming reactive oxygen species. The dimer is a much weaker inhibitor of mitochondrial functions and anthraquinone is almost inactive.

Earler publications also described ultrastructural changes in the mitochondria of psoriatic skin treated with dithranol (25). Such alterations are followed by inhibition of cell respiration (15,26–28). It is likely that other cellular targets are prone to dithranol's reductive power. Evidence has been presented to suggest that the Langerhans cell (LC) is the most sensitive cellular target (29,29a,b): only mild irritation of healthy skin results in strongly swollen mitochondria with broken cristae and sometimes by forming branched and circular Birbeck granules more often with continuity to the LC cytomembrane.

In summary, therefore, dithranol may be considered an inhibitor of cell respiration. The mitochondrial membrane can be imagined as a template for the oxidation that occurs, and as a result dithranol is irreversibly destroyed and the mitochondria inactivated.

Molecules/Cells Involved in Inflammatory Processes

Dithranol has been shown to modulate certain functions of polymorphonuclear leukocytes (PMNLs) in vitro, although discrepancies can be found in the literature.

Depending on experimental conditions, dithranol could enhance stimulus-evoked active oxygen production (30) or, on the contrary, inhibit this production (31,32). However, Anderson (32a) showed increased oxygen uptake and luminol-enhanced chemoluminescence (LECL) in human neutrophils with high concentrations of dithranol. Low doses had no direct effect on LECL, but increased the LECL responses of cells

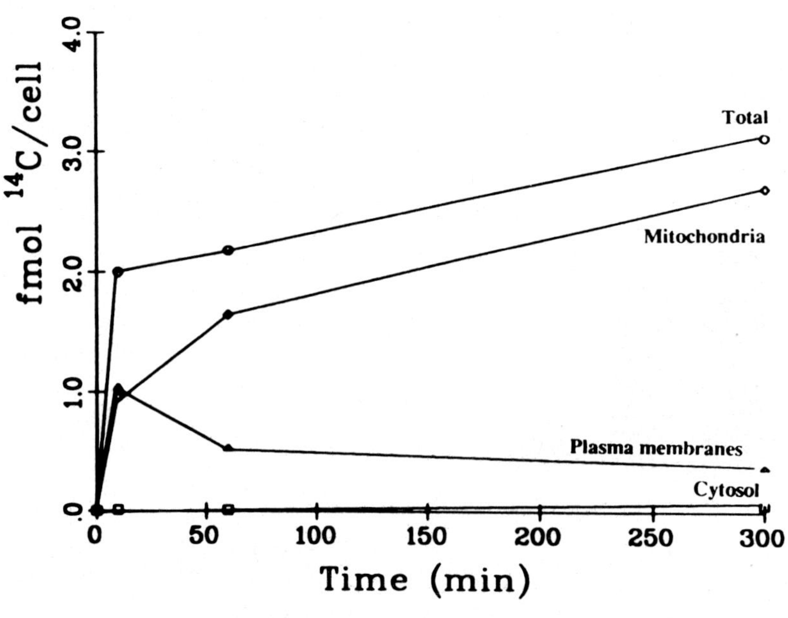

Figure 3 Subcellular distribution of ^{14}C-dithranol in K14 keratinocytes. (Adapted from Ref. 24.)

subsequently stimulated with calcium ionophore and opsonized zymosan. Hegemann et al. (32b) showed an induction of reactive oxygen species (ROS) by dithranol in unstimulated PMNLs. But when the cells were incubated with the drug 46 min before a zymosan or PMA stimulus, the release of ROS was inhibited. They also found inhibition of protein kinase C by dithranol, a key enzyme for the release of ROS (32c–e) and cell proliferation.

Lysosomal enzyme release by activated PMNLs remains unchanged after dithranol treatment (32), or it may be slightly enhanced (30). In contrast, PMNL migration in vitro is inhibited (31,32) by concentrations of the drug likely to be encountered in the skin (33).

Schröder (34) demonstrated that leukotriene production was inhibited in human neutrophils; however, dithranol at its upper limit of solubility (10 μM) was unable to modulate human PMNL 5-lipoxygenase activity (31). Bedord et al. (34a) and Müller and Gawlik (34b) could demonstrate a selective inhibition of epidermal 12-lipoxygenase in vitro. The major lipoxygenase product in the skin is known to be 12-hydroxy-5,8,10,14-eicosatetraenoic acid (12-HETE) (34c), which is, together with free arachidonic acid, dramatically up-regulated in psoriatic skin (34d) and thought to be involved in regulation of cutaneous microcirculation, growth promotion, immune regulation, and chemotaxis for leukocytes, fibroblasts, and keratinocytes (34e,f). Recent work by Müller and Gawlik (34g) demonstrated that reactive oxygen species may be involved in that effect of dithranol: In mouse epidermal homogenate the antioxidants 2,6-di-tert-butyl-4-methylphenol (BHT) or β-carotene or the hydroxyl radical scavenger sodium benzoate protected against dithranol-induced 12-lipoxygenase inhibition (see Fig. 4). The antioxidant enzymes superoxide dismutase and catalase also had a partially preventive effect. But it remains unclear which molecule of the reactive oxygen species generated by dithranol oxidation is responsible for the inhibition of 12-lipoxygenase. In addition, dithranol has been shown to down-regulate the receptor for 12-HETE in the human epidermal cell line SCL-II (34h).

Mrowietz et al. (34i) showed that dithranol also affected proinflammatory activities of human monocytes: It inhibited superoxide-anion generation and enzyme degranulation at low concentrations (0.02 μg/ml), but chemotactic migration was only affected with high doses of the drug (10 μg/ml).

In addition, dithranol reduced the density of CD1a+ Langerhans cells, which are involved in many inflammatory processes in the skin, after application

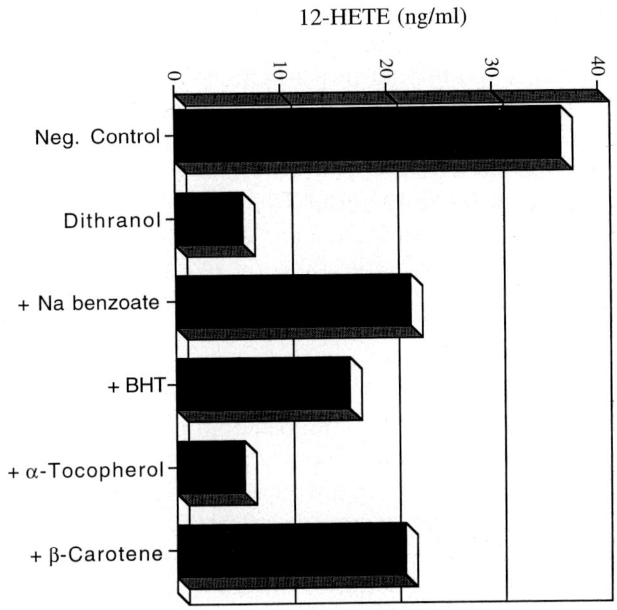

Figure 4 Effects of antioxidants and oxygen radical scavengers on dithranol-induced 12-LO inhibition (34g).

on mouse skin (34j) and ATPase activity on these cells (34k).

Recently Schmidt et al. (34l) made the interesting observation that dithranol induced the activation of the transcription factor NF-κB, known to activate inflammatory genes like cytokines, hemopoietic growth factors, adhesion molecules, and others in response to reactive oxygen species (34m–o), in murine keratinocytes. They suggested that this activation is due to reactive oxygen species, because it could be inhibited by the antioxidants *N*-acetyl-L-cysteine and pyrrolidinedithiocarbamate and is significantly reduced in cells overexpressing catalase.

PHARMACOKINETICS

In Vitro and In Vivo Studies on Human Skin

Qualitative data have been presented to support the presence of free dithranol when applied to human skin. Following topical application of the drug in acetone, Sa e Melo et al. (20) subjected human blister roofs to spectrophotometric analysis; even after 24 hr, some free dithranol was present.

Following topical application of tritium-labeled dithranol on normal skin in vitro, Schalla et al. (35)

found that the flux of radioactivity was related to the applied dose. It was estimated to be 70 pmol/cm^2/hr using 0.1% dithranol in petrolatum.

When the stratum corneum was removed prior to application by tape-stripping, the flux was increased twofold. At higher dose (1%), the flux through normal skin was increased 10-fold. In previous in vivo studies using urinary excretion data, Kammerau et al. (33) confirmed the reservoir function of stratum corneum using 0.1% tritiated dithranol in petrolatum. From autoradiography studies using tritiated dithranol applied to intact human skin in vitro, Selim et al. (36) showed an accumulation of radioactivity in the upper layers of epidermis, after 100-min penetration. This was confirmed by fluorescence microscopy in frozen sections biopsied after local application of dithranol. In this case, the upper layers of epidermis were stained brown. Schaefer, using the horizontal slicing technique (37), found that the concentrations of dithranol in the tape-stripped skin are decreased by a factor of 2–3 on removal of surplus using 10% soap solution, whereas 7–20 times reductions are possible in normal skin. Wang et al. (38) studied the permeation of dithranol in clinically involved and uninvolved psoriatic skin in vitro. They found that dithranol permeated faster through involved psoriatic skin than normal-appearing skin, but large individual variations were noted. They concluded that the stratum corneum is the rate-limiting barrier in normal skin, but in diseased skin the rate of release of the drug from its vehicle is rate-limiting. Wester et al. (39), using psoriatic plaque, observed no increase in penetration into diseased skin.

Newer studies did show an enhanced penetration of dithranol when applied in liposomes on normal skin (39a), but there were also reports on a diminished stability of the drug in liposomal phospholipids when compared to other formulations (39b).

Studies on Animal Skin

The fate in vivo of topically applied dithranol was investigated by Cavey et al. (40) in the skin of the hairless rat, using a specially designed drug-delivery system (polymeric disc). The disc was applied to intact skin as well as to skin that had an impaired barrier function (adhesive tape-stripped). The distribution of the drug was examined after continuous application (24 hr) or at selected times after short contact periods. The exposed skin was extracted with diisopropylether and free dithranol, its dimer and quinone assayed by quantitative HPLC analysis. The incorporation of trace amounts of [^{3}H]dithranol and [^{14}C]dithranol in the vehicle made it possible to quantify the fraction of penetrated drug that was insoluble in ether.

With continuous application to intact skin up to 24 hr (see Fig. 5), extractable dithranol rapidly reached a plateau level (15 min) and was concentrated in the stratum corneum. Substantial dimer formation occurred in both normal and stripped skin. Ether-insoluble material rapidly predominated over soluble material, especially when the stratum corneum was absent. However, on short-contact application (0.5–1.0 hr), ether-soluble material (dithranol in the stratum corneum) was quantitatively predominant in the intact skin. Removal of the disc vehicle after a short contact time resulted in the disappearance of dithranol from the skin. In normal skin, the drug was converted into ether-insoluble material. In the stripped skin, this insoluble fraction remained constant over the duration of the experiment (24 hr).

The insoluble nature of the dithranol breakdown products highlights the fact that it is only possible to wash out excess dithranol from the stratum corneum of noninvolved skin during the first hour or so following application. The time course of dithranol decomposition is relatively rapid both in vitro and in vivo; thus, as the compound permeates through the epidermis, the deposition of the insoluble products is concomitant with oxidation that occurs in the mitochondria of epidermal cells. Thus, absorption of dithranol through hyperproliferating involved skin is autolimiting. In contrast, the relative stability of the drug in the stratum corneum (40) provides adequate time to wash out the excess drug before it can permeate the viable epidermis and be oxidized to give rise to unwanted side effects in noninvolved skin.

These findings are of importance when we will consider the optimum vehicle for short-contact therapy with dithranol.

PHARMACOLOGY AND CLINICAL THERAPY

The fact that there are many treatment schedules for the management of chronic psoriasis with dithranol implies that none is optimal. From pharmacokinetic and clinical data it is obvious that once-daily treatment is sufficient. Despite this, side effects associated with dithranol therapy have been largely documented in the literature.

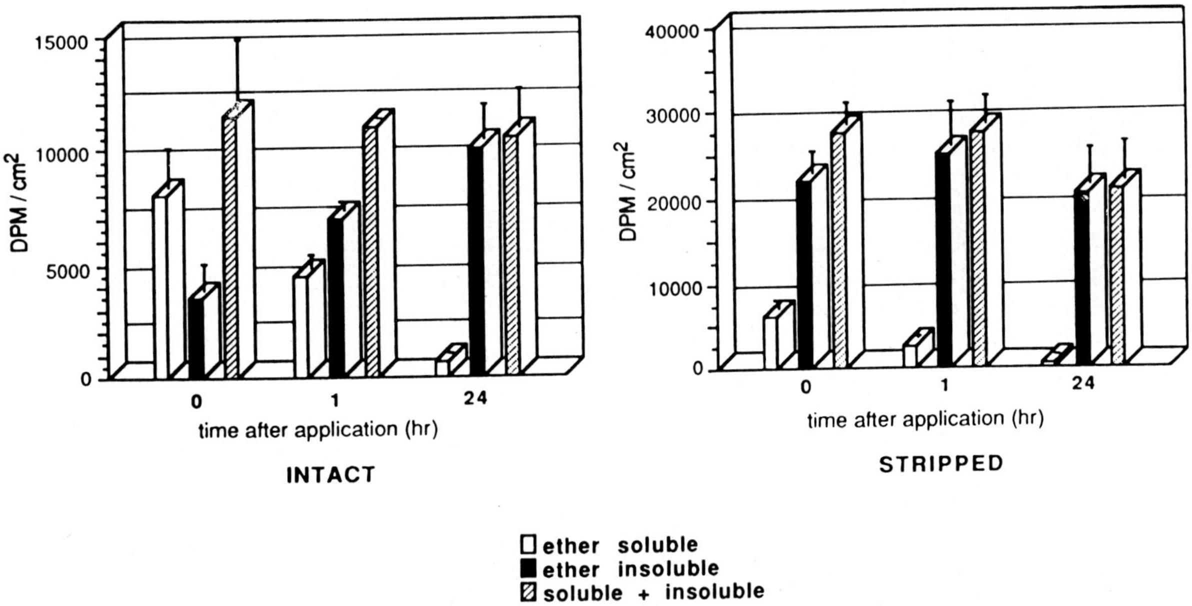

Figure 5 Topical application of [^{14}C]anthralin to the hairless rat: radioactivity dpm per cm^2 skin recovered from the skin as a function of time of application (40).

Adverse Effects

The acute side effects associated with dithranol therapy depend on the concentrations of the drug used. Therefore, the percentages for the undesired effects from the numerous studies vary in a wide range. The most important side effects are staining and irritation of the uninvolved skin. Particularly for the latter, there are individual variations in sensitivity. The erythema reaction peaks 3 days after the first single application, and is not related to the skin type relative to sunburn and tanning. Irritation of the uninvolved skin fades thereafter, even if one continues to apply the same dithranol concentration. This is the reason why the dithranol concentration in the vehicle can be increased according to the individual reaction in the more aggressive treatment regimens.

Rarely, bullae can indicate the development of a bullous pemphigoid or acrobullous eruption with dithranol and other antipsoriatic treatment (41,42). It was thought that irritation induced by dithranol was an essential feature of its mode of action, and in consequence its study would help to find more suitable therapy as well as new drugs. However, it seems that this inflammatory reaction is not a prerequisite for successful clinical responses. Marsden et al. (43) demonstrated that this burning was dose dependent, but this was not related to the therapeutic efficacy (44). Indeed, Mahrle (45) showed that concentrations had to be increased 10-fold for 1-hr applications to obtain a degree of skin inflammation similar to that obtained with a 24-hr application period, in agreement with Kingston and Lowe's study (46).

Furthermore, Paramsothy and Lawrence (47) have shown that there is less dithranol inflammation in psoriatic plaque skin than in neighboring uninvolved skin, as in the earlier results reported by Lawrence et al. (44). Recent results (22a) showing an epidermal hyperproliferation of normal skin after irritation with the drug, which is contrary to its effect on psoriatic lesions, are a contribution to the concept that irritation is not a necessary part in its mode of action. Westerhof et al. (48) showed that in another disease state, vitiligo, there was no statistically significant difference in dithranol irritation in normally pigmented and depigmented skin.

The minimal erythema dose (MED) of dithranol in noninvolved psoriatic skin was 0.012% w/w in chloroform under nonocculsive conditions (49). In petrolatum, the MED is somewhat higher (0.045%). The erythema will maximize in 48–72 hr and subsides after 4–5 days. Besides visual scaling erythema evolution can be followed by skin temperature measurements (50). Brandt and Mustakallio (51) showed that after daily topical applications of dithranol to psoriatic patients over a 3-week period, using a Finn chamber, erythema increased during the first week, and then decreased with further applications. This observation has been confirmed by Farkas et al. (51a), who could show a tolerance reaction in the hyperproliferative human cell line HaCaT after repeated treatment with dithranol: The inhibition of DNA and protein synthesis of the cells 24 hr after a single treatment with 0.3 μM dithranol was higher (38.2% and 32.3%) than in the cells that were pretreated with the same concentration 1 and 3 days before the last treatment (18.4% and 9.1%).

Kersey et al. (52) suggested that the inflammatory response to dithranol could be due to an oxidation metabolite formed by aryl hydrocarbon hydroxylase (AHH), which was induced in humans by dithranol (53). It is suggested that the dithranol irritative response is reduced in patients on cyclosporin therapy (54).

Former results have shown an increase of arachidonic acid and metabolite concentrations in the suction blister fluid of healthy volunteers (55,56) and minipigs (57), which are in one part in contrast to newer findings: an in vitro inhibition of 12-lipoxygenase (34a,b) that would lead to diminished levels of 12-HETE, but would of course not affect prostaglandin synthesis. One can suppose that the capacity of dithranol to produce free radicals, both in solution (58) and in the skin (5), can induce nonspecific peroxidation of arachidonic acid and induce an inflammatory response. It has been suggested (59) that indomethacin, which inhibits prostaglandin synthesis, reduces dithranol-induced erythema. But newer studies (59a,b) showed only a weak or no effect of indomethacin on dithranol inflammation.

Brown discoloration of the uninvolved skin is caused by dithranol metabolites and melanin pigmentation. It is dose dependent, but fades a few weeks after treatment is stopped.

Progress has been made in the reduction of clothes staining with a new formulation (Micanol), which is reported to show a comparable efficacy to known formulations and therefore may be a good alternative for treatment at day-care centers (59c,d).

Other acute side effects of dithranol include itching, stinging, burning, and dryness of the skin. These may to some extent be caused by the vehicle. Folliculitis is rare. Contact allergy has been reported (60–62).

Although animal studies have shown that dithranol can cause side effects in internal organs (63), Gay et al. (64) and Farber and Harris (65) could not find signs of systemic toxicity after long-term topical treatment.

In Sencar mice initiated with dimethylbenzanthracene, topically applied dithranol and some of its derivatives possessed skin-tumor-promoting activity (66). There are no reports of long-term side effects, including the occurrence of skin cancers in humans.

Therapy

With the data about the mode of action and the pharmacokinetics previously described, it is of interest to examine the possibility of maintaining the efficacy of dithranol and reducing its adverse effects (irritation and staining of skin and clothes).

In theory inflammation can be limited by three approaches:

1. Pretreatment or combination therapies
2. Altering dose and time of application (short contact and minutes therapy)
3. Posttreatments and special washing procedures (immediately after application)

Pretreatment or Combination Therapies

Pretreatment with highly potent corticosteroids, PUVA, UVB (67), coal tar, or salicylic acid has alleviated the inflammation reaction associated with the use of dithranol, but none of the approaches has been uniformly successful. Pretreatment together with combination therapy of prednisolone has also been tried without success. The effect of topically or orally applied pharmacological antagonists and anti-inflammatory drugs on sustained erythema induced by topical dithranol was studied. Aspirin, indomethacin, and chlorpheniramine by the oral route as well as scopolamine or betamethasone 17-valerate topically were unable to inhibit erythema induced by MED (49). As mentioned earlier, Kingston and Marks (59) showed that oral pretreatment with indomethacin could reduce erythema produced by dithranol, but more recent results showed no (68) or only weak (59a) effects on the erythema when applied topically and no effect (59b) when applied orally. Ultraviolet B irradiation with 1–2 MED prior to application strongly reduced erythema due to 0.1 and 1% dithranol solutions in chloroform (67). Local application of free radical inhibitors such as DL-tocopherol esters, retinol esters, or butylhydroxyanisole also inhibited the erythema response (69).

Classic Combination Therapies

Ultraviolet Light. The Ingram regimen (70)—combination of dithranol, tar, and UVB—is widely used. When the once-daily use of Lassar paste is not followed by a stronger irritation, the paste is removed in the morning with oil, followed by a tar bath for 20 min and then UV irradiation. The procedure is completed with the application of Lassar paste; the cycle is then repeated the next morning. The additional therapeutic effect of tar and UV is negligible (71). This combination slightly increases the tendency to relapse (72).

Selective UV phototherapy in which the UV lamps have an emission maximum between 310 and 330 nm also has an antipsoriatic effect. Adding this to the commonly used dithranol treatment does not influence the therapeutic efficacy of the latter (73,74).

Because dithranol shows absorption maxima in the shorter-wavelength UV region as well as between 350 and 360 nm depending on the solvent used, it was logical to look for an additional effect of UVA irradiation. Psoriasis could be cleared in a median of 14 days (75), but a comparative trial has not been performed.

The combination of dithranol with PUVA gave better results than either regimen alone (76,77).

Using low dithranol concentrations (0.01–0.05%) in combination with suberythemogenic UVB irradiation, psoriasis could be cleared within 4 weeks (78). In such combination therapy 0.1% is more effective than 0.01% (79).

A combination of short contact dithranol with short-contact coal tar and phototherapy consisting of UVA and UVB, termed UVABA therapy, has been reported (79a) to be effective and to be suitable for day care therapy, because it allows shortened treatment times.

Corticosteroids. Alternating applications of corticosteroids during the day and dithranol at night reduces irritation (65). In this study, contact of the paste to the skin for less than 8 hr was not as effective, indicating that the reduced irritancy could also be due to the shorter application period. Such an interpretation agrees with findings that a combination of dithranol with corticoids is more irritant than dithranol alone under experimental conditions (80) and in a clinical half-side comparison trial (81). Such alternate application modes also resulted in earlier relapses than dithranol alone in a comparative trial (82). However, Monk et al. (83) showed that in patients receiving a mixture of dithranol and clobetasol propionate applied as a cream, there was a faster clearance (14.9 days compared with 18.5 days) and no significant difference in the rate of relapse between these patients and a parallel group receiving dithranol alone.

Short-Contact Therapy

Dithranol penetrates faster and in greater amounts into artificially damaged skin than normal skin. The former was used as a permeability model for parakeratotic psoriatic lesions. If the drug excess is removed by washing with detergent within the first hour of application, the further penetration of dithranol is greatly reduced, particularly in normal skin. This reduction is much less pronounced in the experimental psoriatic lesion (35). This fact is also reflected by the dose- and time-dependent reduction of the erythema formation on normal skin (84).

Schaefer et al. (37) proposed short-contact therapy (SCT) of 1% dithranol for 1 hr on the basis of their studies on the penetration of the drug in normal and stripped skin.

An effective approach to optimize short-contact therapy involves an analysis of the time and dose dependency of the clinical response, with the aim of ascertaining minimum dose and shortest contact times for individual short-contact therapies, since lower dithranol concentrations are needed for therapeutic effectiveness than to produce inflammation/erythema, which is not a prerequisite for therapeutic responses.

Studies by Runne and Kunze (85) as well as by Jones et al. (86) indicate that in comparison to standard dithranol therapy, 1–3% for 10–20 min was superior, and that 0.5–3.0% for 10 min, or 1–3% for 30 min was similarly effective, but that 2–12% for 30 min was less effective.

Marsden et al. (43) found no significant differences in antipsoriatic efficacy using 2% dithranol for 1 hr, or 4% concentration for 30 min, when these regimens were compared to a protocol in which increasing concentrations of 2–8% were applied for a 30-min period. The time of contact for short-contact therapy (usually 20 min or more) can be further reduced to avoid unnecessary skin irritation.

MacDonald and Marks (87) found that contact times of from 5 to 20 min daily for 22 days were sufficient to clear psoriatic plaques (2.0% dithranol plus 0.5% salicylic acid). The margin between the excess concentration in normal skin and therapeutically active drug in diseased areas is reduced by posttreatment washouts. Juhlin and Shroot (88) have indicated the difficulties involved in drug removal using soap.

The washout with 1% potassium hydroxide immediately following application periods of 40 min (0.2–1.6% dithranol) significantly reduced inflammation without any loss of therapeutic efficacy (89). These authors explain that the main reason for this dissociation of inflammatory and therapeutic effects is the different time course of the two reactions. Thus, dithranol inflammation involves continued production of oxygen free radical species of noninvolved skin, whereas the therapeutic effect of dithranol mediated via the same chemistry unaffected by the removal of the drug from the stratum corneum occurs rapidly, within 40 min. This agrees well with Schaefer's original studies on the penetration kinetics of dithranol in skin (90). Chlebarov and Rauh (91) described "on-off" therapy. One-minute contact times are sufficient for psoriatic treatment using 1 or 2% dithranol concentrations compared for 10-min contact times. No problem with inflammation or staining was encountered in the 60 patients under 30-day treatment.

The usefulness of the combination of short-contact therapy with coal tar is controversial. Thus, although Schulze and Steigleder (92) and Young and van Weelden (93) stress the decreased irritation experienced with combinations containing 5–10% coal tar, other groups have been unable to demonstrate such beneficial effects (94). Indeed, Duhra and Ryatt (95) state that neither patients nor nursing staff were in favor of combined short-contact therapy and coal tar therapies.

One postulate for the value of combined preparation of dithranol with 5% coal tar is that over a period of 2 weeks, the concentrations of the former are considerably reduced (96), owing to the rapid formation of nonirritants such as danthron and dithranol dimer in the white petrolatum preparation. A related coal tar effect was also suggested by Lawrence et al. (44): Coal tar pretreatment may induce aryl hydrocarbon hydroxylases. However, Kingston and Lowe (46) stress that this enzyme may not necessarily be involved in the metabolism of dithranol. Indeed, Mahrle's pilot study (45) indicates that increased dithranol degradation caused by coal tar does not reduce its antipsoriatic efficacy to the same extent. However, the concentration of dithranol used in these experiments (1%) was sufficiently high so that even after degradation, there would be enough drug remaining for the treatment to be effective. In other studies (97), UVB was found not to improve short-contact therapy clearance rate, but postponed the relapse.

As mentioned above, recent studies with a combination of short-contact dithranol and coal tar plus UVA/UVB did not get better results than conventional day care therapy, but was less time-consuming (79a).

Gottlieb et al. (97a) suggested recently that combination of short-contact dithranol with cyclosporine improves results in patients who are slow to respond to cyclosporine alone.

The arguments presented here show that through an understanding of the action and skin pharmacokinetics of dithranol, it is possible to reduce the drug's side effects and maintain efficacy. Furthermore, pharmaceutical research can now be directed toward the discovery of drugs even more "user friendly" for the patient and practitioner alike, thus underscoring the place of dithranol as an effective nonsteroidal drug for the management of psoriasis.

Drug Delivery Considerations

Dithranol should be rapidly released from the vehicle and should be stable in the vehicle, both in the tube and in the skin, the latter being necessary to ensure adequate washout of excess drug, since the dimer and dithranol brown are highly insoluble. Several topical formulations of dithranol have been studied, and it was found that release was maximized from petrolatum-type ointments. When creams are applied and the drug as well as the individual components of the formulation are in contact with the skin, it is more difficult to control drug spreading and decomposition, and thus activation. As the side effects of dithranol are manifested on normal-appearing skin, the effect of vehicle on drug concentration in the stratum corneum using the stripping technique was studied (98). The petrolatum-based formulations present the drug high in the skin. Thus, assuming that in the psoriatic lesion drug presence is assured by selecting formulations that release the drug rapidly, it is desirable to have the excess situated high in the uninvolved skin so that adequate washout can be achieved. Because of dithranol's stability in soft and hard paraffin (e.g., Lassar paste) or in degassed petrolatum, these vehicles are often used and recommended, but none is optimal. Cream formulations are available, which are more comfortable for patients, but unfortunately the degree of instability of dithranol in some of these preparations is not acceptable (99). More recently, an emulsifying ointment-based dithranol formulation plus 0.1% w/w ascorbyl palmitate as an antioxidant has been shown to be stable for a long period (52 weeks) compared to Lassar paste (4 weeks) and easier to apply and remove, but further experiences on its clinical efficacy are lacking (99a).

Since the time of Ingram, yellow soft paraffin or mixtures of hard and soft paraffins have been shown to be an effective vehicle for dithranol delivery. The cosmetic inconvenience of these vehicles can be overcome by using petrolatum appropriately thickened to attain patient and nursing staff compliance. In addition, the selection of coingredients should facilitate removal of excess drug by washing. Finally, this formulation does not lead to breakdown in the skin when the individual components are released. In this way, it is possible to control dithranol. This aspect has been elegantly shown in a trial by the use of a cream containing triethanolamine which washed out and deactivated dithranol (100).

Ramsay et al. (101) showed that the dithranol 48-hr irritation response can be significantly reduced if an organic amine is applied to the skin following dithranol application. The same group showed that such a regimen results in maintenance of the clinical effect.

Liposomal preparations have been proposed to enhance the penetration of the drug into the skin (39a), but another group has shown that its stability in liposomes is considerably lower than in paraffin (39b).

Combination Therapy with Salicylic Acid and Urea

The combination of dithranol with keratolytics could increase the flux of the drug into the skin. However, whether this effect plays a role in the treatment of psoriasis is far from clear. Salicylic acid at a certain concentration (0.5%) may act in addition as a stabilizer, preventing the decomposition of dithranol. Using petrolatum as the vehicle, the dithranol concentration is 0.1% and will be increased in the course of therapy to 0.25, 0.5, and, if necessary, 1.0%. Salicylic acid is added in a concentration of 2.0%, but for small areas up to 10% can be used (102).

In Lassar paste and its modifications (65,103) the dithranol concentrations range from 0.1–0.2 to 0.8% and salicylic acid is added at 2%. Lassar paste allows more precise application to the involved areas, but its use is time consuming, and irritation of the surrounding uninvolved skin can still occur. Removal of the paste is facilitated using cream or oil. In practice, the regimen (dithranol-salicylic acid-petrolatum) seems superior to Lassar paste (104).

Treatment of the Scalp

Dithranol can discolor blond hair, especially turning it yellowish. Petrolatum-based formulations are difficult to remove when used on the scalp, and although these preparations are effective in this region, more sophisticated vehicles are need. An O/W vanishing cream is a step in this direction (105).

Maintenance Therapy

Brun et al. (106) showed that if the application of dithranol was continued for 1 month or more following clearance of the lesion, the relapse time was prolonged. Dithranol was applied only to the old lesions. This delay in the onset of relapse has also been reported for PUVA.

Other Indications

Chlbarov et al. (107) described treatment of seborrhoic dermatitis using low concentrations of dithranol (0.1%) for 2–5 min contact, with immediate washoff using warm water. After 4 days, an improvement in one patient was found. An average of 21 days without relapse was found in the 54 patients under treatment.

The side effects at 0.1 and 0.5% were found in only one patient. Naturally, the length of treatment is dependent of the severity of the eczema, ranging from 7–15 days for mild cases to 2–3 weeks for cases with extensive efflorescence. They stressed that applications should be to involved areas only (1% and 10-min contact times). However, they also found that the "on-off" regimen is successful for between 30 and 50% of patients at 2%.

Dithranol is a potent inhibitor of *Pityrosporum orbiculare/ovale* growth in vitro (107a), which is thought to be involved in the pathogenesis of seborrhoic eczema and Koebnerization of psoriasis (107b).

In addition, dithranol has been used in the treatment of alopecia areata (108,108a).

Dithranol, applied as an ointment at 0.25–1.0%, has also been tested in a clinical trial for its effectiveness in mycosis fungoides, which resulted in complete clearing of 6 of 12 patients (108b).

New Derivatives of Dithranol

To diminish irritancy and staining, a number of dithranol derivatives have been investigated. According to Krebs and Schaltegger (109), the minimal structure necessary for antipsoriatic activity is 1-hydroxy-9-anthrone (see Fig. 6). However, this concept has not been fully confirmed in cell biological tests (109a),

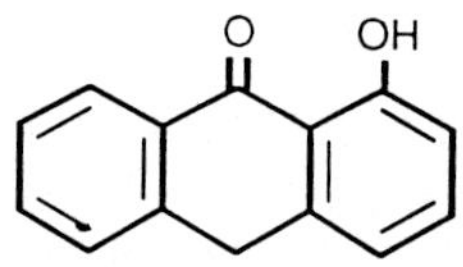

1-hydroxy-9-anthrone
Minimal structure for activity

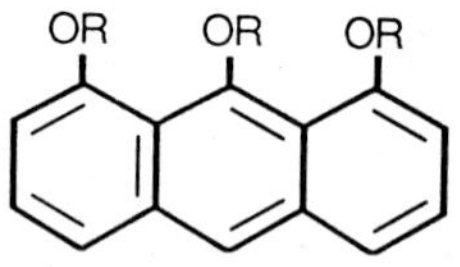

1,8,9-triacetoxy anthracene ($R=CH_3CO$)

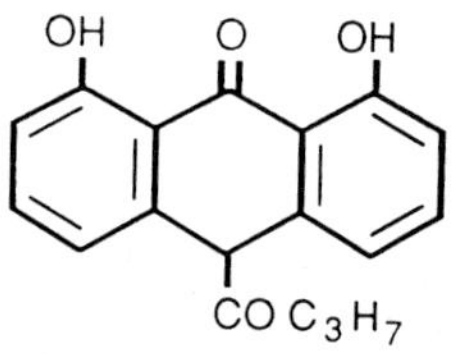

1,8 dihydroxy 10-butyryl-9-anthrone

Figure 6 Structures of dithranol derivatives under study.

which gives way to the search for alternative antipsoriatics not containing that minimal structure. Wiegrebe and Greber (110) studied 1,8,9-triacetoxyanthralin, which is devoid of adverse effects, and they assumed that nonspecific esterases release compounds that correspond to different degrees of acylation on the hydroxyl groups, including dithranol. Mustakallio (50,111) and Brandt and Mustakallio (51) compared single and repeated applications of C_{10}-acylated analogues on psoriatic patients, and they found that the butyryl derivative (butanthrone) is fourfold less irritant than dithranol after daily applications for 3 weeks at a dose of 8 mmol/kg, but is less efficient clinically (111a). Schaltegger et al. (112) showed that in mild conditions of acid hydrolysis C_{10}-acylated derivatives are potential prodrugs of dithranol.

The growth inhibitory and cytotoxic effects of new dithranol derivatives have been investigated by Bonnekoh et al. (109a). Müller and Gawlik (34b) and Müller et al. (112b) tested novel 10-substituted dithranol derivatives and found these substances to be more selective inhibitors of 5-lipoxygenase. Surprisingly, the derivatives with phenolic hydroxyl groups in the aromatic ring could protect, in contrast to dithranol, against lipid peroxidation as it may occur after ROS release by PMNL.

Furthermore, some newer drugs bearing more stable substituents as C_{10} have been described (113). The anti-inflammatory action of these compounds is more pronounced than the antiproliferative effect. Thus, analogue synthesis may be an effective way to separate adverse effects from efficacy; in addition, these substances may provide new classes of compounds for wider clinical indications.

REFERENCES

1. Squire, B. (1877). Lysophanic acid as a remedy in skin diseases. *Br. Med. J.* *1S*:199–200.
2. Shroot, B., Schaefer, H., Juhlin, L., and Greaves, M.W. (1981). Current concepts in the mode of action of anthralin in the treatment of psoriasis. *Br. J. Dermatol.* 105(Suppl 20)3–5.
3. Unna, P.G. (1916). Cignolin als heilmittel der psoriasis. *Dermatol. Wochenscher.* 62:116–137, 151–163, 175–183.
4. Muller, K., and Kappus. (1988). Hydroxyl radical formation by dithranol. *H. Biochem. Pharm.* 37: 4277–4280.
5. Shroot, B., and Brown, C. (1986). Free radicals in skin exposed to anthralin and its derivatives. *Arzneim. Forsch./Drug Res.* 36:1253–1255.
6. Fuchs, J., and Packer L. (1989). Investigations on anthralin free radicals in model systems and in skin of hairless mice. *Clin. Res.* 37:725.
7. Rassner, G. (1972). Enzyme der epidermis. Spezielle aspekte. *Arch. Dermatol. Forsch.* 244:48–52.
8. Hammar, H. (1970). Glyceraldehydephosphate dehydrogenase and glucose-6-phosphate dehydrogenase activities in psoriasis and neurodermatitis and the effect of dithranol. *J. Invest. Dermatol.* 54: 121–125.
9. Raab, W., and Gmeiner, B. (1975). Influence of ultraviolet light, various temperatures and zinc ions on anthralin (dithranol). Biochemical and chemical investigations. *Dermatologia* 150:267–276.
10. Plumier, E., Retzow, A., and Wiegrebe, W. (1982). Untersuchungen zur hemmung der glucose-6-phosphat-dehydrogenase durch dithranol. *Pharm. Z.* 22:2150–2152.
11. Cavey, D., Caron, J.C., and Shroot, B. (1982). Anthralin: chemical instability and glucose-6-phosphate dehydrogenase inhibition. *J. Pharm. Sci.* 71:980–983.
12. Müller, K., Seidel, M., Braun, C., Ziereis, K., and Wiegrebe, W. (1991). Dithranol, glucose-6-phosphate dehydrogenase inhibition and active oxygen species. *Arzneim.-Forsch./Drug Res.* 41: 1176–1181.

13. Raab, W. (1969). Die wirkung externer antipsoriatica auf die gewebsatmung menschlicher und tierishcer haut. *Arch. Klin. Exp. Dermatol.* 234:44–51.
14. Raab, W. (1980). Ingram method: the precursor of photochemotherapy. *Br. J. Dermatol.* 105(Suppl. 20):77–81.
15. Pätel, M. (1981). Calorimetric screening test for dermatologically active drugs on human skin fibroblast cultures. *Theramochim. Acta* 49:123–129.
15a. Hsieh, G.C., and Acosta, D. (1991). Dithranol-induced cytotoxicity in primary cultures of rat epidermal keratinocytes. *Toxicol. Appl. Pharmacol.* 107:16–26.
16. Jacques, Y., and Reichert, U. (1981). Effects of anthralin and analogues on growth and ^{3}H thymidine incorporation in human skin fibroblasts. *Br. J. Dermatol.* 105(Suppl. 20):45.
16a. Gottlieb, A.B., Khandke, L., Krane, J.F., Stainano-Coico, L., Ashinoff, R., and Krueger, J.G. (1992). Anthralin decreases keratinocyte TGF-α expression and EGF-receptor binding in vitro. *J. Invest. Dermatol.* 98:680–685.
16b. Keméy, L., Michel, G., Arenberger, P., and Ruzicka, T. (1993). Down-regulation of epidermal growth factor receptors by dithranol. *Acta Derm. Venereol. (Stockh.)* 73:37–40.
16c. Gottlieb, A.B., Chang, C.K., Posnett, D.N., Fanelli, B., and Tam, J.P. Detection of transforming growth factor α in normal, malignant, and hyperproliferative human keratinocytes. *J. Exp. Med.* 167: 670–675.
16d. Elder, J.T., Fisher, G.J., Lindquist, P.B., Bennett, G.L., Pittelkow, M.R., Coffey, R.J., Ellingsworth, L., Derynck, R., and Voorhees, J.J. (1989). Overexpression of transforming growth factor alpha in psoriatic epidermis. *Science* 243:811–814.
16e. Nanney, L.B., Stoscheck, C.M., Magid, M., and King Jr., L.E. (1986). Altered ^{125}I epidermal growth factor binding and receptor distribution in psoriasis. *J. Invest. Dermatol.* 86:260–265.
16f. Ockenfels, H.M., Nussbaum, G., Schultewolter, T., Burger, P.M., and Goos, M. (1995). Cyclosporin A, FK506 and dithranol alter tyrosine-specific protein phosphorylation an HaCaT keratinocytes. *Arch. Dermatol. Res.* 287:304–309.
17. Clark, J.M., and Hanawalt, P.C. (1982). Inhibition of DNA replication and repair by anthralin or danthron in cultured human cells. *J. Invest. Dermatol.* 79:18–22.
18. Swanbeck, G., and Thyresson, N. (1965). Interaction between dithranol and nucleic acid. A possible mechanism for the effect of dithranol on psoriasis. *Acta Derm. Venereol. (Stockh.)* 45:344–348.
19. Caron, J.C., Eustache, J., Shroot, B., and Prota, G. (1982). On the interaction between anthralin and DNA: a revision. *Arch. Dermatol. Res.* 274: 207–214.
20. Sa e Melo, M.T., Dubertret, L., Prognon, P., Gond, A., Mahuzier, G., and Santus, R. (1983). Physicochemical properties and stability of anthralin in model systems and human skin. *J. Invest. Dermatol.* 80:1–6.
20a. Müller, K., and Gürster, D. (1993). Hydroxyl radical damage to DNA sugar and model membranes induced by anthralin (dithranol). *Biochem. Pharmacol.* 46:1695–1704.
20b. Müller, K., Leukel, P., Mayer, K.K., and Wiegrebe, W. (1995). Modification of DNA bases by anthralin and related compounds. *Biochem. Pharmacol.* 49: 1607–1613.
20c. Healy, E., Reynolds, N.J., Smith, M.D., Campbell, C., Farr, P.M., and Rees J.L. (1994). Dissociation of erythema and p53 protein expression in human skin following UVB irradiation and induction of p53 protein and mRNA following application of skin irritants. *J. Invest. Dermatol.* 103:493–499.
21. Fischer, L.B., and Maibach, H. (1975). The effect of anthralin and its derivatives on epidermal cell kinetics. *J. Invest. Dermatol.* 64:338–341.
22. Lubach, D., and Kietzmann, M. (1988). Effects of treatment with dithranol, etretinate, and a combination of dithranol and etretinate on epidermal metabolism and histology. *Arzneim. Forsch.* 38: 1167–1170.
22a. de Zwart, A.J., de Jong, E.M.G.J., and de Kerkhof, P.C.M. (1992). Topical application of dithranol on normal skin induces epidermal hyperproliferation and increased Ks8.12 binding. *Skin Pharmacol.* 5: 34–40.
22b. Holland, D.B., Wood, E.J., Cunliffe, W.J., and Turner, D.M. (1989). Keratin gene expression during the resolution of psoriatic plaques: effect of dithranol, PUVA, etretinate and hydroxyurea regimens. *Br. J. Dermatol.* 120:9–19.
23. De Young, L.M., Helmes, C.T., Chao, W.R., Young, J.M., and Miller, V. (1981). Paradoxical effect of anthralin on 12-o-tetradecanoylphorbol 13-acetate-induced mouse epidermal ornithine decarboxylase activity, proliferation, and tumor promotion. *Cancer Res.* 41:204–208.
24. Reichert, U., Jaques, Y., Grangeret, M., and Schmidt, R. (1985). Antirespiratory and antiproliferative activity of anthralin in cultured human keratinocytes. *J. Invest. Dermatol.* 84:130–134.
24a. Fuchs, J., Milbradt, R., and Zimmer, G. (1990). Multifunctional analysis of the interaction of anthralin and its metabolites anthraquinone and anthralin dimer with the inner mitochondrial membrane. *Arch. Dermatol. Res.* 282:47–55.
24b. Fuchs, J., Nitschmann, W.H., and Packer, L. (1990). The antipsoriatic compound anthralin influences

bioenergetic parameters and redox properties of energy transducing membranes. *J. Invest. Dermatol.* 94:71–76.

24c. Salet, C., Moreno, G., Morlière, P., and Santus, R. (1991). Effects of anthralin on mitochondrial bioenergetics. *Arch. Dermatol. Res.* 283:186–190.

25. Swanbeck, G., and Lundquist, P. (1972). Ultrastructural changes of mitochondria in dithranol-treated psoriatic epidermis. *Acta Derma. Veneorol. (Stockh.)* 52:94–98.

26. Morlière, P., Dubertret, L., Sa e Melo, M.T., Salet, C., Fosse, M., and Santus, R. (1985). The effects of anthralin (dithranol) on mitochondria. *Br. J. Dermatol.* 112:509–515.

27. Pätel, M., Schaarschmidt, B., and Reichert, U. (1981). Calorimetric and manometric measurements on human skin fibroblasts in culture. *Br. J. Dermatol.* 105(Suppl. 20):60–61.

28. Raab, W., and Patermann, F. (1966). Die wirkung externer antipsoriatika auf die zellatmung. *Arch. Klin. Exp. Dermatol.* 226:144–152.

29. Kanerva, L. (1989). Electron microscopy of the effect of dithranol on healthy and on psoriatic skin. *Clin. Res.* 37:2:676.

29a. Kanerva, L. (1989). Circular and branched Birbeck granules and cytomembrane blebbing in Langerhans' cells after dithranol irritation. *Acta Derm. Veneorol. (Stockh.)* 69:407–409.

29b. Kanerva, L. (1990). Electron microscopy of the effects of dithranol on healthy and on psoriatic skin. *Am. J. Dermatopathol.* 12:51–62.

30. Anderson, R., Lukey, P.T., and Dippenaar, U. (1987). Dithranol mediates pro-oxidative inhibition of polymorphonuclear leukocyte migration and lymphocyte proliferation. *Br. J. Dermatol.* 117: 405–418.

31. Cavey, D. (1989). In vitro models for the evaluation of anti-inflammatory drug action in the skin. In *Pharmacology and the Skin. Non Steroidal Anti-inflammatory Drugs*, Vol. 2. C.N. Hensby and N.J. Lowe (Eds.). Karger, Basel, pp. 44–88.

32. Schröder, J.M., Kosfeld, U., and Christophers, U. (1985). Multifunctional inhibition by anthralin in non-stimulated and chemotactic factor-stimulated human neutrophils. *J. Invest. Dermatol.* 85:30–34.

32a. Anderson, R. (1989). Dithranol-mediated, dose-dependent priming and activation of luminol-enhanced chemiluminescence of human neutrophils in vitro. *Br. J. Dermatol.* 121:1–9.

32b. Hegemann, L., Fruchtmann, R., van Rooijen, L.A.A., Müller-Peddinghaus, R., and Mahrle, G. (1992). The antipsoriatic drug, anthralin, inhibits protein kinase C - implications for its mechanism of action. *Arch. Dermatol. Res.* 284:179–183.

32c. Ohtuska, T., Okamura, N., and Ishibashi, S. (1986). Involvement of protein kinase C in phosphorylation of 46kDa proteins which are phosphorylated in parallel with the activation of NADPH oxidase in intact guinea-pig polymorphonuclear leukocytes. *Biochim. Biophys. Acta* 888:332–337.

32d. Wymann, M.P., von Tscharner, V., Deranleau, D.A., and Baggiolini, M. (1987). The onset of the respiratory burst in human neutrophils. *J. Biol. Chem.* 262:12048–12053.

32e. Nishizuka, Y. (1984). The role of protein kinase C in cell surface signal transduction and tumour promotion. *Nature* 308:693–697.

33. Kammerau, B., Zesch, A., and Schaefer, H. (1975). Absolute concentrations of dithranol and triacetyl-dithranol in the skin layers after local treatment: in vivo investigations with four different types of pharmaceutical vehicles. *J. Invest. Dermatol.* 64: 145–149.

34. Schröder, J.M. (1986). Anthralin (1,8-dihydroxyanthrone) is a potent inhibitor of leukotriene production and LTB4-ω oxidation by human neutrophils. *J. Invest. Dermatol.* 87:624–629.

34a. Bedord, C.J., Young, J.M., and Wagner, B.M. (1983). Anthralin inhibition of mouse epidermal arachidonic acid lipoxygenase in vitro. *J. Invest. Dermatol.* 81:566–571.

34b. Müller, K., and Gawlik, I. (1995). Novel 10-substituted antipsoriatic anthrones as inhibitors of epidermal 12-lipoxygenase and lipid peroxidation in membranes. *Biochem. Pharmacol.* 50: 2077–2083.

34c. Ruzicka, T., Vitto, A., and Printz, M.P. (1983). Epidermal arachidonate lipoxygenase. *Biochim. Biophys. Acta* 751:359–374.

34d. Hammarström, S., Hamberg, M., Samuelsson, B., Duell, E., Stawiski, M., and Voorhees, J.J. (1975). Increased concentrations of nonesterified arachidonic acid, 12L-hydroxy-5,8,10,14-eicostetraenoic acid, prostaglandin $E_{2\alpha}$ in epidermis of psoriasis. *Proc. Natl. Acad. Sci. USA* 72:5130–5134.

34e. Ruzicka, T. (1988). The physiology and pathophysiology of eicosanoids in the skin. *Eicosanoids* 1: 59–72.

34f. Ruzicka, T. (1990). *Eicosanoids and the skin.* CRC Press, Boca Raton, FL.

34g. Müller, K., and Gawlik, I. (1996). Inactivation of mouse epidermal 12-lipoxygenase by anthralin - implications for the role of oxygen radicals. *Biochem. Pharmacol.* 51:1173–1179.

34h. Kemény, L., Gross, E., Arenberger, P., and Ruzicka, T. (1991). Dithranol-induced down-regulation of 12(S)-hydroxyeicosatetraenoic acid [12(S)-HETE] receptors in a human epidermal cell line. *Arch. Dermatol. Res.* 283:333–336.

34i. Mrowietz, U., Falsafi, M., Schröder, J.M., and Christophers, E. (1992). Inhibition of human monocyte functions by anthralin. *Br. J. Dermatol.* 127: 382–386.

34j. Baxter, C.S., Adringa, A., Chalfin, K., and Miller, M.L. (1991). Effect of tumor-promoting agents on density and morphometric parameters of mouse epidermal Langerhans and thy-1+ cells. *Carcinogenesis* 12:1017–1021.

34k. Gruner, S., Zwirner, A., Strunk, D., and Sönnichsen, N. (1992). The influence of topical dermatological treatment modalities on epidermal Langerhans cells and contact sensitization in mice. *Contact Derm.* 26:241–247.

34l. Schmidt, K.N., Podda, M., Packer, L., and Baeuerla, P.A. (1996). Antipsoriatic drug anthralin activates transcription factor NF-κB in murine keratinocytes. *J. Immunol.* 156:4514–4519.

34m. Schreck, R., and Baeuerle, P.A. (1991). A role for oxygen radicals as second messengers. *Trends Cell Biol.* 1:39.

34n. Meyer, M., Schreck, R., Müller, M., and Baeuerle, P.A. (1994). Redox control of gene expression by eukaryotic transcription factors NF-κB, AP-1 and SRF/TCF. In *Oxidative Stress, Cell Activation and Viral Infection.* C. Pasquier (Ed.). Birkhäuser, Basel, pp. 217–235.

34o. Baeuerle, P.A., and Henkel, T. (1994). Function and activation of NF-κB in the immune system. *Annu. Rev. Immunol.* 12:141.

35. Schalla, W., Bauer, E., and Schaefer, H. (1981). Skin permeability of anthralin. *Br. J. Dermatol.* 105(Suppl. 20):104–108.

36. Selim, M.M., Goldberg, L.H., Schaefer, H., Bishop, S.C., and Farber, E.M. (1981). Penetration studies on topical anthralin. *Br. J. Dermatol.* 105(Suppl. 20):101–103.

37. Schaefer, H., Zesch, A., and Stüttgen, G. (1981). Skin permeability. In *Handbuch der Hautund Geschlechtskrankheiten, Ergänzungswerk.* Vol. 1/4B. Springer Verlag, Berlin, pp. 541–886.

38. Wang, J.C.T., Pätel, B.G., Ehmann, C.W., and Lowe, N. (1987). The release and percutaneous permeation of anthralin products, using clinically involved and uninvolved psoriatic skin. *J. Am. Acad. Dermatol.* 16:812–821.

39. Wester, H., Mobayen, M., Ryatt, K., Bucks, D., and Maibach, H. (1986). *In vivo* percutaneous absorption of dithranol in psoriatic patients and normal volunteers. *Clin. Res.* 34:165A.

39a. Gehring, W., Ghyczy, M., Gloor, M., Scheer, T., and Röding, J. (1992). Enhancement of the penetration of dithranol and increase of effect of dithranol on the skin by liposomes. *Arzneim.-Forsch./Drug Res.* 42:983–985.

39b. Mahrle, G., Bonnekoh, B., Ghyczy, M., and Wiegrebe, W. (1991). Stability of anthralin in liposomal phospholipids. *Arch. Dermatol. Res.* 283:483–484.

40. Cavey, D., Dickinson, R., Shroot, B., and Schaefer, H. (1985). The *in vivo* fate of topically applied anthralin in the skin of the hairless rat: a comparison of continuous and short contact application. *Arzneim. Forsch./Drug Res.* 35:605–609.

41. Brun, P., and Baran, R. (1982). Pemphigoide bulleuse induite par la photochimiothérapie du psoriasis. A propos de deux cas, avec revue de la littérature. *Ann. Dermatol. Venereol.* 109:461–468.

42. Kentsch, V., Schalla, W., and Schneider, L. (1981). Die risken der photochemotherapie. *Z. Hautkr.* 56: 1379–1399.

43. Marsden, J.R., Coburn, P.R., Marks, J.P., and Shuster, S. (1983). Response to short term application of dithranol in psoriasis. *Br. J. Dermatol.* 108:243.

44. Lawrence, C.M., Howel, D., and Shuster, S. (1984). The inflammatory response to anthralin. *Clin. Exp. Dermatol.* 9:336–341.

45. Mahrle, G. (1987). Anthralin: new treatment modalities and combination regimens. In *Psoriasis. Stanford Proceedings of the 4th International Symposium* (Farber, E.M., ed.), 1986. Elsevier, pp. 181–187.

46. Kingston, T.P., and Lowe, N.J. (1987). Modification of anthralin irritancy. In *Psoriasis. Stanford Proceedings of the 4th International Symposium* (Farber, E.M., ed.), 1986. Elsevier, pp. 159–171.

47. Paramsothy, Y., and Lawrence, C.M. (1987). Time course and intensity of anthralin inflammation on involved and uninvolved psoriatic skin. *Br. J. Dermatol.* 116:517–519.

48. Westerhof, W., Buehre, Y., Pavel, S., Bos, J.D., Das, P.K., Krieg, S.R., and Siddiqui, A.H. (1989). Increased anthralin irritation response in vitiliginous skin. *Arch. Dermatol. Res.* 281:52–56.

49. Misch, K., Davies, M.W., Greaves, M., and Coutts, A. (1981). Pharmacological studies of anthralin erythema. *Br. J. Dermatol.* 105(Suppl. 20):82–86.

50. Mustakallio, K.K. (1979). Irritation and staining by dithranol (anthralin) related compounds. 1. Estimation with chamber testing and contact thermography. *Acta Derm. Venereol. (Stockh.)* 59(Suppl. 85):125.

51. Brandt, H., and Mustakallio, K.K. (1983). Irriation and staining by dithranol (anthralin) and related compounds 3. Cumulative irritancy and staining during repeated chamber testing. *Acta Derm. Venereol. (Stockh.)* 63:237.

51a. Farkas, B., Bonnekoh, B., and Mahrle, G. (1991). Repeated treatment with dithranol induces a tolerance reaction in keratinocytes in vitro. *Arch. Dermatol. Res.* 283:337–341.

52. Kersey, P., Chapman, P., Rogers, S., Rawlins, M., and Shuster, S. (1981). The inflammatory response to anthralin and its relation to aryl hydrocarbon hydroxylase. *Br. J. Dermatol.* 105(Suppl. 20):64–67.

53. Bickers, D. (1981). Comparative effect of anthralin and coal tar on epidermal aryl hydrocarbon hydroxylase. *Br. J. Dermatol.* 105(Suppl. 20):71.
54. Munro, C., Ransay, B., Lawrence, C., Higgins, E., Marks, J., Friedmann, P., Chadwick, L., Dover, R., Rees, J., Young, S., Matthews, J., Johnson, M., Humphreys, F., and Shuster, S. (1989). Reduction of cutaneous anthralin inflammation by cyclosporin A. *Clinical Res.*37:701A.
55. Barr, R.M., Brain, S.D., Black, A.K., Camp, R.D., Greaves, M.W., Mallet, A.I., and Wong, E. (1983). Lipoxygenase products of arachidonic acid in inflamed skin. *J. Invest. Dermatol.* 80:345.
56. Barr, R.M., Misch, K.J. Hensby, C.N., Mallet, A.I., and Greaves, M.W. (1983). Archidonic acid and prostaglandin level sin dithranol erythema: time course. *Br. J. Clin. Pharmacol.* 16:715–717.
57. Hensby, C.N., Juhlin, L., Chatelus, A., Civier, A., Schaefer, H., Greaves, M.W., Black, A.K., Barr, R.M., and Fourtanier, A. (1982). Mini-pig as a potential alternative for predicting human skin pharmacological reactions. *Int. J. Immunopharmacol.* 4: 352.
58. Martinmaa, J., Vanhal, L., and Mustakallio, K.K. (1978). Free radical intermediates produced by autoxidation of 1,8-dihydroxy-9-anthrone (dithranol) in pyridine. *Experientia* 34:872–873.
59. Kingston, T., and Marks, R. (1981). Irritant reactions to dithranol in normal subjects and psoriatic patients. *Br. J. Dermatol.* 106:725.

59a. Ramsay, B., Rice, N., and Lawrence, C. (1992). The effect of indomethacin on anthralin inflammation. *Br. J. Dermatol.* 126:262–265.

59b. Sheehan-Dare, R.A., Goodfield, M.J.D., and Rowell, N.R. (1991). The effect of oral indomethacin on psoriasis treated with the Ingram regime. *Br. J. Dermatol.* 125:253–255.

59c. Christensen, O.B., Enström, Y., Juhlin, J., Reidhav, I., Svensson, Å., Bjellerup, M., Ridderström, E., Larsson-Styme, B., and Brolund, L. (1992). A novel dithranol formulation in the over night treatment of psoriasis at home. *Acta Derm. Veneorol. (Stockh.).* 172:25–27.

59d. Christensen, O.B., and Brolund, L. (1992). Clinical studies with a novel dithranol formulation (micanol) in combination with UVB at day-care centres. *Acta Derm. Veneorol. (Stockh.).* Suppl. 172:17–19.

60. de Groot, A.C., and Nater, J.P. (1981). Contact allergy to dithranol. *Contact Dermatitis* 7:5–8.
61. de Groot, A.C., Nater, J.P., Bleumink, E., and de Jong, M.C.J.M. (1981). Does DNCB potentiate epicutaneous sensitization to non-related contact allergens? *Clin. Exp. Dermatol.* 6:139–144.
62. Lawlor, F., and Hindons, C. (1982). Allergy to dithranol. *Contact Dermatitis* 8:137–138.
63. Ippen, H. (1959). Toxizität und Stoffwechsel des Cignolins. *Dermatologica* 119:211–220.
64. Gay, M.W., Moore, W.J., Morgan, J.M., and Montes, L.F. (1972). Anthralin toxicity. *Arch. Dermatol.* 105:213–215.
65. Farber, E.M., and Harris, D.R. (1970). Hospital treatment of psoriasis. Modified anthralin program. *Arch. Dermatol.* 101:381–389.
66. DiGiovanni, J., Kruszewski, F.H., Coombs, M.M., Bhatt, T.S., and Pezeshk, A. (1988). Structure-activity relationships for epidermal ornithine decarboxylase induction and skin tumor promotion by anthrones. *Carcinogenesis* 9(8):1437–1443.
67. Juhlin, L. (1981). Factors influencing anthralin erythema. *Br. J. Dermatol.* 105(Suppl. 20):87.
68. Lawrence, C.M., and Shuster, S., (1985). Mechanism of antralin inflammation, 1. Dissociation of response to clabetasol and indomethacin. *Br. J. Dermatol.* 113:107–115.
69. Finnen, M.J., Lawrence, C.M., and Shuster, S. (1984). Anthralin increases lipid peroxide formation in skin and free radical scavengers reduce anthralin irritancy. *Br. J. Dermatol.* 111:717.
70. Ingram, J.T. (1953). Approaches to psoriasis. *Br. Med. J.* 2:591–594.
71. Young, E. (1970). The external treatment of psoriasis. A controlled investigation of the effects of dithranol. *Br. J. Dermatol.* 82:516–520.
72. Seville, R.H. (1975). Simplified dithranol treatment for psoriasis. *Br. J. Dermatol.* 93:205–208.
73. Elbracht, C., and Landes, E. (1983). Untersuchungen über die Wirksamkeit einer kombinierten Psoriasis Behandlung mit Dithranol und UV-B (SUP). *Z. Hautkr.* 58:387–397.
74. Schauder, S., and Mahrle, G. (1982). Kombinierte einstundentherapie der psoriasis mit anthralin und UV-licht. *Hautarzt* 33:206–209.
75. Hindson, C., Diffey, B., Lawlor, F., and Downey, A. (1983). Dithranol-U.V.A. phototherapy (PUVA) for psoriasis: a treatment without dressings. *Br. J. Dermatol.* 108:457–460.
76. Cripps, D.J., and Lowe, N.J. (1979). Photochemotherapy for psoriasis remission times. Psoralens and UV-A and combined photochemotherapy with anthralin. *Clin. Exp. Dermatol.* 4:477–483.
77. Willis, I., and Harris, D.R. (1973). Resistant psoriasis. Combined methoxalen-anthralin therapy. *Arch. Dermatol.* 107:358–362.
78. Montes, L.F., Wilborn, W.H., and Brody, I. (1979). Low strength anthralin in psoriasis. *J. Cutan. Pathol.* 6:445–456.
79. Marley, W.M., Hernandez, A.D., Josephs, J.A., and Dawkins, L. (1982). The effectiveness of low-strength anthralin in psoriasis. *Arch. Dermatol.* 118: 906–908.

79a. Swinehart, J.M. and Lowe, N.J. (1991). UVABA therapy for psoriasis. *J. Am. Acad. Dermatol.* 24: 594–597.

80. Puschmann, M. (1983). Experimentelle untersuchungen zur erythembildung an der gesunden haut durch anthralin. *Arztl. Kosmetol.* 13:207–214.

81. Runne, U., and Kunze, J. (1983). Psoriasis: die praxis der "minuten-therapie" und cignolin. *Z. Hautkr.* 58:219–229.

82. Seville, R.H. (1976). Relapse rate of psoriasis worsened by adding steroids to a dithranol regime. *Br. J. Dermatol.* 25:643–646.

83. Monk, B.E., Hehir, M.E., Clement, M.I., Penmbroke, A.C., and du Vivier, A. (1988). Anthralin-corticosteroid combination therapy in the treatment of chronic plaque psoriasis. *Arch. Dermatol.* 124: 548–550.

84. Puschmann, M., and Schmersahl, P. (1983). Investigations on the side-effects of anthralin and two main impurities on healthy skin. *Z. Hautkr.* 58: 410–416.

85. Runne, U., and Kunze, J. (1982). Short duration (minutes) therapy with dithranol for psoriasis. *Br. J. Dermatol.* 106:135–140.

86. Jones, S.K., Campbell, W.C., and MacKie, Rona M. (1985). Out-patient treatment of psoriasis: short contact and overnight dithranol therapy compared. *Br. J. Dermatol.* 113:331–337.

87. MacDonald, K.J.S., and Marks, J. (1986). Short contact anthralin in the treatment of psoriasis: a study of different contact times. *Br. J. Dermatol.* 114:235–239.

88. Juhlin, L., and Shroot, B. (1985). Detection of anthralin in skin during treatment. *Acta Derm. Venereol. (Stockh.)* 120(Suppl.):27–29.

89. Lawrence, C.M., Shuster, S., Collins, M., and Bruce, J.M. (1987). Reduction of anthralin inflammation by potassium hydroxide and Teepol. *Br. J. Dermatol.* 116:171–177.

90. Schaefer, H., Farber, E.M., Goldberg, L., and Schalla, W. (1980). Limited application period for dithranol in psoriasis. *Br. J. Dermatol.* 102: 571–573.

91. Chlebarov, S., and Rauh, M. (1988). Modified short contact with dithranol in psoriasis vulgaris. *Z. Hautkr.* 63:658–662.

92. Schulze, H.J., and Steigleder, G.K. (1983). Bilateral comparison study on addition of crude coal tar to standard antipsoriatic dithranol ointment. *Z. Hautkr.* 59:654–656.

93. Young, E., and van Weelden, H. (1987). Treatment of psoriasis with a combination of dithranol and coal tar. *Br. J. Dermatol.* 116:281–282.

94. Downey, D.J., and Finlay, A.Y. (1985). Combined dithranol and short contact crude coal tar therapy for psoriasis. *Scott. Med. J.* 30:265.

95. Duhra, P., and Ryatt, K.S. (1988). Lack of additive effect of coal tar combined with dithranol for psoriasis. *Clin. Exp. Dermatol.* 13:72–73.

96. Müller, R., Naumann, E., Detmar, M., and Orfanos, C.E. (1987). Stabilität von cignolin (dithranol) in teerhaltigen salben mit und ohne salicylsäurezusatz. *Hautarzt* 38:107–111.

97. Paramsothy, Y., Collins, M., and Lawrence, C.M. (1988). Effect of UVB therapy and a coal tar bath on short contact dithranol treatment for psoriasis. *Br. J. Dermatol.* 118:783–789.

97a. Gottlieb, S.L., Heftler, N.S., Gilleaudeau, P., Johnson, R. Vallat, V.P., Wolfe, J., Gottlieb, A.B., and Krueger, J.G. (1995). Short-contact anthralin treatment augments the therapeutic efficacy of cyclosporine in psoriasis. *J. Am. Acad. Dermatol.* 33: 637–645.

98. Caron, D., Brzokewicz, A., and Shroot, B. (1989). Libération-pénétration de l'anthraline dans plusieurs formulations *in vivo* chez l'homme. *Ann. Pharmaceut. Franc.* (in press).

99. Caron, J.C., and Shroot, B. (1981b). Determination of anthralin in commercial ointments. *Br. J. Dermatol.* 105(Suppl. 20):57–58.

99a. Weller, P.J., Newman, C.M., Middleton, K.R., and Wicker, S.M. (1990). Stability of a novel dithranol ointment formulation, containing ascorbyl palmitate as an anti-oxidant. *J. Clin. Pharmacol. Ther.* 15: 419–423.

100. Lawrence, C.K., Ramsay, B., Bruce, M., and Shuster, S. (1989). Triethanolamine reduces inflammation in short contact anthralin therapy without loss of therapeutic effect. *J. Invest. Dermatol.* 92:468.

101. Ramsay, B., Lawrence, C.M., Bruce, J.M., and Shuster, S. (1988). Reduction of anthralin inflammation of topical amine compounds. *Br. J. Dermatol.* 118:278.

102. Orfanos, C.E., and Steigleder, G.K. (1976). Psoriasis-therapie mit cignolin (dihydroxyanthranol): das kölner CSV-therapie-schema. *Z. Hautkr.* 51: 473–480.

103. Comaish, S., Smith, J., and Seville, R.H. (1971). Factor affecting the clearance of psoriasis with dithranol (anthralin). *Br. J. Dermatol.* 84:282–289.

104. Runne, U. (1974). Zur anthralin-salizylsäure-therapie der psoriasis. Cignolin-salizyl-säure-Vaseline-behandlung und Lasan-paste im rechts-links-vergleich. *Hautarzt* 25:199–200.

105. Hindson, C. (1980). Treatment of psoriasis of the scalp. An open assessment of 0.1% dithranol in a 17% urea base. *Clin. Trials. J.* 17:131–136.

106. Brun, P., Juhlin, L., and Schalla, W. (1984). Short contact anthralin therapy of psoriasis and maintenance schedule to prevent relapses. *Acta Derm. Venereol. (Stockh.)* 64:174–177.

107. Chlebarov, S., Kunze, J., and Thiele, B. (1988). Dithranol (antralin): ein idealer wirkstoff Reinbeker kolloquium 1988, 39, Beilage Juni.
107a. Bunse, T., and Mahrle, G. (1992). Anthralin is a potent inhibitor of *Pityrosporum orbiculare/ovale* in vitro. *Acta Derm. Venereol. (Stockh.)* 72:72–73.
107b. Rosenberg, E.W., and Noah, P.W. (1988). The Koebner phenomenon and the microbial base of psoriasis. *J. Am. Acad. Dermatol.* 18:151–158.
108. Schmoeckel, C., Weissman, I., Plewig, G., Braun-Falco, O. (1979). Treatment of alopecia areata by anthralin-induced dermatitis. *Arch. Dermatol.* 115: 1254–1255.
108a. Fiedeler, V.C., Wendrow, A., Szpunar, G.J., Metzler, C., and DeVillez, R., (1990). Treatment-resistant alopecia areata. *Arch. Dermatol.* 126:756–759.
108b. Zackheim, H.S. (1992). Evaluation of anthralin for mycosis fungoides. *J. Am. Acad. Dermatol.* 27: 112–113.
109. Krebs, A., and Schaltegger, H. (1969). Untersuchungen zur strukturspezifität der psoriasisheilmittel chrysarobin und dithranol. *Hautarzt* 20: 204–209.
109a. Bonnekoh, B., Tanzer, H., Seidel, M., Geisel, J., Merk, H.F., Mahrle, G., and Wiegrebe, W. (1991). Structure-function relationship of new anthralin derivatives assayed for growth inhibition and cytotoxicity in human keratinocyte cultures. *Arch. Pharm. (Weinheim)* 324:899–906.
109b. Müller, K., Gürsten, D., Piwek, S., and Wiegrebe, W. (1993). Antipsoriatic anthrones with modulated redox properties. *J. Med. Chem.* 36:4099–4107.
110. Wiegrebe, W., and Greber, A. (1979). Untersuchungen zum stoffwechsel antipsoriatisch wirksamer antron-derivate. *Arzneim. Forsch./Drug Res.* 29: 1083–1088.
111. Mustakallio, K.K. (1980). Irritation and staining by dithranol (anthralin) and related compounds. 2. Structure-activity relationships among 10-meso-substituted acyl analogues. *Acta Derm. Venereol. (Stockh.)* 60:169.
111a. Ashton, R.E., Andre, P., Lowe, N.J., and Whitefield, M. (1983). Anthralin: historical and current perspectives. *J. Am. Acad. Dermatol.* 9:173–192.
112. Schaltegger, A., Bloch, U., and Krebs, A. (1982). On the stability of some antipsoriatic active anthralin (dithranol) derivatives. A qualitative high performance liquid chromatography investigation. *Dermatologica* 165:363–368.
113. Hensby, C.N., Shroot, B., Chatelus, A., Cavey, D., Allec, J., and Maignan, J. (1987). In vitro and in vivo anti-inflammatory activities of C10 substituted anthralin derivatives. *Agents Actions* 21:247–249.

31

Topical Corticosteroids

Smita Amin
The Toronto Hospital, Western Division, and University of Toronto, Toronto, Ontario, Canada

Howard I. Maibach
University of California School of Medicine, San Francisco, California

Roger C. Cornell
Scripps Clinic and Research Foundation, La Jolla, California

Richard B. Stoughton[†]
University of California School of Medicine, San Diego, California

Topical glucocorticosteroids are commonly used for psoriasis. The advantages outweigh the disadvantages; other forms of therapy present major and minor problems which are often worse than those presented by topical glucocorticosteroids. The fact that the more potent and superpotent topical steroids are generally the most expensive tends to limit their use and reduces potential topical and systemic side effects. The general utility of glucocorticosteroid formulations in dermatological practice is reflected by the fact that 40–50% of prescriptions by dermatologists are for glucocorticosteroids. Although it has been more than 40 years since their introduction to dermatology, glucocorticosteroids remain "wonder drugs" of therapy.

This chapter covers ways of using these formulations in psoriasis, the role of vehicles in controlling the biological activity of the glucocorticoid, the variation in biological activity of the glucocorticoid formulations, the role of penetration and regional differences in response to glucocorticoid formulations, topical and systemic side effects, and the phenomenon of tachyphylaxis to topical glucocorticoids. Questions about frequency of application, duration of activity, and how these agents work in psoriasis will be discussed.

BACKGROUND

The steroid molecule consists of 17 carbon atoms in four rings. Three of the rings consist of six carbon atoms each and the fourth has five carbon atoms. In 1949, Hench et al. described the effects of cortisone in rheumatoid arthritis. Despite its anti-inflammatory effects in this disorder, cortisone applied topically shows no significant activity, and despite the fact that it penetrates as well as hydrocortisone (Feldmann and Maibach, 1968) and can be converted to hydrocortisone in the skin (Hsia and Hao, 1967). In addition, cortisone and hydrocortisone are interconvertible in the body. It is still unclear why hydrocortisone is clinically effective, whereas cortisone is not, but the low

[†]Deceased.

rate of conversion of cortisone to hydrocortisone in the skin may be an important factor. Subsequent to the development of hydrocortisone, the so-called fluorinated derivatives were shown to have even more potent topical activity than hydrocortisone. Figure 1 shows the steroid ring and the structure of commonly used steroids.

The first synthetic analogues of the naturally occurring cortisone and hydrocortisone were prednisone and prednisolone (Herzog et al., 1955). The addition of a 9-alpha fluoro moiety produced a compound eight times as active as hydrocortisone itself in various anti-inflammatory assays (Fried and Sabo, 1953). These agents, however, greatly increased the mineralocorticoid activity of hydrocortisone. Certain groups such as the alpha-hydroxy, alpha-methyl, and beta-methyl substituted at the 16-position on the steroid molecule greatly reduced the mineralocorticoid activity of the 9-alpha–substituted steroid without significantly affecting its potentiating effect on anti-inflammatory activity.

Subsequently, a wide variety of fluorinated steroids become available which were fluorinated in the 9 and/or 6 positions. The presence of a 16-alpha-hydroxy, 16-alpha-methyl, and 16-beta-methyl has enabled these fluorinated steroids to be used with minimal mineralocorticoid activity and primary glucocorticoid activity. Triamcinolone incorporates the 16-alpha-hydroxy group, dexamethasone the 16-alpha-methyl group, and betamethasone the 16-beta-methyl group.

Subsequently, the masking of hydroxyl groups in the 16- or 17-position by acetonides, valerates, propionates, and other acids has resulted in topical fluorinated glucocorticosteroids which greatly enhance clinical effectiveness compared to topical glucocorticosteroids with 16-alpha-hydroxy, 16-alpha-methyl, and 16-beta-methyl groups alone (Elks, 1976).

Assessment of Activity

Assessments of systemic activity or local anti-inflammatory activity such as inhibition of granuloma growth around foreign bodies are not useful in estimating the activity of a glucocorticoid used as treatment for skin disease by topical application. The most predictive test has been the vasoconstrictor assay (McKenzie, 1962; McKenzie and Stoughton, 1962), which is performed on normal human skin. The site of application of a potent glucocorticoid will blanch 4–7 hr after the original application and remain blanched for 8–48 hr, even after the steroid has been thoroughly washed from the surface. The same blanching can be induced by intradermal injection, takes 2–3 hr to develop, and will last up to 24 hr (Sutton et al., 1971). The original testing was used to compare different glucocorticosteroids dissolved in ethanol to separate the weak from the strong steroids.

Soon after publication of this method, the Glaxo Company worked with McKenzie (McKenzie and Atkinson, 1964) to test 150 glucocorticoids. They found that betamethasone-17-valerate was about 300 times

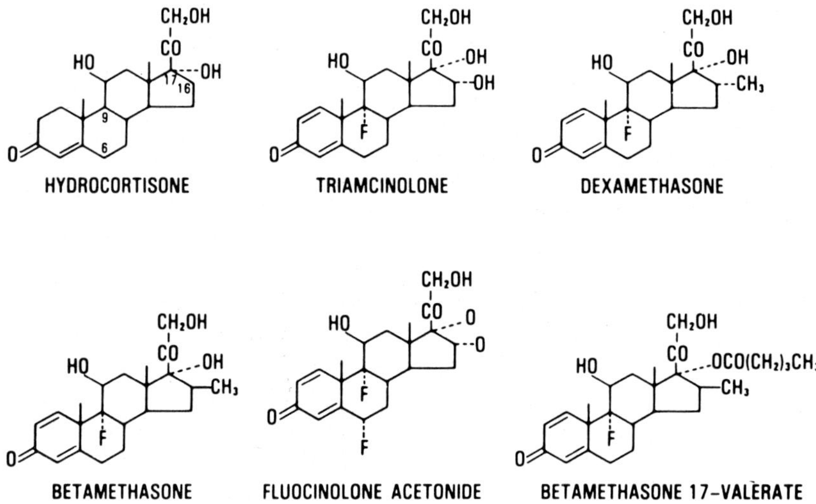

Figure 1 The steroid ring and the structure of commonly used steroids.

as potent as hydrocortisone. This was formulated in a cream ointment, and lotion and made available as Betnovate in England and Valisone in the United States. The dipropionate ester of betamethasone was later made available as Diprosone cream and ointment. The dipropionate formulations proved more potent than the 17-valerate formulations by the vasoconstriction bioassay and by clinical trials. Halog, Lidex, Temovate, Psorcon, Cyclocort, and the majority of glucocorticoid topical formulations have been selected and developed on the basis of screening with the vasoconstrictor assay. The method for applying the vasoconstriction assay to formulations was helpful in this regard (Stoughton, 1972a). Stripped skin that develops erythemas was shown to develop blanching when hydrocortisone was applied (Wells, 1957), and skin made erythematous with a nicotinate ester could be restored to normal color by treating with a glucocorticosteroid (Schlagel and Northam, 1959).

In a 1985 study, Cornell and Stoughton reviewed all their paired comparison clinical studies of topical glucocorticosteroid formulations over the past 15 years. Each pair of formulations was compared in both the vasoconstrictor assay and in a double-blind clinical paired comparison study. There were 21 such paired comparison studies in psoriasis. In 19, the vasoconstrictor assay gave the same results as those found in the paired comparison clinical study. In 2 of the 21 studies, the vasoconstrictor assay did not give the same result as the paired comparison clinical study. These two studies involved hydrocortisone valerate cream (Westcort) and alclometasone cream (Aclovate). Table 1 lists the formulations and the clinical effectiveness as compared to the vasoconstrictor responses for many brand name formulations.

Other workers have found that the vasoconstrictor assay reliably predicts clinical potency of a glucocorticoid formulation (Barry and Woodford, 1978; Gibson J.R., 1984; Barry et al. 1987).

In ranking or discussing the efficacy of topical corticosteroids, often the word "potency" is used. Thus, potency in this chapter means efficacy, even though it has another pharmacological definition. The term potency is used because of its common usage in dermatology. A more costly but important means of evaluating potency (efficacy) of a topical steroid is well-controlled clinical studies. A wide variety of approaches can determine the effectiveness of various topical steroids. Clinical studies comparing one glucocorticosteroid to another or one glucocorticosteroid to its vehicle alone are best performed on steroid-resistant dermatoses and without occlusion. Psoriasis is a particularly well-suited disease to such studies. Bilateral comparison studies, in which a patient applies one agent to the right side of the body and a second agent to the left side of the body, are preferable to so-called parallel or global studies where one group of patients applies one steroid to all involved areas, whereas a second group applied a second steroid or vehicle.

In a paired-comparison study by Cornell and Stoughton (personal observation), glucocorticosteroid formulation A was superior to glucocorticosteroid formulation B in 30 subjects with a p value <0.01. The same formulations were then tested in a parallel study at six different centers in 380 subjects. Formulation A was superior to formulation B at a p value <0.05. Thus, the paired-comparison study of 30 subjects (which took 2 weeks) was a more sensitive test of comparative efficacy in psoriasis than a parallel study of 380 subjects (which took 8 months). If one wishes to evaluate the effectiveness of a topical glucocorticosteroid on a steroid-responsive dermatoses such as psoriasis or eczema, the bilateral paired-comparison study is preferable. Such a clinical study needs intelligent, cooperative, well-instructed patients. Some populations and clinical settings do not fit this type of study.

The site of activity of the glucocorticoid in skin diseases is not known. Probably all cells have specific receptors for glucocorticoids. The topical potency of glucocorticoids correlates fairly well with the ability to combine with receptors on skin cells (Ponec, 1982). There are membrane as well as cytosolic receptors for glucocorticoids. Glucocorticoids may exert their suppressive effects on deoxyribonucleic acid (DNA) synthesis via regulating the flow of Ca^{2+} within the cell (McConkey, 1988). It is well known that DNA synthesis and mitosis are effectively shut down in epidermal cells by topical glucocorticoids (du Vivier et al., 1982). Fibroblast activity is impaired by minute amounts of glucocorticoid (Ponec et al., 1980). Phospholipase A can be inhibited by topical steroids in psoriasis (Hammerstrom et al., 1977); this may be of great importance because of the cascade of inflammatory mediators such as prostaglandins and leukotrienes which results from the delivery of arachidonic acid by phospholipase A. Lipocortin is a protein released from cells by glucocorticoids and may well play a role in regulating phospholipase A activity (Blackwell, 1980).

Table 1 Ranking Formulations Tested[a]

Vasoconstrictor assay	Clinical effectiveness
GROUP I	
Betamethasone diproprionate 0.05% in optimized (OV)	Betamethasone dipropionte 0.05% in OV
GROUP II	
Alclometason ointment 0.05[b]	Amcinonide ointment 0.1%
Amcinonide ointment 0.1%	Betamethasone dipropionate 0.5% in conventional ointment vehicle
Bethamethasone dipropionate 0.05% in conventional ointment vehicle	Desoximetasone emollient cream 0.25%
Desoximetasone emollient cream 0.25%	Diforasone diacetate ointment 0.05% (A-E)
Diforasone diacetate ointment 0.05% (A-E)	Fluocinonide gel 0.05%
Fluocinonide gel 0.05%	Fluocinonide cream 0.05%
Fluocinonide cream 0.05%	Fluocinonide ointment 0.05%
Fluocinonide ointment 0.05%	Halcinonide cream 0.01%
Halcinonide cream 0.01%	
GROUP III	
Betamethasone valerate ointment 0.1%	Betamethasone valerate ointment 0.1%
Betamethasone dipropionate cream 0.05%	Betamethasone dipropionate cream 0.05%
Hydrocortisone valerate cream 0.2%[b]	
GROUP IV	
Fluocinolone acetonide ointment 0.025%	Fluocinolone acetonide ointment 0.025%
GROUP V	
Betamethasone valerate cream 0.1%	Betamethasone valerate cream 0.1%
Flurandrenolide cream 0.05% in self-preserving (SP) vehicle	Flurandrenolide cream 0.05% in SP vehicle
	Hydrocortisone valerate cream 0.2%[b]
GROUP VI	
Desonide (Tridesilon) cream 0.05%	Alclometasone ointment 0.05%[b]
	Desonide (Tridesilon) cream 0.05%
GROUP VII	
Dexamethasone cream 0.1%	Dexamethasone cream 0.1%
Hydrocortisone cream 2.5%	Hydrocortisone cream 2.5%
Hydrocortisone cream 1%	Hydrocortisone cream 1%

[a]Group I was the most potent group and group VII the least potent. Within each group, the compounds are of equal potency, and are listed in alphabetical order.
[b]These formulations showed significant differences in the vasoconstricted assay and clinical effectiveness comparisons.
Source: Cornell & Stoughton (1985).

PERCUTANEOUS PENETRATION

Penetration of a steroid is defined as its ability, after topical application, to find its way through the epidermis and into the dermis. Penetration cannot be equated with potency, since potency refers to the agent's clinical effectiveness. An agent that readily penetrates is not necessarily one that will be potent topically in the treatment of psoriasis, although frequently the ability of an agent to penetrate skin parallels its clinical effectiveness. Some evidence equates activity with ability of the steroid to combine with the steroid receptors on the cells (Ponec et al., 1980; Ponec, 1982).

There are many methods to measure the penetration of a topical agent. Radiolabeled topical steroids have been applied to the epidermis of hairless mouse skin or human skin in in vitro systems and the amount of glucocorticosteroid penetrating measured. In such determinations in vitro chambers are used and the dermis is bathed in saline. The steroid is applied to the epidermis and penetration through the epidermis and into the dermis, and hence the saline bath, can easily be determined.

Other means of measuring the penetration of a topical steroid include excretion of the steroid in vivo. When radiolabeled topical steroids are applied to the epidermis, the blood and urine can be measured to determine if penetration of such an agent has occurred (Malkinson and Ferguson, 1955; Feldmann and Maibach, 1967).

One can also measure penetration of topical glucocorticosteroids by their disappearance from the surface on which they are applied. One can determine residual analysis of a topical steroid by measuring the amount of steroid retained in the stratum corneum. By taking serial strippings of the skin one can measure not only the amount of steroid remaining in the stratum corneum in a specified period after the application, but also the rate of disappearance of the steroid from the surface (Schaffer, 1982).

Chemical assays that actually measure glucocorticosteroids in various layers of the skin have not been widely utilized. While most topical steroids are thought to be primarily active in the upper dermis, it is difficult to measure by chemical means the concentration of a given glucocorticosteroid in the upper dermis, since this would require invasive techniques. As yet, no reproducible assays have been developed to determine the amount of glucocorticosteroid in the lower epidermis or upper dermis, for example, in psoriasis or their steroid-responsive dermatoses.

The penetration of a steroidal agent when applied topically may be enhanced by several factors. A primary consideration is the site of application. A topical steroid applied to the eyelids, for example, will penetrate approximately 4 times as readily as the same quantity of steroid applied to the forehead, 9 times as readily as when applied to the scalp or axilla, and 36–40 times as readily as when applied to the palms and soles (Feldmann and Maibach, 1967). Anything that damages the stratum corneum, including stripping the skin, will increase the penetration of a steroid. Since the stratum corneum can act as a reservoir of a topically applied steroid, eliminating the stratum corneum (whether by artificial means such as with adhesive tape or in disease where the stratum corneum is absent or injured) will only enhance the ability of the steroid to penetrate.

Increasing the humidity of the area treated, such as occlusion with plastic wrap or other occlusive tapes or covering an area to be tested with a vinyl cover may increase penetration (Stoughton, 1972b; Bucks et al., 1988). Increasing temperature will also increase the penetration of a topical glucocorticosteroid. Increasing the concentration of the steroid does not necessarily increase the percentage of its penetration. In fact, as the concentration increases the percentage of applied steroid that penetrates (Stoughton, 1988; Stoughton and Wullich, 1989) may decrease. Thus, one can increase the concentration of hydrocortisone from 1 to 4% and not have any increase in the penetration of hydrocortisone into the skin (Stoughton, 1977). A point is reached at which an increase in concentration does not necessarily result in any net increase in penetration. There is no question that prolonged hydration of the skin is one of the most effective ways to increase a chemical's penetration of the intact stratum corneum, which is why occlusive dressings and tape are so effective. However, patients seem to resist using these coverings on their skin.

ENHANCEMENT OF POTENCY

Many chemical modifications increase the potency of a topical glucocorticosteroid. The acetonide analogue used in triamcinolone, fluocinolone, and flurandrenolide is clearly more potent in these agents than the alcohol base. The valerate ester in betamethasone-17-valerate increases the potency of betamethasone over betamethasone alcohol (McKenzie and Atkinson, 1964). The addition of a 21-acetate moiety to fluocinolone acetonide increases the potency of this agent significantly: fluocinolone acetonide-21-acetate is more potent than fluocinolone acetonide. The acetate moiety results in increased potency compared to a free alcohol moiety on the fluocinole acetonide molecule. The use of these other bases such as butyrates have shown great promise in increasing potency. One cannot equate the presence of a fluoride atom with potency. For example, hydrocortisone butyrate is as potent as triamcinolone acetonide. The latter is fluorinated and the former is not. Many topical fluorinated steroids tested have been found not to be potent and new nonfluorinated steroids currently exist or are being evaluated that shown potency similar to many of the moderately potent fluorinated steroids.

New steroid analogues do not owe their increased potency to enhanced penetration. The increased potency is more likely related to the fact that the fewer absorbed molecules have a greater effect, probably related to affinity for receptors on cells. For example, fluocinolone acetonide penetrates 14 times as well as fluocinolone alcohol, but is 125 times more potent clinically. Betamethasone valerate penetrates no more than betamethasone alcohol, but the former is 625 times as effective as the latter. Thus, a primary way to increase potency is molecular modification of the steroid or a change of the vehicle. The acetonide, valerate, acetate, and butyrate moieties and, to some degree, the benzoate and privalate moieties, enhance clinical effectiveness.

The concentration of the steroidal agent is important in increasing clinical potency to a degree but, as discussed above, a point is reached at which increasing the concentration of an agent does not necessarily increase potency. For example, increasing the concentration of betamethasone-17-valerate from 0.04 to 1.00% in dimethylacetamide results in no increased clinical activity. The authors have determined in clinical studies and vasoconstrictor studies that in a conventional cream vehicle, 2.5% hydrocortisone is no more effective than 1.0% (personal observations). We have investigated the role of increasing concentrations of a glucocorticoid in regard to its bioavailability in the same vehicle (Stoughton and Wullich, 1989). These were all brand name formulations in the United States, Kenalog creams, which have concentrations of triamcinolone acetonide at 0.025, 0.1, and 0.5% all give the same potency as measured by the vasoconstrictor assay in human subjects. Aristocort cream at concentrations of 0.5 and 0.025% gives the same potency or bioavailability. A 20-fold increase in concentration (0.025 to 0.5%) does not increase the potency or bioavailability of triamcinolone acetonide in the cream formulation. Topicort 0.25% cream gives the same potency as Topicort cream 0.05% in the vasoconstrictor assay. However, Synalar cream gives increasing potency with each of the ascending concentrations from 0.01 to 0.025 to 0.2%. Valisone cream at 0.1% is more potent than Valisone cream at 0.01%. This inconsistency of bioavailability with increasing concentration is not surprising considering previous work showing a narrow margin for optimum conditions for maximum penetration of glucocorticoids (Poulsen, 1968).

Another major factor in the potency of a topical steroid is the vehicle. In formulating the steroid one desires a vehicle in which the steroid will be soluble and stable, and that has a satisfactory rate of release, and is able to hydrate the skin (Maibach and Stoughton, 1973).

Topical corticosteroid products can be optimized; that is, their activity can be further enhanced by the use of propylene glycol, such as was done when Diprolene, an optimized vehicle preparation of betamethasone dipropionate, was formulated. In many instances, steroids which are inherently potent have been markedly diminished by the vehicle in which they were used. Dimethylsulfoxide and dimethylacetamide will increase the penetration of a topical steroid (Maibach and Feldmann, 1967), but these are rarely used now because of possible toxicity, odor, and irritation. Azone enhances steroid activity in alcohol solutions when added at 1–2% (Stoughton, 1982). This vehicle is active in enhancing the penetration of many different chemical agents and has to be used at only 1–5% concentrations. Azone is colorless, odorless, tasteless, and nonirritating on human skin, and tests to date show no significant systemic toxicity.

Lotions are particularly poor in conveying the inherent activity of the glucocorticoid. Most lotions evaporate readily, leaving large crystals of glucocorticoid on the skin, which penetrate very poorly. In selecting a proper steroid for the treatment of psoriasis, the physician must consider the degree of involvement, the area of the body to be treated, and many other factors. Potent steroids should not be used on the face, axilla, inguinal area, or other intertriginous areas because of their ability to cause certain side effects such as striae, atrophy, and perioral dermatitis. Ointments are best used on noncovered areas. Creams are best used on covered areas and their effectiveness enhanced by occlusion. As a rule, lotions or aerosols are best used on hair-bearing areas. Some patients with psoriasis are willing to tolerate an ointment in covered areas, and there is no reason why they should not be used in such areas if tolerated by the patient. The patient should be instructed to use the steroid as directed, sparingly, and rub it in gently. Most patients apply far more of the agent topically than is clinically necessary. Patients should be encouraged not to apply the topical agent to normal areas of skin. This is simple when a patient has only scattered large plaques, but obviously it is more difficult for the patient with extensive multiple small guttate lesions. In certain instances, where relatively few but resistant psoriatic plaques are present, steroid-impregnated tape gives very satisfactory results.

The clinician has a wide variety of topical agents to choose from in the treatment of psoriasis. The fact that an agent is clinically more potent does not necessarily mean that it is the steroid of choice. Unfortunately, there is as yet no topical steroid formulation in which clinical potency does not parallel both topical and systemic side effects. Using the vasoconstriction assay as well as clinical studies, one can "rank" topical steroids from most to least potent (Table 2).

TOPICAL SIDE EFFECTS

The clinician must be aware that even if the agent used is "external," side effects may result. The ability

Table 2 Cost of Some Topical Steroids

Steroid		AWP[a]	Range	Vehicle
Lowest potency	(may be ineffective for some indications)			
0.1%	Dexamethasone (Decadron Phosphate, Merck)	$ 15.36		Cream
1.0%[b]	Hydrocortisone, average generic price,	2.21	(1.32 – 5.10)	Cream, ointment
	average brand-name price	5.63	(2.00 – 180.1)	Cream, ointment
	(Cort-Dome, Miles)	18.01		Cream
		45.30		Lotion
2.5%	Hydrocortisone – average generic price,	5.45	(4.26 – 6.88)	Cream, ointment
	average brand-name price	9.93	(7.55 – 11.70)	Cream, ointment
Low potency				
0.01%	Betamethasone valerate (Valison, Schering)	$ 14.76		Cream
0.1%	Clocortolone (Cloderm, Hermal)	20.90		Cream
0.05%	Desonide (Desowen, Owen)	17.76		Cream, ointment
	(Tridesilon, Miles)	18.16		Cream, ointment
0.01%	Fluocinolone acetonide, average generic price	3.19	(2.08 – 4.38)	Cream
0.025%	Triamcinolone acetonide, average generic price,	2.46	(1.25–4.28)	Ointment, cream
		7.55	(7.00 – 8.22)	Lotion
	average brand, name price	8.31	(1.06 – 15.34)	Cream, ointment
	(Aristocort A, Lederle)	15.34		Cream
	(Kenalog, Westwood-Squibb)	25.58		Lotion
Medium potency				
0.025%	Betamethasone benzoate (Uticort, Parke Davis)	$ 25.86		Lotion
0.1%	Betamethasone valerate, average generic price	6.31	(4.06 – 9.26)	Cream, ointment
		9.14	(5.40 – 12.00)	Lotion
	average brand-name price	13.39	(4.18 – 24.84)	Cream, ointment
		18.14	(7.49 – 30.24)	Lotion
0.05%	Desoximetasone, average generic price	14.37		Cream
	(Topicort LP, Hoechst-Roussell)	17.60		Cream
0.025%	Fluocinolone acetonide, average generic price,	4.42	(2.29 – 8.98)	Cream, ointment
	average brand-name price	11.57	(4.88 – 16.54)	Cream, ointment
0.2%	Hydrocortisone valerate (Westcort, Westwood-Squibb)	20.16		Cream, ointment
0.1%	Mometasone furoate (Elocon, Schering)	22.80		Cream, ointment
		23.58		Lotion
0.025%	Halcinonide (Halog, Westwood-Squibb)	23.40		Cream
0.1%	Triamcinolone acetonide, averge generic price	3.09	(1.50 – 4.62)	Cream, ointment
		8.02	(4.88 – 10.95)	Lotion
	average brand-name price	9.18	(1.90 – 19.46)	Cream, ointment
	(Aristocort, Lederle)	15.68		Cream, ointment
	(Aristocort A, Lederle)	19.46		Cream, ointment
	(Kenalog, Westwood-Squibb)	18.98		Cream
0.005%	Fluticasone propionate (Cutivate, Glaxo)	17.04		Ointment
0.05%		17.04		Cream
High potency				
0.1%	Amcinonide (Cyclocort, Lederle)	$ 21.62		Cream, ointment
		33.21		Lotion
0.05%	Betamethasone dipropionate, average generic price,	11.25	(6.80 – 24.48)	Cream, ointment
		11.32	(7.50 – 14.35)	Lotion
	average brand-name price	24.95	(10.76 – 35.56)	Cream, ointment
	(Diprosone, Schering)	37.08		Lotion
0.25%	Desoximetasone, average generic price	19.48	(17.20 – 20.70)	Cream
	(Topicort, Hoechest-Roussel)	23.00		Cream, ointment
0.05%	Diflorasone diacetate (Floreone, Dermik)	22.18		Cream, ointment
	(Maxiflor, Herbert)	21.25		Cream, ointment
0.2%	Fluocinolone (Synalar HP, Syntex)	45.84		Cream

Table 2 *Continued*

Steroid		AWP*[a]	Range	Vehicle
0.05%	Fluocinonide, average generic price	10.47	(7.13 – 15.75)	Cream
	(Lidex, Lidex-E, Syntex)	21.53		Cream, ointment
0.1%	Halcinonide (Halog, Halog-E, Westwood-Squibb)	24.98		Cream, ointment
		40.80		Solution
0.5%	Triamcinolone acetonide, average generic price,	7.10	(4.30 – 10.38)	Cream, ointment
	average brand-name price	27.62	(3.60 – 53.42)	Cream, ointment
	(Aristocort A, Lederle)	53.42		Cream
Super-high potency				
0.05%	Betamethasone dipropionate (Diprolene, Schering)	$ 34.36		Cream, ointment
		40.20		Lotion
0.05%	Clobetasol propionate (Temovate, Glaxo)	23.82		Cream, ointment
0.05%	Diflorasone diacetate (Psorcon, Dermik)	23.05		Ointment
0.05%	Halobetasol propionate (Ultravate, Westwood-Squibb)	34.20		Cream, ointment

[a]Cost to the pharmacist, based on manufacturers' listings in *Drug Topics Red Book* and August 1991 *Update*, for purchase of two 15-g or one 30-g container or 60 mi at average wholesale price; cost to the patient will be higher.
[b]Now available over-the-counter.
Source: *Medical Letter on Drugs and Therapeutics* 1991; 33(857):108–110.

of topical glucocorticosteroids to result in side effects has become more apparent as newer, more potent, steroids have been utilized over the past 10 years. Steroids should be used with caution and, if used on extensive areas of skin, the physician must be aware of potential side effects. Side effects from the use of topical glucocorticosteroids include the following.

Acne

Prolonged treatment with corticosteroids can result in a form of acne characterized by a wave of dense inflamed pustules which may result in crops of comedones. As opposed to acne vulgaris, in this form of acne many lesions are in the same developmental state (Plewig and Kligman, 1973). Scarring following steroid-induced acne is, fortunately, unusual. It may be that the topical steroid, in addition to causing an acneiform eruption, may help to prevent scarring by its anti-inflammatory properties.

Perioral Dermatitis

Discrete papules in the perioral area occur which lack atrophy or telangiectasia. Reports of perioral dermatitis have increased greatly over the past several years secondary to the advent of extremely potent topical steroids (Sneddon, 1972). Unfortunately, many patients who have been given a prescription for a steroid for use on another area of the body assume that it is also effective and safe for use on the face. The physician often needs to take a detailed history to determine that the patient was in fact using a steroid on the face. Treatment consists of discontinuing the steroid and initiating tetracycline. If a patient has been using topical steroids for many months, the perioral dermatitis will flare, severely at times, following discontinuation of the medication. Under these circumstances, it is acceptable to allow the patient to use topical hydrocortisone for a 1–2 month period. This is analogous to not suddenly discontinuing a high dosage of a systemic steroid, but gradually tapering the patient off the steroid using lower dosages.

Rosacea

Potent topical steroids are to be discouraged in the treatment of rosacea. It is frequently difficult to manage a patient with severe rosacea. Patients given potent topical steroids for "psoriasis" on the face may have psoriasis with concomitant rosacea. Initially the symptoms of burning and pustulation are reduced in rosacea, but eventually skin atrophy and telagiectasia result. In patients with mild rosacea using topical steroids, a severe rebound has been described consisting of edema and multiple pustules (Leyden et al., 1974).

Striae and Atrophy

These are common results of the use of potent steroids in certain skin areas. Occasionally atrophy can be severe enough that secondary ulceration occurs (Stevanovic, 1972). The ability of topical steroids to inhibit collagen synthesis by fibroblasts and thus cause atrophy may be the mechanism of steroidal atrophy. Striae and atrophy are worse in areas of sweating and occlusion (Johns and Bower, 1970). Frequently, prior to atrophy the patient complains of pain or burning, followed by thinning of the epidermis and prominent talangiectatic change. Lavker et al. (1986) used human subjects to carefully measure changes in the normal human skin during and after continuous occlusion of clobetasol propionate for 6 weeks. They saw dermal and epidermal atrophy after 3 weeks. Most clinical studies cover 2 weeks of application, so it is not surprising that atrophy is not reported in such clinical studies. They also observed profound changes in the vascular, collagen, and elastic tissue networks. Fibroblasts and mast cells are also profoundly changed by occlusive epidermal applications. In this same report, the investigators detail the recovery process after 6 weeks of occlusive treatment with clobetasol propionate. The epidermis and dermis were quite normal 2 weeks after discontinuing treatment, but the recovery of mast cells was delayed to 3 months.

Purpura

The use of glucocorticosteroids is frequently associated with acquired purpura, particularly in older patients and in areas where the skin is already somewhat thinned, such as on the arms and, to a lesser degree, over the legs. A potent or superpotent steroid may cause atrophy of already somewhat atrophic skin secondary to age and/or actinic change; purpuric lesions after minimal trauma may result. These are often a cause of distress to the patient. While this is usually not an incapacitating problem for the patient, it can cause difficulties for the practicing physician. The topical steroid to be used should be only as potent as necessary and the patient should be warned that it should be used only on areas of involved skin and not rubbed over areas of normal skin.

Glaucoma

The ability of potent topical steroids used around the lids to cause glaucoma is well documented (Cubey, 1976), as is the use of optical steroidal drops (Koss et al., 1972). Potent topical steroids should not be used around the eyelids or on the face in psoriasis.

Bacterial/Fungal Infections

The role of topical glucocorticosteroids in predisposing a patient to bacterial and/or fungal infections is unclear. While topical glucocorticosteroids may not enable fungi to grow, it is not uncommon to see secondary fungi under areas treated by steroids, particularly steroids in ointment vehicles. The ability of tinea to grow in such areas may be related to a slower rate of shedding of stratum corneum because of decreased epidermal turnover. Topical steroids inhibit mitosis and DNA synthesis. In tinea incognito, the infection is not recognized owing in part to a reduction in the inflammatory response. Minimal scaling may be apparent and only after use of a careful potassium hydroxide preparation may organisms be noted (Ive and Marks, 1968).

Allergic Contact Dermatitis

Allergic contact dermatitis occurs with the use of many topical glucocorticosteroids (Alani and Alani, 1972). The allergen is either the steroid itself or the vehicle. In instances where allergic contact dermatitis to a particular steroid is suspected and where the physician wishes to document such sensitivity, find out from the manufacturer all the ingredients of the steroidal vehicle. Individual patch testing to such ingredients will frequently elicit the etiological agent. Unfortunately, topical corticoid allergic contact dermatitis is infrequently diagnosed on morphological grounds. Only by testing with surrogate markers, tixocortal pivalate, bedesonide, and hydrocortisone valerate or butyrate, will the occult allergies in nonresponsive psoriasis and eczematous psoriasis be identified (Wilkinson, 1994). In corticoid-sensitive subjects, prednisone or ACTH injections may elicit generalized dermatitis (Lauerma et al., 1991; Menne et al., 1989).

Both topical and systemic side effects from the use of external glucocorticosteroids occur in infants and children when even less potent steroids are used. For example, children show more profound adrenal suppression with topical steroids of only moderate potency than do their adult counterparts (Feiwel et al., 1969).

SYSTEMIC SIDE EFFECTS

The practicing clinician must be concerned with potential systemic pharmacological effects of such potent steroids on the pituitary-adrenal axis. The potency of a topical steroid may be enhanced by a wide variety of factors, including chemical formulation, concentration, and vehicle. Increase in the humidity by occlusive dressing will increase the penetration of a steroid. The site of application also determines the degree of penetration of a topical agent. Steroids applied to the eyelids and scrotum penetrate far better than the same agent applied to the forehead or scalp. Penetration through the palms and soles is minimal. Topical steroids penetrate diseased stratum corneum more readily than normal skin. The dermatologist should be aware that penetration by the steroid and potential suppression of the pituitary-adrenal axis may be a direct function of the amount of diseased skin treated, the sites of treatment, and whether occlusion is used in conjunction with the topical agent.

Plasma Cortisol Suppression

Scoggins (1962) and Gill and Baxter (1964) demonstrated that plasma cortisol is depressed in patients with extensive psoriasis treated with fluocinolone acetonide 0.025% under occlusion. Scoggins and Kliman (1965) demonstrated a fall in morning plasma cortisol when moderately strong steroids without occlusion were used over very large areas of the body.

Carr and Tarnowski (1968) were unable to show adrenal cortical suppression in a subject with normal skin using large amounts of triamcinolone acetonide 0.1% without occlusion, but they did demonstrate suppression of the pituitary-adrenal axis in a normal subject with as little as 9 mg of triamcinolone acetonide daily applied under a polyethylene film dressing. Conversely, total body treatment in patients with generalized dermatoses led to pituitary-adrenal suppression irrespective of whether occlusive dressings were used. They showed that as little as 2.25 mg of triamcinolone acetonide applied under plastic dressings to the skin of a patient with a generalized dermatosis can suppress urinary 17-hydroxysteroids. Goldman and Cohen (1962) and Rostenberg (1962) were unable to demonstrate alteration of the pituitary-adrenal axis after flurandrenolone acetonide (nonoccluded). March and Kerbel (1964) found similar results when occlusion was used. Monro and Clift (1973) concluded that in the majority of adults using small quantities of moderately strong topical steroid ointments without occlusion there is negligible risk of suppression of the pituitary-adrenal axis. Wilson et al. (1973) found that the vast majority of patients taking betamethasone-17-valerate had normal plasma cortisol levels and were unable to detect any correlation between plasma cortisol level and duration of treatment.

In none of the above-mentioned studies were any of the more recently available potent and superpotent steroids such as halcinonide (Halog), betamethasone dipropionate (Diprosone), fluocinonide (Lidex), desoximetasone (Topicort), or clobetasol propionate (Temorate) used.

Gomez et al. (1977) reported that halcinonide (Halog) cream applied for 5 days suppresses plasma cortisol after topical application both with and without occlusion in patients with extensive psoriasis. No adrenal suppression was noted when halcinonide cream was applied to greater than 50% of the body surface of normal individuals without occlusion. Pituitary-adrenal suppression did occur when this material was applied under occlusion. Betamethasone-17-valerate (Valisone) 0.1% caused suppression of the pituitary-adrenal axis both with and without occlusion in patients with widespread psoriasis, but to a lesser degree than the suppression caused by halcinonide cream. In a larger group of patients treated for 4–6 weeks three or four times a day without occlusion, the authors found no suppression with betamethasone-17-valerate but there was definite adrenal suppression in 2 or 23 patients receiving halcinonide.

Twenty-two patients were treated with desoximetasone emollient cream (Topicort) 0.25 mg% twice daily without occlusion for 6 months. Patients applied the medication to approximately one-third of their body over psoriatic lesions. Plasma cortisol values were decreased to below normal limits in nine patients before the 6-month study was terminated. In four of these, the plasma cortisol spontaneously returned to normal despite therapy. In four other patients, however, the plasma cortisol was still suppressed at the end of 6 months of continual therapy, but returned to normal within 7 days of discontinuation of the medication. In one patient lost to further follow-up at 5.25 months of therapy, the trend at the fourth month was an increase in plasma cortisol to within 1 unit of normal range. Betamethasone-17-valerate 0.1% cream (Valisone) applied twice daily did not suppress plasma cortisol in 23 patients similarly tested. The clinical response to desoximetasone emollient cream was significantly better than to betamethasone valerate cream (Cornell and Stoughton, 1981). This study is the first to approximate closely the way in which many patients with steroid-responsive dermatoses use potent topical steroids, over a long time and without occlusion.

The three class I superpotent agents have all been compared using Food and Drug Administration guidelines on hospitalized patients with psoriasis and eczema. In general, an initial dose of 15 g twice daily is used unoccluded on approximately 30% of the diseased skin over a 7-day period. Three days of baseline plasma cortisol and 24-hr urine determinations of 17-hydroxycorticoids and/or urine cortisols are performed. The study medication is then applied, and on days 6 and 7 of therapy these parameters are repeated and compared with baseline. If suppression occurs, the dose is cut in half and a new group of patients studied. The dose continues to be cut in half until a dose is reached with minimal or no suppression. In general, suppression of the pituitary-adrenal axis parallels clinical effectiveness with the superpotent agents.

Clobetasol propionate (Temovate) suppressed three of four patients when 3.5 g was used twice daily (49 g/week); two of nine patients, when 1.75 g was used twice daily (25 g/week); and one of nine patients, when as little as 1 g was used twice daily (14 g/week). The ointment and cream formulations were equally capable of suppressing the pituitary-adrenal axis. Betamethasone dipropionate in an optimized vehicle (Diprolene) was less suppressive, requiring over 7 g daily (over 49 g/week) to cause a significant reduction in plasma cortisol. Diflorasone diacetate ointment in an optimized vehicle (Psorcon) may have a greater safety profile in that suppression was not seen in a limited number of patients when 15 g was used twice daily over 7 days. It must be stressed that these studies are on relatively few patients over a 7-day period and that additional studies of these compounds when used for several weeks at a time on a large number of patients are in order.

In general, plasma cortisols return to normal 2–3 days after suppression occurs and the topical agent is discontinued. Follow-up metyrapone studies have been normal in virtually all patients who have shown suppression on superpotent agents.

Cushing Syndrome

The typical body habitus in Cushing syndrome consists of moon facies, intracapsular buffalo hump, fat in the mesenteric bed with truncal obesity, and muscle wasting. Increased body weight is often also present. Fatigue and weakness are common complaints. Hypertension, diabetes mellitus, hirsutism, amenorrhea, cutaneous striae, ecchymoses, osteoporosis, and personality change are common in this disorder. The most common cause of Cushing syndrome is adrenal hyperplasia. Adrenal nodular hyperplasia and adrenal neoplasia such as adenomas or carcinomas may also cause Cushing syndrome. Iatrogenic Cushing syndrome due to prolonged use of topical glucocorticosteroids or the prolonged use of systemic steroids or adrenocorticotropin (ACTH) has been reported. It is distinguishable by physical findings from endogenous forms of adrenocortical hyperfunction. Iatrogenic Cushing syndrome is related to the total steroid dosage and duration of therapy. Patients receiving long-term ACTH may have hyperpigmentation as well.

In the endogenous form of Cushing syndrome, the plasma cortisol level is markedly elevated and cannot be suppressed, whereas in the iatrogenic syndrome the plasma cortisol level is decreased. The latter is due to the fact that fluorinated glucocorticosteroids result in a decrease in ACTH production by the pituitary gland and thus a fall in plasma cortisol. The ability of fluorinated glucocorticosteroids to cause significant systemic effects has been reported not only in children, in whom the occurrence of systemic side effects with topical glucocorticosteroids is particularly of concern, but also in adults where frank Cushing syndrome has been reported with topical application and long-term use of potent and superpotent topical steroids such as dexosimetasone emollient cream (Himathongkam et al., 1978) and clobetasol dipropionate. Patients using more than 100 g weekly have shown profound suppression of plasma cortisol (Carruthers et al., 1975) and developed features of Cushing syndrome or withdrawal symptoms of adrenal insufficiency and the development of pustular psoriasis. Pituitary-adrenal suppression has occurred with this agent even when small amounts were applied to nonoccluded normal skin of volunteers (Ortega et al., 1975). Cushing syndrome following the application of hydrocortisone and its derivatives has not been reported. Nonetheless as new hydrocortisone derivatives are developed utilizing new vehicles, one might anticipate topical and systemic side effects. The fact that a glucocorticosteroid is nonfluorinated cannot be equated with an inability to cause either topical or systemic side effects.

Cataracts

Systemic steroids can induce posterior subcapsular cataracts. It is not clear whether topical steroids around the eye can do this. It is difficult to distinguish cataracts that occur spontaneously in atopic dermatitis patients from the posterior subcapsular cataracts resulting from glucocorticoid administration (Castrow, 1981). Only the most mild topical steroids should be used around the eyes.

COMPARISONS OF PITUITARY-ADRENAL EFFECTS

Unfortunately, it is difficult to compare the pituitary-adrenal suppression of various topical steroids. To date no study has used a large number of patients in whom a similar quantity of material was applied to an equal amount of diseased psoriatic skin for the same period of time and where variables such as humidity, occlusion, temperature, and site of application have been consistent. The most potent topical glucocorticosteroids are clinically the most effective, but have the highest incidence of not only topical side effects, but also suppression of the pituitary-adrenal axis.

In evaluating the pituitary-adrenal axis, plasma cortisols are the easiest to measure. While laboratory normals vary, the morning plasma coritsol should be between 5 and 25 μg/100 ml and the evening cortisol less than 10 μg/100 ml. Plasma cortisols, however, only measure basal homeostasis, but are easy to obtain compared to 24-hr urine collections and provide good baseline data.

The ability of a topical glucocorticosteroid to reduce plasma coritsol only measures basal homeostasis. Levels of urinary 17-hydroxy and 17-ketogenic steroids seem to parallel plasma cortisol values, but because of the difficulty in obtaining 24-hr urine samples the plasma cortisol seems to be a good indicator of basla homeostasis of the adrenal gland.

Unfortunately, however, this does not indicate the functional integrity of the pituitary-adrenal axis under conditions of stress. The adrenal gland can be tested directly by the use of naturally occurring or synthetic ACTH. These agents stimulate the adrenal, and one should see at least a fourfold increase in total urinary 17-hydroxy corticosteroid levels after ACTH has been administered. While plasma cortisol has been shown to return to normal quickly even in patients on long-term topical glucocorticosteroid therapy, at times it may be important to measure directly the functional adrenal reserve.

Tests are available to evaluate the pituitary-adrenal axis. Stressful stimuli such as insulin-induced hypoglycemia, intravenous injections of pyrogens, and intravenous injections of vasopressin cause ACTH to increase and, in a normal individual, a brisk increase in the plasma cortisol occurs. Metyrapone (Metopirone) will increase ACTH by inhibiting 11-betahydroxylase. This results in an increased plasma 11-deoxycortisol level which can easily be measured as well as increased total urinary 17-hydroxy corticosteroid. While ACTH tests the adrenal directly, stressful stimuli and metyrapone test the hypothalamic pituitary-adrenal axis.

TACHYPHYLAXIS

Tachyphylaxis describes a diminishing effect of a pharmacological agent as it is repeatedly used to achieve a clinical response. Ephedrine, for example, injected repeatedly intravenously in dogs has a progressively diminishing effect on blood pressure. Potent topical glucocorticosteroids (e.g., Lidex cream) cause vasoconstriction when first applied to human skin, but with subsequent applications the production of vasoconstriction rapidly diminishes. However, after a rest period of a few days the same initial vasoconstrictive effect may be produced again, but will subside if the steroid is continued topically (du Vivier and Stoughton, 1975). Depression of DNA synthesis by topical steroids will also show tachyphylaxis with the continued use of steroids and even allow an increase in DNA synthesis when topical steroids are withdrawn; this may be related to the rebound phenomenon one sees when psoriatic or eczematous patients who "become resistant" to a potent topical steroid after repeated application. A "rebound" phenomenon after systemic steroids have been observed as well. Tachyphylaxis topical steroid suppression of histamine whealing has been described in humans (Singh and Singh, 1986).

If a topical steroid could be given on an intermittent basis, this would have many advantages, including less expense to a patient, more likelihood of patient compliance, since the medication would not need to be applied as frequently, and possibly a decrease in the potential topical and systemic side effects. Once-a-day therapy may be as effective as three-times-daily applications (Fredrikson et al., 1980). Intermittent dosing with clobetasol propionate and other superpotent agents can lead to a prolonged remission if used after initial clearing. In one study (Hradil et al., 1978), 8 of 12 psoriatic patients were kept clear of lesions for 21 weeks by using clobetasol propionate only once a week on any erythematous spots. In a larger study,

75% of 132 psoriatic patients remained in remission using clobetasol propionate only twice a week (Svartholm et al., 1982).

Katz et al. (1988) reported that betamethasone dipropionate in an optimized vehicle applied three times in 1 week kept most of the originally treated and cleared psoriatic lesions from undergoing relapse when the applications were on 2 successive days of the week.

One study of hand eczema compared the relapse rate of the eczema in the 90% of subjects who were cleared by a twice-daily schedule for 71 days. The subjects were maintained on twice-a-week applications of either clobetasol propionate or fluprednidene acetate cream (Moller et al., 1983). Seventy percent of the clobetasol subjects remained free of disease compared with 30% on fluprednidene.

Intralesional steroids in the treatment of psoriasis should be considered, particularly in patients with only a few lesions. Low-solubility steroids such as triamcinolone acetonide may persist for 3–4 weeks when injected intradermally. Triamcinolone hexacetonide, a new intralesional steroid, is even less soluble. The maximum dosage of injected triamcinolone acetonide should not exceed 30 mg total. The atrophy not infrequently seen with intralesional triamcinolone acetonide is often reversible.

GENERICS

In the United States, there has been a surge in sales of generic topical corticosteroids, partly due to a change in government regulations and partly due to the fact that almost all the glucocorticoids used in topical therapy are beyond patent protection.

Comparisons of some of these generics with brand name formulations have revealed that the generics are frequently less potent than the brand name equivalents (Stoughton, 1987; Jackson, 1989). This has been true for formulations containing triamcinolone acetonide, fluocinolone acetonide, betamethasone dipropionate, and betamethasone valerate.

Most of the generics we have tested and found to be inferior are not identical in their vehicle composition to the brand name equivalent (Stoughton, 1988). We have already discussed earlier in this chapter the large influence that vehicle changes can make in the potency of the same steroid at the same concentration, and we suspect these vehicle differences are responsible for the inferior performance of many generics. Until this problem has been rectified, we do not support the use of generics in dermatology. A round table discussion held in January 1992 summarized the scientific issues involved (Maibach, 1992).

CONCLUSIONS

In selecting a topical glucocorticosteroid in the treatment of psoriasis one should use a steroid potent enough to improve or clear the dermatoses. Ointments tend to work better for resistant lesions. In general, twice-daily application is recommended, but as additional information becomes available, daily, alternate-day, or even less frequent therapy may be appropriate. One must remember that a steroid which penetrates is not necessarily the most clinically effective: Penetration cannot necessarily be equated with potency. Thus far no potent topical glucocorticosteroid has been developed in which topical side effects and suppression of the pituitary-adrenal axis do not parallel the agent's clinical effectiveness. The ideal topical glucocorticosteroid would show superior clinical effectiveness but without topical or systemic side effects.

The extensive literature in the field is summarized by Surber (Surber and Maibach, 1992; Surber et al., 1995) and Korting (Korting and Maibach, 1993).

REFERENCES

Alani, M.D., and Alani, S.D. 91972). Allergic contact dermatitis to corticosteroids. *Ann. Allergy* 30:181–185.

Barry, B.W., et al. (1987). Control of the bioavailability of a topical steroid; comparison of desonide creams 0.05% and 0.1% by vasoconstrictor studies and clinical trials. *Clin. Exp. Dermatol.* 12:409–411.

Barry, B.W., and Woodford, R. (1978). Activity and bioavailability of topical steroids. *In vivo* and *in vitro* correlations for the vasoconstrictor test. *J. Clin. Pharmacol.* 3:43–65.

Blackwell, G.J.R., et al. (1980). Macrocortin: a polypeptide causing antiphospholipase effect of glucocorticosteroids. *Nature* 287:147.

Bucks, D.A., McMaster, J.R., Maibach, H.I., and Guy, R.H. (1988). Bioavailability of topically administered steroids: a "mass balance" technique. *J. Invest. Dermatol.* 91(1): 29–33.

Carr, R.D., and Tarnowski, W.M. (1968). Percutaneous absorption of corticosteroids: adrenocortical suppression with total body inuction. *Acta Derm. Venereol.* (*Stockh.*) 48:417–428.

Carruthers, J.A., August, P.J., and Staughton, R.C.D. (1975). Observations on the systemic effect of topical clobetasol propionate (Dermovate). *Br. Med. J.* 4:203–204.

Castrow, F.F. (1981). Atopic cataracts versus steroid cataracts. *J. Am. Acad. Dermatol.* 5:64–66.

Cornell, R., and Stoughton, R.B. (1981). Six-month controlled study of effect of desoximetasone and betamethasone-17-valerate on the pituitary-adrenal axis. *Br. J. Dermatol.* 105:91–95.

Cornell, R.C., and Stoughton, R.B. (1985). Correlation of the vasoconstrictor assay and clinical activity. *Arch. Dermatol.* 121:63–67.

Cubey, R.B. (1976). Glaucoma following the application of corticosteroid to the skin of the eyelids. *Br. J. Dermatol.* 95:207–208.

du Vivier, A., and Stoughton, R.B. (1982). Tachyphylaxis to the action of topically applied corticosteroids. *Arch. Dermatol.* 111:581–583.

du Vivier, A., Phillips, H., and Hehir, M. (1982). Application of glucocorticosteroids. *Arch. Dermatol.* 118:305–308.

Elks, J. (1976). Steroid structure and steroid activity. *Br. J. Dermatol.* 12(Suppl.):3.

Feiwel, M., James, V.H.T., and Barnett, E.S. (1969). Effect of potent topical steroids on plasma cortisol levels of infants and children with eczema. *Lancet* 1:485–587.

Feldmann, R.J., and Maibach, H.I. (1967). Regional variation in penetration of ^{14}C-cortisol in man. *J. Invest. Dermatol.* 48:181–185.

Feldmann, R.J., and Maibach, H.I. (1968). Percutaneous penetration of steroids in man. *J. Invest. Dermatol.* 52: 89–94.

Fredricksson, T., Lassus, T., and Bleeker, J. (1980). Treatment of psoriasis and atopic dermatitis with halcinonide cream applied once and three times daily. *Br. J. Dermatol.* 102:575–578.

Gibson, J.R., Kirsch, J.M., and Darley, E.R. (1984). An assessment of the relationship between vasoconstrictor assay findings, clinical efficacy and skin thinning of effects of a variety of undiluted and diluted corticosteroid preparations. *Br. J. Dermatol.* 111:204–212.

Gill, K.A., and Baxter, D.L. (1964). Plasma cortisol suppression by steroid creams. *Arch. Dermatol.* 89:734–740.

Goldman, L., and Cohen, W. (1962). Total body induction as topical corticosteroid therapy. *Arch. Dermatol.* 85: 266–269.

Gomez, E.C., Kaminester, L., and Frost, P. (1977). Topical halcinonide and betamethasone valerate effects on plasma cortisol. *Arch. Dermatol.* 113:1196–1202.

Hammerstrom, S., Hambert, M., Duell, E., Stawiski, M.A., Anderson, T.E., and Voorhees, J.J. (1977). Glucocorticoid in inflammatory proliferative skin disease reduces arachidonic and hydroxyeicostetraenoic acids. *Science* 197: 994.

Hench, P.S., Kendall, E.C., Slocumb, C.H., and Polley, H.F. (1949). The effect of a hormone of the adrenal cortex and of pituitary adrenocortropic hormone on rheumatoid arthritis. *Mayo Clin. Proc.* 24:181–193.

Herzog, H.L., Nobile, A., Toiksdorf, S., Charney, W., Hershberg, E.G., Perlman, P.L., and Rechet, M.M. (1955). New anti-arthritic steroids. *Science* 121:176.

Himathongkam, T., Dasanabhairochana, P., and Pilchayayothin, N. (1978). Florid Cushing's syndrome and hirsutism by desoximetasone. *J.A.M.A.* 239:430–431.

Hradil, E., Lindstrom, C., and Moller, H. (1978). Intermittent treatment of psoriasis with clobetasol propionate. *Acta Derm. Venereol. (Stockh.)* 58:375–377.

Hsia, S.L., and Hao, Y. (1967). Transformation of cortisone to cortisol in human skin. *Steroid* 10:489.

Ive, F.A., and Markes, R. (1968). Tinea incognito. *Br. Med. J.* 3:149–152.

Jackson, D.B., Thompson, E., McCormack, J., and Guin, J.D. (1989). Bioequivalence (bioavailability) of generic topical corticosteroids. *J. Am. Acad. Dermatol.* 20(5 Pt. 1):791–796.

Johns, A.M., and Bower, B.D. (1970). Wasting of napkin area after repeated use of fluorinated steroid ointment. *Br. Med. J.* 1:347–348.

Katz, H.I., Hien, N.T., Prawer, S.E., et al. (1988). Betamethasone dipropionate in optimized vehicle: intermittent pulse dosing for extended maintenance treatment of psoriasis. 123:1308–1311.

Korting, H.C., and Maibach, H.I. (1993). Topical glucocorticoids with increased benefit/risk ratio. In *Current Problems in Dermatology*, 2nd ed. Vol. 21, Karger, New York.

Koss, M.A., Kolker, A.E., and Becker, B. (1972). Chronic topical corticosteroid use simulating congenital glaucoma. *J. Pediatr.* 81:1175–1177.

Lauerma, A.I., Reitamo, S., and Maibach, H.I. (1991). Systemic hydrocortisone/cortisol induces allergic skin reactions in presensitized subjects. *J. M. Acad. Dermatol.* 24(2 P. 1):182–185.

Lavker, R.M., Schechter, N.M., and Lazarus, G.S. (1986). Effects of topical steroids on human dermis. *Br. J. Dermatol.* 115:101–107.

Leyden, J.J., Thew, M., and Kligman, A.M. (1974). Steroid rosacea. *Arch. Dermatol.* 110:619–622.

McConkey, D.J., et al. (1988). 2,3,7,8-Tetrachlorodibenzo-p-dioxin kills immature thymocytes by Ca^{2+}-mediated endonuclease activation. *Science* 242:256–258.

Maibach, H.I., and Feldman, R. (1967). The effect of DMSO on percutaneous penetration of hydrocortisone in man. *Trans. N.Y. Acad. Sci.* 14:423.

Maibach, H.I., and Stoughton, R.B. (1973). Topical corticosteroids. *Med. Clin. North Am.* 57:1253–1265.

Maibach, H.I. (Ed.) (1992). Bioequivalence of topical preparations. *Int. J. Dermatol.* 31(Suppl. 1):29–33.

Malkinson, F.D., and Ferguson, E.H. (1955). Percutaneous absorption of hydrocortisone 4-C^{14} in two human subjects. *J. Invest. Dermatol.* 25:281–283.

March, C., and Kerbel, G. (1964). Adrenal function after application of topical steroids under occlusive plastic film. *J.A.M.A.* 187:676–678.

McKenzie, A.W. (1962). Percutaneous absorption of steroids. *Arch. Dermatol.* 86:611–614.

McKenzie, A.W., and Atkinson, R.M. (1964). Topical activities of betamethasone esters in man. *Arch. Dermatol.* 89: 741–745.

McKenzie, A.W., and Stoughton, R.B. (1962). Method for comparing percutaneous absorption of steroids. *Arch. Dermatol.* 86:608–610.

Med. Lett. Drugs Ther. (1991) 33 (857):108–110.

Menne, T., Veien, N.K., and Maibach, H.I. (1989). Systemic contact-type dermatitis due to drugs. *Semin. Dermatol.* 8(3):144–148.

Munro, D.D., and Clift, D.C. (1973). Pituitary-adrenal function after prolonged use of topical corticosteroids. *Br. J. Dermatol.* 88:381–385.

Ortega, E., Burdick, K.H., and Segre, E.J. (1975). Adrenal suppression by clobetasol propionate. *Lancet* 1:1200.

Plewig, G., and Kligman, A.M. (1973). Induction of acne by topical steroids. *Arch. Dermatol. Forsch.* 247:29–52.

Ponec, M. (1982). Glucocorticoids and cultured human skin cells: specific intracellular binding and structure-activity relationships. *Br. J. Dermatol.* 107:24–29.

Ponec, M., de Kloet, E.R., and Kempenaar, J.A. (1980). Corticoids and human skin fibroblasts: intracellular specific binding in relation to growth inhibition. *J. Invest. Dermatol.* 75:293–296.

Poulsen, B.J., Young, E., Coquilla, V., Katz, M. (1968). Effect of topical vehicle composition on the in vitro release of fluocinolone acetonide and its acetate ester. *J. Pharm. Sci.* 57:928–933.

Rostenberg, A., Jr. (1962). Clinical evaluation of fluorandrenolone: New steroid in dermatological practice. *J. New Drugs* 1:118–121.

Schaefer, H. (1982). *Skin Permeability.* Springer-Verlag, Berlin, pp. 549–558.

Schlagel, C.A., and Northam, J.I. (1959). Comparative anti-inflammatory efficacy of topically applied steroids on human skin. *Proc. Soc. Exp. Biol. Med.* 101:629.

Scoggins, R.B. (1962). Decrease of urinary corticosteroids following application of fluocinolone acetonide under an occlusive dressing. *J. Invest. Dermatol.* 39:473–474.

Scoggins, R.B., and Kliman, B. (1965). Percutaneous absorption of corticosteroids. *N. Engl. J. Med.* 273:832–840.

Singh, G., and Singh, P.K. (1986). Tachyphylaxis to topical steroids measured by histamine-induced wheal suppression. *Int. J. Dermatol.* 25:324–326.

Sneddon, I. (1972). Perioral dermatitis. *Br. J. Dermatol.* 87: 430–434.

Stevanovic, D.V. (1972). Corticosteroid-induced atrophy of the skin with telangiectsia. *Br. J. Dermatol.* 87: 548–556.

Stoughton, R.B. (1972a). Bioassay system for formulations of topically applied glucocorticosteroids. *Arch. Dermatol.* 106:825–827.

Stoughton, R.B. (1972b). Some bioassay methods for measuring percutaneous absorption. In *Pharmacology and the Skin.* Vol. XII. W. Montagna, R.B. Stoughton, and E.J. Van Scott (Eds.). Appleton-Century-Crofts, New York, pp. 535–545.

Stoughton, R.B. (1977). A perspective of topical corticosteroid therapy. In *Psoriasis: Proceedings of the 2nd International Symposium,* 1976. E. Farber and A.J. Cox (Eds.). Yorke Medical books, New York, pp. 219–225.

Stoughton, R.B. (1982). Enhanced percutaneous penetration with 1-dodecyl-azacycloheptan-2-one. *Arch. Dermatol.* 118:474–477.

Stoughton, R.B., and Wullich, K. (1989). Does increasing the concentration of the same glucocorticoid in brand name products result in greater topical biologic activity. *Arch. Dermatol.* 125(11):1509–1511.

Stoughton, R.B. (1987). Are generic formulation equivalent to trade name topical glucocorticoids? *Arch. Dermatol.* 123:1312–1314.

Surber, C., Itin, P.H., Bircher, A.J., and Maibach, H.I. 91995). Topical corticosteroids. *J. M. Acad. Dermatol.* 32(6):1025–1030.

Surber, C., and Maibach, H.I. (Eds.) (1992). *Topical Corticosteroids.* Karger, Basel.

Sutton, R.M., Feldmann, R.J., and Maibach, H.I. (1971). Vasoconstrictor potency of corticoids: intradermal injection. *J. Invest. Dermatol.* 57(6):371–376.

Wells, G.C. (1957). The effect of hydrocortisone on standard skin surface trauma. *Br. J. Dermatol.* 69:11.

Wilson, L., Williams, D.I., and Marsh, S.D. (1973). Plasma corticosteroid levels in outpatients treated with topical steroids. *Br. J. Dermatol.* 88:373–380.

Wilkinson, S.M. (1994). Hypersensitivity to topical corticosteroids. *Clin. Exp. Dermatol.* 19(1):1–11.

32

Goeckerman Therapy

Lawrence E. Gibson and Harold O. Perry
Mayo Clinic and Mayo Medical School, Rochester, Minnesota

The Goeckerman treatment, consisting of the daily application of crude coal tar followed by ultraviolet B irradiations, was initially employed by William Goeckerman in 1925 (1) for the therapy of patients with generalized psoriasis. It remains a satisfactory treatment for extensive psoriasis, including generalized exfoliative erythroderma, or psoriasis occurring in cosmetically unacceptable or disabling areas such as the face or genital area, or with particularly thick plaques on the hands and feet. Because of the extensive cutaneous involvement of these patients, they were initially hospitalized and to this date, patients who receive the Goeckerman therapy are usually considered to require hospitalization. A modified Goeckerman program has been employed in psoriasis day care centers, and this is referred to specifically as psoriasis day care treatment, or a modified Goeckerman program.

When Goeckerman originated this therapy, he was a member of the staff of the Mayo Clinic. This therapy is used by the present staff at the Mayo Clinic with minor modifications. It is important to emphasize that this therapy is continuous, 24 hr per day as currently practiced at the Mayo Clinic.

APPLICATION OF TAR

For the patient who has never received therapy before, testing for sensitivity and tolerance to tar is done. Trials of specific tar preparations are applied to the abdominal skin and left as an open test for 24 hr to determine any intolerance before a more generalized application of the tar is made. Such trials consist of 3% crude coal tar in petrolatum, 5% Zetar (a refined tar), and 3% Ichthyol and 10% Tween 80 in petrolatum. In those patients who have been treated previously with the Goeckerman therapy, and for whom we have medical records indicating that they tolerate the tar without adverse effects, application of the tar begins as soon after admission as is convenient.

The assistance of a nursing staff well acquainted with the techniques of this therapy is mandatory, as the various phases are carried out by medical personnel under the direction of the physician. Their understanding of the treatment program must be complete to maintain the program in operation 24 hr a day.

Once the patient is recognized as tolerating the tar, the tar is applied to all skin areas, including both normal and involved skin. Tar preparations are not applied to noninvolved intertriginous areas, as these areas sometimes develop irritation because of the close proximity of the skin folds.

If the patient does not have psoriasis in these intertriginous areas, a mild water-soluble lubricant is used in those areas. If a superficial involvement of the skin occurs in such areas, 1% hydrocortisone cream will be employed, and if thicker plaques are present, 0.025–0.05% triamcinolone cream will be used in these areas two to three times daily for a few days. If the intertriginous plaques are sufficiently heavy and it is deemed necessary to have the tar applied to these areas, the patient is asked to personally apply the 3% crude coal tar in petrolatum or Lassar paste, or a tar preparation of 10–20% liquor carbonis detergens in Nivea oil.

Treatment of the scalp parallels that of the skin. Tar ointments are extremely difficult to remove from the hair. Thus, the Goeckerman program has been modified to use either 10 or 20% liquor carbonis detergens in Nivea oil, employing the higher concentration for those patients who have thicker plaques of psoriasis. The preparation will be applied two to three times daily, and even more often if it is necessary to keep the scalp lubricated and thereby free of pruritus.

The technique in applying the liquid to the scalp is to begin at one edge of the scalp, parting the hair and applying the liquid by use of a squeezable lotion bottle with an applicator cap directly onto the scalp and using the fingers to rub the tar solution into the scalp in the parted areas of the hair. Once this is accomplished, the hair is parted 1 cm away and the process repeated until the entire scalp is appropriately treated. As a final measure to ensure adequate application, the margins of the scalp are specifically treated, since frequently the psoriasis is more intense in those areas and the bulk of the hair, as it is parted, tends to prevent application of the tar to the margins.

Tar is usually applied to the skin three times daily but more often if the patient's skin feels dry or he or she experiences excessive itching.

The nurse trained in the technique of tar application recognizes the importance of softening the petrolatum base by rubbing the ointment in the hands rapidly until the friction so generated melts the base. The tar is applied to the entire skin surface beginning at the neck and shoulders and working down over the upper extremities, the trunk, and finally, the lower extremities. This requires that the nurse recognize the hair patterns of growth and always apply the tar in that particular direction as to avoid introducing large amounts into the hair follicles. On the upper arms, this is in a downward motion and over the extensor portions of the forearms, in a more rotating lateral manner. On the trunk, it is easy to recognize the hair pattern and application is usually in a downward movement. The tar is not rubbed back and forth but stroked in one direction only. Although the nurse applies the tar to the greater portion of the skin areas, the patient applies appropriate medication to the genital area.

Over the years, various modifications have been added to the Goeckerman treatment program. Whereas originally 3% crude coal tar in petrolatum was the standard topical therapy, today we sometimes employ 5% concentrations.

To reduce thick hyperkeratotic plaques of psoriasis, in addition to the increased concentration of tar employed, salicylic acid in a concentration of 3–5% is sometimes added. Caution must be exercised when salicylic acid is used. Salicylism from percutaneous absorption can develop if it is used indiscriminately over wide areas. Application is limited to the thick heavy plaques with the use of the standard tar without salicylic acid to the other involved body areas.

A more recent modification utilizes application of anthralin in petrolatum base to areas of thick psoriasis. These applications are usually restricted to areas such as the knees, elbows, anterior legs, and low back when clearing is at a slower rate than the remainder of the psoriatic plaques. One must exercise care in the application of anthralin, restricting this application only to the plaques and sparing the surrounding skin. This is usually accomplished by outlining the plaque with a heavy application of cream base. Generally, a 1% concentration of anthralin is used, and the first application is only for 10–15 min before the anthralin is removed. Application times and concentration can be increased as needed and tolerated. This short-contact anthralin modification is used only in selected cases, as this increases nursing time required for application.

When patients are admitted for generalized erythroderma, the skin reaction may be so acute that the tar may further irritate the exfoliative process. Thus, the patient will be placed in tap water wet dressings to all body areas, applying 0.05% triamcinolone cream to the skin prior to the application of the wet dressings every 3 hr. Such wet dressings are applied to all skin areas for 24–48 hr to reduce the acuity and redness of the erythroderma as well as to decrease the psoriasis. Such treatment for this initial period means that the subsequent tar treatment is much better tolerated.

There may be heavy plaques over the lower legs, palms, and soles. In addition to employing wet dressings for these areas for 48 hr, early during the course of the disease we have found occlusive dressings with steroids to be of benefit. However, occlusion with steroids is used only for a short period, allowing at least 10 days of tar and light therapy following such occlusive therapy before the patient is dismissed. Just as there is a rebound phenomenon in the psoriatic patient when systemic steroids are discontinued, a similar rebound phenomenon may be encountered with topical steroid therapy.

Thick heavy crusts in the scalp sometimes do not respond to the use of the liquor carbonis detergens.

Under those circumstances, a preparation consisting of 20% oil of cade, 10% sulfur, and 5% salicylic acid (20-10-5) in a water-soluble base is employed to the scalp, rubbing it into all areas of the scalp as previously outlined. Some patients find the odor of the oil of cade offensive, but the benefits achieved in removing a thick crust of psoriasis from the scalp make the patient accept this therapy.

At other times, topical therapies to the skin must vary because of the patient's intolerance to tar. The initial trials include Ichthyol and pine tar. If crude coal tar is not tolerated, either of the alternative preparations tolerated are used. Ichthyol 3% with a 10% concentration of a surfactant in zinc oxide ointment works satisfactorily. Pine tar with salicylic acid, each in a concentration of 1–3% in a petrolatum base, may offer a substitute topical therapy when others are not tolerated.

With the application of tar to the body, pajamas are worn as a means of keeping the tar in continual contact with the skin. On the first day, the pajamas are worn, they wick the tar from the skin surface and rapidly become saturated with the tar, and thus frequent application of tar (four or five times) to the patient is required during the first 24 hr to provide a covering of tar to the skin.

For involvement of the hands and feet, cotton dermal gloves and cotton socks are worn as a means of covering these areas and keeping the tar preparation in constant contact with the psoriatic skin.

Internal medications are usually kept to a minimum. The patient with extensive psoriasis frequently itches. Antihistamines and sedative are sometimes of benefit. More frequently used than other antihistamines is hydroxyzine, which has good antipruritic and mild sedative effects. Other antihistamines are employed, depending on the physician's experience.

ULTRAVIOLET LIGHT THERAPY

After the patient has had tar in contact with the skin for 24 hr, the patient's entire skin is exposed to minimal erythema dosages of ultraviolet light on a daily basis. Some tar remaining on the skin provides an increased photosensitizing effect. However, a thick layer of tar would act as a filter and negate the beneficial effect of the ultraviolet light therapy. Thus, prior to the light treatment, excessive tar is removed.

This is accomplished by freely applying with the hands a vegetable oil, either cottonseed or corn oil, to the skin. Applied in a manner similar to the application of the tar, it is left in place long enough to soften any tar that has remained in a dried or caked form. The nurse then will saturate gauze muslin with some additional oil and wipe the skin free of excessive tar. Again, the nurse always wipes in the direction of the pattern of hair growth to avoid introduction of the oils and tars into the hair follicles.

An ultraviolet B (UVB) lamp has traditionally been the source of radiation. A minimal erythema dosage of ultraviolet light is applied daily to the skin. The light technician, another valuable member of the team, has sufficient experience that he or she can assess the skin color of the patient and accurately initiate light therapy with a minimal erythema dosage of ultraviolet light. The beginning dose of UVB is determined mainly by the patient's skin color and previous experience with UVB lights at this institution. The UVB lamps are calibrated often and doses of light are recorded in millijoules. If there is any doubt as to a patient's tolerance of UVB, minimal erythema doses are done prior to institution of total body irradiation. Erythema should develop within 4–6 hr and disappear for the most part by the end of 24 hr. The persistence of some erythema at the end of 24 hr is preferable to administration of an amount of ultraviolet light that does not produce a persistent erythema for 24 hr. The patient's response on any given day forms the basis for judging the dosage of ultraviolet B irradiation the following day.

For application of ultraviolet light, the body is divided into eight regions: two regions on the posterior, two regions on the anterior body exclusive of the head, and two regions on each lateral surface. This technique gives more even distribution of light and allows more or less light to be given to specific regions without overlap. Each of these areas, in turn, is exposed to the ultraviolet light.

If there is involvement of the scalp or on the face, these areas are exposed separately. A paper shield can be cut and fashioned like the brim of a hat to fit over the hair so that the face can be shielded from increased secondary exposure when scalp irradiation is required.

"Spotting" is the process whereby thick heavy plaques of psoriasis are given additional amounts of ultraviolet light. These might occur in the scalp, over the elbows, over the sacral area, the hips, or the knees. The light technician outlines these areas using cotton towels or paper so that just the plaques remain visible for exposure. These areas are given additional amounts of light daily. The dosages of UVB for routine treatment plus these special areas of treatment are charted and the dosage is appropriately increased daily.

CLEANSING THE SKIN

Following ultraviolet light treatment, the patient is returned to his or her room for removal of the tar in a cleansing tub with shampoo. This is thought necessary to remove not only the tar, but also any epithelial debris and bacteria that might have accumulated in the previous 24 hr.

The water temperature is usually between 96 and 103°F, more tepid than warm, so as to avoid the stimulation from a hot bath which might increase the skin's redness and pruritus. Bath oil is routinely added to the bath water to overcome some of the drying effects of frequent bathing. Dial soap is routinely employed for cleansing, although any soap that lathers well is suitable.

The patient is provided with a face cloth so that a lather can be developed from the soap and the skin vigorously washed to remove tar, bacteria, and skin products completely as well as excessive scales from the psoriatic plaques.

Following cleansing of the skin, the scalp is shampooed, at which time the nurse tries to remove manually any thick heavy scales and crusts still adherent to the scalp.

Therapy is arranged so that the cleansing bath and shampoo follow the light treatment followed by reapplication of the tar within an hour after the light treatment. This provides for continuous treatment during 24 hr.

At times, the thick crusts on the scalp are particularly heavy and difficult to manage. Under these circumstances, the scalp preparation, whether tar or other special preparations, is applied several times during the day to soften the "cap" of psoriasis. Shampoos may be given twice or even three times daily to soften the heavy crusts and scales further and remove the debris from the scalp at more frequent intervals than would otherwise be possible.

These cycles of tar application, ultraviolet light administration, and cleansing, followed by reapplication of the tar are carried out daily while the patient is in the hospital for 14–21 days to eradicate 90–95% of the patient's psoriasis. Longer periods of treatment are required for patients who exhibit less response to the treatment.

COMPLICATIONS

There are few complications from the use of the Goeckerman program. Some patients may be sensitive to the tar, but this is rare. Usually, the tar is not tolerated because of the acuity of the psoriasis, but if care is taken to reduce the acute flare of the psoriasis initially with the use of steroids and wet dressings topically for a few days, the tar then is generally tolerated.

Skin color is a determining factor in how much ultraviolet light therapy the patient is able to tolerate. Occasionally, a sunburn will occur, which requires special attention. Topical steroids and wet dressings are applied to the burn area as soon as the patient has an exaggerated reaction to the ultraviolet light. The patient may complain of itching and burning before blistering is perceived. The sooner the wet dressings and steroid creams are applied, the more rapidly the resulting erythema and/or blistering will subside. It may be necessary to use wet dressings and steroids to localized areas for 2–3 days to quiet such a reaction. While wet dressings are used, further tar and ultraviolet light are avoided in those areas. Once the reaction subsides, the ultraviolet light is once again applied to those areas but in a reduced dosage.

Folliculitis may occur. Usually, this is minor and does not require that treatments be interrupted. It is managed by the application of Castellani paint. An alternative is to use Nomland lotion (an alcohol/resorcinal preparation) to the areas of folliculitis to reduce the bacterial flora and promoting healing. Application of either of these preparations to the isolated areas of folliculitis does not preclude tar treatment.

In hirsute individuals, folliculitis of a localized area may occur, for instance over the lower legs. If this becomes severe, the lesions are cultured, antibiotic sensitivity of the bacteria determined, and the appropriate systemic antibiotic administered. With extensive folliculitis tar treatment is withheld until the folliculitis subsides.

Folliculitis occurs most often because of the introduction of the tar into the follicles and the proliferation of endogenous bacteria in the skin. On a rare occasion, the tar becomes contaminated with bacteria and the bacteria are thus introduced onto the patient's skin exogenously. Each patient should use his or her own tar supply to prevent cross-infections from patient to patient.

The fear that tar and light treatments might produce excessive carcinomas of the skin has been of concern.

Table 1 Age Distribution of 123 Psoriatic Patients Treated in 1964 by the Goeckerman Regimen

Age (yrs)	Male patients	Female patients
0–19	3	6
20–29	6	9
30–39	9	10
40–49	14	14
50–59	14	13
60–69	10	8
>70	4	3
Total	60	63

Source: Ref. 3

We recognized that some patients with psoriasis did develop basal cell or squamous cell carcinomas of their skin. Ancillary factors usually had to be considered in addition to the tar and ultraviolet light therapy, including previous arsenic ingestion as well as x-ray irradiation.

In an effort to determine more accurately whether the Goeckerman therapy induced an increased incidence of skin cancer, a 25-year follow-up of patients who have been treated with the Goeckerman therapy was studied. The incidence of carcinoma in this group of patients compared with the normal population as a control showed that the incidence of carcinoma in these patients 25 years later was no greater than would have occurred normally (4). To further corroborate this finding, a 25-year follow-up of atopic patients who had received Goeckerman therapy revealed that the incidence of carcinoma in the second group was, likewise, no greater than that in the normal population (2). Similar experiences have been reported in psoriatic patients treated with UVB in Sweden (5).

Thus, although great concern has been expressed that tar employed therapeutically is a potent carcinogen, there seems little basis for concern when tar is employed under the conditions outlined previously. The total amount of tar used for the average patient receiving 2% crude coal tar (CCT) is approximately 60 g over a 3-week period (6).

RESULTS

Patients treated with the Goeckerman program are ordinarily hospitalized for 2–3 weeks, although variations in the duration of hospital stay occur. To determine the response of patients to the Goeckerman program, a 25-year follow-up study was carried out in 1968 (3).

Table 1 indicates that Goeckerman therapy is satisfactory for all ages. Children tolerate the treatment as well as geriatric patients (Figs. 1 and 2).

An effort was made to assess the duration of remissions before and following the Goeckerman therapy. Table 2 shows that patients who experienced remissions prior to their Goeckerman therapy had a 6-month period of freedom from psoriasis. There was a range as long as 2 years among the male patients in their periods of freedom.

However, in those patients for whom definite information was available, the average length of transmission was as long as 8 years. The median remission was a year for males and 1.4 years for females.

Table 3 indicates the duration of therapy is directly related to the extent of cutaneous involvement when therapy is started. Patients with less than 25% involvement had a shorter hospital stay than those with 75% or more involvement of the skin, even though the plaques may be heavier and isolated in the former group.

The duration of hospitalization seems directly related to the degree of improvement (Table 4). In those patients who experienced 95% or more improvement, the duration of their hospitalization was longer. It would be anticipated that patients with more extensive involvement would require a longer treatment period for resolution of the lesions.

Although these statistics were developed a few years ago, as we continue to administer Goeckerman therapy to psoriatic patients, the beneficial effects and the duration of treatment seem the same.

Most patients who have extensive psoriasis or who are disabled from their disease because of its extent or area of involvement (the genital area, face, hands, and feet), find this treatment to be effective in resolving and bringing their disease into a remission. Some patients find this treatment satisfactory, and they return every year or two as their disease worsens, believing that such treatment permits them a quality of life otherwise not possible.

The Goeckerman regimen remains the major therapeutic approach for patients with extensive or disabling psoriasis seen at the Mayo Clinic. Psoralen and ultraviolet A (PUVA) therapy as well as chemotherapeutic agents are efficacious in given patients under certain circumstances, but the Goeckerman therapy remains the mainstay of therapy for severe and disabling psoriasis.

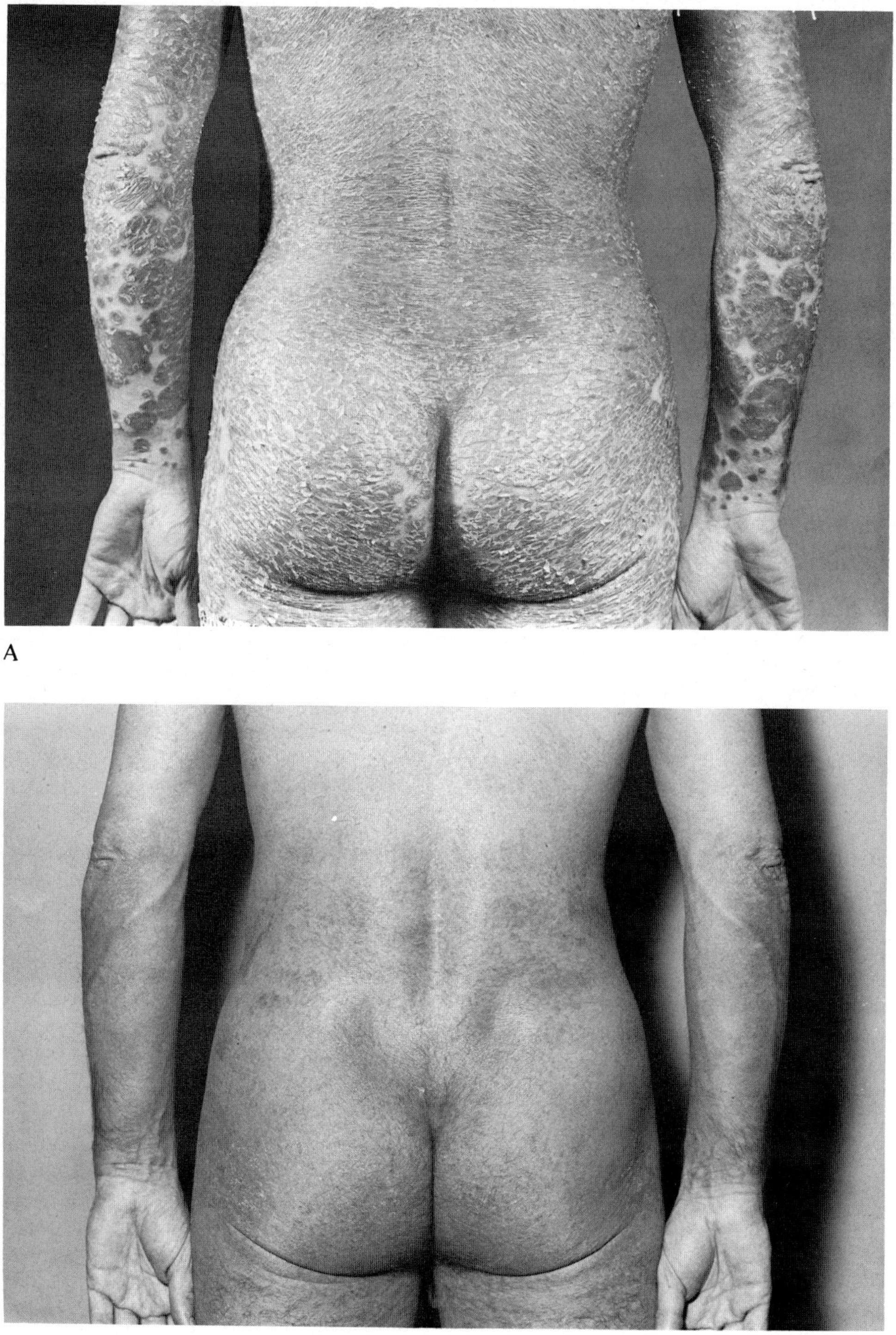

A

B

Figure 1 (A) Back of patient before therapy. (B) After 28 days of treatment with the Goeckerman regimen. Clearing is considered to have occurred when skin lesions are no longer palpable. Hyperpigmentation at sites of previous lesions may be visible.

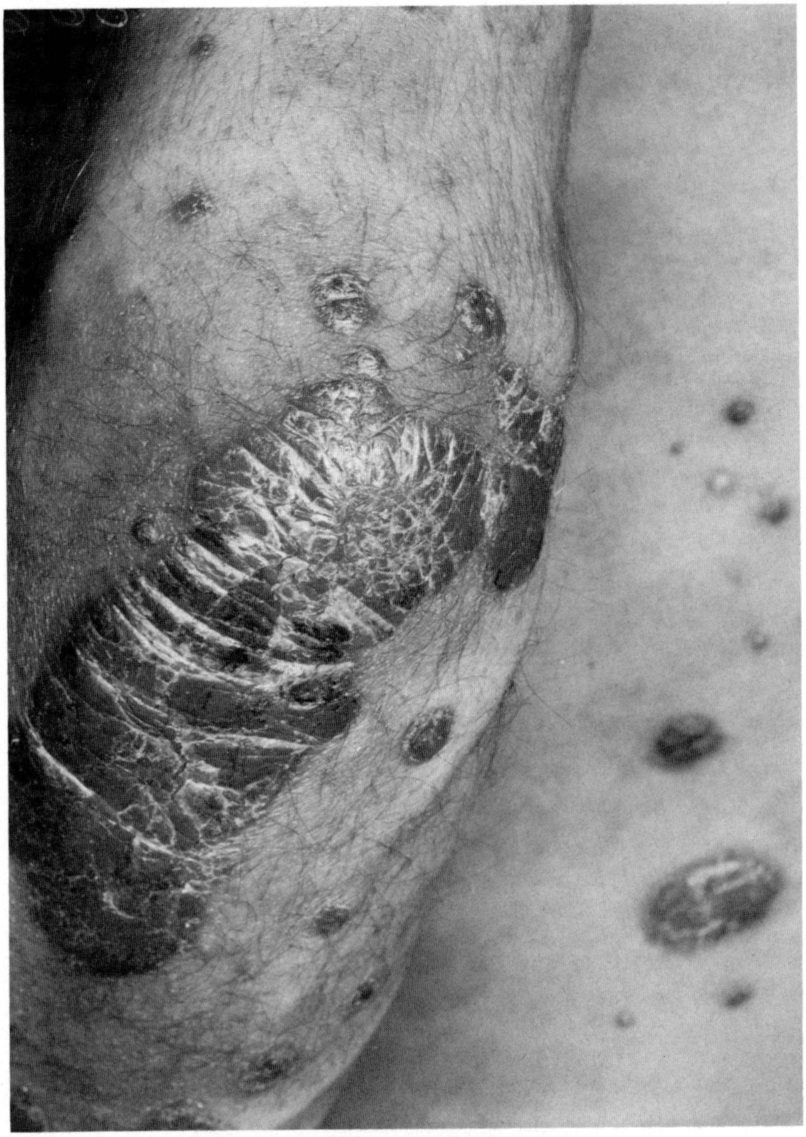

A

Figure 2 Elbow of patient. (A) Before therapy. (B) After 8 days of therapy. (C) After 26 days of therapy with the Goeckerman regimen.

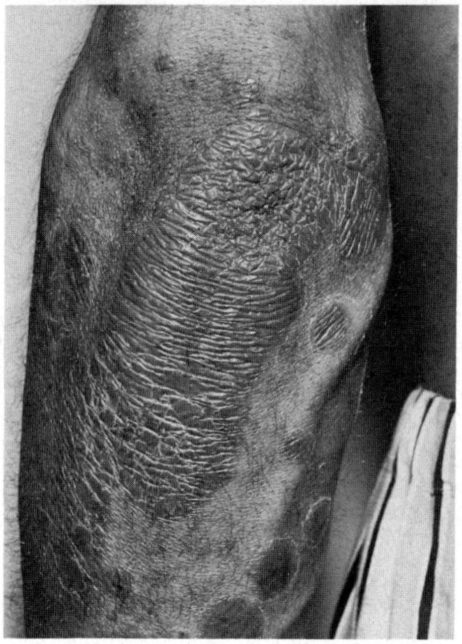

B

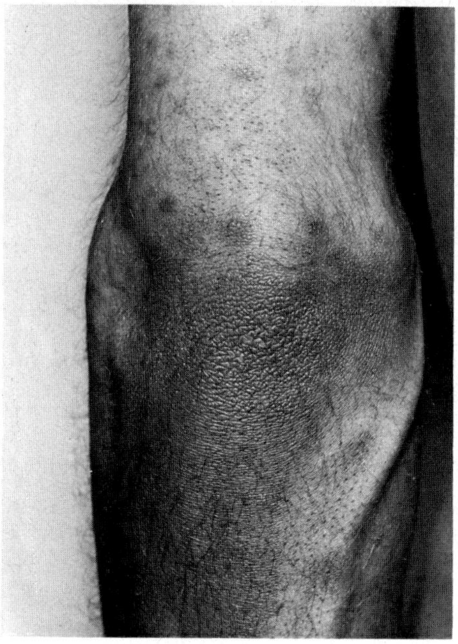

C

Figure 2 Continued.

Table 2 Remissions of Psoriasis Before and After Goeckerman Therapy

	Male patients	Female patients
Before Goeckerman therapy	21	33
without remission	6	11
with remission	15	22
length of remission (yrs)		
average	0.6	0.5
range	0.2–2.0	0.1–1.0
median	0.5	0.5
After Goeckerman therapy	19	20
without remission	0	1
with remission	19	19
length of remission (yrs)		
average	1.7	1.8
range	0.2–8.0	0.5–5.0
median	1.0	1.4

Source: Ref. 3

Table 3 Degree of Cutaneous Involvement Compared with Days of Hospitalization for Psoriatic Patients Treated in 1964

Cutaneous involvement (%)	Hospitalization (days)					
	Male patients			Female patients		
	No.	Average	Range	No.	Average	Range
<25	9	14.4	4–34	15	12.3	6–19
25–49	28	18.7	10–34	36	18.8	9–50
50–74	11	23.8	13–35	7	19.0	15–30
75 or more	9	24.0	13–51	2	42.5	21–64

Source: Ref. 3.

Table 4 Days of Hospitalization Required for Various Degrees of Improvement in Treatment of Psoriasis

Improvement (%)	Hospitalization					
	Male patients			Female patients		
	No.	Average	Range	No.	Average	Range
<71	8	13.0	4–20	6	15.7	9–21
71–85	19	20.4	12–34	17	20.1	9–64
86–95	25	20.2	10–51	28	18.4	6–50
>95	5	24.2	16–35	10	16.1	8–29

Source: Ref. 3

REFERENCES

1. Goeckerman, W.H. (1981). The treatment of psoriasis. *Northwest Med.* 24:229–231.
2. Maughan, W.Z., Muller, S.A., Perry, H.O., Pittelkow, M.R., and O'Brien, P.C. (1980). Incidence of skin cancers in patients with atopic dermatitis treated with coal tar: a 25-year followup study. *J. Am. Acad. Dermatol.* 3:612–615.
3. Perry, H.O., Soderstrom, C.W., and Schulze, R.W. (1968). The Goeckerman treatment of psoriasis. *Arch. Dermatol.* 98:178–182.
4. Pittelkow, M.R., Perry, H.O., Muller, S.A., Maughan, W.Z., and O'Brien, P.C. (1981). Skin cancer in patients with psoriasis treated with coal tar: a 25-year followup study. *Arch. Dermatol.* 117:465–468.
5. Larko, O., and Swanbeck, G. (1982). Is UVB therapy of psoriasis safe? *Acta. Derm. Venereol.* (*Stockh.*) 62(6): 507–512.
6. Muller, S.A., and Perry, H.O. (1984). The Goeckerman treatment in psoriasis: six decades of experience at the Mayo Clinic. *Cutis* 34:265–269.

33

Ambulatory Treatment Centers: United States Experience

Nicholas J. Lowe
Southern California Dermatology and Psoriasis Center, Santa Monica, and UCLA School of Medicine, Los Angeles, California

Pamela S. Lowe
Southern California Dermatology and Psoriasis Center, Santa Monica, California

Ambulatory day care centers to treat patients with moderate to severe psoriasis provide an alternative to hospitalization. This became an important option in the United States beginning in the 1970s to the present, as there has been an increasing demand for cost containment in medical treatment. A well-organized center should be capable of improving or clearing moderate to severe psoriasis without the need for hospitalization or systemic therapy. Even in these days of increasing options in systemic therapy, many patients should not be treated with systemic therapy, and other patients choose not to receive systemic therapy. Therefore, the availability of a comprehensively equipped ambulatory treatment center remains an important option for the psoriatic patient who has failed to improve on outpatient treatment.

The greatest challenge for the 1990s for those who still administer these centers has been the increasing difficulty in getting approval from patients' health insurance programs.

HISTORICAL ASPECTS

Day care centers have been used in other specialties for a number of years—for example, in the treatment of psychiatric illnesses. However, it was not until the 1950s and 1960s, in England and in France (1), that dermatological day care treatment centers were first established. Subsequently psoriasis day care centers were established at the University of California in San Francisco and at Stanford University Medical Center in the early 1970s, and more recently in Chicago, in Dallas, in Santa Monica, in the New York area, in Seattle, and in Ann Arbor, Michigan.

Ambulatory treatment centers are available in several metropolitan areas in various parts of the world, including the United States. These have varying degrees of facilities available for psoriasis treatment.

One of the present difficulties in initiating and organizing such a treatment center in the United States involves the difficulty of obtaining adequate financial reimbursement for this very complex, and staff-intensive therapy. In addition, despite the obvious savings in costs over inpatient care, it is at times difficult to convince private medical insurance companies of the advantages of day care therapy over inpatient care. At present, for example, the costs of inpatient therapy in most hospitals would be at least four times that of ambulatory day care center therapy.

PHYSICAL LOCATION AND FACILITIES

An ideal ambulatory treatment center should be near available hotel accommodations for out-of-town patients.

There should be facilities for a peaceful resting area for patients after topical therapy has been applied.

Food and drink should also be available and those patients staying for a full day of therapy should be provided with facilities for lunch and other refreshments.

It is also important to have facilities for patient entertainment, which includes radios, televisions, video recorders with appropriate cassettes, and patient education videotapes. A quiet room is also desirable, as some patients do not wish to watch or listen to the television and/or radio or be otherwise disturbed. In this quiet area, there should be facilities to allow the patients to read and write if desired.

THERAPEUTIC OPTIONS

A fully equipped ambulatory treatment center should offer a wide range of topical therapies, including:

1. Crude coal tar, with and without salicylic acid
2. Liquor carbonic detergent ointment, with and without salicylic acid
3. Anthralin preparations in different vehicles, i.e., creams, ointments, and pastes in different concentrations ranging from 0.1 to 10%
4. Topical corticosteroid preparations, calcipotriene, emollients, and moisturizing agents
5. A variety of scalp treatment preparations, including lotions and oil-based preparations containing salicylic acid, tar, corticosteroids, and anthralin
6. Appropriate sunscreens for the local protection of the skin during phototherapy
7. Bath delivery of 8-methoxypsoralen for patients receiving bath-water-delivered PUVA, e.g., those with nausea from 8-methoxypsoralen, or those with cataracts
8. Ability to monitor patients on systemic antipsoriatic therapy

THERAPEUTIC EQUIPMENT

The treatment center should be fully equipped with a versatile range of phototherapy equipment, including ultraviolet B (UVB) or UVB plus UVA units for whole-body and localized area treatment units for local areas on the body as well as hand and foot units.

Facilities for application of topical preparations should be available. Bathing and showering areas with appropriately designed space to accommodate handicapped patients are essential. Bathing facilities for water delivery of psoralen for selected patients are valuable.

Facilities for scalp treatment are extremely important, as frequently severe scalp psoriasis can be improved dramatically with the appropriate topical application of agents, including coal tar, salicylic acid, and anthralin preparations, followed by local shampooing and showering.

Recently, a scalp treatment machine (Ocee, Tennessee) has been utilized at our treatment center, which utilizes high-pressure hydrotherapy jets that are valuable for scalp therapy. The machine consists of a chamber that encloses the scalp, which is then exposed to high-pressure liquid jet that contains water plus treatment agents, such as tar and salicylic acid shampoos.

OTHER REQUIREMENTS

Finally, there should be sufficient facilities for the patients to be examined fully by the physician and for the conduct of regular discussion sessions with the day care staff. Some centers conduct psychotherapy and group therapy sessions, which can be very helpful for patients.

PSORIASIS DAY CARE CENTER PERSONNEL

It is important that the medical and nursing personnel in a psoriasis day care center be fully familiar and trained in all aspects of skin disease therapy, and they need to have special competence in the delivery of phototherapy and topical therapy.

The nursing staff should become familiar with treatment and sometimes the personal problems of the patient. They are valuable in acting as a channel for the physician to learn to individualize patient problems.

Our treatment center has two registered nurses and three licensed vocational nurses, in addition to administrative staff. These numbers are necessary to enable adequate staffing as the center is open for 7 A.M. to 7 P.M. Monday through Friday, and also 8 A.M. to 1 P.M. on Saturday.

SPECIFIC TREATMENT PROGRAMS AT THE AMBULATORY TREATMENT CENTER

Anthralin

Anthralin therapy may be conducted either as a short-contact therapeutic approach or as longer-term anthralin application (2). The most frequent form of anthralin therapy at our treatment center is use of short-contact anthralin with rapid increase of the anthralin concentration from 1 to 10% in an ointment base depending on the patient response and absence of irritancy and erythema.

The anthralin is allowed to remain on the affected skin for up to 1 hr; the patient usually has phototherapy prior to the application of anthralin.

For more recalcitrant psoriasis, longer-term application of anthralin in an ointment or paste vehicle, such as Lassar paste (3), is frequently successful in controlling and improving localized areas of psoriasis.

Coal Tar Treatment Programs

Different programs of therapy involving coal tar (4–7) and purified coal tar, usually with ultraviolet phototherapy, are an essential part of many patients' treatment programs at the ambulatory treatment center. These can be all-day programs with coal tar being applied to the entire skin (not just the psoriasis lesions) in the more severely affected patients (8). Other patients with more localized but recalcitrant psoriasis may respond to a shorter contact with tar of approximately 2 hr, followed by ultraviolet phototherapy.

Many patients do not have the available time to stay for a whole day of treatment and will respond well to 2-hr coal tar treatment and phototherapy. It is, however, essential for them to realize that the continuation of a hectic and sometimes stressful work situation may lead to slower improvement in their psoriasis compared to taking a full break from work and full day care therapy.

SOME OPTIONS IN TREATMENT SCHEDULES

The following are some options in treatment schedules:

Full Day Care

7:00 A.M.: Arrive at treatment center. Examination by staff and physician. Application of coal tar and/or anthralin preparation. Application of scalp preparation, if indicated.

8:00 A.M.–12:00 noon: Relax in day care center. Discussion groups. Nursing discussions. Watch educational or entertainment videos.

12:00 noon–1:00 P.M.: Lunch.

1:00 P.M.: Application of anthralin in short-contact mode to selected patients.

2:00 P.M.: Tar oil or oatmeal baths. Removal of tar.

2:30 P.M.: Scalp treatment.

3:00 P.M.: Ultraviolet phototherapy. Leave treatment center to return to home or local accommodation.

In addition to treatments outlined above, the patient should be instructed to apply moisturizers and/or purified tar preparations to the scalp and body overnight, if required, to increase the disease clearance.

Part Day Care Therapy

The above program can be shortened so that the tar stays on the patient for a minimum of 2 hr, should the patient have less severe psoriasis. Anthralin may be applied to escalating concentrations for up to 1 hr.

Other forms of therapy for patients might include substitutions on alternative days of PUVA for ultraviolet phototherapy. This would be particularly useful in a patient in whom there is a previous history of rapid relapse of disease after phototherapy has been stopped and who is considered to be a candidate for PUVA maintenance therapy.

Other patients may be treated with systemic retinoids, e.g., etretinate, acitretin, or methotrexate, to achieve a more rapid clearance of the disease with the day care center therapy. The remission times after such combinations have not been scientifically studied. Patients should be encouraged to use topical treatment at home or in their hotel nightly.

ADVANTAGES OF AMBULATORY TREATMENT CENTERS

The advantages of ambulatory treatment centers include the availability of comprehensive facilities in a single treatment center with appropriately trained nursing staff and medical staff. A *full* range of appropriate treatments is therefore available.

Psoriatic patient interaction with other patients is important to give such a patient a more comprehensive overview of his or her disease and encouragement from the other patients.

Realization by patients that is possible to achieve clearance or a maximal improvement in their psoriasis, followed in many instances by long-term remission, can be reassuring. Some patients are reassured that by having, for example, annual courses of treatment, it is possible to obtain control of psoriasis without the need for systemic therapy.

Patient education is important in any psoriasis treatment program. This includes educational material and discussion groups. Many patients become disillusioned and disappointed by the slowness of response, or a poor response to treatment, and then fail to attend as regularly and as frequently as is required to obtain improvement.

DISEASE SEVERITY CRITERIA FOR DAY CARE CENTER THERAPY

Psoriatic patients need to have significant, severe, disabling, or resistant disease to justify the use of day care center therapy. This is particularly important in view of the present requirements for reimbursement from Medicare, Medicaid, and private insurance carriers. Suggested guidelines are as follows for patient treatment:

- Psoriasis involving more than 25% of body surface or disabling psoriasis with less percentage of involvement, affecting areas such as the face, scalp, hands, feet, and genital area.
- Patients with recalcitrant psoriasis experiencing complications from previous therapy, for example, topical cortisones, PUVA, and methotrexate. Treatment center therapy with coal tars and/or anthralin is a safe and frequently effective alternative to these treatments.
- Illnesses that complicate the use of other forms of systemic therapy in psoriasis, for example, blood dyscrasias, diabetes, or cardiovascular disease.
- Psoriasis that is psychologically and/or physically disabling to limit the patient's daily activities but where the use of systemic therapy is contraindicated.

Some of these criteria are based on those developed for inpatient therapy (9).

CONCLUSION

Ambulatory treatment centers for psoriasis provide an effective additional option that is capable of providing safe and effective forms of treatment. Most treatment programs will take 3–6 weeks, depending on patient response, to achieve maximum improvement or clearance. Careful explanations of therapy and patient education are required to ensure appropriate information being disseminated to the patient and the avoidance of any unanswered questions by the patient.

Such a setting can provide an ideal environment for comprehensive patient care, the education of patients, the education and training of dermatological staff, and the conduct of clinical research.

Some patients are not appropriate candidates because of their personality or attitude toward day care center therapy, and these patients must be carefully screened and offered other options of treatment by the dermatologist.

REFERENCES

1. Grupper, C. (1968). Modifications personnelles du traitment du psoriasis par la methode de Goeckerman. *Bull. Soc. Franc. Dermatol. Syphilol.* 75:585–591.
2. Lowe, N.J., and Ashton, R. (1984). Anthralin and coal tar therapy for psoriasis. *Dermatol. Clin. North Am.* 2(3):389–396.
3. Ingram, J.T. (1953). Approach to psoriasis. *Br. Med. J.* 2:591–594.
4. Goeckerman, W.H. (1925). The treatment of psoriasis. *Northwest Med.* 24:2–9.
5. Lowe, N.J., Wortzman, M.S., Breeding, J., et al. (1982). Coal tar phototherapy for psoriasis reevaluated. *J. Am. Acad. Dermatol.* 8:781–789.
6. Menter, A., and Cram, D. (1983). The Goeckerman regimen in two psoriasis day care centers. *J. Am. Acad. Dermatol.* 9:59–65.
7. Menter, A., and Harrison, P.E. (1994). Psoriasis day care centers. In *Practical Psoriasis Therapy*, 2nd ed. N.J. Lowe (Ed.). Mosby Year Book, St. Louis, pp. 155– 164.
8. Armstrong, R.B. (1984). Modified Goeckerman therapy for psoriasis. *Arch. Dermatol.* 120:313–318.
9. Committee on Psoriasis. (1984). White paper on hospitalization for psoriasis care. *J. Am. Acad. Dermatol.* 10:842–851.

34

Occlusive Therapy of Psoriasis

Joseph B. Bikowski, Jr.
University of Pittsburgh School of Medicine, Pittsburgh, Pennsylvania

Over three decades ago Garb (1) first reported the salutary effects of occlusion in enhancing the healing effects of a topically applied medication. Shortly thereafter Scholtz (2), using fluocinolone acetonide, and Sulzberger and Witten (3), using hydrocortisone, described the therapeutic advantages of a topically applied corticosteroid under a plastic film in the treatment of psoriasis and other corticosteroid-responsive dermatoses. Occlusion (defined as the total prevention of passive transepidermal water loss at the application site) with a pliable plastic film (vinylidine polymer: Saran Wrap, Handi Wrap) has significantly improved the efficacy of topical therapeutic agents. It promotes the rate and amount of percutaneous absorption of pharmacological agents. Although the exact mechanism is not known, it is presumably by altering the degree of hydration of the stratum corneum. This increase in pharmacological effect has been used in studies to assess the potency of many topical corticosteroids and proprietary medicaments (4).

Plastic occlusion treatment, described in dermatology therapeutic texts (5,6), consists of the application of a sheet of plastic film over a topical medication (e.g., corticosteroid, salicylic acid). Plastic gloves are available for the hand, plastic "baggies" for the feet, bathing caps for the head and scalp, sheets of plastic film may be wrapped around the extremities, and large plastic refuse bags may be used for the buttocks and trunk. For total body coverage, vinyl exercise suits ("sauna" suits) are commercially available.

Overnight application of corticosteroids to hydrated skin, under occlusion, may be as effective and far less costly in time and money than twice daily applications of the same medications without occlusion. In the 1960s, various studies (7,8) confirmed the therapeutic efficacy of a corticosteroid (flurandrenolide)-impregnated tape (Cordran Tape).

In the 1970s, Fisher and coworkers (9,10) addressed the issue as to effect of various tape systems, with or without corticosteroids, on the mitotic activity in normal or stripped human epidermis. They concluded that a totally occlusive tape system did not have a more potent pharmacological effect than a non-occlusive tape system. Thus, it might be possible to use a less occlusive system to successfully inhibit hyperproliferative disease processes. The less occlusive system would decrease the frequency of secondary bacterial infection and miliaria and therefore result in increased patient comfort and compliance with occlusive therapy.

The serendipitous observation that a Band-Aid left on a psoriatic lesion for three weeks resulted in clearing at the sites of the adherent portions (11) has introduced the concept that occlusion alone (i.e., without a topical corticosteroid) may be an effective alternative treatment of psoriasis, leading to studies of the application of various tapes, adhesive occlusive dressings, and adhesive dermatological patches.

Therefore, a partially occlusive system with medication, or occlusion alone, without "active ingredient," may be effective treatment for a hyperproliferative disease such as psoriasis.

CLINICAL AND LABORATORY OBSERVATIONS

Numerous clinical trials (11–18) have shown that occlusion alone has definite pharmacological effects and is a safe and effective alternative therapy for the treatment of plaque psoriasis vulgaris in limited size and distribution. Shore (11,12) studied numerous unspecified adhesive tapes with and without topical corticosteroids and demonstrated that most psoriatic plaques either improved or resolved; some remained clear for a month or more after treatment. Tapes with low moisture vapor transmission were more effective than topical emollients and other less occlusive tapes. The prolonged application of tape for 1 week or longer was clearly superior to repeated daily applications (12).

In an attempt to produce an optimal occlusive tape or dressing for psoriasis treatment, numerous products (Table 1) have been evaluated in clinical trials, including adhesive hydrocolloid occlusive dressings (HCD; DuoDERM, Surgihesive, Restore) and an adhesive hydrocolloid dermatological patch (Actiderm).

The HCD (DuoDERM, Surgihesive, Restore) is a lamination of a moisture- and oxygen-impermeable open-cell polyurethane exterior, and a hydrocolloid layer that adheres to the skin. The hydrocolloid is composed of gelatin, pectin, carboxymethylcellulose sodium, and an adhesive (e.g., polyisobutylene). Actiderm consists of a moisture- and oxygen-impermeable polyethylene exterior and a nondispersive hydrocolloid matrix that adheres to the skin; it is designed to be used both alone and over topical medicaments. Hydrocolloid occlusive dressings are designed to be changed every 2–7 days.

In contrast to other tapes and occlusive dressings, the HCD and dermatological patch are initially adherent to the skin (dry tack), but after interaction with cutaneous moisture or wound exudate, a liquid "soup" forms between the dressing and the skin diminishing adhesiveness (wet tack). Because the mechanical trauma of frequently removing an adherent dressing from the skin might incite the appearance of new psoriatic lesions or significantly retard the resolution of existent lesions, reduction of the HCD adhesiveness might therefore be important to minimize the risk of the Koebner (isomorphic) phenomenon via tape-stripping of the skin.

Table 1 Occlusive Dressings Marketed for Psoriasis Treatment

Actiderm (ConvaTac, Princeton, NJ)
DuoDERM (ConvaTac, Princeton, NJ)
Restore Dressings for Psoriasis (Hollister, Libertyville, IL)
Surgihesive (E.R. Squibb & Sons, Princeton, NJ)
Topiclude (Ferndale Laboratories, Inc., Ferndale, MI)

In the study by Friedman (13), the majority of localized plaques of psoriasis achieved improvement (41%) or resolution (47%) with the prolonged application of HCD: DuoDERM and Surgihesive alone were superior to nonoccluded fluocinolone acetonide cream and were equally effective as ultraviolet B radiation therapy for psoriasis.

In a multicenter trial of Actiderm, 37% (17/46) of the psoriatic plaques showed complete clearance and the remainder achieved significant improvement (14). Four patients were withdrawn due to clinical signs of infection (see below).

Gottlieb et al. (15) studied the dermal infiltrate of psoriatic plaques treated with Actiderm. After 2 weeks of therapy, there was clinical improvement of the psoriatic lesions; however, the abnormal presence of HLA DR+ keratinocytes, dermal Langerhans cells, and activated T lymphocytes could still be demonstrated in 75% of patients. The reduction in the scale and induration of the psoriatic plaques with HCD therapy may reflect a normalization of the psoriatic epidermal changes; however, even after 2 weeks of application, the occlusive treatment did not affect the underlying immunopathogenic mechanisms.

David and Lowe (16) compared the Actiderm dermatological patch alone, topical 0.1% triamcinolone acetonide cream (TAC) under the Actiderm patch, TAC under Saran Wrap occlusion, and TAC alone. They observed that the most rapid improvement was achieved with the combination of the dermatological patch plus TAC. After 4 weeks without treatment, the combined TAC and patch therapy retained a more persistent improvement compared to other treated sites.

Lever and Marks (17) determined that occlusion of psoriatic plaques with Actiderm was equivalent to short-contact dithranol, and short-contact dithranol followed by Actiderm occlusion may be more effective than either treatment alone.

Wise et al. (18) demonstrated that after 41 days of treatment, 42% of psoriatic plaques resolved with Restore HCD alone. Complete remission was observed in 29% of lesions treated with corticosteroids of varying potencies without occlusion.

MECHANISM OF ACTION

The precise mechanisms for the clinical improvement of psoriasis under occlusion are unknown. Fry et al. (19) reported reformation of the granular cell layer and reduction of the mitotic rate after treatment of psoriasis with plastic occlusive dressings for 2 weeks. Halprin et al. (20) reported an inhibition of enzyme activities, and Baxter and Stoughton (21) documented a reduction of mitotic index of psoriatic plaques treated with an adhesive tape impregnated with flurandrenolide (Cordan Tape). In these studies, there was no clinical therapeutic evaluation of the psoriatic plaques (19–21).

Other beneficial effects of occlusion on psoriasis may be related to similar pharmacological properties of emollients (22); occlusion with tape or moisturizers may prevent the development of parakeratosis by trapping moisture and hydrating the stratum corneum, and facilitate desquamation by diminishing binding forces between corneocytes (23,24).

Tape-stripping of normal skin may be a good model for psoriasis, since cell cycle parameters and the transepidermal water loss of a psoriatic plaque are of the same order as freshly stripped normal skin (25,26). Fisher and Maibach (25) showed that adhesive tape decreased the mitotic activity of tape-stripped human skin; potent antimitotic effects occurred with semiocclusive and nonocclusive tapes. They observed that complete occlusion was not necessary for the inhibitory influence; part of the hyperproliferative activity in psoriasis may be due to the lack of a normal barrier between the epidermis and the environment. Occlusion may act by establishing an artificial water barrier and/or by reducing traumatic loss of the abnormal stratum corneum (25). Tree and Marks (22) demonstrated similar depression of mitotic activity of tape-stripped mouse skin after application of bland emollients. They believed that topical applications might decrease cell loss by their physical stickiness and the consequence would be a decreased mitotic rate; they concluded that the rate of desquamation not only reflects the rate of cell production, but can independently influence the rate of proliferation.

It has been proposed that the HCD primarily benefit psoriasis by hydration of the stratum corneum. Since the horny layer of psoriasis has a greater transepidermal water loss (TEWL) and a diminished water-holding capacity (26), the reduced amount of unbound water in the pathological horny layer possibly alters the secondary or tertiary structure of the stratum corneum keratin proteins. Trapping and retaining transepidermal water with an occlusive dressing could correct a keratin defect and minimize its effect on the dermal process in the pathogenesis of psoriasis.

Trapping moisture and facilitating desquamation may not be the only factors involved in the clinical efficacy of the HCD in treating psoriasis. Local temperature elevation of the psoriatic plaque due to a possible insulating effect of the HCD may be responsible. Hyperthermia has been shown to be effective in the treatment of psoriasis (27,28).

It is possible that one of the constituents or an unknown ingredient in the adhesive of the HCD may act as a chemical inhibitor that could therapeutically benefit psoriasis. However, chemical inhibition was discounted in tape-stripping studies by Fisher and Maibach (25), and other studies showed beneficial therapeutic effects of materials without an adhesive [e.g., plastic films (19)].

ADVERSE EFFECTS OF OCCLUSIVE DRESSINGS

Undesirable effects from occlusive plastic therapy include infection (bacterial, fungal, or yeast), miliaria, folliculitis, a disagreeable odor from macerated tissue, interference with heat exchange, and an increased tendency to sunburn. Dermal atrophy, striae, and suppression of the hypothalmic-pituitary-adrenal axis (HPA) are associated with corticosteroid under occlusion.

The routine use of occlusion therapy in dermatology has usually been limited by problems with the available materials. Some of the newer adhesive occlusive dressings absorb transepidermal water, and thus minimize skin maceration and discourage the overgrowth of skin microflora, which contrasts with plastic wrap.

Limitations of adhesive occlusive dressing therapy include its use on hair-bearing areas such as the scalp. Also, owing to expense and impracticality, it is not useful for patients with extensive disease because the dressing could be cumbersome, and it could interfere with perspiration.

A significant disadvantage of using tape or an adhesive occlusive dressing is the potential of tape-stripping with subsequent development of the Koebner

Table 2 The Ideal Occlusive Topical Medication Delivery System for Psoriasis

1. Be a one-component system
2. Absorb transepidermal water to avoid maceration
3. Not disperse on hydration
4. Provide little trauma upon removal
5. Be able to conform to contours of the human body to provide excellent surface contact with the skin
6. Have little effect on the microflora to reduce the possibility of secondary infection
7. Be self-adhesive to avoid the need for external fixation
8. Be comfortable, wear evenly, and demonstrate flexibility over joints such as elbows and knees
9. Provide a physical barrier to protect damaged skin from external trauma from scratching, friction, and noxious substances
10. Prevent desiccation
11. Deliver a measured dose of corticosteroid over a given period of time
12. Provide controlled release of the medication for at least 24–72 hr, if not longer, to decrease frequency of application and therefore increase patient compliance with the treatment regimen
13. Essentially limit the corticosteroid absorption to the diseased skin only, thereby preventing possible side effects to normal skin
14. Provide therapeutic and cost-effectiveness by decreasing frequency of application, limiting medication amount, and applying to diseased skin only
15. Be cosmetically acceptable and elegant with ease of use to encourage patient compliance

phenomenon (29,30). The Auspitz sign was noted in two plaques upon removal of the HCD (DuoDERM), and was probably due to the adhesiveness of the HCD (9). The Koebner phenomenon was observed in four plaques treated with HCD, conforming to the distribution of the dressing (13). The exact mechanism for the local psoriatic exacerbation was not known. Evaluation for cutaneous delayed hypersensitivity was negative, and bacterial cultures did not reveal a particular organism associated with the exacerbation of the psoriasis. It is possible that the dry-tack was not sufficiently reduced and tape-stripping occurred upon removal of the HCD (29,30). Perhaps permitting the dressing to remain on the plaque for longer than 7 days would then be a project for future studies.

Clinical infection has been associated with an adhesive hydrocolloid occlusive dermatological patch (Actiderm). In contrast, infection was not noted in 26 patients studied with DuoDERM, and bacterial cultures did not reveal a particular organism associated with the exacerbation of the psoriasis (13). Rajka et al. (31) and Cherry et al. (32) demonstrated significant increases in the density of *Staphylococcus aureus* and lipophilic diptheroids after occlusion of psoriatic skin with a plastic film. Normal skin (33) and psoriatic plaques (32) did not demonstrate increases in bacterial colony counts with a HCD (Actiderm).

OPTIMAL PROPERTIES OF OCCLUSIVE DRESSINGS

Advantages for occlusive dressing therapy of localized psoriasis include cost-effectiveness, convenience, reduction of plaque itching, and protection of the psoriatic plaque with the reduction of trauma.

At this time, a particular tape, occlusive dressing, or dermatological patch with optimal properties remains to be determined. Table 2 lists the desired characteristics of an ideal occlusive topical medication delivery system for psoriasis.

FUTURE APPLICATIONS OF OCCLUSIVE DRESSINGS

Clinical studies have demonstrated that the prolonged application of tape (11,12,23), an occlusive dressing (13,18), or a dermatological patch (14–17) alone is an effective therapeutic modality for patients with limited psoriasis.

The psoriatic scale was expediently diminished in all plaques treated with HCD. Elimination of plaque scale was noted within 2 weeks (two HCD dressing changes) and preceded improvement of plaque induration and erythema by many weeks (13,15,16).

Because of the salutary keratolytic effect of HCD, combined therapeutic trials with other psoriatic medications are warranted.

In future studies, the development and elucidation of optimal treatments are of importance where occlusion may act together with other therapies such as 5-fluorouracil (34), arachidonic acid (35), 1, 25-dihydroxyvitamin D_3 (36), anthralin (17,37), topical steroids (12,16,38), and chlorpromazine (39).

Considering that there have been significant advances in the technology of providing controlled delivery of drugs to the dermis or systemic circulation (40), the development of an optimized dressing, a dermatological patch, or a dermatological drug delivery system in the treatment of limited psoriasis vulgaris may be available in the not too distant future.

REFERENCES

1 Garb, J. (1960). Nevus verrucosus unilateralis cured with podophyllin ointment. *Arch. Dermatol.* 81: 606–609.
2. Scholtz, J.R. (1961). Topical therapy of psoriasis with fluocinolone acetonide. *Arch. Dermatol.* 84: 1029–1030.
3. Sulzberger, M.B., and Witten, V.H. (1961). Thin pliable plastic films in dermatologic therapy. *Arch. Dermatol.* 84:1027–1028.
4. Marriott, C., and Martin, G.P. (1988). Preclinical results of a new dermatological patch used in conjunction with topical corticosteroids including the blanching response. In *Beyond Occlusion: Wound Care Proceedings.* T.J. Ryan (Ed.). Royal Society of Medicine International Congress and Symposium Series No. 136. Royal Society of Medicine, London, pp. 25–34.
5. Camisa, C. (1994). Occlusive dressings. In *Psoriasis.* Blackwell Scientific Publications, Boston, pp. 185–186.
6. Arndt, K.A. (1995). *Manual of Dermatologic Therapeutics.* 5th ed. Little, Brown, Boston, p. 302.
7. Goldman, L., Igelman, J.M., and Kitzmiller, K.W. (1967). Clinical investigative studies with flurandrenolone tape. *Cutis* 3:367.
8. Fields, R.J., and Magpantay, R. (1968). Studies with flurandrenolone tape. *Med. Ann. D.C.* 37:272.
9. Fisher, L.B., Maibach, H.I., and Trancik, R.J. (1978). Variably occlusive tape system and the mitotic activity of stripped human epidermis, effects with and without hydrocortisone. *Arch. Dermatol.* 114:727–729.
10. Fisher, L.B., Maibach, H.I., and Trancik, R.J. (1978). Effects of occlusive tape systems on the mitotic activity of epidermis, with and without corticosteroids. *Arch. Dermatol.* 114:384–386.
11. Shore, R.N. (1985). Clearing of psoriatic lesions after the application of tape. *N. Engl. J. Med.* 312:246.
12. Shore, R.N. (1986). Treatment of psoriasis with prolonged application of tape. *J. Am. Acad. Dermatol.* 15: 540–542.
13. Friedman, S.J. (1987). Management of psoriasis vulgaris with a hydrocolloid occlusive dressing. *Arch. Dermatol.* 123:1046–1052.
14. Telfer, N.R., Ryan, T.I., Blanc, D., et al. (1988). Results of a multicenter trial of Actiderm in the treatment of plaque psoriasis. In *Beyond Occlusion: Dermatology Proceedings.* T.J. Ryan (Ed.). Royal Society of Medicine International Congress and Symposium Series No. 137. Royal Society of Medicine, London, pp. 53–56.
15. Gottlieb, A.B., Cohen, S.R., and Carter, D.M. (1988). Efficacy of Actiderm in the treatment of psoriasis. In *Beyond Occlusion: Dermatology Proceedings.* T.J. Ryan (Ed.). Royal Society of Medicine International Congress and Symposium Series No. 137. Royal Society of Medicine, London, pp. 25–34.
16. David, M.D., and Lowe, N.J. (1989). Psoriasis therapy: comparative studies with a hydrocolloid dressing, plastic film occlusion, and triamcinolone acetonide cream. *J. Am. Acad. Dermatol.* 21:511–514.
17. Lever, L., and Marks, R. (1988). Actiderm and Dithranol in the treatment of chronic plaque psoriasis. In *Beyond Occlusion: Dermatology Proceedings.* T.J. Ryan (Ed.). Royal Society of Medicine International Congress and Symposium Series No. 137. Royal Society of Medicine, London, pp. 67–70.
18. Wise, It., Jarmoszuk, I., Finn, S., and Zeitz, Il. (1988). *Comparison of Hydrocolloid Dressing to Topical Steroids in Psoriasis.* American Academy of Dermatology Summer Session, New York, December.
19. Fry, L., Almeyda, L., and McMinn, R.M.H. (1970). Effects of plastic occlusive dressings on psoriatic epidermis. *Br. J. Dermatol.* 82:458–462.
20. Halprin, K.M., Fukui, K., and Ohkawara, A. (1969). Flurandrenolone (Cordran) tape and carbohydrate metabolizing enzymes. *Arch. Dermatol.* 100:336–341.
21. Baxter, D.L., and Stoughton, R.B. (1970). Mitotic index of psoriatic lesions treated with anthralin, glucocorticosteroids and occlusion only. *J. Invest. Dermatol.* 54:410–412.
22. Tree, S., and Marks, R. (1975). An explanation for the "placebo" effect of bland ointment bases. *Br. J. Dermatol.* 92:195–198.
23. Shore, R.N. (1985). *Response of Psoriasis to Occlusion with Tape: An Update.* American Academy of Dermatology 44th Annual Meeting. Psoriasis Symposium, Las Vegas, December.
24. Marks, R. (1984). Topical therapy for psoriasis: general principles. *Dermatol. Clin. North. Am.* 2:383–388.
25. Fisher, L.B., and Maibach, H.I. (1972). Physical occlusion controlling epidermal mitosis. *J. Invest. Dermatol.* 59:106–108.

26. Tagami, H., and Yoshikuni, K. (1985). Interrelationship between water-barrier and reservoir functions of pathologic stratum corneum. *Arch. Dermatol.* 121: 642–645.
27. Urabe, H., Nishitani, K., and Kohda, H. (1981). Hyperthermia in the treatment of psoriasis. *Arch. Dermatol.* 117:770–774.
28. Orenberg, E.K., Deneau, D.G., and Farber, E.M. (1980). Response of chronic psoriatic plaques to localized heating induced by ultrasound. *Arch. Dermatol.* 116:893–897.
29. Jablonska, S., Chowaniec, O., Beutner, E.H., et al. (1982). Stripping of the stratum corneum in patients with psoriasis. *Arch. Dermatol.* 118:652–657.
30. Miller, R.A.W. (1982). The Koebner phenomenon. *Int. J. Dermatol.* 21:192–197.
31. Rajka, G., Aly, R., Bayles, C., et al. (1981). The effect of short-term occlusion on the cutaneous flora in atopic dermatitis and psoriasis. *Acta Derm. Venereol. (Stockh.)* 161:150–153.
32. Cherry, G.W., Cherry, C.A., Telfer, N.R., et al. (1988). Bacterial growth under Actiderm and Saran Wrap applied to psoriatic plaques. In *Beyond Occlusion: Dermatology Proceedings.* T.J. Ryan (Ed.). Royal Society of Medicine International Congress and Symposium Series No. 137. Royal Society of Medicine, London, pp. 45–51.
33. Lilly, H.A., and Lawrence, J.C. (1988). The effect of Actiderm dermatological patch and Saran Wrap on the bacteriological flora of skin. In *Beyond Occlusion: Dermatology Proceedings.* T.J. Ryan (Ed.). Royal Society of Medicine International Congress and Symposium Series No. 137. Royal Society of Medicine, London, pp. 35–41.
34. Perlman, D.L., Youngberg, B., and Engelhard, C. (1986). Weekly pulse dosing schedule fluorouracil: a new topical therapy for psoriasis. *J. Am. Acad. Dermatol.* 15:1247–1252.
35. Hebborn, P., Jablonska, S., Beutner, E.H., et al. (1988). Action of topically applied arachidonic acid on the skin of patients with psoriasis. *Arch. Dermatol.* 124: 387–391.
36. Smith, E.L., Pincus, S.H., Donovan, L., and Holick, M.F. (1988). A novel approach for the evaluation and treatment of psoriasis. Oral or topical use of 1,25-dihydroxyvitamin D_3 can be safe and effective therapy for psoriasis. *J. Am. Acad. Dermatol.* 19:516–528.
37. Williamson, D.M. (1983). Treatment of chronic psoriasis by Psoradrate (0.1% dithranol in a 17% urea base) applied under occlusion. *Clin. Exp. Dermatol.* 8: 287–290.
38. Jaeger, L. (1986). Psoriasis treatment with betamethasone dipropionate using short-term occlusion. *Acta Derm. Venereol. (Stockh.)* 66:84–97.
39. Knopf, B., Wollina, U., Zollmann, C., et al. (1988). Therapeutic modification of chronic stable psoriasis lesions by a chlorpromazine ointment and occlusive dressings. *Dermatol. Monatsschr.* 174:151–155.
40. Syhaw, J.E., Prevo, M.E., and Amkraut, A.A. (1987). Testing of controlled-release transdermal dosage forms. Product development and clinical trials. *Arch. Dermatol.* 123:1548–1556.

35

Vitamin D: Rationale and Potential Mechanism of Action

Elke M.G.J. de Jong
University Hospital Nijmegen, Nijmegen, The Netherlands

Ole Baadsgaard
University of Copenhagen, Gentofte Hospital, Copenhagen, Denmark

Vitamin D has been interesting to dermatologists since 1985, when patients were reported in the literature who were cured from psoriasis by oral or topical administration of vitamin D_3 (1–4). They were not the first patients treated with vitamin D_3 for skin disease. Already in the decade between 1930 and 1940 patients were treated with oral vitamin D_3. It was applied not only in psoriasis, but also in eczema, acne, lupus vulgaris, pemphigus vulgaris, and scleroderma (5). Probably due to its side effects and the availability of other treatments, the therapeutic use of vitamin D_3 was not further developed.

In 1985, the renewed application of vitamin D_3 coincided with the recent development of knowledge about effects of vitamin D in vitro. It was shown that vitamin D_3 inhibits proliferation and increases differentiation of various cell types in vitro [keratinocytes, HL60 cells (a human monoblastic leukemia cell line), U937 cells (a human promyelocytic leukemia cell line), fibroblasts, and breast cancer cells] (6–10).

This has led to a wave of investigations and applications of various types of vitamin D. Especially, the development of analogues with less calciotropic effects has increased application in skin disease.

PHYSIOLOGY OF VITAMIN D

Vitamin D is produced in the skin under the influence of ultraviolet light in the UVB range, and is taken up from food via the intestine. In the epidermis, a precursor is present (7-dehydrocholesterol), which is converted to previtamin D_3 under the influence of sunlight of 290–300 nm. Further conversion of vitamin D_3 occurs under the influence of the skin temperature.

This vitamin D_3 is transported by a vitamin D–binding protein present in the blood. This vitamin D_3 is not active. In order to become active two hydroxylation steps are necessary. The first occurs in the liver where 25-OH-vitamin D_3 is formed. The second takes place in the kidney, where 1α,25$(OH)_2$ vitamin D_3 or active vitamin D_3 or calcitriol is formed.

The kidney possesses a 24-hydroxylase as well, so that 24,25 $(OH)_2$ vitamin D_3 is formed in vivo also. Hydroxylation seems to be possible in other organs and cells as well (e.g., placenta, bone, macrophages, and even keratinocytes) (11).

Receptors for 1α,25 $(OH)_2$ vitamin D_3 are reported in many cells, not only in the classic target organs such as bone, parathyroid, and gut, but in virtually all cell types including keratinocytes, T lymphocytes, B lymphocytes, monocytes, macrophages, fibroblasts, and in neutrophils (12,13). Inactivation takes place via thermic conversion in the skin to lumisterol and tachysterol, probably also via a mitochondrial catabolic cascade.

MODE OF ACTION

1α,25 $(OH)_2$ vitamin D_3 exerts its effects via more than one mechanism: nuclear and nonnuclear mechanisms. It is bound to a cytosolic receptor that is transported to the nucleus, modulating transcription of proteins, and is involved in calcium homeostasis and growth control (14). This receptor belongs to the steroid receptor superfamily, which consists of a family of nuclear receptors for steroid hormones (glucocorticosteroids, estrogens, thyroid hormone, vitamin D, and vitamin A).

Nuclear Mechanisms

Vitamin D_3 binds to the vitamin D receptor (VDR). This complex binds to VDR response elements present in the promoter region of target genes for vitamin D_3. It is now known that for, example, the retinoid X-receptor influences the response and nuclear binding of vitamin A, D_3, and thyroid hormone. Therefore, cross-talks between these substances are possible (15). The DNA-binding domain of the nuclear receptor superfamily is characterized by two zinc finger-like motifs. The DNA response elements that these receptors bind to are similar in sequence and organization. Recently, it was shown that the vitamin D_3 receptor communicates vitamin D_3-mediated signals together with the other members of the nuclear receptor superfamily. For this interaction between members of the steroid receptor superfamily a novel structural domain has been identified that is conserved within the members of the nuclear receptor superfamily and may function in transactivation of cognate genes (16). Interaction with the retinoid-X receptor-alpha (RXR-alpha) has been reported by several authors. RXR-alpha interacts directly with and enhances the binding of nuclear receptors conferring responsiveness to vitamin D_3 and thyroid hormone (15). RXR-alpha is a dimerization partner for the vitamin D_3 receptor. RXR-alpha has been postulated to enhance tight binding of VDR with vitamin D response elements (17). The expression of the high-affinity vitamin D receptor is susceptible to various control mechanisms. It has been demonstrated in mouse fibroblasts that the vitamin D_3 receptor is up-regulated by calcipotriol and 1α,25-dihydroxyvitamin D_3 (18). It was shown that 1α,25-dihydroxyvitamin D_3 at a 10 nM concentration induced up-regulation of the receptor in nontransformed fibroblasts. In transformed cell lines up-regulation could not be induced (19). In human monocytes up-regulation of the vitamin D_3 receptor has also been demonstrated (20). The expression of the vitamin D receptor has been shown to be 4.5-fold increased in rapidly proliferating endothelial cells, compared to density arrested cells, which suggests that the expression of this receptor can be modulated by factors involved in growth control (21). The vitamin D receptor proved to be up-regulated by protein kinase C activation and this was prevented by sphingosine (21). The expression of the VDR is susceptible to various control mechanisms. Its effect consists of:

- Inhibition of transcription of the MYC-oncogene in HL60 cells (22)
- Inhibition of transcription of gene regulatory proteins (such as CMYC and CFOS) (23,24)
- Induction of transcription of α-protein kinase C and β-protein kinase C (25)
- Enhancement of transcription of insulin growth factor 1 receptors (26)
- Increased expression of fibronectin (27)

Nonnuclear Mechanisms

Increase of intracellular calcium within 90 sec after addition of 1α,25 $(OH)_2$ vitamin D_3 is seen in keratinocytes (28). Because of the speed of the reaction and because cycloheximide did not inhibit this, no protein synthesis is involved. In addition, cGMP is elevated (29).

Intracellular Signaling

The nuclear effects of active vitamin D_3 and the more immediate induction of a transmembrane calcium influx result in modulation of intracellular signaling.

It has been shown that 1α,25-dihydroxyvitamin D_3 enhances the production of inositol triphosphate, 1,2-diacylglycerol, and induces an increase of intracellular calcium. Vitamin D_3 promotes the translocation of protein kinase C from the cytosolic to the membrane position (30). To what extent the nuclear mechanisms or the transmembrane signaling effect of active vitamin D_3 is responsible for its biological effects is difficult to establish.

The physiological relevance of protein kinase C as an intermediary stage between vitamin D_3 action and epidermal differentiation is evident from the observation that inhibition of protein kinase C causes marked suppression of 1α,25-dihydroxyvitamin D_3–induced formation of cornified envelopes (20).

The biochemical effects resulting from an increase of the intracellular calcium concentration are diverse. Increasing the extracellular calcium concentration in keratinocyte cultures will result in keratinization. An increase of the intracellular calcium concentration occurs during differentiation of these cells (31).

Vitamin D_3 exerts many effect on various cell types in vitro as well as in vivo. These are summarized in Table 1.

Table 1 Effects of Vitamin D on Cell Types In Vitro

Cell types	Effects
Keratinocytes	IL-8 ↓
	CMYC ↓ CFOS ↓
	Proliferation ↓
	Differentiation ↑
	Transglutaminase ↑ in culture, ↓ in vivo
	Inositol triphosphate ↑
	1,2-diacylglycerol ↑
	Protein kinase C ↑
	Involucrin ↑ in culture, ↓ in vivo
	Keratin 16 ↓, 18 ↓, 2 ↑, 5 ↑, 10 ↑
	Filaggrin ↓ in vivo
	TGF-β ↑—> proliferation ↓
	IL-6 ↓
	TNFα =
Fibroblasts	Proliferation ↓
	IL-8 ↓
T lymphocytes	Activation by
	IL-1 ↓, IL-2 ↓, IL-6 ↓
	IL-2 receptors ↓
	IFN gamma ↓ GM-CSF ↓
B lymphocytes	IgG and IgM production ↓
Macrophages/ monocytes	IL-1 ↑, IL-6 ↓, IL-8 ↓, TNFα ↓
	PGE_2 ↑
	IF ↑
	Cytotoxicity ↑ differentiation ↑
	Granuloma formation ↑ proliferation ↓
	Giant cell formation ↑
	Hydrogen peroxide production ↑
	HLA-DR ↓
	CD14 ↑
	CD23 ↓
Neutrophils	AA release ↓ migration ↓
	Phagocytosis ↓
	PAF ↑
	Proliferation ↓
	Differentiation ↑

IN VIVO EFFECTS IN PSORIASIS

Treatment of patients with psoriasis with orally applied 1α,25 $(OH)_2$ vitamin D_3 has a narrow safety range but is effective (3). Oral 1α (OH) vitamin D_3 was effective as well (1).

Topical treatment with 1α,25 $(OH)_2$ vitamin D_3 initially seemed to be unsuccessful, but this proved to be a problem of vehicle used. Systemic side effects have to be treated (32). Topical 1α,24 $(OH)_2$ vitamin D_3 is equipotent to 1α,25 $(OH)_2$ vitamin D_3 in effects on kertinocyte growth (33). Less hypercalcemia is induced (34). Kato et al. showed improvement in 10 patients out of 15 (4). Gerritsen et al. treated 10 patients with tacalcitol 4 μg/g; 8 of 10 patients showed marked improvement (35).

Topical treatment with the vitamin D_3 analogue calcipotriol has been widely used and has proven beneficial. Even high-dose studies showed quite moderate side effects. Calcipotriol has the advantage of being 100× less calciotropic. It binds to the same receptor as 1α,25 $(OH)_2$ vitamin D_3 but is rapidly metabolized. It is used as monotherapy, but is also effective in combination therapy with corticosteroids (36), dithranol (37), ultraviolet (38,39), and cyclosporin (40).

Epidermal proliferation, abnormal keratinization, and cutaneous inflammation are key features of the psoriatic lesion. Vitamin D_3 analogues have been shown to modulate these features in vitro. However, to what extent these features are relevant to the antipsoriatic efficacy remains to be elucidated. Several studies have been carried out to assess changes of epidermal growth, differentiation, and inflammation during treatment of psoriatic plaques with vitamin D_3 analogues.

During treatment of psoriatic plaques with calcipotriol in ointment (50 μg/g) it was shown that the accumulation of polymorphonuclear leukocytes decreases already during the first week of treatment; the number of cycling epidermal cells showed a reduction after 2 weeks of treatment; after 4 weeks of treatment the number of keratin 16–positive cells and the number of T lymphocytes decreased significantly (41). The number of CD14 cells and Langerhans cells remained unaffected during treatment with calcipotriol (41). A quantification of these changes by flow cytometry revealed a highly significant reduction of the percentage of cells in SG_2M phase and a highly significant reduction of the number of keratin 16–positive cells. However, also in those patients who showed complete clinical resolution of the psoriatic plaques, the percentages of keratin 16–positive cells

Table 2 In Vivo Effects of Calcipotriol, Calcitriol, and Tacalcitol

	Calcipotriol 50 μg/g 2dd	Calcitriol 3 μg/g 2 dd	Tacalcitol 4 μg/g 1 dd
Ki67 (proliferation)	+	+	+
Keratin 16	±/+	Not done	+
Involucrin	Not done	+	+
Filaggrin	Not done	+	+
PMN	+	+	+
T-lymphocytes	±	+	+
Monocytes/macrophages	−	Not done	+
Langerhans cells	−	Not done	−

and cells in SG_2M phase remained well above the normal range (42). During treatment of psoriatic plaques with calcipotriol a reduction of the number of keratin 16– and keratin 17–positive cells and a normalization of the number of keratin 5– and keratin 10–positive cells have been shown (43–45). However, calcipotriol treatment of psoriatic plaques did not result in a modification of ornithine decarboxylase activity (46). During treatment with calcipotriol a reduction of CD4+ T cells and a preponderance of CD8+ T cells were induced (47). Most studies agree that calcipotriol induces pronounced changes in epidermal behavior, leaving the mononuclear infiltrate largely unaffected (44,47,48). However, one study suggests a relative persistence of the epidermal phenomena (47). Compared to the effects of betamethasone valerate, calcipotriol induced a reduction of epidermal growth and differentiation characteristics to the same extent (42). During treatment of psoriatic plaques with calcipotriol, a decline of staining intensity of interleukin-6, but not of TNF-alpha, was observed in lesional and clinically uninvolved skin (49).

Studies have been carried out during treatment with 1α,25-dihydroxyvitamin D_3 in ointment (3 μg/g) and 1α,24-dihydroxyvitamin D_3 in ointment (4 μg/g). Similar changes as seen during calcipotriol applications were observed during these treatments (32,35). In addition, involucrin, filaggrin, and transglutaminase were studied. Involucrin decreased, filaggrin increased, and transglutaminase increased. ICAM-1 and PAL-E, a staining for vascular endothelium, tend to decrease. Remarkably, during treatment with 1α,25-dihydroxyvitamin D_3 and 1α,24-dihydroxyvitamin D_3, a reduction of the accumulation of T lymphocytes and monocytes was seen, in contrast to the inconspicuous modulation induced by calcipotriol (32,35). Systemic treatment of psoriatic patients with 1α-hydroxyvitamin D_3 resulted in inhibition of keratinocyte proliferation and a reduction of keratin 16 expression (50).

It can be concluded that a reduction of epidermal proliferation and a decrease of the number of polymorphonuclear leukocytes are the most prominent changes during treatment of psoriatic plaques with vitamin D_3 analogues (Table 2).

FUTURE ASPECTS OF USE OF VITAMIN D_3 AND ANALOGUES

Other indications for the use of vitamin D_3 and analogues are currently being investigated. Topical use for malignancies such as breast cancer metastases, T-cell lymphoma of the skin, HIV-related psoriasis, or generalized pustular psoriasis may be of benefit (51–54). Also, treatment of pityriasis rubra pilaris with calcipotriol was shown to be an effective approach (55). A beneficial effect of topical calcipotriol on congenital ichthyosis was shown as well (56).

New vitamin D_3 analogues will become available with a shift of their working mechanisms toward antiproliferative or anti-inflammatory actions, and it is expected that the indication for use will extend in the future.

REFERENCES

1. Morimoto, S., and Kumahara, Y. (1985). A patient with psoriasis cured by 1α-hydroxyvitamin D_3. *Med. J. Osaka Univ.* 35–51.
2. Morimoto, S., Onishi, T., Imanaka, S., Yukahawa, H., Kazuka, T., Kitano, Y., Yoshikawa, K., and Kumahara, Y. (1986). Topical administration of 1,25-

dihydroxyvitamin D_3 for psoriasis: report of five cases. *Calcif. Tissue Int.* 38:1119–1122.
3. Morimoto, S., Yoshikawa, K., Kozuka, T., Kitano, Y., Imanaka, S., Fukuo, K., and Kamahara, Y. (1986). *Br. J. Dermatol.* 115:421–429.
4. Kato, T., Rokugo, M., Terui, T., and Tagami, H. (1986). Successful treatment of psoriasis with topical application of active vitamin D_3. *Br. J. Dermatol.* 115: 431–433.
5. Reed, C.I., Struck, H.C., and Steck, I.E. (1939). Other therapeutic applications of vitamin D. In *Vitamin D Chemistry, Physiology, Pharmacology, Pathology, Experimental and Clinical Investigations.* I.C. Reed, H.C. Struck, and I.E. Steck (Eds.). University of Chicago Press, Chicago, pp. 312–313.
6. Smith, E.L., Walworth, N.C., and Holick, M.F. (1986). Effect of 1α,25-dihydroxyvitamin D_3. *Endocrinology* 86:709–714.
7. Tanaka, H., Habe, E., Miyaura, C., Kuribayashi, T., Konno, K., Ishii, Y., and Suda, T. (1982). 1α,25-dihydroxy-cholecalciferol and a human meyloid leukaemia cell line (HL60). The presence of a cytosol receptor and induction of differentiation. *Biochem. J.* 204:713–719.
8. Oberg, F., Bolling, J., and Nilsson, K. (1993). Functional antagonism between vitamin D_3 and retinoic acid in the regulation of CD14 and CD23 expression during monocytic differentiation of U-937 cells. *J. Immunol.* 150:3487–3495.
9. Eil, C., and Marx, J.S. (1981). Nuclear uptake of 1,25-dihydroxyl[^{3}H]cholecalciferol in dispersed fibroblasts cultured from normal human skin. *Proc. Natl. Acad. Sci. USA* 78:2562–2566.
10. Abe, J., Nakano, T., Matsumoto, T., Ogata, E., and Ikeda, K. (1991). A novel vitamin D_3 analogue, 22-oxa-1,25-dihydroxyvitamin D_3, inhibits the growth of human breast cancer in vitro and in vivo without causing hypercalcemia. *Endocrinology* 129:832–837.
11. Avioli, L.V., and Haddai, J.G. (1984). The vitamin D family revisited. *N. Engl. J. Med.* 1:47–49.
12. Stumpf, W.E., Sar, M., Reid, F.A., Tanaka, Y., and DeLuca, H.F. (1979). Target cells for $1,25(OH)_2D_3$ in intestinal tract, stomach, kidney, skin, pituitary and parathyroid. *Science* 206:1188–1190.
13. Haussler, M.R. (1986). Vitamin D receptors: nature and function. *Annu. Rev. Nutr.* 6:527–562.
14. Franceschi, R.T., Simpsom, R.U., and DeLuca, H.F. (1981). Binding proteins for vitamin D metabolites: serum carriers and intracellular receptors. *Arch. Biochem. Biophys.* 210:1–13.
15. Kliewer, S.A., Umesono, K., Manglsdorf, D.J., and Evans, R.M. (1992). Retinoid X receptor interacts with nuclear receptors in retinoic acid, thyroid hormone and vitamin D_3 signalling. *Nature* 355:446–449.
16. Maksymowych, A.B., Hsu, T.C., and Litwack, G. (1992). A novel, highly conserved structural motif is present in all members of the steroid receptor superfamily. *Receptor* 2:225–240.
17. Brugge, Th., Polh, J., Lonnoy, O., and Stunnenberg, H.G. (1992). RXR-alpha, a promiscuous partner of retinoic acid and thyroid hormone receptors. *EMBO J.* 11:1409–1418.
18. Trydal, T., Lillehang, J.R., Aksnes, R.R., and Aarskog, D. (1990). Regulation of cell growth, C myc RNA, and 1,25-dihydroxyvitamin D_3 receptor in C3H/10T1/2 mouse embryo fibroblasts by calcipotriol and 1,25 dihydroxyvitamin D_3. *Acta Endocrinol.* (Copenh.) 126: 75–79.
19. Trydal, T., Lillehang, J.R., Aksnes, J.R., and Aarskog, D. (1990). Effect of 1,25-dihydroxyvitamin D_3 on growth, homologous receptor and c-*myc* regulation in C3H/10T1/2 cells. *Mol. Cell Endocrino.* 74:191–202.
20. Merke, J., Nawrot, M., Hugel, J., Szabo, A., and Ritz, E. (1989). Evidence for in vivo upregulation of $1,25(OH)_2$ vitamin D_3 receptor in human monocytes. *Calcif. Tissue Int.* 45:255–256.
21. Merke, J., Milde, P., Lewicka, S., Hugel, U., Klaus, G., Mangelsdorf, D.J., Haussler, M.R., Rauterberg, E.W., and Ritz, E. (1989). Identification and upregulation of 1,25-dihydroxyvitamin D_3 receptor activity and biosynthesis of 1,25-dihydroxyvitamin D_3. Studies in cultured bovine aortic endothelial cells and human dermal capillaries. *J. Clin. Invest.* 83:1903–1915.
22. Zhou, J.Y., Norman, A.W., Akashi, M., Uskokovic, M.R., Aurrecoechea, J.M., Dauben, W.G., Okamura, W.H., and Koeffler, H.P. (1991). Development of a novel 1,25 $(OH)_2$-vitamin D_3 analogue with potent ability to induce HL-60 cell differentiation without modulating calcium metabolism. *Blood* 78:75–82.
23. Sebag, M., Gulliver, W., and Kremer, R. (1994). Effects of 1,25 dihydroxyvitamin D_3 and calcium on growth and differentiation and on c-fos and p53 gene expression in normal human keratinocytes. *J. Invest. Dermatol.* 103:323–329.
24. Trydal, T., Lillehaug, J.R., Aksnes, L., and Aarskog, D. (1992). Regulation of cell growth, c-myc mRNA, and $1,25\text{-}(OH)_2$ vitamin D_3 receptor in C3H/10T1/2 mouse embryo fibroblasts by calcipotriol and 1,25-$(OH)_2$ vitamin D_3. *Acta Endocrinol.* 126:75–79.
25. Obeid, L.M., Okazaki, T., Karolak, L.A., and Hannun, Y.A. (1990). Transcriptional regulation of protein kinase C by 1,25-dihydroxyvitamin D_3 in HL-60 cells. *J. Biol. Chem.* 265:2370–2374.
26. Nakajima, S., and Seino, Y. (1990). 1,25 Dihydroxyvitamin D_3 increases insulin-like growth factor I receptors in clonal osteoblastic cells. *Endocrinology* 126: 2088–2094.
27. Dean, D.C. (1989). Expression of the fibronectin gene. *Am. J. Respir. Cell Mol. Biol.* 1:5–10.
28. Bittiner, B., Bleehen, S.S., and MacNeil, S. (1991). 1α,25-$(OH)_2$-Vitamin D_3 increases intracellular cal-

cium in human keratinocytes. *Br. J. Dermatol.* 124: 230–235.
29. Barsony, J., and Marx, S.J. (1988). A very rapid receptor mediated action of 1,25-dihydroxyvitamin D_3: increase of intracellular cyclic GMP in human skin fibroblasts. In *Vitamin D. Molecular, Cellular and Clinical Endocrinology.* Walter, de Gruyter & Co., Berlin.
30. Yada, Y., Ozeki, T., and Meguro, S. (1989). Signal transduction in the onset of terminal keratinocyte differentiation induced by 1,25-dihydroxyvitamin D_3: role of protein kinase C translocation. *Biochem. Biophys. Res. Commun.* 163:1517–1522.
31. Sharpe, G.R., Gillespie, J.I., and Greenwell, J.R. (1990). Changes in intracellular free calcium of human keratinocytes during differentiation and stimulation with EGF. *Br. J. Dermatol.* 122:269–270.
32. Gerritsen, M.J.P., Rulo, H.F.C., Vlijmen-Willems, I. van, Erp, P.E.J. van, and Kerkhof, P.C.M. van. (1993). Topical treatment of psoriatic plaques with 1,25 dihydroxyvitamin D_3: a cell biological study. *J. Dermatol.* 128:666–673.
33. Kwarra, S., Hatta, N., and Hirone, K. (1989). Effect of externally applied 1α,24(R)-$(OH)_2D_3$ on the kinetics of epidermal keratinocytes in the psoriasis focus. *Jpn. J. Dermatol.* 13:99.
34. Matsunaga, T., Yamamato, and Mimura, H. (1990). 1,24 (R)-Dihydroxyvitamin D_3, a novel active for of vitamin D_3 with activity for inducing epidermal differentiation but decreased hypercalcaemic activity. *J. Dermatol.* 17:135–142.
35. Gerritsen, M.J.P., Boezeman, J.B.M., Vlijmen-Willems, I.M.J.J. van, and Kerkhof, P.C.M. van. (1994). The effect of tacalcitol (1,24$(OH)_2D_3$) on cutaneous inflammation, epidermal proliferation and keratinization in psoriasis, a placebo-controlled, double-blind study. *Br. J. Dermatol.* 131:57–63.
36. Cunliffe, W.J., Henderson, C.A., Holden, C.A., Maddin, W.S., Ortonne, J.P., and Young, M. (1992). Comparative study of calcipotriol (MC903) ointment and betamethasone-17-valerate ointment in patients with psoriasis vulgaris. *J. Am. Acad. Dermatol.* 26:736–743.
37. Berth-Jones, J., Chu, A.C., Dodd, W.A.H., Ganpule, M., Griffiths, W.A.D., Haydey, R.P., Klaber, M.R., Murray, S.J., Rogers, S., and Jurgensen, H.J. (1992). A multicentre, parallel-group comparison of calcipotriol ointment and short-contact dithranol therapy in chronic plaque psoriasis. *Br. J. Dermatol.* 127: 266–271.
38. Kragballe, K. (1990). Combination of topical calcipotriol (MC903) and UVB radiation for psoriasis vulgaris. *Dermatologica* 181:211–214.
39. Frappaz, A., and Thivolet, J. (1993). Calcipotriol in combination with PUVA: a randomized double blind placebo study in severe psoriasis. *Eur. J. Dermatol.* 3: 351–354.
40. Grossman, R.M., Thivolet, J., Claudy, A., Souteyrand, P., Guilhou, J.J., Thomas, P., Amblard, P., Belaich, S., Belilvosky, C. de, Brassinne, M. de la, Martinet, C., Bazex, J.A., Beylot, C., Combemale, P., Lambert, D., Ostojic, A., Denoeux, J.P., Lauret, Ph., Vaillant, L., Weber, M., Pamphile, R., and Dubertret, L. (1994). A novel therapeutic approach to psoriasis with combination calcipotriol ointment and very low-dose cyclosporine: results of a multicenter placebo-controlled study. *J. Am. Acad. Dermatol.* 31:68–74.
41. Jong, E.M.G.J. de, and Kerkhof, P.C.M. van de. (1991). Simultaneous assessment of inflammation and epidermal proliferation in psoriatic plaques during long term treatment with vitamin D_3 analogue MC903: modulations and interrelations. *Br. J. Dermatol.* 124: 221–229.
42. Mare, S. de, Jong, E.M.G.J. de, and Kerkhof, P.C.M. van de. (1990). DNA content K_s 8.12 binding of the psoriatic lesion during treatment with the vitamin D_3 analogue MC903 and betamethasone. *Br. J. Dermatol.* 123:291–295.
43. Holland, D.B., Roberts, S.G., Russell, A., Wood, E.J., and Cunliffe, W. (1990). Changes in epidermal keratin levels during treatment of psoriasis with the topical vitamin D_3 analog MC903. *Br. J. Dermatol.* 122:284.
44. Jong, E.M.G.J. de, Vlijmen, I.M.J.J. van, Erp, P.E.J. van and Ramaekers, F.C.S. (1991). Keratin 17: a useful maker in psoriatic therapies. *Arch. Dermatol. Res.* 283: 480–482.
45. Berth-Jones, J., Fletcher, A., and Hutchinson, P.E. (1991). Epidermal cytokeratin and immunocyte responses during treatment of psoriasis with Calcipotriol. In *Vitamin D: Gene Regulation, Structure Function Analysis, Clinical Application.* A.W. Norman, R. Bouillon, M. Thomass (Eds.). De Gruyter, Berlin, pp. 424–425.
46. Arnold, W.P., and Kerkhof, P.C.M. van de. (1991). The induction of epidermal ornithine decarboxylase following tape stripping is inhibited by a topical vitamin D_3 analogue (MC903). *Br. J. Dermatol.* 125:6–8.
47. Malet, R.B., Coulson, I.H., Purkis, P.E., Leigh, I.M., and Holden, C.A. (1990). An immunohistological analysis of changes in the immune infiltrate and keratin expression in psoriasis treated with calcipotriol compared with betamethasone ointment. *Br. J. Dermatol.* 123:837.
48. Verburgh, C.A., and Nieboer, C.A. (1989). Local application of vitamin D derivative MC903 in psoriasis: influence on cellular infiltrate, Langerhans cells and keratinocyte markers. *J. Invest. Dermatol.* 93:310.
49. Oxholm, A., Oxholm, P., Staberg, B., and Bendtzen, K. (1989). Expression of interleukin-6-like molecules and tumour necrosis factor after topical treatment of psoriasis with a new vitamin D analogue (MC 903). *Acta Derm. Venereol.* 69:385–390.

50. Holland, D.B., Wood, E.J., Roberts, S.J., West, M.R., and Cunliffe, W.J. (1989). Epidermal keratin levels during oral 1-alpha-hydroxyvitamin D_3 treatment for psoriasis. *Skin Pharmacol.* 2:68–76.
51. Bower, M., Colston, K.W.K., Stein, R.C., Hedley, A., Gazet, J.-C., Ford, H.T., and Coombers, R.C. (1991). Topical calcipotriol treatment in advanced breast cancer. *Lancet* 337:701–702.
52. Mackie, P.S., Hickish, T., Mortimer, P., Sloane, J., and Cunningham, D. (1993). Calcipotriol and regression in T-cell lymphoma of skin. *Lancet* 342:172.
53. Gray, J.D., Bottomley, W., Layton, A.M., Cotterill, J.A., and Monteiro, E. (1992). The use of calcipotriol in HIV-related psoriasis. *Clin. Exp. Dermatol.* 17: 342–343.
54. Berth-Jones, J., Bourke, J., Bailey, K., Graham-Brown, R.A.C., and Hutchinson, P.E. Generalized pustular psoriasis: response to topical calcipotriol. *Br. Med. J.* 305:868–869.
55. Kerkhof, P.C.M. van de, and Steijlen, P.M. (1994). Topical treatment of pityriasis rubra pilaris with calcipotriol. *Br. J. Dermatol.* 130:675–678.
56. Kragballe, K., Steijlen, P.M., Henning Ibsen, H., Kerkhof, P.C.M. van de, Esmann, J., Halkier Sorensen, L., and Buhl Axelsen, M. (1995). Efficacy, tolerability, and safety of calcipotriol ointment in disorders of keratinization. *Arch. Dermatol.* 131:556–560.

36

Vitamin D Analogues in the Treatment of Psoriasis

John Y.M. Koo, Charles Gambla, and Jaeho Lee
University of California Medical Center, San Francisco, California

John Siebenlist
University of Texas, San Antonio, Texas

Vitamin D is best known for its role in calcium homeostasis through regulation of intestinal calcium absorption, reabsorption of calcium from the kidneys, and bone mineralization. Over 60 years ago, oral vitamin D in high doses was used for the treatment of psoriasis based on the idea that improvement of psoriasis with exposure to sunlight might be due to an increased production of vitamin D_3 in the skin (1). Ultimately, this treatment lost favor because the results were inconsistent and no more efficacious than other more established treatments and, additionally, many patients developed hypercalcemia as a side effect. Then, in 1985, while studying the effects of 1α-hydroxy-vitamin D_3 in patients with osteoporosis, Japanese scientists quite serendipitously discovered marked improvement of psoriasis in a patient (2). This again refueled interest in vitamin D_3 as a possible treatment for psoriasis. At about the same time, the discovery of a vitamin D receptor in the skin led to the understanding that skin is a specific target tissue for vitamin D_3. Since that time, many of the molecular mechanisms and functions of vitamin D, specifically in the skin, have been studied. 1,25(OH)2 D_3, and its analogues have proven to be an effective and relatively safe weapon in the armory for treating psoriasis.

MECHANISM OF ACTION

Vitamin D_3 is absorbed from the gut and synthesized in human skin by ultraviolet irradiation of 7-dehydrocholesterol. After two successive hydroxylations in the liver and kidney, respectively, the most biologically active form, 1,25(OH)2 D_3 or calcitriol, is produced. It is this form which mediates the biological effect in vivo. Calcitriol demonstrates a direct effect on calcium metabolism by increasing the absorption of calcium in the gut and possibly in the distal tubules of the kidney and by mobilizing skeletal calcium stores. This increase of calcium (and indirectly phosphorus) promotes the mineralization of bone. Calcitriol and many other vitamin D_3 analogues have also demonstrated modulation of biological function in many cell types not associated with calcium regulation. As with many other cells, most skin cells (keratinocytes, fibroblasts, Langerhans cells, monocytes, and T and B lymphocytes) possess a nuclear receptor termed vitamin D receptor (VDR) (3–5). The discovery of this receptor furthered investigation of the functional role of calcitriol in areas other than calcium metabolism. In vitro, calcitriol has been shown to induce very specific changes in the epidermal architecture decreasing cellular proliferation and increasing cellular differentiation (5). Other studies have found calcitriol also to be a moderately potent immunomodulator (6). These characteristics suggest vitamin D_3 and its analogues would be effective treatment for a disease, such as psoriasis, characterized by hyperproliferation and inflammation.

MODULATION OF CELLULAR DIFFERENTIATION AND PROLIFERATION

Two basic cellular mechanisms appear to be responsible for the action of these hormones. The first, a nuclear mechanism, is brought about by vitamin D_3 binding an intracellular VDR found in most cells of the skin (4,5). The VDR is structurally similar to the family of steroid receptors, including estrogen, glucocorticoid, and thyroid receptors. Its expression appears to be promoted by increased levels of vitamin D_3. Each of these receptors has three binding domains: a steroid-binding domain, a receptor-binding domain allowing interaction between receptors of the same family, and a DNA-binding domain (4). After binding of vitamin D_3 to the VDR, the VDR complex binds in the cell nucleus to specific DNA sequences, termed vitamin D–response elements, present in the promoter region of target genes (3–5). This binding response modulates the transcription of the target genes producing a response by the cell. The second cellular mechanism involves an influx of calcium into the cell, brought about by calcitriol enhancing rapid hydrolysis of phosphatidyl inositol phosphate, resulting in increased intracellular calcium levels (4). The increase in intracellular calcium in response to vitamin D_3 is quite rapid, occurring within 90 sec, much too quickly to be compatible with transcription (4,5). Additionally, it is not affected by cyclohexamide, indicating that protein synthesis is not involved (4). Together, these two mechanisms function to decrease proliferation and increase differentiation of the target cells. In vitro, calcitriol appears to stimulate the differentiating pathways within the suprabasalar cells demonstrated by increased levels of transglutaminase and involucrin (markers of epidermal cell differentiation) and cornified envelope formation (5). This enhanced differentiation appears to be correlated with increased production of inositol triphospate, 1,2-diacylglycerol, and protein kinase C via the nuclear pathway and increased intracellular calcium levels. Both activation of protein kinase C and increased intracellular calcium levels are associated with enhanced keratinization and cornified envelope formation (2). The antiproliferative action of vitamin D_3 has yet to be elucidated.

MODULATION OF INFLAMMATION

As mentioned previously, monocytes, along with B and T lymphocytes, have demonstrated VDRs. Recently, vitamin D_3 and its analogues have been discovered to have potent immunoregulatory action disrupting several pathways of the inflammatory response. And, just as with the modulation of keratinocytes, both nuclear and nonnuclear mechanisms are involved. Vitamin D_3 inhibits T-cell proliferation by suppressing the response of T lymphocytes to interleukin-1 (3–6) subsequently decreasing the production of immunoglobins by these cells. Vitamin D_3 also inhibits production of interleukin-2 and -6 and interferon-γ, potent mediators of the inflammatory response (4,6). Additionally, suppressor T-cell activity is enhanced and cytotoxic and natural killer cell formation is inhibited (4).

CALCITRIOL

Calcitriol (1,25-dihydroxyvitamin D_3) is the physiologically active form of vitamin D_3. Treatment of plaque-type psoriasis with calcitriol, both orally and topically, has been successful but safety concerns have been raised owing to calcitriol's potent calcemic effect. Calcitriol's major physiological actions, increased absorption of calcium from the gut and kidney and mobilization of calcium from bone, are important to calcium homeostasis. Thus, many feel the value of calcitriol for treating psoriasis is limited owing to the possibility of side effects such as hypercalcemia, hypercalciuria, nephrocalcinosis, nephrolithiasis, and a reduction in bone mineral density secondary to its calcemic effect (5). Recently, Perez et al. (7), in a single-center, double-blind, right/left comparison, placebo-controlled study, showed topical calcitriol to be an effective treatment compared to placebo for plaque-type psoriasis in 84 patients, with 96% showing some improvement over 2.4 months while applying 15 μg/g of vehicle/day. The most common side effect seen with vitamin D_3 and its analogues is perilesional irritation, but in this study, none was noted in any of the patients. Additionally, a long-term (12 month), large-area-application (15 μg/g up to 10 g/day), follow-up study in 22 patients showed 91% of patients experienced significant improvement in their psoriasis and no cutaneous adverse events or statistically significant changes in either 24-hr urinary calcium or serum calcium levels.

In another study by this same group (2), a single-center open trial of oral calcitriol in 85 patients with moderate plaque psoriasis, 88% had some improvement in their disease, and 62% of those had moderate to complete clearance with dosages ranging from 0.5 to 3.0 μg/day over a 3-year period. Equally as important, therapy with oral calcitriol was found to be safe in regard to hypercalcemia, hypercalciuria, reduction of bone mineral density, nephrolithiasis, and calcinosis. Using oral calcitriol, serum calcium level rose an average of 3.6% and the 24-hr excretion of urinary calcium rose 148% but both were within a normal range. Despite the increase in urinary calcium, only two patients of 55 were found to have kidney stones by ultrasonography. No signs of nephrocalcinosis were seen. Creatinine clearance decreased 13.4%, but inulin and PAH clearance did not change from baseline. Therefore, although creatinine clearance decreased, the glomerular filtration rate and renal tubular function were preserved. Finally, bone mineral density analysis did not show any statistically significant change from baseline for up to 2 years of treatment with calcitriol. Oral calcitriol was found to be especially efficacious in treating erythrodermic and generalized psoriasis with minimal plaque thickness. This treatment is not recommended for patients with idiopathic hypercalciuria or mild renal failure. And, although oral calcitriol was found to be safe in this particular study, frequent monitoring of blood and urinary calcium levels along with yearly renal ultrasounds was recommended (2).

VITAMIN D_3 ANALOGUES

Science has been able to manipulate vitamin D_3 analogues to enhance antipsoriatic characteristics and limit calcemic side effects by slightly altering their structure. Most of the alteration is done by modifying side chains of calcitriol. Numerous analogues exists but by far the most frequently studied and most successful has been calcipotriol.

UPDATE ON THE USE OF CALCIPOTRIENE (DOVONEX) OINTMENT

Calcipotriene, also called calcipotriol in Europe (Dovonex), is an analogue of vitamin D, which is modified to minimize the systemic effects in terms of altering calcium metabolism. It is known to have less than 1/200 of the effect of calcitriol, in terms of its effect on calcium metabolism. This is accomplished partially by the fact that calcipotriene, even though binding well to keratinocyte nuclear receptors, does not bind as efficiently as calcitriol to vitamin D–binding proteins and, once in circulation, is metabolized faster than calcitriol.

In terms of the overall efficacy of calcipotriene ointment in the treatment of psoriasis, one of the latest comparison studies involved a comparison between calcipotriene ointment and fluocinonide ointment (Lidex) in a series of two multicenter, double-blind studies (8). In one of the multicenter studies involving 106 patients, by week 2 calcipotriene ointment performed better than fluocinonide ointment in terms of decreasing plaque elevation (p = 0.043) and scaling (p = 0.003). By week 4, calcipotriene ointment was better than fluocinonide ointment in terms of erythema and overall severity (p = 0.002) and global improvement over baseline (p = 0.004). Although more side effects were noted with calcipotriene ointment as compared to fluocinonide ointment in terms of lesional and perilesional irritation, no patients discontinued calcipotriene ointment during the trial owing to side effects. In the other multicenter, double-blind comparison study, by week 1 calcipotriene ointment scored better than fluocinonide ointment in terms of decreases in plaque elevation (p = 0.002), and the rest of the findings were generally consistent with those of the first multicenter study.

Using calcipotriene ointment in the usual clinical setting, one does not always find the efficacy demonstrated by the above multicenter, double-blind comparison studies. Probably the most important difference between the clinical studies and actual clinical practice is the degree to which patients comply with the twice-per-day regimen prescribed. Calcipotriene ointment works better twice per day than once per day, but in real life, not all patients are compliant. This is in contrast to clinical studies where, if a patient proves to be noncompliant, he or she is promptly eliminated from the study.

In the package insert for calcipotriene ointment in the United States, there is no absolute restriction in terms of how much calcipotriene ointment can be used at any single time. However, the package inserts in many other countries, including England and Canada, contain a firm and explicit restriction of using no more than 100 gr/week of calcipotriene. Adherence to this restriction is important since there is a small, but finite, chance of developing hypercalcemia, possibly symptomatic, if patients use more than 100 gr/week of calcipotriene ointment. These cases have not only occurred among psoriasis patients, but were also noted among patients with ichthyosis (another calcipotriene-responsive hyperproliferative skin disorder) who used more than 100 gr/week of calcipotriene ointment (9,10). Because of several case reports of hypercalcemia resulting from excessive use of calcipotriene ointment, a clinical study was performed in England whereby patients with extensive psoriasis were purposely asked to use 200 gr of calcipotriene ointment for one week, followed by 300 gr of calcipotriene the second week. The calcipotriene was then discontinued (11). In this 2-week study, the patients noted 71% improvement in the Psoriasis Area and Severity Index (PASI) scores. However, mean 24-hr urine calcium rose from 4.79 mmol/24 hr to 7.27 mmol/24 hr ($p < 0.0001$) and there was also a statistically significant increase in serum calcium from 2.26 mmol/L to 2.32 mmol/L ($p < 0.005$). Both serum and urine calcium levels returned to normal after calcipotriene ointment was discontinued. Even though the patients in this study did very well in terms of improving their psoriasis in only 2 weeks, the well-documented increase in both serum and urine calcium levels underscores the importance of observing the 100 gr/week limitation when prescribing calcipotriene ointment in the usual clinical setting. Therefore, for patients with widespread psoriasis, calcipotriene ointment probably should not be the main therapeutic modality. However, even for patients who are being treated with systemic agents like methotrexate or phototherapy, such as PUVA therapy, calcipotriene ointment can be used to speed up the improvement in localized, recalcitrant areas of psoriasis such as on the elbows or shins.

The other main side effect of calcipotriene is lesional and perilesional irritation. In some clinical studies, up to 15–20% of the patients using calcipotriene ointment for the first time have experienced some local irritation, which might have been, in some cases, a stinging or burning sensation rather than a visible rash. However, most patients find this type of reaction is both mild and transient and quickly become accustomed to it. However, 2–3% of patients in the clinical study situation had to discontinue the use of calcipotriene ointment because of persistent irritation. Even though the authors are unaware of any systematic, clinical studies looking for ways to overcome this problem in this 2–3% of patients, both the authors' experience and that of many clinicians seems to indicate persistent irritant dermatitis from calcipotriene ointment may be overcome by making the skin accustomed to this agent. This is empirically performed by having the patient first make sure the irritant dermatitis completely resolves with or without the use of other medications such as topical steroids. Second, patients are instructed to dilute calcipotriene ointment 1:1 with Vaseline ointment or any other pure grease in the palms of their hands right before application. If this 1:1 dilution still irritates the skin, the calcipotriene ointment is diluted further by the use of a 2:1 or even a 3:1 dilution with Vaseline ointment until a concentration is found where the patient can use the diluted form of calcipotriene without experiencing irritation. Once that concentration is determined, the patient is instructed to use this diluted formulation for several weeks before trying a higher concentration again. Using this technique, it has been noted by many clinicians, including the authors, that the patient can eventually use full-strength calcipotriene ointment, even though he experienced significant and persistent irritation the first time he tried using calcipotriene ointment. Almost all irritation noted with calcipotriene ointment represents irritant dermatitis rather than true allergic contact dermatitis. Since irritant dermatitis usually has a "threshold effect," it is reasonable that one can use the medication without getting irritation if it is used in low enough concentrations to be below this threshold and allows the skin to become accustomed to this agent, just as is done with patients who become irritated with higher concentrations of tretinoin cream (Retin-A) or anthralin (Drithocreme). It is important to dilute calcipotriene ointment with pure grease and not with creams or lotions because calcipotriene ointment is formulated in an alkaline pH of 8 and can therefore be inactivated by any vehicle that is acidic in formulation, including salicylic acid. Finally, it is important to have the patient mix the pure grease and calcipotriene ointment just before application since, if they are premixed, calcipotriene ointment can possibly be inactivated over time.

One of the benefits of calcipotriene ointment is it does not have typical steroid side effects such as skin atrophy or adrenal suppression. In a clinical research setting, calcipotriene ointment has been used for 6 months on noninvolved skin; after this 6-month usage, no decrease in the thickness of the epidermis or papillary dermis was noted compared to normal-looking skin not exposed to calcipotriene ointment over this 6-month period (12). A 1-year study on the use of calcipotriene ointment for psoriasis patients has been published from Canada and Europe and has been presented but not yet published from the United States

(13). According to a clinical study involving the continuous use of calcipotriene ointment for 1 year in Canada, Europe, and the United States, the maximum benefit from calcipotriene ointment for psoriasis is not seen until calcipotriene has been used for approximately 16 weeks. Also, as a group, tachyphylaxis is not seen. In other words, the PASI score improves and stays improved; it does not go back up as would be expected if, over time, a large number of patients developed tachyphylaxis to this agent. The urine calcium excretion stays within normal limits, even if patients use calcipotriene ointment continuously for 1 year, as long as they do not have renal problems and do not use more than 100 gr of calcipotriene ointment per week.

Calcipotriene has been safely and effectively used for a pediatric population in multicenter studies performed in Europe, including one in England where 66 children as young as 3 years old were involved. In this British pediatric study, using calcipotriene ointment at the frequency of twice-per-day application, the mean PASI score decreased from 6.1 to 2.63 after 8 weeks. There was no significant change in mean ionized calcium from baseline to 2 weeks or 8 weeks of treatment and no values above the normal reference range were recorded (14). However, a safe amount of calcipotriene ointment to be used per week has not been defined for any particular pediatric age group. Therefore, if calcipotriene ointment is used in the pediatric age group, the authors recommend checking serum or 24-hr urine calcium to be sure hypercalcemia does not occur. The authors also have the mothers of pediatric patients keep track of how much calcipotriene ointment is used week by week, and if the usage is stable and there is no evidence of hypercalcemia, the frequency of checking serum or 24-hr urine calcium can be diminished.

Occlusion is also known to enhance the efficacy of calcipotriene (15). However, occlusion may also enhance the penetration of calcipotriene and, therefore, if large areas of the body are occluded, it is recommended that the patient's serum calcium be checked. In addition, occlusion may increase the probability of developing irritation from calcipotriene ointment. Therefore, the patient should be firmly convinced she can use calcipotriene ointment without irritation before attempting to occlude. On the other hand, the use of occlusion may be critical in making the treatment efficacious for hard-to-treat areas such as in the hyperkeratotic psoriatic involvement of the palms and soles. Calcipotriene ointments appears to have synergistic properties when combined with either ultraviolet light B or PUVA therapy (16–18). However, a recent poster presentation by Dr. Mark Lebwohl and his colleagues at Mt. Sinai Medical Center in New York City indicated that ultraviolet light A may destroy calcipotriene if UVA is applied right after the application of calcipotriene ointment. Also, a small number of patients may develop burning sensations if calcipotriene ointment is applied right before exposure to either UVB or UVA. For these reasons, it is best to have calcipotriene ointment applied *after* the light therapy and not right before.

Calcipotriene ointment has also been used in many HIV-related psoriatic cases (19). It is reasonable to use calcipotriene ointment in HIV cases since calcipotriene ointment is not known to be an immunosuppressant and has demonstrated usefulness in treating localized, recalcitrant psoriatic lesions in these populations, such as hyperkeratotic psoriasis on the palms and soles resembling Reiter's disease, so typical of HIV-related psoriasis.

Finally, in clinical usage of calcipotriene ointment, it is now a common practice to combine calcipotriene ointment with superpotent topical steroids trying to maximize the speed of improvement while minimizing the amount of both calcipotriene ointment and superpotent topical steroid required. Multicenter clinical studies have shown the combination of calcipotriene ointment and Ultravate ointment, one used in the morning and the other at night, resulted in twice as much complete clearance of psoriasis after 2 weeks' usage as compared to use of only Ultravate ointment twice per day (20). The greatest advantage in the clinical use of calcipotriene ointment is its lack of side effects typically associated with the use of topical steroids, such as skin atrophy and adrenal suppression. Also, calcipotriene ointment does not seem to be associated with the problem of tachyphylaxis as frequently as topical steroids. All of these advantages make calcipotriene ointment a more ideal agent for long-term use in keeping psoriasis under control. However, for short-term use, patients used to the quick therapeutic action of superpotent topical steroids tend to complain about the relatively slower response typically noted from the use of calcipotriene ointment. This is especially true in regard to the persistence of erythema since calcipotriene ointment does not have the vasoconstrictive effective of topical steroids. Therefore, in view of the strengths and weaknesses as mentioned above, it is reasonable to use calcipotriene ointment in combination with superpotent topical steroids in the initial stages (first 2–3 weeks) of treatment to maximize the response rate, at the same time minimizing the amount of either agent used, since both the strongest of the superpotent topical steroids and calcipotriene have limitations in the amounts one can use per week.

Eventually, it is desirable to discontinue the use of topical steroids altogether, avoiding long-term steroid side effects such as skin atrophy or tachyphylaxis, simply using the calcipotriene ointment for maintenance. If a clinician cuts off the use of superpotent topical steroids "cold turkey," there can be a risk of recurrence or even rebound from the sudden discontinuation of superpotent topical steroids. Therefore, in between the combination use and the use of calcipotriene ointment as a monotherapy for maintenance, most clinicians find it wise to have an intermediate step where the use of superpotent topical steroid is gradually decreased. Most often, this takes the form of "pulse therapy," whereby the superpotent topical steroid is used only on weekends and the calcipotriene ointment is used twice per day on weekdays. This second phase of pulse therapy can go on as long as necessary for the psoriatic lesions to become almost invisible; the patient is then switched over to calcipotriene ointment used as a monotherapy for maintenance. Eventually, the frequency of usage of calcipotriene ointment can be decreased to once per day or even less, i.e., once every other day, and eventually discontinued if the maintenance treatment is successful and there is no hint of recurrence of psoriasis.

UPDATE ON EFFICACY AND SAFETY OF CALCIPOTRIENE 0.05% CREAM: U.S. DATA

Method

The efficacy and safety of calcipotriene cream 0.05% in the treatment of psoriasis was studied in two pivotal studies, DE127-025 and DE127-027. These were randomized, double-blind, parallel-group, vehicle-controlled studies in patients with moderate to severe plaque psoriasis. The DE127-025 study involved 190 subjects (96 vehicle and 94 calcipotriene cream) and the DE127-027 study involved 172 evaluable subjects (87 vehicle and 85 calcipotriene cream 0.05%). Calcipotriene cream or vehicle was applied twice daily for 8 weeks and the subjects were evaluated at weeks 0, 1, 2, 4, 6, and 8. Erythema, scaling, plaque elevation, overall disease severity, and physician's global assessment were performed.

Efficacy Measures

In study DE127-025, at the week 1 evaluation, the calcipotriene cream group demonstrated significant improvement over the vehicle group in plaque elevation and overall disease severity ($p \leq 0.036$). By the week 2 evaluation, all four measures favored calcipotriene cream and remained highly significant through week 8 ($p \leq 0.002$). By week 8, in terms of the physician's global assessment, 51% of the subjects in the calcipotriene cream group were rated "completely clear," "almost clear," or "marked improvement," compared with only 10% of the subjects in the vehicle group being rated in these categories.

The results from the DE127-027 study were similar in that by week 1, calcipotriene cream was satistically superior to its vehicle ($p = 0.002$) and remained significantly in favor of the calcipotriene cream through week 8 of treatment. In terms of the physician's global assessment, at week 8, 47% of the subjects in the calcipotriene cream group were rated "completely clear," "almost clear," or "marked improvement," as compared to only 24% of the subjects in the the vehicle group who were rated within these categories.

Adverse Events

Combining the two studies, 39.3% of the calcipotriene cream 0.05% subjects reported at least one adverse event, compared to 45.6% of those in the vehicle group. In terms of adverse events thought to be related to the study medication, 28.9% of the vehicle group and 31% of the calcipotriene cream group reported adverse events thought to be related to the study medication. The three most common adverse events reported were lesional irritation/follicultis, facial irritation/dermatitis, and worsening of psoriasis—17.4% of those in the vehicle group reported lesional irritation/follicultis compared with 13.2% of those in the treated group; 1.1% of the vehicle group reported facial irritation/dermatitis compared with 6.9% of the treated group. Finally, psoriasis worsened in 6.3% of the vehicle group and 3% of the treated group. The other events thought to be related to the study medication, occurring at a rate of ≥1%, for the calcipotriene cream and vehicle groups, respectively, were melanosis (rates 1% vs. 0.4%), rash (rates 1% vs. 0%), and dryness of the skin (rates 1.2% vs. 0%). Analysis of the adverse events by demographics revealed a statistically significant differenece in the frequency of reporting adverse effects according to gender and race.

Female subjects reported adverse events more frequently than male subjects ($p = 0.030$) and Caucasian patients reported more adverse effects than non-Causasian patients ($p = 0.004$). These differences by gender and race were consistent in both the active and vehicle-treated subjects, suggesting differences in race and gender were independent of treatment modality used. Twenty-four of 183 subjects receivng vehicle dropped out due to adverse events, while 11 of 179 subjects receiving calcipotriene 0.05% cream dropped out due to adverse events. In terms of laboratory abnormalties, no consistently out-of-range values were noted among the subjects who received calcipotriene 0.05% cream. More specifically, four subjects who received calcipotriene 0.05% cream were noted to have isolated instances of hypercalcemia, but none of these findings persisted despite continuation of treatment.

Comparison of Calcipotriene Cream 0.05% Versus Calcipotriene Ointment 0.05%

Overall, the efficacy of calcipotriene cream was similar to that of calcipotriene ointment, although, as expected for a cream formulation, calcipotriene cream 0.05% was slightly less effective in treating plaque psoriasis than the ointment formulation. After 8 weeks of twice-per-day usage of calcipotriene ointment in clinical trials, global physician's assessment showed 70% rated as havng achieved "marked improvement" or better and 10% as having achieved "complete clearance." A similar 8-week, twice-per-day application of calcipotriene cream in clinical trials resulted in approximately 50% being rated "markedly improved" or better, and 4% achieving "complete clearance." However, the fact that the cream is more cosmetically acceptable may lead to better compliance, which may easily overcome this slight difference in efficacy. Also, as expected for a cream formulation, calcipotriene 0.05% cream had a slightly higher rate of stinging, irritation, and erythema (lesional irritation/folliculitis) compared to the ointment formulation. However, once again, the cosmetic benefit preceived by the patient may outweigh the risk of a slightly higher rate of stinging, irritation, and erythema side effects.

In view of the better efficacy of the ointment and the better cosmetic acceptability of the cream, if calcipotriene is to be used as a monotherapy, the optimal usage for those not willing to apply the ointment formulation in the morning due to its greasiness appears to be use of the cream formulation in the morning and ointment formulation at night, rather than use of the cream formulation twice per day.

UPDATE ON SCALP CALCIPOTRIENE SOLUTION: U.S. DATA

Method

Two pivotal efficacy and safety studies for calcipotriene scalp solutions were conducted in the United States by Bristol-Myers Squibb (i.e., Westwood-Squibb) Pharmaceutical Corporation. These studies were designated DE127-031 and DE127-032. They were double-blind, dose-ranging, vehicle-controlled studies. Subjects were treated twice daily for 8 weeks with calcipotriene 50 μg/ml, 25 μg/ml, or vehicle. The calcipotriene solution tested by Bristol-Myers Squibb in the United States and Leo Pharmaceutical Products in Europe differed only in the amount of menthol they contained—the American formulation contained 0.8 mg/ml menthol while the Leo formulation contained 1.0 mg/ml menthol. When these two protocols are combined, 159 evaluable subjects were treated with calcipotriene solution 50 μg/ml, 158 subjects were treated with calcipotriene 25 μg/ml, and 157 subjects were treated with vehicle. A maximum of one 60-ml bottle per week was dispensed to each subject during the course of each study. The average total consumption for all treatment groups was 202 gr of solution per subject. No statistical difference in consumption was observed between the two treatment groups.

Efficacy Measures

Scaling, erythema, plaque elevation, overall disease severity, and pruritus were evaluated at baseline and at day 4, and weeks 1, 2, 4, 6, and 8. The primary efficacy parameter was overall disease severity. A physician's global assessment was also performed using a seven-point scale at each postbaseline visit.

For study SE127-031, statistically significant differences in pairwise comparisons were found from week 1 through week 8 favoring both calcipotriene solution 50 μg/ml and 25 μg/ml over vehicle ($p \leq 0.023$). For subjects rated "completely clear" or "almost clear" by week 8, 29% of the calcipotriene solution 50 μg/ml subjects were in this category, compared with 25% of the calcipotriene 25 μg/ml subjects, and only 6% of the vehicle subjects.

For study DE127-032, similar findings were noted favoring both calcipotriene solution 50 μg/ml and 25 μg/ml over vehicle ($p \leq 0.017$) from week 2 through week 8. By week 8, 32% of the calcipotriene solution 50 μg/ml subjects were rated "completely clear" or "almost clear," compared with 28% of the calcipotriene solution 25 μg/ml subjects and only 12% of the vehicle subjects.

Comparing the two groups with different calcipotriene solution concentrations, in study DE127-031, calcipotriene solution 50 μg/ml was more effective than the calcipotriene solution 25 μg/ml in reducing scaling, erythema, plaque elevation, overall disease severity, and pruritus from week 1 through the end of the study (except for pruritus, a difference was noticed starting in week 2). In study DE127-032, the same pattern was seen from week 2 through week 8. Consistently, calcipotriene solution 50 μg/ml compared with vehicle reduced symptoms and signs of scalp psoriasis earlier than calcipotriene 25 μg/ml compared with vehicle.

In short, efficacy outcome supports the use of calcipotriene solution 50 μg/ml twice daily, for the optimal treatment of moderate to severe psoriasis of the scalp.

Adverse Events

When the data from DE127-031 and DE127-032 were combined, the overall frequency of reported adverse effects was roughly similar between the calcipotriene solution 50 μg/ml group and the calcipotriene solution 25 μg/ml group and those who were treated with vehicle. The number of subjects reporting at least one adverse event was 98 of 159 subjects (61.6%) in the calcipotriene solution 50 μg/ml group, 88 of 158 subjects (55.7%) in the calcipotriene solution 25 μg/ml group, and 97 of 157 subjects (61.8%) in the vehicle group. The two most frequently reported adverse effects considered related to the treatments were burning/stinging/tingling and the appearance of a rash. With respect to the burning/stinging/tingling, a 22.6% frequency was noted among the calcipotriene solution 50 μg/ml group, a 23.4% frequency was seen in the calcipotriene solution 25 μg/ml group, and a 21.7% frequency was seen in the vehicle group. The rate of rash was highest in the calcipotriene solution 50 μg/ml group, with a 11.3% frequency; lowest in the vehicle group, with a 4.5% frequency; and intermediate in the calcipotriene solution 25 μg/ml group, with a 7.6% frequency. The other adverse effects occurring at rates greater than 1% were worsening of psoriasis, pruritus, dryness of the skin, skin irritation, and contact dermatitis. A single occurrence of hypercalcemia was noted in one subject in the calcipotriene solution 25 μg/ml group.

Facial irritation was assessed independently of other adverse reactions. Combining the two studies, facial irritation occurred in 26 subjects (16.4%) in the calcipotriene solution 50 μg/ml group, 17 subjects (10.8%) in the calcipotriene solution 25 μg/ml group, and seven subjects (4.5%) in the vehicle group. Seven subjects each from the calcipotriene solution 25 μg/ml group and the calcipotriene solution 50 μg/ml group and nine subjects from the vehicle group discontinued the studies due to adverse events. None of the observed laboratory abnormalities were thought to be related to the study medication except for one isolated occurrence of hypercalcemia in the calcipotriene solution 25 μg/ml group.

As compared with the largest European study conducted by Leo Pharmaceutical Products comparing calcipotriene solution 50 μg/ml with betamethasone 17-valerate 0.1% solution, the frequency of reporting adverse effects seems to be higher among American subjects than among European subjects. For example, as stated earlier, combining DE127-031 and DE127-032, 61.6% of the subjects reported at least one adverse event. This is in contrast with the above-mentioned European study where only 38.1% of 299 patients treated with calcipotriene solution 50 μg/ml reported at least one adverse event. The frequency of reporting of the adverse events for those on the vehicle was also approximately half as much among the Europeans compared with the American subjects (29.8% vs. 61.8%). Among all the demographic variables assessed in DE127-031 and DE127-032, the most impressive demographic difference resulting in statistically significant differences in reports of adverse effects was gender. Consistently among all three treatment groups, female subjects reported adverse effects more frequently than the male subjects and the difference was statistically significant ($p = 0.011$).

1a, 24-DIHYDROXYVITAMIN D_3 (TACALCITOL)

Tacalcitol, another side-chain derivative of calcitriol, has demonstrated powerful in vitro action inducing cell division and inhibiting cell proliferation similar to calcipotriol. In vitro comparison with calcitriol shows topical tacalcitol has increased receptor affinity (21), greater inhibition of keratinocyte proliferation (22), and equal inhibition of T-cell-mediated antibody production (23), although no significant effect on the polymorphonuclear cells was seen (22). Other studies have found tacalcitol to have less effect on calcium metabolism than calcitriol (24). In Japan, where it has been available for approximately 3 years in ointment form, tacalcitol has proven to be effective and well-tolerated with only 1% of patients having irritation to their skin (25) compared to 15–20% with calcipotriol, although only 2–3% of these continue to have persistent irritation. In a recent multicenter, placebo-controlled, double-blind study with 122 Caucasian subjects, Van De Kerkhof et al. (25) reported tacalcitol to be superior to placebo in decreasing desquamation, induration, and erythema using 4 μg/g. Only 12.3% of all patients complained of skin irritation and it was unclear whether the irritation was caused by the vehicle or tacalcitol because irritation was reported in both the treatment and placebo groups. Overall, tacalcitol appears to be effective in treated moderate plaque psoriasis and is possibly less irritating than calcipotriol although adequate side-to-side comparative efficacy and safety studies remain to be done.

KH 1060

Another analogue, again produced by side-chain alteration, has shown extensive immunosuppressive activity (4), along with potent effects on cellular proliferation and differentiation. Other work with this analogue has shown KH 1060 is effective not because of its affinity for the VDR but because of its ability to stabilize the VDR-KH1060 complex protecting its degradation by enzymes in vivo (26).

As more studies are performed with vitamin D analogues, it is becoming increasingly evident that each analogue has a specific mechanism of action for the treatment of psoriasis. In other words, a particular side-chain alteration may enhance the differentiation-inducing ability but not the affect the antiproliferative effect or the immunomodulatory capacity of a vitamin D analogue (4). In addition, other analogues have demonstrated a predilection for the nuclear or non-nuclear pathway for activation of action. Some of these analogues show almost no binding to the VDR but strongly stimulate influx of calcium, thus eliciting cellular change. In the future, one can expect development of even more specifically designed vitamin D analogue molecules with efficacy for psoriasis.

REFERENCES

1. Kragballe, K., (1995). Vitamin D_3 analogues. *Dermatol. Clin.* 13:835–839.
2. Perez, A., Raab, R., Chen, T.C., et al. (1996). Safety and efficacy of oral calcitriol (1,25-dihydroxyvitamin D_3) for the treatment of psoriasis. *Br. J. Dermatol.* 134: 1070–1078.
3. Kragballe, K. (1992). Treatment of psoriasis with calcipotriol and other vitamin D analogues. *J. Am. Acad. Dermatol.* 27:1001–1008.
4. Van Der Kerkhof, P.C.M. (1995). Biological activity of vitamin D analogues in the skin, with special reference to antipsoriatic mechanisms. *Br. J. Dermatol.* 132: 675–682.
5. Kragballe, K. (1995). Calcipotriol: a new drug for topical psoriasis treatment. *Pharm. Toxicol.* 77:241–246.
6. Bagot, M., Charue, D., Lescs, M.C., Pamphile, R. and Revuz, J. (1994). Immunosuppressive effects of 1,25-dihydroxyvitamin D_3 and its analogue calcipotriol on epidermal cells. *Br. J. Dermatol.* 130:424–431.
7. Perez, A., Raab, R., Chen, T.C., et al. (1996). Safety and efficacy of topical calcitriol (1,25-dihydroxyvitamin D_3) for the treatment of psoriasis. *Br. J. Dermatol.* 134:238–246.
8. Bruce, S., Epinette, W.W., Funicella, T., Ison, A., et al. (1994). Comparative study of calcipotriene (MC903) ointment and fluocinonide ointment in the treatment of psoriasis. *J. Am. Acad. Dermatol.* 31(5 pt 1):755–759.
9. Hoeck, H.C., Laurberg, G., and Laurbert P. (1994). Hypercalcemic crisis after excessive topical use of a vitamin D derivative. *J. Intern. Med.* 235:281–282.
10. Dwyer, C., and Chapman, R.S. (1991). Calcipotriol and hypercalcemia. *Lancet* 2:338:764 (letter).
11. Bourke, J.F., Berth-Jones, J., Iqbal, S.J. and Hutchinson, P.E. (1993). High-dose topical calcipotriol in the treatment of extensive psoriasis vulgaris. *Br. J. Dermatol.* 129:74–76.
12. Kragballe, K., Fogh, K. and Sogarrd, H. (1991). Long-term efficacy and tolerability of topical calcipotriol in psoriasis: results of an open study. *Acta Derm. Venereol. (Stochk.)* 71:475–478.
13. Berth-Jones, J., Bourke, J.F., Iqbal, S.J., and Hutchinson, P.E. (1993). Urine calcium excretion during treatment of psoriasis with topical calcipotriol. *Br. J. Dermatol.* 129:411–414.
14. Darley, C.R., Cunliffe, W.J., Green, C.M., Hutchinson, P.E., Klaber, M.R., and Downes, N. (1996). Safety and efficacy of calcipotriol ointment (Dovonex) in treating children with psoriasis vulgaris. *Br. J. Dermatol.* 135(3):390–393.

15. Bourke, J.F., Berth-Jones, J., and Hutchinson, P.E. (1993) Occlusion enhances the efficacy of topical calcipotriol in the treatment of psoriasis vulgaris. *Clin. Exp. Dermatol.* 18:504–506.
16. Kragballe, K. (1990). Combination of topical calcipotriol (MC903) and UVB radiation for psoriasis vulgaris. *Dermatologica* 181:211–214.
17. Speight, E.L. and Farr, P.M. (1994). Calcipotriol improves the response of psoriasis to PUVA. *Br. J. Dermatol.* 130:79–82.
18. Frappaz, A., and Thivolet, J. (1993). Calcipotriol in combination with PUVA: a randomized double blind placebo study in severe psoriasis. *Eur. J. Dermatol.* 3: 351–354.
19. Gray, J.D., Bottomley, W., Layton, A.M. Cotteril, J.A., and Monteriro, E. (1992). The use of calcipotriol in HIV-related psoriasis. *Clin. Exp. Dermatol.* 17: 342–343.
20. Lebwohl, M.G., Siskin, S.B., Epinette, W., Breneman D., Funicella, T., Kalb, R., and Moore, J. (1996). Multicenter trial of calcipotriene ointment and halobetasol ointment compared to either agent alone for the treatment of psoriasis. *J. Am. Acad. Dermatol.* 35:268–269.
21. Matsunaga, T., Yamamato, M., and Mimura, H. (1990). 1,24 (R)-dihydroxyvitamin D_3, a novel active form of vitamin D_3, with high activity for inducing epidermal differentiation but decreased hypercalcaemic activity. *J. Dermatol.* 17:135–142.
22. Kato, T., Terui, T., and Tagami, H. (1987). Topically active vitame D_3 analogue, 1α,24-dihydroxycholecalciferol has an antiproliferative effect on the epidermis of guinea pig sking. *Br. J. Dermatol.* 117: 528–530.
23. Komoriya, K., Nagata, I., Tsuchimoto, M., et al. (1985). 1,25-Dihydroxyvitamin D_3 and 1,24-dihydroxyvitamin D_3 suppress in vitro antibody response to T cell dependent antigen. *Biochem. Biophys. Res. Commun.* 127:753–738.
24. Veyron, P., Pamphile, R., Binderup, L., and Touraine, J.L. Two novel vitamin D analogues, KH11060 and CB 966, prolong skin allograft survival in mice.
25. Van De Kerkhof, P., Werfel, T., Haustein, U.F., Luger, T., et al. (1996). Tacalcitol ointment in the treatment of psoriasis vulgaris: a multicentre, placebo-controlled, double-blind study on efficacy and safety. *Br. J. Dermatol.* 135:758–765.
26. Van Den Bemd, G-J, Pols, H., Birkenhager, J.C., and Van Leeuwen, J. Conformational change and ehanced stabilization of the vitamin D receptor by the 1,25-dihydroxyvitamin D_3 analog KH1060.

37

Clinical Experience with Vitamin D Analogues

David J. Hecker and Mark Lebwohl
Mount Sinai School of Medicine, New York, New York

Although topical steroids have long been considered the mainstay of topical treatment in psoriasis, problems with their long-term use include the development of tachyphylaxis and such adverse effects as cutaneous atrophy, telangiectasia, striae, and hypopigmentation. This has led to the development of a new class of safer topical medications for psoriasis: the vitamin D analogues. Calcipotriene, or calcipotriol (as it is called outside the United States), is a vitamin D_3 analogue that inhibits proliferation and induces differentiation of keratinocytes with very little effect on calcium metabolism systemically (1,2). With the hope that in vitro results would translate into efficacy in vivo, clinical studies were launched and in 1994 calcipotriene was approved for topical use in the United States. Numerous clinical trials have compared calcipotriene to most of the other available treatments for psoriasis. The new medication was found more effective than betamethasone valerate (3), fluocinonide ointment (4), and anthralin (5). As might be expected for a topical medication, however, calcipotriene was not able to induce total clearing in nearly as many psoriasis study patients as more aggressive treatments, such as methotrexate or PUVA (6,7). Clinical trials with calcipotriene resulted in either marked improvement or total clearing of psoriasis in 53–69% of patients studied, while as many as 20% of these patients had little or no improvement (4,8).

CALIPOTRIENE VERSUS TOPICAL STEROIDS

Based on the above clinical trials, dermatologists cannot guarantee patients that psoriasis will clear with the prescribed use of calcipotriene. They can, however, provide their patients with a reasonable alternative to current therapies with this new medication. For example, many problems associated with the use of topical steroids are avoided with calcipotriene. Localized adverse reactions to topical steroids, particularly with measures that increase overall absorption such as occlusion, excessive application, and long-term use, can create very undesirable cosmetic results for patients. Potentially more serious is the small risk of suppressing the hypothalamic-pituitary-adrenal (HPA) axis with topical corticosteroids. In contrast, calcipotriene therapy possesses none of the above undesirable effects, and may even protect against the localized steroid-induced effects on skin by its observed ability to thicken the dermis (9). Problems with tachyphylaxis (reduced efficacy with long-term use) were not observed in clinical trials of the use of calcipotriene up to 1 year (10). In addition, the vitamin D_3 analogue does not suppress the HPA axis, thus making its use in pediatric patients a good alternative to topical steroids (11).

CALCIPOTRIENE VERSUS ANTHRALINS AND TARS

Calcipotriene has compared to anthralin therapy, with a more significant clinical improvement of psoriatic plaques (5). The same result has been found in comparison to tar (12). In addition, unlike calcipotriene, both anthralin and tar preparations are known for their tendency to stain the skin, clothing, and furniture. Calcipotriene was first approved only in its ointment form, which is greasy but much more cosmetically acceptable than therapies such as anthralin and tar, which actually stain skin and fabrics. Calcipotriene cream and solution have also been shown to be nonstaining and cosmetically acceptable to patients, although these preparations are in early stages of development, and we are not aware of comparative trials with tars or anthralin (13).

ADVERSE EFFECTS

Two potential problems with the use of calcipotriene are localized cutaneous side effects and hypercalcemia. It has been shown that up to 20% of patients may experience localized irritation at the site of calcipotriene application (14). Most often seen on the face and in intertriginous areas such as the axillae and groin, this adverse effect closely resembles an irritant contact dermatitis and not an allergic reaction (15). Since the face and intertriginous areas are also particularly sensitive to local cutaneous side effects of topical steroids, it would be useful to have an alternative agent for these sites. Calcipotriene should therefore be applied cautiously on the face and in intertriginous areas, and patients should be warned of possible irritation. The irritation subsides upon discontinuation of calcipotriene, and unlike medications that cause allergic contact dermatitis, calcipotriene can be reintroduced when the irritant reaction has resolved.

Likewise, limits should be set for the amount of calcipotriene applied to the body, to avoid the reported possibility of hypercalcemia (16). Reports are inconsistent, however, regarding the maximum amount of calcipotriene that can safely be applied without affecting calcium metabolism. Bourke et al. reported a significant elevation in both mean 24-hr urinary calcium and mean serum calcium in 10 patients treated with 200 g of calcipotriene for 1 week followed by 300 g the second week, although all of the patients were asymptomatic (17). Another patient was described to have developed symptomatic hypercalcemia after 1 week of treatment with 200 g of topical calcipotriene (16). Several articles have been published describing hypercalcemia or hypercalciuria in patients who have used 100 g or less of the vitamin D_3 analogue per week (18,19). Mortensen et al. found normal values for a number of metabolic parameters, including serum calcium, phosphate, alkaline phosphatase, parathyroid hormone, calcitonin, vitamin D concentrations, urinary calcium and phosphate, and creatinine clearance, in patients treated with no more than 95.4 g of calcipotriene over a 3-week period (20). Based on the conflicting results of published case reports, it is currently suggested that patients routinely use 100 g or less of the 0.05% ointment each week to avoid clinically significant hypercalcemia (19). Laboratory monitoring with urine and serum calcium determinations should be considered in patients with renal disease and parathyroid disease.

COMBINATION THERAPY WITH CALCIPOTRIENE

A common practice in the treatment of psoriasis is to combine different therapies for an additive or synergistic effect, calcipotriene has been studied in combination with other topical medications, phototherapy, and systemic agents. The theoretical protective effect calcipotriene may have on the localized atrophy caused by topical steroids may be used to counteract an irritant contact dermatitis caused by calcipotriene. Topical medications with a low pH such as salicylic acid, on the other hand, may be a deterrent to the therapeutic effects of calcipotriene, as Kragballe found that the vitamin D_3 analogue is significantly degraded when exposed to an acidic pH (8). Considering the instability of calcipotriene, it may be prudent to alternate the preparation with other topical medications for maximal efficacy. For example, calcipotriene ointment could be applied on weekdays and topical steroids applied on weekends, or one agent applied in the morning and the other in the evening.

Conflicting reports have been published regarding the combination of calcipotriene with UVB phototherapy. While Kragballe described no significant difference in improvement between patients treated with topical calcipotriene in conjunction with UVB radiation and those treated with calcipotriene alone (21), Kerscher et al. found that the combination of narrowband UVB light with calcipotriene had an additive effect (22). The combination of UV light and calcipotriene was superior to monotherapy with calcipotriene. Clinicians need to be aware, however, of the potential problems associated with this treatment regimen. There have been reports of calcipotriene's ability to absorb UVB, thus lowering the radiation's efficacy (23). Patients should thus apply the topical medication after their light treatment to avoid this undesirable effect. In an additional report, phototesting was performed on three psoriasis patients who have developed photosensitivity reactions after being treated with a combination of calcipotriene and UVB phototherapy (24). Testing verified that the psoriatic plaques treated with calcipotriene were more sensitive to UVB radiation than untreated skin. It should be noted that these three patients were already on UVB phototherapy for a period of time before calcipotriene was added to their regimen. Those patients who were applying calcipotriene before beginning a regimen of phototherapy (11 patients) never reported a burn, while four of 11 patients who added calcipotriene to a regimen of UVB radiation reported photosensitivity reactions. Thus, calcipotriene may increase the risk of burning in patients already on high doses of UVB by lowering the minimal erythema dose. Further studies examining the risk/benefit ratio of this combination therapy are needed.

More promising studies have been performed on the effects of combining calcipotriene with PUVA. Both the number of PUVA treatments and the cumulative dose of UVA needed for clearing are reduced when calcipotriene is added to PUVA (25). As with UVB, care must be taken to apply calcipotriene after PUVA treatment but for a different reason than with UVB light. Patients treated with UVA radiation with calcipotriene already on their skin have had the applied ointment analyzed by high-performance liquid chromatography, showing a decrease in the concentration of the active ingredient (26).

Vitamin D analogues have an important role in the treatment of psoriasis, but dermatologists must be aware of both its maximum potential and possible limitations. Calcipotriene has a quite different efficacy profile than topical steroids. Despite problems with long-term or cumulative use, ultrapotent topical steroids initially work very fast and effectively in clearing psoriatic plaques. Calcipotriene, on the other hand, is generally safe to use in the chronic setting provided the patient does not exceed the 100 g/week limitation. Efficacy with this vitamin D_3 analogue, though, is more limited, with up to 30% of patients studied experiencing limited or no improvement, while approximately 60% experience clearing or significant improvement (8,9). Those who have been on topical steroids before considering application of calcipotriene should be warned not to abruptly discontinue the steroids due to the possibility of a rebound flare of their psoriasis. Plaques treated with calcipotriene often initially show an increase in peripheral scaling before noticeable improvement is seen, thus deceptively looking worse before improving. Care should also be taken when applying the vitamin D analog to the face and intertriginous sites on the body, the areas most susceptible to localized irritation from the medication.

Although calcipotriene is a relatively new psoriasis treatment, it has had a major impact on the therapy of psoriasis. New preparations of calcipotriene such as a cream and a solution for the scalp, both less greasy in consistency than their ointment counterpart, should add to the acceptability of this new class of topical medications in the treatment of chronic plaque psoriasis.

REFERENCES

1. Kragballe, K., and Wildfang, I.L. (1990). Calcipotriol (MC903), a novel vitamin D3 analogue, stimulates terminal differentiation and inhibits proliferation of cultured human keratinocytes. *Arch. Dermatol. Res.* 228: 164–167.
2. Binderup, L., and Bramm, E. (1988). Effects of a novel vitamin D analogue MC903 on cell proliferation and differentiation in vitro and on calcium metabolism in vivo. *Biochem. Pharmacol.* 37:889–895.
3. Cunliffe, W.J., Claudy, A., Faririss, G., et al. (1992). A multicenter comparative study of calcipotriol and betamethasone 17-valerte in patients with psoriasis vulgaris. *J. Am. Acad. Dermatol.* 26:736–742.
4. Bruce, S., Epinette, W.W., Funicella, T., et al. (1994). Comparative study of calcipotriene (MC903) ointment and fluocinonide ointment in the treatment of psoriasis. *J. Am. Acad. Dermatol.* 31(part 1):755–759.
5. Berth-Jones, J., Chu, A.C., Dodd, W.A., et al. (1992). A multicentre, parallel group comparison of calcipotriol ointment and short contact dithranol therapy in chronic plaque psoriasis. *Br. J. Dermatol.* 127: 266–271.
6. Weinstein, G. (1983). Three decades of folic acid antagonists in dermatology. *Arch. Dermatol.* 119: 525–527.
7. Parrish, J.A., Fitzpatrick, T.B., Tanenbaum, L., and Pathak, M.A. (1974). Photochemotherapy of psoriasis

with oral methoxsalen and long wave ultraviolet light. *N. Engl. J. Med.* 291:1207–1211.
8. Kragballe, K. Vitamin D3 analogues. *Dermatol. Clin.* 13(4):835–839.
9. Levy, J., Gassmiller, J., Schroder, G., Audring, H., and Sonnichsen, N. (1994). Comparison of the effects of calcipotriol, prednicarbate and clobetasol 17-propionate on normal skin assessed by ultrastound measurement of skin thickness. *Skin Pharmacol.* 7: 231–236.
10. Ramsey, C.A., Berth-Jones, J., Brundin, G. et al. (1994) Long term use of tropical calcipotriol in chronic plaque psoriasis. *Dermatology* 189:260–264.
11. Darley, C.R., Cunliffe, W.J., Ferguson, J. Hutchinson, P.E., and Laber, M.R. (1993) Safety and efficacy of calcipotriol ointment (Dovonex) in treating children with psoriasis vulgaris. *Br. J. Dermatol.* 129(Suppl. 46):133.
12. Tham, S.N., Lun, K.C., and Cheong, W.K. (1994) A comparative study of calcipotriol ointment and tar in chronic plaque psoriasis. *Br. J. Dermatol.* 131: 673–677.
13. Green, C., Ganpule, M., Harris, D., et al. (1994). Comparative effects of calcipotriol (MC903) solution and placebo (vehicle of MC903) in treatment of psoriasis of the scalp. *Br. J. Dermatol.* 130:483–487.
14. Kragballe, K. (1989). Treatment of psoriasis by topical application of the novel cholecalciferol analogue calcipotriol (MC903). *Arch. Dermatol.* 125:1647–1652.
15. Serum, J., and Fullerton, A. (1994). Safety and skin irritation with vitamin D. In *Programs and Abstracts of the Sixth International Psoriasis Symposium*, July 20–24, Chicago.
16. Dwyer, C., and Chapman, R.S. (1991). Calcipotriol and hypercalcaemia. *Lancet* 338:764–765.
17. Bourke, J.F., Berth-Jones, J., Iqbal, S.J., and Hutchinson, P.E. (1993). High-dose topical calcipotriol in the treatment of extensive psoriasis vulgaris. *Br. J. Dermatol.* 129:74–76.
18. Berth Jones, J., Boruke, J.F., Iqbal, S.J., and Hutchinson, P.E. (1993). Urine calcium exretion during treatmentof psoriasis with topical calcipotriol. *Br. J. Dermatol.* 129:411–414.
19. Hardman, K.A., Heath, D.A., and Nelson, H.M. (1993). Hypercalcaemia associated with calcipotriol (Dovonex) treatment. *Br. Med. J.* 306:896.
20. Mortensen, L. Kragballe, K., Wegmann, E., Schifter, S., Risteli, J., and Charles, P. (1993). Treatment of psoriasis vulgaris with topical calcipotriol has no short term effect on calcium bone metabolism. *Acta Derm. Venereol. (Stockh).* 73:300–304.
21. Kragballe, K. (1990). Combination of topical calcipotriol (MC903) and UVB radiation for psoriasis vulgaris. *Dermatologica* 181:211–214.
22. Kerscher, M., Volkenandt, M., Plewig, G., et al. (1993). Combination phototherapy of psoriasis with calcipotriol and narrow band UVB. *Lancet* 343:923.
23. Kornreich, C., Zheng, Z.S., Zhen Xue, G., and Prystowsky, J. (1995). UV absorbance of topical agents commonly used in psoriasis treatment. *J. Invest. Dermatol.* 104(Suppl.):691.
24. McKenna, K.E., and Stern, R.S. (1995). Photosensitivity associated with combined UV-B and calcipotriene therapy. *Arch. Dermatol.* 131:1305–1307.
25. Speight, E.L. and Farr, P.M. (1994). Calcipotriol improves the response of psoriasis to PUVA. *Br. J. Dermatol.* 130:79–82.
26. Hecker, D., Martinez, J., Sapadin, A., Patel, B., and Lebwohl, M. (1995). Effects of topical calcipotriene on transmission of ultraviolet light and effect of ultraviolet light on the stability of calcipotriene. *J. Invest. Dermatol.* 104(Suppl.):659.

38

Combination Therapies: Dovonex and Phototherapy

Alan K. Silverman
Professional Practice, Dallas, Texas

M. Alan Menter
Psoriasis Center, Baylor University Medical Center, Dallas, Texas

Calcipotriene (calcipotriol, MC903) is an active synthetic (side-chain-modified) vitamin D_3 analog that was approved for the topical treatment of mild to moderate plaque psoriasis in the United States in 1994 (1–3). Topical administration of vitamin D and its analogs has been shown to inhibit the proliferation of fibroblasts and keratinocytes, modulate inflammation, and induce terminal epidermal differentiation (4). Receptors for calcitriol have been found in bone, intestine, pancreas, breast, pituitary, gonads, mononuclear cells, activated T lymphocytes, and skin (5–7).

Monotherapy using calcipotriene is effective in treatment of mild to moderate psoriasis. During phase IV clinical trials in the United States, Dovonex (MC 903/calcipotriene) was used to treat limited (less than 20% total body surface area), stable plaque psoriasis. After 8 weeks of treatment, 70% of calcipotriene-treated patients showed 75% or greater improvement compared with only 19% of vehicle-treated patients (8).

As is the fate of most newly approved drugs for psoriasis, Dovonex has subsequently been utilized in a number of so-called combination regimens—synergistic combinations of different therapeutic agents developed to maximize clinical responses while minimizing side effects and toxicities. Preliminary reports suggest that calcipotriene-UVB (narrow band) and calcipotriene-PUVA combinations may be more effective than UVB or PUVA individually. It seems reasonable to use Dovonex (or tar or anthralin) as an adjunct to phototherapy, photochemotherapy, or systemic therapy (retinoids, methotrexate, etc.) if its use decreases the total cumulative UV dose or the total dose of systemic medication required for clearing. The only caveat is the recent report by McKenna and Stern (9) that in addition to causing irritation and burning, Dovonex may cause photosensitivity during UVB phototherapy.

DOVONEX: COMPARISON TO OTHER TOPICAL MONOTHERAPIES

Dovonex is a reasonably effective topical medication for treatment of stable plaque psoriasis, comparable in efficacy to midpotency topical corticoids such as betamethasone-17-valerate (10,11) and superior to fluocinonide (12). Calcipotriol solution (50 μg/ml) has been shown to be useful in treatment of scalp psoriasis, superior to placebo (vehicle) (13), but not as effective as betamethasone-17-valerate solution (1 mg/ml) (14).

Berardesca et al. compared Dovonex to clobetasole by measuring transepidermal water loss (TEWL) and laser Doppler velocimetry (LDV), and correlated these findings with subjective assessment of clinical changes (using PASI). TEWL and LDV were used to monitor restoration of barrier function and normalization of blood flow, respectively, in psoriatic plaques of 24 male patients during 3 weeks of treatment. Levels of TEWL decreased more rapidly with clobetasol, but the final result did not differ significantly in the two treatment groups. The results correlated well with the PASI score. However, the use of TEWL and LDV measurements in development of new drugs and in clinical research and their correlation with indices of clinical improvement have yet to be clearly established (15).

The effect of combining occlusion with topical calcipotriol was studied in 48 patients with symmetrical chronic plaque psoriasis affecting the limbs in a single-blind, right/left comparison study. One group treated one side with calcipotriol alone and the opposite side with calcipotriol plus occlusion; the other group treated one side with placebo plus occlusion and the opposite side with calcipotriol plus occlusion. In the first group, the mean improvements were 40% for calcipotriol alone and 61% for calcipotriol plus occlusion. In the second group, occlusion plus placebo produced no significant change. The combination of calcipotriol plus occlusion was significantly better than calcipotriol alone (16).

Nielsen reported that it was impossible to distinguish between lesions treated with Dovonex or Dermovate (clobetasole) ointment occluded with Contreet (hydrocolloid dressing) after three applications of medication over a period of 12 days (17).

Dovonex has been shown to be as effective as, if not slightly superior to, anthralin (18).

The antipsoriatic efficacy, tolerability, and safety of calcipotriol ointment were compared with those of tar (coal tar solution BP 15% v/w in aqueous cream) in a right/left, randomized, investigator-blinded, controlled study of 30 patients with plaque-type psoriasis. The differences from baseline between the two treatments were statistically significant in favor of calcipotriol. Improvement with calcipotriol was rapid in the first 2 weeks of treatment; with tar, significant improvement occurred only after 4 weeks of treatment. Seven patients developed irritation on the calcipotriol-treated side; no adverse effects were noted on the tar-treated side (19).

DOVONEX: ADVERSE REACTIONS

Adverse reactions to Dovonex during large, vehicle-controlled trials in the United States include rash, erythema, pruritus, and burning (8). In comparison studies with fluocinonide, the most common adverse events were a burning sensation and pruritus. The most distressing side effect of Dovonex is local irritation in up to 20% of patients, which is unfortunate since the most sensitive areas (face, axilla, and groin) are traditionally the most difficult areas to clear in patients with severe psoriasis. Kokelj et al. reported that three of nine patients treated with calcipotriol and heliotherapy developed pigmented patches at the sites of calcipotriol applications that lasted for months (20).

Long-term use of Dovonex has been shown to be safe and effective, and the frequency of adverse effects such as irritation does not increase with the duration of treatment (21). In an open, prospective study of 12 months' duration, calcipotriene completely cleared 26% of subjects (who then used Dovonex intermittently); the remaining patients required continuous treatment with Dovonex (22).

Dovonex does not cause side effects that have been associated with prolonged use of topical corticosteroids (e.g., atrophy, striae, tachyphylaxis, rebound). Dovonex causes dermal thickening, with histological features of an irritant reaction (subacute dermatitis) (23).

There is just one report of generalized pustular psoriasis precipitated by Dovonex (24). However, the reaction occurred 2 weeks after starting Dovonex in a woman with previously stable plaque psoriasis; i.e., it is possible that this represented an allergic contact reaction with Koebnerization.

In mixed epidermal cell lymphocyte reactions, both Dovonex and cyclosporin A have synergistic effects on inhibition of lymphocyte proliferation in mixed epidermal cell lymphocyte reactions. Bagot et al. reported that combination Dovonex-cyclosporin (2 mg/kg) induced disappearance of psoriatic lesions (25). Additional studies showed complete clearing of 90% improvement in PASI in 50% of patients treated with calcipotriol and cyclosporin, in comparison with 11.8% of patients treated with placebo (calcipotriol vehicle) and cyclosporin (26).

Immunohistological studies show that before treatment with calcipotriene, lesional infiltrates were composed mainly of T cells and there was decreased expression of CD1 on the intraepidermal Langerhans cells. ICAM-1 and EGF receptor were present throughout the epidermis. After 2 weeks of calcipotriene, there were significantly fewer CD4 T cells in the dermis and an increased number of intraepidermal CD1+ Langerhans cells. ICAM-1 expression on lesional keratinocytes was reduced in all patients and changes were concurrent with moderate clinical improvement of the lesions. The results suggest that in early stages of the clinical response to calcipotriol, there is an immunomodulating effect of the drug associated with variable decreases in kertinocyte expression of markers of activation (27).

Boisseau-Garsaud et al. reported that oral calcitriol was beneficial in treatment of five patients with severe psoriasis, four of who had erythrodermic or pustular psoriasis, and two of whom had concomitant hypocalcemia. Doses ranged from 0.5 μg to 1 μg given once daily at bedtime for approximately 1 month (28). While oral calcitriol would appear to be an interesting therapeutic solution to the problem of treating pustular psoriasis and hypocalcemia, there is currently insufficient data to justify its use.

CONTACT DERMATITIS

Allergic contact sensitization to all of the fat-soluble vitamins can occur. Yip and Goodfield were the first to report contact dermatitis to MC903 but not the vehicle (29). Vilaplana et al. patch-tested 100 volunteers to calcipotriol cream. Only one of 100 patients patch-tested showed slight irritation to Dovonex by day 2, which had completely disappeared by day 4 (30). Bruynzeel et al. reported that cross-sensitization to other vitamin D analogs occurred in a patient with allergic sensitivity to calcipotriol (31).

de Groot reported positive patch test reactions to calcipotriol 10 and 2 μ/ml isopropanol. He suggested that patients with severe apparent irritation from calcipotriol ointment as well as those who exacerbate during treatment be evaluated for contact sensitivity to calcipotriol or to other ingredients in the vehicle including propylene glycol (32). Steinkjer also reported a case of contact sensitivity to calcipotriol, performed a dilution series of calcipotriol in isopropanol, and suggested that 2 μg/ml might be a suitable concentration for patch testing (33).

It is interesting that a topical medication known to have a wide variety of immunodulatory functions can function as a contact sensitizer.

DOVONEX-UVB PHOTOTHERAPY

The role of Dovonex in UVB phototherapy is still not clear. Efficacy may depend on the type of regimen used and other variables, including type of phototherapy (erythemogenic vs. suberythemogenic), wavelength (broad-band UVB vs. narrow-band UVB), and timing of application (topical Dovonex absorbs UVC and UVB light).

Kragballe initially observed that the combination of Dovonex and UVB was not more effective than UVB alone (34). Dovonex was assessed in combination with suberythemogenic UVB using a bilateral comparison study approach. Patients were treated twice daily with Dovonex on both sides and with UVB on one side using suberythemogenic doses three times weekly for 8 weeks. No statistically significant difference was found between monotherapy and combination therapy.

In a subsequent preliminary report, Kerscher et al. (35) found that narrow-band 311-nm UVB combined with Dovonex was more effective than Dovonex alone. Twenty patients with stable plaque psoriasis were treated in a left-right trial using Dovonex with 311-nm UVB. Psoriatic plaques on both halves of the body were treated with Dovonex twice daily; lesions on one half were treated with 311-nm UVB. After only 2 weeks, differences in response were seen. There was a mean PASI reduction of 68% in patients receiving combination therapy, compared to 36% with Dovonex alone. These findings of increased efficacy using the combination of Dovonex and narrow-band UVB were statistically significant, in contrast to the smaller trial by Kragballe (34) using broad-band UVB. The investigators believed that narrow-band UVB was more effective because it was less erythemogenic and could be administered more aggressively (36).

Hofmann and Schirle (37) treated 40 patients either with Dovonex alone or in combination with phototherapy. After 4 weeks of treatment, psoriasis had cleared in 11 of 18 patients using Dovonex alone, and in 20 of 22 patients who had received either Dovonex+UVB or Dovonex+UVA+B.

Kornreich et al. (38) reported that Dovonex absorbs UVB and should therefore be applied only after and not immediately before phototherapy. Recently, Lebwohl et al. (39) reviewed the "blocking potential" of various topical preparations prior to phototherapy. They showed that preparations containing tar or salicyclic acid, or thickly applied petrolatum or emollients, can block UVB. In a subsequent letter, Marsico and Dijkstra (40) discussed the transmission of UVB through Dovonex in comparison to light mineral oil. This showed a significant decrease in UVB irradiation through Dovonex ointment. Their recommendation of applying mineral oil to psoriatic plaques before exposure to UVB with subsequent application of Dovonex ointment after the light treatment was seconded by Lebwohl in a reply (41). Exposure to UVA also reduces the concentration of Dovonex as determined by HPLC (42), so Dovonex must likewise be applied after UVA exposure and not before.

PHOTOSENSITIVITY DURING DOVONEX-UVB PHOTOTHERAPY

McKenna and Stern (9) described photosensitivity developing in a small number of patients receiving UVB phototherapy for chronic plaque psoriasis. Photosensitivity developed only after Dovonex was added to the regimen, only in areas to which Dovonex had been applied, and only in patients who had started using Dovonex after initiation of phototherapy. Photosensitivity occurred without changes in UVB dosage or frequency of treatment. The time from starting Dovonex therapy to the development of photosensitivity ranged from 4 to 28 days and the number of UVB exposures during this period varied between one and 12 treatments. The mean UVB dose at burning was 1114 mJ/cm^2. Twenty-two patients had used Dovonex in combination with UVB therapy of a total of 103 UVB-treated patients during the period when the adverse events occurred. Half of these patients started Dovonex therapy prior to starting treatment with UVB. However, cases of photosensitivity occurred only in the remaining half of the patients in whom Dovonex was added during UVB therapy.

Combined therapy was continued or resumed in two patients by reduction of the UVB dose. In three cases, phototesting confirmed greater photosensitivity to Dovonex-treated skin than to petrolatum-treated skin. Reactions were limited to plaques exposed to UVB to which Dovonex had been applied and occurred in patients who were tolerating these doses of UVB prior to the addition of Dovonex. None of the patients had previously experienced burning with UVB alone. Two patients had received comparable UVB doses while being treated over at least a 10-year period.

These patients developed a sunburn-like reaction limited to plaques to which Dovonex had been applied, with the exception of one patient whose reaction was limited only to the arms (treated plaques on the legs did not react). Burning and stinging began within 24 hr of the preceding UVB treatment and lasted 2–3 days, interfering with sleep. Two patients who had the highest UVB dose prior to starting Dovonex were able to use Dovonex for 28 and 14 days, respectively, before burning. The other two patients had lower cumulative UVB doses prior to starting Dovonex and were able to use Dovonex for 6 and 4 days, respectively, before burning. Two patients were able to resume calcipotriene when the UVB dose was diminished.

Allergy and primary irritation were thought to be unlikely as treatment was restarted in two patients without any problems (after substantial reductions in the UVB dose, however). It is possible that Dovonex alters the inflammatory response to UVR in areas of active psoriasis. The fact that one patient who developed burning following a single UVB exposure and after only 4 days of Dovonex use tends to discount suppositions based on changes in skin thickness, melanization, and the like. Phototesting showed that calcipotriene caused a greater erythemogenic response than did emollient in three patients, which was dose related. However, Hecker et al. (42) found that the minimal erythema dose (MED) was unaffected by application of calcipotriene either immediately before or the evening before phototherapy with UVA or UVB.

DOVONEX-PUVA PHOTOTHERAPY

Yu et al. (43) suggested that vitamin D_3 and its analogs (including EB1089, MC903) could inhibit growth of squamous cell cancers and associated hypercalcemia. Since a major concern of PUVA therapy is development of skin cancer, combined therapy using Dovonex might suppress or reduce the risk of cutaneous malignancy during PUVA therapy.

PUVA combination therapy has as its goal the minimization of total radiation exposure, treatment times, and treatment frequency—all of which help reduce overall incidence of cutaneous malignancy and other long-term toxic effects.

When used in conjunction with PUVA, Dovonex has been show to reduce the number of treatments and the total number of joules per cubic meter required for clearing. The effect of Dovonex was studied in 13 patients with plaque-type psoriasis who were about to start twice-weekly PUVA, using a bilateral comparison protocol (44). There was median reduction in UVA dose of 26.5% for Dovonex compared with placebo, and with the exception of one patient, the improved response was not associated with earlier relapse. Over half the patients had used calcipotriol previously without achieving clearance.

In each patient, from the start of PUVA treatment, two plaques on symmetrical body sites were selected for assessment. Dovonex ointment was applied to one site twice daily, and placebo to the other. Response was assessed weekly for 6 weeks using PASI and assessment of blood flux with scanning laser-Doppler velocimetry. Eleven patients completed the study: in nine the calcipotriol-treated plaque either cleared before the placebo-treated plaque or was consistently judged to be better. From the third week of the trial, mean blood flux was significantly lower in the calcipotriol-treated plaques than in those treated with placebo. In seven patients whose psoriasis was clear in at least one plaque at the end of the study period, there was a median reduction in UVA dose of 26.5% for calcipotriol compared with placebo. With the exception of one patient, the improved response was not associated with earlier relapse.

In a large multicenter, randomized, double-blind, parallel-group trial, Frappaz and Thivolet (45) studied the effect of using calcipotriol or vehicle beginning 2 weeks prior to PUVA. Patients initially received 2 weeks of Dovonex or placebo ointment, followed by double-blind combination therapy (initiation of PUVA) for 10 weeks. Pretreatment with Dovonex followed by PUVA significantly reduced cumulative UVA dose, number of treatments required for clearance, and time to clinical improvement. Two weeks of combination treatment was more effective than 8 weeks of monotherapy with ointment alone. The most common adverse event was lesional/perilesional irritation, which occurred at about the same frequency in the combined therapy group (17%) as in the placebo-treated group. No photosensitization or phototoxicity was observed. Erythema was infrequent in both treatment groups with no significant difference between the two.

As is the case with UVB, exposure to UVA reduces the concentration of Dovonex as determined by HPLC, so Dovonex should not be applied immediately before phototherapy. Hecker et al. also reported that the MED for UVA and UVB was unaffected by calcipotriene (42). Thick application of Dovonex can increase the MED, possibly by reducing transmission of UVR.

CONCLUSION

Topical vitamin D analogs have potent effects on cutaneous inflammation, differentiation, and proliferation without causing hypercalcemia. Dovonex has been shown to be effective monotherapy for mild to moderate plaque psoriasis and is equivalent or superior to anthralin, tar, and mid- to high-potency topical steroids. Occlusion may increase the efficacy of Dovonex monotherapy.

Dovonex appears to be an effective part of combination regimens including narrow-band UVB and PUVA, but this assertion is based on a relatively small number of studies done to date. Since a small number of patients have developed photosensitivity, Dovonex should be started 2–3 weeks prior to initiating phototherapy. If Dovonex is added to an ongoing phototherapy regimen, the UVB dose should be adjusted as recommended by McKenna and Stern.

For treatment of plaque-type psoriasis, combination Dovonex-UVB and Dovonex-PUVA seem to produce better results than single-modality therapy. No conclusions can yet be drawn regarding Dovonex-phototherapy combinations for localized psoriasis (e.g., palmar-plantar), or for pustular and erythrodermic psoriasis, or the effects of combination therapy on psoriatic arthritis.

Dovonex can induce contact sensitization, and patients who receive combination regimens including Dovonex should be evaluated for allergic contact dermatitis if sudden psoriasis flares occur.

At this time, there is no literature regarding Dovonex-retinoid-phototherapy regimens. As retinoid-PUVA (Re-PUVA) combination is commonly used in psoriasis, adding Dovonex for recalcitrant areas may be worthy of consideration. There already is experimental evidence that retinoids work synergistically with vitamin D_3 analogs to inhibit growth of leukemic cell lines (46).

ACKNOWLEDGMENT

We would like to thank Shari Landa for her review, and assistance.

REFERENCES

1. Kragballe, K., Beck, H.I., and Sogaard, H. (1988). Improvement of psoriasis by a topical vitamin D_3 analogue (MC903) in a double-blind study. *Br. J. Dermatol.* 119(2):223–230.
2. Holick, M.F. (1989). Will 1,25-dihydroxyvitamin D_3, MC903 and their analogues herald a new pharmacologic era for the treatment of psoriasis? *Arch. Dermatol.* 125(12):1692–1697.
3. Kragballe, K. (1989). Treatment of psoriasis by the topical application of the novel cholecalciferol analogue calcipotriol (MC 903). *Arch. Dermatol.* 125(12): 1647–1652.

4. Gerritsen, M.J., Rulo, H.F., Van Vlijmen-Willems, I., Van Erp, P.E., and van de Kerkhof, P.C. (1993). Topical treatment of psoriatic plaques with 1,25-dihydroxyvitamin D_3: a cell biological study. *Br. J. Dermatol.* 128(6):666–673.
5. Holick, M.F. (1993). Active vitamin D compounds and analogues: a new therapeutic era for dermatology in the 21st century. *Mayo Clin. Proc.* 68(9):925–927.
6. Morimoto, S., Yoshikawa, K., Kozuka, T., Kitano, Y., Imanaka, S., Fukuo, K., Koh, E., and Kumahara, Y. (1986). An open study of vitamin D_3 treatment in psoriasis vulgaris. *Br. J. Dermatol.* 115(4):421–429.
7. DeLuca, H.F. (1984). The metabolism, physiology, and function of vitamin D. In *Vitamin D: Basic and Clinical Aspects*. R. Kumar (Ed.). Martinus Nijhoff, The Hague, pp. 1–68.
8. Highton, A., Quell, J. (1995), and the Calcipotriene Study Group. Calcipotriene ointment 0.005% for psoriasis: a safety and efficacy study. *J. Am. Acad. Dermatol.* 32(1):67–72.
9. McKenna, K.E., and Stern, R.S. (1995). Photosensitivity associated with combined UV-B and calcipotriene therapy. *Arch. Dermatol.* 131:1305–1307.
10. Cunliffe, W.J., Berth-Jones, J., Claudy, A., Fairiss, G., Goldin, D., Gratton, D., Henderson, C.A., Maddin, W.S., and Ortonne, J.P. (1992). Comparative study of calcipotriol (MC 903) ointment and betamethasone 17-valerate ointment in patients with psoriasis vulgaris. *J. Am. Acad. Dermatol.* 26(5 Pt. 1):736–743.
11. Kragballe, K., Gjertsen, B.T., De Hoop, D., Karlsmark, T., van der Kerkhof, P.C., Larko, O., Neiboer, C., Roed-Petersen, J., Strand, A., and Tikjob, G. (1991). Double-blind, right/left comparison of calcipotriol and betamethasone valerate in treatment of psoriasis vulgaris. *Lancet* 337(8735):193–196.
12. Bruce, S., Epinette, W.W., Funicella, T., Ison, A., Jones, E.L., Loss, R., Jr., McPhee, M.E., and Whitmore, C. (1994). Comparative study of calcipotriene (MC 903) ointment and fluocinonide ointment in the treatment of psoriasis. *J. Am. Acad. Dermatol.* 31(5 Pt. 1):755–759.
13. Green, C., Ganpule, M., Harris, D., Kavanagh, G., Kennedy, C., Mallett, R., Rustin, M., and Downes, N. (1994). Comparative effects of calcipotriol (MC903) solution and placebo (vehicle of MC903) in the treatment of psoriasis of the scalp. *Br. J. Dermatol.* 130(4): 483–487.
14. Klaber, M.R., Hutchinson, P.E., Pedvis-Leftick, A., Kragballe, K., Reunala, T.L., van de Kerkhof, P.C., Johnsson, M.K., Molin, L., Corbett, M.S., and Downess, N. (1994). Comparative effects of calcipotriol solution (50 micrograms/ml) and betamethasone 17-valerate solution (1 mg/ml) in the treatment of scalp psoriasis. *Br. J. Dermatol.* 131(5):678–683.
15. Berardesca, E., Vignoli, G.P., Farinelli, N., Vignini, M., Distante, F., and Rabbioso, G. (1994). Non-invasive evaluation of topical calcipotriol versus clobetasol in the treatment of psoriasis. *Acta Derm. Venereol.* 74(4):302–304.
16. Bourke, J.F., Berth-Jones, J., and Hutchinson, P.E. (1993). Occlusion enhances the efficacy of topical calcipotriol in the treatment of psoriasis vulgaris. *Clin. Exp. Dermatol.* 18(6):504–506.
17. Nielsen, P.G. (1993). Calcipotriol or clobetasole propionate occluded with a hydrocolloid dressing for treatment of nummular psoriasis. *Acta Derm. Venereol.* 73(5):394.
18. Berth-Jones, J., Chu, A.C., Dodd, W.A., Ganpule, M., Griffiths, W.A., Haydey, R.P., Klaber, M.R., Murray, S.J., Rogers, S., and Jurgensen, H. J. (1992). A multicentre, parallel-group comparison of calcipotriol ointment and short-contact dithranol therapy in chronic plaque psoriasis. *Br. J. Dermatol.* 127(3):266–271.
19. Tham, S.N., Lun, K.C., and Cheong, W.K. (1994). A comparative study of calcipotriol ointment and tar in chronic plaque psoriasis. *Br. J. Dermatol.* 131(5): 673–637.
20. Kokelj, F., Lavaroni, G., Perkan, V., and Plozzer, C. (1995). Hyperpigmentation due to calcipotriol (MC 903) plus heliotherapy in psoriatic patients. *Acta Derm. Venereol.* 75:307–309.
21. Poyner, T., Huges, I.W., Dass, B.K., and Adnitt, P.I. (1993). Long-term treatment of chronic plaque psoriasis with calcipotriol. *J. Dermatol. Treat.* 4:173–177.
22. Ramsay, C.A., Berth-Jones, J., Brundin, G., Cunliffe, W.J., Dubertret, L., van de Kerkhof, P.C., Menne, T., and Wegmann, E. (1994). Long-term use of topical calcipotriol in chronic plaque psoriasis. *Dermatology* 189(3):260–264.
23. Levy, J., Gassmuller, J., Schroder, G., Audring, H., and Sonnichsen, N. (1994). Comparison of the effects of calcipotriol, prednicarbate and clobetasol 17-propionate on normal skin assessed by ultrasound measurement of skin thickness. *Skin Pharmacol.* 7(4): 231–236.
24. Georgala, S., Rigopoulos, D., Aroni, K., and Stratigos, J.T. (1994). Generalized pustular psoriasis precipitated by topical calcipotriol cream. *Int. J. Dermatol.* 33(7): 515–516.
25. Bagot, M., Grossman, R., Pamphile, R., Binderup, L., Charue, D., Revuz, J., and Dubertret, L. (1994). Additive effects of calcipotriol and cyclosporine A: from in vitro experiments to in vivo applications in the treatment of severe psoriasis. *C.R. Acad. Sci. Ser. Iii Sci. Vie* 317(3):282–286.
26. Grossman, R.M., Thivolet, J., Claudy, A., Souteyrand, P., Guilhou, J.J., Thomas P., Amblard, P., Belaich, S., de Belilovsky, C., de la Brassinne, M., et al. (1994). A novel therapeutic approach to psoriasis with combination calcipotriol ointment and very low-dose cyclosporine: results of a multicenter placebo-controlled study. *J. Am. Acad. Dermatol.* 31(1):68–74.

27. Mozzanica, N., Cattaneo, A., Schmitt, E., Diotti, R., and Finizi, A.F. (1994). Topical calcipotriol for psoriasis–an immunohistologic study. *Acta Derm. Venereol.* 186:171–172.
28. Boisseau-Garsaud, A.M., Legrain, V., Hehunstre, J.P., Maleville, J., and Taieb, A. (1993). Treatment of psoriasis by oral calcitriol. A study of 5 cases and review of the literature. *Ann. Dermatol. Venereol.* 120(10): 669–674.
29. Yip, J., and Goodfield, M. (1991). Contact dermatitis from MC 903, a topical vitamin D_3 analogue. *Contact Derm.* 25(2):139–140.
30. Vilaplana, J., Mascaro, J.M., Lecha, M., and Romaguera, C. (1994). Low irritancy of 2-day occlusive patch test with calcipotriol cream. *Contact Derm.* 30(1):45–46.
31. Bruynzeel, D.P., Hol, C.W., and Neiboer, C. (1992). Allergic contact dermatitis to calcipotriol. *Br. J. Dermatol.* 127(1):66.
32. de Groot, A.C., (1994). Contact allergy to calcipotriol. *Contact Derm.* 30(4):242–243.
33. Steinkjer, B. (1994). Contact dermatitis from calcipotriol. *Contact Derm.* 31(2):122.
34. Kragballe, K. (1990). Combination of topical calcipotriol (MC 903) and UVB radiation for psoriasis vulgaris. *Dermatologica* 181(3):211–214.
35. Kerscher, M., Volkenandt, M., Plewig, G., and Lehmann, P. (1993). Combination phototherapy of psoriasis with calcipotriol and narrow-band UVB. *Lancet* 342(8876):923.
36. Kerscher, M., Lehmann, P., and Plewig, G. (1994). Combination phototherapy of psoriasis with calcipotriol and narrow-band UVB light. *Photodermatol. Photoimmunol. Photomed.* 10:86.
37. Hofmann, C., and Schirle, S. (1993). Topical treatment of psoriasis with calcipotriol. Report of clinical experience. *Fortschr. Med.* 111(35–36):562–564.
38. Kornreich, C., Zheng, Z.S., Xue, G.Z., et al. (1994). UV absorbance of topical agents commonly used in psoriasis treatment. *J. Invest. Dermatol.* 104:691 (abstract).
39. Lebwohl, M., Martinez, J., Weber, P., and DeLuca, R. (1995). Effects of topical preparations on the erythemogenicity of UVB: implications for psoriasis phototherapy. *J. Am. Acad. Dermatol.* 32(3):469–471.
40. Marsico, E., and Dijkstra, J. (1996). UVB blocking effect of calcipotriene ointment 0.005%. *J. Am. Acad. Dermatol.* 34:539–540.
41. Lebwohl, M. (1996). Reply. *J. Am. Acad. Dermatol.* 34:540.
42. Hecker, D., Martinez, J., Spadin, A., Patel, B., and Lebwohl, M. (1995). Effect of topical calcipotriene on transmission of ultraviolet light and effect of ultraviolet light on the stability of calcipotriene. *J. Invest. Dermatol.* 104(4):659.
43. Yu, J., Papvasiliou, V., Rhim, J., Goltzman, D., and Kremer, R. (1995). Vitamin D analogs: new therapeutic agents for the treatment of squamous cancer and its associated hypercalcemia. *Anti-cancer Drugs* 6(1): 101–108.
44. Speight, E.L., and Farr, P.M. (1994). Calcipotriol improves the response of psoriasis to PUVA. *Br. J. Dermatol.* 130(1):79–82.
45. Frappaz, A., and Thivolet, J. (1993). Calcipotriol in combination with PUVA: a randomized double blind placebo study in severe psoriasis. *Eur. J. Dermatol.* 3: 351–354.
46. Defacque, H., Dornand, J., Commes, T., Cabane, S., Sevilla, C., and Marti, J., (1994). Different combinations of retinoids and vitamin D_3 analogs efficiently promote growth inhibition and differentiation of myelomonocytic leukemia cell lines. *J. Pharmacol. Exp. Ther.* 271(1):193–199.

39

Safety of and Skin Irritation with Vitamin D

Jørgen Serup
Leo Pharmaceutical Products, Copenhagen, Denmark

Only two analogues of vitamin D_3 are available for topical use. Calcipotriol (USAN name calcipotriene, MC903) is registered in more than 70 countries including the United States as a 50 $\mu g/g$ prescription pharmaceutical for BID application. Tacalcitol, the 1,24-dihydroxy analogue of vitamin D_3, has been available in Japan for a few years as a 2 $\mu g/g$ formulation to be applied BID. Recently the analogue became registered in some European countries as a 4 $\mu g/g$ formulation for QD application. The genuine vitamin D hormone 1,25-dihydroxy-D_3 (calcitriol) is not used because of the risk of hypercalcemia. Thus, the knowledge about cutaneous tolerability of D vitamins is based mainly on studies on calcipotriol simply because of the widespread use of this analogue.

Irritation (Latin *irritare*, "to incite or provoke") is often defined as an inflammatory adverse reaction, which may occur as an acute event or on a cumulative basis following repeated applications, the latter being the typical situation in clinical use of topicals. Clinical signs and symptoms per se do not allow a clear-cut differentiation between irritant and allergic events or between events related to the active substance in a formulation or constituents of the vehicle. Thus, a more detailed evaluation depends on further testing, detailed case history, and so forth, combined with past experience as reported in the literature.

Irritants may be divided into corrosive and noncorrosive irritants, and into mild and strong irritants (1). Classification of irritation was recently reviewed including the role of modern bioengineering techniques such as evaporimetry with measurement of transepidermal water loss (TEWL) to characterize corrosiveness (2).

Irritation elicited by topicals is intuitively considered a single-component problem, which is a simplification. Substance penetration into skin strongly depends on the vehicle as a whole and its delivery of the active substance via a transepidermal or an adnexal route or both. Irritation may easily be elicited by two or more constituents creating clinical irritation by additive or synergistic effects. Additionally, the sensitivity of diseased and nondiseased skin may vary, and anatomical site, race, age, and sex are other individual-related variables contributing to the complexity of clinical irritation.

The sum of all these factors may or may not allow some characteristic clinical situations of known etiology to be defined.

In the present chapter the various clinical and experimental aspects of skin irritation elicited by D vitamins will be reviewed including guidance on how to handle problem cases. Systemic safety is covered in other chapters.

D VITAMINS: TYPE AND PROFILE OF IRRITANCY

Irritation elicited by D vitamins is dominated by redness. In patch test reactions elicited by 1,25-dihydroxy-D_3, calcipotriol, and the potent analogue KH1060, erythema and increase in redness by colorimetry and increase in cutaneous blood flow by laser Doppler flowmetry are prominent. Clinically doubtful and 1+ reactions are common, while edema, papules, and skin thickening noted on high-frequency ultrasonography is found only in the relatively few advanced reactions (3,4). TEWL is normally increased only in advanced reactions secondary to inflammation. It was demonstrated that the special ointment vehicle with propylene glycol and alkaline pH needed for D vitamins for stability reasons is itself slightly irritant and increases TEWL (14). Sodium laryl sulfate (SLS), the standard corrosive irritant, elicits much stronger reactions and markedly increased TEWL in comparison with calcipotriol, other D vitamins, and the ointment base. The irritant profile of D vitamins in human skin is dominated by vascular reactions and redness in contrast to normal TEWL and minor edema.

Thus, D vitamins are generally weak irritants of the noncorrosive type dominated by vascular reactions with erythema. This simple pattern of irritation following single application may, of course, be modified in various ways in practical use depending on other variables.

The profile of irritancy was found identical in hairless guinea pigs. Screening of a large number of different D-vitamin analogues in vitro and in vivo by the hairless guinea pig model indicates that irritation, as therapeutic efficacy, is not straightforwardly dependent on vitamin D–receptor affinity. There is an overall positive correlation between irritancy in the guinea pig, in vitro antiproliferative effect, and keratinocyte differentiation in cell culture systems, however, with exceptions. Vascular effects of irritation correlate with reactive epidermal hyperplasia response in experimental animals. 1.25-Dihydroxy-D_3, calcipotriol, and tacalcitol are equally irritant in hairless guinea pigs (5).

It is unclear whether irritation from D vitamins represents a separate mechanism of action or whether it shares a signaling pathway with the therapeutic response, i.e., the antipsoriatic effect. Skin penetration data obtained with a range of analogues and formulations and clinical data have, nevertheless, indicated that better permeation in vitro, better efficacy, and less irritation clinically are correlated and dependent on the formulation. A predominantly adnexal route of penetration and more direct access to the vasculature seem to be associated with both increased irritation and a poorer therapeutic outcome.

FREQUENCY OF IRRITATION DURING TOPICAL TREATMENT WITH D VITAMINS

Calcipotriol is, as already mentioned, the only analogue which has been extensively used and studied and which therefore may serve as a basis for conclusions (6). In 11 published studies from 1989 to 1995, skin irritation/total number of local adverse events were recorded in 4–25% of patients during short-term and long-term use; however, only 1–3.6% dropped out because of irritation (7). Irritation was typically noted in 10–15% of the patients in these detailed studies of the ointment formulation, conducted for registrational purposes. Irritation was mainly manifested as *lesional and perilesional irritation* (Fig. 1). Irritation typically appeared as cumulative irritation during the first 4–6 weeks of treatment.

However, these disciplined studies may not be realistic with regard to routine use in the clinic because the studies operate with fixed regimens, strict control, and registration of any kind of adverse event with little or no room for doctors' normal adjustment of treatment in cases with potential irritation and foreseeable increased risk.

A postmarketing surveillance study of 1664 patients conducted in Germany by 339 dermatologists showed 4.7% drug-related adverse events and efficacy results in accordance with the protocol studies (8). This incidence may be more universal. Nevertheless, since irritation depends on a number of individual related factors and medical practice, it is expected that the incidence will vary from country to country and from clinic to clinic.

INTRAPERSON VARIATION OF SENSITIVITY

Quite early it became clear that the face is especially vulnerable to irritation (Fig. 2). D vitamins, being lipophilic, are expected to penetrate the skin in this region via the adnexal route and target the vasculature, as was demonstrated for tacalcitol using microautoradiography (9). However, facial skin may also be especially sensitive to irritation because of the high density of microvessels in the skin serving for thermoregulation. The percutaneous absorption of cal-

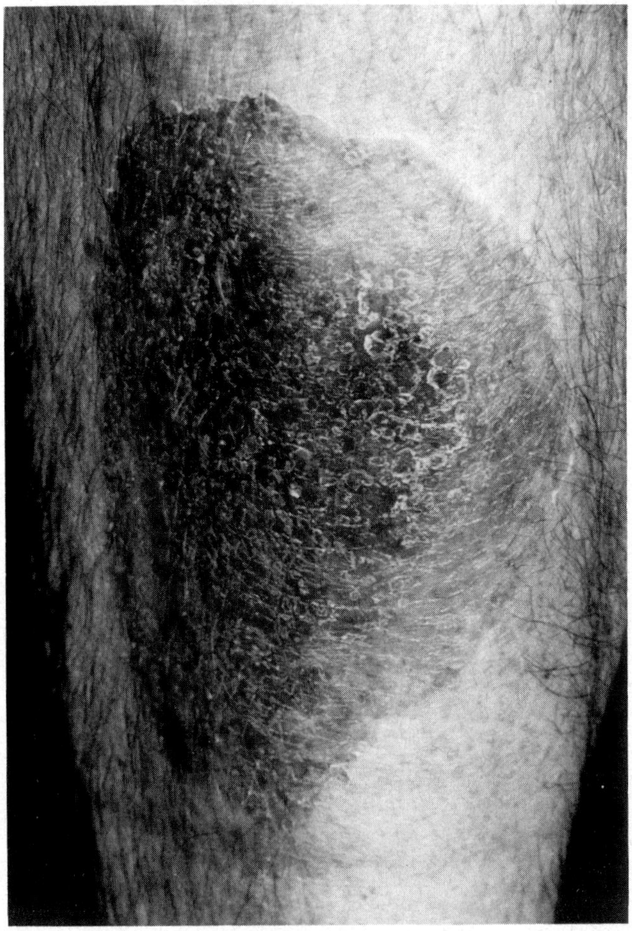

Figure 1 A case of lesional and perilesional irritation during vitamin D (calcipotriol) topical treatment.

cipotriol does not, however, appear increased on the scalp in comparison to truncal skin. Detailed information about D vitamins and their penetration in various anatomical sites is not available. Studies with radiolabeled calcipotriol have indicated a percutaneous absorption of 1–5% in truncal skin.

Calcipotriol and D vitamins are not expected to penetrate the nail plate in significant amounts because of protein binding by keratin and the hydrophilic character of the nail.

There appears to be a well-defined threshold of irritation in a given patient in a given body region simply because perilesional irritation is sharply demarcated, typically with a scaly demarcation line. Thus, it should be possible to lower the dose in a given patient to a level under this threshold of irritation. Study of radiolabeled calcipotriol has not indicated any difference in percutaneous absorption through plaque skin versus intact skin; however, such study does not automatically reflect intraepidermal drug levels, the drug-to-cell contact, or cellular responsiveness. The possible change in penetration of D vitamins and dermal distribution in a plaque during the course of healing, where the plaque successively undergoes a change from a relatively hydrophilic condition with increased TEWL to a more lipophilic stage, is unknown.

INTERPERSON VARIATION OF SENSITIVITY

Groups of healthy individuals, psoriatics never treated with D vitamins, psoriatics treated with calcipotriol with and without adverse dermatitis, and eczema patients show the same sensitivity to D-vitamin irritation when patch-tested with calcipotriol on the back (4). Doubtful and 1+ reactions are quite common irrespective of the group. Surprisingly, there was only a minor trend of patients with previous dermatitis to calcipotriol to react more strongly, and all groups showed overlap in reactivity and no difference versus healthy volunteers. There was no correlation with complexion or with skin type.

The various clinical studies with calcipotriol have indicated that the irritation is widely age independent; however, old skin may be more sensitive. It is possible that skin chronically exposed to sun, such as in the Mediterranean countries, is less sensitive to vitamin D irritation (10). This might be a result of sun-induced epidermal thickening. The various studies have indicated no influence of gender on sensitivity to vitamin D irritation. No study of racial difference in sensitivity has been published.

Thus, there is no definite predictor of risk of D-vitamin irritation except, possibly, past bad experience and old age.

SEVERE IRRITATION AND SUSPECTED ALLERGY

A few reports of severe cases of allergy to either calcipotriol or tacalcitol have appeared in the literature (11–16). Some of these patients were carefully evaluated with patch testing using dilution series in isopropanol, repeated testing after a period, repeat open application test, and by other means.

The diagnostic evaluation of suspected allergy is difficult because irritant patch test reactions to D vi-

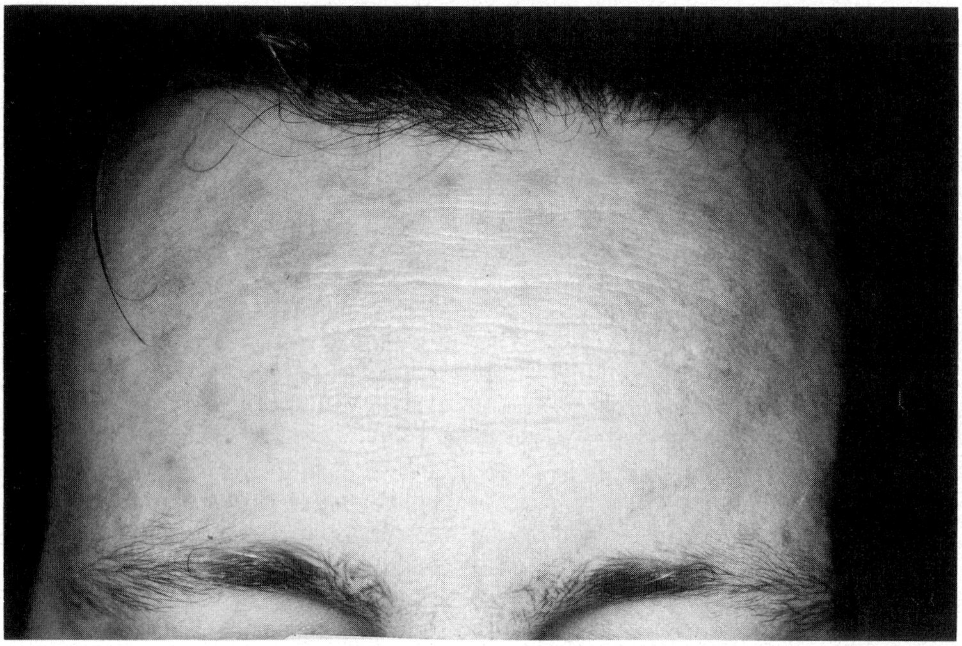

Figure 2 A case of facial irritation due to unintended transfer of calcipotriol to the face.

tamins are papular and even papulovesicular and may mimic positive allergic reactions, although the former may show a characteristic scaly demarcation on the day 7 reading. Those patients who develop a severe adverse dermatitis during treatment with a topical D vitamin may have a spontaneous or preexisting low threshold to irritation to D vitamins.

Allergy patch testing with the substance and the ointment vehicle is generally not recommended because the vehicle may itself be a mild irritant and create false positive readings or contribute to reactivity when occlusively applied. In a recent study 179 healthy volunteers never treated with topical D vitamins were patch-tested with a dilution series of calcipotriol from 50 to 0.016 μg/ml in isopropanol buffered to alkaline pH (17). Doubtful reactions were common and varied with concentration in a dose-dependent manner; however, 1+ reactions were found even at low doses. Only 2+ reactions showed a lower threshold of nonreactivity at 2 μg/ml confirmed by colorimetric measurement of redness and laser-Doppler scanning with measurement of cutaneous blood flow. The study indicated that allergy patch test in suspected cases of allergy to calcipotriol should be conducted with occlusive chambers (48 hr occlusion, 72 hr reading) with calcipotriol 2 μg/ml in isopropanol buffered to alkaline pH, and only 2+ reactions (marked erythema and moderate edema with papules and possibly vesicles) taken as indicative of allergic sensitization. Reading 1+ reactions as allergy would lead to a high percentage of false positive conclusions. Most of the case reports of allergy or possible allergy to D vitamins would not be concluded to be allergic according to the criteria resulting from the detailed study of 179 healthy individuals. Allergy patch testing with D vitamins is the classic problem of testing a local irritant where irritant reactions mimic allergic reactions. The patient's history may or may not be helpful because cumulative irritation will typically become manifest after a period of some weeks. In the testing of problem cases, a repeat open application test (antecubital skin, BID for 7 days) with the product and if possible with the vehicle may be helpful (18). In case of a positive patch test indicative of allergic sensitization, the test should always be repeated after a minimum of 3 months to establish that it is reproducible over time.

The testing mentioned is, of course, interesting only as an instrument to search the reason and mechanism behind the adverse dermatitis. Clinical manifestations, patient history, and a repeat open application test with the product used will normally suffice for the practicing dermatologist to decide whether a given patient can continue with or reapply a topical D vitamin. It is a general clinical experience that patients intolerant on some occasions may often tolerate calcipotriol later since aggravating factors seemingly have declined spontaneously in the meantime.

HOW TO HANDLE IRRITATION

Manifest Irritation (Table 1)

Patients with mild and potential irritation may interrupt treatment for a few days or a short period, and then the treatment typically can be reinstituted or used at a lower dose to create hardening (QD, weekend free, etc.) or meet with the patient's lower threshold at that particular period. The doctor should ensure the correct usage of the drug by the patient, including thin-layer application and hand washing after application.

In severe irritation and inflammation the topical D vitamin should be stopped and a topical corticosteroid instituted. Whether the topical D vitamin may be tried again after a period must depend on the precise history, the availability of alternative therapies, and so forth. As mentioned earlier, it is general experience that an individual's sensitivity to irritation varies over time (months), and treatment may easily be tolerated on a later occasion, following reassurance about correct use. Proper allergy testing should be conducted if allergic sensitization is in question.

Table 1 How to Handle Irritation During Topical D Vitamin Therapy

Manifest
1. Mild/potential
Pause
Thin-layer application
Reinstitute lower dose and create hardening (QD, weekends free, etc.)
Be sure of correct usage by patient
2. Severe
Pause
Topical corticosteroid
Prevention. There is no valid predictor of risk.
Inform patient
Ensure compliance
Hand wash after application
Corticosteroid combination possible

Prevention of Irritation (Table 1)

There is no valid predictor of risk or irritation except perhaps old age and past bad experience (see above). It is of course important to inform the patient about proper application to affected lesions only, in a thin layer and with hand washing after application to avoid unintended transfer to the face. Corticosteroid combination therapy from the start of therapy to lower the risk of irritation and possibly improve efficacy is possible. Studies of fixed combinations of calcipotriol and topical steroids have indicated a reduction in the incidence of irritation during such continuous combination. It has not been studied whether a regimen with calcipotriol 5 days a week and corticosteroids on the weekends has a lower irritation rate.

D VITAMINS, LIGHT, AND PHOTOSENSITIVITY

"Photosensitivity" is a poorly used term. Irritation may occur during combined topical treatment with D vitamin and light (PUVA and UVB) for several reasons:

1. *Phototoxicity.* The causative substance absorbs light and transfers the energy or reacts in the excited state with cellular components.
2. *Photoallergy.* Initiation as (1); however, reactions are mediated via an immune mechanism.
3. *Single or cumulative irritation due to the D vitamin* (chemical irritation).
4. *Single or cumulative irritation due to light* (burn).
5. *Trivial addition/synergy* of two irritants.
6. *Ointment/cream vehicle effects* with increase of absorbed light dose and subsequent burn.
7. *D-vitamin therapeutic effect with reduction of scaling* (a physical light filter) and subsequent burn.

D-vitamin compounds contain a conjugated triene system that is able to absorb ultraviolet light in the UVB and UVC range. Nevertheless, calcipotriol ointment recovered from the skin surface (by scraping with a wooden spatula) showed no degradation of the active substance following treatment with UVB while UVA resulted in a decrease of approximately 25% (19). The decrease in calcipotriol following UVA in the lower epidermis and at the basal cell layer is probably less because scattering and absorption of light in the outer epidermis. Suction blister studies and measurement of drugs in the blister fluid have not been performed. Calcipotriol is degraded in vitro to 5,6-*trans*-calcipotriol, which is known to be nontoxic and less biologically active than calcipotriol. The standard phototoxicity and photoallergy testing in humans required for registration purposes did not indicate phototoxicity or photoallergy problems related to calcipotriol. Calcipotriol and other D-vitamin products are not expected to have any sun-blocking or UVB-absorbing effect under realistic clinical use because of the very low concentration of the analogues in marketed creams and ointments (calcipotriol 0.005%, tacalcitol 0.0002–4%).

Clinical studies on calcipotriol in combination with UVB and PUVA did *not* indicate increased risk of adverse irritant dermatitis in comparison with the range of studies conducted on calcipotriol monotherapy, and no special risk of burn (20–22). The studies did not indicate a lower incidence of irritation if calcipotriol was applied after light. Postmarketing surveillance includes only a few reports of "photosensitivity" to calcipotriol despite the widespread use of this topical, and no special incidence in regions with much sun. Thus, neither experimental studies nor clinical research and practical experience indicate a general problem with phototoxicity/photoallergy of calcipotriol or other D-vitamin analogues albeit isolated cases of obscure nature might occur in widespread use and exposure of large groups of patients.

McKenna and Stern reported four cases of burn reactions occurring when calcipotriol was added to ongoing UVB therapy (23). Two patients continued the treatment after reduction of the UVB dose and tolerated the combination. It is likely that patients with recalcitrant psoriasis with unsatisfactory response to ongoing aggressive UVB may develop burn if calcipotriol is added without reducing the UVB dose (see schematic drawing, Fig. 3). As part of therapeutic efficacy the drug reduces scaling, which is a physical light filter, with the consequence that the absorbed UVB dose in the treated lesions increases.

Table 2 Calcipotriol and Light

Calcipotriol is neither phototoxic nor photoallergic in the strict sense
Light overdose may arise in recalcitrant patients already on light therapy if calcipotriol is added without reducing the light dose.

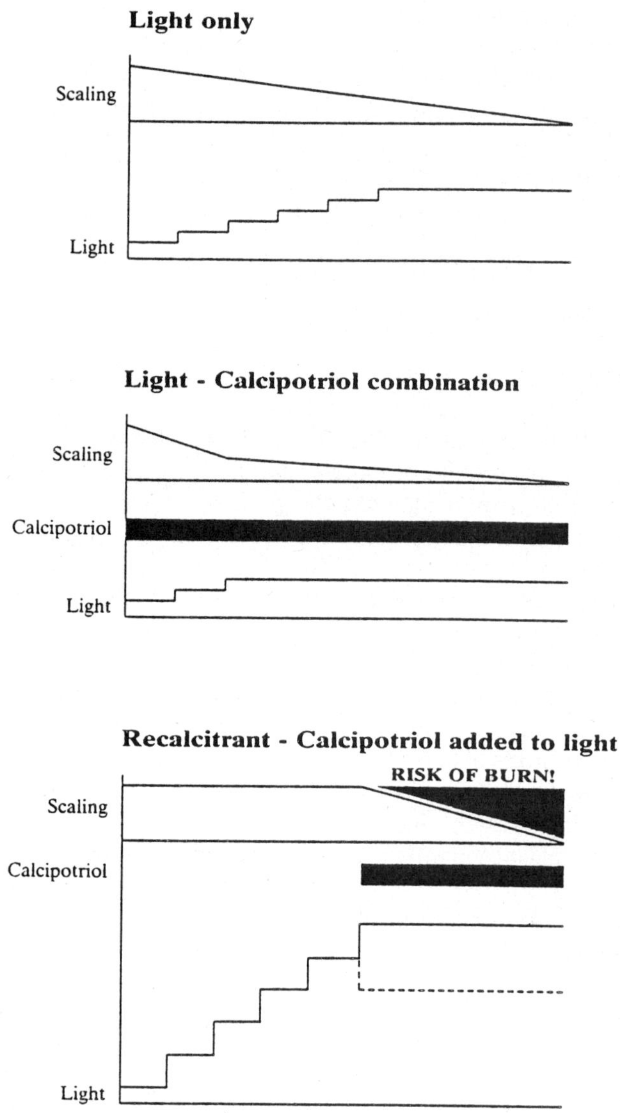

Figure 3 Phototherapy combined with topical vitamin D (calcipotriol) (22). Recalcitrant psoriasis on aggressive UVB may have a special risk of burn when topical vitamin D is added unless light dose is reduced.

Light therapy is practiced in different ways in different clinics and there is no universal standard of lamps and bulbs used. Light also has a risk of burn, which is difficult to control. The single most important factor in keeping the risk of adverse irritation and burn low in topical D-vitamin and light combination therapy seems to be that the topical is applied at a fixed time of day relative to the light exposure (either before or after) and at a constant dose so that the dose of light remains the only major treatment variable for the doctor to decide upon. As mentioned, recalcitrant patients already on aggressive UVB may have special risk of burn.

OCCLUSIVE TREATMENT WITH D-VITAMIN ANALOGUES AND IRRITATION

Patch test occlusion to healthy skin results in many doubtful reactions, some 1+ reactions, and a few 2+ reactions (4). Testing with small and large chambers shows similar results and the occluded area appears of no major importance to reactivity. Psoriasis plaque test with repeated applications during 1–2 weeks can be successfully performed with calcipotriol with no special risk of irritation. This could indicate that a plaque is in fact less sensitive to irritation. Studies with occlusive treatment of psoriasis plaques using either a hydrocolloid dressing or overnight application with a plastic film, using calcipotriol ointment, showed that such treatment is possible although the risk of irritation may be increased (24,25).

REFERENCES

1. Kligman, A.M. and Wooding, W.M. (1967). A method for the measurement and evaluation of irritants on human skin. *J. Invest Dermatol.* 49:78–94.
2. Serup, J. (1995). The spectrum of irritancy and applications of bioengineering techniques. In *Irritant Dermatitis.* P. Elsner and H.I. Maibach (Eds.). Karger, Basel, 1995, vol. 23, pp. 131–143.
3. Fullerton, A., and Serup, J. (1994). Characterization of irritant patch test reactions to 1.25 vitamin D_3 and the D-vitamin analogue calcipotriol. ESCD 2nd Congress, Barcelona, October 6–8 (abstract).
4. Fullerton, A., Avnstorp, D., Agner, T., Dahl, J.C., Olsen, L.O., and Serup, J. (1996). Patch test study with calcipotriol ointment in different patient groups, including psoriatic patients with and without adverse dermatitis. *Acta Derm. Venereol. (Stockh.)* 76: 194–202.
5. Fullerton, A., and Serup, J. (1996). Irritative potential of 1.25-dihydroxyvitamin D_3, 1.25-dihydroxyvitamin D_3 and calcipotriol studied in a guinea pig model. *J. Invest. Dermatol.* 1:112 (abstract).
6. Kragballe, K. (1994). Vitamin D and derivatives. In *Psoriasis.* L. Dubertret (Ed.). ISED, Brescia, pp. 123–134.
7. Berth-Jones, J. (1996) Calcipotriol in dermatology, a review and supplement. *Br. J. Clin. Pract.* 83:(Suppl.) 1–32.
8. Friedmann, D., Schnitker, J., and Schroeder, G. (1995). Efficacy and tolerability of calcipotriol ointment, proven in the course of a drug monitoring in 1664 patients. ESDR Symposium: Vitamin D, Actions and Applications in Dermatology, Århus, Denmark, April 27–29 (abstract).
9. Ohta, T., Okabe, D., Azuma, Y., and Kiyoki, M. (1996). In vivo microautoradiography of [^{3}H]1,24(OH)$_2$ D_3 (tacalcitol) following topical application to normal rats and in vitro metabolism in human keratinocytes. *Arch. Dermatol. Res.* 288:188–196.
10. Vilaplana, J., Mascaro, J.M., Lecha, M., and Romaguera, C. (1994). Low irritancy of 2-day occlusive patch test with calcipotriol. *Contact Derm.* 30:45.
11. Yip, J., and Goodfield, M. (1991). Contact dermatitis from MC903, a topical vitamin D_3 analogue. *Contact Derm.* 25:139.
12. Bruynzeel, D.P., Hol, C.W., and Nieboer, C. (1992). Allergic contact dermatitis to calcipotriol. *Br. J. Dermatol.* 127:66.
13. de Groot, A.C. (1994). Contact allergy to calcipotriol. *Contact Derm.* 30:242–243.
14. Steinkjaer, B. (1994). Contact dermatitis from calcipotriol. *Contact Derm.* 31:122.
15. Molin, L. (1996). Contact dermatitis after calcipotriol and patch test evaluation. *Acta Derm. Venereol. (Stockh.)* 76:163–164.
16. Kimura, K., Katayama, I., and Nishioka, K. (1995). Allergic contact dermatitis from tacalcitol. *Contact Derm.* 33:441–442.
17. Fullerton, A., Vejlstrup, E., Roed-Peterson, J., Jensen, S.B., and Serup, J. (1987). The calcipotriol dose-irritation relationship. 48-hour occlusive testing in healthy volunteers using Finn chambers. *Br. J. Dermatol.*, in press.
18. Hannuksela, M., and Salo, H. (1986). The repeated open application test (ROAT). *Contact Derm.* 14: 221–227.
19. Lebwohl, M., Martinez, J., Weber, P., and DeLuca, R. (1995). Effects of topical preparations on the erythemogenicity of UVB: Implications for psoriasis phototherapy. *J. Am. Acad. Dermatol.* 32:469–471.
20. Kragballe, D. (1990). Combination of topical calcipotriol (MC903) and UVB radiation for psoriasis vulgaris. *Dermatologica* 181:211–214.
21. Kokelj, F., Lavaroni, G., and Guadagnini, A. (1995). UVB plus calcipotriol (MC903) therapy for psoriasis vulgaris. *Acta Derm. Venereol. (Stockh.)* 75:386–387.
22. Frappaz, A., and Thivolet, J. (1993). Calcipotriol in combination with PUVAa: a randomized double blind placebo study in severe psoriasis. *Eur. J. Dermatol.* 3: 351–354.
23. McKenna, K.E., and Stern, R.S. (1995). Photosensitivity associated with combined UV-B and calcipotriene therapy. *Arch. Dermatol.* 131:1305–1307.

24. Nielsen, P.G. (1993). Calcipotriol or clobetasol propionate occluded with a hydrocolloid dressing for treatment of nummular psoriasis. *Acta Derm. Venereol. (Stockh.)* 73:394.

25. Bourke, J.F., Berth-Jones, J., and Hutchinson, P.E. (1993). Occlusion enhances the efficacy of topical calcipotriol in the treatment of psoriasis vulgaris. *Clin. Exp. Dermatol.* 18:504–506.

Part VI

PHOTOTHERAPY

40

UVB Phototherapy

Charles R. Taylor, Elissa J. Liebman, and Bernhard Ortel
Harvard Medical School and Massachusetts General Hospital, Boston, Massachusetts

Despite continued progress toward an elucidation of the genetic and pathophysiological pathways involved in psoriasis, a definitive cure remains elusive. Current treatments are aimed at amelioration of symptoms. Ultraviolet (UV) therapy, also known as "UVB phototherapy," is considered after failure of topical therapy or when disease covers at least 20% of body surface area. Generally, phototherapy treatments have two main phases, namely, "clearing," or those treatments designed to effect a remission, and "maintenance," or those treatments given after a patient clears in an effort to keep the patient clear.

We shall focus on the treatment of psoriasis in this chapter, but UVB phototherapy has numerous other dermatological applications. It is useful in the induction of tolerance for the idiopathic photodermatoses, especially polymorphous light eruption (PMLE) (1), and slightly less so for actinic prurigo, hydroa vacciniforme, chronic actinic dermatitis, and solar urticaria (2). It can also be used successfully for atopic dermatitis (3), pruritus (4), eosinophilic pustular folliculitis (5,6), pityriasis rosea (7), parapsoriasis, and HIV-associated pruritic papular eruption (8). These applications, however, will not be addressed here.

TREATMENT

Determination of Minimal Erythema Dose

UVB therapy usually commences with the determination of a safe initial dose of radiation. There are two ways to determine the starting level. The simplest method designates an initial dose according to the patient's skin type or phototype (9), namely, an assignment of patient sun sensitivity based on history (Table 1). Although this method is convenient, it is not highly recommended because skin type is not always a reliable predictor of actual photosensitivity. Therefore, this technique may lead to the use of inappropriate UVB doses, either too strong potentially causing burns or too weak possibly resulting in treatment failure.

The most highly regarded procedure for choosing initial UVB doses involves determination of the patient's minimal erythema dose (MED). The MED is obtained by using a piece of flexible plastic or self-adhesive aluminum foil with several holes cut into it. Often there are eight holes, each 1 cm^2. This template is preferentially placed on gluteal skin, which is usu-

Table 1 UVB Dosimetry According to Skin Type

Skin type	Skin response	Initial UVB dose (mJ/cm^2)
I	Always burn, never tan	10–20
II	Always burn, sometimes tan	20
III	Sometimes burn, always tan	30–40
IV	Never burn, always tan	40
V	Moderately pigmented	50–60
VI	Darkly pigmented	60

Source: Ref. 9.

ally the area of greatest UV sensitivity, and all other areas of the body are shielded from UVB. Each test site is exposed to an increasing dose of UVB, the range chosen according to the patient's skin type. Both arithmetic and geometric increments of irradiation may be employed for MED determination (Table 2). A geometric progression is preferred because it more accurately reflects the biological erythema response and covers a wider dose range. The patient is reexamined 24 hr later to assess the erythema reaction. The MED is defined as the lowest UVB dose that produces uniform pink erythema with distinct borders 24 hr after exposure. By knowing the MED, one can carefully choose a therapeutic starting dose according to the protocols described below, thus avoiding burns.

Therapeutic Regimens

After determination of the MED, patients continue treatment using a variety of protocols. To clear, a minimum of two treatments per week must be used. In the United States, so-called TIW (i.e., thrice weekly) and BIW (i.e., twice weekly) protocols using a broad-spectrum UVB source are common. Either protocol may be used as they are equally effective, requiring approximately 25 treatments to clear. Often social factors such as job and distance from the treatment center dictate which clearing protocol to follow. Generally, treatments are separated by at least 48 hr in the TIW protocol and 48–72 hr in the BIW schedule. One widely used TIW protocol (Table 3), sometimes referred to as the UVB3 protocol, begins at 80% of the MED. The second treatment delivers 100% of the MED in the first phase; patients then put on their undergarments, exposing only their arms and legs to an additional 10% of the MED. From the third treatment onward, the total body dose continues to escalate, but in incrementally smaller percentages. Extremities continue to receive incrementally larger percentages of additional exposures until 50% of the total body dose is reached. Because the face is exposed to daily UV radiation (UVR) and is often free of disease, most physicians shield it during treatment or limit its exposure to 40 mJ/cm^2 or less. Exceptions may be made for cases of scalp psoriasis extending onto the forehead.

Depending on how the patient reacts to the last treatment, the physician decides whether to increase the dose according to the protocol, hold the treatment at the previous level, or omit one treatment altogether. If the patient experienced no erythema from the last irradiation, the dose is increased to the next level. If the erythema is mild, nonpainful, and transient, the same dose is given again. If the erythema was painful, that treatment is omitted.

In BIW protocols, subsequent irradiations are also determined according to the severity and duration of

Table 2 Range of UVB Doses (in mJ/cm^2) for Determining MED

Skin type	Arithmetic	Geometric
I, II	5, 10, 15, 20, 25, 30, 35, 40	5, 7, 10, 14, 20, 28, 40, 56
III, IV	10, 20, 30, 40, 50, 60, 70, 80	7, 10, 14, 20, 28, 40, 56, 80
V, VI	30, 40, 50, 60, 70, 80, 90, 100	14, 20, 28, 40, 56, 80, 112, 160

Arithmetic rows use a fixed dose increase; geometric rows increase doses by a constant factor (e.g., $\sqrt{2}$).

Table 3 Typical UVB-TIW Treatment Protocol

Treatment number	Total body dose[a]	Additional exposure to extremities[b]
1	80% of MED	0
2	MED	10%
3	+50% of prior day	20%
4	+40%	30%
5	+30%	50%
6	+20%	50%
7	+19%	50%
8	+18%	50%
9	+17%	50%
10	+16%	50%
11–18	+15%	50%
19	+12%	50%
20	+10%	50%
21	+8%	50%
22	+6%	50%
23	+4%	50%
24	+2%	50%
25	0	50%

[a]UVA doses are increased according to this schedule if the latest exposure did not cause erythema. Increments from treatment 3 onward reflect a percentage increase over the last treatment. For example, the 4th treatment is 140% that of the 3rd treatment.
[b]Extremity doses are expressed as additional percentage of the total body dose given that same day.

erythema caused by the previous dose (Table 4). The first dose administered is a standard percentage of the MED, often 80%. Subsequent treatments are increased by 40%, 20%, or 0%. If the patient does not develop erythema, the dose is raised by 40%. If mild erythema is present for a few hours after treatment and resolves within 24 hr, the dose is raised by 20%. If the erythema was mild, but persistent at 24 hr, the previous dose is administered. However, if the patient's skin remains erythematous and sensitive, treatment is temporarily discontinued.

The possibility of daily UVB treatment exists because the peak of erythema is between 8 and 24 hr. In some American centers, daily irradiations are given to hospitalized patients. These protocols start at a specified fraction of the MED with daily increments of 17% as long as the previous treatment did not cause erythema.

When patients miss treatments due to illness or vacation, the chosen protocol is temporarily abandoned. A safe rule-of-thumb is to decrease the last dose by 10% for each UVB treatment missed. In practical terms, a patient coming 2–3 times per week who misses one week of therapy may be safely given a dose that is 25% less than the previous dose given. For 2 and 3 weeks missed, the decreases are 50% and 75%, respectively. Those who have missed a month of treatment usually need to restart the protocol from the beginning.

MAINTENANCE AND REMISSION

Maintenance

Maintenance philosophy varies around the world; moreover, the efficacy and requirements of maintenance are controversial. In Europe, many dermatologists avoid maintenance therapy, while in America some continue treatment for years after clearing. These differences may in part be related to insurance issues because it has become increasingly difficult to hospitalize patients with psoriasis in the United States and every effort is made to keep patients outside the hospital. It is generally felt that maintenance therapy keeps patients clear of disease.

Table 4 Typical UVB-BIW Protocol

Treatment number	No erythema[a]	Transient erythema[b]	Persistent erythema[c]
1–10	40%	20%	0%
11–20	30%	15%	0%
21+	20%	10%	0%

[a]If no erythema is present, increase dose by 40%.
[b]If erythema is present within a few hours after treatment and resolves within 24 hr, increase dose by 20%. However, if erythema is present within a few hours after treatment and stays for 24 hr, use the previous dose.
[c]If the skin is still erythematous and sensitive, defer treatment.

A few problems exist with maintenance UVB therapy. Treatment becomes time-consuming and interferes with the patient's quality of life. As more maintenance treatments are given, cumulative UVB doses rapidly increase, thus risking premature aging and photocarcinogenesis. Also, as the patient undergoes less frequent UVB exposure, tolerance is lost. Taylor and Stern found that 3 weeks after discontinuation of UVB therapy, tolerance fades to approximately half of the last UVB dose (10). Presumably, loss of skin pigmentation and stratum corneum thickening renders patients more susceptible to developing uncomfortable burns (10). Such problems may be overcome by switching patients to maintenance PUVA therapy, which may be given as seldom as once a month with fewer erythema problems as tolerance lasts much longer. More multicenter trials are necessary to quantify the long-term risks and answer questions about the role of maintenance therapy.

Maintenance therapy is instituted in a fairly standard way. Generally, once clear, patients decrease the frequency of UVB treatments while maintaining the last dose given at the time of clearing. If the patient had been on a TIW protocol, 1 month at BIW is usually given and then 1 month at QW, holding the final dose constant. Usually, UVB cannot be given any less than once a week as tolerance is lost rather rapidly and problems with burning arise. Depending on the patient's previous experience, the season of the year, social factors, and geographic factors, treatment may be discontinued.

Remission

In one study (11), the issue of remission time following UVB phototherapy was addressed. Those who received maintenance therapy experienced a statistically longer period of remission. The results of this study suggest that maintenance UVB phototherapy may be beneficial.

How long patients remain clear after discontinuing UVB therapy is quite variable. Other factors bearing on a flare are elusive. Furthermore, there is no good evidence that any one protocol is more successful than another for generating longer remissions. However, in comparison with PUVA, UVB seems slightly less likely to induce long-term remissions (12).

UVB TOXICITY

Acute Side Effects

The short-term problems patients are most likely to note include erythema of "sunburn," dry skin with pruritus, occasional phototoxic blisters, and an increased frequency of recurrent herpes labialis. Moderate painful erythema resulting from overexposure is treated with topical corticosteroids. Systemic nonsteroidal anti-inflammatory agents and corticosteroids have also proven useful for severe cases. Subacute effects such as pruritus and dry skin respond well to intensified lubrication with bland emollients after lukewarm baths.

Chronic Side Effects

Long-term phototherapy toxicities include photoaging and carcinogenesis. UVB is a known carcinogen in humans and animals; however, its carcinogenic potential seems to be less potent than that of PUVA therapy (13). Stern and Laird (14) conducted a 13-year study of 1380 patients with psoriasis who had a history of either treatment with PUVA or both PUVA and prior UVB phototherapy. This study failed to show a relationship between UVB phototherapy and nonmelanoma skin cancer. However, the authors strongly caution that future studies may reveal an increased risk of nonmelanoma skin cancer with UVB phototherapy.

In 1990, Stern (15) also examined the relationship between men treated with PUVA and UVB phototherapy and subsequent development of cutaneous tumors in the genital area. The study examined 892 men over a 12-year period and found that patients using UVB radiation had a 4.6 times higher risk of developing tumors in genital skin. Therefore, male patients should always shield their genital area during UV exposure (15).

UVB ACTION SPECTRUM

General Principles

The action spectrum describes the efficacy of a radiation-induced process as a function of wavelength (16). In terms of irradiating psoriatic skin, the therapeutic efficacy has been compared with the erythemogenic potential of ultraviolet radiation. Below 290 nm the erythemogenic potential is much higher than any antipsoriatic effect. Between 295 and 365 nm the action spectrum for erythema induction and therapeutic efficacy in psoriasis are very similar. This action spectrum is well covered by the emission of standard UVB fluorescence sources, which emit between 295 and 350 nm with a peak at 305 nm. In the UVA range, erythemogenic doses are also therapeutically relevant, but such doses are 1000 times higher than in UVB phototherapy and therefore not practical without psoralen sensitization.

Narrow-Band Phototherapy

It has been shown (16,17) that wavelengths around 305–315 nm are most efficient for clearing psoriasis. To remove shorter wavelengths, which are relatively more erythemogenic than therapeutic, radiation sources are chosen that eliminate wavelengths below 295 nm. One approach has been use of the so-called selective UV phototherapy (SUP), which uses the spectrum of a high-pressure mercury lamp that has additional emission peaks between 295 and 330 nm (18). However, a half-sided comparison with PUVA demonstrated superiority of the latter (19). A more recent successful development is the availability of a narrow-band UVB fluorescent tube (Philips TL-01), which emits a high, distinct peak at 311–312 nm with minor spikes at 304 and 334 nm. Several recent studies (20,21) show that the TL-01 source is superior to broad-band UVB for clearing psoriasis. Both SUP and narrow-band UVB are currently used as loose synonyms for the TL-01 lamp. Narrow-band phototherapy has a higher ratio of therapeutic to erythemogenic activity, resulting in increased efficacy, reduced incidence of burning, and longer remissions (17,20). However, if the same number of bulbs per box is used, the new system requires twice the irradiation time compared to the broad-band tubes, resulting in more inconvenience to patient, technician, and treatment center. Adding more bulbs to each treatment cubicle overcomes this problem, but creates problems with additional heat production and increased need for ventilation systems (22). Currently, 100-W tubes are available that allow the phototherapist to deliver narrow-band UVB treatments in irradiation times comparable to those of traditional, broad-band UVB.

In 1988, van Weelden et al. (23) compared TL-01 with TL-12 bulbs in a paired study of 10 psoriatic patients. The new lamp was found to be therapeutically superior in nine of the 10 patients. In 1992, Picot et al. (21) conducted a left-right comparative study of 15 patients with symmetrical psoriasis. The patients were treated 3 times a week with both lamps; one lamp was used on one side of the body and one lamp was used on the other. In a randomized, double-blind fashion, the investigators determined the percentage response of the psoriatic plaques on the 10th and 20th exposure. By the 10th treatment, they found no significant difference between the two sides; however, by the 20th treatment, the psoriasis cleared to a greater extent with the TL-01 bulbs. In addition, they noted more frequent episodes of burning with the broad-spectrum lamps than with the narrow-spectrum tubes. While the endpoints used in this study are subject to question, namely comparison of progress by treatment number, as opposed to number of treatments to clear, distinct narrow-band UVB advantages prevailed. A 1990 study by van Weelden et al. (24) compared narrow-band UVB phototherapy to PUVA photochemotherapy using oral 8-MOP in 10 patients. That study concluded that BIW narrow-band UVB phototherapy and PUVA photochemotherapy are equally effective.

Currently, narrow-band phototherapy is used primarily in Europe. The treatment protocol is very similar to the schedules used for broad-spectrum UVB. For example, treatments begin at 70–80% of the patient's MED. Doses are increased by 40% if there is no erythema present from the previous treatment and 20% if there is slight erythema. If there is more than slight erythema, but no painful burn, the same dose is given as for the last treatment. If there is a mild burn, the dose is decreased by 50%, while for a severe burn, one dose is omitted (20). Treatment schedules vary between 3 and 5 times a week.

Recently, four cases of unusual blistering occurred with narrow-band UVB phototherapy (25). Two asymptomatic and two painful episodes of blistering developed at the site of psoriatic lesions in the middle of a treatment course. These blisters are different from those that develop during PUVA therapy after minor trauma because they lack erythema, resolve spontaneously, and occur only on treated psoriatic plaques rather than on normal skin.

Controversy exists as to the relative carcinogenicity of the narrow-band versus broad-band UVB treatment. Van Weelden et al. (23) conducted a study with albino hairless mice examining the tumor induction times for the TL-12 broad-band bulbs compared to the TL-01 narrow band ones on the basis of equal acute responses. The mice were irradiated every day and the experiments were stopped when most of the tumors were larger than 4 mm. They found that narrow-band phototherapy resulted in longer induction times for tumors smaller than 1 mm. In contrast, for larger tumors there was no difference in induction times between the two systems. Two studies (26,27) showed the risk with TL-01 is probably greater. Since each study used different mouse models, irradiation regimens, starting doses, and endpoints, no definitive conclusion can be drawn yet. Because the erythema action spectrum is believed to parallel the one for carcinogenesis, one might suspect TL-01 bulbs to be less carcinogenic because less erythemogenic wavelengths are involved.

Like broad-band UVB, narrow-band UVB phototherapy has other dermatological applications besides psoriasis. It may also be used to treat photodermatoses and atopic dermatitis. Additional applications will likely occur in the future.

LIGHT SOURCES

Metal Halide Lamps

Two types of UVB light sources are used for the treatment of psoriasis: high-pressure metal halide lamps and fluorescent bulbs. Hot quartz lamps were frequently used during the beginning of UVB phototherapy, but have fallen out of favor owing to their excessive production of ozone and heat. Metal halide lamps gained popularity over the hot quartz lamps primarily because of their ability to provide a more continuous UVR spectrum, which may be achieved by using the same source with long-pass filters to deliver UVA, UVB, or both. However, these lamps are basically point sources and need good paraboloid reflectors to provide even dose distribution for larger areas. For whole-body irradiation, lamps need to be stacked in columns or be evenly distributed over a bed. With metal halide sources, both heat and ozone production require special ventilation. However, most of the sources have recently become available as ozone-free lamps.

Fluorescent Lamps

Today, fluorescent lamps are the most commonly used light source for UVB phototherapy. The bulbs are composed of a low-pressure mercury discharge source within a thin glass tube coated with a phosphor. The spectral emission depends on the phosphor coating, which absorbs 254-nm radiation emitted from the low-pressure mercury vapor. Once excited, the phosphor reemits energy at a longer wavelength as fluorescence. Therapeutic lamps are sold as 2-, 4-, and 6-ft-long tubes. The longer the bulb, the higher its intensity. UVB lamps generally emit a continuous spectrum of UVR throughout UVB (280–320 nm) extending into UVA (320–400 nm), thus covering the therapeutic action spectrum for psoriasis. Typically, broad-band UVB bulbs emit approximately 60% of their output in UVB and 40% in UVA. The narrow-band fluorescent tube Philips TL-01 has been discussed in detail above.

Fluorescent lamps have gained favor among dermatologists for UVB phototherapy because they are relatively inexpensive, very effective, and cover a large field size with low heat production. They can be mounted either as open banks or as enclosed cabinets. One disadvantage is that with time the fluorescent intensity and spectral distribution of the lamps change. After 500 hr of use, the lamps produce only 70–80% of their original output and must be replaced after approximately 1000 hr (28). In addition, the ends of each bulb emit 10–30% less radiation than the central portion. This difference may cause problems in treating the distal portion of the lower extremities and the upper torso or head, if exposed, in tall individuals.

Heliotherapy

Heliotherapy refers to the use of the sun in the treatment of skin disease. The sun is the oldest source of UVB and it works well for the treatment of psoriasis if used carefully and correctly, but it is unpredictable. Generally, the climatic conditions in moderate zones limit the therapeutic exposures to summer months. In subtropical and tropical areas, solar exposure is more plentiful, but social conditions generally restrict total body exposure. The Dead Sea is a popular location for heliotherapy of psoriasis and other dermatoses. Since it is below sea level, mostly longer wavelengths reach the ground while shorter wavelengths are dissipated (29–32). The diminution of the shorter UVB wavelengths results in an improved fit of the solar spectrum to the therapeutic action spectrum. In addition, patients soak in sea water, which helps remove UV-absorbing substances from the skin and thus increases the effectiveness of heliotherapy. Rest and relaxation likely contribute to the treatment's success. On the other hand, the sudden withdrawal of such combined benefits once the patient departs from the Dead Sea may predispose to early relapses.

Home UVB Therapy

For the highly motivated, intelligent, and responsible patient who is unable to make regular visits to a qualified treatment center, the physician may consider making a home UVB panel available. In some countries, this arrangement can only be done by prescription. With proper documentation, some insurance companies will pay for a home panel because, although expensive, in the long run it is more economical. Because only a single panel of four 6-ft-long bulbs is typically provided, the patient has to expose front and back sequentially, and occasionally the sides when the disease is extensive. This inconvenience is further aggravated by the comparatively lower intensity of just four bulbs. Consequently, exposure times are long. Patients are usually treated according to an incrementally increased protocol based on time. Some units have safety features so that patients cannot treat themselves without regular supervision. Generally, treatments are given daily. After a specified number of exposures, some units do not operate until the patient sees the physician again for an assessment. If indicated, the physician will provide the patient with a code number or key for reactivation of the radiation source. Giving a patient access to a home unit is potentially a prescription for unsupervised therapy with risks to patient and doctor alike. Informed consent and careful follow-up are essential.

Dosimetry

Dosimetry is essential to deliver the correct amount of UV exposure. This is especially important when using fluorescent bulbs because of their shorter life. Radiometers are used to measure the amount of UV emitted from each phototherapy unit. They have specific spectral sensitivity and this should be matched with the radiation source. The following formula is used to determine the amount of time for UV exposure.

$$\frac{\text{Dose desired (mJ/cm}^2\text{)}}{\text{Output measured (mW/cm}^2\text{)}} = \text{time (sec)}$$

Many units have built-in radiometers and electronically regulate exposure times on-line according to the actual measured output.

ADJUNCTIVE AGENTS

Tar

Both adjunctive and combination strategies are directed at an accelerated clearing phase and a reduced cumulative UVB exposure. UVB can often clear psoriasis more effectively if it is used with a topical agent. The oldest adjunctive agent is tar. In 1925, Goeckerman began using crude coal tar to enhance the beneficial effects of UV irradiation (33,34). Currently, tar is seldom used in the United States. Patients dislike it because it is messy, stains skin, clothing, and bathtubs, and has an unpleasant odor. Consequently, dermatologists have turned to other adjunctive agents to enhance UVB phototherapy.

Emollients

Emollients have become a popular alternative to tar. In some studies they have proven equally effective (35) and are better tolerated by patients. Recently, a single-blind, controlled study (36) looked at patients with stable plaque psoriasis. Patients were treated unilaterally with a lubricating base prior to UVB while they received UVB exposure alone on the other side. Higher improvement rates occurred on the sides treated with the lubricating base.

However, not all lubricating bases are beneficial in phototherapy. Lebwohl et al. (37) demonstrated that tars and salicylic acid may absorb UVB if they are not thoroughly removed before phototherapy. Thick applications of petrolatum and emollient creams can also reduce UVB penetration. However, clear liquid emollients and mineral oil can be used effectively in conjunction with phototherapy. Controversy exists over the use of coconut oil as a lubricating base. Although coconut oil does not significantly absorb UVB or UVA and does not affect minimal erythema or minimal phototoxic doses, it does not enhance the efficacy of narrow-band UVB or PUVA therapy (38). Further studies are needed to explore this issue fully.

Anthralin

Anthralin is also used as a topical adjunct in UVB phototherapy. Widely used in Europe and less so in the United States, it has received mixed reviews in the literature. Some studies (39) advocate its use in conjunction with broad-band UVB. In contrast, others do not believe its use is worthwhile (40,41). However, it has recently proved quite effective in combination with narrow-band UVB phototherapy (42).

Corticosteroids

Topical corticosteroids are sometimes used in conjunction with phototherapy. They are most beneficial when used to treat the early symptomatic stages of psoriasis. Studies (43,44) have shown that steroids used together with UVB cause an initial rapid improvement of the disease. However, the effect plateaus, and by the time of clearing, there is no difference between plaques treated with steroids and UVB and those treated with UVB alone. Combinations of UVB with corticosteroids may actually produce unstable clearing and mislead the therapist into initiating the maintenance phase prematurely, resulting in early relapse (43,44). Hence, they do not seem to make major contributions to the phototherapy of psoriasis. Generally, their use is discouraged.

Calcipotriene

Calcipotriene (45,46) is a synthetic vitamin D analog that has been used in the United States to treat psoriasis since 1994. It can be used alone or in combination with UVB phototherapy or PUVA. A 1995 study by Kokelj et al. (47) compared UVB to UVB plus calcipotriene in an open right-left comparison study with 4 weeks of treatment. Nearly 90% of the patients had greater improvement of those psoriatic plaques treated with UVB plus topical calcipotriene than those treated with UVB alone.

Lesional or perilesional irritation is the most common side effect of calcipotriene therapy. Four reactions involving burning and blistering have been reported with this treatment (48). Therefore, it has been suggested that calcipotriene plus UVB be used with caution (48). Vitamin D analogs have also been used successfully with narrow-band TL-01 bulbs, with the combination proving more effective than the topical therapy alone (49).

Soaks

Some treatment centers have their patients take a warm water bath prior to UVB therapy. This primarily serves to hydrate the skin and to loosen psoriatic plaques. However, Momtaz et al. (50) reported that soaks may result in a change in the optical properties of the stratum corneum and cause the skin to be more sensitive to UVB. Therefore, lower doses of UVB may be required for clearing. Nevertheless, the magnitude of the resultant benefit is not justified if considerable effort has to be expended to do the soaks prior to UVB exposure.

COMBINATION THERAPIES

UVB plus Psoralen Photochemotherapy

UVB is frequently combined with a number of different therapies such as PUVA, methotrexate, and retinoids. The advantage of utilizing such combinations is to reduce the patient's long-term cumulative UV exposure. The combination of UVB and PUVA has been shown to be very effective (51). Momtaz and Parrish (51) studied 11 patients with papular and/or plaque-type psoriasis involving at least 25% of their body surface area. They treated the patients three times a week with both UVA and UVB 2 hr after the oral administration of 0.6 mg/kg of 8-MOP. All of the patients cleared after five to 20 treatments.

A more recent 1993 (52) study compared the effects of narrow-band UVB monotherapy versus narrow-band UVB plus PUVA in a small group of patients. Ninety percent experienced clearing more rapidly with combination therapy. However, although UVB/PUVA combination therapy reduces cumulative doses of either irradiation alone, the carcinogenic potential of treatments combining UVB and PUVA is not clear.

Methotrexate

A combination of methotrexate and UVB therapy has proven effective in patients with severe disease (53). It is beneficial because the combined use of methotrexate and UVB reduces the peak UVB dose at clearing and thus the maintenance dose; hence, there is reduced cumulative UVB exposure. However, an increased carcinogenic hazard of the UVB/MTX combination also has to be considered.

Treatments begin with 3 weeks of oral methotrexate, which is then integrated with standard UVB phototherapy. After clearing, both the UVB frequency and methotrexate doses are slowly tapered. Eventually, the methotrexate is discontinued and the UVB is used as maintenance therapy.

Retinoids

Systemic retinoids may also be used in conjunction with UVB phototherapy. Etretinate was formerly the drug of choice. Recently, acitretin, a major metabolite of etretinate, has become available in Europe and was FDA-approved in 1996. This drug is preferred because it has the same therapeutic profile as etretinate, but its half-life is 50 hr compared to 100 days for etretinate (54). A 1991 study (55) found that patients treated with acitretin plus UVB experienced faster clearing than those treated with UVB alone. Extreme caution must be used in women of childbearing age because of the high teratogenic potential of retinoids. In addition, retinoids can cause mucocutaneous toxicity, hyperlipidemia, and abnormal liver function tests (55). Besides the favorable therapeutic effect of this combination, retinoids have an apparent cancer-protective effect, which may reduce the long-term carcinogenic potential of UVB even more than by just reducing cumulative UVB exposures.

MECHANISMS

While most of the UVB is absorbed by the epidermis, some penetrates to the papillary dermis. When nucleic acids and certain amino acids absorb UVB, they become electronically excited and may engage in photochemical reactions such as photobinding, photocrosslinking or photoxidization (56). Clearly, UVB exposure induces nucleic acid photoproducts, especially pyrimidine dimers. In the stratum corneum, *trans*-urocanic acid absorbs UVB and isomerizes to the *cis* form. Although these photochemical reactions occur within fractions of seconds, the biological consequences may not become apparent until years later. Moreover, UVB-induced events occur in both the epidermis and dermis, potentially affecting a multitude of cells such as keratinocytes, Langerhans cells, endothelial cells, mast cells, and lymphocytes. Consequently, the biological effects of UVB-induced reactions are quite complicated and not completely understood.

UVB exposure is known to cause a reduction of DNA synthesis (57,58). Therefore, it can be used to suppress the accelerated DNA synthesis found in psoriatic epidermal cells. A more detailed explanation of how UVB and UVB-induced DNA damage interfere with cell division has recently been developed. The tumor suppressor gene product p53 has been demonstrated to be up-regulated after UVB exposure. It is involved in control of the cell cycle via regulation of the WAF 1/CIP 1 gene (59). This mechanism may be relevant for the reversal of the shortened cell cycle in keratinocytes of psoriatic epidermis. The UVB-induced alteration of cell cycle control mechanisms is also important for apoptosis, which is seen in skin after UVB exposure ("sunburn cells"), and the control of skin carcinogenesis (60).

Well established in both the murine and human systems, immunosuppression by UVB is relevant in skin photocarcinogenesis and in the clearing of psoriasis (61). There is some controversy about whether *cis*-urocanic acid or DNA is involved in these immunosuppressive effects of UVB. However, important mediators are felt to be the epidermal-derived cytokines interleukin (IL)-10 and IL-4 (62). UVB exposure has also been shown to alter the expression and excretion of a number of cytokines, namely IL-1, IL-4, IL-6, IL-8, IL-10, granulocyte-macrophage colony-stimulating factor (GM-CSF), and tumor necrosis factor-alpha (TNF-α) (61). Altered expression of cytokine and growth factor receptors has also been demonstrated in psoriatic epidermis. The interaction of epidermal keratinocytes and infiltrating activated lymphocytes seems to play an important role in active psoriatic lesions and cytokines mediate some of these interactions. UVB exposure likely modulates cytokine patterns, thus conceivably altering such interactions and interfering with pathophysiological pathways.

The involvement of arachidonic acid, prostaglandins, and histamine in the development of UVB-induced skin erythema has also been demonstrated (63). The suppression of cyclooxygenase has been found to reduce UVB-induced erythema. However, the release of arachidonic acid products may also be a consequence of cytokine activation (64).

Finally, cellular-molecular signaling events have been described after UVR exposure in vitro. For example, UVR has been shown to induce tyrosine phosphorylation of the epidermal growth factor receptor (65). Additional cellular signaling pathways that activate transcription factors upon UVR exposure have been identified (66). Some of the pathways are shared by stress response events and may be involved in the activation of protective cellular mechanisms. One important aspect of these UVR effects is that they are independent of DNA damage and even are activated cells without nuclei (67).

Our increased knowledge of the reaction patterns in psoriasis on the molecular level has opened new approaches to understanding how UVB affects psoriatic skin lesions. The primary target may still be the nuclear DNA in epidermal keratinocytes and endothelial and/or infiltrating leukocytes. The secret of successful phototherapy may lie in the repeated controlled UVB-induced release of prostaglandins, leukotrienes, and cytokines that modulate the altered interactions between epidermal cells and leukocytes. The improved understanding of cell cycle control by p53 suggests a sophisticated DNA damage-dependent mechanism regulating keratinocyte balance between apoptotic death, survival, and carcinogenesis. Antipsoriatic effects secondary to UVB immunomodulation, urocanic acid isomerization, or DNA damage-independent transcriptional activation are all possible therapeutic mechanisms, but the complex interplay is far from being understood.

In summary, our current knowledge about both the mechanisms involved in the pathogenesis of psoriasis and about UVB photobiology allows more opportunity for speculation. However, the precise mechanisms by which repeated UVB exposure leads to clearing of psoriatic skin await clarification.

UVB PHOTOTHERAPY AND HIV DISEASE

In 1985 the first patient with AIDS and psoriasis was reported (68). The relationship between the two diseases has been well documented in the literature of the last decade. However, it is still unknown if psoriasis is more frequent among HIV-infected individuals than in the general population. The two diseases have a paradoxical relationship because HIV results in immunosuppression and psoriasis usually resolves with immunosuppressive treatments (69). HIV's effect on the immune system may trigger the exacerbation or onset of psoriasis. HIV infects and depletes CD4+ helper T cells and epidermal Langerhans cells (70,71). The virus infects, but does not necessarily kill, the cells. It is able to alter the cell's gene expression patterns and cause abnormalities in the growth or function of the cell (70). It is known that HIV causes dysregulation of both cellular and humoral immunity, disturbing the delicate balance of cytokines. This disruption of cytokine pattern is currently believed to trigger psoriasis (72). Occasionally, the psoriasis of patients with very low CD4 counts spontaneously resolves, possibly because of the AIDS patient's inability to produce the cytokines needed for epidermal hyperproliferation. Such a phenomenon is seen in other terminally ill patients as well.

Psoriasis in HIV-infected individuals usually resists treatment with standard therapies such as topical steroids. Often UVB phototherapy or PUVA has to be employed to help these patients. Controversy exists over the safety of such treatments in immunosuppressed patients. In 1988, Valerie et al. (73) reported that 254 nm UVR or sunlight was capable of inducing the HIV promoter (73,74). Later, Morrey et al. (75) used transgenic mice to show activation of the HIV-1 long terminal repeat (LTR) by both UVB and PUVA.

Clinically, HIV patients seem to do well with UV therapy in spite of these data. Meola et al. (76) examined five HIV-infected individuals with psoriasis and one with pruritus prior to and after UVB treatments. CD4+ counts, CD4+/CD8+ ratios, β_2-microglobulin, and HIV-1 p24 antigen concentrations were quantified to monitor the effects of phototherapy. After 21 and 42 treatments, there were no statistically significant changes in the laboratory data. In addition, all patients improved without developing opportunistic infections or malignancies. Long-term studies are needed to evaluate further the risk/benefit ratio of phototherapy in HIV-infected patients.

UVB phototherapy has numerous dermatological therapeutic applications besides psoriasis in the HIV-infected population. A common chronic dermatosis of the HIV population, pruritic papular eruption (PPE), is characterized by chronic pruritus and a widespread eruption. Because the itching is so intense, excoriations, prurigo-like nodules, and postinflammatory hyperpigmentation ensue. Pardo et al. (8) reported that TIW phototherapy is effective in decreasing the pruritis, papules, and dermal inflammation. There was no significant alteration in the patient's systemic immune status except a minor local effect expressed as a decrease in the number of infiltrating T lymphocytes in treated areas (8).

Eosinophilic pustular folliculitis (EPF) is another HIV-related dermatological disorder that may be confused with PPE. While PPE and EPF are similar histologically, the former is characterized by papules and pustules that coalesce to form polycyclic plaques. Buchness et al. (6) reported six cases of AIDS-associated EPF that responded to UVB phototherapy.

FUTURE UVB THERAPY

Future UVB therapy will likely be geared toward increasing the effectiveness and decreasing the side effects of UVR. Physicians will begin to decrease the total treatment number, reduce the amount of superfluous radiation exposure, and narrow the UVB wavelengths to the most beneficial ones. Treatments that are more selective for the involved skin will likely evolve. One possibility involves applying high-potency substantive sunscreen, which is more adherent to uninvolved skin than psoriatic skin, prior to UVB exposures. Conceivably, such an approach should lessen harmful side effects. Another possible development in UVB therapy may be the incorporation of an oral medication into current protocols. If such a drug were highly selective for hyperproliferating epidermal tissue, UVB radiation might be more selectively geared toward the psoriatic skin, resulting in a form of "photodynamic UVB therapy." With further research, UVB phototherapy will undoubtedly become safer and provide psoriasis patients with longer-lasting benefits for a shorter time investment.

REFERENCES

1. Addo, H.A., and Sharma, S.C. (1987). UVB phototherapy and photochemotherapy (PUVA) in the treatment of polymorphic light eruption and solar urticaria. *Br. J. Dermatol.* 116:539–547.
2. Keahey, T.M., Lavker, R.M., Kaidbey, K.H., Atkins, P.C., and Zweiman, B. (1984). Studies on the mechanism of clinical tolerance in solar urticaria. *Br. J. Dermatol.* 110:327–338.
3. Jekler, J., and Larkö, O. (1990). Combined UVA-UVB phototherapy for atopic dermatitis: a paired-comparison study. *J. Am. Acad. Dermatol.* 22:49–53.
4. Gilchrest, B.A., Rowe, J.W., Brown, R.S., Steinman, T.I., and Arndt, K.A. (1979). Ultraviolet phototherapy of uremic pruritus: long-term results and possible mechanisms of action. *Ann. Intern. Med.* 91:17–21.
5. Porneuf, M., Guillot, B., Barneon, G., and Guilhou, J.J. (1993). Eosinophilic pustular folliculitis responding to UVB therapy. *J. Am. Acad. Dermatol.* 29:259–260.
6. Buchness, M.R., Lim, H.W., Hatcher, V.A., Sanchez, M., and Soter, N.A. (1987). Eosinophilic pustular folliculitis in the acquired immunodeficiency syndrome. Treatment with ultraviolet B phototherapy. *N. Engl. J. Med.* 318:1183–1186.
7. Arndt, K.A., Paul, B.S., Stern, R.S., and Parrish, J.A. (1983). Treatment of pityriasis rosea with UV radiation. *Arch. Dermatol.* 119:381–382.
8. Pardo, R.J., Bogaert, M.A., Penneys, N.S., Byrne, G.E., and Ruiz, P. (1992). UVB phototherapy of the pruritic papular eruption of the acquired immunodeficiency syndrome. *J. Am. Acad. Dermatol.* 26:423–428.
9. Fitzpatrick, T.B. (1975). Soleil et Peau. *J. Med. Esth.* 2:33–34.
10. Taylor, C.R., and Stern, R.S. (1991). Magnitude and duration of UV-B induced tolerance. *Arch. Dermatol.* 127:673–677.
11. Stern, R.S., Armstrong, R.B., Anderson, T.F., Bickers, D.R., Lowe, N.J., Harber, L., Voorhees, J., and Parrish, J.A. (1986). Effect of continued ultraviolet B phototherapy on the duration of remission of psoriasis: a

randomized study. *J. Am. Acad. Dermatol.* 15:546–522.
12. Hönigsmann, H., Calzavara-Pinton, P.G., and Ortel, B. (1994). Phototherapy and photochemotherapy. In *Psoriasis.* L. Dubertret (Ed.). ISED, Brescia, Italy, pp. 135–150.
13. Studniberg, H.M., and Weller, P. (1993). PUVA, UVB, psoriasis, and nonmelanoma skin cancer. *J. Am. Acad. Dermatol.* 29:1013–1022.
14. Stern, R.S., and Laird, N. (1994). The carcinogenic risk of treatments for severe psoriasis. *Cancer* 73: 2759–2764.
15. Stern, R.S. (1990). Genital tumors among men with psoriasis exposed to psoralens and ultraviolet A radiation (PUVA) and ultraviolet B radiation. *N. Engl. J. Med.* 322:1093–1097.
16. Parrish, J.A., and Jaenicke, K.F. (1981). Action spectrum for phototherapy of psoriasis. *J. Invest. Dermatol.* 76:359–362.
17. Fisher, T., Alsins, J., and Berne, B. (1984). Ultraviolet action spectrum and evaluation of ultraviolet lamps for psoriasis healing. *Int. J. Dermatol.* 23:633–637.
18. Steigleder, G.K., Orfanos, C.E., and Pullman, H. (1979). Retinoid-SUP-Therapie de Psoriasis. *Z. Hautkr.* 54:19–23.
19. Hönigsmann, H., Fritsch, P., and Jaschke, E. (1977). UV-Therapie der Psoriasis. Halbseitenvergleich zwischen oraler Photochemotherapie (PUVA) und selektiver UV-Phototherapie (SUP). *Z. Hautkr.* 52: 1078–1082.
20. Green, C., Ferguson, J., Lakshmipathi, T., and Johnson, B.E. (1988). 311 nm UVB phototherapy—an effective therapy for psoriasis. *Br. J. Dermatol.* 119: 691–696.
21. Picot, E., Meunier, L., Picot-Debeze, M.C., Peyron, J.L., and Meynadier, J. (1992). Treatment of psoriasis with a 311-nm UVB lamp. *Br. J. Dermatol.* 127: 509–512.
22. Larkö, O. (1989). Treatment of psoriasis with a new UVB lamp. *Acta Derm. Venereol. (Stockh.)* 69: 357–359.
23. Van Weelden, H., Baart de la Faille, H., Young, E., and van der Leun, J.C. (1988). A new development in UVB phototherapy of psoriasis. *Br. J. Dermatol.* 119: 11–19.
24. Van Weelden, H., Baart de la Faille, H., Young, E., and van der Leun, J.C. (1990). Comparison of narrow-band UVB phototherapy with PUVA photochemotherapy in the treatment of psoriasis. *Acta Derm. Venereol. (Stockh.)* 70:212–215.
25. George, S.A., and Ferguson, J. (1992). Lesional blistering following narrow-band (TL-01) UVB phototherapy for psoriasis: a report of four cases. *Br. J. Dermatol.* 127:445–446 (letter).
26. Flindt-Hansen, H., McFadden, N., Eeg-Larsent, T., and Thune, P. (1991). Effect of a new narrow-band UVB lamp on photocarcinogenesis in mice. *Acta Derm. Venereol. (Stockh.)* 71:245–248.
27. Gibbs, N.K., Traynor, N.J., MacKie, R.M., Cambell, J., Johnson, B.E., and Ferguson, J. (1995). The phototumorigenic potential of broad-band (270–350 nm) and narrow-band (311–313 nm) phototherapy sources cannot be predicted by their edematogenic potential in hairless mouse skin. *J. Invest. Dermatol.* 104:359–363.
28. Anderson, T. (1990). Light sources in photomedicine. In *Clinical Photomedicine.* H. Lim and N. Soter (Eds.). Marcel Dekker, New York, pp. 37–58.
29. Sapeika, N. (1976). Treatment of psoriasis at the Dead Sea. *S. Afr. Med. J.* 50:2021.
30. Schamberg, I.L. (1978). Treatment of psoriasis at the Dead Sea. *Int. J. Dermatol.* 17:524–525.
31. Avrach, W.W. (1977). Climatotherapy at the Dead Sea. In *Psoriasis: Proceedings of the 2nd International Symposium.* E.M. Farber and A.J. Cox (Eds.). Yorke Medical Books, New York, p. 258.
32. Goldberg, L.H., and Kushelevsky, A. (1977). Ultraviolet light measurements at the Dead Sea. In *Psoriasis: Proceedings of the 2nd International Symposium.* E.M. Farber and A.J. Cox (Eds.). Yorke Medical Books, New York, p. 461.
33. Goeckerman, W.H. (1925). The treatment of psoriasis. *Northwest Med.* 24:229—231.
34. Goeckerman, W.H. (1931). Treatment of psoriasis: continued observation on the use of crude coal tar and ultraviolet light. *Arch. Dermatol.* 24:446–450.
35. Petrozzi, J.W., and Reyes, O.D.L. (1982). Ultraviolet phototherapy in psoriasis with hydrophilic ointment alone or crude coal tar. *Arch. Derm. Res.* 272:257–262.
36. Berne, B., Blom, I., and Spangberg, S. (1990). Enhanced response of psoriasis to UVB therapy after pretreatment with a lubricating base. *Acta Derm. Venereol. (Stockh.)* 70:474–477.
37. Lebwohl, M., Martinez, J., Weber, P., and DeLuca, R. (1995). Effects of topical preparations on the erythemogenicity of UVB: implications for psoriasis therapy. *J. Am. Acad. Dermatol.* 32:469–471.
38. George, S.A., Bilsland, D.J., Wainwright, N.J., and Ferguson, J. (1993). Failure of coconut oil to accelerate psoriasis clearance in narrow-band UVB phototherapy or photochemotherapy. *Br. J. Dermatol.* 128:301–305.
39. Bowers, R.E., Dalton, D., Fursdon, D., and Knoweldon, J. (1966). The treatment of psoriasis with UVR, dithranol paste and tar baths. *Br. J. Dermatol.* 78: 273–281.
40. Brun, P., Juhlin, L., and Schalla, W. (1984). Short contact anthralin therapy of psoriasis with and without UV-irradiation and maintenance schedule to prevent relapses. *Acta Derm. Venereol. (Stockh.)* 64:174–177.
41. Boer, J., and Smeenk, G. (1986). Effect of short-contact anthralin therapy on ultraviolet B irradiation of psoriasis. *J. Am. Acad. Dermatol.* 15:198–204.

42. Storbeck, K., Holzle, E., Schhurer, N., Lehmann, P., and Plewig, G. (1993). Narrow band UVB (311 nm) versus conventional broad-band UVB with and without dithranol in phototherapy for psoriasis. *J. Am. Acad. Dermatol.* 28:227–231.
43. Larkö, O., Swanbeck, G., and Svartholm, J. (1984). The effects on psoriasis of clobetasol propionate used alone or in combination with UVB. *Acta Derm. Venereol.* (*Stockh.*) 64:151–154.
44. Horwitz, S.N., Johnson, R.A., Sefton, J., and Frost, P. (1985). Addition of a topically applied corticosteroid to a modified Goeckerman regimen for treatment of psoriasis: effect on duration of remission. *J. Am. Acad. Dermatol.* 13:784–791.
45. Kragballe, K., and Iverson, L. (1993). Calcipotriol. A new topical antipsoriatic. *Dermatol. Clin.* 11:137–141.
46. Kragballe, K. (1992). Treatment of psoriasis with calcipotriol and other vitamin D analogues. *J. Am. Acad. Dermatol.* 27:1001–1008.
47. Kokelj, F., Lavaroni, G., and Guadagnini, A. (1995). UVB versus UVB plus calcipotriol (MC 903) therapy for psoriasis vulgaris. *Acta Derm. Venereol.* (*Stockh.*) 75:386–387.
48. McKenna, K.E., and Stern, R.S. (1995). Photosensitivity associated with combined UVB and calcipotriene therapy. *Arch. Dermatol.* 131:1305–1307.
49. Kerscher, M., Lehmann, P., and Plewig, G. (1994). Combination phototherapy of psoriasis with calcipotriol and narrow band UVB light. *Lancet* 342:923.
50. Momtaz, T.K., Tanghetti, E., and Parrish, J.A. (1983). Effect of warm water soaks on phototherapy of psoriasis. *Clin. Res.* 31:589.
51. Momtaz, T.K., and Parrish, J.A. (1984). Combination of psoralens and ultraviolet B in the treatment of psoriasis vulgaris: a bilateral comparison study. *J. Am. Acad. Dermatol.* 10:481–486.
52. Sakuntabhal, A., Diffey, B.I., and Farr, P.M. (1993). Response of psoriasis to psoralen-UVB photochemotherapy. *Br. J. Dermatol.* 28:296–300.
53. Paul, B.S., Momtaz, T.K., Stern, R.S., Arndt, K.A., and Parrish, J.A. (1982). Combined methotrexate-ultraviolet B therapy in the treatment of psoriasis. *J. Am. Acad. Dermatol.* 7:758–762.
54. Ruzicka, T.R., Sommerburg, C., Braun-Falco, O., Köster, W., Lengen, W., Lensing, W., Letzel, H., Meigel, W.N., Paul, E., Przybilla, B., Steinert, M., Winzer, M., and Wiskemann, A. (1990). Efficiency of acitretin in combination with UVB in the treatment of severe psoriasis. *Arch. Dermatol.* 126:482–486.
55. Lowe, N.J., Prystowsky, J.H., Bourget, T., Edelstein, J., Nychay, S., and Armstrong, R. (1991). Acitretin plus UVB therapy for psoriasis comparisons with placebo plus UVB and acitretin alone. *J. Am. Acad. Dermatol.* 24:591–594.
56. Anderson, R.R., and Parrish, J.A. (1982). Optical properties of human skin. In *The Science of Photomedicine.* J.D. Regan and J.A. Parrish (Eds.). Plenum Press, New York, pp. 3–17.
57. Kramer, D.M., Pathak, M.A., Kornhauser, A., and Wisekmann. (1974). Effects of ultraviolet radiation on biosynthesis of DNA in guinea pig skin. *J. Invest. Dermatol.* 62:388–393.
58. Epstein, W.L., Fukuyama, K., and Epstein, J.H. (1969). Early effects of ultraviolet light on DNA synthesis in human skin in vivo. *Arch. Dermatol.* 100:84–89.
59. Liu, M., and Pellingo, J.C. (1995). UV-B/A irradiation of mouse keratinocytes result in p53-mediated WAF-1/CIP-1 expression. *Oncogene* 10:1955–1960.
60. Brash, D.E., Rudolph, J.A., Simon, J.A., Lim, A., McKenna, G.J., Baden, H.P., Halperin, A.J., and Ponten, J. (1991). A role for sunlight in skin cancer: UV-induced p53 mutations in squamous cell carcinoma. *Proc. Natl. Acad. Sci. U.S.A.* 88:10124–10128.
61. Ulrich, S.E. (1995). Modulation of immunity by ultraviolet radiation: key effects of antigen presentation. *J. Invest. Dermatol.* 105:305–365.
62. Rivas, J.M., and Ullrich, S.E. (1994). The role of IL-4, IL-10, and TNF-alpha in the immune suppression induced by ultraviolet radiation. *J. Leukoc. Biol.* 56: 769–775.
63. Black, A.K., Findiam, N., Greves, M.W., and Hensby, C.N. (1980). Time course changes in levels of arachidonic acid and prostglandins D2, E2, F2 in human skin following ultraviolet B irradiation. *Br. J. Clin. Pharmacol.* 10:453–457.
64. Grewe, M., Trefzer, U., Ballhorn, A., Gyufko, K., Henninger, H., and Krutmann, J. (1993). Analysis of the mechanism of ultraviolet (UV) B radiation-induced prostaglandin E2 synthesis by human epidermoid carcinoma cells. *J. Invest. Dermatol.* 101:528–531.
65. Warmuth, I., Harth, Y., Matsui, M.S., Wang, N., and DeLeo, V.A. (1994). Ultraviolet radiation induces phosphorylation of the epidermal growth factor receptor. *Cancer Res.* 54:374–376.
66. Sachsenmaier, C., Radler-Pohl, A., Zinck, R., Nordheim, A., Herrlich, P., and Rahnsdorf, H.J. (1994). Involvement of growth factor receptors in the mammalian UVC response. *Cell* 78:963–972.
67. Devary, Y., Rosette, C., DiDonato, J.A., and Karin, M. (1993). NF-KB activation by ultraviolet light not dependent on a nuclear signal. *Science* 261;1442–1445.
68. Johnson, T.M., Duvic, M., Rapini, R.P., and Rios, A. (1985). Acquired immunodeficiency syndrome exacerbates psoriasis. *N. Engl. J. Med.* 313:1415 (letter).
69. Duvic, M., Crane, M.M., Conant, M., Mahoney, S.E., Reveille, J.D., and Lehrman, S.N. (1994). Zidovudine improves psoriasis in human immunodeficiency virus-positive males. *Arch. Dermatol.* 130:447–451.
70. Stingl, G., Rappersberger, K., Tschachler, E., Garner, S., Groh, V., Mann, D.L., Wolff, K., and Popovic, M. (1990). Langerhans cells in HIV-1 infections. *J. Am. Acad. Dermatol.* 22:1210–1217.

71. Mahoney, S.E., Duvic, M., Nickoloff, B.J., Minshall, M., Smith, L.C., Griffiths, C.E., Paddock, S.W., and Lewis, D.E. (1991). Human immunodeficiency virus transcripts identified in human immunodeficiency virus related psoriasis and Kaposi's sarcoma lesions. *J. Clin. Invest.* 88:174–185.
72. Kadunce, D.P., and Krueger, G.G. (1995). Pathogenesis of psoriasis, current concepts. *Dermatol. Clin.* 13: 723–737.
73. Valerie, K., Delers, C., Bruck, C., Thiriart, H., Rosenberg, C., Debouck, C., and Rosenberg, M. (1988). Activation of human immunodeficiency virus type 1 by DNA damage in human cells. *Nature* 333:78–81.
74. Zmudzka, B.Z., and Beer, J.Z. (1990). Activation of human immunodeficiency virus by ultraviolet radiation. *Photochem. Photobiol.* 52:1153–1162.
75. Morrey, J.D., Bourn, S.M., Bunch, T.D., Jackson, M.K., Sidwell, R.W., Barrows, L.R., Daynes, R.A., and Rosen, C.A. (1991). In vivo activation of human immunodeficiency virus type 1 long terminal repeat by UV type A (UV-A) light plus psoralen and UV-B light in the skin of transgenic mice. *J. Virol.* 65:5045–5051.
76. Meola, T., Soter, N.A., Ostreicher, R., Sanchez, M., and Moy, J.A. (1993). The safety of UVB phototherapy in patients with HIV infection. *J. Am. Acad. Dermatol.* 29:216–220.

41

Oral Psoralen Photochemotherapy

Bernhard Ortel, Elissa J. Liebman, Herbert Hönigsmann,* and Charles R. Taylor
Harvard Medical School and Massachusetts General Hospital, Boston, Massachusetts

HISTORY

The concept of photochemotherapy or the therapeutic use of a chemical in conjunction with radiation has existed for more than 3000 years. Its first use was documented in ancient Hindu scriptures. Healers used psoralen derived from the seeds of the bavachee plant in combination with natural sunlight to repigment vitiligo (1–3). The plant was also described as a remedy for vitiligo in Buddhist scriptures from approximately A.D. 200 and in 10th-century Chinese manuscripts (1–3). Another psoralen-containing plant named *Ammi majus*, which grows in the Egyptian Nile Valley, was used with sunlight to treat vitiligo from the 13th to the 20th century A.D. (1–3). In 1947, extracts from this plant were analyzed, revealing three crystalline compounds as active phototoxic agents: ammoidin or 8-methoxypsoralen (8-MOP), ammidin or 8-isoamylenoxypsoralen, and majudin or 5-methoxypsoralen (5-MOP) (4–6). That same year clinical trials with the purified compounds for the treatment of vitiligo began (7–9). In 1951, 8-MOP was first made available in the United States (2). One decade later, researchers tested the use of topical and oral 8-MOP with UVA to treat psoriasis (10). Finally, psoralen photochemotherapy, as it is commonly applied today, was introduced in 1974 when investigators at the Massachusetts General Hospital reported complete clearing in 21 psoriatic patients treated with systemic 8-MOP followed by a newly developed, high-intensity UVA radiation provided by Sylvania (11). The acronym PUVA was introduced by this same group of investigators. In its broadest terms, PUVA refers to the combination of any psoralen (P) with ultraviolet A (UVA) radiation (320–400 nm). However, the Food and Drug Administration (FDA) did not approve PUVA until 1982 after extensive clinical trials. Subsequently, PUVA progressed to become a mainstream therapy for psoriasis. PUVA can be used to treat all variants of psoriasis. Generally, it is recommended for patients with psoriasis covering at least 20% body surface area after intensive topical treatments and UVB phototherapy fail.

Since PUVA has proven its high efficacy in the treatment of psoriasis, it has been employed in a variety of cutaneous disorders. Currently, PUVA is being used for nearly 30 indications. It remains one of the best treatments for vitiligo and for inducing tolerance in patients with idiopathic photodermatoses such as polymorphic light eruption (PMLE) (12). Additional indications include mycosis fungoides (13,14), atopic dermatitis (15,16), pityriasis lichenoides (17,18), eosinophilic pustular folliculitis (19), pityriasis alba (20), generalized granuloma anulare (21), urticaria pigmentosa (22,23), lichen planus (17,24,25), graft-versus-host disease (26–28), and most recently morphea (29,30). This chapter, however, focuses on PUVA as a specific therapy for psoriasis. It is also confined to

*University of Vienna Medical School, Vienna, Austria.

regimens employing oral psoralens, since topical psoralen sensitization is described in another chapter.

PSORALENS

Psoralens are naturally occurring, linear tricyclic furocoumarins found in a variety of plants such as citrus fruits, celery, figs, and parsnips. Although some psoralens are still obtained from natural sources (e.g., 5-MOP), most are produced synthetically. While numerous substituted psoralens and related furocoumarins have been synthesized and tested in vitro and in vivo, the three most commonly used psoralens are 8-methoxypsoralen (8-MOP), 5-methoxypsoralen (5-MOP), and 4,5′,8-trimethylpsoralen (TMP) (Fig. 1). At present, 8-MOP is the most widely prescribed psoralen for the treatment of psoriasis in the United States. However, because it causes less nausea and vomiting, 5-MOP is quickly gaining popularity in Europe. TMP is a synthetic furocoumarin primarily employed orally in the treatment of vitiligo, especially in conjunction with the sun for so-called "PUVA-Sol" therapy. Topical application of this preparation by bath water delivery has been used extensively in Scandinavia for psoriasis (31). Several angelicins (angular furocoumarins) and substituted psoralens (e.g., pyridopsoralen) have been tested and reported to produce less erythema with good antipsoriatic activity (32,33). Unfortunately, they have been available in limited quantities, thus preventing widespread clinical trials. Long-term studies of their efficacy are eagerly awaited.

8-MOP Pharmacokinetics

The understanding of psoralen pharmacokinetics is essential to the proper administration of PUVA. 8-MOP is hepatically metabolized using cytochrome P_{450} enzymes (34) and is excreted into the urine 12–24 hr after ingestion. Small changes in dose can significantly alter plasma levels because the drug undergoes a significant first-pass effect (35).

A significant problem with oral 8-MOP administration is the great intraindividual and interindividual variation of psoralen blood levels after the administration of equal oral doses (36). This variability is due to numerous factors influencing the drug's intestinal absorption such as the concurrent presence of food, the liver's capacity to metabolize psoralens, and the exact type of pharmaceutical preparation. Successful therapy requires adequate, reproducible plasma psoralen concentrations (37,38). The timing between psoralen ingestion and UVA administration is essential because skin phototoxicity correlates well with 8-MOP's peak serum level (39,40). Bonnot et al. (41) compared patients treated with standard PUVA (UVA irradiation 2 hr after 8-MOP ingestion) with patients treated using a protocol where the irradiations were precisely coordinated with the individual time and magnitude of the maximal 8-MOP plasma level. Patients in the latter group needed 27% fewer exposures and had a 38% reduction in the cumulative UVA dose needed for clearing. While such a protocol has the potential to decrease long-term PUVA consequences, it is prohibitively time-consuming and expensive.

Oxsoralen, in its original galenic preparation of 8-MOP crystals in hard gelatin capsules, has been largely replaced by a liquid preparation of 8-MOP in soft gelatin capsules. It is marketed as Oxsoralen-Ultra in the United States and similar preparations are available worldwide. It has slightly different pharmacokinetics with peak plasma levels 1 hr after ingestion, whereas the older crystalline preparations do not peak until 2 hr. With the liquid capsules, the peak concentrations of 8-MOP are higher and show a lesser degree of intraindividual variation (39). However, the higher plasma levels result in an increased incidence of short-term side effects such as nausea, vomiting, and weakness.

5-MOP

5-MOP differs structurally from 8-MOP in the position of the methoxy group on the coumarin ring. It is less water-soluble and has an intestinal absorption rate of only 25% that of 8-MOP. This reduced uptake of oral 5-MOP can be partially compensated for by an increased dosage, namely, 1.2–1.5 mg/kg body weight (42,43).

5-MOP is more rapidly metabolized, with a serum half-life of 1 hr (44). Its distinct advantage is a much lower incidence of short-term side effects such as nausea, vomiting, pruritus, and phototoxicity (45). Crystalline as well as liquid preparations in capsules are available for oral administration outside the United States. Similar to methoxsalen, 5-MOP reaches its peak plasma concentration 1 hr after ingestion of liquid preparations (43). On the other hand, 5-MOP causes higher degrees of pigmentation and requires greater cumulative UVA doses (45). Calzavara-Pinton et al. (45) compared the efficacy and tolerability of 8-MOP and 5-MOP in 25 patients with skin phototypes

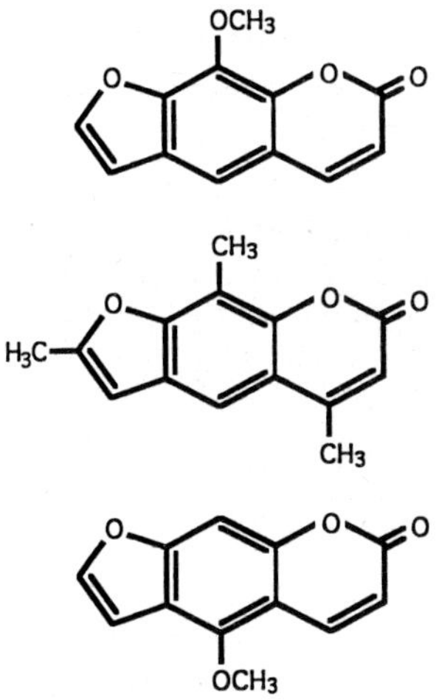

Figure 1 Structures of psoralens used in photochemotherapy.

III and IV with relapsing plaque-type psoriasis. During the first year of the study, patients were treated with 8-MOP (0.6 mg/kg), and relapses with 5-MOP (1.2 mg/kg) in the second year. Patients needed the same number of treatments with either psoralen, but higher cumulative doses of UVA were required for courses with 5-MOP.

A new micronized tablet of 5-MOP has been developed. There are early claims for its higher bioavailability, increased efficacy, decreased adverse effects, and a reduced cumulative UVA burden (46). Only after more clinical trials will definitive conclusions be reached.

Trimethoxypsoralen (TMP)

TMP is a synthetic psoralen with minimal gastrointestinal absorption. Peak serum concentration is reached 2 hr after ingestion. While plasma levels after oral administration are not sufficient to allow psoriasis treatment, they are adequate for vitiligo therapy (47). For psoriasis, TMP is efficiently and predominantly used via bath-water delivery (31).

Finally, there is evidence that psoralen dosing based on body surface area is more accurate than when based on weight alone (48). However, psoralen doses determined by weight and by body surface area tend to be the same unless body habitus is at the extremes of the range seen in routine practice.

Little is known about interactions between psoralens and other drugs. Reduced 8-MOP plasma levels with concomitant phenytoin treatment (49) may be explained by the induction of hepatic enzymes by phenytoin. Similar modifications may be expected with barbiturates and alcohol, but data are not available.

ACTION SPECTRUM

The PUVA action spectrum is defined as the effectiveness of clearing psoralen-sensitized psoriasis as a function of wavelength. Currently, broad-band, high-intensity UVA sources ranging from 320 to 400 nm with a peak emission at 352 nm are typically used in PUVA. However, recent advances may change this methodology. The action spectrum for psoralen-sensitized delayed erythema, once believed to be optimally induced at 365 nm (50), has been demonstrated to peak around 330 nm (51–54). Although therapeutic responses to PUVA seem to correlate well with erythemogenicity, the waveband dependency had to be established for therapeutic activity. Farr et al. (55) made a paired comparison of the antipsoriatic activity of fluorescent tubes with different emission spectra. Two hours after the administration of oral 8-MOP (0.6 mg/kg), the extremities of each patient were treated thrice weekly for 6 weeks with a pair of three different radiation sources. The lamp with a peak emission of 325 nm was felt to be superior to the ones with maximal outputs at 352 or 370 nm. Another study using oral 8-MOP plus monochromatic radiation showed that 335 nm was twice as effective as 365 nm in terms of its erythemogenicity and antipsoriatic efficacy (56). The experimental use of narrow-band (311 nm) UVB has demonstrated higher efficacy after both oral and bath-water delivery of 8-MOP than for 311 nm UVB alone (57). Since the Philips TL-01 lamp has a high therapeutic efficacy by itself, the relative contributions and interactions of UVB and photoactivated psoralen are not understood. Psoralens form crosslinks at any of the clinically investigated wavelengths. The contribution of unsensitized UV effects to the efficacy of PUVA treatment varies greatly with the applied spectra. Conceivably, optimized narrow-spectrum light sources may be developed to lower the cumulative UVA dose for PUVA, which is an important factor of its carcinogenic potential.

LIGHT SOURCES

Light sources for PUVA include fluorescent and metal halide lamps. Fluorescent lamps are composed of a low-pressure mercury arc discharge source encased in phosphor-coated glass (58,59). This coating determines the emission spectrum. The mercury arc discharge source releases radiation that is absorbed by the phosphor, which undergoes excitation, reemitting energy at a longer wavelength via fluorescence (58). Standard PUVA fluorescent light sources have an emission range from 320 to 400 nm, peaking at 352 nm and emitting less than 0.5% UVB and less than 1% visible light. The benefits of fluorescent light sources are their lower cost, large field size, and relatively low heat production. One disadvantage is that they emit 10–30% less energy at the ends than in the middle portion of the tubes, possibly reducing treatment efficacy for the distal lower extremities and the head in tall patients. In addition, in a busy practice the lamps may need to be replaced 2–3 times per year because they retain only 70–80% of their original output after 500 hr and generally need replacing after 1000 hr (59).

Metal halide lamps are medium- to high-pressure mercury arcs housed within quartz. The type of filter used with each lamp determines its emission spectrum. With exchangeable filters, these lamps may be used as UVB as well as UVA units. The advantage of these sources is that they have very high, stable outputs, resulting in shorter treatment times. Several lamps may be stacked to form a column. However, because these lamps are point sources, they need good paraboloid reflectors to produce an even irradiance distribution. Because metal halide lamps may produce a lot of heat and some of them ozone, they need good ventilation systems.

The use of UVB wavelengths in psoralen photochemotherapy has been advocated by a few phototherapists in the past (60). Recent publications have readdressed this issue and demonstrated that photochemotherapy works if psoralen is activated by UVB (61,62). Narrow-band (311 nm) UVB has been effectively used with both topical and oral 8-MOP (57). It appears that the combination of topical 8-MOP and narrow-band UVB phototherapy is the better of the two. The role of this fluorescent light source in psoralen photosensitization remains to be determined. Some concern has been expressed over the simultaneous presence of UVB-induced DNA photoproducts and psoralen-DNA photoadducts.

Dosimetry

Careful dosimetry is essential for proper and standardized PUVA therapy, especially if patients switch treatment centers that may use different units and methods. Precise dosimetry measurements ensure correct therapy and prevent unnecessary over- or underexposures. Today most UVA cabinets contain built-in radiometers, which measure the radiation emitted and automatically report the time for exposure. Changes in output during the irradiation will result in an automatically adjusted treatment time. Regular recalibration of such systems is required.

ERYTHEMA AND PIGMENTATION

PUVA therapy results in erythema and subsequent pigmentation of the skin. PUVA erythema peaks 48–96 hr after irradiation as opposed to UVB erythema, which peaks at 12–24 hr. In addition, PUVA erythema is more enduring, sometimes lasting 3 weeks after exposure. The amount of pigmentation produced by PUVA therapy depends on the patient's constitutive (i.e., genetic) and facultative (i.e., inducible) abilities as suggested by the skin phototype (Table 1) (63). Skin phototyping categorizes individuals according to their erythema and pigmentation responses following 1 hr of ambient high-noon sun exposure on the first bright, sunny summer day without sun protection. Individuals who tan easily are also more prone to develop darker PUVA-induced pigmentation.

GETTING STARTED

If a psoriatic patient seems suitable for receiving PUVA therapy, contraindications have to be excluded. These include pregnancy, breastfeeding, age under 12 years, and unspecified and drug photosensitivity disorders. Patients with a history of multiple skin cancers or with genetic disorders such as xeroderma pigmentosum are not eligible for PUVA. The history of treatment with ionizing radiation or arsenicals also increase the lifetime risk of developing skin cancer and

Table 1 Skin Phototypes

I	Always burn, never tan
II	Always burn, sometimes tan
III	Sometimes burn, always tan
IV	Never burn, always tan
V	Moderately pigmented
VI	Darkly pigmented

Source: Ref. 63.

such patients should receive PUVA only if there is no treatment alternative. Lupus erythematosus and other autoimmune diseases such as bullous pemphigoid may worsen with PUVA. Therefore, a negative ANA screen is also advised. Hepatotoxicity is not considered a risk, but in people with increased liver function parameters an altered psoralen metabolism has to be considered.

Once a patient is selected for PUVA, the physician has to make sure that the patient understands the hazards of the combined action of the drug and UVA radiation. Particular emphasis should be placed on persistent eye protection during and after therapeutic exposure. A baseline eye examination to screen for cataracts is performed and should be repeated annually. Patients must be taught to avoid accidental sun exposure whether direct or indirect, such as through a window, to their skin during the same period. Patients should also be informed about the increased risk of developing nonmelanoma skin carcinomas associated with prolonged PUVA with high cumulative UVA exposures. Finally, patients have to sign a consent form detailing all of the above risks.

DETERMINATION OF MINIMAL PHOTOTOXICITY DOSE

The best way to begin PUVA therapy is to determine the patient's minimal phototoxic dose (MPD). It ensures that the patient will receive a starting UVA dose that is neither too high resulting in phototoxicity nor too low causing ineffective therapy. One or 2 hr after the administration of oral psoralen, a template is placed on the patient's buttocks, as the area of greatest UV sensitivity. The template consists of six to eight areas of at least 1 cm^2, which can each be exposed to increasing doses of UVA. Visual assessment of the erythema response is performed at 72 hr using a grading scale (Table 2). The MPD is the lowest dose that produces pink erythema with distinct borders 72 hr after exposure (64). A fraction of this dose (e.g., 50–80%) is frequently used as a starting dose in PUVA therapy.

Table 2 Grading Scale of the Phototoxic Response to PUVA

Scale	Degree of erythema
0	No erythema
Trace	Miminal perceptible erythema
+1	Light pink erythema
+2	Marked erythema, red in color, but not edematous
+3	Fiery red erythema with edema and tenderness
+4	Violaceous red erythema accompanied by marked edema, blistering, and tenderness

The individual threshold value (1+) is called the minimal phototoxic dose (MPD).

PROTOCOLS

Since the introduction of PUVA in 1974, numerous protocols have been used. Although they are slightly different, they share the same basic principle of using regularly repeated PUVA exposures. Reasons for choosing a particular protocol may often lie in practicality and established local custom rather than in a critical evaluation of the respective advantages of any one protocol. Generally, PUVA protocols have two phases: (1) the clearing phase aiming at psoriasis suppression and (2) maintenance characterized by a tapering to a minimal number of regular visits in an effort to maintain and extend remission. This chapter will describe two classic protocols, the so-called American and European schedules as well as current modifications. The American protocol is derived from the initial study by Parrish et al. (11) and was documented on a large number of patients by Melski et al. in the 16-center US Cooperative Clinical Trial (USCCT) (65). Almost simultaneously, the European protocol was developed by the Vienna group (66) and was similarly investigated in a large group of psoriatics (67).

American Versus European PUVA

As suggested by their names, the American and European PUVA protocols are largely practiced on opposite sides of the Atlantic Ocean. The customs are solidly rooted and controversy abounds regarding advantages of each protocol (Table 3). For example, in the USCCT (65) 1139 patients were treated according to the American protocol outlined wherein the initial UVA dose was based on patient's skin phototype while subsequent doses were increased in fixed, rigid increments. Treatments were given either two or three times a week. For comparison, in the study by Henseler et al. (67) 3175 patients were treated with a more flexible and aggressive European protocol, utilizing four weekly treatments. Both trials cleared psoriasis in the same percentage of patients. However, the U.S. protocol required 7 more weeks to clear and resulted

Table 3 Comparison Between the EPS and USCCT Trials

	EPS	USCCT
Number of patients	3175	1139
How initial dose is determined	Minimal phototoxic dose testing	Skin phototype
Number of weekly treatments	4	2 or 3
Increments	Individualized and flexible	Predetermined and fixed
% of patients with marked improvement of complete clearing	88.8%	88.0%
Weeks of treatment required for clearing	5.7	12.7
Median number of exposures	20	25
Cumulative UVA dose (J/cm^2)	96	245

Source: Adapted from Ref. 65 and 67.

in a higher number of exposures and a higher cumulative UVA dose. These results suggest that the European protocol may be superior to its American counterpart. Its accelerated treatment schedule ultimately saves patients time, effort, and money. It also decreases the cumulative UVA burden. Consequently, this protocol may ultimately incur less long-term risk of carcinogenesis and photoaging, as seems to be reflected in the reports of PUVA carcinogenesis (see below). Except on an inpatient basis, many American physicians do not employ the European schedule because of the difficulty of treating a patient four times a week during the clearing phase.

American PUVA Protocol

American protocols are generally rigid and cautious. As already mentioned, they also tend to require more treatments and result in a higher cumulative UVA dose. For clearing, one can choose between either a twice-a-week (BIW) or a thrice-a-week (TIW) schedule. Typical protocols begin with UVA irradiations of 70–80% of the baseline MPD. However, some centers use the patients' skin phototype to determine the starting dose, as shown in Table 4. The patient receives the UVA exposure 1 or 2 hr after psoralen ingestion, depending on which formulation is used. The UVA doses are increased, held the same, or omitted depending on the amount of erythema produced by the prior visit. If there was no erythema from the last treatment, increments are 0.5–1.0 J/cm^2 per session. If the erythema was mild and short-lived, the dose is held the same. If there was persistent erythema, one treatment may be omitted. Generally, it requires 20–25 treatments to clear psoriasis regardless of whether BIW or TIW frequency is used. If the patient has significant disease on the extremities, additional exposures may be given to those areas. After the appropriate dose is delivered to the total body, patients then put on their undergarments (top and bottom), exposing only their arms and legs to an additional dose. Patients with skin phototype I and II are exposed to an extra 1 J/cm^2 of UVA with subsequent treatment increments of 0.5 J/cm^2 as tolerated. Those with skin phototypes III–VI begin with an extra dose of 3 J/cm^2 with increments of 1 J/cm^2 per treatment as tolerated. Most skin phototypes I/II individuals are held at a maximum total body dose of 8–12 J/cm^2, while skin phototypes III/IV and V/VI patients are allowed to reach maximum UVA doses of 12–16 J/cm^2 and 16–20 J/cm^2, respectively.

European PUVA Protocol

The original European protocol involved four treatments a week, with intermissions on Wednesdays and weekends. MPD testing is invariably performed and

Table 4 Skin Phototype–Dependent Dosimetry (J/cm^2)

Skin phototype	Initial dose	Increments
I	1.5	0.5
II	2.5	0.5
III	3.5	0.5–1.0
IV	4.5	1.0
V	5.5	1.0
VI	6.5	1.0–1.5

For BIW and TIW schedules according to the American protocol, skin type–dependent starting UVA exposures and fixed dose increments are employed.

the starting dose is 70–80% of the MPD, not 100% as used in the original EPS study (67). The physician decides to increase, hold the same, or omit irradiations depending on the degree of erythema caused by the previous exposure. During the clearing phase, increments are made every other visit to avoid cumulative phototoxicity induced by exposures on consecutive days. Additional exposures of, for example, the extremities are not done routinely. The advantage of this aggressive schedule is that it generally requires fewer treatments (around 15) and uses lower doses of radiation (4–12 J/cm^2). The difficulty with this method is that the patient has to visit the center 4 times a week. In addition, this protocol may result in a higher frequency of phototoxic side effects than the American protocol.

Modified PUVA Protocols

Currently, there exists numerous variations of the original American and European protocols. One modified European protocol uses weekly repeated MPD testing to determine UVA threshold doses throughout the clearing phase (68). Treatments are given twice weekly 72 hr apart. Patients take either Oxsoralen-Ultra or Oxsoralen and receive the first dose of UVA either 1 or 2 hr later, respectively. The first UVA dose is based on a fixed percentage of the patient's baseline MPD. During this same visit, the patient has a second graded test exposure for MPD determination after the therapeutic irradiation. When the patient returns 72 hr later for the next treatment, this MPD is assessed. The patient is then given the initial dose plus the highest UVA exposure that did not result in erythema. For example, assume the baseline MPD was 4 J/cm^2, and the initial dose was 80%, or 3.2 J/cm^2. Immediately after the first treatment, the following MPD series is performed: 1, 2, 3, 4, 5, 6, 7, and 8 J/cm^2. The test site shows no reaction up to 4 J/cm^2, trace erythema at 5 J/cm^2, and the MPD at 6 J/cm^2. The highest test dose that did not produce erythema was 4 J/cm^2. Therefore, the dose to be given on the day of the second visit would be 3.2 J/cm^2 (the dose given on day 1) plus 4 J/cm^2 for a total dose of 7.2 J/cm^2. On the third visit, assuming there was no erythema from the previous treatment, UVA is increased by 1 J/cm^2 and another MPD test is performed. Generally the MPDs are done only for the first 2–3 weeks of PUVA therapy. The objective is to reach optimally therapeutic doses quickly and safely. Once patients reach approximately 10 J/cm^2 MPD testing is no longer necessary and doses are increased 0.5–1.0 J/cm^2 per treatment as tolerated.

MAINTENANCE THERAPY

Maintenance philosophy varies around the world. The rationale behind maintenance is based on the USCCT report (65). The patients whose psoriasis cleared were divided into four groups. The first received one treatment a week, while the second had one treatment every other week, and the third received treatment every third week. The fourth group did not receive any maintenance therapy. Only 27% of the first group flared, compared to 30, 34, and 62% of the other groups, respectively. Therefore, the use of short-term maintenance regimes is recommended by many therapists. Maintenance therapy generally leads to a period of remission of 6–12 months (65).

In Europe, many dermatologists avoid extended periods of maintenance therapy. Commonly, the final UVA exposure of the clearing phase is used for maintenance therapy consisting of BIW treatments for 1 month, followed by once-weekly treatments for another month before PUVA is discontinued (69). The UVA dose used in maintenance is usually kept constant. In contrast, some American dermatologists follow initially the same kind of tapering, but continue often to as low as once a month for a prolonged period. For patients who have a history of relapsing severely on PUVA cessation, they may choose to continue treatment for years after clearing. One problem with once-monthly maintenance is that about every 4 months the PUVA dose must be decreased by approximately 10% to avoid burns due to gradual loss of tolerance.

These differences may in part be related to insurance issues because it has become increasingly difficult to hospitalize patients with psoriasis in the United States and every effort is made to keep patients out of the hospital. While it is generally felt that maintenance therapy keeps patients clear of disease, the current trend is to shorten maintenance regimes to decrease the patient's cumulative UVA exposure.

If a patient experiences a minor relapse of disease during maintenance therapy, one might increase the frequency of treatments rather than raise the UVA dose. If the irradiation is increased, the patient may become more tolerant without necessarily helping the disease to clear. If the psoriasis flare is severe enough, the patient should revert to a clearing protocol.

COMBINATION PROTOCOLS

To enhance the efficacy of PUVA and minimize its side effects, PUVA is frequently employed in combination with a number of other agents. For example, PUVA is frequently combined with oral retinoids (etretinate or isotretinoin), which is called chemophotochemotherapy or re-PUVA (70–73). PUVA can also be combined with UVB (74), methotrexate, interferon, calcipotriol, or, in rare instances, cyclosporin (75). The rationale behind all these combination therapies is to clear psoriasis more efficiently with fewer treatments, lower cumulative UVA doses, and a distribution of the various risk categories. Combined protocols are discussed in detail in other chapters of this book.

PUVA AND PREGNANCY

Photobound psoralens are mutagenic, carcinogenic, and produce sister chromatid exchanges (76). In contrast to their dramatic biological effects, two recent studies have confirmed the long-held impression that PUVA is not a potent teratogen in humans (77,78). Stern and Lange (77) documented the pregnancy outcomes of the 1380 patients enrolled in a PUVA follow-up study. They documented 258 delivered infants whose father or mother had received PUVA treatment prior to birth. Two of the infants were stillbirths and one had Down's syndrome. One of the stillbirths occurred in a woman exposed to PUVA throughout all three trimesters. The case of Down's syndrome occurred in the child of a woman who did not use PUVA during her pregnancy. These data support the view that PUVA is not teratogenic. Gunnarskog et al. (78) conducted a similar study in Sweden, which analyzed 1205 infants born to psoriatic women who were pregnant either before, during, or after PUVA therapy. They found that none of the infants exposed to PUVA treatment of the mother during gestation had any congenital malformation. Of the infants conceived after cessation of PUVA, 3.2% had congenital malformations. For those infants born prior to the initiation of PUVA, 3.6% had congenital malformations. Both of these rates were below the average 4.8% rate in the general population. Hence, these birth defects cannot be assumed to have been caused by PUVA. However, the study did find that a large percentage of infants were born with low birth weights. Seven percent of the infants born in women who conceived after terminating PUVA had a low birth weight and an additional 7% were born prematurely. Five percent of the infants born before PUVA was initiated were low in birth weight and 7% of the infants exposed to PUVA during gestation were also below average weight. This study similarly concluded that there was no evidence that PUVA therapy caused congenital malformations; however, there may be an association between low birth weight and PUVA. Although they did not establish an association between PUVA and risk of congenital malformations, both studies advise against pregnant women undergoing therapy. In fact, current practice highly recommends that all women on PUVA use birth control.

SIDE EFFECTS OF PUVA

Acute Side Effects

Like any medical treatment, PUVA therapy may result in both acute and chronic side effects. The most common acute problems are gastrointestinal side effects, such as anorexia, nausea, and vomiting. Such problems may be overcome by ingesting 8-MOP with food. Many patients report that ginger ale and ginger snaps help alleviate the nausea. Patients also commonly complain of headaches, dizziness, lightheadedness, depression, and insomnia. If they are severe, these CNS complaints may require a slight reduction of the 8-MOP dose. In general, most of these strategies mitigate the side effects of oral psoralen by lowering the plasma psoralen levels.

Patients may also experience unwanted symptoms of psoralen phototoxicity such as blisters, excessive erythema, pruritus, and skin pain (79). Unfortunately, there is no ideal treatment for painful PUVA erythema and most patients must wait 1–3 weeks for it to abate. In the interim, patients may derive partial benefit from cool baths, lubrication, aspirin, antipruritics, and topical steroids. Capsaicin has also been reported to help decrease PUVA itch (80). For those patients who experience very severe pruritus, phenytoin 150 mg BID may relieve symptoms (81). It is important to identify the cause of the excessive phototoxicity. Besides UVA overdosages, photosensitizing medications such as tetracyclines, phenothiazides, sulfa drugs, and thiazide diuretics may lead to inadvertent additive phototoxicity. Patients should be screened for all concurrent medications to prevent accidental phototoxicity before PUVA actually starts and before each treatment.

Rare side effects include asthma exacerbation (82), drug fever (83), widespread maculopapular eruption (84), photo-onycholysis (85), friction blisters (86), hypertrichosis (87), and urticaria (88). While it is not a true side effect of PUVA, phytophotodermatitis occasionally occurs (89). Phytophotodermatitis is the interaction of a psoralen-containing plant or plant substance with UVA on the skin to produce phototoxicity, which may blister, and resolve with long-lasting hyperpigmentation. For example, a bartender who handles limes may experience an unexpected burning episode on the hands due to the presence of residual psoralens from the lime peels while he is on PUVA.

With 5-MOP, side effects are much less pronounced, even if the dose is increased to 1.2–1.5 mg/kg body weight to compensate for the lesser gastrointestinal absorption (43). 5-MOP rarely leads to phototoxic side effects but may induce a peculiar asymptomatic rash that may resemble polymorphic light eruption (43).

Chronic Side Effects

Cutaneous Aging

Premature photoaging may be a consequence of high cumulative UVA exposure associated with long-term PUVA therapy. It results in damage to collagen and elastin, which are essential components of the skin's extracellular matrix (90,91), thereby weakening the structural integrity of the skin. It is not clear if this effect is mediated by UVA alone, or if psoralen phototoxicity adds to cutaneous aging.

Ophthalmological Risk

Since 1974, the PUVA follow-up study has been monitoring a group of 1380 patients. Recently, the ophthalmology examinations of 1235 of these patients before and after 10 years of PUVA were compared (92). There was no significant association between the risk of ocular lens abnormality and the PUVA dose. In fact, this study failed to find a relationship between the level of PUVA exposure and the risk of cataract formation. However, a higher incidence of cataracts was found in the PUVA cohort as compared to the incidence in the general population. The study concludes that as long as patients are compliant with the ocular protection, there is no dose-dependent increased risk of ocular lens changes.

Recently, Calzavara-Pinton et al. (93) examined the ocular side effects of PUVA in patients who refused to use eye protection. Over a 4-year period, 82 patients who did not protect their eyes were compared to 749 patients who wore UVA-blocking sunglasses. They found that of those who refused to wear the glasses, 25.6% developed conjunctival hyperemia and 24.4% had decreased lacrimation. In contrast, 0.7% of the compliant group developed conjunctival hyperemia and only 0.1% experienced decreased lacrimation. None of the patients in the study developed decreased visual acuity, lens opacities, or lesions of the vitreous body and fundus.

At present, it is recommended that patients wear UVA-opaque glasses for at least 24 hr after psoralen ingestion. These shades should be worn both outside and inside when near windows. For ambient light exposure wrap-around glasses are favored. While patients are undergoing irradiation, they may put on smaller goggles to prevent "raccoon eyes."

Cancer

The risk of developing nonmelanoma skin carcinoma is one of the more significant side effects of PUVA. Long-term use of PUVA has been clearly associated with increased risk to develop cutaneous squamous cell carcinoma (94–99) and basal cell carcinoma (97–100). However, more recent observations indicate that there is only an increased risk of squamous cell but not basal cell carcinomas (101). One study (97) also indicated a higher risk of lung, colon, and renal cancer in psoriatics after PUVA, but this needs confirmation. There have also been case reports (102) of malignant melanoma occurring during PUVA treatment, but there is no documentation of increased risk of melanoma associated with PUVA.

Stern (103) found a specific increase of cutaneous carcinomas in the genital skin of male PUVA patients. This led to the recommendation to shield the genital area during UVA exposure. A survey among 11 European centers with 32,599 patients did not show such a risk (104). Although an increased risk for nonmelanoma skin carcinomas was also reported by European centers, the magnitude of the risk increase is smaller. This has been attributed to the reduced cumulative UVA doses associated with the European PUVA protocol. Controversy also exists about the specific role of PUVA in skin carcinogenesis, namely, whether PUVA is a cocarcinogen or a complete carcinogen, and the magnitude of the effect in comparison with other carcinogens. However, it is currently agreed that PUVA increases the risk of nonmelanoma skin carcinomas. Current therapeutic efforts are aimed at minimizing the cumulative exposure, which is the determining factor for skin cancer risk, by modifying existing treatment schedules and practice of maintenance therapy.

MECHANISM OF ACTION

Psoralens require activation by ultraviolet radiation to become therapeutically effective. Therefore, the photochemical psoralen reactions are confined to the epidermis and the upper dermis, as far as UVA penetrates. The psoralen absorbs a photon and enters an electronically excited state (triple state via single excited state) from which it reacts with molecules in its environment. Traditionally, the focus has been on photochemical reactions with DNA (105,106). Here, the psoralen is first intercalated in the dark and can upon irradiation form both monofunctional and bifunctional adducts with the DNA. Psoralens that can form bifunctional adducts (crosslinks) are therapeutically more active in psoriasis, although monofunctional psoralens have shown therapeutic activity after topical application (32,33). Although most detail is known about psoralen-DNA photoreactions, other photoproducts of 8-MOP may contribute to the therapeutic effect (107,108). Excited psoralens may also react with molecular oxygen generating reactive oxygen species. These may cause cell membrane damage and activation of the cyclooxygenase and arachidonic acid metabolic pathways. At present it is not clear how much different photochemical pathways and specific photoproducts contribute to the antipsoriatic activity.

The observation that DNA-psoralen crosslinks inhibit DNA replication is supported by the current view of cell cycle control via p53 and its regulation by DNA damage. This insight into these cellular molecular mechanisms has helped to elucidate the pathway by which psoralen phototoxicity affects cellular kinetics. This, however, does not mean that keratinocytes are the only target of such consequence of psoralen photochemistry.

Psoralen photosensitization results in altered expression of cytokines and their receptors (109). Epidermal Langerhans cells are reduced for a prolonged period by clinical PUVA exposures (110). The strong suppressive effect of activated psoralens on lymphocytes (111–113) is best exemplified by the high efficacy of PUVA in the treatment of cutaneous T-cell lymphoma. In a recent study (114), bath PUVA was shown to revert the pathologically altered pattern of keratinocyte differentiation markers and to reduce the proliferative cell population by 73%. HLA-DR expression was markedly reduced in treated skin. Infiltrating lymphocytes were strongly suppressed by PUVA, with variable effects on different T-cell subsets. The same group could also demonstrate that PUVA is far more potent in inducing apoptosis in lymphocytes than in keratinocytes although the antiproliferative effect is similar in both cell types (115). This study indicates that PUVA readily induces apoptotic cell death in lymphocytes. This observation may explain the high efficacy in mycosis fungoides as well as in psoriasis.

Recent advances have improved our understanding of different cellular molecular pathways induced by psoralen photochemistry (116). The interactions and relative contributions of these factors to therapeutic effects in psoriasis and other disease are yet to be understood.

IMMUNOLOGICAL EFFECTS

PUVA and HIV Disease

The treatment of HIV-positive psoriatic patients remains a challenge. Although the incidence of psoriasis is not increased in this population (117), the disease usually has an atypical appearance and proves recalcitrant to conventional therapy. In addition, many of the usual treatments such as topical steroids may cause more harm than benefit. Therefore, PUVA may be the treatment of choice, especially if UVB phototherapy fails. However, PUVA causes immunosuppression and may theoretically exacerbate the HIV infection. Zmudzka et al. (118,119) have reported the activation of the HIV-1 gene promoter with both UVB and PUVA. In addition, Valerie et al. (120) activated the HIV long terminal repeat by DNA damage using UV irradiation. Consequently, PUVA may influence HIV disease progression.

A recent pilot study (121) examined the effect of PUVA on AIDS patients, all of whom had CD4+ counts under 50 cells/ml. Patients were treated for 2 months with PUVA. On days 0, 14, 30, and 60, the patient's HIV-1 burden was measured. The researchers did not find an increase in any of the HIV-1-related parameters nor did they find any worsening of clinical HIV disease. They concluded that PUVA is a safe therapeutic option for those psoriatics infected with HIV. More data are needed in this area before PUVA can be generally declared safe and recommended for the treatment of immunosuppressed individuals. The issue of HIV and psoriasis is further explored in another chapter.

PUVA and Autoimmune Disease

Although they are a rare complication of PUVA therapy, autoimmune diseases have been reported to be precipitated during or after treatment. Both bullous pemphigoid (122–126) and lupus erythematosus (127,128) have been reported to flare with PUVA therapy.

CONCLUSION

While photochemotherapy has existed for thousands of years, PUVA has evolved to its sophisticated, versatile present-day form only over the last score of years. PUVA is highly efficacious for psoriasis as well as for a number of other disorders. It requires careful attention to detail, especially to patient selection, dosimetry, and follow-up. Variables such as psoralen type, radiation source, irradiation protocol, and maintenance plan allow for flexibility of treatment. Patients and therapists must be mindful of the short- and long-term side effects of PUVA. While existing strategies attempt to minimize side effects, maximize clearance rates, and prolong remission periods, future therapies will likely become less time-consuming and more selective, targeting the involved skin, while protecting adjacent normal skin.

REFERENCES

1. Roelandts, R. (1991). The history of photochemotherapy. *Photodermatol. Photoimmunol. Photomed.* 8: 184–189.
2. Fitzpatrick, T.B., and Pathak, M.A. (1959). Historical aspects of methoxsalen and other furocoumarins. *J. Invest. Dermatol.* 31:229–231.
3. Pathak, M.A., and Fitzpatrick, T.B. (1992). The evolution of photochemotherapy with psoralens and UVA (PUVA): 2000 B.C. to 1992 A.D. *J. Photochem. Photobiol. B: Biol.* 14:3–22.
4. Fahmy, I.R., and Abu-Shady, H. (1947). *Ammi majus* Linn: pharmacognostical study and isolation of crystalline constituent, ammoidin. *Q. J. Pharmacol.* 20: 281–291.
5. Fahmy, I.R., Abu-Shady, H., Schonberg, A., and Sina, A. (1947). A crystalline principle from *Ammi majus* L. *Nature* 160:468–469.
6. Fahmy, I.R., and Abu-Shady, H. (1948). *Ammi majus* Linn: The isolation and properties of ammoidin, ammidin and majudin, and their effects in the treatment of leukoderma. *Q. J. Pharmacol.* 21:499–503.
7. El-Mofty, A.M. (1948). A preliminary clinical report on the treatment of leucoderma with *Ammi majus* Linn. *J. Egypt. Med. Assoc.* 31:651–665.
8. El-Mofty, A.M. (1952). Further study on treatment of leucoderma with *Ammi majus* Linn. *J. Egypt Med. Assoc.* 35:1–28.
9. El-Mofty, A.M. (1952). Observations on the use of *Ammi majus* Linn in vitiligo. *Br. J. Dermatol.* 64: 431–441.
10. Oddoze, L., Temime, P., Marchand, J.P., and Benne, M. (1967). L'association meladinine per os et rayons UV dans le traitement du psoriasis. *Bull. Soc. Fr. Dermatol. Syph.* 74:609–610.
11. Parrish, J.A., Fitzpatrick, T.B., Tanenbaum, L., and Pathak, M.A. (1974). Photochemotherapy of psoriasis with oral methoxsalen and longwave light. *N. Engl. J. Med.* 291:1207–1211.
12. Gschnait, F., Hönigsmann, H., Brenner, W., Fritsch, P., and Wolff, K. (1978). Induction of UV light tolerance by PUVA in patients with polymorphous light eruption. *Br. J. Dermatol.* 99:293–295.
13. Gilchrest, B.A., Parrish, J.A., Tanenbaum, L., Haynes, H.A., and Fitzpatrick, T.B. (1976). Oral methoxsalen photochemotherapy of mycosis fungoides. *Cancer* 38:683–689.
14. Hönigsmann, H., Konrad, K., Gschnait, F., and Wolff, K. (1976). Photochemotherapy of mycosis fungoides. In *Book of Abstracts*, VIIth International Congress of Photobiology, Rome, p. 222.
15. Gschnait, F., Hönigsmann, H., Konrad, K., and Fritsch, P. (1977). Photochemotherapie (PUVA) bei Neurodermatitis. *Z. Hautkr.* 52:1219–1224.
16. Morison, W.L., Parrish, J.A., and Fitzpatrick, T.B. (1978). Oral psoralen photochemotherapy of atopic eczema. *Br. J. Dermatol.* 98:25–30.
17. Brenner, W., Gschnait, F., Hönigsmann, H., and Fritsch, P. (1978). Erprobung von PUVA bei verschiedenen Dermatosen. *Hautarzt* 29:541–544.
18. Boelen, R., Faber, W., Lambers, J., and Cormane, R. (1982). Long term follow-up of photochemotherapy in pityriasis lichenoides. *Acta Derm. Venereol (Stockh.)* 62:442–444.
19. Breit, R., and Röcken, M. (1991). Klassische Form einer eosinophilen pustulösen Follikulitis. Erfolgreiche Therapie mit PUVA. *Hautarzt* 42:247–250.
20. Zaynoun, S., Jaber, L., and Kurban, A. (1986). Oral methoxsalen photochemotherapy of extensive pityriasis alba. *J. Am. Acad. Dermatol.* 15:61–65.
21. Kerker, B., Huang, C., and Morison, W.L. (1990). Photochemotherapy of generalized granuloma anulare. *Arch. Dermatol.* 126:359–361.
22. Christophers, E., Gschnait, F., Hönigsmann, H., Wolff, K., and Langner, A. (1978). PUVA treatment for urticaria pigmentosa. *Br. J. Dermatol.* 98: 701–702.
23. Vella-Briffa, D., Eady, R., James, M., Gatti, S., and Bleehen, S. (1983). Photochemotherapy (PUVA) in the treatment of urticaria pigmentosa. *Br. J. Dermatol.* 109:67–75.
24. Ortonne, J., Thivolet, J., and Sannwald, C. (1978). Oral photochemotherapy in the treatment of lichen planus. *Br. J. Dermatol.* 99:77–88.

25. Gonzalez, E., Momtaz, T., and Freedman, S. (1984). Bilateral comparison of generalized lichen planus treated with psoralens and ultraviolet A. *J. Am. Acad. Dermatol.* 10:958–961.
26. Hymes, S., Morison, W.L., and Farmer, E. (1985). Methoxsalen and ultraviolet A radiation in treatment of chronic cutaneous graft-versus-host reaction. *J. Am. Acad. Dermatol.* 12:30–37.
27. Atkinson, K., Weller, P., and Ryman, W. (1986). PUVA therapy for drug-resistant graft-versus-host disease. *Bone Marrow Transplant.* 1:227–236.
28. Volc-Platzer, B., Hönigsmann, H., Hinterberger, W., and Wolff, K. (1990). Photochemotherapy improves chronic graft-versus-host disease. *J. Am. Acad. Dermatol.* 23:220–228.
29. Scharffetter-Kockhanek, K., Goldermann, R., Lehmann, P., Holzle, E., and Goerz, G. (1995). PUVA therapy in disabling pansclerotic morphoea of children. *Br. J. Dermatol.* 132:830–831 (letter).
30. Kerscher, M., Volkenandt, M., Meurer, M., Lehmann, P., Plewig, G., and Rocken, M. (1994). Treatment of localized scleroderma with PUVA bath photochemotherapy. *Lancet* 343:1233 (letter).
31. Calzavara-Pinton, P.G., Ortel, B., Hönigsmann, H., Zane, C., and DePanfillis, G. (1994). Safety and effectiveness of an aggressive and individualized bath-PUVA regimen in the treatment of psoriasis. *Dermatology* 189:256–259.
32. Tanew, A., Ortel, B., and Hönigsmann, H. (1988). 5-Methoxypsoralen and other new furocoumarins in the treatment of psoriasis. In *Light in Biology and Medicine.* R. Douglas, J. Moan, and F. Dall'Acqua (Eds.). Plenum Press, New York, pp. 183–188.
33. Dubertret, L., Averbeck, D., and Bisagny, E. (1985). Photochemotherapy using pyridopsoralens. *Biochimie* 67:417–422.
34. Bickers, D., and Pathak, M. (1984). Psoralen pharmacology: studies on metabolism and enzyme induction. *Natl. Cancer Inst. Monogr.* 66:77–84.
35. Brickl, R., Schmid, J., and Koss, F.W. (1984). Pharmacokinetics and pharmacodynamics of psoralens after oral administration: considerations and conclusions. *Natl. Cancer Inst. Monogr.* 66:63–67.
36. Herfst, M.J., and de Wolff, F.A. (1983). Intraindividual and inter-individual variability in 8-methoxypsoralen kinetics and effect in psoriatic patients. *Clin. Pharmacol. Ther.* 34:117–124.
37. Andrew, E., Nilsen, A., Thune, P., and Wilk, I. (1981). Photochemotherapy in psoriasis. Clinical response and 8-MOP plasma concentrations at two levels. *Clin. Exp. Dermatol.* 6:591–600.
38. Swanbeck, G., Eriksson, H., Ehrneb, M., Wallin, I., and Jonsson, L. (1979). Serum concentrations and phototoxic effects of methoxypsoralen in patients with psoriasis. *Clin. Pharmacol. Ther.* 25:478–480.
39. Hönigsmann, H., Jaschke, E., and Nitsche, V. (1982). Serum levels of 8-methoxypsoralen in two different drug preparations. Correlation with photosensitivity and UVA dose requirements for photochemotherapy. *J. Invest. Dermatol.* 79:233–236.
40. McLellan, J., Fisher, C., Farr, P.M., Diffey, B.L., and Cox, N.H. (1991). The relationship between plasma psoralen concentration and psoralen-UVA erythema. *Br. J. Dermatol.* 124:585–590.
41. Bonnot, D., Beani, J.C., Boitard, M., Reymond, J.L., Beriel, H., and Amblard, P. (1994). Determination of 8-methoxypsoralen kinetics: a relevant factor in the treatment of psoriasis by psoralen plus ultraviolet A therapy. *Photodermatol. Photoimmunol. Photomed.* 10:33–37.
42. Kornhauser, A., Wamer, W.G., and Giles, A.L. (1982). Psoralen phototoxicity: correlation with serum and epidermal 8-methoxypsoralen and 5-methoxypsoralen in the guinea pig. *Science* 217: 733–735.
43. Tanew, A., Ortel, B., Rappersberger, K., and Hönigsmann, H. (1988). 5-methoxypsoralen (Bergapten) for photochemotherapy. *J. Am. Acad. Dermatol.* 18: 333–338.
44. Treffel, P., Renaud, A., Humbert, P., Makki, S., Faivre, B., and Agache, P.E. (1990). Chronopharmacokinetics of 5-methoxypsoralen. *Acta Derm. Venereol.* 70:515–517.
45. Calzavara-Pinton, P.G., Ortel, B., Carlino, A., Hönigsmann, H., and De Panfilis, G. (1992). A reappraisal of the use of 5-methoxypsoralen in the therapy of psoriasis. *Exp. Dermatol.* 1:46–51.
46. Aubin, F., Makki, S., Humbert, P., Muret, P., and Agache, P. (1994). Treatment of psoriasis with a new micronized 5-methoxypsoralen tablet and UVA radiation. *Arch. Dermatol. Res.* 286:30–34.
47. Stolk, A., Siddiqui, A.H., and Cormane, R.H. (1981). Serum levels of trimethylpsoralen after oral administration. *Br. J. Dermatol.* 104:443–445.
48. Sakunthabai, A., Matthews, J.N.S., and Farr, P.M. (1994). Improved prediction of the minimal phototoxic dose in PUVA therapy. *Br. J. Dermatol.* 130: 604–609.
49. Staberg, B., and Hueg, B. (1985). Interaction between 8-methoxypsoralen and phenytoin. Consequence for PUVA therapy. *Acta Derm. Venereol.* 65:553–555.
50. Pathak, M.A. (1961). Mechanism of psoralen photosensitization and in vivo biological action spectrum of 8-methoxypsoralen. *J. Invest. Dermatol.* 37: 397–406.
51. Cripps, D.J., Lowe, N.J., and Lerner, A.B. (1982). Action spectra of topical psoralens: a re-evaluation. *Br. J. Dermatol.* 107:77–82.
52. Young, A.R., and Magnus, I.A. (1981). An action spectrum for 8-MOP-induced sunburn cells in mammalian epidermis. *Br. J. Dermatol.* 104:451–458.

53. Kaidbey, K.M. (1985). An action spectrum for 8-MOP-sensitized inhibition of DNA synthesis in vivo. *J. Invest. Dermatol.* 85:98–101.
54. Ortel, B., and Gange, R. (1990). An action spectrum for the elicitation of erythema in skin persistently sensitized by photobound 8-methoxypsoralen. *J. Invest. Dermatol.* 94:781–785.
55. Farr, P.M., Diffey, B.L., and Matthews, J.N. (1991). The action spectrum between 320 and 400 nm for clearance of psoriasis by psoralen photochemotherapy. *Br. J. Dermatol.* 124:443–448.
56. Brücke, J., Tanew, A., Ortel, B., and Hönigsmann, H. (1991). Relative efficacy of 335 and 365 nm radiation in photochemotherapy of psoriasis. *Br. J. Dermatol.* 124:372–374.
57. Ortel, B., Perl, S., Kinaciyan, T., Calzavara-Pinton, P.G., and Hönigsmann, H. (1993). Comparison of narrow-band (311 nm) UVB and broad-band UVA after oral and bath-water 8-methoxypsoralen in the treatment of psoriasis. *J. Am. Acad. Dermatol.* 29: 736–740.
58. Harber, L., and Bickers, D. (1989). Artificial ultraviolet light sources: clinical applications. In *Photosensitivity Diseases: Principles of Diagnosis and Treatment*, 2nd ed. L. Harber and D. Bickers (Eds.). W.B. Saunders, Philadelphia, pp. 142–159.
59. Anderson, T. (1990). Light sources in photomedicine. In *Clinical Photomedicine.* H. Lim and N. Soter (Eds.). Marcel Dekker, New York, pp. 37–58.
60. Fisher, T., Alsins, J., and Berne, B. (1984). Ultraviolet action spectrum and evaluation of ultraviolet lamps for psoriasis healing. *Int. J. Dermatol.* 23:633–637.
61. Sakuntabhai, A., Diffey, B.L., and Farr, P.M. (1993). Response of psoriasis to psoralen-UVB photochemotherapy. *Br. J. Dermatol.* 128:296–300.
62. Cox, N.H., Farr, P.M., and Diffey, B.L. (1989). A comparison of the dose-response relationship for psoralen-UVA erythema and UVB erythema. *Dermatology* 125:1653–1657.
63. Fitzpatrick, T.B. (1975). Soleil et Peau. *J. Med. Esth.* 2:33–34.
64. Wolff, K., Gschnait, F., Hönigsmann, H., Konrad, K., Parrish, J.A., and Fitzpatrick, T.B. (1977). Phototesting and dosimetry for photochemotherapy. *Br. J. Dermatol.* 96:1–10.
65. Melski, J., Tanenbaum, L., Parrish, J.A., Fitzpatrick, T.B., and Bleich, H. (1977). Oral methoxsalen photochemotherapy for the treatment of psoriasis: a cooperative clinical trial. *J. Invest. Dermatol.* 68: 328–335.
66. Wolff, K., Hönigsmann, H., Gschnait, F., and Konrad, K. (1975). Klinische Erfahrungen bei 152 Patienten. *Deutsch. Med. Wochenschr.* 100:2471–2477.
67. Henseler, T., Wolff, K., Hönigsmann, H., and Christophers, E. (1981). Oral 8-methoxypsoralen photochemotherapy of psoriasis. The European PUVA Study: a cooperative study among 18 European centers. *Lancet* 1:853–857.
68. Carabott, F.M., and Hawk, J.L.M. (1989). A modified dosage schedule for increased efficiency in PUVA treatment of psoriasis. *Clin. Exp. Dermatol.* 14: 337–340.
69. Wolff, K., and Hönigsmann, H. (1981). Clinical aspects of photochemotherapy. *Pharmacol. Ther.* 12: 381–418.
70. Fritsch, P., Hönigsmann, H., Jaschke, E., and Wolff, K. (1978). Augmentation of oral methoxsalen photochemotherapy with an oral aromatic retinoic acid derivative. *J. Invest. Dermatol.* 70:178–182.
71. Heidbreder, G., and Christophers, E. (1979). Therapy of psoriasis with retinoid plus PUVA: clinical and histologic data. *Arch. Derm. Res.* 264:331.
72. Hönigsmann, H., and Wolff, K. (1983). Isotretinoin-PUVA for psoriasis. *Lancet* 1:236 (letter).
73. Tanew, A., Guggenbichler, A., Hönigsmann, H., Geiger, J.-M., and Fritsch, P. (1991). Photochemotherapy of severe psoriasis without or in combination with acitretin: a randomized double-blind comparison study. *J. Am. Acad. Dermatol.* 25:682–684.
74. Momtax, T.K., and Parrish, J.A. (1984). Combination of psoralens and ultraviolet A and ultraviolet B in the treatment of psoriasis vulgaris. *J. Am. Acad. Dermatol.* 10:481.
75. Petzlbauer, P., Hönigsmann, H., Langer, K., Anegg, B., Strohal, R., Tanew, A., and Wolff, K. (1990). Cyclosporin A in combination with photochemotherapy (PUVA) in the treatment of psoriasis. *Br. J. Dermatol.* 125:641–647.
76. Lambert, B., Bredberg, A., McKenzie, W., and Sten, M. (1982). Sister chromatid exchange in human populations: the effect of smoking, drug treatment, and occupational exposure. *Cytogen. Cell Genet.* 33: 62–67.
77. Stern, R., and Lange, R. (1991). Outcomes of pregnancies among women and partners of men with a history of exposure to methoxsalen photochemotherapy (PUVA) for the treatment of psoriasis. *Arch. Dermatol.* 127:347–350.
78. Gunnarskog, J., Kallen, A., Lindelof, B., and Sigurgeirsson, B. (1993). Psoralen photochemotherapy and pregnancy. *Arch. Dermatol.* 129:320–323.
79. Roelandts, R., and Stevens, A. (1990). PUVA-induced itching and skin pain. *Photodermatol. Photoimmunol. Photomed.* 7:141–142.
80. Burrows, N., And Norris, P. (1994). Treatment of PUVA-induced skin pain with capsacin. *Br. J. Dermatol.* 131:584–585 (letter).
81. Morison, W.L. (1991). PUVA Therapy. In *Phototherapy and Photochemotherapy of Skin Disease*, 2nd ed., W.L. Morison (Ed.). Raven Press, New York, pp. 93–131.

82. Anderson, C.D., Fröndin, T., and Skogh, M. (1984). Unusual adverse effects of 8-methoxypsoralen: bronchial reaction during photochemotherapy (PUVA). *J. Am. Acad. Dermatol.* 10:298.
83. Berg, M. (1989). Drug fever caused by 8-methoxypsoralen. *Photodermatology* 6:149–150.
84. Cox, N., and Rogers, S. (1989). Cutaneous drug eruption caused by 8-methoxypsoralen. *Photodermatology* 6:96–97.
85. Baran, R., and Juhlin, L. (1978). Drug-induced photooncholysis. *J. Am. Acad. Dermatol.* 17:1012–1016.
86. Friedman, P., Coburn, P., and Dahl, M. (1987). PUVA-induced blisters, complement deposition, and damage to the dermoepidermal junction. *Arch. Dermatol.* 123:1471–1477.
87. Rampen, F. (1983). Hypertrichosis in PUVA-treated patients. *Br. J. Dermatol.* 109:657–660.
88. Moller, H. (1990). Contact and photocontact allergy to psoralens. *Photodermatol. Photoimmunol. Photomed.* 71:43–44.
89. Roelandts, R., Lonche, J., and Degreff, H. (1985). Phytophotodermatitis-like lesion induced by PUVA. *Photodermatology* 2:40–43.
90. Talwar, H.S., Griffiths, C.E., Fisher, G.J., Hamilton, T.A., and Voorhees, J.J. (1995). Reduced type I and type III procollagens in photodamaged adult human skin. *J. Invest. Dermatol.* 105:285–290.
91. Lavker, R.M. (1979). Structural alteration in exposed and unexposed aged skin. *J. Invest. Dermatol.* 73: 59–66.
92. Stern, R. (1994). Ocular lens findings in patients treated with PUVA. *J. Invest. Dermatol.* 103: 534–538.
93. Calzavara-Pinton, P.G., Carlino, A., Manfred, E., Semeraro, F., Zane, C., and DePanfilis, G. (1994). Ocular side effects of PUVA-treated patients refusing eye sun protection. *Acta Derm. Venereol. (Stockh.)* (Suppl.) 186:164–165.
94. Stern, R., Laird, N., and Melski, J. (1984). Cutaneous squamous cell carcinoma in patients treated with PUVA. *N. Engl. J. Med.* 310:1156–1161.
95. Stern, R., Lange, R., and Members of the PUVA Follow-Up Study. (1988). Non-melanoma skin cancer occurring in patients treated with PUVA five to ten years after first treatment. *J. Invest. Dermatol.* 91: 120–124.
96. Stern, R. (1992). Risks of cancer associated with long-term exposure to PUVA in humans: current status—1991. *Blood Cells* 18:91–99.
97. Lindelof, B., Sigurgeirsson, B., and Tegner, E. (1991). PUVA and cancer: a large scale epidemiological study. *Lancet* 338:91–93.
98. Weinstock, M., Coulter, S., Bates, J., Bogaars, H., Larson, P., and Burmer, G. (1995). Human papillomavirus and widespread cutaneous carcinoma after PUVA photochemotherapy. *Arch. Dermatol.* 131: 701–704.
99. Bruynzeel, I., Bergman, W., Hartevelt, H., Kenter, C., Van De Velde, E.A., Schothorst, A., and Suurmond, D. (1991). High single-dose European PUVA regimen also causes an excess of nonmelanoma skin cancer. *Br. J. Dermatol.* 124:49–55.
100. Chuang, T-Y., Heinrich, L.A., Schultz, M.D., Reizner, G.T., Kumm, R.C., and Cripps, D.J. (1992). PUVA and skin cancer. A historical cohort study on 492 patients. *J. Am. Acad. Dermatol.* 26:173–177.
101. Stern, R.S., and Laird, N. (1994). The carcinogenic risk of treatments for severe psoriasis. *Cancer* 73: 2759–2764.
102. Marx, J., Auerbach, R., Possick, P., Myrow, R., Gladstein, A., and Kopf, A. (1983). Malignant melanoma in situ in two patients treated with psoralens and ultraviolet A. *J. Am. Acad. Dermatol.* 9:904–911.
103. Stern, R., and Members of the PUVA Follow-Up Study. (1990). Genital tumors among men with psoriasis exposed to psoralens and ultraviolet A radiation (PUVA) and ultraviolet B radiation. *N. Engl. J. Med.* 332:1093–1097.
104. Wolff, K., and Hönigsmann, H. (1991). Genital carcinomas in psoriasis patients treated with photochemotherapy. *Lancet* 1:439 (letter).
105. Musajo, L., and Rodighiero, G. (1970). Studies on the photo-C4-cyclo-addition reactions between skin-photosensitizing furocoumarins and nucleic acids. *Photochem. Photobiol.* 11:27–35.
106. Musajo, L., Rodighiero, G., Colombo, Torlone, V., and Dall'Acqua, F. (1965). Photosensitizing furocoumarins: interaction with DNA and photoinactivation of DNA containing viruses. *Experientia* 21:22–24.
107. Schmitt, I., Chimenti, S., and Gasparro, F. (1995). Psoralen-protein photochemistry—the forgotten field. *J. Photochem. Photobiol. B: Biol.* 27:101–105.
108. Bordin, F., Carlassare, F., Busuline, L., and Bacci-chetti, F. (1993). Furocoumarin photosensitization induces DNA-protein crosslinks. *Photochem. Photobiol.* 58:133–136.
109. Neuner, P., Charvat, B., Knobler, R., Kirnbauer, R., Schwarz, A., Luger, T., and Schwarz, T. (1994). Cytokine release by peripheral blood mononuclear cells is affected by 8-methoxypsoralen plus UVA. *Photochem. Photobiol.* 59:182–188.
110. Koulu, L., Söderström, K., and Jansen, C. (1984). Relation of antipsoriatic and Langerhans cell depleting effects of systemic psoralen photochemotherapy: a clinical, enzyme histochemical and electron microscopic study. *J. Invest. Dermatol.* 82:591–593.
111. Okamoto, H., Horio, T., and Maeda, M. (1987). Alteration of lymphocyte functions by 8-methoxypsoralen and long-wave ultraviolet radiation. II. The effect of in vivo PUVA on IL-2 production. *J. Invest. Dermatol.* 89:24–26.

112. Strauss, G., Bridges, B., Greaves, M., Hall-Smith, P., Price, M., and Vella-Briffa, D. (1980). Inhibition of delayed hypersensitivity in skin (DNCB test) by 8-methoxypsoralen photochemotherapy. Possible basis for pseudo-promoting action in skin carcinogenesis. *Lancet* 2:556–559.
113. Moscicki, R., Morison, W.L., Parrish, J.A., Bloch, K., and Colvin, R. (1982). Reduction of the fraction of circulating helper-inducer T cells identified by monoclonal antibodies in psoriatic patients treated with long-term psoralen/ultraviolet A radiation (PUVA). *J. Invest. Dermatol.* 79:205–208.
114. Vallat, V., Gilleaudeau, P., Battat, L., Wolfe, J., Nabeya, R., Heftler, N., Hodak, E., Gottlieb, A., and Krueger, J. (1994). PUVA bath therapy strongly suppresses immunological and epidermal activation in psoriasis: a possible cellular basis for remittive therapy. *J. Exp. Med.* 180:283–296.
115. Johnson, R., Staiano-Coico, L., Austin, L., Cardinale, I., Nabeya-Tsukifuji, R., and Krueger, J. (1996). PUVA treatment selectively induces a cell cycle block and subsequent apoptosis in human T-lymphocytes. *Photochem. Photobiol.* 63:566–571.
116. Gasparro, F. (1996). Psoralen photobiology: recent advances. *Photochem. Photobiol.* 63:553–557.
117. Coldiron, B., and Bergstresser, P. (1989). Prevalence and clinical spectrum of skin diseases in patients infected with human immunodeficiency virus. *Arch. Dermatol.* 125:357–361.
118. Zmudzka, B.Z., and Beer, J.Z. (1990). Activation of human immunodeficiency virus by ultraviolet radiation. *Photochem. Photobiol.* 52:1153–1162.
119. Zmudzka, B.Z., Strickland, A.G., and Miller, S.A. (1993). Activation of the HIV promoter by UVA radiation in combination with psoralens or angelicins. *Photochem. Photobiol.* 58:226–232.
120. Valerie, K., Delers, A., and Bruck, C. (1988). Activation of human immunodeficiency virus type 1 by DNA damage in human cells. *Nature* 333:78–81.
121. Horn, T., Morison, W.L., Farzadegan, H., Zmudzka, B., and Beer, J. (1994). Effect of psoralen plus UVA radiation (PUVA) on HIV-1 in human beings: a pilot study. *J. Am. Acad. Dermatol.* 31:735–740.
122. Thomsen, K., and Schmidt, H. (1976). PUVA-induced bullous pemphigoid. *Br. J. Dermatol.* 95: 568–569.
123. Abel, A.E., and Bennett, A. (1979). Bullous pemphigoid. Occurrence in psoriasis treated with psoralen plus long-wave ultraviolet radiation. *Arch. Dermatol.* 115:988–989.
124. Bastian, P., Drobacheff, C., and Laurent, R. (1990). Pemphigoides bulleuses declenchees par la puvatherapie. *Ann. Dermatol. Venereol.* 117:73–82.
125. Weber, P.J., and Salazar, J.E. (1989). Bullous eruption in a psoriatic patient. Bullous pemphigoid and psoriasis. *Arch. Dermatol.* 125:693–694.
126. Perl, S., Rappersberger, K., Födinger, D., Anegg, B., Hönigsmann, H., and Ortel, B. (1996). Bullous pemphigoid induced by PUVA therapy. *Dermatology* 193: 245–247.
127. Neumann, C. (1987). Induktion eines subakuten Lupus erythematodes durch Psoralen-UV-A-Therapie. *Z. Hautkr.* 62:1523–1524.
128. Dowdy, M.J., Nigra, T.P., and Barth, W.F. (1989). Subacute cutaneous lupus erythematosus during PUVA therapy for psoriasis: case report and review of the literature. *Arthritis Rheum.* 32:343–346.

42

Hand and Foot PUVA

Torkel Fischer
National Institute for Working Life, Solna, Sweden

Psoriasis and pustulosis palmoplantaris (PPP) of the palms and soles are recalcitrant dermatoses and a therapeutic challenge. The introduction of PUVA treatment was followed by an initial optimism with positive reports of healing also in the treatment of hand and foot psoriasis, but this was followed by a period of skepticism and reports that PUVA treatment of palms and soles was more or less ineffective (1–8).

Our present modified view is that it is more difficult to achieve a therapeutic response on palms and soles than in other parts of the body, but that both PUVA and retinoid-PUVA (RePUVA) are effective treatments in many patients with plaque psoriasis and PPP and that these treatments should be considered especially in hand disease (9–14).

Oral PUVA (2,4–8,10–14), topical PUVA (1,3,8,11,15), bath PUVA (3,11), and RePUVA (9,10,16) are all worth trying. They need skill and patience, and the time of treatment until healing may be long. Indications and contraindications are the same as with other types of PUVA and RePUVA treatments.

SENSITIZATION TECHNIQUE

Oral Sensitization

The same standard schedule of photosensitization is followed in palm and sole disease as that used for psoriasis in other areas of the body, i.e., 0.4–0.6 mg of 8-methoxypsoralen (8-MOP)/kg body weight 1–2 hr prior to irradiation.

Topical Sensitization

The photosensitization obtained differs with different vehicles used for the psoralens. Most commonly, 8-MOP is included in either ointment, cream, lotion, or oil bases in a concentration of 0.1–1.0% (1,3,8,11,17). A psoralen preparation of 0.1–1.0% is applied to the affected skin area 0.25–2 hr prior to the irradiation (1,3,11,17). Polyethylene bag occlusion may be used (18). Topical sensitization may also be obtained with 8-MOP water soaks. Hands and feet are then submerged in 2 L of 8-MOP solution 2.5 mg/L for 30 min. Treatment with 0.1% MOP in hydrophilic ointment or 50% isopropanol applied sparingly over hands and soles resulted in undetectable plasma levels of 8-MOP (19). The mean serum level of 8-MOP 60 min after completion of hand and foot soaks was 2.5 ± 0.5 ng/ml compared with 95.75 ± 10.43 ng/ml after oral 8-MOP, 0.5 mg/kg (20). No reports have yet been published on the short-contact sensitization reported to be effective in psoriasis of palms and soles.

Bath Sensitization

Both 8-MOP and trioxsalen (trimethylpsoralen, TMP) are effective. The hand or foot bath is prepared by adding 6 ml of an alcoholic solution of either 0.1% 8-MOP or 0.05% TMP to 10 L of hot tap water (about

102°F). Shake the bottle with psoralen solution well before use because small crystals may remain undissolved in it. The concentration of psoralen in the baths thus obtained are 0.6 mg/L with 8-MOP and 0.3 mg/L with TMP (3,16).

RADIATION SOURCES

With oral sensitization, UVA is the irradiation of choice. With TMP sensitization, either UVA or UVB irradiation may be used. If UVB tubes are used, then the irradiation dose is evaluated according to the UVA part of the lamp spectrum. 8-MOP has a lower topical sensitizing capacity than TMP, and therefore UVA lamps should be used after this type of sensitization. The special hand and foot PUVA irradiation panels developed that deliver 5–15 mW/cm^2 in the UVA range are suitable for this kind of treatment. Details of topical treatment are discussed in another chapter.

As is the case with PUVA treatment of hand eczema, whole-body irradiation may be most effective in healing palm and sole psoriasis and PPP (21).

RADIATION DOSAGE

Treatments are preferably given three to five times weekly until clearing or to the point of maximum improvement. Dose increments should not be planned more frequently than once a week. If irritation or pain develops, the dose should be kept constant; in case of a severe reaction, it is advisable to reduce the dose 30%, or to make a pause in the treatment.

Maintenance starts with treatments once a week and intervals are successively expanded to once a month, whatever is necessary to keep the disease under control. Maintenance treatment is usually performed with the last UVA dose of the clearing phase, and if this dose is irritant, it should be reduced by 30%. During maintenance doses are often subsequently reduced as treatment intervals increase (9).

Oral Sensitization

As a rule, psoriasis of palms and soles can be treated with somewhat higher irradiation doses as compared to psoriasis in ordinary skin. Start with 2.5 J/cm^2 UVA (1.0–4.5 J/cm^2 depending on skin type). The UV dose is increased weekly. Choose increment steps of 0.5–1.0 J/cm^2 to a joule dose of 6–28 J/cm^2 (6,10,12,14).

Topical Sensitization

The following dose schedule is suggested after 8-MOP sensitization. Ultraviolet A irradiation is started at a dose of 0.25–0.8 J/cm^2 and the dose is increased weekly with 0.1–0.2 J/cm^2 up to 1 J/cm^2, and then with increment steps of 0.3–0.5 J/cm^2 depending on the clinical response. The maximum dose is in the range of 12 J/cm^2 (1,3,8,17).

After sensitization with water soaks and immediate irradiation the initial UVA dose recommended is 0.25 J/cm^2, with subsequent increments of 0.25 J/cm^2 until 1.0 J/cm^2 and then increments of 0.5–1.0 J/cm^2. The range of maximum UVA dosage reported per treatment was 3.5–17.5 J/cm^2, and the range of cumulative UVA required for maximal improvement was 45–388 J/cm^2 with a mean of 165 J/cm^2 (20).

Bath Sensitization

Patients should be irradiated within 15 min after the bath when the photosensitivity is maximal With 8-MOP, the same schedule can be used as with topical sensitization (3). With TMP bath sensitization, the initial dose of UVA to be used is 0.1–0.4 J/cm^2, with dose increments of 0.1–0.2 J/cm^2 until 4–6 J/cm^2 or untoward effects begin to occur (11,16).

RePUVA TECHNIQUES

Oral etretinate is so far the only retinoid that has been reported to be used in conjunction with PUVA for the treatment of psoriasis of palms and soles. Etretinate is given in a conventional dose 4–14 days before the start of the PUVA treatment (0.6–1.0 mg/kg body weight per day). The higher dose is reduced after 14 days to 0.6 mg/kg/day. The psoralens are given according to the same schedule as described for the various techniques of oral and topical application. Retinoids do not change the phototoxicity threshold of psoralens, and the same UV doses are recommended with PUVA and RePUVA (9). Burning is an indication for temporary withdrawal of the PUVA or for a dose reduction (9,14).

HEALING

With all the different kinds of PUVA treatments, about half of the patients respond with significant improvement or healing. It is not definite whether the oral or the topical PUVA is the superior method to treat psoriasis of palms and soles. RePUVA seems to give better healing results than PUVA only, and 80–100% improvement/healing has been reported with this technique.

Plaque psoriasis responds somewhat better to PUVA treatment than do pustulovesicular types (1). Hand lesions heal more easily than those of the foot.

Improvement may already be apparent after 2–4 weeks of treatment, but may be late, and before considering the treatment a failure, PUVA or RePUVA should be given for at least 12 weeks. The treatment period until healing may be 18 weeks or more.

Oral PUVA

Menné reported complete healing in seven of 12 patients with PPP and in 10 of 12 patients with palm and sole psoriasis after a mean of 16 treatments within a month (4).

Mizuno et al. found improvement in all of their four patients with PPP; in three of them the hands cleared completely (5).

Morison et al. successfully cleared 18 of 20 patients, five with pustular psoriasis, five with plaque psoriasis, three with palmoplantar psoriasis, and five with endogenous eczema within 40–60 days and 14–22 treatments. The two patients who did not clear both had pustular psoriasis; one ceased treatment because of nausea, the other improved (6).

Murray et al. treated randomly on one side 22 patients with bilateral symmetrical PPP. The treated side cleared completely in 12 patients (8).

Lawrence et al. cleared five of nine patients with hyperkeratotic psoriasis or PPP within a mean of 59 days of treatment. Two patients remained clear for 6 months and the other three for an average of 12 weeks (10).

In 13 patients with PPP, Lassus et al. found partial but no complete healing after 2 weeks of treatment (11).

Ågren-Jonsson and Tegner treated 40 patients with palmoplantar psoriasis. Thirty-six had palmar lesions, which cleared in 31 cases. After 2 years, nine of them were still completely healed. Plantar lesions healed less satisfactorily and only five of 34 patients healed; however, most patients had long-standing improvement (12).

Moseley and Lever reported nine patients with PPP, two on palms and seven on soles. After 1 month, three patients had improved, no change was observed in five, and deterioration occurred in one; after 3 months, four patients showed improvement and two no change (13).

Rosén et al. have reported healing in three of 12 patients treated with oral psoralen and unilateral UVA radiation. The unirradiated control side improved but did not heal in any patient (14).

Topical PUVA

Beneficial results from topical treatment were reported when psoralen was applied 1–2 hr before UVA irradiation, while no benefit was found when the psoralen was applied just prior to irradiation (1,3,5,8,15,22,23). Konya et al. found a lag time of approximately 40 min after hands and feet were immersed in methoxsalen solution before maximum UVA sensitivity was reached (24). The vehicle affects the penetration and the greatest penetration occurs with solutions and emulsions (25).

Abel et al. treated 14 patients with plaque psoriasis and 14 with vesiculopustular dermatosis with topical PUVA. In the first group, nine responded with considerable improvement, as evidenced by flattening of the plaques, decreased scaling and erythema, and decreased vesicle and pustule formation. Of these, two healed completely. In the second group, seven demonstrated considerable improvement, and of these three had complete healing. The disease had maximum therapeutic response within 12–40 weeks of treatment. During the healing phase of the palmoplantar vesiculopustular psoriasis vesiculopustules continued to develop. Patients who missed the maintenance usually flared within a month to a year (1).

Murray et al. treated 15 patients with persistent PPP with topical 8-MOP and UVA. Seven of them cleared completely, six were much improved, and two improved (8).

Jansén and Malmiharju treated five patients with PPP topically with 8-MOP ointment and got no response in four and exacerbation in one (3).

Lassus et al. improved their group of 28 PPP patients with topical 8-MOP and UVA, but complete healing occurred in only four patients after 12 weeks of treatment (11).

Coleman et al. found in 11 patients with moderate to severe palmoplantar psoriasis who had been resistant to previous topical therapies that the condition of one patient cleared completely, and seven showed good improvement. The range of treatments required for maximal improvement was 14–43 with a mean of 28 (20).

Hawk and Grice compared oral or topical PUVA of chronic hand and foot dermatoses, mostly psoriasis and PPP. There were broadly similar success rates for the two groups. Eight of 13 patients cleared completely and three had significant improvement with oral PUVA, 11 of 23 cleared, and seven had significant improvement with topical PUVA. The mean number of treatments and treatment durations and relapse rates were comparable in the two groups (17).

Layton et al. made a placebo-controlled study of the effect of topical MOP emulsion used 10 min prior to UVA in 27 patients with PPP. There was little difference in the overall improvement of the hands and feet in both the active and placebo-treated areas (23).

Bath PUVA

Jansén and Malmiharju used 8-MOP bath and UVA treatment in eight patients with PPP. One had a good response, two moderate, three no response, and two exacerbation of the disease (3).

Lassus et al. found no complete healing but significant improvement in their group of 18 patients with PPP treated with TMP bath PUVA for 12 weeks (11).

RePUVA

Fritsch et al. cleared 12 patients with severe palmoplantar psoriasis with 7 ± 3 treatments of etretinate plus PUVA within 12.8 ± 5.5 days requiring 2.14 ± 17.3 J/cm^2. The total energy for clearing was considerably lower with the RePUVA regimen and the healing much faster than with ordinary oral PUVA (9).

Lawrence et al. treated 10 patients with palmoplantar psoriasis or PPP with etretinate-PUVA and all cleared in a mean of 30 days. Two patients remained clear after 6 months, the other eight remained clear for an average of 9 weeks (10).

Rosén et al. cleared 14 of 18 PPP patients with etretinate-PUVA within a mean of a little less than 3 months (14).

In 20 patients with PPP, Matsunami et al. compared topical PUVA, oral etretinate, or combined PUVA and etretinate. Re- and Re-PUVA-treated sites improved and/or cleared more rapidly and had longer remission periods than PUVA-treated sites (18).

Comparisons Between Treatments

Murray et al. found similar results with oral and topical psoralen on PPP, but their numbers were too small for a reliable comparison. They found that oral psoralen was more convenient, as pigmentation was regular and burns infrequent.

Patients with classic PPP and well-separated pustules responded better than those with vesicles. Those with thick scaling were more resistant (8).

In the treatment of patients with plaque psoriasis and vesiculopustular psoriasis, Abel et al. found that it was more difficult to achieve a therapeutic response to topical PUVA for psoriasis on the palms and soles than on other parts of the body, and that vesiculopustulosis responded less well than palmoplantar plaque type of psoriasis (1).

Jansén and Malmiharju compared topical 8-MOP PUVA to 8-MOP bath PUVA; both gave poor results and healing frequency was too low to allow comparative conclusions (3).

Lawrence et al. found etretinate-oral PUVA superior to oral PUVA only. The healing was more rapid; palmoplantar psoriasis healed better than PPP (10).

Lassus et al. found etretinate (not in combination with PUVA) to be superior to systemic PUVA, trioxsalen bath PUVA, and topical 8-MOP PUVA. The three PUVA treatments gave significant improvement but low frequency of complete healing with 12 weeks of treatment. There was no significant difference between the PUVA treatments (11).

Rosén et al. gave 30 patients either etretinate or placebo at random and, after 2 weeks, oral psoralen plus UVA radiation to one hand or one foot; 14 of the 18 hands or feet cleared with the combined etretinate-PUVA treatment, three of these 18 patients cleared on etretinate only, and there was complete healing in three of the 12 hands and feet given PUVA only. The patients were given a mean of 25 and 29 treatments, respectively (range 9–42 treatments), for a mean of 76 and 83 days (range 24–139 days) (14).

SIDE EFFECTS

Short-Term Effects

Morison et al. and Coleman et al. report erythema in a surprisingly high number of their patients. One patient stopped the treatment. Other investigators report one or a few patients with symptomatic erythema (1,3,6,20). Helm and Dijkstra noted a phototoxic reaction in the early treatment course on the lateral aspect and the instep of one foot (26). One of Rosén's 14 patients showed signs of polymorphic light eruption on the dorsum of a treated foot (14).

Abel et al. observed initial mild pruritus in 12 of 28 patients for 1–2 days, which was relieved by emollients or cold water. Several reports mention that pruritus, dryness, and itch are problems in a few patients, especially at the start of the treatment (1,4,6,11,20).

Smarting, tenderness, and burning discomfort occurs occasionally. With topical psoralen treatment, this may be caused by accidental painting of previously untreated skin. Burning is, however, also reported with oral psoralen (1,8,14).

Blistering may develop within or adjacent to the lesions, especially in topical treatment. Abel et al. found severe blistering in located areas in two of 28 patients. This side effect may be related to inadvertent sun exposure (1,3,14).

Ågren-Jonsson and Tegner found subungual petechia in one of their 40 patients (12).

Fritsch et al. mention that three patients (4.5%) of their whole group, including 12 PPP patients, demonstrated slight photoonycholysis (9).

The Koebner phenomenon and exacerbation as evidenced by an advancing margin of the psoriasis at the junction of thicker palmar or plantar skin has been reported in a few instances (1,3,6). This indicates that different UV doses must be administered depending on the degree of skin thickness. Zinc oxide paste applied around the margins of the lesions prevents this problem (1).

Localized hyperpigmentation occurred to some degree in all patients on hands and feet, but was not prominent on palms and soles (1). Morison et al. found that two of their 20 patients developed scattered hyperpigmentation. They also found postinflammatory depigmentation in four of their patients as the disease cleared (6). Rosén et al. found brown macules in two of 39 patients (14).

Nausea and to some extent headache and dizziness of varying intensity occurred in 5–50% of the patients on oral psoralen. Expected retinoid side effects occur in the frequency as with other types of retinoid treatments.

Long-Term Effects

Long-term side effects of palmoplantar PUVA treatment have so far not been investigated separately, but are not expected to differ from those of PUVA in other areas of the body.

REFERENCES

1. Abel, E., Goldberg, L.H., and Farber, E.M. (1980). Treatment of palmoplantar psoriasis with topical methoxsalen plus long-wave ultraviolet light. *Arch. Dermatol.* 116:1257–1261.
2. Bruynzeel, D.P., and Boonk, W.J. (1980). Zur PUVA-therapie von chronischen Dermatosen der Handflächen und Fussolen. *Z. Hautkr.* 55:523–529.
3. Jansén, C.T., and Malmiharju, T. (1981). Inefficacy of topical methoxsalen plus UVA for palmoplantar pustulosis. *Acta Derm. Venereol. (Stockh.)* 61:354–356.
4. Menné, T (1976). Behandling med 8-metoksypsoralen og langbølget ultraviolet lys. *Ugeskr. Laeg.* 138: 3119–3122.
5. Mizuno, N., Uematsu, S., and Ohno, M. (1976). Methoxsalen and irradiation. Treatment for pustulosis palmaris et plantaris. *Arch. Dermatol.* 112:883–884.
6. Morison, W.L., Parrish, J.A., and Fitzpatrick, T.B. (1978). Oral methoxsalen photochemotherapy of recalcitrant dermatoses of the palms and soles. *Br. J. Dermatol.* 99:297–302.
7. Murray, D., and Warin, A.P. (1979). Photochemotherapy for persistent palmoplantar pustulosis (PPP). *Br. J. Dermatol.* 101(Suppl. 17):13.
8. Murray, D., Corbett, M.F., and Warin, A.P. (1980). A controlled trial of photochemotherapy for persistent palmoplantar pustulosis. *Br. J. Dermatol.* 102: 659–663.
9. Fritsch, P.O., Hönigsmann, H., Jaschke, E. et al. (1978). Augmentation of oral methoxsalen photochemotherapy with an oral retinoic acid derivative. *J. Invest. Dermatol.* 70:178–182.
10. Lawrence, C.M., Marks, J., Parker, S. et al. (1984). A comparison of PUVA-etretinate and PUVA placebo for palmoplantar pustular psoriasis. *Br. J. Dermatol.* 110: 221–226.
11. Lassus, A., Lauharanta, J., and Eskelinen, A. (1985). The effects of etretinate compared with different regimens of PUVA in the treatment of persistent palmoplantar pustulosis. *Br. J. Dermatol.* 11(2):455–459.
12. Ågren-Jonsson, S., and Tegner, T.E. (1985). PUVA therapy for palmoplantar pustulosis. *Acta Derm. Venereol. (Stockh.)* 65:531–535.
13. Moseley, H., and Lever, R. (1985). Assessment by a quantitative technique of UVA and PUVA in the treatment of palmoplantar pustulosis. *Photodermatology* 2: 322–326.
14. Rosén K., Mobacken, H., and Swanbeck, G. (1987). PUVA, etretinate, and PUVA-etretinate therapy for pustulosis palmoplantaris. *Arch. Dermatol.* 123: 885–889.

15. Weber, G. (1974). Combined 8-methoxsalen and black light therapy of psoriasis. *Br. J. Dermatol.* 90:317–323.
16. Fischer, T., and Alsins, J. (1976). Treatment of psoriasis with trioxsalen baths and dysprosium lamps. *Acta Derm. Venereol. (Stockh).* 56(5):383–390.
17. Hawk, J.L., and Grice, P.L. (1994). The efficacy of localized PUVA therapy for chronic hand and foot dermatoses. *Clin. Exp. Dermatol.* 19(6):479–482.
18. Matsunami, E., Takashima, A., and Mizuuo, N. (1990). Topical PUVA, etretinate, and combined PUVA and etretinate for palmoplantar pustulosis: comparison of therapeutic efficacy and the influences of tonsillar and dental focal infections. *J. Dermatol.* 17(2):92–96.
19. Pham, C.T., and Koo, J.Y. (1993). Plasma levels of 8-methoxypsoralen after topical paint PUVA. *J. Am. Acad. Dermatol.* 28(3):460–466.
20. Coleman, W.R., Lowe, N.J., David, M., et al. (1989). Palmoplantar psoriasis: experience with 8-methoxypsoralen soaks plus ultraviolet A with the use of a high-output metal halide device. *J. Am. Acad. Dermatol.* 20(6):1078–1082.
21. Sjövall, P. (1988). Ultraviolet radiation and allergic contact dermatitis. An experimental and clinical study. Thesis, Department of Dermatology, Lund University, General Hospital, Malmö, Sweden, pp. 33–35.
22. Lakshmipathi, T., Gould, P.W., Mackenzie, I., et al. (1977). Photochemotherapy in the treatment of psoriasis. *Br. J. Dermatol.* 96:587–593.
23. Layton, A.M., Sheehan-Dare, R., and Cunliffe, W.J., (1991). A double-blind, placebo-controlled trial of topical PUVA in persistent palmoplantar pustulosis. *Br. J. Dermatol.* 124(6):581–584.
24. Konya, J., Diffey, B.L., and Hindson, T.C. (1992). Time course of activity of topical 8-methoxypsoralen on palmoplantar skin [letter]. *Br. J. Dermatol.* 127(6): 654–656.
25. Gazith, J., Schalla, W., Bauer, E., et al. (1978). 8-Methoxypsoralen (8-MOP) in human skin: penetration kinetics. *J. Invest. Dermatol.* 71:126–130.
26. Helm, T.N., and Dijkstra, J.W. (1991). Topical (bathwater) PUVA therapy. *J. Am. Acad. Dermatol.* 24 (6 Pt. 1):1035 (letter).

43

Topical PUVA and Bath PUVA

Torkel Fischer
National Institute for Working Life, Solna, Sweden

HISTORY

Many plants, particularly those of the Umbelliferae and Rutacae families, contain photosensitizing substances, usually psoralens. Their sap will photosensitize human skin to longwave ultraviolet radiation (UVA). Both occasional and occupational exposure to their sap coupled with outdoor activities can result in burns. Erythema, edema, and blisters form after 8–48 hr; this is followed by disfiguring pigmentation.

Psoralens have a high biological potency and exposure to sap with approximately 1 ppm psoralen may photosensitize sufficiently strongly to produce burns. The psoriasis-healing properties of psoralen plus UV radiation were described by Allyn in 1962, but were forgotten for a decade (1). In 1972–1974, there was an intense period of successful topical PUVA treatment (2–6). These topical PUVA treatments had undesirable side effects, such as uneven and cosmetically disfiguring pigmentation. In 1974, topical PUVA was surpassed by oral PUVA (7). Bath PUVA has been used in combination with oral PUVA on a large-scale basis for more than 20 years in Scandinavia (8,9). This simple, effective, low-risk treatment together with other methods to sensitize topically has gained increasing popularity in the last 10 years (10–32) and bath PUVA is particularly recommended to older patients (25).

BACKGROUND

Molecular and cellular events occurring with topical PUVA do not differ from those with oral PUVA. There are differences in the photosensitizing capacity between psoralens of different chemical structure (33). Two psoralens are currently in routine topical use, trioxsalen (4,5,8-trimethylpsoralen, TMP), and methoxsalen (8-methoxypsoralen, 8-MOP).

The most potent oral photosensitizing psoralen, 8-MOP, is less effective topically than TMP (34). This difference is especially pronounced with TMP and 8-MOP bath sensitization (8). This may be due to differences in water/lipid solubility (35), or to differences in the metabolism of TMP and 8-MOP (36,37).

The photosensitivity obtained with topical psoralens is dependent on the vehicle. There are conflicting reports regarding the optimal vehicle for topical 8-MOP sensitization: Gazith and co-workers (38) report isopropanol solution and an emulsion to be most effective, finding increasing penetration with increasing polarity, whereas Kaidbey and Kligman (39) report optimal photosensitivity with hydrophilic ointment. Suhonen (40) preferred petrolatum and a foundation cream. TMP photosensitizes in lipophilic ointment (35,41) and with this vehicle it is possible to obtain the same photosensitization as with bath treatment.

8-MOP concentration in the horny layer after topical application of an alcohol solution is at least 100 times higher than in the living epidermis; the horny layer is thought to act as a barrier. The concentration of psoralen commonly used in topical preparations is 0.05–0.15%, sometimes 1.0%. The application of 1% 8-MOP ointment to half the body surface results in the same blood levels and total amount absorbed as with oral administration (42). After whole-body topical application of 0.15% 8-MOP emulsion, plasma levels of 8-MOP were comparable to those found with oral treatment (43). Whole-body application with topical 8-MOP paint, emulsion, cream, or ointment plus UVA seems thus to have no advantages in eliminating systemic side effects and has its main use for localized treatment (30).

With TMP baths, the concentration gradient from the horny layer to living epidermis is 10:1. The average amount of TMP absorbed into the skin from a 50-mg TMP bath is 0.03 mg (44). The typical plasma value of TMP after such a bath is 1–2 ng/ml at the onset of a treatment series, but this falls to about 10% of the initial value after 4–6 weeks. The cause of this decrease is unknown, but it is probably due to decreased absorption as the skin heals (44–46). The plasma concentrations with TMP bath treatments are about the same as those obtained with oral TMP. The TMP serum values are about 1% of those with oral 8-MOP treatment. There are no reports of systemic photosensitization or of systemic side effects with TMP bath treatment (9). 8-MOP baths give plasma concentrations of psoralen of 2.6–10 ng/ml, which is a benefit as compared to oral plasma levels of 95–360 ng/ml (15,24,28,47). These observations imply that systemic absorption of psoralen from 8-MOP bath is minimal.

The photosensitivity action spectra of topical 8-MOP and TMP are within the 313–365-nm range, with a maximum between 330 and 340. The spectral sensitivity does not differ significantly from that with oral sensitization (34). After application of 8-MOP or TMP in an ointment, cream, or alcohol solution, there is a gradual increase in photosensitivity during the first hour. The sensitivity is maximal after 1–2 hr and remains high for several hours unless the substance is removed from the skin surface (5,38,48). Washing with soap and water or removing the ointment with blotting paper results in a rapid decrease in the photosensitivity. Four hours later, none is demonstrable (35); otherwise the activity persists for more than 24 hr (8).

Topical sensitization with 1% 8-MOP in ethanol-acetone-propylene glycol and immediate irradiation with doses smaller than the 2-hr minimal phototoxic dose (MPD) result in healing of psoriasis with low risk of erythema. In an animal model, immediate irradiation suppressed deoxyribonucleic acid (DNA) synthesis as much as PUVA in the 2-hr model (49).

After psoralen bath, photosensitivity is maximal immediately after the bath and persists unchanged for 15 min. One hour after the bath, the sensitivity has dropped 25% of the maximum value, and at 24 hr none is demonstrable (8).

TECHNIQUE

Sensitization

Alcohol Solutions, Emulsions, Oils, and Ointments

Apply 8-MOP or TMP in a suitable vehicle to the skin area to be treated. Irradiate when photosensitivity is maximal 1 hr after application. Immediate irradiation may be tried (49). Cleanse the skin with soap and water immediately after irradiation to decrease the photosensitivity (41).

Trioxsalen (TMP) Bath

A solution is prepared by dissolving 0.05% (0.5 mg/ml) TMP in ethanol. Small crystals remain undissolved; the solution must be shaken before use. TMP is colorless; adding 0.05% methylene blue to the solution will give the bath a faint blue color, indicating the type of bath to avoid radiation errors. The bath is prepared from 100 ml of this TMP-alcohol stock solution added to 150 L of water (37–38°C) (50 mg TMP/bath = 0.3 mg TMP/L). The patient, except for the head, is immersed for 10–15 min. It is possible to treat the face by wetting it with a sponge during the bath. Normally this should be avoided because of the risk of burning from outdoor UV exposure. Irradiate the patient within 15 min after the bath (8,9).

8-Methoxsalen (8-MOP) Bath

Crystalline 8-MOP is dissolved in 95% ethanol to a 0.5–1.0% solution. This stock solution is further diluted into 80–150 L liter of water (37–38°C) to a concentration of 1.8–5 mg 8-MOP/L (10–15,19,28), exceptionally 0.3–0.5 mg 8-MOP/L (50,51). The patient is immersed for 15–30 min; otherwise the technique is the same as with TMP baths. For bathing suite delivery, where the patient is enclosed in a polyethylene bag with 4 L liquid for 15 min, concentrations of 0.5 and 3.75 mg 8-MOP/L have been used (31,32).

Radiation Sources

Ultraviolet A, UVA/UVB, and most UVB lamps can be used with TMP bath PUVA. For 8-MOP baths with their weaker UV sensitization, UVA lamps are preferred (52,53). The erythema and probably also the psoriasis healing obtained with UVB and topical PUVA are additive. The best radiation sources are those with maximal output in the 330–340 range. Only insignificant amounts of irradiation below 300 nm should be accepted (52). TMP bath sensitization results in 5–20 times stronger photosensitization than oral administration. Consequently, the ratio between PUVA and UVB sensitivity is increased, and the PUVA effect will dominate the combined treatment more than with oral PUVA. With most common UVB lamps (e.g., Sylvania UV-6 and UV-21, Westinghouse Sun Lamp, and Philips TL-12), the TMP-PUVA and UVB will result in about equal proportions of erythema-producing and healing effects. With 8-MOP baths fluorescent tubes with wavelength maximal at 311 nm (Philips TL-01) proved to be superior to UVA radiation (54).

Radiation Dosage

Individual factors such as type and activity of the psoriasis, skin type and skin pigmentation, light tolerance of the skin, systemic disease, and medication must be considered. Interindividual differences in phototoxic reactivity are prominent. With bath PUVA, an increase in bath temperature tends to increase the photosensitization (51).

At any given time the patient has a limited therapeutic radiation dose interval: a minimum irradiation dose necessary to induce healing, but also a maximum dose that must not be exceeded or untoward side effects will ensue, such as phototoxic reactions followed by a Koebner reaction and aggravation of the psoriasis. The range of this dose interval is 0.3–3.0 minimal erythema doses (MED). The dose providing the most rapid healing is usually 0.5–1.0 MED. Doses as low as 0.3 MED have been reported to have significant healing effect. In patients with pustular, inverse, and erythrodermic psoriasis, this therapeutic interval is often narrow and the radiation dose must be determined with care and skill (8,53).

Initial Dose

The minimal phototoxic dose is a good indicator of the correct radiation dose. A starting dose of 0.3–0.5 times the MPD determined on the gluteal area is recommended. The mean phototoxic dose in 10 patients tested on the untanned buttocks after a single 8-MOP bath (3 mg/L) was 3.5 J/cm^2 (range 1.2–6.4 J/cm^2), and half that dose with daily repeated baths (10). A somewhat lower starting dose is normally used, namely 0.2–0.5 J/cm^2. The typical starting radiation dose in individuals photosensitized with TMP baths and skin type I–II, is 0.2–0.3 J/cm^2 UVA or -AB, and for skin types II–IV, 0.4–0.6 J/cm^2 (55).

With UVA/UVB and UVAB radiation sources, both UVA and UVB effects must be considered. A correct dose is obtained by adding the PUVA and the UVB effects, the sum being the same joule dose as with UVA treatment (52).

With topical PUVA, especially with the TMP baths, there are often irradiation times of a few seconds, which can be difficult to administer correctly. A light tube solarium does not have a stable radiation output until after about 10 sec have passed. Discover the exact amount of energy emitted from the solarium during each of the first 10 sec. The best equipment is a unit with automatic joule dosing.

Dose Increment

After a single PUVA treatment, the phototoxic erythema peaks at 3 days.

Repeated daily PUVA treatments are additive and result in a phototoxic peak at 5–7 days. The additive effect is not caused by persistence of psoralen in the skin (23,24,56). An overdose is thus recognized on the third day after single treatment, and a 3-day interval must be allowed to observe this reaction and plan the dose schedule accordingly. Dose increment steps of 40% are normally well tolerated. In the standard schedule, irradiation doses are increased every third day until the appearance of a slight irritation. Now the dose is kept constant or increments are made on a weekly basis.

The normal increment schedule with TMP bath sensitization and treatments 3–5 days a week is 0.1–0.2 J/cm^2 once a week. The maximum dose of 1–2 J/cm^2 is usually reached within 6–8 weeks.

For topical 8-MOP and 8-MOP bath PUVA the normal recommendation is increments of 0.1–0.25 J/cm^2 until a dose of 0.5–1.0 J/cm^2, and then increments of 0.5–1.0 J/cm^2 until erythema threshold, which may be as high as 15 J/cm^2 (13). If scheduled treatment results in more than minimal erythema, the exposure should be reduced 30% until further treatments no longer produce this reaction.

Maintenance

Maintenance treatment once or twice a week will normally keep the psoriasis stable/healed. We try to stop maintenance therapy 1–2 months after healing. Patients with rapid and constant relapses can be kept on long-term maintenance treatment once every 1–2 weeks. In the first months of this treatment, the maximum dose of clearing is well tolerated, but this may be followed by a period of irritation and erythema. The maintenance dose should then be decreased 40%. If relapses occur during the maintenance, the patient is returned to the clearing schedule.

Special Types of Psoriasis

The dose schedule described above applies to plaque psoriasis. Pustular, inverse, and erythodermic psoriasis have narrow therapeutic radiation dose intervals and must be treated with extreme care; however, they often respond favorably to low radiation doses. In extreme cases, the initial radiation dose after the TMP bath can be as low as 0.01–0.02 J/cm^2, and the maximum dose after 6–8 weeks' treatment 0.1–0.2 J/cm^2.

Topical treatment of hand and foot psoriasis and PPP is described in another chapter.

Transfer Factors of Radiation Dose Between Different Types of UV Treatment

Changing treatment from topical PUVA to other types of radiation treatment can result in dosage problems (57). Table 1 shows conversion factors of UV doses between various common types of UV radiation treatments. The regimens are detailed in Table 2. The actual dose for a patient to be transferred is multiplied by the transfer factor to give the new dose. This table is approximate and must be used with caution as the dose is influenced by the spectral wavelength distribution between light tubes of different manufacture. The spectral sensitivity of the UV meters has to be considered as it influences the transfer factors. There may also be different protective mechanisms in the skin between PUVA and UVB. Especially patients who have been on treatment schedules for more than 4 weeks and are moderately tanned experience irritation both when changed from PUVA to UVB and vice versa. In such cases, it is advisable to reduce to half the calculated dose.

Table 1 Radiation Dosage Transformation for Different Common Types of UV Treatment

	TMP bath PUVA	Oral 8-MOP PUVA	UVB	Coal tar bath/UVB
TMP bath PUVA	X	18	1.0	0.8
Oral 8-MOP PUVA	0.06	X	0.06	0.05
UVB	1.0	18	X	0.8
Coal tar bath/UVB	1.2	22	1.2	X

Multiply the actual joule dosage by the transformation factor to obtain the desired joule dosage.

PRECAUTIONS

Patient Selection

Patients below age 16 years are infrequently accepted for topical PUVA treatment. Light-sensitive patients must be treated with great care. Other reasons for exclusion are pregnancy, cardiac disease, systemic lupus erythematosus (SLE), and history of skin cancer and melanoma. Alcohol abuse will often cause an unstable psoriasis difficult to treat with UV and PUVA (56).

Systemic medication must be carefully controlled regarding light-sensitizing properties.

Skin Protection

Topically photosensitized skin must be protected against daylight for at least 6 hr after sensitization. Psoralen creams, oils, ointments, etc., have to be cleansed with soap and water after irradiation; otherwise the skin must be protected for at least 24 hr. Daylight that has passed through window glass still photoactivates psoralens. Topical sunscreens with high UVA protection factor are of value. The hands of the nursing staff who apply psoralen to the patients must be protected by plastic or rubber gloves. Do no forget to protect the patients' hands and ankles, where most accidental burns occur.

Eye Protection and Systemic Controls

With extensive topical application of psoralen solutions, lotions, creams, and ointments, the same rules

Table 2 Treatment Regimens

	Pretreatment	Radiation Source	Evaluation (UV meter/range)
TMP bath PUVA	Bath: 50 mg TMP in 150 L water	UVA: Sylvania "PUVA" Philips TL 09, or equivalent	Waldman: UVA
Oral 8-MOP PUVA	Orally: 0.6 mg 8-MOP/kg body weight		
UVB	None	UVB: Sylvania UV-6, Philips TL-12, Westinghouse, "sun lamp"	Waldman: UV6
Coal tar bath/UVB	Bath 100 ml liquor carbonic detergent or 20 ml Balnetar in 150 L water		

regarding eye protection and systemic controls as described with oral PUVA are recommended. No eye protective measures are necessary with bath PUVA because the tissue levels of psoralen are low. Antinuclear antibody test is recommended to exclude subclinical lupus erythematosus, but no other laboratory investigations are required prior to PUVA bath.

HEALING

Ordinary Psoriasis

The normal healing time with topical PUVA is 2–8 weeks. A correct radiation dose schedule is essential and results in identical healing with UVA and combined UVA/UVB treatment (8,58).

Treatment scheduled five times a week will result in a slightly more rapid healing than if given two to three times a week. Radiation dosage close to the MPD will produce the most rapid healing (56).

Immediate healing results after topical treatment with 8-MOP in alcohol solutions, emulsions, oils, or ointments plus UVA are 50–85% (2–6,27,59–61). Most of these treatment modalities were abandoned with the advent of oral PUVA but are presently regaining interest for localized psoriasis.

TMP baths plus UVA or UVA/UVB have been routine psoralen therapy since 1974 in Uppsala, Sweden. About 900 psoriasis patients have been treated, many repeatedly. Only a few have undergone longer periods of maintenance treatment. Patients with more extensive psoriasis have been carefully followed up (62,63). Healing of psoriasis, defined as disappearance of infiltration and scaling and a normalization of the outer structure of the skin, was reached in 85% of the patients and the typical UVA dose to healing is 11 J/cm^2. These healing results and those of maintenance treatment agree with other reported series of PUVA bath treatment (9,46,64,65).

8-MOP bath PUVA is less phototoxic than TMP bath PUVA. Healing results of 60–100%, an equal or lower healing effect than with oral 8-MOP PUVA, have been reported (11,13,14,29). There have been speculations that the 8-MOP bath treatment has a better relationship between psoriasis healing and tissue damage (29,53).

During maintenance with topical PUVA, it is possible to keep about 80% of the patients in good or excellent condition. Without such therapy 90% relapse within a year; the mean remission time is 4 months (27,65). In total the results do not differ significantly from long-term results reported with oral PUVA (29,58,66,67).

Pustular, Inverse, Erythrodermic, and Photosensitive Psoriasis

Half of the patients with pustular, inverse, erythrodermic, and light-sensitive psoriasis respond favorably to TMP bath photochemotherapy. Their aggressive psoriasis often shows high isomorphic reactivity, and radiation overdose is poorly tolerated.

Failures

Poor results or failure with topical PUVA treatment are in the 5–20% range. The irradiation dose is critical and a therapeutic irradiation dose interval may be missing. Therapy failures frequently occur in patients of the following groups:

1. Psoriasis of high isomorphic reactivity, for example, the pustular, inverse, or erythrodermic variety.
2. Light-sensitive psoriasis, which most often has a background of polymorphic light eruption (PLE), more seldom lupus erythematosus or transient acantholytic disease. Patients with PLE respond to UV testing with an initial erythema reaction followed by a Koebner response, but repeated radiation may result in healing.
3. Increased photosensitivity due to photosensitizing drugs.
4. High alcohol intake combined with a strong pathological response to UV radiation (56).

COMBINATION TREATMENT

There are no contraindications to the combination of topical PUVA with other types of psoriasis therapy. Topical PUVA in combination with UVB has already been discussed.

Topical Treatment

Topical corticosteroids in combination with topical PUVA will sometimes result in areas of blanching, which disappear after a few more treatments. The healing obtained with topical PUVA and corticosteroids will relapse more rapidly than with single PUVA treatment. This drawback can be diminished by withdrawal of the corticosteroids after the initial treatment period. Topical corticosteroids rapidly ameliorate phototoxic reactions and should be used liberally for this purpose.

There are no publications so far regarding combined topical PUVA and coal tar treatment.

Topical anthralin and topical PUVA act synergistically. Resistant cases of psoriasis may be treated with topical PUVA followed by conventional anthralin pastes (6). Pretreatment with topical PUVA will decrease the initial irritative erythema reaction of anthralin in the same way as UVB.

Systemic Treatment

There are a few reports on systemic therapy with cytostatic agents and topical PUVA. Our own experience with patients treated with methotrexate in combination with TMP-PUVA bath has been good. These patients have often had a severe psoriasis, difficult to handle, with a narrow therapeutic irradiation interval. They were somewhat less tolerant to UV radiation than patients with ordinary psoriasis and the radiation had to be given with care (68). There have been no immediate flares of the type reported by Möller with methotrexate and UVB after the discontinuation of the phototherapy, but a rebound flare 4–12 weeks after withdrawal of methotrexate will occur in almost all patients (69).

Retinoids act just as favorably when combined with TMP-PUVA baths as with oral PUVA. Rapid healing is obtained and the patients with severe, recalcitrant psoriasis often heal within a week (70,71). Radiation doses may need to be somewhat reduced as compared to the standard schedule. The retinoids should be administered in a normal oral dose of 0.6–1.0 mg etretinate/kg body weight per day, with a dose reduction to 0.4–0.6 mg/kg/day after 14 days. The retinoid therapy should be given 4–14 days prior to PUVA to have a stable drug level and avoid irradiation mistakes, with unpredictable photosensitivity. Combined oral etretinate plus 8-MOP ointment PUVA also compares favorably with 8-MOP ointment PUVA or etretinate only (27).

SHORT-TERM SIDE EFFECTS

The short-term side effects with topical PUVA are rare and include phototoxic reactions, pigmentary disturbances, itching, stinging, isomorphic reactions, and contact sensitization.

Phototoxic Side Effects

A slight generalized erythema will appear in almost all patients after 5–8 days of treatment. More pronounced erythema and edema, often in areas with thin skin, is reported to occur with the same frequency as with oral PUVA (11,13,14,29). With a well-trained staff accustomed to dose the UV correctly, painful erythema and blistering reactions are rare (8,65). Linear phototoxic erythema has been reported corresponding to the bath level (72).

Patients must be carefully instructed concerning daylight exposure of sensitized skin after the treatment. Sunscreens which filter UVA give some protection against psoralen photosensitization (73). The photosensitivity after a TMP bath decreases rapidly and is just 25% of the peak value after 1 hr (8). This sensitivity, however, is still five times higher than with oral sensitization. The skin thus remains strongly sensitized for 1–2 hr after the bath, and as little as 10–15 min of sun exposure may induce severe redness, swelling, and even blistering during the initial weeks of treatment. Later the skin becomes more tolerant to sun.

Uneven Pigmentation and Distant Rash

The application of topical PUVA to small areas may result in an unattractive patchy pigmentation, but this can be overcome by whole-skin application of psoralen cream or oil. The areas not immersed in TMP bath will remain untanned, but the bath will otherwise produce even sensitization and tanning. Untanned individuals often react with a 1–2-cm-wide zone of increased sensitivity around psoriasis plaques during the first weeks of treatment. There is first a zone of increased erythema followed by progressive pigmentation, which disappears after 6–8 weeks of continued treatment.

Occasionally, well-delineated and circumscribed areas of erythema develop at distant, uninvolved sites. These reactions usually appear early in the treatment series, but sometimes they are delayed and followed by superficial blistering. These reactions will disappear after a week of continued treatment with slightly reduced radiation doses. One or 2 weeks of UVB pretreatment before topical PUVA will reduce this effect. As a rule, the original sites of psoriasis heal with some hyperpigmentation, which may persist for a long time.

Itching and Stinging

Slight itching and stinging in the skin are common initial complaints. More pronounced itching is reported in a few percent of the PUVA-bath patients (11,13,14,29). The reaction, which resembles that after sun bathing, disappears after 1 or 2 days and is diminished by a cool shower and application of topical corticoids. Severe itching and stinging necessitate interruption of topical PUVA in a few patients. We have had no problems with the persistent pain described with oral PUVA (74).

Isomorphic (Koebner) Reaction

The isomorphic type of reaction is usually the result of UV overdoses or pathological light sensitivity. Most such reactions heal with continued treatment.

Contact Sensitivity

In regard to their frequent topical use there are few reports of psoralen contact sensitivity and photoallergy (8,75–79). Suppression of the immune system by UV radiation during and after the treatment may contribute to contact sensitivity. We have had two cases of proven contact sensitivity to psoralen. One patient was sensitized to 8-MOP after topical application and had positive patch test reactions to both 8-MOP and TMP. The other patient was sensitized to TMP bath. The patient was patch test sensitive to TMP but not to 8-MOP. Photoallergic reactions to psoralens are uncommon (8,78).

Systemic Side Effects

Topical PUVA treatment is not complicated by nausea, headache, dizziness, or other immediate systemic reactions (65). Elevation of liver transaminsases has been reported in one patient from application of 1% methoxypsoralen lotion over the total body surface (80). Positive ANA was found in 6/56 patients treated with topical 8-MOP PUVA but not found in patients treated with etretinate plus topical PUVA (27).

LONG-TERM SIDE EFFECTS

Possible long-term side effects of topical PUVA include actinic damage to the skin, mutagenesis, carcinogenesis, ocular hazards, and immunological changes.

Actinic Damage

Degenerative Changes

Animal experiments show degenerative changes in collagen and elastic tissue with both oral and topical PUVA. There are no indications that radiation doses resulting in equal actinic damage will give different long-term degenerative changes with these two types of treatment. Väätäinen et al. found no degenerative changes or long-term effects of topical PUVA on collagen metabolism (81); Oikarinen et al., however, noticed slightly decreased proliferation rate and slightly increased collagen synthesis in topical PUVA–treated patients (82).

Pigmentary Disturbances

There is a risk of uneven pigmentation of the mottling type described with oral PUVA after long-term topical

PUVA treatment and high radiation doses (83). Poskitt et al. have reported a case of patchy speckled pigmentation after bath PUVA (84) and Miller has reported a case with a severe type of pigmentary disturbance (85). None was found in the 5- and 9-year controls of our first 149 TMP bath-PUVA patients (62). Lentiginosis induced by 8-MOP ointment PUVA was found in 42% of 214 Japanese patients, comparable to the figure reported with oral PUVA (86).

Mutagenesis and Carcinogenesis

Both oral and topical PUVA involve a risk of skin cancer (87). The mechanism is promotive rather than inductive. Earlier treatments with arsenials and/or x-ray act as inducers of skin carcinoma with an increased risk for patients earlier treated this way. TMP and 8-MOP are equally mutagenic in *Escherichia coli* (88).

Early animal experiments with discordant DNA damage aroused the suspicion that topical PUVA was more carcinogenic than oral PUVA (89–91). In recent lifelong studies in mice using epitoxic doses of UVA, topical 8-MOP plus UVA caused malignant skin lesions, but topical trioxsalen plus UV-A did not (92,93).

Two recent Scandinavian studies indicate that the long-term risks with TMP bath PUVA are lower than with oral PUVA. In the Finnish study of 527 patients with a mean follow-up time of 10.8 years and an average cumulative UVA dose of 66 J/cm^2, 26 cancer cases were observed versus 30 expected (94). Lindelöf et al., in a study of patients from four Swedish dermatology clinics, compared the expected number of skin cancers in 597 patients treated with trioxsalen bath PUVA (average observation period 8.7 years) and 2378 patients treated with oral 8-MOP PUVA (average observation period 6 years). A total of 18 cancers of the skin were reported in the two groups (expected number 3.1). The bath PUVA group had no increased risk of skin cancer in contrast to the three centers using oral PUVA, which all had increased risk (63). A study of Takashima et al. in long-term control of 214 Japanese PUVA-treated patients, sensitized with 8-MOP 0.3% in an ointment or lotion base, found no actinic keratoses and just one case of multiple superficial basaliomas (86). This is substantially less than normally reported with oral PUVA.

Ocular Changes

The risk of ocular changes must be low as no eye problems have yet been reported with bath PUVA.

Immunological Changes

Topical PUVA has interesting effects on the skin immune system, which may be both advantageous and disadvantageous and could be one possible factor in its therapeutic effect (50,95–97).

REFERENCES

1. Allyn, B. (1962). Studies on phototoxicity in man and laboratory animals. Presented at the 21st Annual Meeting of the American Academy of Dermatology, Chicago, 1962.
2. Mortazavi, S.A.M., and Oberste-Lehn, H. (1973). Lichtsensibilatoren und ihre therapeutischen Fähigkeiten. *Z. Hautkr.* 49:1–9.
3. Tronnier, H., and Schule, D. (1973). Zur dematologischen Therapie von Dermatosen mit langwelligem UV nach photosensibilisienung der Haut mit Methoxsalen. *Z. Hautkr.* 48:385–393.
4. Walter, J.F., and Voorhees, J.J. (1973). Psoriasis improved by psoralen plus black light. *Acta Derma. Venereol. (Stockh.)* 53:469–472.
5. Weber, G. (1974). Combined 8-methoxsalen and black light therapy of psoriasis. *Br. J. Dermatol.* 90:317–323.
6. Willis, I., and Harris, D.R. (1973). Resistant psoriasis. Combined methoxsalen-anthralin therapy. *Arch. Dermatol.* 107:358–362.
7. Parrish, J.A., Fitzpatrick, T.B., Tanenbaum, L. et al. (1974). Photochemotherapy of psoriasis with oral methoxsalen and long-wave ultraviolet light. *N. Engl. J. Med.* 291:1207–1211.
8. Fischer, T., and Alsins, J. (1976). Treatment of psoriasis with trioxsalen baths and dysprosium lamps. *Acta Derm. Venereol. (Stockh.)* 56(5):383–390.
9. Hannuksela, M., and Karvonen, J. (1978). Trioxsalen bath plus UVA effective and safe in the treatment of psoriasis. *Br. J. Dermatol.* 99:703–707.
10. Calzavara-Pinton, P.G., Ortel, B., Carliuo, A.M. et al. (1993). Phototesting and phototoxic side effects in bath PUVA. *J. Am. Acad. Dermatol.* 28(4):657–659.
11. Calzavara-Pinton, P.G., Ortel, B., Hönigsmann, H. et al. (1994). Safety and effectiveness of an aggressive

and individualized bath-PUVA regimen in the treatment of psoriasis. *Dermatology* 189:256–259.
12. Collins, P., and Rogers, S. (1990). 8-Methoxypsoralen bath PUVA clears psoriasis after failure of oral PUVA. *Clin. Exp. Dermatol.* 15(4):320 (letter).
13. Collins, P., and Rogers, S. (1991). Bath-water delivery of 8-methoxypsoralen therapy for psoriasis. *Clin. Exp. Dermatol.* 16(3):165–167.
14. Collins, P., and Rogers, S. (1992). Bath-water compared with oral delivery of 8-methoxypsoralen PUVA therapy for chronic plaque psoriasis. *Br. J. Dermatol.* 127(4):392–395.
15. David, M., Lowe, N.J., Halder R.M. et al. (1990). Serum 8-methoxypsoralen (8-MOP) concentrations after bath water delivery of 8-MOP plus UVA. *J. Am. Acad. Dermatol.* 23(5 Pt 1):931–932.
16. Grattan, C.E., Carmichael, A.J., Shuttleworth, G.J., et al. (1991). Comparison of topical PUVA with UVA for chronic vesicular hand eczema. *Acta Derm. Venereol.* 71(2):118–122.
17. Hawk, J.L., and Grice, P.L. (1994). The efficacy of localized PUVA therapy for chronic hand and foot dermatoses. *Clin. Exp. Dermatol.* 19(6):479–482.
18. Helm, T.N., and Dijkstra, J.W. (1991). Topical (bath-water) PUVA therapy. *J. Am. Acad. Dermatol.* 24(6 Pt 1):1035 (letter).
19. Kerscher, M., Lehmann, P., and Plewig, G. (1994). PUVA-Bad-Therapie. *Hautartz* 45:526–528.
20. Konya, J., Diffey, B.L., and Hindson, T.C. (1992). Time course of activity of topical 8-methoxypsoralen on palmoplantar skin. *Br. J. Dermatol.* 127(6):654–656 (letter).
21. Layton, A.M., Sheehan-Dare, R., and Cunliffe, W.J. (1991). A double-blind, placebo-controlled trial of topical PUVA in persistent palmoplantar pustulosis. *Br. J. Dermatol.* 124(6):581–584.
22. Matsunami, E., Takashima, A., and Mizuno, N. et al. (1990). Topical PUVA, etretinate, and combined PUVA and etretinate for palmoplantar pustulosis: comparison of therapeutic efficacy and the influences of tonsillar and dental focal infections. *J. Dermatol.* 17(2):92–96.
23. Ortel, B., (1993). [Long-term effect of psoralens?]. *Hautarzt* 44(4):249.
24. Pham, C.T., and Koo, J.Y. (1993). Plasma levels of 8-methoxypsoralen after topical paint PUVA. *J. Am. Acad. Dermatol.* 28(3):460–466.
25. Rogers, M.B. (1988). Standard oral versus bath-psoralens plus ultraviolet A. *J. Am. Acad. Dermatol.* 19(2 Pt 1):368 (letter).
26. Sheehan-Dare, R.A., Goodfield, M.J., and Rowell, N.R. (1989). Topical psoralen photochemotherapy (PUVA) and superficial radiotherapy in the treatment of chronic hand eczema. *Br. J. Dermatol.* 121(1):65–69.
27. Takashima, A., Sunohara, A., Matsunami, E., et al. (1988). Comparison of therapeutic efficacy of topical PUVA, oral etretinate, and combined PUVA and etretinate for the treatment of psoriasis and development of PUVA lentigines and antinuclear antibodies. *J. Dermatol.* 15(6):473–479.
28. Thomas, S.E., O'Sullivan, J., and Balac, N. (1991). Plasma levels of 8-methoxypsoralen following oral or bath-water treatment. *Br. J. Dermatol.* 125(1):56–58.
29. Lowe, J.N., Weingarten, D., Bourget, T. et al. (1986). PUVA therapy for psoriasis: comparison of oral and bath-water delivery of 8-methoxypsoralen. *J. Am. Acad. Dermatol.* 14:754–760.
30. Hallman, C.P., Koo, J.Y., Omohundro, C. et al. (1994). Plasma levels of 8-methoxypsoralen after topical paint PUVA on nonpalmoplantar psoriatic skin. *J. Am. Acad. Dermatol.* 31(2):273–275.
31. Pai, S., and Srinvas, C.R. (1994). Bathing suit delivery of 8-methoxypsoralen for psoriasis: a double blind, placebo-controlled study. *Int. J. Dermatol.* 33:576–578.
32. Streit, V., Wiedow, O., and Christophers, E. (1994). Innovative Balneotherapie mit reduzierten Badevolumiuna: Folienbäder. *Hautarzt* 45:140–144.
33. Pathak, M.A., and Fitzpatrick, T.B. et al. (1977). Phototherapeutic photobiological and photochemical properties of psoralens. In *Seventh International Congress on Photobiology.* Plenum Press, New York.
34. Cripps, D.J., Lowe, N.J., and Lerner, A.B. (1982). Action spectra of topical psoralens: a reevaluation. *Br. J. Dermatol.* 107:77–82.
35. Väätäinen, N. (1980). Phototoxicity of topical psoralen. *Acta Derm. Venereol.* (*Stockh.*) 60:327–331.
36. Mandula, B.B., Pathak, M.A., and Dudek, G. (1976). Identification of a metabolite of 4,5′,8-methylpsoralen. *Science* 193:1131.
37. Ros, A.-M., Wennersten, G., Wallin, J. et al. (1988). Concentration of trimethylpsoralen in blood and skin after oral administration. *Photodermatology* 5:121–125.
38. Gazith, J., Schalla, W., Bauer, E. et al. (1978). 8-methoxypsoralen (8-MOP) in human skin: penetration kinetics. *J. Invest. Dermatol.* 71:126–130.
39. Kaidbey, K.H., and Kligman, A.M. (1974). Topical photosensitizers. Influence of vehicles on penetration. *Arch. Dermatol.* 110:868–870.
40. Suhonen, R. (1976). Photoepicutaneous testing. Influence of the vehicle, occlusion time and concentration of test substance on the results. *Contact Derm.* 2:218–226.
41. Hannuksela, M., and Kokkonen, E.-L. (1985). Short contact trioxsalen cream PUVA. *Photodermatology* 2:398–400.
42. Kammerau, B., Zesch, A., and Schaefer, H. et al. (1976). Penetration, permeation and resorption of 8-methoxypsoralen. *Arch. Dermatol. Res.* 255:31–42.

43. Neild, V.S., and Scott, L.V. (1982). Plasma levels of 8-methoxypsoralen in psoriatic patients receiving topical 8-methoxypsoralen. *Br. J. Dermatol.* 106:199–203.
44. Väätäinen, N., and Taskinen, J. (1981). Penetration of trioxsalen into skin from trioxsalen bath. *Arch. Dermatol. Res.* 270:157–158.
45. Fischer, T., Hartvig, P., and Bondesson, U. (1980). Plasma concentrations after bath treatment and oral administration of trioxsalen. *Acta Derm. Venereol. (Stockh.)* 60(2):177–179.
46. Salo, O.P., Lassus, A., and Taskinen, J. (1981). Trioxsalen bath plus UVA treatment of psoriasis. Plasma concentrations of the drug and clinical results. *Acta Derm. Venereol. (Stockh.)* 61:551–554.
47. Coleman, W.R., Lowe, N.J., David, M. et al. (1989). Palmoplantar psoriasis: experience with 8-methoxypsoralen soaks plus ultraviolet A with the use of a high-output metal halide device. *J. Am. Acad. Dermatol.* 20(6):1078–1082.
48. Meffert, H., Anderson, K.E., and Sönnichsen, N. (1984). Phototoxicity and antipsoriatic effect of a topical methoxypsoralen solution in relation to the application time. *Photodermatology* 1:191–194.
49. Danno, K., Toda, K., Ishida, H. et al. (1982). Topical methoxsalen followed immediately by long-wave UV irradiation. *Arch. Dermatol.* 118:471–473.
50. Vallat, V.P., Gilleaudeau, P., Battat, L. et al. (1994). PUVA bath therapy strongly suppresses immunological and epidermal activation in psoriasis: a possible cellular basis for remittive therapy. *J. Exp. Med.* 180: 283–296.
51. Jansen, C.T. (1988). Water temperature effect in bath-PUVA treatment. *J. Am. Acad. Dermatol.* 19(1 Pt 1): 142–143.
52. Fischer, T., Alsins, J., and Berne, B. (1984). Ultraviolet-action spectrum and evaluation of ultraviolet lamps for psoriasis healing. *Int. J. Dermatol.* 23(10): 633–637.
53. Koulu, L.M., and Jansén, C.T. (1988). Antipsoriatic, erythematogenic, and Langerhans cell marker depleting effect of bath-psoralens plus ultraviolet A treatment. *J. Am. Acad. Dermatol.* 18:1053–1059.
54. Ortel, B., Perl, S., Kinacyan, T. et al. (1993). Comparison of narrow band (311 nm) UVB and broad-band UVA after oral or bath-water 8-methoxypsoralen in the treatment of psoriasis. *J. Am. Acad. Dermatol.* 29: 736–740.
55. Fischer, T., and Juhlin, L. (1977). Trioxsalen bath and ultraviolet light treatment of psoriasis. *Arch. Dermatol.* 113(6):852 (letter).
56. Fischer, T. (1977). *Studies on UV-Light Treatment of Psoriasis.* University of Uppsala, Uppsala.
57. Berne, B., and Fischer, T. (1984). Conversion factors for ultraviolet radiation dosage with different types of ultraviolet therapy. *Photodermatology* 1(6):307–310.
58. Petrozzi, J.W., Kaidbey, K.K., and Kligman, A.M. (1977). Topical methoxsalen and blacklight in the treatment of psoriasis. *Arch. Dermatol.* 115:436–439.
59. Petrozzi, J.W., Barton, J.O., and Kligman, A.M. (1979). Topical methoxsalen administration and sunlamp fluorescent irradiation in psoriasis. *Arch. Dermatol.* 115:436–439.
60. Rodermund, O.E., and Stein, G. (1975). Zur Therapie de Psoriasis. *Fortscher. Med.* 93:1484–1487.
61. Schaefer, H., Vivell, K., Kentsch, V. et al. (1976). Simplification of local therapy of psoriasis with 8-methoxypsoralen. *Br. J. Dermatol.* 94:363–367.
62. Berne, B., Fischer, T., Michaelsson, G. et al. (1984). Long-term safety of trioxsalen bath PUVA treatment: an 8-year follow-up of 149 psoriasis patients. *Photodermatology* 1(1):18–22.
63. Lindelöf, B., Sigurgeirsson, B., Tegner, E. et al. (1992). Comparison of the carcinogenic potential of trioxsalen bath PUVA and oral methoxsalen PUVA. A preliminary report. *Arch. Dermatol.* 128(10): 1341–1344.
64. Väätäinen, N., Hannuksela, M., and Karvonen, J. (1981). Long-term local trioxsalen photochemotherapy in psoriasis. *Dermatologica* 163:229–231.
65. Turjamaa, K., Salo, H., and Reunala, T. (1985). Comparison of trioxsalen bath and oral methoxsalen PUVA in psoriasis. *Acta Derm. Venereol. (Stockh.)* 85:86–88.
66. Melski, J.W., Tannenbaum, L., Parrish, J.A. et al. (1977). Oral methoxsalen photochemotherapy for the treatment of psoriasis: a cooperative clinical trial. *J. Invest. Dermatol.* 68:328–335.
67. Roenigk, H.H., Farber, E.M., Storrs, F. (1979) Photochemotherapy for psoriasis. A clinical cooperative study of PUVA-48 and PUVA-64. *Arch. Dermatol.* 115:576–579.
68. Lahkshmipathi, T., Gould, P.W., Mackenzie, L.A. et al. (1977). Photochemotherapy in the treatment of psoriasis. *Br. J. Dermatol.* 96:587–593.
69. Möller, H. (1969). Reactivation of acute inflammation by methotrexate. *J. Invest. Dermatol.* 52:437–441.
70. Michaëlsson, G., Norén, P., and Vahlquist, A. (1978). Combined therapy with oral retinoid and PUVA baths in severe psoriasis. *Br. J. Dermatol.* 99:221–222.
71. Väätäinen, N., Hollmen, A., and Fräki, J.E. (1985). Trimethylpsoralen bath plus ultraviolet A combined with oral retinoid (etretinate) in the treatment of severe psoriasis. *J. Am. Acad. Dermatol.* 12:52–55.
72. George, S.A., and Ferguson, J. (1992). Unusual pattern of phototoxic burning following trimethylpsoralen (TMP) bath photochemotherapy (PUVA). *Br. J. Dermatol.* 127(4):444–445 (letter).
73. Kawada, A., Hiruma, M., Noda, T., et al. (1989). An evaluation of broad-spectrum sunscreens against topical PUVA-induced erythema. *Acta Derm. Venereol.* 69(4):335–337.

74. Tegner, E. (1979). Severe skin pain after PUVA treatment. *Acta Derm. Venereol.* (Stockh.) 59:467–468.
75. Sidi, E., and Bourgeois-Gavardin, J. (1953). Mise au point du traitement du vitiligo par L'ammi Majus. *Presse Med.* 61:436–440.
76. Fulton, J.E., and Willis, I. (1968). Photoallergy to methoxsalen. *Arch. Dermatol.* 98:445–450.
77. Plewig, G., Hofmann, C., and Braun-Falco, O. (1978). Photoallergic dermatitis from 8-methoxypsoralen. *Arch. Dermatol. Res.* 261:201–211.
78. Ljunggren, B. (1977). Psoralen photoallergy caused by plant contact. *Contact Derm.* 3:85–90.
79. Takashima, A., Yamamoto, K., Kimura, S. et al. (1991). Allergic contact and photocontact dermatitis due to psoralens in patients with psoriasis treated with topical PUVA. *Br. J. Dermatol.* 124(1):37–42.
80. Park, Y.M., Kim, T.Y., Kim, H.O. et al. (1994). Reproducible elevation of liver transaminases by topical 8-methoxypsoralen. *Photodermatol. Photoimmunol. Photomed.* 10:261– 263.
81. Väätäinen, N., Oikarinen, A., and Kuutti-Savolainen, E.-R. (1980). The effects of long term PUVA treatment on collagen metabolism in human skin. *Arch. Dermatol. Res.* 269:99–104.
82. Oikarinen, A., Ala-Kokko, L., Tamminen, M. et al. (1990). Effect of long-term PUVA treatment of psoriasis on the collagen and elastin gene expression and growth of skin fibroblasts in vitro. *Br. J. Dermatol.* 123(5):621–630.
83. Gschnait, F., Wolff, K., Honigsmann, H. et al. (1980). Long term photochemotherapy: histopathological and immunofluorescence observations in 243 patients. *Br. J. Dermatol.* 103:11–22.
84. Poskitt, B.L., Wilkinson, J.D., and Wojnarowska, F.T. (1993). Patchy speckled PUVA pigmentation. *J. R. Soc. Med.* 86:665–666.
85. Miller, R.A. (1982). Psoralens and UV-A-induced stellate hyperpigmented freckling. *Arch. Dermatol.* 118: 619–620.
86. Takashima, A., Matsuami, E., Yamamoto, K. et al. (1990). Cutaneous carcinoma and 8-methoxypsoralen and ultraviolet A (PUVA) lentigines in Japanese patients with psoriasis treated with topical PUVA: a follow-up study of 214 patients. *Photodermatol. Photoimmunol. Photomed.* 7(5):218–221.
87. Hönigsmann, H., Wolff, K., Gschnait, F. et al. (1980). Keratoses and nonmelanoma skin tumors in long-term photochemotherapy (PUVA). *J. Am. Acad. Dermatol.* 3:406–414.
88. Kirkland, D.J., and Creed, K.L. (1993). Comparative bacterial mutagenicity studies with 8-methoxypsoralen and 4,5′,8-trimethylpsoralen in the presence of near ultraviolet light and in the dark. *Mutat. Res.* 116:73–82.
89. Griffin, A.C., (1959) Methoxsalen in ultraviolet carcinogenesis in the mouse. *J. Invest. Dermatol.* 32: 367–372.
90. Urbach, F. (1959). Modification of ultraviolet carcinogenesis by photoactive drugs. *J. Invest. Dermatol.* 32:373–378.
91. Hakim, R.E., Griffin, A.C., and Knox, J.M. (1960). Erythema and tumor formation in methoxsalen treated mice exposed to fluorescent light. *Arch. Dermatol.* 82: 572–577.
92. Hannuksela, M., Stenbäck, F., and Lahti, A. (1986). The carcinogenic properties of topical PUVA: a lifelong study in mice. *Arch. Dermatol. Res.* 278:347–351.
93. Hannuksela, M., and Karvonen, J. (1989). Carcinogenicity of trioxsalen bath PUVA. *J. Am. Acad. Dermatol.* 21(4 Pt 1):813–814 (letter).
94. Hannuksela, A., Pukkala, E., Hannuksela, M. et al. (1995). Cancer incidence among Finnish trioxsalen bath PUVA treated psoriatic patients (1977–1993). *Nouv. Dermatol.* 14(Suppl 1):26–27.
95. Guo, Z., Okamoto, H., Damo, K. et al. (1992). The effects of non-interval PUVA treatment on Langerhans cells and contact hypersensitivity. *J. Dermatol. Sci.* 3(2):91–96.
96. Larmi, E. (1989) PUVA treatment inhibits nonimmunologic immediate contact reactions to benzoic acid and methyl nicotinate. *Int. J. Dermatol.* 28(9): 609–611.
97. Ullrich, S.E., Alcalay, J., Applegate, L.A. et al. (1989). Immunosuppression in phototherapy. *Ciba Found. Symp.* 146:131–139.

44

PUVA and Skin Cancer

Henry H. Roenigk, Jr.
Northwestern University Medical School, Chicago, Illinois

HISTORICAL ASPECTS

The efficacy of psoralen and ultraviolet A (PUVA) in the treatment of psoriasis has been repeatedly and convincingly demonstrated since its introduction in 1974. The short-term laxicities have been well documented, and strategies to avoid such adverse effects as phototoxic reactions have been developed. Long-term effects of any treatment are far more difficult to document. A few multicenter studies were initiated at the onset of PUVA therapy to monitor its chronic toxicity (1–4). Although chronic effects of PUVA therapy such as premature aging changes of the skin were expected and noted, the main concern was the carcinogenic potential of PUVA. The initial multicenter studies have now had up to 13 years of follow-up (5–9), and other additional centers have reported on their experience with the chronic toxicity of PUVA (10–15). Thus, the past 20 years have yielded sufficient worldwide experience to make it possible to draw some conclusions about the associated risk of epidermal and melanocytic tumors from PUVA therapy.

EXPERIMENTAL CARCINOGENICITY OF PUVA

Photocarcinogenesis is an old concept, dating back to the 1890s when Unna first noted that persons with extensive actinic damage developed skin cancer (16). In the 1940s, it was demonstrated that ultraviolet (UV) radiation could induce skin cancer in rodents (17). Action spectrum investigations have shown that UVB is more effective than UVA in inducing epithelial carcinomas in hairless mice (18), and that this corresponds with the absorption spectrum of deoxyribonucleic acid (DNA) (19). Psoralens intercalate with epidermal DNA and form mono- and bifunctional adducts (20,21) as well as crosslinks between DNA strands (22) and an increase in sister chromatic exchanges (23) in human epidermal cells exposed to UVA radiation. These effects could be expected to translate into an increase in epidermal tumors with PUVA exposure. PUVA induction of carcinogenesis in hairless mice had been demonstrated as early as 1958 (24,25).

A new concept in the etiopathogenesis of epidermal carcinoma is the effect of ultraviolet radiation on the immune system (26). It appears that ultraviolet radiation not only directly damages DNA, but also may induce a cell-mediated immunity in skin, leading to a "tolerance" of sunlight-induced tumors (27). Although originally described as an effect of UVB, many immunomodulating properties of PUVA have now also been demonstrated. These include depressed delayed-type hypersensitivity (28,29), decreased Langerhans cell number, and abnormal morphology (30,31), alteration in number and proportion of circulating T lymphocytes (32–34), and inhibition of lymphoid cell DNA synthesis (35).

Thus, there has been ample experimental evidence that PUVA is a cutaneous carcinogen in an animal model. What remained to be determined was whether this was also true for human patients undergoing PUVA therapy for psoriasis. Questions to be addressed if PUVA carcinogenicity was established included time to onset of tumors; the relationship between dose, therapy schedules, and development of tumors; and assessment of risk versus benefit of this form of therapy for psoriasis patients.

REVIEW OF CLINICAL LONG-TERM STUDIES

Four large cooperative studies have undertaken long-term follow-up for the detection of nonmelanoma skin cancers in PUVA-treated psoriasis patients (1–4). All of the centers have published updated findings extending their original observations to 5–13 years of follow-up (5–9a).

One criticism of these types of studies has been the lack of a proper control group (36). There is no large group of moderately severe to severe psoriatics who have been followed for long periods of time for the development of epidermal tumors and who have *not* received PUVA therapy. The incidence of tumors calculated in these studies was compared with the incidence of basal cell carcinoma (BCC) and squamous cell carcinoma (SCC) American skin cancer survey (37) and adjusted for age. It has long been speculated, however, that psoriasis patients may have an inherently increased susceptibility to developing skin cancer because of the hyperproliferative nature of their disease. In an attempt to clarify this possible bias in such studies, Stern et al. (38) analyzed a subgroup involved in a national skin cancer survey and found a twofold increase in the incidence of BCC, but no such increase in SCC for psoriatic patients. Thus, although ideally all large clinical trails would have a proper control group, great efforts have been made to remove other confounding variables that could falsely elevate the incidence of SCC in psoriasis patients treated with PUVA. These factors include age, exposure to other cutaneous carcinogens, and inherent susceptibility of psoriatics to skin cancer.

Incidence of Squamous Cell Carcinoma in PUVA Patients

Stern et al.'s update in 1984 (5) of the 16-center U.S. prospective study was the first to show a substantial dose-related increase in the incidence of SCC in 1380 patients after an average follow-up of 68 months, suggesting that PUVA is a primary carcinogen. Stern et al.'s (9a) most recent update in 1994 continues to show a significant increase in SCC in one-fourth of patients exposed to high doses of PUVA. Metastatic disease developed in seven patients with SCC. High-dose exposure to methotrexate is associated with a twofold increase in risk of SCC but Stern et al. did not demonstrate any interaction between PUVA and methotrexate. There is no associated risk of SCC with long-term exposure to UVB or topical tar. They concluded that long-term exposure to PUVA and methotrexate significantly increased the risk of SCC in patients with psoriasis. Tanew et al. (7), from Austria, published follow-up observations of 297 patients after an average 63 months. They concluded that the increased observed incidence of SCC was due to exposure of patients with these tumors to arsenic and ionizing radiation, confirming previous observations that PUVA could act as a tumor promoter (1). In 1987, Henseler et al. (8) reported their findings from 1643 patients followed prospectively for an average of 96 months, and like Tanew, they found that the majority of patients with SCC had been exposed to another carcinogen. In 1989, the 16-center U.S. study extended their observations to include 10 years of follow-up and demonstrated an 11-fold increase in risk for SCC in patients with more than 260 treatments as compared with patients with less than 160 treatments (6). The PUVA-48 cooperative group's update (9) was the first major study to confirm this finding of a substantial increase in the incidence of SCC that was independent of other carcinogenic risk factors on studying a group of 551 psoriasis patients for an average follow-up of 57 months.

In addition, three Scandinavian (10–12), one Japanese (13), one British (14), and one German (15) study have reported on their experience. Lindskov (11) followed 134 patients for an average of 43 months and reported a high incidence of SCC. Importantly, however, 97% of this study population had another major risk factor such as exposure to ionizing radiation or arsenic or a history of previous skin cancer.

On the other hand, Eskelinen et al. (10) in studying 1047 patients for an average of 50 months, Ros et al. (12) with 250 patients followed for 49 months, Torinuki and Tagami (13) with 108 patients followed for 48 months, Cox et al. (14) with 95 patients followed for 96 months, and Barth et al. (15) with 6820 patients followed for 50 months all found no increased incidence of SCC in their PUVA-treated populations.

Takashima et al. (15a) reported on 214 Japanese patients treated with topical PUVA and no SCC. Lever and Fan (15b), from Britain examined 54 patients with greater than 2000 J/cm^2. Ten patients (19%) had developed SCC. In a case-control study of PUVA patients with SCC, Lindelof and Sigargeirsson (15c) also found that prior treatment with methotrexate increased the risk of developing SCC. In a comparison of oral and bath PUVA by Lindelof et al. (15d) in Sweden there was less carcinogenic risk with trioxsalan baths than oral PUVA.

Another study from one institution in the United States (15e) reported again an increased risk of SCC in high-dose PUVA patients. A large Swedish follow-up of 4799 patients from 1974–1985 showed dose-dependent risk of SCC (15f).

Possible reasons for the discrepancy of the observation by the 16-center U.S. study (5,9a) and the PUVA-48 cooperative group's (9) findings of an increase in tumor initiation of SCC and these other studies are the higher average cumulative dosages of the American studies, the lower cumulative sun exposure and incidence of skin cancer in the European population, the minimal phototoxic dosage testing followed by more aggressive PUVA schedules widely practiced in Europe, and the greater concomitant European use of retinoids with PUVA, which may have antitumor properties. An attempt to sort out some of these variables and understand these discrepancies is aided by a closer look at the data.

Cumulative Dosage and Squamous Cell Carcinoma

The demographics of some of these studies is presented in Table 1; the finding of greatest import is the relationship between cumulative joules and development of SCC (Table 2). Only three centers had mean cumulative J/cm^2 dosages of greater than 1000: Stern's (5) with a median dosage of 1500, Tanew's (7) with a mean dosage of 1065, and Forman and Roenigk's (9) with a mean dosage of 1861. However, 38–50% of the Stern and the PUVA-48 patients achieved greater than 1000–1500 J/cm^2, whereas only 16% of Tanew's patients did so. Thus, a smaller number of patients in Tanew's study shared a larger dosage burden. The total number of patients (and hence the "pool" of potential tumor-bearing patients) with high J/cm^2 dosages is very different–690 patients in Stern's study versus only 48 in Tanew's study had dosages higher than the mean. It would be difficult to demonstrate a statistical increase of skin tumors with such a small population of 48 patients at risk. In Stern's most recent study (9a) they divided patients into low, medium, and high PUVA doses based on number of treatments and not total J/cm^2.

All four major cooperative centers did show an increased risk in the incidence of SCC in their high-dose (>1500 J/cm^2) as compared with their low-dose (<1500 J/cm^2) group (see Table 2). In the Stern (5), Eskelinen (10), and Forman and Roenigk (9) groups, an almost twofold increase is noted (5.3% SCC in the high-dose group vs. 2.1% in the low-dose group for Stern, 1.5% vs. 0, for Eskelinen, and 2.4% vs. 1.2% for Forman and Roenigk). Tanew et al. (7) and Henseler et al. (8) both show a greater than sixfold increase in SCC (6.3% in the high-dose group vs. 1.2% in the low-dose group for Tanew and 6.8% vs. 0.5% for Henseler).

Lindskov's study (11), although smaller, was the only other one to find an appreciable incidence of SCC, but information about the relative dosage of the tumor versus nontumor group was unavailable. It should be noted, however, that more than 75% of the tumor populations of Tanew, Henseler, and Lindskov had other carcinogenic exposures and the incidence of SCC in Eskelinen's group was very low overall (Tables 3 and 4). Thus, Stern (5) and Forman and Roenigk (9) have been the only studies with a significant number of patients with high cumulative dosages and at least one-half of the tumor population free of other significant carcinogenic risk factors such as exposure to ionizing radiation or arsenic or a history of previous skin cancer. Studies in the past five years (15a–f) have tended to confirm these observations on the development of more SCC in patients with high-dose PUVA exposure.

Another way to prove that PUVA has a primary role in tumor initiation is to demonstrate a dose-risk relationship. This was clearly shown in Stern's study (9a) in which the high-dose PUVA group had a 25%, or 5.9-fold, increase in incidence of SCC as compared with the low-dose group; an increase of such magnitude could not be based on chance alone. Although Forman and Roenigk (9) could not demonstrate a statistically significant dose-risk relationship (probably owing to a much smaller population size), there was a distinct trend of increasing tumors with increasing J/cm^2 dosages in their study population.

Thus, it appears that one of the most important determinants in the development of SCC is cumulative dosage of PUVA. This correlates with the fact that the

Table 1 PUVA Centers, Demographics, and Incidence of Skin Cancer

Center	No. patients	Average follow-up (months)	Average age (years)	% Skin type I + II	% BCC	% SCC
Stern (5)	1380	68.4	44	29	4.5	4.8
Tanew (7)	297	63.1	48	34	1.0	2.0
Henseler (8)	1643	96.0	49	29	1.1	1.1
Eskelinen (10)	IW7	50.88	40	[b]	0.2	0.1
Lindskov (11)	134	43.0	52	34	5.2	3.7
Ros (12)	250	49,4[a]	47	10	0	0
Torinuki (13)	108	48.0[a]	45	0[a]	0	0.9
Cox (14)	95	[b]	54	48	0	4.2
Barth (15)	6820[a]	50.4	[b]	[b]	0	0
PUVA-48 (9)	551	57.2	49	33	2.4	1.6

[a]Approximation derived from data given in the paper.
[b]Data not given.

incidence of SCC in the general population rises steadily with age (37); i.e., with higher cumulative sun exposure. This relationship will most likely be increasingly borne out as larger numbers of patients receive high doses and are followed for longer periods of time.

Incidence of Basal Cell Carcinoma in PUVA Patients

The data on the incidence of BCC in PUVA patients is less dramatic than that for SCC. While many studies have found an increased risk of BCC in their PUVA populations, the increase was dependent on the presence of other carcinogenic risk factors such as exposure to ionizing radiation or arsenic or previous skin cancer. Many of the centers found a negligible incidence of BCC in their subgroup of PUVA without other risk factors (see Table 3) when compared with the incidence of BCC in the general population, whereas all had substantial numbers of tumors in the subgroup of patients with other risk factors. In the PUVA-48 cooperative study (9), 6% of such at-risk patients developed BCC, supporting the concept that PUVA is an efficient tumor promoter with respect to BCC.

The U.S. 16-center study's most recent update (6), however, shows a dose-dependent increase in the relative risk for developing BCC. They found a relative risk of developing BCC to increase consistently from 1.3 for patients with less than 160 treatments to 6.9 for patients with greater than 260 treatments. These recent studies (9a) confirm no relationship between dose and anatomical distribution. While this is modest compared to the 11-fold relative risk for SCC in patients with greater than 260 treatments, the dose-risk relationship suggests that PUVA may be a tumor initiator with respect to BCC as well as a tumor promoter.

Another factor to consider when evaluating these data is the finding that psoriatics have a twofold increase in the incidence of BCC (38). In addition, recent epidemiological studies by Robinson (39) reveal that one-third of nonpsoriatic patients with BCC will develop another tumor within a 5-year period. Thus, the development of BCC in a PUVA patient with a history of BCC in the previous 5 years should not be attributed to therapy.

PUVA as Tumor Promoter

The first report in 1979 by the 16-center U.S. study showed an increase in SCC, which was dependent on the preexistence of other carcinogenic risk factors in psoriasis patients undergoing PUVA such as arsenic or radiation exposure or a previous history of skin cancer (1). Their subsequent report (5) emphasized the role of PUVA as a tumor initiator, as discussed above, as well as a tumor promoter. Many of the subsequent studies have confirmed the tumor-promoting effect of PUVA, an effect that seems to appear earlier and with less cumulative joules than its tumor-initiating effect.

In all four major cooperative centers, the incidence of both BCC and SCC was increased two to six times in the group with an identifiable risk factor (see Table 3). In breaking down the data by individual risk group

Table 2 PUVA Centers, UVA Dosage, and Skin Cancer

Center	Mean J/cm²	>1500 J/cm²			<1500 J/cm²		
		% Total	% BCC	% SCC	% Total	% BCC	% SCC
Stern (5)	1500[a]	50[b]	2.4[b]	5.3[b]	50[b]	3.3[b]	2.1[b]
Tanew (7)	1065	16.2[b]	0	6.3	83.8	1.2	1.2
Henseler (8)	745	9.0	2.0[b]	6.8	91.0	0.9[b]	0.5
Eskelinen (10)	499[b]	6.5[b]	1.5[b]	1.5	93.5[b]	0.1[b]	0
Lindskov (11)	351[b]	[c]	[c]	[c]	[c]	[c]	[c]
Ros (12)	735[b]	13.6[b]	0	0	76.4[b]	[c]	[c]
Torinuki (13)	388[b]	3.7[b]	0	0	96.3[b]	0	1.0
Cox (14)	333	8.0[b]	0	26.3	92.0[b]	0	2.3
Barth (15)	[c]	[c]	[c]	[c]	[c]	[c]	[c]
PUVA-48 (9)	1861	37.6	3.4	2.4	62.4	1.7	1.2

[a]Median.
[b]Derived approximation.
[c]Data not given.

(see Table 4), it can be seen that the incidence of SCC could be as high as 6% (5,9) in the group with previous exposure to radiation and as high as 9% (7) in the group exposed to arsenic.

It appears fairly clear that patients with a history of exposure to arsenic or therapeutic ionizing radiation, or those with already advanced actinic damage as evidenced by history of previous BCC or SCC, are at greatly increased risk of subsequent development of BCC or SCC if undergoing PUVA therapy, and that these tumors are likely to appear sooner and at a lower cumulative dose than in those patients without such risk factors. Recent studies (9a,15c) have suggested that prior exposure to methotrexate may increase the risk of developing SCC in PUVA-treated psoriatics.

Incidence of Malignant Melanoma in PUVA Patients

There has been tremendous concern that long-term PUVA therapy could increase the risk of malignant melanoma. This concern is based on the biological effects of PUVA as well as the epidemiology of melanoma.

Table 3 PUVA Centers and Relationship of Risk Factors with Development of Skin Cancer

Center	With risk[a]			Without risk			Tumor + risk/tumor	
	% Total	% BCC	% SCC	% Total	% BCC	% SCC	% BCC	% SCC
Stern (1,5)c	29.6	4.7	6.2	70.4	4.4	4.2	31[b]	38[b]
Tanew (7)	37.7	2.7	4.5	62.3	0	0.5	100	83
Henseler (8)	20.7	4.4	5.3	79.3	0.2	0.3	81	78
Eskelinen (10)	12.6	0.8	0	87.4	0.1	0.1	50	0
Lindskov (11)	97.0	5.4	3.7	3.0	0	25.0	100	80
Ros (12)	40.0	0	0	60.0	0	0	0	0
Torinuki (13)	0.9	0	100.0	99.1	0	0	0	100
Cox (14)	16.9	[d]	[d]	83.1	[d]	[d]	[d]	[d]
Barth (15)	[d]	[d]	[d]	[d]	[d]	[d]	[d]	
PUVA-48 (9)	15.1	6.0	3.6	84.9	1.7	1.3	63	50

[a]Risk defined as exposure to therapeutic ionizing radiation or arsenic or history of previous skin cancer.
[b]Estimating using data given in the paper.
[c]Information on arsenic risk not available.
[d]Data not given.

Table 4 PUVA Centers and History of Arsenic Exposure, Exposure to Ionizing Radiation, and Previous Skin Cancer

	Arsenic			Radiation			Cancer		
Center	% Total	% BCC	% SCC	% Total	% BCC	% SCC	% Total	% BCC	% SCC
Stern (1,5)	a	a	a	26.8	4.1	5.9	2.8	10.3	7.7
Tanew (7)	18.5	3.6	9.1	25.6	2.6	1.3	a	a	a
Henseler (8)	12.8[b]	6.2	5.7	7.9[b]	1.6	4.7	a	a	a
Eskelinen (10)	12.2	0.8	0	0.4	0	a	0	0	0
Lindskov (11)	14.0	21.4	5.3	80.0	5.6	3.7	3.0	75.6	0
Ros (12)	19.6	0	0	20.4	0	0	a	a	a
Torinuki (13)	0	0	0	0.9	0	100.0	0	0	0
Cox (14)	4.2	a	a	11.6	a	a	1.1	a	a
Barth (15)	a	a	a	a	a	a	a	a	a
PUVA-48 (9)	0.9	0	0	12.9	5.6	2.8	0.9	20.0	0

[a]Data not given.
[b]Some patients exposed to arsenic + x-ray.

As discussed previously, PUVA is mutagenic as well as immunosuppressive. It has been postulated that this mutagenicity may apply to melanocytes as well as epidermal cells. Proliferation and morphological abnormalities of melanocytes have been reported in PUVA patients studied by electron microscopy (40–42). Collections of atypical melanocytes have been noted histologically in PUVA lengigines (43–45). It has been speçulated that the immunological tolerance to the formation of epidermal tumors induced by PUVA may extend as well to melanocytic tumors (46).

It is well known that the incidence of and mortality from malignant melanoma is highest in geographical regions closest to the equator (47–49), a finding that has been used to support the concept that ultraviolet radiation plays a major role in its pathogenesis.

The clinical evidence has thus far not substantiated the fear that melanoma is increased in PUVA patients. Although there are case reports of melanoma in PUVA patients (46,50,51), there are no clearly documented instances of PUVA lentigines evolving into melanoma (52). As noted by Marx et al. (46), as of 1983 approximately 75,000 psoriatic patients had received PUVA therapy, and of this population (based on the 1973–1976 age-adjusted incidence of melanoma in the United States) four melanomas per year would be expected. Far less cases than these expected have been reported. In addition, the U.S. 16-center study found three cases of malignant melanoma in 1380 patients over a 10-year period (6), the PUVA-48 cooperative group (9) found one case in 551 patients over a 6-year period (6), and the European cooperative group (8) found one case in 1643 patients over 8 years. Although this represents a twofold increase in the incidence of melanoma over that expected in these populations, this increase is not of sufficient magnitude to be causally related to PUVA exposure. Stern et al. in 1997 (52a) has for the first time revealed an increased risk of malignant melanoma in the 16-center study. The risk is greatest in patients with more than 200 PUVA treatments.

In summary, although PUVA can induce pigmented lesions with atypical histology, these lesions have not been shown to be precursors of invasive melanoma. One long-term clinical study has supported the relationship between PUVA therapy and malignant melanoma. However, more years of follow-up will probably be required before the nature of the relationship between PUVA and melanoma can be established with certainty. Caution and careful follow-up are indicated.

Anatomical Location of PUVA-Associated Tumors

Some of the long-term clinical studies have shown an increased proportion of squamous cell carcinoma located on non-sun-exposed areas. Five of nine of the patients with SCC in the PUVA-48 cooperative group (9) had SCC on a site other than head/neck or dorsal upper extremities, including two scrotal lesions. In U.S. 16-center study, only 12% of the SCC patients had lesions on the head or neck (6). High percentages of tumors on non-sun-exposed areas were also found in other cooperative centers (7,8). This is much higher percentage than that expected in the general population, in which 70–80% of SCC is found on sun-exposed areas (37). Alteration of these site predilections appears attributable to PUVA. No such dramatic change in anatomical location has been noted for PUVA-associated BCC.

Skin Type and Risk of Skin Cancer

Both of the cooperative studies demonstrating an increase in PUVA-associated SCC independent of other carcinogenic risk factors show a mildly elevated increase in the incidence of SCC in skin types I and II versus that for skin types III and IV (6,9). This difference was not statistically significant in the PUVA-48 cooperative group (9) and appeared to hold only for medium cumulative dosages (160–259 exposures) and not for low (<160 exposures) or high (>260 exposures) dosages in the U.S. 16-center study (6). This may be due to the fact that the relative increased risk of SCC in burning skin types is overwhelmed by the much stronger risk factor of total exposure in the higher-dosage group.

Biological Activity of PUVA-Associated Epidermal Tumors

The squamous cell carcinomas that have been reported thus far in PUVA-treated psoriatics have not exhibited a biological aggressiveness or anaplasia markedly different from solar-induced SCC. Of the nine patients found to have squamous cell carcinoma in the PUVA-48 cooperative group, all were treated surgically, there were no metastases, and none have recurred (9). Of the 96 patients who developed SCC in the U.S. 16-center study, only two developed metastases and one patient died (53). This would be comparable to the 0.5–2.0% incidence of metastases noted for SCCs arising in a solar keratosis and much lower than the incidence of distant spread from de novo SCC, which is unknown but has been estimated to be as high as 18% (54). Their most recent studies show seven patients with metastatic SCC.

Systemic Carcinogenicity of PUVA

The U.S. 16-center study has documented a statistically increased incidence of colonic and central nervous system cancer in their cohort of 1380 PUVA-treated psoriasis patients (53). They found no increased incidence of leukemia or lymphoma. They speculated that this increase may be due to increased surveillance of a closely monitored population and what are often occult malignancies. Also, it is unknown whether the increased exposure to tar and petrolatum could account for the increase in central nervous system tumors. Further studies to determine the nature of the association between PUVA and internal malignancies will need to be undertaken to elucidate these relationships.

CONCLUSIONS

Many cooperative and single centers have undertaken long-term clinical studies to determine the risk of developing skin cancer from PUVA therapy since its introduction as a treatment for psoriasis in 1974. Many of these studies have now reported their findings for 5–13 years of follow-up.

The most dramatic finding has been the dose-related increased incidence of squamous cell carcinoma first reported by Stern et al. in 1984 (5) and 1994 (9a) and confirmed by Forman and Roenigk in 1989 (9). Although some other studies worldwide have found a similar increase, only a few had patient populations with a mean cumulative dosage of 2000 J/cm^2 or greater, as had these American studies. Most of these studies did find an increased incidence of SCC in patients treated with PUVA who also had other known carcinogenic risk factors (such as exposure to therapeutic ionizing radiation or arsenic or previous skin cancer), a tumor-promoting effect that is demonstrated earlier and at lower dosages than the tumor-initiating effect of PUVA in patients without other risk factors.

The 13-year follow-up of Stern's U.S. 16-center study also reported a modest but increased dose-related incidence of basal cell carcinoma (9a), a finding that has been confirmed by other centers. Some other studies have demonstrated a definite tumor-promoting effect of PUVA on BCC in patients with other carcinogenic risk factors (exposure to radiation or arsenic or previous skin cancer). A statistical analysis of skin cancer patients has shown a twofold increase in the incidence of BCC in patients with psoriasis, raising the possibility that psoriatics have an inherent tendency to develop these tumors (38).

There is new evidence from Stern's 16-center study to support an increased incidence of malignant melanoma in patients treated with PUVA.

The squamous cell carcinomas induced by PUVA appear more frequently on non-sun-exposed areas than those found in the general population. However, the biological aggressiveness of the PUVA-associated SCCs is similar to that found in SCCs arising from solar keratoses, in that their metastatic potential is low and they are easily treated with local surgical procedures without recurrence. The exception to this would be the relatively high number of scrotal SCCs found, which have a higher metastatic potential because of their anatomical location.

There appears to be a modest increase in the risk of developing SCCs in patients with type I or II skin at medium cumulative dosages, an effect not seen in very-high-dose groups because the risk from the cumulative dose overwhelms the smaller increased risk from skin type.

The U.S. 16-center study found an increased incidence of colonic cancer and central nervous system tumors in PUVA patients, a finding that has not yet been confirmed by any other group.

It appears that after 20 years of experience with PUVA therapy the therapeutic-to-toxic ratio remains favorable for patients with moderate to severe psoriasis. Although there is an increased risk of cutaneous squamous cell carcinoma, the risk may be decreased by excluding patients with a history of exposure to therapeutic ionizing radiation or arsenic or a previous history of skin cancer, along with careful shielding of noninvolved skin, particularly of the scrotum. In addition, dose-sparing regimens, such as those based on minimum phototoxic dosage testing with aggressive schedules but fewer overall treatments and joules, may prove to be tumor sparing. Patients who receive less than 1500 J/cm^2 cumulatively probably are at low risk. In addition, increasing concomitant use of systemic retinoids and the use of rotational therapy may reduce the incidence of skin cancer in these psoriatic patients.

REFERENCES

1. Stern, R.S., Thibodeau, L.A., Kleinerman, R.A., et al. (1979). Risk of cutaneous carcinoma in patients treated with oral methoxsalen photochemotherapy for psoriasis. *N. Engl. J. Med.* 300:800–813.
2. Honigsmann, H., Wolff, K., Gschnait, F., et al. (1980). Keratoses and non-melanoma skin tumors in long-term photochemotherapy (PUVA) *J. Am. Acad. Dermatol.* 3:406–414.
3. Henseler, T., Honigsmann, H., Wolff, K., et al. (1981). Oral 8-methoxypsoralen photochemotherapy of psoriasis: the European PUVA study: a cooperative study among 18 European centers. *Lancet* 1:853–857.
4. Roenigk, H.H., Jr., and Caro, W.A. (1981). Skin cancer in the PUVA-48 cooperative study. *J. Am. Acad. Dermatol.* 4:319–324.
5. Stern, R.S., Laird, N., Melski, J., et al. (1984). Cutaneous squamous cell carcinoma in patients treated with PUVA. *N. Engl. J. Med.* 310:1156–1161.
6. Stern, R.S., Lange, R., et al. (1988). Non-melanoma skin cancer occurring in patients treated with PUVA five to ten years after first treatment. *J. Invest. Dermatol.* 91:120–124.
7. Tanew, A., Honigsmann, H., Ortel, B., et al. (1986). Non-melanoma skin tumors in long-term photochemotherapy treatment of psoriasis. *J. Am. Acad. Dermatol.* 15:960–965.
8. Henseler, T., Christophers, E., Honigsmann, H., et al. (1987). Skin tumors in the European PUVA study. *J. Am. Acad. Dermatol.* 26:108–116.
9. Forman, A.B., Roenigk, H.H., Jr., Caro, W.A., and Magid, M.L. (1989). Skin cancer in the PUVA-48 Cooperative Study. *Arch. Dermatol.* 125:515–519.

9a. Stern, R.S., Laird, N., et al. (1994). The carcinoma risk of treatments for severe psoriasis. *Cancer* 73: 2759–2764.

10. Eskelinen, A., Halme, H., Lassus, A., and Idanpaan-Hekkila, J. (1985). Risk of cutaneous carcinoma in psoriatic patients treated with PUVA. *Photodermatology* 2:10–14.
11. Lindskov, R. (1981). Skin carcinomas and treatment with photochemotherapy (PUVA). *Acta Derm. Venereol. (Stockh.)* 61:141–145.
12. Ros, A., Wennersten, G., and Lagerholm, B. (1983). Long-term photochemotherapy for psoriasis: a histopathological and clinical follow-up study with special emphasis on tumor incidence and behavior of pigmented lesions. *Acta. Derm. Venereol. (Stockh.)* 63: 215–221.
13. Torinuki, W., and Tagami, H. (1988). Incidence of skin cancer in Japanese psoriatic patients treated with either PUVA, Goeckerman regimen or both therapies: a 100-year follow-up study. *J. Am. Acad. Dermatol.* 18:1273–1281.
14. Cox, N.H., Jones, S.K., Downey, D.J., et al. (1987). Cutaneous and ocular side-effects of oral photochemotherapy: results of an 8-year follow-up study. *Br. J. Dermatol.* 116:145–152.
15. Barth, J., Meffert, H., et al. (1987). 10 Jahre PUVA-therapie in der DDR-analyse zum langzeitrisiko. *Z. Klin. Med.* 42:889–892.

15a. Takashima, A., Matsunami, Z., Yamamoto, K., Ketajima, S., and Mizano, N. (1990). Cutaneous carcinoma and 8-methoxypsoralen and ultraviolet A (PUVA) lentigenes in Japanese patient with psoriasis treated with topical PUVA; a follow-up of 214 patients. *Photodermatol. Photoimmunol. Photomed.* 7(5):218–221.

15b. Lever, L.R., and Fan, P.M. (1994). Skin cancers or premalignant lesions occur in half of high dose PUVA patients. *Br. J. Dermatol.* 13(2):215–219.
15c. Lindelof, B., and Sigargeirsson, B. (1993). PUVA and cancer: a case control study. *Br. J. Dermatol.* 129(1): 39–41.
15d. Lindelof, B., et al. (1992). Comparison of the carcinogenic potential of trioxsalan bath PUVA and oral methoxsalan PUVA: a preliminary report. *Arch. Dermatol.* 128(10):1341–1344.
15e. Chuang, T.X., et al. (1992). PUVA and skin cancer. A historical cohort study on 492 patients. *J. Am. Acad. Dermatol.* 26:173–177.
15f. Lindelof, B., et al. (1991). PUVA and cancer: a large scale epidemiological study. *Lancet* 338(8759):91–93.
16. Unna, P.G. (1894). *Die Histopathologic der Hautkrankheiten.* A. Hirschwald, Berlin.
17. Rusch, H.P., Kline, B.Z., and Bauman, C.A. (1941). Carcinogenesis by UV rays with reference to wavelength and energy. *Arch. Pathol.* 371:135–146.
18. Forbes, P.D., et al. (1982). Simulated stratospheric ozone depletion and increased UV radiation: effects on photocarcinogenesis in hairless mice. *Cancer Res.* 42:2796.
19. Rothman, R.H., and Setlow, R.B. (1979). An action spectrum for cell killing and pyrimidine dimer formation in Chinese hamster V-79 cells. *Photochem. Photobiol.* 29:57.
20. Musajo, L., and Rodighiero, G. (1970). Studies on the photo-C4-cycll-addition reactions between skin-photosensitizing coumarins and nucleic acids. *Photochem. Photobiol.* 11:27.
21. Pathak, M.A., and Kramer, D.M. (1969). Photosensitization of skin in vivo by furocoumarins. *Biochim. Biophys. Acta* 195:197.
22. Johnston, B.H., Johnson, M.A., Moore, C.B., et al. (1977). Psoralen-DNA photoreaction: controlled production of mono- and diadducts with nanosecond ultraviolet laser pulses. *Science* 197:906.
23. West, M.R., Johansen, M., and Faed, M.J.W. (1982). Sister chromatid exchange frequency in human epidermal cells in culture treated with 8-methoxypsoralen and long-wave UV radiation. *J. Invest. Dermatol.* 78:67.
24. Griffin, A.C., et al. (1958). The wavelength effect upon erythemal and carcinogenic response in psoralen treated mice. *J. Invest. Dermatol.* 31:289.
25. Urbach, F. (1959). Modification of ultraviolet carcinogenesis by photoactive agents. *J. Invest. Dermatol.* 32:372.
26. Kripke, M.L. (1986). Immunology and photocarcinogenesis. *J. Am Acad. Dermatol.* 14:149–155.
27. Kripke, M.L., and Morrison, W.L. (1985). Modulation of immune function by UV radiation. *J. Invest. Dermatol.* 85(1s):635–665.
28. Briffa, D.V., Parker, D., Tosca, N., Turk, J.L., and Greaves, M.W. (1981). The effect of photochemotherapy (PUVA) on cell mediated immunity in the guinea pig. *J. Invest. Dermatol.* 77:377–380.
29. Strauss, G.H., Greaves, M., Price, M., Bridges, B.A., Hall-Smith, P., and Vella-Buffa, D. (1980). Inhibition of delayed hypersensitivity reaction in skin (DNCB test) by 8-methoxy psoralen photochemotherapy. *Lancet* 2:556.
30. Okamoto, H., and Horio, T. (1981). The effect of 8-methoxypsoralen and long-wave ultra violet light on Langerhans cell. *J. Invest. Dermatol.* 77:345–346.
31. Ree, K. (1982). Reduction of Langerhans cells in human epidermis during PUVA therapy: a morphometric study. *J. Invest. Dermatol.* 78:488–492.
32. Morison, W.L., Parrish, J.A., Block, K.J., and Krugler, J.F. (1979). Transient impairment of peripheral blood lymphocyte function during PUVA therapy. *Br. J. Dermatol.* 101:391–397.
33. Clayton, R., Valdimarsson, H., and Fry, L. (1979). The effect of PUVA treatment on multiple lymphocytes. *Br. J. Dermatol.* 100:225–226
34. Moscichi, R.A., Morison, W.L., Parrish, J.A., Black, K.J., and Colvin, R.B. (1982). Reduction of the fraction of circulating helper-induced T-cells identified by monoclonal antibodies in psoriatic patients treated with long-term psoralen/ultraviolet-A radiation (PUVA). *J. Invest. Dermatol.* 79:205–208.
35. Kraemer, K.H., Waters, H.L., Cohen, L.I., et al. (1981). Effects of 8-methoxypsoralen and ultraviolet radiation on human lymphoid cells in vitro. *J. Invest. Dermatol.* 76:80–87.
36. Halprin, K.M. (1980). Psoriasis, skin cancer and PUVA. *J. Am. Acad. Dermatol.* 2:334–339.
37. Fears, T.R., and Scotto, J. (1982). Changes in skin cancer morbidity between 1971–1972 and 1977–1978. *J. Natl. Cancer Inst.* 69:365–370.
38. Stern, R.S., Scotto, J., and Fears, T.R. (1985). Psoriasis and susceptibility to nonmelanoma skin cancer. *J. Am. Acad. Dermatol.* 12:67–73.
39. Robinson, J.K. (1987). Risk of developing another basal cell carcinoma, a 5-year prospective study. *Cancer* 60:118–120.
40. Hashimoto, K., Kohda, H., Tmakin, M., et al. (1978). Psoralen-UVA treated psoriatic lesions. *Arch. Dermatol.* 114:712–722.
41. Zelickson, A.S., Mottax, J.H., and Muller, S.A. (1979). Melanocyte changes following PUVA therapy. *J. Am. Acad. Dermatol.* 1:422–430.
42. Rhodes, A.R., Stern, R.S., and Melski, J.W. (1983). The PUVA lentigo: an analysis of predisposing factors. *J. Invest. Dermatol.* 81:459–463.
43. Nakagawa, H., Rhodes, A.R., Monitaz, T.K., et al. (1984). Morphologic alterations of epidermal melanocytes and melanosomes in PUVA lentigines: a com-

parative ultrastructural investigation of lentigines induced by PUVA and sunlight. *J. Invest. Dermatol.* 82: 101.

44. Gschnait, F., Wolff, K., Hönigsmann, H., et al. (1980). Long-term photochemotherapy: histopathological and immunofluorescence observations in 243 patients. *Br. J. Dermatol.* 103:11–22.

45. Ros, A., Wennersten, G., and Lagerholm, B. (1983). Long-term photochemotherapy for psoriasis: a histopathological and clinical follow-up study with special emphasis on tumor incidence and behavior of pigmented lesions. *Acta Derm. Venereol.* (*Stockh.*) 63: 215–221.

46. Marx, J.L., Averbach, R., Possick, P., et al. (1983). Malignant melanoma in vitro in two patients treated with psoralens and ultraviolet A. *J. Am. Acad. Dermatol.* 9:904–911.

47. Lancaster, H.O. (1970). Some geographical aspects of mortality from melanoma in Europeans. *Med. J. Aust.* 2:846–851.

48. Elwood, J.M., Lee, I.A.H., Walter, S.D., et al. (1974). Relationship of melanoma and other skin cancer mortality to latitude and ultraviolet radiation in the United States and Canada. *Int. J. Epidemiol.* 3: 325–331.

49. Crombie, I.K. (1929). Variation of melanoma incidence with latitude in North America and Europe. *Br. J. Cancer* 40:774–781.

50. Forrest, J.B., and Forrest, T.H. (1980). Malignant melanoma arising during drug therapy for vitiligo. *J. Surg. Oncol.* 12:337.

51. Kemmett, D., Reshad, H., and Baker, H. (1984). Nodular malignant melanoma and multiple squamous cell carcinomas in a patient treated by photochemotherapy for psoriasis. *Br. Med. J.* 289:1498.

52. Stern, R.S. (1986). PUVA carcinogenesis after ten years: prospect and retrospect. *Photodermatology* 3: 257–260.

52a. Stern, R.S., Nichols, K.T., Vakeon, L.H. (1997). Malignant melanoma in patients treated for psoriasis with methoxsalen and ultraviolet A radiation (PUVA). *N. Engl. J. Med.* 336:96–101.

53. Stoll, H.L., and Schwartz, R.A. (1987). Squamous cell carcinoma. In *Dermatology-General Medicine.* 3rd ed. T.B. Fitzpatrick, et al. (Eds.). McGraw-Hill, New York, p. 753.

54. Stern, R.S., Lange, R., et al. (1988). Cardiovascular disease, cancer and cause of death in patients with psoriasis: 10 year prospective experience in a cohort of 1380 patients. *J. Invest. Dermatol.* 91:197–201.

45

Combination and Rotational Therapy for Psoriasis

Henry H. Roenigk, Jr.
Northwestern University Medical School, Chicago, Illinois

There are many different choices that a physician has to treat patients with psoriasis. Frequently, the disease is so mild that topical corticosteroid, tar, and lubrication are all that is needed. The Goeckerman treatment with tar and ultraviolet B (UVB) phototherapy which was traditionally an in-hospital therapy is now done in psoriasis day care centers or as outpatient therapy three to five times per week. Psoralen and ultraviolet A (PUVA) has become a standard form of therapy which clears about 90% of patients, but has the long-term risk of the development of skin cancer and of photoaging skin. Retinoids are most effective in pustular or erythrodermic psoriasis. The response in plaque-type psoriasis is so slow that patients often give up because of distressing cutaneous side effects. Methotrexate is a valuable drug for clearing psoriasis, but because of the high incidence of liver damage from chronic use there are limits on its safety for long-term use in psoriasis. Cyclosporine is a highly effective drug in clearing psoriasis, but, again, the long-term toxicity to the kidneys or the development of skin cancer or lymphoma could hamper its long-term use in psoriasis.

Because many of our systemic therapies for psoriasis have side effects that limit their usefulness, dermatologists have turned to combining therapies to try to achieve the same effectiveness but at a lower dosage of each component of the combination (1).

WHAT IS COMBINATION AND ROTATIONAL THERAPY?

The National Psoriasis Foundation recently sponsored a conference on psoriasis combination and rotational therapy. The proceedings from that conference (1a) have helped to define what has become a more common plan in the management of long-term psoriasis.

Combination Therapy

Although single agents are likely to limit side effects, decrease costs, and improve compliance of patients, there are situations in which combination therapies are useful. These include failed therapy with single agents, limiting toxicities of individual agents by decreasing the dosages used for combination, emergence of toxicity to a single agent, and tapering patients off an individual drug.

Rotational Therapy

This facilitates long-term treatment and minimizes chronic toxicity by rotating to different treatment regimens before significant "individual drug" toxicities occur.

In combination therapy, a lower dosage of each agent is used and usually one agent is discontinued after the psoriasis has cleared and the open agent used as maintenance therapy. The long-term use of both components is sometimes necessary because of resistance to treatment or instability of the psoriasis.

PUVA COMBINATIONS

PUVA and Topical Therapies

Therapy with PUVA is very effective when used alone to clear psoriasis. The only form of topical therapy usually recommended is lubrication with Vaseline or other moisturizers. Early in the development of PUVA, combinations with other topical agents were studied. Topical corticosteroids seemed to accelerate the clearing of lesions patients being treated with PUVA compared with lubrication and PUVA. The rebound flares of psoriasis when topical steroids are used can result in shorter remissions while patients are on maintenance PUVA therapy. Tars and anthralin topically can be beneficial additive therapy for thicker plaques of psoriasis to make them more responsive to PUVA. These agents are photo-sensitizing and therefore can result in UVA burns.

Calcipotriene (Vitamin D ointment) in combination with PUVA results in faster clearance and reduced UVA dosage (1B).

PUVA and Retinoid Therapy

Systemic retinoids have added another important agent to the treatment of disorders of keratinization which includes psoriasis. Two agents are currently available for use as treatment. Isotretinoin (Accutane) is generally used for severe cystic acne vulgaris and disorders of keratinization, such as ichthyosis, Darier disease, and other dermatoses. Isotretinoin has a short half-life and has been found to be only partly effective in psoriasis. The effect of isotretinoin on combination with PUVA or UVB for psoriasis is controversial (2,3). The aromatic retinoid etretinate (Tegison) was developed specifically for psoriasis and has been most effective in erythroderma and pustular (localized and generalized) forms (4). It is also effective in plaque psoriasis when used alone, but it is much more effective when combined with UVB or PUVA therapy (5).

The metabolite of etretinate (acetretin, Soritane®) has been proven to have the same effects as etretinate, but it has a short half-life, and thus can be used in women of childbearing age (6).

Since photochemotherapy with 8-methoxypsoralen and UVA (PUVA) represents a powerful tool to control psoriasis, it appeared logical to combine it with retinoids with the aim of reducing its potential long-term hazards.

The retinoid PUVA (RePUVA) combination was the first simultaneous used by Fritsch, in 1978 (7,8). The main advantages of this combination are an acceleration of the response rate of psoriatic lesions in the clearing treatment phase of PUVA, a reduction of the number of individual treatments to obtain clearing, and the clearing of patients who cannot be brought into remission by PUVA alone. Probably the most important advantage is the fact that the total cumulative dose of UVA (J/cm^2) necessary to achieve clearing can be cut to approximately 50% of what would be required in conventional PUVA therapy (9).

The combination of PUVA and etretinate is the most extensively investigated regimen. The original observations on the efficacy of this treatment were soon confirmed by Frenk (10), Grupper and Berretti (11), Heidbreder and Christophers (12), Lauharanta (13), and Orfanos (14). Considerable information has now accumulated on other retinoids and psoralens used in such combinations.

All of these studies on retinoid/PUVA combinations were done in Europe, since the United States was late in approving retinoids as a monotherapy for psoriasis. No official trials have been done in the United States using the combination of PUVA and Tegison or Soritane.

The most commonly used treatment is to start with Tegison in a dose of 1 mg/kg per day or less 7 to 10 days prior to PUVA therapy. Both Tegison and PUVA are then concomitantly given until complete clearing of psoriasis lesions is obtained. Then the dose of Tegison is reduced and eventually stopped, whereas the PUVA is continued once per week or less for long-term maintenance. The substitution of isotretinoin for Tegison has been equally effective in some studies, but not as effective in others (2,3). The combinations with acetretin and PUVA are equally effective to etretinate and PUVA. This combination has been effective also in both pustular and erythrodermic psoriasis.

Another method of combining retinoids and PUVA is for "PUVA-resistant" patients. Sometimes PUVA patients require large doses of PUVA (25–30 J/cm^2) treatment given three times per week and they are still not under control. In this situation, the PUVA is reduced by one-third the dose and Tegison 1 mg/kg per day is added simultaneously. This will accelerate clearing, and then the dose of Tegison can be reduced to 25–50 mg/day long term in combination with PUVA. This could also reduce the long-term risk of developing skin cancer from PUVA.

A combination of trimethylpsoralen-bath-PUVA and etretinate has been successfully used by Michaelson (15) and Vaatainen (16). As with oral PUVA, the UVA dose requirements for clearing psoriasis are reduced by about 50% compared with bath-PUVA monotherapy, provided that etretinate is administered 3–14 days before PUVA in a daily oral dose of 0.5–1.0 mg/kg body weight and maintained throughout the entire clearing phase.

In summary RePUVA or the induction with systemic retinoids and then clearing combined with PUVA seems to be the most popular combination and most effective with evidence of lowered incidence of side effects.

PUVA and UVB Phototherapy

The combination of PUVA plus UVB therapy has been used primarily in an aggressive hospital setting. The routine is usually done as follows:

Monday:	PUVA
Tuesday:	UVB
Wednesday:	PUVA
Thursday:	UVB
Friday:	PUVA
Saturday:	UVB
Sunday:	Rest

This can result in more rapid clearing of psoriasis than with PUVA alone, but there is the risk of UVB burn added to the PUVA therapy as the dose increases. Usually the PUVA is used for long-term maintenance. One disadvantage of this combination is if the UVB phototherapy results in rapid tanning which blocks the effect of PUVA.

PUVA and Methotrexate

In the PUVA-methotrexate (MTX) regimen, MTX is administered alone initially, then combined with PUVA, after which PUVA alone is used for maintenance therapy (17). The main advantage of using this combination is the marked reduction possible in the total cumulative exposure to UVA radiation during the clearance phase of therapy and during the maintenance phase of PUVA therapy, thus reducing long-term UVA radiation side effects.

This combination is certainly effective and the number of treatments with PUVA and MTX may be reduced to one-half of that of PUVA alone. It should, however, be borne in mind that the possibility exists of a synergistic effect on tumor promotion (18) and that MTX may increase light sensitivity, which again may lead to phototoxic reactions. Prolonged phototoxic reactions have also been reported.

PUVA and Cyclosporine

Cyclosporine crisis therapy has been advocated by some as an effective therapy for severe cases of generalized flares of psoriasis or erythroderma and instability of psoriasis (19,20). The decision as to whether to continue long-term low-dose cyclosporine will depend on toxic side effects, especially renal function decrease due to cyclosporine (21). Switching to PUVA therapy for long-term maintenance is a viable option. Since one side effect of cyclosporine is skin cancer, the long-term combination of PUVA and cyclosporine is not advisable.

Cyclosporine (5 mg/kg per dose) for 2 weeks, followed by combination PUVA and cyclosporine until clearance, was found to be as effective as Re-PUVA in terms of the number of treatments to clear psoriasis and duration of treatment (21a). However, the overall exposure to UVA radiation was much higher in the cyclosporine-treated patients. With the added risk of skin-cancer from both agents this combination is not recommended.

PUVA and Interferons

Interferons alone have been used in psoriasis and have not been proven effective. The combination of PUVA plus interferons have been shown to be highly effective in clearing mycosis fungoides (22). It results in clearing of lesions equal to PUVA alone but with fewer total joules per square centimeter. The long-term benefit of adding interferons to PUVA therapy for mycosis fungoides are yet to be determined. It could result in more long-term control of mycosis fungoides than PUVA alone. The combination of PUVA and interferons has not been tried in psoriasis. There are a considerable number of side effects from the intramuscular use of interferon, which is usually given three times weekly. Interferon alone has not been effective in psoriasis.

NONPUVA SYSTEMIC COMBINATIONS

Retinoids and Methotrexate

Methotrexate has been combined with etretinate in the treatment of severe, generalized, pustular psoriasis when the disease is unaltered by MTX or etretinate alone (23,24). Methotrexate is used in this combination only during the acute phase of the disease; the MTX dosage is then tapered and etretinate alone is used during the chronic (maintenance) phase. Rapid remission of the acute phase is often achieved with this combination, with eventual clearing of the skin. The rapid clearing of pustular psoriasis by MTX during the acute phase allows time for etretinate to exert its effect and permits the sole use of etretinate in the chronic phase of treatment. By utilizing these therapeutic modalities together, it is possible to obtain a rapid and prolonged clinical response with few toxic side effects.

van der Veen et al. (23), Adams (24), and Rosenbaum and Roenigk (24) have described the benefits of combining etretinate and methotrexate. Zachariae (25), however, warned against the combination because of the development of a severe toxic hepatitis after etretinate was given to a 47-year-old woman, who had been on MTX for 10 years, and who had an almost normal liver biopsy the year before. Etretinate has in some cases been reported to cause hepatitis; however, there is no proof that etretinate alone would not have given the same symptoms. These are two potentially hepatotoxic drugs in which an interaction in the liver could very well take place. From a pharmacological viewpoint, displacement from albumin should give rise to increased toxicity.

Since the original reports, other patients have benefited from the combination of etretinate and methotrexate, including patients with pustular psoriasis and Reiter disease. Zachariae (27) has since used the treatment with good results in therapy-resistant cases of pustular psoriasis or psoriasis vulgaris, and without observing further cases of toxic hepatitis. Methotrexate and etretinate may be tried in severely affected psoriatics when either drug fails. Start with a low etretinate dose of from 25 mg twice weekly and build up to a dose of 25 mg daily combined with doses of MTX 15 mg weekly by the divided intermittent oral dosage. For the first 2–3 months, before adding etretinate perform weekly laboratory controls, including liver enzymes, leukocyte, and platelet counts, even when the patient has been on MTX for long periods. Serum triglycerides and cholesterol are checked after 1 month.

Retinoids and UVB

The combination of retinoids and UVB allows an improved percentage of clearing compared with results for the two methods used separately. It has allowed treatment of patients unresponsive to other regimens (UVB, PUVA, etretinate), with a reduction in parameters for clearing and good general tolerance. This method has the same efficacy as PUVA or RePUVA, but it eliminates the psoralen administration, and thus any possibility of chronic side effects theoretically attributable to prolonged and repeated PUVA.

Grupper and Berretti have summarized their own clinical experience (5). They have treated more than 50 patients with severe or refractory psoriasis with UVB in combination with etretinate. Methods were entirely analogous with those previously described (28,29); however, results have been disappointing by comparison with other studies as well as by comparison with their usual results with PUVA, and especially RePUVA. Only 40% of patients showed clearing; the time to clearing was always greater than that with RePUVA, and they were particularly impressed by the high frequency (50%) of phototoxic effects, which frequently required withdrawal of treatment. They currently reserve the retinoid-UVB combination for particularly RePUVA-resistant cases, in which addition of UVB frequently can be a deciding factor, since it provides clearing without a major increase in total energy amount and psoralen or etretinate dosage.

Trials in the United States have studied the combination of Acetretin and UVB phototherapy (29a). Results show there is an advantage to combining UVB and Acetretin over UVB alone.

Cyclosporine and Retinoids

Cyclosporine has been advocated for crisis therapy to get severe unstable psoriasis under control (19). Once clearing is achieved, then long-term maintenance therapy with retinoids (Tegison, Soritane) may be a useful combination. Retinoids may be introduced once the psoriasis is stabilized by cyclosporine (20). The usual dose of 0.5–1.0 mg/kg per day is used and the dose of cyclosporine is gradually reduced. Eventually the cyclosporine is discontinued and the long-term retinoid therapy is continued as monotherapy in the lowest effective dose.

Meinardi and Bos (32) evaluated this combination using etretinate at initial doses of 0.2 mg/kg per day to 1 mg/kg per day. The preliminary results of this treatment combination suggest that at higher dosages, etretinate did show a modest cyclosporine-sparing effect, but it did not represent a major advance over cyclosporine monotherapy. Other studies (32a) have shown variable efficacy.

Cyclosporine and Methotrexate

Patients who have been on long-term cyclosporine therapy will frequently show signs of renal function abnormalities. If these become of concern, then cyclosporine needs to be discontinued. One option if hematological and hepatic function are normal is MTX therapy. Methotrexate can have toxic effects if renal function is abnormal. Hospitalization with careful monitoring of renal function, MTX serum levels, and hematological parameters can result in the rapid conversion of a patient well controlled with cyclosporine (but with renal function abnormalities) to MTX therapy for long-term control (30). Switching systemic agents which have different target organs for toxic effects has certain advantages.

Cyclosporine and UVB

Meinazdi and Bos (32) conducted a study to evaluate alternate treatment schedules either alone or in combination with other therapies in an effort to minimize the drug's nephrotoxicity. A pilot study in which cyclosporine A was combined with UVB did not show any cyclosporine A–sparing effects. The possible synergistic effects of cyclosporine A and UVB on the induction of tumor formation also makes this combination undesirable.

Methotrexate and UVB

In the MTX-UVB regimen, MTX is administered alone initially, then combined with UVB, after which the patient is maintained on UVB (31). The combination of MTX and UVB is so effective in clearing psoriasis that relatively low doses of MTX and UVB can be used, thus reducing the long-term cumulative toxicity of each. There has been no report of reactivation or prolongation of UVB-induced erythema by MTX administration, but this effect is possible.

The enhancement of skin cancer risk as mentioned with the PUVA-MTX combination (18) needs to be considered with this combination.

REFERENCES

1. Roenigk, H.H., Jr. (1986). *Combination Therapies for Psoriasis. An Overview.* Psoriasis Symposium IV. Elsevier Scientific Publishing Co., Inc., pp. 233–239.

1a. Mentor, M.A., See, J.A., Amend, W.J.C. Ellis, C.M., Kraeger, G.F., Lebwohl, M., Morrison, W.L., et al. (1996). Proceedings of the psoriasis combination and rotational therapy conference. *J. Am. Acad. Dermatol.* 34(2)315–321.

2. Gibsteine, C., and Roenigk, H.H. (1985). Oral isotretinoin followed by psoralens and ultraviolet for psoriasis. *J. Am. Acad. Dermatol.* 13:153–155.

3. Honigsmann, and Wolfe, K. (1983). Isotretinoin-PUVA for psoriasis. *Lancet* 1:236.

4. Orfanos, C.E., Braun-Falco, O., Forbes, E.M., Grupper, G., Polano, M.K., and Schuppli, R. (Eds). (1981). *Retinoids—Advances in Basic Research and Therapy.* Springer Verlag, New York.

5. Grupper C., and Berretti, C. (198). Retinoid combinations. In *Psoriasis.* H.H. Roenigk and H.I. Maibach (Eds.). Marcel Dekker, Inc., New York, pp. 637–644.

6. Lowe, N.J., Roenigk, H., and Voorhees, J.J. (1988). Etretinate appropriate use in severe psoriasis. *Arch. Dermatol.* 124(4):527–528.

7. Fritsch, P.O., Honigsmann, H., Jaschke, E., and Wolff, K. (1978). Augmentation of oral methoxsalen. Photochemotherapy with an oral retinoid acid derivative. *J. Invest. Dermatol.* 70:178–182.

8. Fritsch, P., Honigsmann, H., Jaschke, E., and Wolff, K. (1978). Augmentation of oral methoxsalen. Photochemotherapie bei psoriasis: steigerung der wirksamkeit durch ein orales aromatisches retinoid. Klinische orfahrungen bel 134 patienten. *Disch. Med. Wochenschr.* 103:1731–1736.

9. Wolff, K., and Fritsch, P.O. (1982). Retinoid-PUVA chemophotochemotherapy. In *Psoriasis.* E. Farber, A.J. Cox, L. Nall, and P.H. Jacobs (Eds.). Grune & Stratton, New York, pp. 211–219.

10. Frenk, E. (1989). Traitement du psoriasis par l'association d'un retinoide oranotigie et de la photochemotherapy oral 8-methorpsoraline. *Praxis* 69:221–224.

11. Grupper, C., and Berretti, B. (1981). Treatment of psoriasis by oral PUVA-therapy combined with aromatic retinoid. *Dermatologica* 162:404–413.

12. Heidbreder, G., and Christophers, E. (1979). Therapy of psoriasis with retinoid plus UVA. *Arch. Dermatol. Res.* 264:331–337.

13. Lauharenta, J., Javakonski, T., and Lassas, A. (1981). A clinical evaluation of the effects of an aromatic retinoid (Tegison) combination of retinoid and PUVA and PUVA alone in severe psoriasis. *Br. J. Dermatol.* 104:325–332.

14. Orfanos, C.E., Pullman, H.J., Sterry, W., and Kanzig, M. (1978). Retinoid-PUVA (Repuva): Septemische

kombentions-bhandburg bei psoriasis. *Hantarzi* 53: 494–545.

15. Michaelson, Noren, P., and Vahlquist, A. (1978). Combined therapy with oral retinoid and PUVA baths in psoriasis. *Br. J. Dermatol.* 99:221–222.
16. Väätäinen, Hollmen, A., and Fraki, J.E. (1985). Trimethylpsoralen bAth plus ultraviolet A combined with retinoid (etretinate) in the treatment of severe psoriasis. *J. Am. Acad. Dermatol.* 12:52–55.
17. Morison, W.L., et al. (1982). Combined methotrexate PUVA therapy in the treatment of psoriasis. *J. Am. Acad. Dermatol.* 6:46–51.
18. Fitzsimmons, C., Long, J., and Mackie. (1983). Synergistic carcinogenic potential of methotrexate and PUVA in psoriasis (letter). *Lancet* 1:235–236.
19. Picascia, D.D., Gardern, J.M., Freinkel, R.K. and Roenigk, H. (1988). Resistant severe psoriasis controlled with systemic cyclosporin therapy. *Transplant. Proc.* 20(3 Suppl. 3):58–62.
20. Picascia, D.D., Garden, J.M., Feinkel, R.K., and Roenigk, H.H. (1987). Treatment of resistant severe psoriasis with systemic cyclosporin. *J. Am. Acad. Dermatol.* 17(3):408–414.
21. Dieterle, A., Abeywickrama, K., and von Graffenried, B. (1988). Nephrotoxicity and hypertension in patients with autoimmune disease treated with cyclosporine. *Transplant. Proc.* 20(3 Suppl. 4):349–355.

21a. Petzeltover, P., Honigsmann, H., Longer, K., et al. (1990). Cyclosporins A in combinations with photochemotherapy (PUVA) in the treatment of psoriasis. *Br. J. Dermatol.* 123:641–647.

22. Springer, E., Rosen, S., and Roenigk, H.H. (1989). Interferon alpha-2A combined with photochemotherapy for cutaneous T-cell lymphoma. *J. Invest. Dermtol.* 92(3):521 (abstract).
23. van der Veen, E., et al. (1982). MTX and etretinate as concurrent therapies in severe psoriasis. *Arch. Dermatol.*118(9):660–662.
24. Rosenbaum, M.M., and Roenigk, H.H. (1984). Treatment of generalized pustular psoriasis with etretinate (RO 10-0359) and methotrexate. *J. Am. Acad. Dermatol.* 10:357–361.
25. Adams. J.D. (1983). Concurrent MTX and etretinate therapy for psoriasis (letter). *Arch. Dermatol.* 119(10): 793.
26. Zachariae, H., (1983). MTX and etretinate as concurrent therapies in the treatment of psoriasis (letter). *Arch. Dermatol.* 119(10):793.
27. Zachariae, (1986). Combination cystotoxic therapy. In *Psoriasis: Proceedings of the 4th International Symposium.* E.M. Farber, Cox, and Jacobs (Eds.). Elsevier Scientific Publishing Co., pp. 240–247.
28. Orfanos, C.E., Pulmann. H., Steigleder, G.K., and Block, P.II. (1979). Oral retinoid and UVB radiation: a new alternative treatment for psoriasis on an outpatient basis. *Acta Derm. Venereol. (Stockh.)* 59: 241–244.
29. Lubach D., Edmuller, J., and Rahm-Hoffman, L.A. (1980). Kombinierte retinoid-and-UV-phototherapie bei pustulosis subcornealis (Sneddon-Wilkinson). *Hautarzi* 31(10):545–547.

29a. Lowe, N.J., Prystrosky, J.H.. Boarget, T. et al. (1991). Acetretin plus UVB therapy for psoriasis. *J. Am. Acad. Dermatol.* 24:591–594.

30. Foreman, A., Gold, M., and Roenigk, H.H. (1989). Methotrexate and cyclosporine therapy for psoriasis. *Arch. Dermatol.* in press.
31. Paul, B.S., et al. (1982). Combined methotrexate-Ultraviolet B therapy in the treatment of psoriasis. *J. Am. Acad. Dermatol.* 7:758–762.
32. Meinardi, M.M., and Bos, J.D. (1988). Cyclosporin maintenance therapy in psoriasis. *Transplant. Proc.* 20(3 Suppl. 4):42–49.

32a. Brechtel, B., Wellenreuther, U., Toppe, E. et al. (1994). Combination of etretinate with cyclosporine in the treatment of sever recalcitrant psoriasis. *J. Am. Acad. Dermatol.* 30:1023–1024.

46

Climatotherapy of Psoriasis

Louis Weinrauch
Bell Dermatology Associates, Jerusalem, Israel

> One should praise the Dead Sea. . . . Its water is bitter, and no living creatures inhabit it. In many places, the sea spits out masses of asphalt. This brings healing to the human body and is, therefore, included in many medical prescriptions. (Joseph Flavius: The Jewish War IV.8.4)

Climatotherapy (Gr. *klima* + G. *therapeia*) is explained by *Dorland's Illustrated Medical Dictionary* as the treatment of disease by means of a favorable climate. Climatotherapy, including balneo-, helio-, and thalassotherapy, treatment methods widely in use throughout the world for centuries for almost all illnesses, is in a continuous decline in our modern times.

Their real boom was in the years before and between the two world wars, especially in Europe (both Western and Eastern sides, including the Soviet Union). It seems that spas and sanatoriums have been replaced by interferons and cyclosporines.

The syllabus of many medical schools in Europe has included, and to date still includes, topics such as balneology and medical climatology. For some reason, this European approach has never reached the United States.

In spite of the decreasing popularity of climato- and balneotherapy in almost all the medical fields, it seems that the interest of the dermatological community (physicians and patients as well) in this direction is continuing to rise.

It is impossible to discuss the effect of climatotherapy in skin diseases without mentioning first of all psoriasis. There is no other disease in general and skin disease especially that is so much affected by the climate as psoriasis. Perhaps only certain rheumatic ailments treated by balneotherapy may claim some equality in effectiveness (1,2). The advantages in psoriasis are that the results are objectively measurable and visible, whereas in all other illnesses mostly subjective parameters are detected and described. However, little has been written and published in the medical literature about the healing effect of the climate in psoriasis. To the best of my knowledge there is not even one controlled study dealing with this effect in spite of the impressive results achieved. In discussing the effect of climatotherapy in psoriasis, three major elements have to be taken into consideration: sun, sea, and air.

The conservative approach in the therapy of psoriasis is based mostly on phototherapy achieved by artificial sources of energy. Numerous scientific articles have been written discussing this form of treatment and elucidating the principles involved that are presently being defined. Concurrent with this knowledge, much more is now understood about the photobiological mechanisms and the ultraviolet (UV) spectrum, phototherapy having progressed today into a well-accepted form of treatment in most medical centers. In climatotherapy, the artificial UV lamps are replaced by a natural UV emitter, the sun. Solar radiation, the basic thermal and light energy source for the earth's surface, provides the climatological balance to which humans and all other living organism have been adapted. A very large portion of this solar radiation falls in the visible (400–700 nm) and infrared (>700 nm) wavelengths and only a small portion of the incoming solar input lies in the short wave spectrum (<400 nm).

The incoming flux of natural ultraviolet radiation is very high and would be fatal if it were allowed to reach the earth's surface. Most of this radiation is absorbed by the very thin ozone layer, so that only small traces of ultraviolet B manage to reach the earth's surface, producing sunburn, skin aging, and cutaneous cancer. Under normal circumstances, the solar UVB and UVA dosages received at the equatorial latitudes are almost 10 times those at high latitudes. The same increase of radiation is also measurable at high altitudes.

Many of the biological effects of UVA, such as tanning and erythema, required a greater radiant exposure dose than do those of shorter wavelengths, such as UVB. Even though UVA is 200–2000 times less erythematogenic than UVB, the role of UVA in producing sunburn reactions cannot be ignored because of the high UVA irradiance presence in solar radiation and because of the existence of additive or augmentative interreactions between these two wavelengths.

The major effects of UVB and UVA are as follows:

UVB	UVA
Immediate erythema	Delayed erythema
Delayed tanning	Immediate tanning

Selective ultraviolet phototherapy (SUP), combining the healing effects of those two spectrums, first described in the European literature is currently gaining popularity and many phototherapy centers are applicating this conception.

The clinical improvement of psoriasis following sun exposure is a well-established basis for the various phototherapy and photochemotherapy methods used in the treatment of this disease. It has been suggested that the psoriatic therapeutic response spectrum may parallel the action spectrum for delayed erythema for all portions of the UV spectrum that penetrate the psoriatic plaque. However, it is the erythematous response of the normal skin of the psoriatic patients that limits the exposure and frequency periods of phototherapy. Such overexposure to a UV radiation source may cause severe sunburn reaction and even may induce the undesirable Koebner phenomenon.

Climatotherapy benefitting psoriasis patients from the sun exposure is popular at the Mediterranean shores of Spain, Italy, and Yugoslavia, the North Sea and at several California and Florida beaches (3–6).

The most well-known center for climatotherapy of psoriasis is the Dead Sea. Because of its unique elevation, the treatment at the Dead Sea mainly consists of the patients being exposed to an UV spectrum of long-wave light found naturally in high intensity in that area of the world, and, in addition, a sea very rich in natural minerals and a relaxing atmosphere.

The Dead Sea is the lowest point in the world. It is more than 1200 feet (396 m) below sea level with a barometric pressure of 800 mm Hg and a resulting high oxygen pressure. It is extremely arid and hot in the summer with an average monthly temperature range from 16 to 34°C (61 to 93°F); 54°C (129°F) has been recorded during the midday in the summer. Despite the high temperature, the summertime relative humidity is very low, about 35–45% and the mean annual rainfall is only between 50 and 75 mm. The sun shines almost constantly more than 300 days a year, and the majority of UVB sunburning rays are filtered out by the thick atmosphere layer caused by the natural depression together with the haze resulting from the extreme evaporation of the sea. Therefore, a greater exposure to the longer wavelength UVB and UVA rays is allowed.

Ultraviolet B is further diminished relative to UVA because of the greater diffraction of shorter wavelengths. This factor accounts for the reduced danger of sunburn and for the longer exposure times possible at the Dead Sea as compared to other locations.

The Dead Sea is not only the lowest place on the face of the earth, but also the world's most hypersaline natural lake with an average salinity of 30%. For thousands of years water has flowed through the Jordan River into the Dead Sea, a terminal lake, and evaporates into the desiccated air, leaving the salts to accumulate in the lake. These salts are at an average of 300 g/kg compared with those from the Jordan River of 15 g, from the ocean 35 g, or from the Great Salt Lake in Utah with an average between 200 and 270 g/kg. A comparison of the chemical composition of waters from these different sources is given in Table 1.

The chemical character of the Dead Sea water is unique. Compared with waters from marine origin they are enriched in calcium, magnesium, potassium, and bromide and depleted in sodium, sulfate, and car-

Table 1 Comparison of Chemical Composition of Waters from Different Sources

	Cations (%)				Anions (%)			
	Potassium	Calcium	Magnesium	Natrium	Bromide	Bicarbonate	Sulfate	Chloride
Dead Sea 300 g/kg	7	16	40	37	2	<1	<1	97
Jordan River 15g/kg	7	27	20	46	<1	17	9	73
Mediterranean Sea 35 g/kg	3	3	10	84	<1	<1	12	87
Great Salt Lake 200–270 g/kg	7	<1	<10	83	<1	<1	11	89

bonate. Such a composition could not have evolved from evaporating seawater or from the major river system.

Has this unique composition of the Dead Sea bitter waters any influence on the healing effect of psoriasis? There is not yet a clear-cut answer to this question. The water alone is not enough in clearing the psoriatic lesions. One may claim that bathing in a supersaturated brine may increase the keratolytic effect of the scales and also that the salt crystals that accumulate on the skin cause an enhancement of the UV radiation (7).

The third relevant supportive factor in the climatotherapy of psoriasis at the Dead Sea is bromine, which occurs in significant concentrations in both Dead Sea waters and air, and which is known to have a sedative effect on the stress-induced psoriasis.

The unpolluted allergen-free desert air in this region of the world is very rich in gaseous bromine, 20-fold higher than that in the vicinity city of Jerusalem. With 2400 ng/m^3 in the air, and assuming normal inhalation of 20 m^3 daily, this high gaseous bromine level may account for the up to 0.05 mg/day of bromine intake.

The Dead Sea brine contains about 2.3 g/liter of bromine, so that bathing in it is enough for minute amounts to penetrate into the normal, but especially into the damaged psoriatic skin, and from there into the circulation.

In addition, the drinking water in the Dead Sea area is three times more rich in bromine as compared to rural inland areas, and this accounts for the third source of bromine intake of the Dead Sea residents.

And last, but not least, psychotherapeutic influences certainly play a role in the patients' overall improvement at the Dead Sea. In contrast to the conventional therapy for psoriasis, both topical and systemic, as well as in- or outpatients, the treatment at the Dead Sea is simplicity itself, mostly natural and without unpleasant side effects. Patients are required to lie in the sun for increasing periods of time at the shoreline solarium, bathe in the mineral-rich sea, and to breathe the bromine-enriched atmosphere.

The only topical medications used are for lubrication and keratolytic purposes. Tar in ointments and shampoos is added in selected patients, primarily for its UV-potentiating effect. It is understandable that no topical or systemic glucocorticosteroids, no systemic retinoids or antimytotic agents, and no additional artificial radiation is used. The minimum recommended stay at the Dead Sea is 3 weeks and preferably a period of 4 weeks. Even though clearing may be achieved after 2 weeks in some patients, many of them did not show significant improvement until the third or fourth week and have to work very hard, sunbathing the entire day in order to achieve their goal.

Grouped together for several weeks in an informal, pleasant, and relaxed atmosphere allows those affected with this chronic skin disease to discuss and share similar frustrations and apprehensions.

The economical aspect of climatotherapy in psoriasis has to be taken into consideration (8). An average treatment at one of these resorts (including air travel) costs between one-third to one-half of the same period of hospitalization (9). This is the reason why sick funds and insurance companies prefer to send patients for climatotherapy instead of paying exorbitant hospital fees.

About two-thirds of the psoriatics leave the Dead Sea spas clear or much improved, whereas in only 2% of these no change or deterioration is reported (10,11). Naturally, the more resistant cases, those with erythroderma, pustular, or palmoplantar psoriasis have a much lower success rate (12).

It is superfluous to say that no one has been cured of his psoriasis at the Dead Sea. Since the biblical days of Sodom and Gomorrah there are no more miracles in this part of the world. On the other hand, climatotherapy is as effective as any of the other psoriasis treatments used on hundreds of thousands of patients every year in hospitals and clinics throughout the world. Most of these patients have already attempted all of the conventional and less conventional therapies, and finally chose a more simple, agreeable, and less deleterious form of treatment—climatotherapy.

REFERENCES

1. Milivaskii, A.I., Losev, V.B., Perelmuter, D.L., Ryzhkova, M.A., and Nereviatkin, G.K. (1989). The efficacy of health resort treatment of psoriatic arthritis at Yevpatoriya. *Vest. Dermatol. Venerol.* 1:42–44.
2. Sukenik, S., Giryes, H., Halevy, S., Neumann, L., Flusser, D., and Buskila, D. (1994). Treatment of psoriatic arthritis at the Dead Sea. *J. Rheumatol.* 21:1305–1309.
3. Hartung, J. (1969). Ultraviolet therapy at the North Sea coast. In *The biologic Effects of Ultraviolet Radiation.* F. Urbach (Ed.). Pergamon Press, Oxford, pp. 657–661.
4. Molin, L. (1971). Climate therapy of Swedish psoriatics on Hvar, Yugoslavia. *Acta Derm. Venereol. (Stockh.)* 52:155–160.
5. Menger, W. (1989). Indications and successes of climate therapy of children. *Offentl. Gesundheidswes.* 51: 470–476.
6. Snellman, E., Jansen, C.T., Lauharanta, J., and Kolari, P. (1992). Solar ultraviolet (UV) radiation and UV doses received by patients during four-week climate therapy periods in the Canary Islands. *Photodermatol. Photoimmunol. Photomed.* 9:40–43.
7. Boer, J., Schothorst, A.A., Boom, B., Hermans, J., and Suurmond, D. (1982). Influence of water and salt solutions on UVB irradiation of normal skin and psoriasis. *Arch. Dermatol. Res.* 273:247–259.
8. Sander, H.M., Morris, L.F., Phillips, C.M., Harrison, P.E., and Menter, A. (1993). The annual cost of psoriasis. *J. Am. Acad. Dermatol.* 28:422–425.
9. Weinrauch, L. (1996). The cost of psoriasis treatment at the Dead Sea. *Int. J. Dermatol.* 35:150.
10. Abels, D.J., and Kattan-Byron, J. (1985). Psoriasis treatment at the Dead Sea: a natural selective ultraviolet phototherapy. J. Am. Acad. Dermatol. 12: 639–643.
11. Abels, D.J., Rose, T., and Bearman, J.E. (1995). Treatment of psoriasis at a Dead Sea dermatology clinic. *Int. J. Dermatol.* 34:134–137.
12. Holubar, K., Weinrauch, L., Leibovici, V., and Siladji, S. (1986). Climatotherapy of psoriasis at the Dead Sea. *J. Am. Acad. Dermatol.* 15:1299–1301.

Part VII

SYSTEMIC THERAPY

47

Systemic Corticosteroids

Arto Lahti
University of Oulu, Oulu, Finland

Howard I. Maibach
University of California School of Medicine, San Francisco, California

Systemic corticosteroids became widely available to dermatologists at the beginning of the 1950s. The first preparations were ACTH, cortisone, hydrocortisone acetate, prednisolone, and later the fluoroderivative of prednisolone, triamcinolone. Soon they also were used in psoriasis therapy.

EFFECTIVENESS

It became evident that systemically administered corticosteroids powerfully influenced the different manifestations and course of psoriasis. Case reports and small series appeared.

The First Report of the Medical Research Council (1954) described seven patients with widespread exfoliative psoriasis, treated with ACTH and cortisone (dosage varied from 100 to 150 mg cortisone or 50 to 100 IU ACTH daily). All but one patient clearly improved during therapy; the tendency to relapse during therapy or soon after drug withdrawal was noticed.

In another group of 13 patients with severe psoriasis, ACTH therapy (1.5 months) proved effective in 11, leading to complete or almost complete clearance of plaques in 9. Improvement of joint systems was marked. Lesion recurrence during treatment, especially with dosage reduction or within 1 month after therapy, was noticed in 11 of the 13. One patient had fatal generalized pustular psoriasis when ACTH was discontinued (Fergusson and Dewar, 1957).

Shelley and Harun (1958) used triamcinolone in the treatment of 60 patients in doses of 12–16 mg daily orally. In 36, response was prompt and obvious; within a week, scaling and erythema diminished; within 2–4 weeks lesions in some completely cleared. Upon cessation of treatment or reduction of dosage, however, lesions regularly returned. Disease in the remaining 24 patients failed to respond.

The most important long-term trial is that by Hollander and co-workers (1959), who studied the effect of oral triamcinolone (6–16 mg/day) on psoriatic arthritis and skin lesions. They observed the patients for two years. Nine of their 17 patients showed virtually complete clearing and 4 patients showed 50–75% clearing of lesions within the first 2 months. In all but 2 of the 17, joint symptoms were better controlled by triamcinolone than by previous therapy with other corticoids or with other treatments. Those two patients were returned to prednisolone treatment; their joint symptoms improved but their psoriasis relapsed promptly and was worse than before triamcinolone. After 1 year, 3 of the 15 patients continuing triamcinolone therapy experienced partial relapse of lesions. Triamcinolone therapy was interrupted in five patients during the first year, and relapse in lesions and arthritis was prompt and troublesome. Those who substituted prednisolone experienced little relapse in arthritis but skin lesions relapsed severely. At the end of 2 years, 14 of the 17 patients remained on triamcinolone. Partial relapse in lesions was noted in nearly every patient; but in 9 of the 14, the skin lesions were definitely less marked and widespread than before triamcinolone. In spite of at least partial relapse in skin symptoms, 12 of the 14 were satisfied with their joint symptoms and preferred triamcinolone to other corticoids used and wished to continue therapy.

Cohen and Baer (1960) and Mardsen (1961) found orally administered triamcinolone more effective than methyl prednisolone and prednisolone in their psoriasis patients. It was also stated that intralesional injections of triamcinolone in persistent localized areas of psoriasis may be a worthwhile therapeutic procedure.

In spite of this wave of enthusiasm for triamcinolone in psoriasis, we have no double-blind studies comparing this drug to other corticoids. There is little scientific basis for choosing triamcinolone over the more standard prednisone or prednisolone.

DISADVANTAGES

The initial effect of systemic corticosteroid therapy is impressive but recurrence of skin lesions during therapy usually requires larger corticoid dosages. If dosage is lowered or tapered off, relapse seems the rule. Many dermatologists have the impression that when psoriasis has relapsed after systemic corticosteroid therapy in its plaque or exfoliative erythrodermic pattern, it can be more severe than before therapy and can be more unresponsive to other treatments (Champion, 1966). However, controlled studies on these questions have not been found.

It seems possible that systemic and even intensive topical therapy with corticosteroids can convert the ordinary plaque-type psoriasis into the pustular type. In a study of 104 patients with generalized pustular psoriasis (GPP), Baker and Ryan (1968) found that 37 received corticoids systemically for various reasons before the first attack of GPP. In 21 instances, pustulosis appeared within a few days or weeks after reduction or complete withdrawal of the corticoid. Therefore, 20% of the patients in this large series were regarded as having corticoid-provoked GPP.

According to these results and further studies, the authors concluded that systemic corticosteroid therapy has a significant risk of converting nonpustular forms of psoriasis into pustular ones, localized pustular forms into severe GPP, and can also perpetuate psoriatic erythroderma and GPP (Baker, 1976; Baker and Ryan, 1968; Boyd and Menter, 1989; Ryan and Baker, 1969, 1971).

Baker and Ryan (1968) noted the possibility that their patients were highly selected; perhaps less severely involved psoriatics may not have developed GPP. Their clinical judgment led them, and most other dermatologists to discount this likelihood. Unfortunately, because controlled trials in appropriately matched patient populations were not performed, we lack scientific certainty on this point.

SYSTEMIC EFFECTS

In addition to its effect on the course of psoriasis itself, systemic corticosteroid therapy has many well-defined effects on metabolic processes.

Short courses of prednisolone (30–60 mg/day for 10–14 days as a single morning dose) or intramuscular triamcinolone acetonide when used occasionally and for acute dermatoses are unlikely to cause serious complications (Storrs, 1979). However, their chronic use is associated with the well-known risks and side effects of all systemic corticosteroid therapy: suppression of hypothalamic-pituitary-adrenal axis, osteoporosis, diabetogenesis, increased susceptibility to infections, cushingoid habitus, moon face, skin atrophy, striae, cataracts, and purpura. These side effects have been reviewed in detail elsewhere (Axelrod, 1976; Fine, 1979a,b; Storrs, 1979).

INTRAMUSCULAR INJECTION

Numerous highly skilled dermatologists (Arnold, 1978; Rees, 1981) with vast clinical experience insist that appropriate dosages of intramuscular triamcinolone acetonide have a good result with little or no significant side effects. Others (Storrs, 1979, 1981; Thiers, 1980) are far less enthusiastic, believing that the frequency of side effects contraindicates their repeated use. Controlled trials of efficacy and safety necessary to document the merits of either position do not exist. This is unfortunate as many qualified dermatologists exist in the former group; they believe that this dosage schedule should not be denied to patients on a theoretical basis if, in fact, the regimen is well-tolerated.

CONCLUSIONS

No controlled studies have been published on systemic corticosteroid therapy of psoriasis. However, based on case reports, clinical experience, and judgment of most dermatologists, the following generalizations appear justified.

Systemic corticosteroid therapy is not indicated for ordinary plaque-type psoriasis. Although it may temporarily induce clearing, severe rebound may occur. These exacerbations tend to be worse and more difficult to treat than the initial eruption.

Systemic corticosteroid therapy may be indicated in fulminating GPP, especially if methotrexate is contraindicated (because of preexisting severe liver disease or bone marrow hypoplasia), or if GPP is complicated by malabsorption and difficult metabolic disturbances.

In severe psoriatic arthritis, systemic corticosteroids are sometimes indicated for a short time if the therapeutic effect of other drugs such as anti-inflammatory analgesics and gold is not satisfactory.

In some exceptional cases of psoriatic erythroderma, when the widespread cutaneous inflammation produces high-output heart failure, edema, hyperpyrexia, or other serious metabolic disturbances, corticosteroids can rapidly reduce inflammation and therefore may be justified as a life-saving measure.

When systemic corticosteroid therapy is indicated, prednisolone as a single morning dose or on an alternate-day schedule has been preferred to intramuscular preparations (Storrs, 1979, 1981; Thiers, 1980). However, some dermatologists regard the use of long-acting intramuscular steroids, usually triamcinolone acetonide, at least as safe and physiological as prednisolone (Arnold, 1978; Rees, 1981). We await appropriately controlled studies to document this position scientifically.

REFERENCE

Arnold, H.L. (1978). Systemic steroid therapy with intramuscularly injected triamcinolone. *South. Med. J.* 71: 102–107.

Axelrod, L. (1976). Glucocorticoid therapy. *Medicine* 55: 39–65.

Baker, H. (1976). Corticosteroids and pustular psoriasis. *Br. J. Dermatol.* 94(Suppl. 12):83–88.

Baker, H., and Ryan, T.J. (1968). Generalized pustular psoriasis: a clinical and epidemiological study of 104 cases. *Br. J. Dermatol.* 80:771–793.

Boyd, A.S., and Menter, A. (1989). Erythrodermic psoriasis: precipitating factors, course, and prognosis in 50 patients. *J. Am. Acad. Dermatol.* 21:985–991.

Champion, R.H. (1966). Treatment of psoriasis. *Br. Med. J.* 2:993–995.

Cohen, H.H., and Baer R.L. (1960). Triamcinolone and methyl prednisolone in psoriasis: comparison of their intralesional and systemic effects. *J. Invest. Dermatol.* 34: 271–275.

Fergusson, A.G., and Dewar, W.A (1957). Observations on steroid therapy in psoriasis. *Br. J. Dermatol.* 69:57–60.

Fine, R.M. (1979a). The systemic use of corticosteroids in dermatology. Part I, basic aspects. *Progr. Dermatol.* 13(3):1–8.

Fine, R.M. (1979b). The systemic use of corticosteroids in dermatology. Part II, practical aspects. *Progr. Dermatol.* 13(4):1–4.

Hollander, J.L., Brown, E.M., Jessar, R.A., Udell, L., Cooperband, S., and Smukler, N.M. (1959). The effect of triamcinolone on psoriatic arthritis. A two year study. *Arthritis Rheum.* 2:513–525.

Mardsen, C.W. (1961). Oral steroid therapy in psoriasis vulgaris: a comparison of triamcinolone, methyl prednisolone and dexamethasone. *Br. J. Dermatol.* 73:103–106.

Medical Research Council Report. Panel on dermatological applications of ACTH and cortisone. (154). *Br. Med. J.* 2:1307–1313.

Rees, R.B. (1981). Oral vs. parenteral corticosteroids: a clinical controversy. *J. Am. Acad. Dermatol.* 5:602–604.

Ryan, T.J., and Baker, H. (1969). Systemic corticosteroids and folic acid antagonists in the treatment of generalized pustular psoriasis. Evaluation and prognosis based on the study of 104 cases. *Br. J. Dermatol.* 81:134–145.

Ryan, T.J., and Baker H. (1971). The prognosis of generalized pustular psoriasis. *Br. J. Dermatol.* 85:407–411.

Shelley, W.B., and Huran, J.S. (1958). The treatment of psoriasis and other dermatoses with triamcinolone (Aristocort). *JAMA* 167:959–964.

Storrs, F.J. (1979). Use and abuse systemic corticosteroid therapy. *J. Am. Acad. Dermatol.* 1:95–105.

Storrs, F.J. (1981). Intramuscular corticosteroids: a second point of view. *J. Am. Acad. Dermatol.* 5:600–602.

Thiers, B. (1980). Steroids, gold, hydroxychloroquine. *J. Am. Acad. Dermatol.* 3:320–324.

48

Topical Corticosteroid Occlusion Therapy: Psoriasis

Yung-Hian Leow and Howard I. Maibach
University of California School of Medicine, San Francisco, California

Plastic occlusive dressings have been used as therapeutic enhancement since 1961 (1). Subsequently more elegant occlusive dressings that require less frequent changing have been developed. This chapter reviews the data on occlusion therapy for psoriasis therapy (Table 1).

OCCLUSION THERAPY

In 1970, Fry et al. (2) demonstrated that plastic occlusive dressings on psoriatic lesions decreased the high mitotic rates of epidermal basal cells and caused a restoration of the granular layer, which was often absent or partially formed in classic psoriatic histopathological specimens. Baxter and Stoughton, utilizing plastic film alone, showed therapeutic efficacy in psoriasis (3). Fisher and Maibach (4), using cellophane tape-stripped skin as a hyperproliferative model for the hyperproliferative aspect of psoriasis, demonstrated that by applying an adhesive, occlusive tape (Blenderm) over this wounded skin, the mitotic activity of the hyperproliferative epidermis was reduced. In 1985, Shore noted that occlusion with a Band-Aid on a psoriatic plaque cleared the lesion after 3 weeks (5).

Occlusion Dressing Alone

Subsequently Shore applied various tapes and occlusive dressings on multiple psoriatic lesions in a dozen patients; many lesions cleared completely, some as long as 1 month after treatment, but most cleared partially. He observed that continuous occlusion for 1 week or longer was superior to repeated daily application; waterproof tape was more effective than less occlusive tapes (5).

Friedman (6) evaluated the clinical efficacy of an adherent hydrocolloid occlusive dressing (HCD) (duoDERM) composed of a lamination of a moisture and oxygen-impermeable open-cell polyurethane exterior and an inner hydrocolloid layer that adhered to the skin. In a 10-week study on 26 patients with plaque-type psoriasis, he demonstrated that the HCD alone, changed weekly, was therapeutically comparable to erythemogenic ultraviolet B therapy and superior to twice daily application of fluocinolone acetonide cream.

Occlusion Dressing with Topical Corticosteroid

Occlusion therapy with topical corticosteroid increases the endpoint dilution penetration 100-fold when utilized in vasoconstriction studies (7). However, actual human in vivo penetration studies reveal an enhancement factor of only 10-fold on the forearm with occlusion for 96 hr (8). Its superb efficacy enhancement is often marred by the possible local and systemic side effects (9). Hence the search for an effective, safe, and convenient occlusive delivery system for topical corticosteroid, with minimal side effects, remains a holy grail.

Table 1 Summary of Studies

Type of Psoriasis	Number of patients	Treatment response	Side effects	Ref.
PV	26	HCD > FCA, = UVB	Koebner phenomenon (4) Offensive odor (3)	6
PV	38	HCD + TAC > HCD > TAC	Pain/tenderness (1) Worsen (2)	10
PV	23	HCD + BV (all healed)	None	11
PV	21	HCD + BV > BV > HCD	Irritation (5) Sterile pustules (1)	12
PV	189	HCD + corticoid cream > corticoid cream alone	Erythema (5) Itch (1) Folliculitis (1) Burning/ erythema (1)	13
PPPU LPP	19	HCD + TAC > CLP	Loose dressing (2) Sweating under dressing (1)	14
PV PPP PPPU	62	Complete clearance (60)	Folliculitis (3)	15
PV	40	HCD + TAC > TAC > TAC + plastic dressing	Irritation (7)	16
PV	19	OCD + Flu > Flu = OCD > control	Folliculitis (5) Offensive odor (3) Itch (1)	17
PV	10	HCD + CLP > CLP	Not stated	18
PV	10	HCD + CLP > HCD + BV > HCD + TAC > HCD + HC	Not stated	19

PV, psoriasis vulgaris; PPPU, palmoplantar pustulosis; LPP, localized pustular psoriasis; PPP, palmoplantar psoriasis; HCD, hydrocolloid occlusive dressing; FCA, flucinolone acetonide; UVB, ultraviolet B therapy; TAC, triamcinolone acetonide; BV, betamethasone valerate; CLP, clobetasol propionate; OCD, occlusive dressing; Flu, flucinonide ointment; HC, hydrocortisone. (>) better results than; (=) comparable to; (+) with. Numbers in parentheses represent the number of patients.

David and Lowe (10) investigated the efficacy of a HCD (Actiderm) in 38 psoriatic patients with a bilateral paired-comparison method. They compared the clinical responses of patients treated with HCD alone, 0.1% triamcinolone acetonide cream alone, triamcinolone acetonide under HCD occlusion, and triamcinolone acetonide under polyethylene film occlusion (Saran). Best results were achieved in patients receiving triamcinolone acetonide cream under HCD occlusion. There was no significant difference between patients treated with the HCD alone and with corticosteroid cream under plastic film occlusion, but the posttreatment clinical improvement was more sustained in the former group.

Juhlin (11) treated eight patients with clobetasol propionate, betamethasone valerate 0.1% triamcinolone 0.1%, and hydrocortisone 1%, under occlusion with HCD (Actiderm) for 1 week. Areas treated with the first three preparations showed clinical clearance in four patients and the other four had only mild residual erythema at the end of treatment. In another 23 psoriatic patients, he treated their lesions with 0.1% betamethasone valerate under occlusion, which was changed weekly till healing. However, some patients (the number was not specified) also received ultraviolet B treatment at the same time. All lesions healed after 2 weeks of treatment and relapses occurred after 4–8 weeks in most. No side effect was documented. The author felt that with the use of topical corticosteroid under HCD, there was no added advantage in prescribing the most potent corticosteroid for treating psoriatic plaques and it could be used as an adjunct to other treatment modalities like phototherapy to prevent relapses.

Wilkinson and Ohayon (12) treated 21 patients with chronic plaque-type psoriasis, with betamethasone valerate 0.1% cream under HCD occlusion (Actiderm) versus cream alone and HCD alone. Significant resolution of lesions treated with HCD and corticosteroid cream was observed, compared with lesions treated with either agent on its own.

A total of 189 patients with psoriasis vulgaris from 22 centers were enlisted in a multicenter, paired comparison study (13). Psoriatic plaques were treated with a twice-daily application of a corticosteroid cream (triamcinolone acetonide 0.1%, betamethasone valerate 0.1%, or halcinonide 0.1%) alone, while another plaque in the same patient was treated with the same cream under HCD occlusion (Actiderm). After 3 weeks, there was significant improvement in all clinical parameters of erythema, induration, scaling, and fissuring in the occlusion group, compared with the group treated with corticosteroid alone. Improvement was sustained throughout the 4-week posttreatment period. Eight patients reported adverse reactions: mild erythema (five), pruritus (one), mild folliculitis (one) and bruising/erythema (one).

Kragballe and Larsen (14), conducting a randomized, open, prospective right-left comparison study in 19 patients with palmoplantar pustulosis and localized pustular psoriasis, compared the therapeutic response of using a HCD (Actiderm) over a medium-potency corticosteroid (triamcinolone acetonide 0.1% cream) with that of a high-potency corticosteroid (clobetasol propionate 0.05% cream) alone. The dressing was changed every 3 days, while the cream was applied twice daily in the latter group. Complete clinical clearance was documented in 63% of the patients in the former group, but in only 21% of the patients in the latter. Four weeks after treatment, most lesions reverted to their pretreatment status, though lesions treated with occlusion and topical corticosteroids showed a slight improvement in erythema score. No atrophy was detected.

Volden (15) treated 25 patients with chronic plaque-type psoriasis, 18 patients with palmoplantar psoriasis, and 19 patients with palmoplantar pustulosis, with clobetasol propionate lotion under HCD occlusion (Duoderm/Duoderm Extra Thin). Dressings were changed weekly until total clearance. All patients with plaque-type psoriasis achieved complete remission after an average of 12 days (range: 1–6 weeks). Seventeen of the 18 patients with palmoplantar psoriasis achieved complete remission after an average of 2.5 weeks (range: 1–5 weeks). Eighteen of the 19 patients with palmoplantar pustulosis achieved complete remission after an average of 2.2 weeks (range: 1–7 weeks). Four patients, three patients, and six patients in each respective group had relapse during the posttreatment follow-up period (range: 1–8 months). The author estimated that as this form of treatment required less frequent application of topical corticosteroids, the total amount of topical corticosteroids used was reduced to 1/20 to more than 1/100 times, of the amount of cream used when applied daily.

Van de Kerkhof et al. (16) compared the therapeutic efficacy and tolerance of topical treatment with triamcinolone acetonide 0.1% under a HCD (Duoderm E), triamcinolone acetonide 0.1% alone, HCD alone, and triamcinolone acetonide under plastic semiocclusive dressing (Opsite IV 3000), in 40 patients with psoriasis. Both occlusive dressings were well-tolerated by study subjects, though seven patients complained of irritation while using either occlusive dressing. Nonetheless, topical corticosteroid under HCD achieved the best clinical improvement and was superior to plastic occlusive dressing.

Griffiths et al. (17), comparing the clinical therapeutic responses in 19 patients with plaque-type psoriasis, performed a 3-week study comparing the efficacy of using twice-daily application of 0.05% flucinonide ointment, weekly application of occlusion dressing (Topiclude) alone, weekly application of fluocinonide ointment with occlusion dressing, and control (no treatment). The combination of topical corticosteroid and occlusion produced significantly more improvement than either treatment alone, though there was no significant difference between the efficacy of occlusion alone or fluocinonide ointment alone. Four weeks after cessation of treatment, psoriatic plaques treated with occlusion alone or combined fluocinonide and occlusion were still significantly improved.

With the use of noninvasive bioengineering methods (TCM-2-oxygen monitor, laser-Doppler flowmetry, and thermocouples), Broby-Johansen and Kristensen (18) demonstrated, in 10 patients with chronic plaque-type psoriasis, that treatment with clobetasol propionate cream under occlusion with a HCD (Comfeel), reduced the oxygen consumption and blood flow significantly after 24 hr of treatment. These findings showed a good correlation with improvement in clinical scores. However, treatment with clobetasol propionate alone only achieved marginal improvement after 7 days' treatment.

The same investigators (19) also studied the antipsoriatic effect of various topical corticosteroid (1% hydrocortisone, 0.1% triamcinolone acetonide, 0.1% betamethasone-17-valerate cream, and 0.05% clobetasol propionate), under occlusion with HCD (Comfeel), in 10 patients with chronic plaque-type psoriasis. Noninvasive bioengineering techniques (ultrasound skin thickness, laser-Doppler flowmetry, and colorimetry) and clinical scoring were used to assess the therapeutic responses. After 1 week, they observed a decline in blood flow, a decrease in skin thickness, normalization of color approaching that of normal skin, and improvement of clinical scores. They noted that there was direct correlation between treatment response (both clinical and with noninvasive methods) and the potency of topical corticosteroid used.

MECHANISM OF ACTION OF OCCLUSION THERAPY

Despite the encouraging clinical experiences with these dressings, the exact mechanism of action of prolonged occlusion in the improvement of psoriasis remains speculative (Table 2).

Fry et al. (2) reported the restoration of the granular cell layer and reduction of the mitotic rate after 2 weeks of plastic occlusive therapy. Baxter and Stoughton also documented a reduction in the mitotic index of psoriatic plaque treated with an adhesive tape (3). Fisher and Maibach (4) postulated that occlusion restored an artificial water barrier to the damaged skin, thus resulting in a reduction of *water vapor loss*. Halprin et al. (20) reported that suppression of the enzyme activity of carbohydrate metabolism and local temperature elevation probably also account for some of the beneficial effects of occlusive therapy (21,22).

Various investigators tried to address the issue by looking at the immunohistochemical changes that occurred with occlusion. With the use of flow cytometry, Gottlieb et al. (23) observed a modest decrease in the keratinocyte growth fraction in occluded psoriatic plaques, but could not detect a reduction in other immunological markers.

Van Vlijmen-Willems et al. (24) found that 3 weeks' treatment with HCD also modestly decreased the suprabasal expression of keratin 16 (epidermal proliferation), the number of cycling epidermal cells, and the number of polymorphonuclear leukocytes and T lymphocytes.

However, Griffith and Wilkinson (9) were unable to demonstrate a change in the immunohistological markers in 10 patients who had 1-week treatment with an occlusive dressing (Topiclude) alone. Lotti (25) felt that immune mechanism was not the predominant pathogenic mechanism in psoriasis and reported that there was a marked reduction in the activity of epidermal plasminogen activator in occluded psoriatic plaques.

There have also been numerous studies exploring the molecular changes in the skin as a barrier to water loss. However, these studies are not designed specifically to investigate the psoriasis model and almost all studies use rodents as the prototype. Grubauer et al. (26) and Proksch et al. (27) demonstrated that artificial repair with a water-impermeable membrane on acetone-damaged skin in hairless mice reduced an expected increase in the biosynthesis of epidermal lipids (cholesterol, fatty acids, and total nonsaponifiable lipids) and an increase in DNA synthesis. Wood et al. found that occluding the damaged (acetone and tape-stripped) skin of hairless mice with latex glove reduced the epidermal pool of IL-1- α (28). In the human model, Proksch et al. demonstrated that occlusion with water-impermeable latex wrap reduced epidermal cellular proliferation (reduced Ki-S_3 cell density) in skin damaged by acetone, cellophane tape stripping, and sodium dodecylsulfate (29).

CONCLUSION

Should occlusion therapy with topical corticosteroids be used in psoriasis? Despite the relatively few minor side effects reported in most clinical studies, the inherent possible side effects that may arise from inap-

Table 2 Possible Mechanism of Action of Occlusion Therapy

Possible mechanism of action	Ref.
Reduction of water vapor loss	4
Reduction of an expected increase in the biosynthesis of epidermal lipids	26
Reduction of an increase in DNA synthesis	27
Reduction of epidermal cellular proliferation	29

propriate use of topical corticosteroids still exist. It is not a panacea for psoriasis, as relapse may occur quickly. However, the obvious advantages of less frequent application of topical medication and change of dressing will certainly improve compliance in patients.

Under the supervision of an experienced dermatologist and with the development of more efficacious, convenient, and cosmetically acceptable occlusive dressings, this treatment modality can certainly be recommended as a short-term adjuvant therapy to other forms of treatment for patients with plaque-type psoriasis, palmoplantar psoriasis, localized pustular psoriasis, and palmoplantar pustulosis.

REFERENCES

1. Sulzberger, M.B., and Witten, V.H. (1961). Thin pliable plastic films in topical dermatologic therapy. *Arch. Dermatol.* 84:1027.
2. Fry, L., Almeyda, J., and McMinn, R.M.H. (1970). Effect of plastic occlusive dressings on psoriatic epidermis. *Br. J. Dermatol.* 82:458–462.
3. Baxter, D.L., and Stoughton, R.B. (1970). Mitotic index of psoriatic lesions treated with anthralin, glucocorticosteroid and occlusion only. *J. Invest. Dermatol.* 54:410–412.
4. Fisher, L.B., and Maibach, H.I. (1972). Physical occlusion controlling epidermal mitosis. *J. Invest. Dermatol.* 59:106–108.
5. Shore, R.N. (1985). Clearing of psoriatic lesions after the application of tape. *N. Engl. J. Med.* 312:246.
6. Friedman, S.J. (1987). Management of psoriasis vulgaris with a hydrocolloid occlusive dressing. *Arch. Dermatol.* 123:1046–1052.
7. McKenzie, A.W., and Stoughton, R.B. (1962). Method for comparing percutaneous absorption of steroids. *Arch. Dermatol.* 86:608.
8. Feldman, R.J., and Maibach, H.I. (1965). Penetration of ^{14}C hydrocortisone through normal skin. The effect of stripping and occlusion. *Arch. Dermatol.* 19: 661–666.
9. Griffith, W.A.D., and Wilkinson, J.D. (1992). Topical therapy. In *Rook/Wilkinson/Ebling Textbook of Dermatology.* R.H. Champion, J.L. Burton, and F.J.G. Ebling (eds.). Blackwell Scientific Publications, Oxford, pp. 3037–3084.
10. David, M., and Lowe, N.J. (1989). Psoriasis therapy: comparative studies with a hydrocolloid dressing, plastic film occlusion, and triamcinolone acetonide cream. *J. Am. Acad. Dermatol.* 21:511–514.
11. Juhlin, L. (1989). Treatment of psoriasis and other dermatoses with a single application of a corticosteroid left under a hydrocolloid dressing for one week. *Acta Derm. Venereol. (Stockh.)* 69:355–357.
12. Wilkinson, R.D., and Ohayon, M. (1990). Therapeutic response to a dermatologic patch and betamethasone valerate 0.1 percent cream in the management of chronic plaques in psoriasis. *Cutis* 45:468–470.
13. The Actiderm Multi-Center Study Group. (1990). A trial of the actiderm dermatological patch and topical corticosteroids in the treatment of psoriasis vulgaris. *Cutis* 46:84–88.
14. Kragballe, K., and Larsen, G.F. (1991). A hydrocolloid occlusive dressing plus triamcinolone acetonide cream is superior to clobetasol cream in palmo-plantar pustulosis. *Acta Derm. Venereol. (Stockh.)* 71:540–542.
15. Volden, G. (1992). Successful treatment of chronic skin diseases with clobetasol propionate and a hydrocolloid occlusive dressing. *Acta Derm. Venerol. (Stockh.)* 72:60–71.
16. Van de Kerkhof, P.C.M., Chang, A., Van der Walle, H.B., Van Vlijmen-Willems, I., Boezeman, J.B.M., and Hujigen-Tijdink, R. (1994). Weekly treatment of psoriasis with a hydrocolloid dressing in combination with triamcinolone acetonide. *Acta Derm. Venereol. (Stockh.)* 74:143–146.
17. Griffiths, C.E.M., Tranfaglia, M.G., and Kang, S. (1995). Prolonged occlusion in the treatment of psoriasis: a clinical and immunohistologic study. *J. Am. Acad. Dermatol.* 32:618–622.
18. Broby-Johansen, U., and Kristensen, J.K. (1989). Antipsoriatic effect of local corticosteroids—O_2-consumption and blood flow measurements compared to clinical parameters. *Clin. Exp. Dermatol.* 14: 137–140.

19. Broby-Johansen, U., Karlsmark, T., Petersen, L.J., and Serup, J. (1990). Ranking of the antipsoriatic effect of various topical corticosteroids applied under a hydrocolloid dressing—skin thickness, blood-flow and colour measurements compared to clinical assessments. *Clin. Exp. Dermatol.* 15:343–348.
20. Halprin, K.M., Fukui, K., and Ohkawara, A. (1969). Flurandrenolone (Cordran) tape and carbohydrate metabolizing enzymes. *Arch. Dermatol.* 100:336–341.
21. Urabe, H., Nishitani, K., and Kohda, H. (1981). Hyperthermia in the treatment of psoriasis. *Arch. Dermatol.* 117:770–774.
22. Orenberg, E.K., Deneau, D.G., and Farber, E.M. (1980). Response of chronic psoriatic plaques to localized heating induced by ultrasound. *Arch. Dermatol.* 116:893–897.
23. Gottlieb, A.B., Staiano-Coico, L., Cohen, S.R., Varghese, M., and Carter, D.M. (1990). Occlusive hydrocolloid dressings decrease keratinocyte population growth fraction and clinical scale and skin thickness in active psoriatic plaques. *J. Dermatol. Sci.* 1:93–96.
24. Van Vlijmen-Willems, I.M.J.J., Chang, A., Boezeman, J.B.M., and Van De Kerkhof, P.C.M. (1993). The immunohistochemical effect of a hydrocolloid occlusive dressing (duoDERM E) in psoriasis vulgaris. *Dermatology* 187:257–262.
25. Lotti, T. (1996). Occlusive treatment in psoriasis: how does it work? *J. Am. Acad. Dermatol.* 35:283.
26. Grubauer, G., Elias, P.M., and Feingold, K.R. (1989). Transepidermal water loss: the signal for recovery of barrier structure and function. *J. Lipid Res.* 30: 323–333.
27. Proksch, E., Feingold, K.R., Man, M-Q., and Elias, P.M. (1991). Barrier function regulates epidermal DNA synthesis. *J. Clin. Invest.* 87:1668–1673.
28. Wood, L.C., Elias, P.M., Calhoun, C., Tsai, J.C., Grunfeld, C., and Feingold, K.R. (1996). Barrier disruption stimulates interleukin-1 α expression and release from a pre-formed pool in murine epidermis. *J. Invest. Dermatol.* 106:397–403.
29. Proksch, E., Brashch, J., and Sterry W. (1996). Integrity of the permeability barrier regulates epidermal Langerhans cell density. *Br. J. Dermatol.* 134:630–638.

49

Methotrexate

Henry H. Roenigk, Jr.
Northwestern University Medical School, Chicago, Illinois

Howard I. Maibach
University of California School of Medicine, San Francisco, California

INTRODUCTION

Systemic drugs to control severe generalized psoriasis have long been a goal of dermatologists. Early drugs such as arsenic and systemic corticosteroids have resulted in serious adverse reactions and are generally not used today. The first use of antimetabolic drugs ushered in a new era in the treatment of psoriasis. In 1951, Gubner et al. (1) noted the rapid clearing of psoriatic skin lesions that fortuitously occurred in a patient treated with aminopterin for rheumatoid arthritis. Clinical experience developed with aminopterin (2), but this drug was later replaced by a more stable derivative, methotrexate (3), which was used in cyclic dosages with fewer severe side effects than aminopterin (4). Other antimetabolic drugs, such as hydroxyurea, azathioprine, azaribine, mycophenolic acid, and thioguanine, have been used in psoriasis, but they have not matched the standard of methotrexate, which has remained the most effective treatment despite its many side effects. Psoralen and ultraviolet A (PUVA) therapy, systemic retinoids, and cyclosporine have challenged methotrexate as the best systemic treatments for psoriasis.

Therapy with PUVA has proven to be highly effective with almost no internal side effects; the only concerns are photoaging of the skin and skin cancer. Cyclosporine is another new drug that may be even more effective than methotrexate, but it also has significant internal toxicity which still must be monitored carefully.

The first guidelines on methotrexate therapy, published in 1972 (5,6), were followed by FDA approval. The most recent official guidelines were published in 1982 (7) and 1988 (8). We have summarized the current literature on the increased use of methotrexate in rheumatoid arthritis in a recent review (8) and editorial (9). Methotrexate was approved for treatment of rheumatoid arthritis in 1988, and guidelines published by the American College of Physicians (10) differed from dermatology guidelines in not requiring a liver biopsy before starting treatment. Recent revised guidelines by rheumatologists also differ in recommendations on following liver toxicity resulting from methotrexate. The recent revision of the dermatology methotrexate guidelines (11) contains updated recommendations for the use of methotrexate in the treatment of psoriasis.

MECHANISM OF ACTION

Antimetabolites are synthetic substances that by their chemical nature resemble essential metabolites. They compete with the natural substances for specific enzymes; usually the antimetabolite has a substantially greater affinity for a specific enzyme than for the natural substitute.

Methotrexate (MTX) (4-amino-10-methylpteroylglutamic acid) is a folic acid antagonist. A structural analog of folic acid and a potent inhibitor of the enzyme dihydrofolate reductase, methotrexate catalyzes the formation of dihydrofolic and tetrahydrofolic acid from folic acid. Tetrahydrofolic acid is the precursor of $N^{5,10}$-methylenetetrahydrofolic acid, an essential cofactor in the conversion of deoxyuridylic to thymidylic acid. Thymidylic acid is required for deoxyribonucleic acid (DNA) synthesis. There may also be direct inhibition of thymidylate synthetase. In humans methotrexate appears to inhibit DNA synthesis to a greater extent than ribonucleic acid (RNA) synthesis; this can result in cell death if methotrexate is present during the S phase of the cell cycle.

Methotrexate at low dosages is well absorbed from the gastrointestinal tract, with peak serum levels occurring in 1–2 hr. Parenteral administration is followed by rapid absorption and plasma levels related to drug dosage. Most of the drug is excreted by the kidneys, but small amounts remain for weeks, distributed particularly in the kidneys and liver. Repeated daily dosages, even in small amounts, result in more sustained serum levels, greater tissue exposure, and retention, and thus greater toxicity than if given in single, higher doses. Methotrexate is bound to plasma protein by drugs such as sulfonamides, salicylates, diphenylhydantoin, and others, and results in increased toxicity. Cell kinetic studies in psoriasis (4) indicated that one factor in the pathogenesis of psoriasis is a rapidly proliferating epidermis, with more cells in the S phase than normal skin. Methotrexate can reverse this process and bring epidermal proliferation back to normal.

INDICATIONS

Moderate to severe psoriasis can be treated with several modalities, including phototherapy, photochemotherapy (PUVA), retinoids, or methotrexate. These guidelines are directed to use of methotrexate in treatment of psoriasis. To minimize the toxicity of systemic therapy, combination or rotational therapy should be considered in the management of psoriasis.

The decision to administer methotrexate for the treatment of psoriasis should be individualized. Each patient should be evaluated with reference to disease severity, discomfort, incapacity, and general medical and psychological status. Methotrexate is indicated in the symptomatic control of recalcitrant psoriasis not responsive to topical therapy or other systemic therapies such as PUVA or retinoids. The diagnosis of psoriasis and the need for methotrexate therapy should be established by dermatological consultation. In general, these patients should have severe psoriasis that may be ruining their lives physically, emotionally, or financially. Examples of candidates for methotrexate therapy are patients with:

- Moderate to severe psoriasis
  - Psoriatic erythroderma
  - Psoriatic arthritis, moderate to severe
  - Acute pustular psoriasis, von Zumbusch type
- Localized pustular psoriasis
  - Psoriasis that affects certain areas of the body to the extent that normal function and employment are prevented
  - Psoriasis that has not responded to phototherapy, PUVA, and retinoids

RELATIVE CONTRAINDICATIONS

Methotrexate treatment may not be viable in the presence of:

- Any abnormalities in renal function, which may require other therapy or a marked reduction in the dose (see Appendix A)
- Significant abnormalities in liver chemistry
- Pregnancy or nursing (absolute contraindications)
- Male or female fertility (conception must be avoided during methotrexate therapy and afterward for at least 3 months in the male or one ovulatory cycle in the female)
- Hepatitis, active or recent
- Cirrhosis
- Severe anemia, leukopenia, or thrombocytopenia
- Excessive alcohol consumption
- Active infectious disease (e.g., tuberculosis, pyelonephritis)
- Unreliability on the part of the patient

Circumstances may arise in which contraindications must be waived, such as when the benefits can be expected to outweigh the risks of methotrexate therapy in an individual patient.

PREMETHOTREXATE EVALUATION

The premethotrexate evaluation starts with the history and physical examination. Laboratory tests consist of the following studies:

Complete blood count with differential and platelet count (quantitative)
Renal function
Serum creatinine
BUN
Urinalysis
Creatinine clearance or estimate (see Appendix A), particularly in elderly patients
Liver chemistry
AST (SGOT)
ALT (SGPT)
Alkaline phosphatase
Bilirubin
Albumin
Hepatitis A, B, and C serology test
HIV antibody determination in patients at risk for AIDS

EARLY-TREATMENT LIVER BIOPSY: ANALYSIS AND RECOMMENDATIONS

A thorough history and physical examination will identify some patients with preexisting risk factors for liver disease. Liver chemistry tests will identify only *some* patients with existing liver disease. The most reliable test of liver damage remains the needle biopsy of the liver. This should be performed by specially trained, experienced individuals. In most studies examining patient populations with psoriasis before methotrexate treatment, fibrosis or cirrhosis has been found by liver biopsy when not otherwise anticipated by history, physical examination, or laboratory tests.

Risk Factors for Liver Disease

There is controversy on the issue of whether an early-treatment liver biopsy is necessary when starting patients on methotrexate. We believe that the decision on the need for this early biopsy can be influenced by whether there are preexisting risk factors in the patient.

The following risk factors should be specifically sought in evaluating psoriasis patients for methotrexate treatment. The presence of any of these factors to a significant degree would be important in considering an early-treatment liver biopsy.

1. History of past or current excessive alcohol consumption. (Methotrexate toxicity is associated with a history of total lifetime alcohol intake before methotrexate therapy. The exact amount of alcohol that confers risk is unknown and differs among individuals.)
2. Persistent abnormal liver chemistry studies.
3. History of liver disease, including chronic hepatitis B or C.
4. Family history of inheritable liver disease.
5. Diabetes mellitus (probably of secondary importance).
6. Obesity (probably of secondary importance).
7. History of significant exposure to hepatotoxic drugs or chemicals (probably of secondary importance).

Liver Biopsy Recommendations in Patients with No Risk Factors

In the absence of significant risk factors, it is rare to develop life-threatening liver disease with the first 1.0–1.5 g of methotrexate. Therefore, if a physician is confident that significant risk factors are absent, a liver biopsy is not necessary until the patient has been treated with 1.0–1.5 g of methotrexate.

Liver Biopsy Recommendation in Patients with Risk Factors

In patients with risk factors, it is advisable that a liver biopsy be done, when feasible, at or near the beginning of methotrexate therapy. A small percentage of patients will not continue to take methotrexate after 2–4 months because of adverse effects or lack of clinical effectiveness, or for other reasons. Therefore, the early treatment liver biopsy might be postponed until after this initial period. If long-term therapy is anticipated, the initial biopsy should be performed in patients with risk factors. No information is available to suggest that a short or several-month period of methotrexate treatment will cause clinically significant liver disease. A liver biopsy might not be indicated:

1. In elderly patients
2. During acute illness
3. When there are medical contraindications for liver biopsy (e.g., cardiac instability, prolonged bleeding times or prothrombin time)
4. In patients with limited life expectancy

CONTINUING LABORATORY STUDIES

During methotrexate treatment, the following tests should be carried out:

1. Complete blood cell count with differential and platelet count (quantitative) weekly for the first 2 weeks, then biweekly for next month, and then approximately monthly depending on WBC count and stability of patient
2. Renal function studies—BUN and serum creatinine at 3–4-month intervals
3. Liver chemistries—ALT, AST, alkaline phosphatase, serum albumin every 4–8 weeks (more frequent liver chemistry monitoring in lieu of an initial liver biopsy)
4. More frequent monitoring may be useful in the following circumstances:
   During initial treatment
   When increasing dosage
   During episodes of increased risk of elevated methotrexate blood levels (e.g., dehydration, impaired renal function, addition of or increased concomitant medications such as NSAIDs)

INTERPRETATION OF LABORATORY STUDIES

A significant reduction in leukocyte or platelet counts necessitates reduction or temporary discontinuation of methotrexate therapy. The maximum depression of the leukocyte and platelet counts usually occurs 7 to 10 days after a dose of methotrexate. Leukopenia (leukocyte count <3500) continuing beyond 1 week deserves special attention. It may be advisable to discontinue methotrexate for 2 to 3 weeks. Thrombocytopenia (platelet count <100,000 mm^3) may also necessitate methotrexate discontinuation. Consider immediate administration of folinic acid 20 mg in cases of leukopenia and thrombocytopenia (see "Overdosage").

If liver chemistry tests are called for, they should be obtained at least 1 week after the last methotrexate dose. The reason is that liver chemistry values are frequently elevated 1 to 2 days after methotrexate therapy. If a significant, persistent abnormality in liver chemistry develops, withhold methotrexate therapy for 1 to 2 weeks and repeat the battery of liver chemistry tests. Liver chemistry values should return to normal in 1 to 2 weeks. If a significantly abnormal liver chemistry persists for 2 to 3 months, a liver biopsy should be considered.

STARTING TREATMENT

The details of when and how to start and follow a patient on methotrexate can best be given by presenting a hypothetical case.

Mr. Jones is 56 years old and has a 20-year history of psoriasis which has generally been confined to the elbows and knees. In the past 6 months the disease has become more generalized, now covering almost 50% of his body. He is also developing psoriatic arthritis in a few joints in his hands. Outpatient therapy consisting of a topical fluorinated corticosteroid and a tar gel was attempted. Aspirin was given for the arthritis. After a 6-week trial at home there was little response of his skin lesions; the arthritis was worse and not controlled by aspirin. The patient was admitted to the hospital, where he stayed for 4 weeks while receiving a full Goeckerman treatment consisting of tar or lubrication followed by gradually increasing UVB phototherapy. During hospitalization, routine laboratory studies (except liver biopsy) were obtained. The patient was discharged with his psoriasis cleared and his arthritis controlled on a nonsteroidal anti-inflammatory agent. He was instructed to come back frequently for outpatient UVB but because of work obligations he is unable to do so.

One month after hospitalization Mr. Jones returns; his psoriasis is starting to flare again and his arthritis is not controlled with the nonsteroidal anti-inflammatory drug. He does not want to go to the hospital again. You discuss the choices of systemic therapy, including photochemotherapy, retinoids, and methotrexate. After he has heard the risks and benefits of each, you both decide he would be best managed on methotrexate. Aspirin and nonsteroidal anti-inflammatory drugs are stopped. Repeat CBC, platelet count, and SMA-20 are performed.

A test dose of methotrexate, two 2.5-mg tablets (total 5 mg), is given and results of the CBC and platelet count are checked the next day and are normal. One week later, the full dose of 15–25 mg (six to 10 tablets) is given orally. The patient returns each week for the first 6 weeks to have a CBC and platelet count before taking his next dose of methotrexate. Clearing of skin lesions begins after the third week, and by 6 weeks his skin is almost clear.

The arthritis is also much better controlled than with any previous medication. It is anticipated that long-term methotrexate therapy will be necessary. Because the patient has no risk factors, a liver biopsy is not performed at this time.

Weekly visits are now changed to monthly visits. The WBC and platelet counts are performed at a convenient lab near his work or home at weekly to biweekly intervals. The lab is instructed to give the result to the patient, and he is to mail it to the physician. A reliable patient can thus monitor this critical aspect of drug response. The methotrexate dosage is lowered by 2.5 mg about every month until a dosage of 10–15 mg (four to six tablets) once weekly is reached, which keeps the patient's skin and arthritis under control. A few remaining skin lesions are easily controlled with topical or intralesional steroids. Results of liver function tests are checked every 3 months. The dosage is continually lowered until psoriasis flares again. Then the dosage is increased slightly to control the process. Some patients require as little as 5–10 mg once weekly to biweekly.

At one follow-up visit, the patient's SGPT level is abnormal. In a discussion with the patient, it is discovered that the liver function tests were performed the day after his taking methotrexate. The repeat SGPT test is done at least 1 week after the patient takes methotrexate, and the results return to normal. If the SGPT level had been persistently abnormal, we would have recommended a liver biopsy. The patient continues on methotrexate for several years under close supervision, reducing and even stopping the drug during the summer months while on vacation and getting extra UVB. After a cumulative dosage of 1.5 g, we recommended a liver biopsy. This specimen showed moderate fatty infiltration, anisonucleosis, and mild periportal inflammation. We continue to administer methotrexate but repeat the liver function tests more frequently and recommend a repeat liver biopsy after only 1 g more of cumulative dosage.

After several years of methotrexate therapy—and with a moderate amount of alcohol consumption, against our orders—a repeat liver biopsy after a total cumulative dose of over 4 g now shows severe fibrosis. Methotrexate is now discontinued and alternative forms of systemic therapy are discussed with the patient.

LIVER BIOPSY DURING METHOTREXATE THERAPY

Deciding Whether Liver Biopsy Is Necessary

One of the most difficult issues that has persisted over the last 35 years of methotrexate use is the recognition of liver damage in a small percentage of patients and how to test for this damage. The liver biopsy has been the most definitive test for severe liver disease, and many publications about psoriatic patients have attempted to develop recommendations on its role in the safe use of methotrexate over the long term.

In the past decade, methotrexate has become a very popular treatment for rheumatoid arthritis; today it is undoubtedly being used in many more patients with rheumatoid arthritis than with psoriasis. The past history of potential liver damage from methotrexate in some patients with psoriasis has sensitized the rheumatology community to look for evidence of liver disease in their rheumatoid arthritis patients receiving methotrexate.

With methotrexate being used in large numbers of patients with rheumatoid arthritis, many studies have been conducted and analyzed to approach the methotrexate liver issue in this population. As discussed elsewhere, rheumatoid arthritis patients appear to have substantially lower incidences of advanced liver changes compared to psoriasis patients. Thus, the concern and/or need for periodic liver biopsies in rheumatoid arthritis patients has been much less than in the psoriasis populations. We stress that the reasons for differences in liver disease related to methotrexate in these two disease populations remain unclear. The American College of Rheumatology has sponsored a Subcommittee on Hepatitic Toxicity and methotrexate to evaluate the risks of methotrexate therapy in their patients and to provide recommendations about monitoring patients for liver toxicity (9,10). The subcommittee recommends a pretreatment liver biopsy only for patients with extensive prior alcohol consumption, persistent abnormal liver function tests, and/or chronic hepatitis B or C infection. During methotrexate treatment, frequent liver function tests at 1- to 2-month intervals should be obtained. If these laboratory tests are abnormal five or six times in a year of methotrexate treatment, indicating persistent liver test abnormalities, then a liver biopsy is performed. According to the recommendations, several test abnormalities are required over the year to minimize the number of liver biopsies since sporadic and random abnormal liver function test results are routinely found in as many as 30% of patients. Kremer et al. (10) indicate that only four or five patients in 100 will have recurrent elevations in serum transaminase tests (the most sensitive test) and be candidates for liver biopsies. Limiting the liver biopsy to these patients will substantially reduce costs and the risk of adverse events associated with liver biopsy.

In psoriasis, all data indicate a higher incidence of advanced liver changes than in rheumatoid arthritis patients receiving methotrexate. Whiting-O'Keefe et al. (1991) (see "Risks of Liver Biopsy" section of references) suggest a 2.5- to 5.0-fold difference in psoriasis patients having liver changes. With this perspective it remains necessary to have a greater degree of vigilance in methotrexate-treated psoriatic patients requiring liver biopsies as suggested in these guidelines.

Many of the liver methotrexate studies have suggested that significant alcoholic usage leads to more severe liver changes in association with methotrexate. In a meta-analysis of 635 patients in 15 studies, Whiting-O'Keefe et al. have analyzed the risks of advanced liver changes in psoriatic and rheumatoid arthritis patients with and without alcohol usage. On average, 6.7% of patients progress one histological grade (using the scale developed by Roenigk et al.) for every 1000 mg of methotrexate. Advanced changes, grades IIIB and IV (moderate to severe fibrosis or cirrhosis), appear in 0.9% of patients for every 1000 mg of methotrexate. The data of Whiting-O'Keefe et al. show that there is a 20% chance of progressing one grade after 3 g of methotrexate. Their calculations suggest that one in 35 patients will develop advanced liver changes.

When alcohol intake is considered, heavy drinkers (>100 g/wk) have advanced changes in 13/73 patients (171.8%), while nondrinkers and light drinkers (<100 g/wk) are in the 4.5–5.0% range. However, the data indicate that there is a slightly lower incidence of advanced changes in rheumatoid arthritis patients compared to psoriasis patients (9/334 vs. 23/299, $p =$ 0.005). Whiting-O'Keefe et al. thus conclude there is a 2.5 to 5.0 times greater risk in heavy alcohol users. This confirms the long-held impression that heavy alcohol drinkers should have limited exposure to methotrexate, particularly over the long term.

The liver biopsy is not an innocuous procedure and certainly elicits patient anxiety. Fortunately, in psoriatic patients, the risks have tended to be lower than in patients with other diseases. The risks include subcapsular hemorrhage, gall bladder perforation, pneumothorax, and hemoperitoneum. Most of the adverse events occur in patients with internal abnormalities related to other diseases. The risks of liver biopsy have been summarized by Kremer et al. (10), who estimate the frequency of liver biopsy complications to be 1.5 per 1000 procedures. Adverse events to biopsies entail additional medical and occasionally surgical procedures, thereby increasing the overall costs. The cost of a liver biopsy ranges from $1000 to 1500, or even higher. Kremer et al. (10) have calculated that if the cumulative risk of clinically significant liver disease is 1%, the cost would be $100,000 for each case found. Thus, liver function tests should be used judiciously to minimize the need for liver biopsies.

In the presence of normal findings on liver chemistry tests, history, and physical examination, the decision to perform or omit liver biopsies while giving treatment with methotrexate should be made in each case after consideration of the relative risk (see Appendix A). However, in most patients with no risk factors of liver disease, the first liver biopsy would be done at approximately 1.0–1.5 g of cumulative methotrexate (Table 1).

If the first liver biopsy shows no significant abnormalities, repeat liver biopsies are recommended at intervals of approximately 1.5 g cumulative methotrexate (Table 1).

When cumulative doses of methotrexate reach 4.0 g or above, the liver biopsy should be repeated with every additional 1.0–1.5 g (see "Liver Toxicity" in Appendix A). In patients having persistent significant abnormalities in liver chemistry values, a liver biopsy is indicated. A follow-up liver biopsy is recommended after 0.5–1.0 g cumulative methotrexate dose (or approximately 6 months).

The length of treatment required to achieve a cumulative methotrexate dose of 1.5 g is related to the weekly dose if used on a regular basis For example:

Weekly dose (mg)	Months to 1.5 g
7.5	50
15	25
25	15

Classification of Liver Biopsy Findings

The following is a classification of pathological changes that may be detected on liver biopsy. Recommendations concerning the continuation or discontinuation of methotrexate therapy are based on these pathological changes. Interpretation should be done by persons with special competence in drug-induced liver abnormalities. A connective tissue or reticular stain is required to distinguish fibrosis.

Grade I: Normal; fatty infiltration, mild; nuclear variability, mild; portal inflammation, mild.

Grade II: Fatty infiltration, moderate to severe; nuclear variability, moderate to severe; portal tract

Table 1 Guidelines on When to Perform Liver Biopsy

Liver biopsy	Approximate cumulative methotrexate dose (g)
No risk factors	
First	1.0–1.5
Repeat	3.0
Repeat	4.0
Risk factors	
First	2–4-month therapy
Repeat	1.0–1.5
Next repeat	3.0
Following repeat	4.0

expansion, portal tract inflammation, and necrosis, moderate to severe.

Grade IIIA: Fibrosis, mild. (Portal fibrosis here denotes formation of fibrotic septa extending into the lobules. Slight enlargement of portal tracts without disruption of limiting plates or septum formation does not put the biopsy specimen in grade III.)

Grade IIIB: Fibrosis, moderate to severe.

Grade IV: Cirrhosis (regenerating nodules as well as bridging of portal tracts must be demonstrated).

Clinical Interpretation of Liver Biopsy Results

The decision regarding continuation or discontinuation of methotrexate therapy is made after liver biopsy. The following recommendations are based on liver abnormality:

1. Patients with grade I or II changes may continue to receive methotrexate therapy
2. Patients with grade IIIA change may continue to receive methotrexate therapy but should have a repeat liver biopsy after approximately 6 months of methotrexate therapy. Consider alternative therapy.
3. Patients with grades IIIB and IV changes should not be given further methotrexate therapy. Exceptional circumstances, however, may require continued methotrexate therapy, with careful follow-up liver biopsies (see Appendix A).

COMMONLY USED DOSAGE SCHEDULES

1. Single weekly oral, intravenous, intramuscular, or subcutaneous dosage schedule
2. Intermittent oral schedule of three divided doses over a 36-hr period each week (Q 12 hr × 3 in one week)

The oral administration can be tablets or carefully measured parenteral solution (0.1 ml of 50 mg/2 ml parenteral solution is equivalent to 2.5 mg oral). According to the results of published studies, the two schedules have equal effectiveness.

Studies indicate that when a certain amount of drug is given in one dose, there are fewer toxic effects than when the same total amount is dispensed in daily doses over an extended period of 5 to 7 days. Cellular therapeutic effect versus cellular toxicity is governed, in part, by the duration of cell–drug contact. Because of the increased toxicity, a daily oral dose schedule should not be used.

SPECIFIC DOSAGE RECOMMENDATION

Dosages cited below pertain to the average adult weighing 70 kg. An initial test dose of 2.5–5.0 mg should be used first to detect any unusual sensitivity to toxic effects. A similar test dose should be used in patients off methotrexate for several years. Maximal myelosuppression usually occurs within 7 to 10 days. Regular methotrexate dosage may be initiated 1 week later if laboratory studies are normal. Special caution should be used in dosing patients with reduced renal function, particularly the elderly and patients on some nonsteroidal anti-inflammatory drugs. Sulfa drugs and/or trimethoprim should never be used together with methotrexate.

1. Weekly single, oral, intramuscular, intravenous, or subcutaneous dose schedule
   a. The range of oral dosages ordinarily is 7.5 to 30 mg/wk. The weekly dose may be increased gradually (2.5 mg to 5.0 mg/wk) with appropriate monitoring of the blood counts. Occasional patients will need a maximum of 50 mg/wk.
   b. The range of intramuscular, subcutaneous, or rapid ("push") intravenous dosage ordinarily is 7.5 mg to 50 mg/wk, with occasional patients needing titration to a maximum of 75 mg/wk. Intravenous drips of methotrexate should not be used. As the

total dose is gradually increased, blood cell counts should be more frequently monitored.

2. Divided oral dose schedule
   a. 2.5 to 5.0 mg at 12-hr intervals for three doses each week
   b. Gradual increase by 2.5 mg/wk permissible with appropriate monitoring of the blood cell counts
   c. Total dose ordinarily not to exceed 30 mg/wk

All schedules should be continually tailored to the individual patient. Patients on any schedule should have dosage reduced and rest periods increased to the greatest possible extent. The goal is not necessarily to achieve complete clearing of psoriasis, but rather to achieve adequate control at the lowest possible dosage and with the longest rest period off methotrexate treatment. The use of methotrexate may permit the return to other therapies; this course should be encouraged.

FOLIC AND FOLINIC ACID SUPPLEMENTS

It has been suggested in studies on small numbers of patients that concomitant administration of folic acid (1–5 mg/d) reduces side effects such as nausea and megaloblastic anemia without diminishing the efficacy of methotrexate. Additional studies with folinic acid administered on days when methotrexate is not given also resulted in a reduction in methotrexate side effects such as nausea without reducing its beneficial effects.

ROTATIONAL THERAPY

All forms of therapy (phototherapy, photochemotherapy, methotrexate, oral retinoids) for moderate to severe psoriasis have varying degrees of long-term toxicity. To minimize long-term toxicity of any of these modalities when used as monotherapy, the rotational therapy concept entails switching from one modality to another prior to reaching a cumulative toxic range. In the case of methotrexate, the first concern of chronic toxicity is liver disease, which may occur at about 1.0–1.5 g of cumulative dose. Thus, if methotrexate is discontinued at about 1.0–1.5 g and patients rotated to another modality, one can minimize the risk of long-term liver changes by providing a "rest period" off methotrexate for several years. There are several rotational therapy choices: photochemotherapy, phototherapy, retinoids, cyclosporine. There may be patient benefit–risk issues in which alternative therapies may not be as favorable as methotrexate.

COMBINATION THERAPIES

Although serious adverse reactions can occur when methotrexate is combined with other drugs, some drug combinations with methotrexate may have beneficial effects and reduce potential toxicity from both drugs.

Topical therapy should be encouraged in psoriatic patients taking methotrexate to minimize the dosage. Patients tend to rely on methotrexate and forget about effective topical and intralesional corticoids, tars, vitamin D analogs, and even a full Goeckerman regimen in those whose disease exacerbates while on methotrexate.

Methotrexate combined with PUVA results in clearing at a lower amount of UVA than with PUVA alone. Patients have been treated with a 3-week course of methotrexate followed by a combination of UVB and methotrexate.

Methotrexate has been combined with retinoids to give a more rapid clearing of severe generalized pustular psoriasis than possible with each drug alone. Since each of these two drugs has the potential to produce hepatotoxicity, they should be used together only for short periods with careful monitoring of liver function tests.

OVERDOSAGE

Two leading causes of acute methotrexate toxicity are impaired renal function that prevents excretion of normal doses of methotrexate and concomitant administration of trimethoprim or trimethoprim-sulfamethoxazole (Bactrim, Septra, and generic).

Leucovorin calcium (citrovorum factor or folinic acid) is the only antidote for the hematological toxic effects of methotrexate. When an overdose of methotrexate is suspected for any reason, including minimal renal compromise, the patient should be given leucovorin immediately. An immediate leucovorin dose of 20 mg (10 mg/m^2) should be given parenterally or orally, and subsequent doses should be given every 6 hr, parenterally or orally, as tolerated by the patient. As the time interval between methotrexate administration and the initiation of leucovorin treatment increases, the effectiveness of leucovorin in counteracting the hematological toxicity of methotrexate decreases. Serum methotrexate levels should be measured as soon as possible after overdose is suspected, and further leucovorin doses adjusted accordingly. Serum methotrexate levels should be measured initially and every 12 to 24 hr, and leucovorin should be continued until the methotrexate concentration is less than 10^{-8} M (0.01 μM). Subsequent leucovorin dosing should be adjusted in the following fashion:

Serum methotrexate level (M)	Leucovorin dose every 6 hr (mg)
5×10^{-7}	20
1×10^{-6}	100
2×10^{-6}	200
$>2 \times 10^{-6}$	Proportionately increased

Because the oral absorption of leucovorin appears to reach a plateau at doses of 25 to 50 mg, any dose of leucovorin >25 mg should be given parenterally. When an overdose of methotrexate is suspected for any reason, including minimal renal impairment or other cause of reduced methotrexate clearance, leucovorin must be continued for extended periods. However, a prompt oral dose is preferable to a delayed parenteral dose. The physician using methotrexate should have leucovorin in the office. If the patient needs hospitalization, start oral leucovorin before admission. If the serum creatinine concentration 24 hours after overdose is 350% greater than the baseline creatinine concentration, the intravenous dose of leucovorin should immediately be increased to 100 mg/m^2 every 3 hours until the serum methotrexate concentration is below 1×10^{-8} M. In cases of massive overdose, hydration and urinary alkinization may be necessary to prevent precipitation in the renal tubules of methotrexate, its metabolites, or both. After a documented or suspected overdose, whether or not treated with leucovorin, patients must be closely monitored for the development of hematological or other toxic effects. Further treatment with methotrexate or other similarly toxic agents should be postponed until the development of toxic effects has been ruled out.

ADVERSE REACTIONS

The most commonly reported adverse reactions to the doses of methotrexate used in the treatment of psoriasis include malaise, gastrointestinal-tract effects, headaches, and leukopenia. The severity of side effects is, in general, dose-related. Adverse reactions reported during the use of methotrexate include the following:

1. General fatigue; headaches; chills and fever; dizziness
2. Skin—pruritus; pain; urticaria; mild, reversible alopecia; ecchymosis; acute ulcerations of psoriatic lesions; reactivation of phototoxic responses; given within a few days after ultraviolet irradiation, may reactivate on acute sunburn response.
3. Blood—bone marrow depression; leukopenia leading to decreased resistance to infection; anemia; thrombocytopenia; bleeding and megaloblastic anemia
4. Gastrointestinal system—ulcerative stomatitis; nausea and anorexia; less frequently, hepatotoxicity, pharyngitis, diarrhea, vomiting, enteritis
5. Urogenital system—azotemia; microscopic hematuria; cystitis; transient oligospermia; defective spermatogenesis; defective oogenesis; teratogenesis; menstrual dysfunction; nephropathy
6. Nervous system—headaches; dizziness; drowsiness; blurred vision; acute depression

DRUG INTERACTIONS

The use of any drug in addition to methotrexate should be carefully evaluated. Potentially interacting drugs are listed in Table 2. Drug interactions are most likely to be clinically relevant problems in patients with low renal function. Interactions with nonsteroidal anti-inflammatory drugs have been reported with low doses of methotrexate (7.5 mg/wk). When introducing or increasing the dose of nonsteroidal anti-inflammatory drugs, additional monitoring is indicated. Numerous other drug interactions have been studied. In particular, theophylline levels should be followed when administering methotrexate to patients on theophylline (Glyson-Barnhart et al., 1991—see "Drug Interactions" section of references). Plasma prothrombin times should also be followed when administering methotrexate to patients on warfarin anticoagulants such as coumadin, and platelet counts should be monitored frequently. Because of potentially significant additive pharmacological effects, patients receiving methotrexate should not be treated

Table 2 Drugs That May Interact with Methotrexate to Increase Toxicity

Mechanism	Drugs[a]
Decreased renal elimination of methotrexate	Nephrotoxins (e.g., aminoglycosides, cyclosporin)
	Salicylates
	Phenylbutazone
	Sulfonamides
	Probenecid
	Cephalothin
	Penicillins
	Colchicine
	Many nonsteroidal anti-inflammatory drugs (naproxyn, ibuprofen and others)
Additive or synergistic toxicity	Trimethoprim-sulamethoxazole[b]
	Ethanol
	Pyrimethamine
	Triamterene
Displacement of methotrexate from plasma protein binding	Salicylates
	Probenecid
	Barbiturates
	Phenytoin
	Retinoids
	Sulfonamides[b]
	Sulfonylureas
	Tetracycline
Intracellular accumulation of methotrexate	Probenecid
	Dipyridamole
Hepatotoxicity	Retinoids
	Ethanol

[a]For a more complete list, see Evans and Christensen (1985) in the "Drug Interactions" section in the reference list. Methotrexate-associated toxic effects (gastrointestinal effects, leukopenia, thrombocytopenia) have been observed in patients treated concomitantly with these drugs. Evidence for drug interaction between methotrexate and the other drugs listed in this table are from in vitro studies. The clinical significance of some of these interactions in psoriasis is not known.
[b]Absolute contraindication.

with trimethoprim or trimethoprim-sulfamethoxazole; the latter alone can cause toxic effects in bone marrow.

APPENDIX A: ADDITIONAL INFORMATION ON GUIDELINES FOR USE OF METHOTREXATE IN PSORIASIS*

General reviews of the use of methotrexate in psoriasis have been published by Roenigk et al. (7), Weinstein (1977), Weinstein (1983), Hanno et al. (1980), Greaves and Weinstein (1995), Kremer et al. (10). General reviews of the use of methotrexate in rheumatoid arthritis include Letendre et al. (1985), Klippel and Decker (1985), and Willkens (1983).

Liver Toxicity

Hepatotoxicity resulting from methotrexate therapy for psoriasis remains the most significant long-term issue. The position paper of the Health and Public Policy Committee of the American College of Physicians (9) states that, in patients with rheumatoid arthritis, pretreatment biopsies should be done only if the patient has preexisting liver disease. In contrast to patients with rheumatoid arthritis, abnormal liver histological findings appear to be more common in patients with psoriasis, for unknown reasons. In psoriasis

*References for the Appendixes follow the numbered references and are organized by section.

patients, liver chemistry studies and liver scans are helpful but have not been uniformly predictive of fibrosis and cirrhosis before or during methotrexate therapy (Weinstein et al., 1973; Reese et al., 1974; Zachariae et al., 1975; Van de Kerkhof et al., 1985; Miller et al., 1985; Coulson et al., 1987; Mitchell et al., 1987; Newman et al., 1989; O'Connor et al., 1989. Therefore the need for liver biopsy remains an important but somewhat controversial issue.

The international cooperative study (Weinstein et al., 1973) involved 550 patients, 81 of whom had both pre- and postmethotrexate liver biopsies. With large cumulative doses of methotrexate (>2.2 g), there was no significant increase in the incidence of cirrhosis but there was an overall small increase in fibrosis. Evaluation of single postmethotrexate liver biopsy specimens showed a 3% incidence of cirrhosis. Additional studies have reported small increases in cirrhosis in limited populations.

The data reported by Zachariae and Nyfors suggest that longer exposure (years) to methotrexate or higher cumulative doses of methotrexate, or both, lead to a higher incidence of cirrhosis. Nyfors (1977) and Zachariae et al. (1980) reported the highest rate of fibrosis/cirrhosis with cumulative methotrexate dose (4 g) in a large group. No other studies, including the International Cooperative Study, have adequate data to support the data of Nyfors and Zachariae showing a much higher incidence of cirrhosis. Nor do other studies have adequate patient experience in these dose ranges to confirm the results from Scandinavia (Nyfors and Zachariae et al.) in other medical or geographic environments. All studies indicate that the incidence of cirrhosis is low with a total dose of methotrexate <1.5 g.

Zachariae et al. (1980), Zachariae and Sogaard (1987), and Zachariae et al. (1996) have provided evidence suggesting that the clinical course of cirrhosis induced by methotrexate is often nonaggressive; in fact, many of these patients have been continued on methotrexate therapy without worsening of liver biopsy findings. Deaths resulting from hepatic damage in psoriatic patients after long-term treatment with methotrexate have occurred but appear to be very uncommon. Reported deaths (Coe and Bull, 1968; Pai et al., 1973) occurred mainly in the era before the present appreciation of the importance of evaluating both renal and liver function relative to methotrexate therapy. Other methotrexate induced severe liver disease or deaths have involved patient or physician misuse or abuse of methotrexate and failure to follow the methotrexate guidelines.

Renal Function

Ninety percent of methotrexate is excreted in the urine in 24 hr. Minimal renal insufficiency, often seen in elderly patients, can be associated with severe methotrexate toxicity, requiring that this drug be used with great caution, if at all, in patients with renal disease. The lower the creatinine clearance, the greater the circulating half-life of methotrexate and the potential for toxic effects. Since methotrexate is not excreted in a linear fashion, minor changes in methotrexate dose or renal function can result in major toxicity. Methotrexate is not eliminated by dialysis. In healthy patients under the age of 60, serum creatinines less than 1.5 indicate adequate renal function. The 24-hr creatinine clearance tests are more sensitive and could be used for initial work-up. In elderly patients or patients with reduced muscle mass, creatinine clearance can be calculated from the Cockroft-Gault formula:

$$\frac{(140 - \text{age in years}) \times (\text{weight in kg})}{\text{Serum creatinine (mg/100 ml)} \times 72}$$

For women, multiply by 0.85.

Methotrexate should be used with caution in patients whose creatinine clearance is less than 50 ml/mm. Extreme care should be used in patients with a creatinine clearance under 30 ml/mm, and alternative therapy considered.

Pulmonary Toxicity

Methotrexate-induced pneumonitis should be considered whenever a patient receiving the drug develops a persistent, dry, nonproductive cough, dyspnea, or both. The diagnosis of methotrexate-associated lung disease is a diagnosis of exclusion; infection must always be considered. Methotrexate should be discontinued, at least temporarily. Systemic corticosteroids may be effective in controlling the acute pneumonitis.

Methotrexate-associated pulmonary disease has been described as an acute pneumonitis and as a more chronic, indolent process that may evolve. These complications appear to be much rarer in psoriasis than in rheumatoid arthritis, possibly because of an association with rheumatoid lung. The pathophysiology of methotrexate-induced pneumonitis and risk factors for development of the process are currently inadequately understood. The development of pulmonary complications is not necessarily related to the weekly or cumulative dose of methotrexate. Chest x-ray studies and pulmonary function tests are of questionable value in predicting patients at risk for pneumonitis.

Pharmacokinetics

The absorption of methotrexate is impaired in some psoriatic patients, and it displays great interpatient variation. Although studies with cancer patients showed complete absorption of oral methotrexate at doses less than 30 mg/m^2, the absorption in patients with psoriasis is incomplete and unpredictable even at low doses. There is also increased incidence of malabsorptive enteropathy in patients with psoriasis (Hendel et al., 1982). Dose-dependent absorption of oral methotrexate has been demonstrated, with lower doses (less than 30 mg/m^2) absorbed more completely than higher doses. This observation suggests the presence of a saturable intestinal absorption mechanism (Evans and Christensen, 1985; Hendel, 1985). The drug should be taken on an empty stomach because concurrent food, especially milk-based meals, may decrease its bioavailability [Roenigk, 1988 (Ref. 8)]. At doses used in psoriasis, more than 80% of the drug is absorbed after intramuscular administration [Roenigk et al., 1988 (Ref. 8)]. Recent studies have indicated that food may have no effect on the absorption of methotrexate (Kozloski et al., 1992; Oguey et al., 1992).

After intravenous administration, methotrexate is distributed initially within a volume of 18% body weight, then within a volume of 76% of body weight, corresponding to those of extracellular space and total body water, respectively (Bleyer, 1978). Approximately 50% of the drug in serum is reversibly bound to albumin (Hendel, 1985; Menard et al., 1980). Following intravenous administration, methotrexate is distributed in a triphasic fashion (Hendel, 1985; Jones et al., 1986 ("Liver Toxicity" section of references); Menard et al., 1980). The first-phase half-life of less than 1 hr corresponds to the distribution of drug into the body fluids, while the half-lives of the second phase (2 to 3 hr) and the terminal phase (8 to 10 hours) reflect renal clearance and probably the combined effects of drug being released from peripheral compartments, enterohepatic circulation, and renal tubular reabsorption, respectively (Bleyer, 1978; Hendel, 1985). It is the prolongation of this terminal phase that increases the toxicity of methotrexate. Higher doses of methotrexate have been shown to produce higher but not directly proportional concentrations of methotrexate in tissues. At equilibrium, the greatest concentrations of the drug are in the kidneys, gallbladder, spleen, liver, and skin (Anderson et al., 1970).

Although three metabolic pathways have been described for methotrexate, their clinical significance has not been established. Two of the metabolities—2,4,diamino-10-methyl pteroic acid and 7-hydroxymethotrexate—are seen only after high-dose methotrexate therapy and have not been reported at doses used in psoriasis (78; Hendel, 1985). Methotrexate is also converted intracellularly to polyglutamyl metabolites containing two to five glutamyl groups in gamma peptide linkage (Hendel, 1985; Menard et al., 1980). These polyglutamate derivates are potent inhibitors of dihydrofolate reductase and form slowly dissociable complexes with the enzyme (Hendel, 1985; Jolivet et al., 1983). Intracellularly, the polyglutamates are retained preferentially over methotrexate, and the glutamyl groups are cleaved before methotrexate is released from the tissue into plasma (Bleyer, 1978; Hendel, 1985). The rate of disappearance of the polyglutamates from the intracellular-bound fraction and the free fraction decreases with increasing chain length, suggesting a slower dissociation of the longer-chain metabolites from the enzyme (Jolivet et al., 1983). The slower dissociation of the longer-chain polyglutamates from dihydrofolate reductase could lead to the replacement of methotrexate on the enzyme by the polyglutamates as successive doses of methotrexate are administered. Since over 90% of the polyglutamates present in the epidermis of rats were shown to be of chain length greater than two glutamyl groups, this may explain the prolonged skin/plasma ratio of antifolate activities seen after methotrexate doses (Zimmerman et al., 1984). If the same phenomenon occurs in the epidermis of human skin, it may be possible to decrease the frequency of methotrexate dosing in psoriasis.

Methotrexate is excreted primarily as unchanged drug by the kidneys through a combination of glomerular filtration and active tubular transport (Hendel, 1985). The tubular reabsorption of methotrexate is saturated at a plasma concentration of 1 mg/L, resulting in increased clearance of the drug (Hendel and Nyfors, 1984). The increase in clearance reaches its peak at the saturation point of tubular secretion, which has been reported to occur after doses as low as 100 mg. From that point on, clearance decreases with increasing methotrexate plasma concentration. However, at doses used in psoriasis, the saturation of the tubular secretory mechanism is unlikely to occur.

Liver Chemistry Tests and Scans

The search for noninvasive tests to detect early fibrosis, or any precirrhosis change, is of importance to dermatologists as well as to rheumatologists and hepatologists. Reports in the literature usually deal with liver disease in patients who are not receiving methotrexate, e.g., patients with hepatitis or cystic fibrosis. Not only are these reports variable in their predicted ability to detect fibrosis and/or cirrhosis, but they cannot be carried over to the methotrexate situation.

The most discussed test in the last few years is the serum aminoterminal type III procollagen propeptide (PIIIP). Zachariae et al. (1991—in "Liver Toxicity" section of references) published the study most applicable to our situation and found that, in the absence of psoriatic arthritis, increased PIIIP indicated liver fibrogenesis. However, it was a poor predictor of cirrhosis and failed to support their conclusion that, with a normal PIIIP, liver biopsies can be reduced to a minimum. This still leaves open the question of what constitutes a "minimum." The PIIIP test may be a useful adjunct in decision-making as threshold total methotrexate doses are reached when liver biopsy is being considered. However, at the present time it should not be relied on as we rely on the liver biopsy. With psoriatic arthritis, 38% of Zachariae's patients had elevated PIIIP.

Mitchell et al. (1987) found that neither PIIIP nor standard liver tests were able to identify patients with significant liver damage. This remains a good summation of the situation and represents the opinions of the authors of the methotrexate guidelines. An article in a nondermatological journal expressed the same view (Gilbert et al., 1990).

Magnetic resonance imaging is of no value as a screening procedure for detecting methotrexate-induced liver damage (Rademacher et al., 1987). Personal experience with ultrasonography has also shown a lack of sensitivity and predictability in detecting liver disease (Geronemus et al., 1982—in "Liver Toxicity" section of references). The paper by Geronemus et al. deals with technetium scans and *not* ultrasonography. Many studies have evaluated the possible usefulness of ultrasound in the detection of methotrexate-induced hepatic damage. Favorable results were obtained by Miller et al. (1985) and Coulson et al. (1987) but were not corroborated by Mitchell et al. (1987) or Hultcranz and Gabrielsson (1993). At present, results are not sufficiently consistent to recommend the routine use of ultrasonography as a substitute for liver biopsies.

A recent modification of radionucleotide imaging called "dynamic hepatic scintigraphy" (DHS), which measures the portal venous contribution to the total hepatic blood flow, may reduce the number of liver biopsies required for patients receiving methotrexate. Abnormal DHS gave a low (25%) predictive value for fibrosis in a study by McHenry et al. (1992). The predictive value of a normal scan for absent or mild fibrosis was high (98.5%), although the predictive value of an abnormal scan for moderate or severe fibrosis was only 25% (McHenry et al., 1992). Thus, DHS appears to have considerable promise in identifying patients with no significant fibrosis, but cannot be relied on to grade the severity of liver damage. The combination of PIIIP measurements with DHS had only limited additional value above that of DHS alone, according to VanDooren-Greebe et al. (1996) in the best study on hepatic scintigraphy. This indicates that DHS may be of value in detecting early methotrexate-induced liver damage.

Imaging methods and various serum determinations will have to become more sensitive before they can detect early fibrosis.

Malignancy

Cases have been reported of malignancies developing in patients treated with methotrexate for psoriasis, often in combination with other agents (IARC Working Group, 1981). No excess of cancer was found in two studies of patients who received methotrexate for psoriasis (Bailin et al., 1975; Nyfors and Jensen, 1983) or as treatment for choriocarcinoma (Bagshawe, 1976). The relationship between methotrexate treatment and subsequent malignancy has been investigated in a cohort of 457 patients treated for trophoblastic tumors (Rustin et al., 1983). A case–control study of treatment for psoriasis has also been performed (Stern et al., 1982, 1994) that looks at the relationship of skin cancer and PUVA. The latest results showed a significant relationship between high levels of exposure to methotrexate and risk of squamous cell carcinoma (SCC) with PUVA. It was not modified by other exposures or level of exposure to PUVA. A Swedish study (Lindelof, 1993) also found a similar association between methotrexate and SCC in PUVA patients.

There have been case reports (Zimmer-Galber, 1994; Kenysmore, 1992) of patients with rheumatoid arthritis treated with methotrexate developing non-Hodgkin's lymphoma. A case–control study found no association between rheumatoid arthritis, methotrexate, and hematological malignancy (Moder, 1995). Methotrexate, of course, is the drug of choice in the treatment of selected internal malignancies.

Reproductive Effects

Methotrexate has produced chromosomal damage in bone marrow cells in treated patients (Krogh Jensen, 1967; Krogh Jensen and Nyfors, 1979; Melnyk et al., 1971) but not in peripheral lymphocytes (Voorhees et al., 1969; Melnyk et al., 1971; Krogh Jensen and Nyfors, 1979). Experience with previously treated patients revealed no excess of fetal abnormalities in subsequent pregnancies (Van Thiel et al., 1970; Ross, 1976; Walden and Bagshawe, 1976). Methotrexate is an abortifacient and may be teratogenic if taken during pregnancy (Milunsky et al., 1968; Powell and Ekert, 1971; Kozlowski et al., 1990). Male patients who have been treated with methotrexate at the time of conception have had partners who produced normal offspring (Weinstein, 1977; Perry, 1983). Pregnancy is an absolute contraindication to treating psoriasis with methotrexate.

In men methotrexate can produce reversible oligospermia. Just as in women, there is no evidence of abnormal offspring subsequent to using methotrexate. After discontinuing methotrexate, women should wait two menstrual cycles before becoming pregnant to be sure they were not already pregnant while on methotrexate. Men should wait 3 months before impregnating their partner to get past the 74 days needed for sperm development.

AIDS and Methotrexate

Methotrexate treatment for patients with HIV-associated psoriasis should be limited to those with severe, extensive disease in whom topical and other systemic therapies have failed. Such patients should also receive prophylactic medications for opportunistic infections. Controlled studies of long-term survival are not available. Many of these patients are on sulfa trimethoprin, which should not be used with methotrexate.

Pustular Psoriasis

Patients with generalized pustular psoriasis (von Zumbusch's type) need special attention. With good supportive care, including attention to rehydration, some patients can be followed until clearing without active systemic therapy. A search for infection, drug etiological factors, or both, is necessary. The combination of systemic corticosteroids and methotrexate may increase the risk of further illness and death (Ryan and Baker, 1969). Oral retinoid treatment is the choice for acute pustular psoriasis, alone or in combination with low-dose methotrexate. Methotrexate therapy for pustular psoriasis should be initiated only when the patient is adequately hydrated, with low-doses of methotrexate and careful monitoring of leukocytes and differential counts. Methotrexate should rarely be administered more often than once a week, regardless of the severity of the illness. Dosage increments should be gradual.

APPENDIX B: PATIENT INSTRUCTIONS

Your physician has started you on methotrexate, a potent medicine that can be very effective in treating severe psoriasis. It usually shows initial benefit in 6 to 8 weeks. However, it can cause side effects that occasionally can be serious. Most side effects can be detected *before* they become serious, and for that reason your physician will keep you under close supervision, arranging regular visits and laboratory tests. For your safe treatment, it is important that you carry out your physician's instructions faithfully and promptly report any side effects or symptoms you may develop.

How To Take Methotrexate

Methotrexate is given *weekly*, rather than daily. This is different from most medications. This schedule is critical! The weekly dose is taken as either a single or a divided dose. Taking methotrexate more often or changing the dose schedule in any way can result in serious side effects. If doses are taken too often, notify your physician immediately. If an accidental overdose occurs, an antidote is necessary and must be given as early as possible. Other medicines you are taking may result in an increase in side effects or a decrease in the effectiveness of methotrexate. Tell your physician about *all* the medicines you are taking, whether they are prescription or nonprescription medicines. *Do not begin or change the dosage of any medicine* without first checking with your physician. This is especially true of aspirin, aspirin-like drugs (the so-called nonsteroidal anti-inflammatory drugs), and antibiotics such as Bactrim, Septra, or generic equivalents.

Unrelated medical conditions, especially dehydration, can also increase the risk of methotrexate toxicity. Abdominal upset, when accompanied by significant vomiting, diarrhea, or decreased fluid intake, can lead to dehydration. Excessive thirst may be a symptom of dehydration. Notify your physician if these symptoms develop.

Alcoholic beverages (including beer and wine) will increase some of the side effects, including the chance of liver damage, and should be avoided altogether.

Side Effects

Side effects can occur *at any time* during your treatment. Periodic laboratory tests, such as blood tests, are essential, and sometimes other types of tests arranged by your physician are necessary for the continued safe use of methotrexate. Your cooperation is essential.

The most common side effects caused by methotrexate are fatigue; loss of appetite; nausea (but rarely vomiting); diarrhea; abnormal blood, kidney, or liver test results (the periodic blood tests will check for this); or sores or ulcers in the mouth. If these or other problems trouble you, or if you develop any signs of infection or unusual bleeding, notify your doctor promptly, *before* your next dose of methotrexate is due. These side effects are usually temporary, but changes in dose are frequently required.

Methotrexate is known to cause birth defects and may cause miscarriage or stillbirth, especially in the first 3 months of pregnancy. Pregnant women *must not* take methotrexate, and women of childbearing age *must not* become pregnant while taking methotrexate. An abortion must be considered if one becomes pregnant while on methotrexate. Adequate contraceptive measures are necessary during therapy and for several months thereafter. Consult your physician before considering pregnancy.

A side effect of long-term therapy may be the development of scarring (fibrosis or cirrhosis) in the liver. At times it may be necessary to take a small specimen of liver tissue with a needle (a liver biopsy) to determine whether scarring is present. If and when to do a liver biopsy is a matter of discussion between you and your physician.

In addition, very rarely in psoriasis patients, methotrexate can cause a lung reaction similar to pneumonia. The symptoms are usually fever, cough (often dry and hacking), and shortness of breath (which can become severe). Should you develop such symptoms, notify your physician promptly.

Summary

1. *Follow your physician's instructions carefully.*
2. Take your methotrexate *weekly*, not daily, in one or three doses as directed.
3. Notify your physician *at once* if an accidental overdose is suspected.
4. Notify your physician *at once* if you develop fever, cough, or shortness of breath.
5. If any side effects develop or any symptoms of dehydration occur, notify your physician *before* the next dose of methotrexate.
6. Do not begin or change any medicines without first checking with your physician.
7. Avoid alcoholic beverages.
8. Obtain the tests ordered by your physician.
9. Avoid pregnancy while taking methotrexate and for 3 months after concluding treatment.

Keep this medicine out of the reach of children, and remember that it has been prescribed for your current medical problem. It must not be given to other people.

REFERENCES

1. Gubner, R., August, S., and Ginsberg, V. (1951). Therapeutic suppression of tissue reactivity: effect of aminopterin in rheumatoid arthritis and psoriasis. *Am. J. Med. Sci.* 221:176–182.
2. Rees, R.B., Bennett, J.H., and Bostick, W.L. (1955). Aminopterin for psoriasis. *Arch. Dermatol.* 72:133–143.
3. Edmundson, W.F., and Guy, W.B. (1958). Treatment of psoriasis with folic acid antagonist. *Arch. Dermatol.* 78(2):200–203.
4. Weinstein, G.D., and Frost, P. (1968). Abnormal cell proliferation in psoriasis. *J. Invest. Dermatol.* 50: 254–259.
5. Roenigk, H.H., Jr., Maibach, H.I., and Weinstein, G. (1972). Guidelines on methotrexate therapy for psoriasis. *Arch. Dermatol.* 105:363–365.
6. Roenigk, H.H., Jr., Maibach, H.I., Weinstein, G. (1973). Methotrexate therapy for psoriasis—revision of guidelines. *Arch. Dermatol.* 108:36–42.
7. Roenigk, H.H., Jr., Auerbach, R., Maibach, H.I., and Weinstein, G.D. (1982). Methotrexate guidelines—revised. *J. Am. Acad. Dermatol.* 6:145–155.
8. Roenigk, H.H., Jr., Auerbach, R., Maibach, H.I., and Weinstein, G.D. (1988). Methotrexate in psoriasis: revised guidelines. *J. Am. Acad. Dermatol.* 19:145–156.
9. Health and Public Policy Committee, American College of Physicians (1987). Position paper: methotrexate in rheumatoid arthritis. *Ann. Intern. Med.* 107:418–419.
10. Kremer. J.M., Alancon, G.S., Lightfoot, R.W., et al. (1994). Methotrexate for rheumatoid arthritis: suggested guidelines for monitoring liver toxicity. *Arthritis Rheum.* 37(3):316–328.

11. Roenigk, H.H., Jr., Auerbach, R., Maibach, H.I., Weinstein, G.D., and Lebwohl, M. (1998). *J. Am. Acad. Dermatol.* Accepted.

General Reviews

Greaves, M.W., and Weinstein, G.D. (1995). Drug therapy, treatment of psoriasis. *N. Engl. J. Med.* 332(9):581–588.

Hanno, R., Gruber, G.G., and Owen L.G., et al. (1980). Methotrexate in psoriasis: a brief review of indications, usage, and complications of methotrexate therapy. *J. Am. Acad. Dermatol.* 2:171–174.

Klippel, J.H., and Decker, J.L. (1985). Methotrexate in rheumatoid arthritis. *N. Engl. J. Med.* 312:853–854.

Letendre, P.W., DeJong, D.J., and Miller, D.R. (1985). The use of methotrexate in rheumatoid arthritis. *Drug Intell. Clin. Pharm.* 19(5):349–358.

Liem, W., McCullough, J.L., and Weinstein, G.D. (1995). Effectiveness of topical therapy for psoriasis: results of national survey. *Cutis* 55:306–310.

Peckham, P.E., Weinstein, G.D., and McCullough, J.L. (1987). The treatment of severe psoriasis: a national survey. *Arch. Dermatol.* 123(10):1301–1307.

Roenigk, H.H., Jr., Haserick, J.R., and Curtis, G.H. (1983). Methotrexate for psoriasis. *Cleve. Clin. Q.* 50(2): 101–105.

Roenigk, H.H., Jr., and Maibach, H.I. (1990). Methotrexate. In: *Psoriasis.* 2nd ed. H.H. Roenigk and H.I. Maibach (Eds.). Marcel Dekker, New York, pp. 563–575.

Roenigk, H.H., Jr. (1990). Methotrexate and liver biopsies—is it really necessary? *Arch. Intern. Med.* 150(4):733–734.

Roenigk, H.H., Jr. (1994). Methotrexate therapy. In *Psoriasis.* L. Dubertret (ed.). ISSED, Brescia, Italy, pp. 161–162.

Tung, J.P., and Maibach, H.I. (1990). The practical use of methotrexate in psoriasis. *Drugs* 40(5):697–712.

Weinstein, G.D. (1977). Methotrexate. *Ann. Intern. Med.* 86(2):199–204.

Weinstein, G.D. (1983). Commentary: three decades of folic acid antagonists in dermatology. *Arch. Dermatol.* 119(6): 525–527.

Willkens, R.F. (1983). Reappraisal of the use of methotrexate in rheumatic disease. *Am. J. Med.* 75(4B):19–25.

Liver Toxicity

Ashton, R.E., Millward-Sadler, G.H., and White, J.E. (1982). Complications in methotrexate treatment of psoriasis with particular reference to liver fibrosis. *J. Invest. Dermatol.* 79(4):229–232.

Coe, R.O., and Bull, F.E. (1968). Cirrhosis associated with methotrexate treatment of psoriasis. *JAMA* 206(7): 1515–1520.

Coulson, I.H., McKenzie, J., Neild, V.S., et al. (1987). A comparison of liver ultrasound with liver biopsy histology in psoriatics receiving long-term methotrexate therapy. *Br. J. Dermatol.* 116(4):491–495.

Geronemus, R.G., Auerbach, R., and Tobias, H. (1982). Liver biopsies v. liver scans in methotrexate-treated patients with psoriasis. *Arch. Derm.* 118(9):649–651.

Gilbert, S.C., Klintmalm, G., Menter, A., et al. (1990). Methotrexate-induced cirrhosis requiring liver transplantation in three patients with psoriasis: a word of caution in light of the expanding use of this "steroid-sparing" agent. *Arch. Intern. Med.* 150(4):889–891.

Hendel, J., Poulsen., H., Nyfors, B., et al. (1985). Changes in liver histology during methotrexate therapy of psoriasis correlated to the concentration of methotrexate and folate in erythrocytes. *Acta Pharmacol. Toxicol.* 56(4):321–326.

Hilsden, R.J., Urbanski, S.J., and Swain, M.G. (1995). Endstage liver disease developing with use of methotrexate in heterozygous alpha 1-antitrypsin deficiency. *Arthritis Rheum.* 38(7):1014–1018.

Hoffmeister, R.T., (1983). Methotrexate therapy in rheumatoid arthritis: 15 years experience. *Am. J. Med.* 75(6A): 69–73.

Jones, S.K., Aherne, G.W., Campbell, M.J., et al. (1986). Methotrexate pharmacokinetics in psoriatic patients developing hepatic fibrosis. *Arch. Dermatol.* 122(6): 666–669.

Kremer, J.M., and Lee, J.K. (1986). The safety and efficacy of the use of methotrexate in long-term therapy for rheumatoid arthritis. *Arthritis Rheum.* 29(7):822–831.

Lanse, S.B., Arnold, G.L., Gowans, J.D., et al. (1985). Low incidence of hepatotoxicity associated with long-term, low-dose oral methotrexate in treatment of refractory psoriasis, psoriatic arthritis, and rheumatoid arthritis: an acceptable risk/benefit ratio. *Dig. Dis. Sci.* 30(2):104–109.

Mackenzie, A.H. (1985). Hepatotoxicity of prolonged methotrexate therapy for rheumatoid arthritis. *Cleve. Clin. Q.* 52(2):129–135.

McHenry, P.M., Bingham, E.A., Callender, M.E., et al. (1992). Dynamic hepatic scintigraphy in the screening of psoriatic patients for methotrexate-induced hepatotoxicity. *Br. J. Dermatol.* 127(2):122–125.

Miller, J.A., Dodd, H., and Rustin, M.H., et al. (1985). Ultrasound as a screening procedure for methotrexate-induced hepatic damage in severe psoriasis. *Br. J. Dermatol.* 113(6):699–705.

Mitchell, D., Johnson, R.J., Testa, H.J., et al. (1987). Ultrasound and radionuclide scans—poor indicators of liver damage in patients treated with methotrexate. *Clin. Exp. Dermatol.* 12(4):243–245.

Mitchell, D., Smith, A., Rowan, B., et al. (1990). Serum type III procollagen peptide, dynamic liver function tests and hepatic fibrosis in patients receiving methotrexate. *Br. J. Dermatol.* 122(1):1–7.

Newman, M., Auerbach, R., Feiner, H., et al. (1989). The role of liver biopsies in psoriatic patients receiving long-term methotrexate treatment. *Arch. Derm.* 125:1214–1228.

Nyfors, A., (1977). Liver biopsies from psoriatics related to methotrexate therapy. 3. Findings in post-methotrexate liver biopsies from 160 psoriatics. *Acta Pathol. Microbiol.* 85(4):511–518.

Nyfors, A., and Poulsen, H. (1976). Liver biopsies from psoriatics related to methotrexate therapy. 2. Findings before and after methotrexate therapy in 88 patients: a blind study. *Acta Pathol. Microbiol.* 84(3):262–270.

O'Connor, T.G., Olmstead, E.M., and Zug, K. (1989). Detection of hepatotoxicity associated with methotrexate therapy for psoriasis. *Arch. Derm.* 125:1209–1217.

Pai, S.H., Werthamer, S., and Zak, F.G. (1973). Severe liver damage caused by treatment of psoriasis with methotrexate. *N.Y. State J. Med.* (21):2585–2587.

Reese, L.T., Grisham, J.W., Aach, R.D., et al. (1974). Effects of methotrexate on the liver in psoriasis. *J. Invest. Dermatol.* 62(6):597–602.

Reynolds, F.S., and Lee, W.M. (1986). Hepatotoxicity after long-term methotrexate therapy. *South. Med. J.* 79(5): 536–539.

Robinson, J.K., Baughman, R.D., Auerbach, R., et al. (1980). Methotrexate hepatotoxicity in psoriasis: consideration of liver biopsies at regular intervals. *Arch. Dermatol.* 116(4):413–415.

Roenigk, H.H., Jr., Auerbach, R., Bergfeld, W.F., et al. (1977). A cooperative prospective study of the effects of chemotherapy of psoriasis on liver biopsies. In *Psoriasis.* E.M. Farber and A.J. Cox (eds.). Proceedings of the Second International Symposium. Yorke Medical Books, New York, pp. 243–248.

Tobias, H., and Auerbach, R. (1973). Hepatotoxicity of long-term methotrexate therapy for psoriasis. *Arch. Intern. Med.* 132(3):391–396.

Tolman, K.G., Clegg, D.O., Lee, R.G., et al. (1985). Methotrexate and the liver. *J. Rheumatol.* 12(12):29–34.

Van de Kerkhof, P.C., Hoefnagels, W.H., van Haelst, U.J., et al. (1985). Methotrexate maintenance therapy and liver damage in psoriasis. *Clin. Exp. Dermatol.* 10(3):194–200.

Weinstein, A., Marlowe, S., Korn, J., et al. (1985). Low-dose methotrexate treatment of rheumatoid arthritis: long-term observations. *Am. J. Med.* 79(3):331–337.

Weinstein, G.D., Roenigk, H.H., Jr., Maibach, H.I., et al. (1973). Psoriasis-liver-methotrexate interactions. *Arch. Dermatol.* 108:36–42.

Zachariae, H. (1984). Cytostatic treatment of psoriasis: present status. *Acta Dermatol. Venereol.* 113:127–130.

Zachariae, H., Grunnet, E., and Sogaard, H. (1975). Liver biopsy in methotrexate-treated psoriatics: a reevaluation. *Acta Dermatol. Venereol.* 55:291–296.

Zachariae, H., Kragballe, K., and Sogaard, H., (1980). Methotrexate-induced liver cirrhosis: studies including serial liver biopsies during continued treatment. *Br. J. Dermatol.* 102:407–412.

Zachariae, H., Kragballe, K., Thestrup-Pedersen, K., et al. (1980). Antigens in methotrexate-induced liver cirrhosis. *Acta Dermatol. Venereol.* 60:165–166.

Zachariae, H., and Sogaard, H. (1987). Methotrexate-induced liver cirrhosis: a follow-up. *Dermatologica* 175(4):178–182.

Zachariae, H., Sogaard, H., and Heickendorff. H. (1996). Methotrexate-induced cirrhosis: clinical, histological and serological studies: a further 10-year follow-up. *Dermatology* 192(4):343–346.

Zachariae, H., Aslam, H.M., Bjerring, P., et al. (1991). Serum aminoterminal propeptide of type III procollagen in psoriasis and psoriatic arthritis: relation to liver fibrosis and arthritis. *J. Am. Acad. Dermatol.* 25(1):50–53.

Renal Function

al-Awadhi, A., Dale, P., and McKendry, R.J. (1993). Pancytopenia associated with low-dose methotrexate therapy: a regional survey. *J. Rheumatol.* 20(7):1121–1125.

Cockcroft, D., and Gault, M.H. (1976). Prediction of creatinine clearance from serum creatinine. *Nephron* 16: 31–41.

Hendel, J., and Nyfors, A. (1984). Nonlinear renal elimination kinetics of methotrexate due to saturation of renal tubular reabsorption. *J. Clin. Pharmacol.* 26:121–124.

Kennedy, C., and Baker, H. (1976). Renal function in methotrexate-treated psoriatics [letter]. *Br. J. Dermatol.* 94(6): 702–703.

Kremer, J.M., Petrillo, G.F., and Hamilton, R.A. (1995). Pharmacokinetics and renal function in patients with rheumatoid arthritis receiving a standard dose of oral weekly methotrexate: association with significant decreases in creatinine clearance and renal clearance of the drug after 6 months of therapy. *J. Rheumatol.* 22(1): 38–40.

Kristensen, L.O., Weismann, K., and Hutters, L. (1975). Renal function and the rate of disappearance of methotrexate from serum. *Eur. J. Clin. Pharmacol.* 8(6):439–444.

Rheumatoid Arthritis Clinical Trial Archive Group (1995). The effect of age and renal function on the efficacy and toxicity of methotrexate in rheumatoid arthritis. *J. Rheumatol.* 22(2):218–223.

Van Den Berg, H.W., Murphy, R.F., and Kennedy, D.G. (1980). Rapid plasma clearance and reduced rate and extent of urinary elimination of parenterally administered methotrexate as a result of severe vomiting and diarrhea. *Cancer Chemother. Pharmacol.* 4(1):47–48.

Weismann, K. (1977). Methotrexate therapy for psoriasis in elderly patients with impaired renal function. *Acta Dermatol. Venereol.* 57(2):185.

Drug Interactions

Aherne, G., Piall, E., Marks, V., et al. (1978). Prolongation and enhancement of serum methotrexate concentrations by probenecid. *Br. Med. J.* 1(6120):1097–1099.

Beck, H.I., and Foged, E.K. (1983). Toxic hepatitis due to combination therapy with methotrexate and etretinate in psoriasis. *Dermatologica* 167(2):94–96.

Bourke, R.S., Chheda, G., Bremer, A., et al. (1975). Inhibition of renal tubular transport of methotrexate by probenecid. *Cancer Res.* 35(1):110–116.

Combe, B., Edno, L., Lafforgue, P., et al. (1995). Total and free methotrexate pharmacokinetics, with and without piroxicam in rheumatoid arthritis patients. *Br. J. Rheumatol.* 34(5):421–428.

Hansten, P.D., and Horn, J.R. (1986). Methotrexate and nonsteroidal antiinflammatory drugs. *Drug Interactions Newsl.* 6:41–44.

Hendel, J., and Nyfors, A. (1984). Nonlinear renal elimination kinetics of methotrexate due to saturation of renal tubular reabsorption. *J. Clin. Pharmacol.* 26:121–124.

Lafforgue, P., Monjanel-Mouterde, S., Durand, A., et al. (1993). Is there an interaction between low doses of corticosteroids and methotrexate in patients with rheumatoid arthritis? A pharmacokinetic study in 33 patients. *J. Rheumatol.* 20(2):263–267.

Larsen, F.G., Nielsen-Kudsk, F., Jakobsen, P., et al. (1990). Interaction of etretinate with methotrexate pharmacokintics in psoriatic patients. *J. Clin. Pharmacol.* 30(9): 802–807.

Rooney, T.W., Furst, D.E., Koehnke, R., et al. (1993). Aspirin is not associated with more toxicity than other nonsteroidal anti-inflammatory drugs in patients with rheumatoid arthritis treated with methotrexate. *J. Rheumatol.* 20(8):1297–1302.

Schroder, H., and Ostergaard, J.R. (1994). Interference of high-dose methotrexate in the metabolism of valproate? *Pediatr. Hematol. Oncol.* 11(4):445–449.

Thomas, M.H., and Gutterman, L.A. (1986). Methotrexate toxicity in a patient receiving trimethoprim-sulfamethoxazole. *J. Rheumatol.* 13(2):44–51.

Tracy, T.S., Krohn, K., Jones, D.R., et al. (1992). The effects of a salicylate, ibuprofen, and naproxen on the disposition of methotrexate in patients with rheumatoid arthritis. *Eur. J. Clin. Pharmacol.* 42(2):121–125.

Tracy, T.S., Worster, T., Bradley, J.D., et al. (1994). Methotrexate disposition following concomitant administration of ketoprofen, piroxicam and flurbiprofen in patients with rheumatoid arthritis. *Br. J. Clin. Pharmacol.* 37(5): 453–456.

Vanderveen, E.E., Ellis, C.N., Campbell, J.P, et al. (1982). Methotrexate and etretinate as concurrent therapies in severe psoriasis. *Arch. Dermatol.* 118(9):660–662.

Wallace, C.A., Smith, A.L., and Sherry, D.D. (1993). Pilot investigation of naproxen/methotrexate interaction in patients with juvenile rheumatoid arthritis. *J. Rheumatol.* 20(10):1764–1768.

Zachariae, H. (1984). Methotrexate and etretinate as concurrent therapies in the treatment of psoriasis. *Arch. Dermatol.* 120(2):155.

Combination and Rotational Therapy

Bensen, W., Tugwell, P., Roberts, R.M., et al. (1994). Combination therapy of cyclosporine with methotrexate and gold in rheumatoid arthritis (2 pilot studies). *J. Rheumatol.* 21(11):2034–2038.

Haagsma, C.J., van Riel, P.L., de Rooij, D.J., et al. (1994). Combination of methotrexate sulphasalazine vs methotrexate alone: a randomized open clinical trial in rheumatoid arthritis patients resistant to sulphasalazine therapy. *Br. J. Rheumatol.* 33(11):1049–1055.

Shiroky, J.B. (1995). Combination of sulphasalazine and methotrexate in the management of rheumatoid arthritis-view based on personal clinical experience. *Br. J. Rheumatol.* 34(suppl 2):109–112.

Stern, R.S., and Laird, N. (1994). The carcinogenic risk of treatments for severe psoriasis: photochemotherapy follow-up study. *Cancer* 73(11):2759–2764.

Tugwell, P., Pincus, T., Yocum, D., et al. (1995). Combination therapy with cyclosporine and methotrexate in severe rheumatoid arthritis: the Methotrexate-Cyclosporine Combination Study Group. *N. Engl. J. Med.* 333(3): 137–141.

Weinstein, G.D., and White, G. (1993). Rotational approach to therapy for moderate to severe psoriasis. *J. Am. Acad. Dermatol.* 28(3):454–459.

Adverse Reactions

Altz-Smith, M., Kendall, L.G., Jr., and Stamm, A.M. (1987). Cryptococcosis associated with low-dose methotrexate for arthritis. *Am. J. Med.* 83(1):179–181.

Edelman, J., Russel, A.S., Biggs, D.F., et al. (1983). Methotrexate levels, a guide to therapy? *Clin. Exp. Rheumatol.* 1(2):153–156.

Lambert, R.E., and Kaye, B.R. (1987). Methotrexate and the acquired immunodeficiency syndrome. *Ann. Intern. Med.* 106(5):773.

MacKinnon, S.K., Starkebaum, G., and Willkens, R.F. (1985). Pancytopenia associated with low dose pulse methotrexate in the treatment of rheumatoid arthritis. *Semin. Arthritis Rheum.* 15(2):119–126.

Mallory, S.B., and Berry, D.H. (1986). Severe reactivation of sunburn following methotrexate use. *Pediatrics* 78(3): 514–515.

Marks, C.R., Willkens, R.F., Wilske, K.R., et al. (1984). Small-vessel vasculitis and methotrexate. *Ann. Intern. Med.* 100(6):916.

Okamoto, H., Fukuda, A., Mizuno, K., et al. (1994). Reactivation of phototoxicity test for psoralens plus ultraviolet A by low-dose methotrexate. *Photodermatol. Photoimmunol. Photomed.* 10(3):134–136.

Westwick, T.J., Sherertz, E.E., McCarley, D., et al. (1987). Delayed reactivation of sunburn by methotrexate: sparing of chronically sun-exposed skin. *Cutis* 39(1):49–51.

Winchester, R., Bernstein, D.H., Fischer, H.D., et al. (1987). The co-occurrence of Reiter's syndrome and acquired immunodeficiency. *Ann. Intern. Med.* 106(1):19–26.

Folic Acid

Hills, R.J., Ive, F.A. (1972). Folinic acid rescue used routinely in psoriatic patients with known methotrexate "sensitivity." *Acta Dermatol. Venereol.* 72(6):438–440.

Jobanputra, P., Hunter, M., Clark, D., et al. (1995). An audit of methotrexate and folic acid for rheumatoid arthritis: experience from a teaching centre. *Br. J. Rheumatol.* 34(10):971–975.

Morgan, S.L., Baggott, J.E., Vaughn, W.H., et al. (1994). Supplementation with folic acid during methotrexate therapy for rheumatoid arthritis: a double-blind, placebo-controlled trial. *Ann. Intern. Med.* 121(11):833–841.

Risks of Liver Biopsy

Albert, D.A., Rimon, D., and Silverstein, M.D. (1988). The diagnosis of polyarteritis nodosa. I. A literature-based decision analysis approach. *Arthritis Rheum.* 31(9): 1117–1127.

Piccinino, F., Sagnelli, E., and Pasquale, G., et al. (1986). Complications following percutaneous liver biopsy: a multicentre retrospective study on 68,276 biopsies. *J. Hepatol.* 2:165–173.

Whiting-O'Keefe, Q.E., Fye, K.H., and Sack, K.D. (1991). Methotrexate and histologic hepatic abnormalities: a meta-analysis. *Am. J. Med.* 90(6):711–716.

Pulmonary Toxicity

Akoun, G.M., Gauthier Rahman, S., Mayaud, C.M., et al. (1987). Leukocyte migration inhibition in methotrexate-induced pneumonitis: evidence for an immunologic cell-mediated mechanism. *Chest* 91(1):96–99.

Carson, C.W., Cannon, G.W., Egger, M.J., et al. (1987). Pulmonary disease during the treatment of rheumatoid arthritis with low dose pulse methotrexate. *Semin. Arthritis Rheum.* 16(3):186–195.

Elsasser, S., Dalquen, P., Solar, M., et al. (1989). Methotrexate-induced pneumonitis: appearance four weeks after discontinuation of treatment. *Am. Rev. Respir. Dis.* 140(4):1089–1092.

Hargreaves, M.R., Mowat, A.G., and Benson, M.K. (1992). Acute pneumonitis associated with low dose methotrexate treatment for rheumatoid arthritis: report of 5 cases and review of published reports. *Thorax* 47(8):628–633.

Leduc, D., De-Vuyst, P., Lheureux, P., et al. (1993). Pneumonitis complicating low-dose methotrexate therapy for rheumatoid arthritis: discrepancies between lung biopsy and bronchoalveolar lavage findings. *Chest* 104(5): 1620–1623.

Mulherin, D., Cummiskey, J.M., Doyle, G.D., et al. (1992). Methotrexate pneumonitis in rheumatoid arthritis—a dramatic response to treatment. *Br. J. Rheumatol.* 31(5): 356–357.

Phillips, T.J., Jones, D.H., and Baker, H. (1987). Pulmonary complications following methotrexate therapy. *J. Am. Acad. Dermatol.* 16(2 pt 1): 373–375.

Phillips, T.J., Wallis, P.J., D.H., et al. (1986). Pulmonary function in patients on long-term, low-dose methotrexate. *Br. J. Dermatol* 115(6):657–662.

Pourel, J., Guillemin, F., Fener, P., et al. (1991). Delayed methotrexate pneumonitis in rheumatoid arthritis. *J. Rheumatol.* 18(2):303.

Sostman, H.D., Matthay, R.A., Putman, C.E., et al. (1976). Methotrexate-induced pneumonitis. *Medicine Baltimore* 55(5):371–388.

Pharmacokinetics

Aherene, G.W., and Quinton, M. (1981). Techniques for the measurement of methotrexate in biological samples. *Cancer Treat. Rep.* 65(suppl 1):55–60.

Bertino, J.R. (1982). Clinical pharmacology of methotrexate. *Med. Pediatr. Oncol.* 10(4):401–411.

Campbell, M.A., Perrier, D.G., Dorr, R.T., et al. (1985). Methotrexate: bioavailability and pharmacokinetics. *Cancer Treat. Rep.* 69(7–8):833–838.

Edelman, J., Biggs, D.F., Jamali, F., et al. (1984). Low-dose methotrexate kinetics in arthritis. *Clin. Pharmacol. Ther.* 35(3):382–386.

Evans, W.E., and Christensen, M.L. (1985). Drug interactions with methotrexate. *J. Rheumatol.* 12(12):15–20.

Fulton, R.A., Oxholm, A., and Thomsen, K. (1986). Megaloblastic anemia and methotrexate treatment. *Br. J. Dermatol.* 114:267–269.

Hendel, J. (1985). Clinical pharmacokinetics of methotrexate in psoriasis therapy. *Dan. Med. Bull.* 32(6):329–337.

Hendel, L., Hendel, J., Johnsen, A., et al. (1982). Intestinal function and methotrexate absorption in psoriatic patients. *Clin. Exp. Dermatol.* 7(5):491–497.

Hendel, J., and Nyfors, A. (1985). Impact of methotrexate therapy on the folate status of psoriatic patients. *Clin. Exp. Dermatol.* 10(1):30–35.

Hendel, J., and Nyfors, A. (1984). Nonlinear renal elimination kinetics of methotrexate due to saturation of renal tubular reabsorption. *Eur. J. Clin. Pharmacol.* 26(1): 121–124.

Jolivet, J., Cowan, K.H., Curt, G.A., et al. (1983). The pharmacology and clinical use of methotrexate. *N. Engl. J. Med.* 309(18):1094–1104.

Kozloski, G.D., DeVito, J.M., Kisicki, J.C., et al. (1992). The effect of food on the absorption of methotrexate sodium tablets in healthy volunteers. *Arthritis Rheum.* 35(7):761–764.

Langleben A., Hollomby D., and Hand R., (1982). Case report: management of methotrexate toxicity in an anephric patient. *Clin. Invest. Med.* 5(2–3):129–132.

Maricic, M., Davis, M., and Gall, E.P. (1986). Megaloblastic pancytopenia in a patient receiving concurrent methotrexate and trimethoprim-sulfamethoxazole treatment. *Arthritis Rheum.* 29(1):133–135.

Oguey, D., Kolliker, F., Gerber, N.J., et al. (1992). Effect of food on the bioavailability of low-dose methotrexate in patients with rheumatoid arthritis. *Arthritis Rheum.* 35(6): 611–614.

Zackheim, H.S. (1992). Subcutaneous administration of methotrexate. *J. Am. Acad. Dermatol.* 26(6):1008.

Liver Chemistry Tests and Scans

Coulson, I.H., McKenzie, J., Neild, V.S., et al. (1987). A comparison of liver ultrasound with liver biopsy histology in psoriatics receiving long-term methotrexate therapy. *Br. J. Dermatol.* 116(4):491–495.

Hulcrantz, R., and Gabrielsson, N., (1993). Patients with persistent elevation of aminotransferases: investigation with ultrasonography, radionuclide imaging and liver biopsy. *J. Intern. Med.* 233(1):7–12.

McHenry, P.M., Bingham, E.A., Callender, M.E., et al. (1992). Dynamic hepatic scintigraphy in the screening of psoriatic patients for methotrexate-induced hepatotoxicity. *Br. J. Dermatol.* 127(2):122–125.

Miller, J.A., Dodd, H., Rustin, M.H., et al. (1985). Ultrasound as a screening procedure for methotrexate-induced hepatic damage in severe psoriasis. *Br. J. Dermatol.* 113: 699–705.

Mitchell, D., Johnson, R.J., Testa, H.J., et al. (1987). Ultrasound and radionuclide scans—poor indicators of liver damage in patients treated with methotrexate. *Clin. Exp. Dermatol.* 12(4):243–245.

Rademacher, M., Web, J.A., Lowe, D.G., et al. (1987). Magnetic resonance imaging as a screening procedure for methotrexate induced liver damage. *Br. J. Dermatol.* 117(3):311–316.

VanDooren-Greebe, R.J., Kuipers, A.L., Buijs, W.C., et al. (1996). The value of dynamic heptic scintigraphy and serum aminoterminal propeptide of type III procollagen for early detection of methotrexate-induced hepatic damage in psoriasis patients. *Br. J. Dermatol.* 134:481–487.

Malignancy

Bagshawe, K.D. (1976). Risk and prognostic factors in trophoblastic neoplasia. *Cancer* 38(3):1373–1385.

Bailin, P.L., Tindall, J.P., Roenigk, H.H., Jr., et al. (1975). Is methotrexate therapy for psoriasis carcinogenic? A modified retrospective-prospective analysis. *JAMA* 232(4):359–362.

Kenysmore, S.F., Hall, B.D., Alter, N.B., Rice, Jr. (1992). Association of methotrexate, rheumatoid arthritis, and lymphoma: report on 2 cases and literature review. *J. Rheumatol.* 19(9):1462–1465.

IARC (International Agency for Research on Cancer) Working Group (1981). Methotrexate. *IARC Monogr. Eval. Carcinog. Risk. Chem. Hum.* 26:267–292.

Lindelof, B., Siegersson B. (1993). PUVA and cancer: a case control study. *Br. J. Dermatol.* 129:39–41.

Moder, K.G., Tefkie A., Cohen, M.D. (1995). Hematologic malignancies and use of methotrexate in rheumatoid arthritis: a retrospective study. *Am. J. Med.* 99(3):276–281.

Nyfors, A., and Jensen, H. (1983). Frequency of malignant neoplasms in 248 long-term methotrexate-treated psoriatics: a preliminary study. *Dermatologica* 167(5): 260–261.

Rustin, G.J., Rustin, F., Dent, J., et al. (1983). No increase in second tumors after cytotoxic chemotherapy for gestational trophoblastic tumors. *N. Engl. J. Med.* 308(9): 473–476.

Stern, R.S., Zierler, S., and Parrish, J.A. (1982). Methotrexate used for psoriasis and the risk of noncutaneous or cutaneous malignancy. *Cancer* 50(5):869–872.

Stern, R.S., Laird N. (1994). The carcinogenic risk of treatments for severe psoriasis *Cancer* 73:2759–2764.

Zimmer-Galber, I., Lie, J.T. (1994). Choroidal infiltrates as the initial manifestation of lymphoma in rheumatoid arthritis after treatment with methotrexate. *Mayo Clinic Proc.* 69(3):258–261.

Reproductive Effects

Grunnet, E., Nyfors, A., and Hansen, K.B. (1977). Studies on human semen in topical corticosteroid-treated and in methotrexate-treated psoriatics. *Dermatologica* 154(2): 78–84.

Jensen, M.K. (1967). Chromosome studies in patients treated with azathioprine and amethopterin. *Acta Med. Scand.* 182(4):445–455.

Jensen, M.K., and Nyfors, A. (1979). Cytogenetic effects of methotrexate on humans cells in vivo: comparison between results obtained by chromosome studies on bone-marrow cells and blood lymphocytes and by the micronucleus test. *Mutat. Res.* 65(5):339–343.

Kozlowski, R.D., Steinbrunner, J.V., MacKenzie, A.H., et al. (1990). Outcome of first-trimester exposure to low-dose methotrexate in eight patients with rheumatic disease. *Am. J. Med.* 88(6):589–592.

Melnyk, J., Duffy, D.M., and Sprikes, R.S. (1971). Human mitotic and meiotic chromosome damage following in vivo exposure to methotrexate. *Clin. Genet.* 2(1):28–31.

Milunsky, A., Graef J.W., and Gaynor, M.F., Jr. (1968). Methotrexate-induced congenital malformations. *J. Pediatr.* 72(6):790–795.

Morris, L.F., Harrod, M.J., Menter, M.A., et al. (1993). Methotrexate and reproduction in men: case report and recommendations. *J. Am. Acad. Dermatol.* 29(5 pt 2): 913–916.

Perry, W.H. (1983). Methotrexate and teratogenesis. *Arch. Dermatol.* 119(11):874–875.

Powell, H.R., and Ekert, H. (1971). Methotrexate-induced congenital malformations. *Med. J. Aust.* 2(21): 1076–1077.

Ross, G.T. (1976). Congenital anomalies among children born to mothers receiving chemotherapy for gestational trophoblastic neoplasms. *Cancer* 37(2):1043–1047.

Van Thiel, D.H., Ross, G.T., and Lipsett, M.B. (1970). Pregnancies after chemotherapy of trophoblastic neoplasms. *Science* 169(952):1326–1327.

Voorhees, J.J., Janzen, M.K., Harrell, E.R., and Chakraborti, S.G. (1969). Cytogenetic evaluations of methotrexate-treated psoriatic patients. *Arch. Dermatol.* 100:269–274.

Walden, P.A., and Bagshawe, K.D. (1976). Reproductive performance of women successfully treated for gestational trophoblastic tumors. *Am. J. Obstet. Gynecol.* 125(8):1108–1114.

Weinstein, G.D. (1977). Methotrexate. *Ann. Intern. Med.* 86: 199–204.

AIDS and Methotrexate

Duvic, M., Johnson, T.M., Rapini, R.P., et al. (1987). Acquired immunodeficiency syndrome–associated psoriasis and Reiter's syndrome. *Arch. Dermatol.* 123(12): 1622–1632.

Maurer, T.A., Zackheim, H.S., Tuffanelli, L., et al. (1994). The use of methotrexate for treatment of psoriasis in patients with HIV infection. *J. Am. Acad. Dermatol.* 31: 372–375.

Pustular Psoriasis

Hoffman, T.E., and Watson, W. (1978). Methotrexate toxicity in the treatment of generalized pustular psoriasis. *Cutis* 21(1):68–71.

Horiguchi, M., Takigawa, M., Imamura, S. (1981). Treatment of generalized pustular psoriasis with methotrexate and colchicine. *Arch. Dermatol.* 117(12):760.

Hubler, W.R., Jr. (1984). Familial juvenile generalized pustular psoriasis. *Arch. Dermatol.* 120(9):1174–1175.

Rosenbaum, M.M., and Roenigk, H.H., Jr. (1984). Treatment of generalized pustular psoriasis with etretinate (Ro 10-9359) and methotrexate. *J. Am. Acad. Dermatol.* 102: 357–361.

Ryan, T.J. and Baker, H.S. (1969). Systemic corticosteroids and folic acid antagonists in the treatment of generalized pustular psoriasis: evaluation and prognosis based on the study of 104 cases. *Br. J. Dermatol.* 91(12):134–145.

50

Hydroxyurea

Stephen Wright and Brian Gemzik
Abbott Laboratories, Chicago, Illinois

HISTORY

Hydroxyurea was first synthesized in 1869 (1). It occurs as a white crystalline powder, which is essentially tasteless. Hydroxyurea is a simple molecule, which was investigated as a potential anticancer drug 70 years ago when it was shown to be capable, in large doses, of inducing anemia, megaloblastic bone marrow changes, and leukopenia I rabbits (2). Interest then lapsed until anticancer activity was again demonstrated in experimental animals in 1960 (3), leading to a resurgence of interest among oncologists (4,5) and many subsequent publications. Its use in psoriasis was described in a single patient by Yarbro in 1969 (6), and the first controlled study in a group of 10 patients was published in 1970 (7).

PHARMACOLOGY/TOXICOLOGY

Hydroxyurea inhibits DNA synthesis by direct inhibition of ribonucleotide reductase, presumably through the nonenzymatic formation of a nitroxyl radical (8). This reductase reduces ribonucleotides to deoxyribonucleotides and its activity is thought to depend on a cation radical of tyrosine at its active site. This unusual radical is stabilized by two molecules of nonheme ferric iron and oxygen and can be scavenged by hydroxyurea, which results in activation of the enzyme. In this manner, hydroxyurea is an inhibitor of cell turnover and is specific for the S phase of the cell cycle.

The clinical pharmacokinetics of hydroxyurea have not been extensively studied (9–12). In practice, dosages are adjusted based on potential hematological effects rather than pharmacokinetic considerations. Following a therapeutic oral dose, peak plasma concentrations are typically reached within 2 hr with an elimination half-life of less than 6 hr. Plasma concentrations show a large degree of interindividual variability. Hydroxyurea is readily bioavailable in humans and distributes in appreciable concentrations to tissues as well as to cerebrospinal fluid and breast milk (13,14). Clearance by the kidney appears to be the primary route of elimination in animals and humans. 10–90% of an administered dose is mostly recovered as hydroxyurea in the urine within 48 hr. Studies in rodents indicate enzymatic reduction of hydroxyurea to urea by the liver and kidney (15,16).

Hematopoietic toxicity is the dose-limiting effect of hydroxyurea (17,18). Abnormal elevations in enzymes indicative of liver toxicity, most notably serum transaminase levels, have been reported. In one case, hepatitis was found to be recurrent upon rechallenge with drug (19). Elevations of serum creatinine and urea nitrogen, and proteinuria have been reported at relatively high dosages (20). However, two cases of renal failure occurred in elderly patients following chronic therapy for polycythemia vera (21).

Positive results of hydroxyurea in a number of in vivo and in vitro assays of mutagenicity are consistent with its mechanism of action as an inhibitor of DNA synthesis. Genotoxicity mediated by reactive oxygen species formed during biotransformation of hydroxyurea has also been suggested (22,23). Treatment of chronic myeloproliferative disorders with hydroxyurea has been associated with chromosomal abnormalities and a potential increased risk of acute leukemia (24–26).

Hydroxyurea demonstrated little or no carcinogenic potency in mice or rats treated with 125 or 250 mg/kg by intraperitoneal injection three times a week for 6 months followed by an additional year without treatment (27). A lack of tumorigenicity was reported in a study in which mice were treated weekly with 500 mg/kg by intraperitoneal injection for 1 year (28). However, neither of these studies adequately establishes the lack of carcinogenic potential of hydroxyurea in rodents or risk for chronic therapeutic use.

Hydroxyurea is a teratogen in all animal species in which it has been evaluated (29). Fetal growth retardation and malformations were observed in rhesus monkeys following maternal treatment at an oral dosage of 100 mg/kg/day during the period of major organogenesis (30,31). However, several cases of pregnancy with successful outcomes have been reported during therapeutic use of hydroxyurea (32–35). In addition, reproductive competence has been reported for males while on chronic hydroxyurea therapy (36).

CLINICAL EXPERIENCE

The first reports that hydroxyurea might have efficacy in the treatment of psoriasis came in 1969 (6,37) when three cases of refractory psoriasis were reported to have responded well to hydroxyurea. Subsequently, a controlled study of 10 patients treated with 500 mg twice daily for 4 weeks confirmed the efficacy of hydroxyurea in refractory psoriasis (7). In this crossover study, patients continued with hydroxyurea at the end of the study, and the authors suggested that the maximum response occurred after 6 weeks of therapy. After treatment was stopped, several patients remained in long-term remission. Soon afterward, Rosten reported somewhat less favorable results in 12 patients with refractory psoriasis treated with doses between 1.5 and 2 g daily (38). Only half the patients improved: two failed to do so even after 8 weeks of treatment and 4 of 12 patients had to stop the drug because of drug-related adverse events.

The first large-scale study was reported by Moschella and Greenwald in 1973 (39). Sixty patients with severe incapacitating psoriasis were given intermittent courses of hydroxyurea over 18 months. Unfortunately, treatment was not blinded in any way, and was prescribed according to a protocol that titrated duration of therapy with hydroxyurea against clinical response and the occurrence of adverse events. Although these patients had all been refractory to previous treatment, including methotrexate in many cases, results with hydroxyurea were good: 63% of the patients had a "good to excellent" response within 6 weeks of therapy at 500 mg twice daily. In this study, "good to excellent" was defined as better than 60% of lesions clearing. A poor response occurred in 17% of patients. Those patients who responded generally maintained their response over an 18-month treatment period. Hydroxyurea was given in treatment courses that lasted between 4 and 12 weeks and were repeated as and when the patient relapsed. Results in pustular psoriasis were not generally as good as in patients with psoriasis vulgaris.

The authors drew attention to a flu-like syndrome occurring in six patients, and interestingly, to one case of fixed drug eruption that they attributed to hydroxyurea. There was no evidence of hepatotoxicity in these patients.

Overall, 15% of patients had to be withdrawn from treatment owing to drug-related adverse events. The authors concluded that the drug was toxic enough to be reserved for patients with extensive psoriasis who required a rapid response to therapy without the need for hospitalization.

By 1976, 19% of 510 dermatologists surveyed indicated that they used hydroxyurea in the treatment of psoriasis, compared with 52% who used methotrexate (40).

More long-term experience of hydroxyurea was reported by Baker, who reported less enthusiastically on more than 100 patients treated for up to 6–8 years (41). He stressed the lack of gastrointestinal side effects or hepatotoxicity seen even with this prolonged treatment. Clinical response in 63% of patients was judged to be worthwhile to excellent in the short term, although Baker reported in a previous edition of this book that long-term therapy was maintained in only a few of these because of side effects, relapse while on hydroxyurea, or therapeutic failure (42).

A further contribution to defining the place of hydroxyurea in the therapy of psoriasis came with the publication of a long-term study of 85 patients in 1989. Layton et al. found a satisfactory response to treatment in 61% of patients, a figure remarkably similar to those reported earlier (43). While significant hematological abnormalities (anemia and/or leukopenia and/or thrombocytopenia) developed in 35% of patients, these were always reversible within 6–8 weeks on reducing the dose or on stopping therapy altogether.

Pustular Psoriasis

There has been no systematic study of the effect of hydroxyurea on pustular psoriasis. Stein et al. reported good results in an open study of four patients with generalized pustular psoriasis of the von Zumbusch type (44). In these patients, both the cutaneous and systemic manifestations of GPP improved, but treatment was limited to only a few weeks. Moschella and Greenwald reported very limited success in two patients with generalized pustular psoriasis, and no success at all in two patients with pustular psoriasis of the palms and soles (39). The lack of therapeutic efficacy of hydroxyurea in therapy of palmoplantar pustular psoriasis is confirmed by Hattel and Sondergaard (45).

Psoriatic Erythroderma

In one patient with generalized exfoliative psoriasis of 2 years' duration, an impressive clinical response was seen (39). The response was maintained for several months until bone marrow toxicity compelled withdrawal of the drug.

Topical Use of Hydroxyurea

Encouraging results were reported by Zackheim et al. with 10 and 15% hydroxyurea in a cream base (46). When used under continuous occlusion, hydroxyurea cream was significantly better than base cream alone, and local irritation developed in very few patients. However, there was little if any effect without the use of occlusive wraps, and the authors concluded that topical hydroxyurea would be of limited use in the treatment of psoriasis.

Hydroxyurea in Combination

The combination of more than one chemotherapeutic agent seems an attractive option, with the possibility of enhancing efficacy without increasing toxicity. In the field of solid tumor chemotherapy, hydroxyurea is synergistic in vitro with cisplatin, floxuridine, and 5-fluorouracil, although convincing evidence of this synergy in vivo is lacking (8). Sauer treated 14 patients with a combination of methotrexate, up to 12.5 mg weekly, and hydroxyurea, 500 mg daily, with a treatment duration between 3 and 22 months (47). Response was considered "adequate" in 13/14 patients, although there is no description of what defines an "adequate" response. The results were encouraging enough for the authors to recommend further studies. None have been reported. The questionnaire study reported by Bergstresser et al. (40) showed that a number of dermatologists use hydroxyurea in combination with systemic corticosteroids. Unfortunately, no clinical results of this combination have been reported. In the experience of this author, the combination of hydroxyurea with methotrexate is no longer used.

Wright et al. studied hydroxyurea in combination with etretinate in therapy-resistant patients (48). We achieved a satisfactory clinical response in long-term therapy in about 50% of patients.

Hydroxyurea in Other Indications

Enthusiasm for the use of hydroxyurea in the chemotherapy of solid tumors has waxed and waned since the drug was first introduced into clinical use, and today it is not used routinely in the therapy of any solid tumor. Its most promising future in this field may lie in the apparent ability of the drug to increase the rate of loss of resistance to other agents, notably cisplatin, by its inhibitory action on ribonucleotide reductase, and consequent enhancement of cisplatin cytotoxicity (49).

Interestingly, this biochemical effect of hydroxyurea has led to the drug being tested in several large-scale clinical trials in human immunodeficiency virus disease, where it may be synergistic with antiviral agents (50).

Hydroxyurea is used in the treatment of both acute and chronic myelogenous leukemia, and myeloproliferative syndromes (17). Polycythemia rubra vera is now routinely treated with hydroxyurea. Charache et al. (32) reported hydroxyurea to be highly effective in preventing sickle cell crises in sickle cell disease, probably by increasing the production of fetal hemoglobin in red cells.

Adverse Reactions to Hydroxyurea

The use of hydroxyurea is limited by its hematological toxicity. It induces a dose-related megaloblastic erythropoiesis in all patients within a few days of the start of treatment (51). This is believed to occur because of impaired DNA synthesis in the presence of continuing RNA synthesis, which results in large red cells with a reduced capacity for cell division. In general, the macrocytosis seen in all patients will resolve within 6–8 weeks of ceasing treatment, but has been observed to persist for 6 months (43). A mild to moderate anemia is common. Reduced white cell counts occur less often, but may be severe, and thrombocytopenia occurs in as few as 2% of treated patients. The bone marrow suppression associated with the mechanism of action of the drug is always reversible.

Apart from these predictable hematological effects, the most common side effect is probably an influenza-like symptom complex, with low-grade fever, malaise, and muscle aches (39). It has been described in association with a cutaneous vasculitis (52). With the higher doses of 1.5–2 g daily used by Rosten, lassitude, vertigo, headache, mouth ulceration, epistaxis, and rectal hemorrhage were reported (38). Libido was affected in one 53-year-old woman; the effect was evident three times when the drug was withdrawn and restarted. A recent report suggests that patients treated with hydroxyurea in the long term may develop anti-DNA and antiphospholipid antibodies (53), in one case apparently progressing to a syndrome indistinguishable from systemic lupus erythematosus (54).

A variety of cutaneous adverse reactions have also been reported. Some of these are clearly attributable to hydroxyurea. Generalized pigmentation is described in up to 44% of patients after long-term therapy (55) and both horizontal and vertical pigmented bands have been described in the fingernails (56). The pigment stains positive for melanin. Although there has been one report of increased melanocyte-stimulating hormone in association with hydroxyurea-induced hyperpigmentation, in fact the mechanism of pigmentation is believed to be local rather than systemic (57). Diffuse alopecia occurs, which is reversible when the drug is stopped (58). Cutaneous erosions have been reported rarely.

Cutaneous ulcers of the lower leg have been reported in elderly patients receiving hydroxyurea for the treatment of myelogenous leukemia (59). In one series, 82% of the ulcers healed when the drug was stopped, suggesting a casual relationship (60).

SUMMARY

In 1973, Leavell et al. (61) published the results of a postal survey they conducted among U.S. dermatologists. At that time, when asked to compare it with methotrexate, they reported that hydroxyurea was believed to be less effective, but was safer, with fewer side effects. In the quarter-century since that survey was published, it seems unlikely that views will have changed much. Hydroxyurea has undoubted antipsoriatic efficacy in up to 60% of therapy-resistant patients at a dose of 1.0–1.5 g daily. Its potency is undoubtedly less than that of methotrexate. When the daily dose exceeds 1.5 g, side effects are inevitable. The bone marrow suppression caused by hydroxyurea is always reversible over a period of a few weeks, and there have been no deaths reported due to the drug. While this relative lack of serious toxicity may seem to be a major advantage, it is counterbalanced by the undoubtedly narrow margin between the dose associated with therapeutic efficacy and that associated with toxicity.

REFERENCES

1. Dresler, E.F.C., and Stein, R. (1869). Uber den hydroxylharnstoff. *Liebig Ann. Chem.* 150:242–252.
2. Rosenthal, F., Wislicki, L., and Kollek, L. (1928). Uber die beziehungen von schwersten blutgiften zu abbauprodukten des eiweisses; ein beitrag zum entsehungsmechanismus der perniziosen anemie. *Klin. Wochenschr.* 7:972–977.
3. Stock, C.C., Clarke, D.A., Phillips, F.S., et al. (1960). Sarcoma 180 screening data. *Cancer Res.* 20:193–381.
4. Stearns, B., Losee, K.A., and Bernstein, J. (1963). Hydroxyurea: a new type of potential anti-tumor agent. *J. Med. Chem.* 6:201.
5. Yarbro, J.W., Kennedy, B.J., and Barnum, C.P. (1965). Hydroxyurea inhibition of DNA synthesis in ascites tumour. *Pro. Natl. Acad. Sci. U.S.A.* 53:1033–1035.
6. Yarbro, J.W. (1969). Hydroxyurea in the treatment of refractory psoriasis. *Lancet* 2:846–847.
7. Leavell, U.W., and Yarbro, J.W. (1970). Hydroxyurea: a new treatment for psoriasis. *Arch. Dermatol.* 102: 144–150.
8. Yarbro, J.W. (1992). Mechanism of action of hydroxyurea. *Semin. Oncol.* 19(Suppl. 9):1–10.
9. Rosner, F., Rubin, H., and Parise, F. (1971). Studies on the absorption, distribution and excreation of hydroxyurea (NSC-32065). *Cancer Chemother. Rep.* 55: 167–173.
10. Davidson, J.D., and Winter, T.S. (1963). A method of analyzing for hydroxyurea in biological fluids. *Cancer Chemother. Rep.* 27:97–110.

11. Bolton, J., Woods, L.A., Kaung, D.T., and Lawton, R.L. (1965). A simple method of colorimetric analysis for hydroxyurea (NSC-32065). *Cancer Chemother. Rep.* 46:1–5.
12. Creasey, W.A., Capizzi, R.L., and DeConti, R.C. (1970). Clinical and biochemical studies of high-dose intermittent therapy of solid tumors with hydroxyurea. *Cancer Chemother. Rep.* 54:191–193.
13. Beckloff, G.L., and Lerner, H.J., Frost, D., et al. (1965). Hydroxyurea in biologic fluids: dose-concentration relationship. *Cancer Chemother. Rep.* 48:57–58.
14. Sylvester, R.K., Lobell, M., Teresi, M., et al. (1987). Excretion of hydroxyurea into milk. *Cancer* 60: 2177–2178.
15. Colvin, M., and Bobo, V.H. (1970). The enzymatic reduction of hydroxyurea to urea by mouse liver. *Cancer Res.* 30:1516–1519.
16. Adamson, R.H., Ague, S.L., Hess, S.M., and Davidson, J.D. (1965). The distribution, excretion and metabolism of hydroxyurea-C^{14}. *J. Pharmacol. Exp. Ther.* 150:322–327.
17. Donehower, R.C. (1992). An overview of the clinical experience with hydroxyurea. *Semin. Oncol.* 19(Suppl. 9): 11–19.
18. Boyd, A.S., and Neldner, K.H. (1991). Hydroxyurea therapy. *J. Am. Acad. Dermatol.* 25:518–524.
19. Samuals, M.L., and Howe, C.D. (1964). Renal abnormalities induced by hydroxyurea (NSC-32065). *Cancer Chemother. Rep.* 40:9–13.
20. Heddle, R., and Calvert, A.F. (1980). Hydroxyurea induced hepatitis. *Med. J. Aus.* 1:121.
21. Sharon, S., Tatarsky, I., and Ben-Ariah, Y. (1986). Treatment of polycythemia vera with hydroxyurea. *Cancer* 57:718–720.
22. Rossberger, S., and Andrae, U. (1985). DNA repair synthesis induced by *N*-hydroxyurea, acetohydroxamic acid, and *N*-hydroxyurethane in primary rat hepatocyte cultures: comparative evaluation using the autoradiographic and the bromodeoxyuridine density-shift method. *Mutat. Res.* 145:201–207.
23. Andrae, U. (1984). Evidence for the involvement of cytochrome P-450-dependent monooxygenase(s) in the formation of genotoxic metabolites from *N*-hydroxyurea. *Biochem. Biophys. Res. Commun.* 118: 409–415.
24. Weinfeld, A., Swolin, B., and Westin, J. (1994). Acute leukemia after hydroxyurea therapy in polycythemia and related disorders: prospective study of efficacy and leukaemogenicity with therapeutic implications. *Eur. J. Haematol.* 52:134–139.
25. Diez-Martin, J.L., Graham, D.L., Pettit, R.M., and Dewald, G.W. (1991). Chromosome studies in 104 patients with polycythemia vera. *Mayo Clin Proc.* 66: 287–299.
26. Siver, R.T. (1995). Hydroxyurea and sickle cell crises. *N. Engl. J. Med.* 33:1008–1009.
27. Weisburger, E.K. (1977). Bioassay program for carcinogenic hazards of cancer chemotherapeutic agents. *Cancer* 40:1935–1949.
28. Muranyi-Kovacs, I., and Rudali, G. (1972). Comparative study of carcinogenic activity of hydroxyurea and urethane n XVII/G mice. *Rev. Eur. Etudes Clin. Biol.* 17:93–95.
29. Murphy, M.L., and Chaube, S. (1964). Preliminary survey of hydroxyurea (NSC-32065) as a teratogen. *Cancer Chemother. Rep.* 40:1–7.
30. Theisen, C.T., Fradkin, R., and Wilson, J.G. (1973). Teratogenicity of hydroxyurea in rhesus monkeys. *Teratology* 7:A–29.
31. Wilson, J.G., Scott, W.J., Ritter, E.J., et al. (1975). Comparative distribution and embryotoxicity of hydroxyurea in pregnant rats and rhesus monkeys. *Teratology* 11:168–178.
32. Charache, S., Terrin, M.L., Moore, R.D., et al. (1995). Effect of hydroxyurea on the frequency of painful crises in sickle cell anemia. *N. Engl. J. Med.* 332: 1317–1322.
33. Tertian, G., Tchernia, G., Papiernik, E., and Elefant, E. (1992). Hydroxyurea and pregnancy. *Am. J. Obstet. Gynecol.* 166:1868.
34. Cinkotai, K.I., Wood, P., Donnai, P., and Kendra, J. (1994). Pregnancy after treatment with hydroxyurea in a patient with primary thrombocythaemia and history of recurrent abortion. *J. Clin. Pathol.* 47:769–770.
35. Patel, M., Dukes, I.A.F., and Hull, J.C. (1991). Use of hydroxyurea in chronic myeloid leukemia during pregnancy: a case report. *Am. J. Obstet. Gynecol.* 165: 565–566.
36. Triadou, P., Maier-Redelsperger, M., Krishnamoorty, R., et al. (1994). Fetal haemoglobin variations following hydroxyurea treatment in patients with cyanotic congenital heart disease. *Nouv. Rev. Fr. Hematol.* 36: 367–372.
37. Yarbro, J.W., and Leavell, U.W. (1969). Hydroxyurea: a new agent for the management of refractory psoriasis: *J. Kentucky Med. Assoc.* 67:899.
38. Rosten, M. (1971). Hydroxyurea: a new antimetabolite in the treatment of psoriasis. *Br. J. Dermatol.* 85: 177–181.
39. Moschella, S.L., and Greenwald, M.A. (1973). Psoriasis with hydroxyurea: an 18 month study of 60 patients. *Arch. Dermatol.* 107:363–368.
40. Bergstresser, P.R., Schreiber, S.H., and Weinstein, G.D. (1976). Systemic chemotherapy for psoriasis. A national survey. *Arch. Dermatol.* 112:977–981.
41. Baker, H. (1982). Hydroxyurea for psoriasis. In *Psoriasis. Proceedings of the 3rd International Symposium.* E.M. Farber and A.J. Cox (Eds.). Grune & Stratton, New York, p. 119.

42. Baker, H. (1985). Hydroxyurea. In *Psoriasis*. H.I. Maibach, and H.H. Roenigk (eds.). Marcel Dekker, New York, pp. 451–455.
43. Layton, A.M., Sheehan-Dare, R.A., Goodfield, M.J.D., and Cotterill, J.A. (1989). Hydroxyurea in the management of therapy resistant psoriasis. *Br. J. Dermatol.* 121:647–653.
44. Stein, K.M., Shelley, W.B., and Weinberg, R.A. (1971). Hydroxyurea in the treatment of pustular psoriasis. *Br. J. Dermatol.* 85:81–85.
45. Hattel, T., and Sondergaard, J. (1974). Pustulosis palmaris et plantaris treated with hydroxyurea. *Acta Derm. Venereol. (Stockh.)* 54:152–154.
46. Zackheim, H.S., Karasek, M.A., and Cox, A.J. (1972). Topical hydroxyurea and psoriasis. *J. Invest. Dermatol.* 58:24–27.
47. Sauer, G.C. (1973). Combined methotrexate and hydroxyurea therapy for psoriasis. *Arch. Dermatol.* 107: 369–370.
48. Wright, S., Baker, H., and Warin, A.P. (1990). Treatment of psoriasis vulgaris with a combination of etretinate and hydroxyurea. *J. Dermatol. Treat.* 1:211–213.
49. Albain, K.S., Swinnen, L.J., Erickson, L.C., et al. (1992). Cytotoxic synergy of cisplatin with concurrent hydroxyurea and cytarabine: summary of an in vitro model and initial clinical pilot experience. *Semin. Oncol.* 19:102–109.
50. Voelker, R. (1995). Cancer drug may join AIDS arsenal. Medical news and Perspectives. *J.A.M.A.* 274:523.
51. Bergsagel, D.E., Frenkel, E.P., Alfrey, C.P., and Thurman, W.G. (1964). Megaloblastic erythropoiesis induced hydroxyurea. *Cancer Chemother. Rep.* 40: 15–17.
52. Roe, L.D., and Wilson, J.W. (1973). Hydroxyurea therapy. *Arch. Dermatol.* 108:426–427.
53. Layton, A.M., and Cotterill, J.A. (1992). Hydroxyurea induced collagen disease. *Br. J. Dermatol.* 120(Suppl. 40):35 (abstract).
54. Layton, A.M., Cotterill, J.A., and Tomlinson, I.W. (1993). Hydroxyurea-induced lupus erythematosus. *Br. J. Dermatol.* 121:687–688.
55. Dahl, M., and Comaish, J.S. (1972). Long-term effects of hydroxyurea in psoriasis. *Br. Med. J.* 4:585–587.
56. Gropper, C.A., Don, P.C., and Sadjadi, M.M. (1993). Nail and skin hyperpigmentation associated with hydroxyurea therapy for polycythemia vera. *Int. J. Dermatol.* 32:731–733.
57. Hendrix, J.D., and Greer, K.E. (1992). Cutaneous hyperpigmentation caused by systemic drugs. *Int. J. Dermatol.* 31:458–465.
58. Kennedy, B.J., Smith, R., and Goltz, R.W. (1975). Skin changes secondary to hydroxyurea therapy. *Arch. Dermatol.* 111:183–187.
59. Nguyen, T.V., and Margolis, D.J. (1993). Hydroxyurea and lower leg ulcers. *Cutis* 52:217–219.
60. Montefusco, E., Alimena, G., Gastaldi, R., et al. (1986). Unusual dermatologic toxicity of long-term therapy with hydroxyurea in chronic myelogenous leukemia. *Tumori* 72:317–321.
61. Leavell, U.W., Mersack, I.P., and Smith, C. (1973). Survey of the treatment of psoriasis with hydroxyurea. *Arch. Dermatol.* 107:467.

51

6-Thioguanine

Herschel S. Zackheim, Richard G. Glogau, and David A. Fisher
University of California, San Francisco, California

Howard I. Maibach
University of California School of Medicine, San Francisco, California

6-Thioguanine (6-TG), a purine analog closely related to two other purine analogs, 6-mercaptopurine and azathioprine (Fig. 1), is mainly used for induction and maintenance therapy in acute myelogenous leukemia. The principal mechanism of action is inhibition of purine synthesis and interconversions by 6-TG ribonucleotide. Clearance is primarily hepatic. Myelosuppression is the most frequent toxicity (1).

We first described our experience with 6-TG in psoriasis in 1982 (2), and our most recent publication appeared in 1994 (3).

DRUG ADMINISTRATION

6-TG is available as 40-mg tablets (Burroughs Wellcome). All daily doses were given as an undivided dose.

A number of dosage schedules have been used during the long period of this study. For patients in an acute generalized flare a daily dose appears to be the most dependable in achieving rapid suppression of disease activity. The initial daily dose is 40 mg. If the response is inadequate and laboratory values remain within normal limits, this is increased after 2 weeks to an alternating daily dose of 40 mg and 80 mg. After an additional 2 weeks the dose is increased to 80 mg daily as needed and tolerated. Our maximum daily dose is 160 mg. Most patients respond to a daily dose of 80 mg.

For patients with stable but resistant disease the daily dose or a twice-weekly schedule given on days 1 and 3 (preferred by one of us, RG) can be used. The twice-weekly schedule usually starts at 80 mg and is gradually increased every 2 weeks by 20-mg increments as needed and tolerated. The highest dosage given twice weekly is 280 mg. Most patients respond to 120 or 160 mg twice weekly. Other schedules include five consecutive daily or thrice-weekly doses.

Since 6-TG is not FDA-approved for treatment of psoriasis, patients are asked to sign an informed consent form.

LABORATORY STUDIES

A baseline complete blood count (CBC) and liver and kidney function tests are obtained. During the period of dose escalation CBCs are repeated weekly and chemistries every 2 or 4 weeks. After a stable dose is reached, CBCs are repeated every 2–4 weeks and chemistries every 1–3 months, depending on the values.

STATISTICAL METHODS

"Effective maintenance" is defined as maintaining a level of response judged by both patient and physician to be sufficiently good to warrant continuing treatment. The duration of response (period of effective maintenance) was calculated from the date of starting treatment and was determined by the Kaplan-Meier method. The log-rank and Wilcoxon tests were used to test for homogeneity of duration of response distributions for sex and difference in age.

RESPONSE TO TREATMENT

Plaque-Type Psoriasis

The response to treatment in 76 patients with plaque-type psoriasis is indicated in Figure 2. This Kaplan-Meier plot reflects all causes of treatment failure including inadequate response, intolerable side effects, or patient withdrawal for any reason. The median duration of response was 33 months. At 24 months 58% of the patients were still effectively maintained by 6-TG. Statistical analysis failed to reveal a significant difference in response between men versus women, and between those below and above age 50.

Palmoplantar Pustular Psoriasis

Six patients with palmoplantar pustular psoriasis were effectively maintained with 6-TG for periods of 2, 7, 9, 11, 13, and 36 months (median 10 months). The most frequent dose was 80 mg daily, although both lower and higher doses were used.

SIDE EFFECTS (Table 1)

Myelosuppression

Myelosuppression was the most frequent side effect, affecting 39 patients (47.5%) and causing treatment failure in 17 patients (20.7%). Leukopenia was the most common form, involving 34 patients (41.5%). Anemia occurred in nine patients (11.0%), and thrombopenia in seven patients (8.5%).

Two severe episodes occurred. A 41-year-old woman who was not properly monitored experienced pancytopenia, which required blood transfusions. She recovered rapidly. A 45-year-old man had total agranulocytosis from which he soon recovered without need for transfusion.

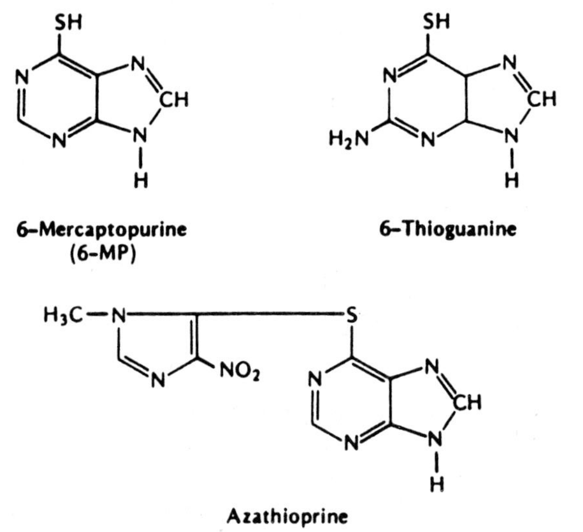

Figure 1 Structures of 6-mercaptopurine, 6-thioguanine, and azathioprine. (From Ref. 3.)

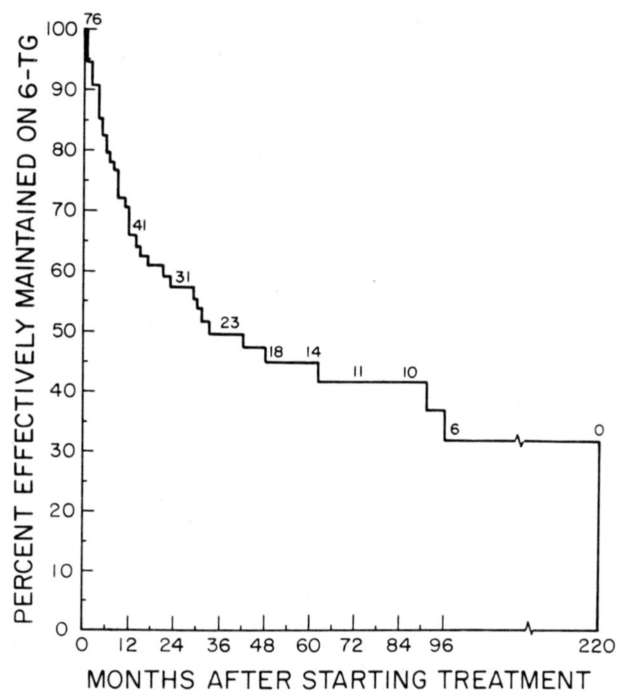

Figure 2 Duration of response for 76 patients with plaque-type psoriasis treated with 6-thioguanine. Numbers on plot indicate number of patients still managed by 6-thioguanine at various time periods. (From Ref. 3.)

Table 1 Side Effects in 82 Patients Treated with 6-Thioguanine

	Frequency		Causing treatment failure	
	No. of patients	%	No. of patients	%
Myelosuppression	39	47.5	17	20.7
Elevated liver enzymes[a]	15	25.0	6	10.0
Gastrointestinal	10	12.2	2	2.4
Multiple skin cancers	4	4.9	0	0
Drug eruption	2	2.4	2	2.4
Herpes zoster	2	2.4	0	0
Warts	2	2.4	0	0
Acute hepatitis	1	1.2	1	1.2
Cirrhosis with ascites[b]	1	1.2	1	1.2
Other[c]	6	7.3	0	0

[a]Transaminase values were obtained in 60 patients.
[b]Had prior advanced fibrosis.
[c]One patient each: furunculosis, mucositis, flu-like symptoms, hot flashes, "bloating around eyes," vertigo.

Hepatotoxicity

An increase in serum transaminase levels (AST or ALT) occurring at least twice was the second most common complication, involving 15 of 60 (25%) patients who had such determinations. This caused treatment failure in six patients (10%). Four of 22 patients (18.2%) who had no prior treatment with methotrexate experienced increased transaminase levels as contrasted to 10 of 33 patients (30.3%) with elevated enzymes who had prior treatment with methotrexate.

A 52-year-old man had an episode of acute hepatitis from which he recovered uneventfully. A 65-year-old woman with a long history of ethanol abuse and prior treatment with methotrexate with early cirrhosis developed frank cirrhosis and ascites while on 6-TG.

Liver biopsies were obtained in 12 patients. Four patients had both pre- and posttreatment biopsies, and eight had only posttreatment biopsies. There was no evidence of fibrosis or other significant change with the exception of the 65-year-old woman who had prior early cirrhosis. The principal reason for the small number of liver biopsies is that a number of gastroenterologists refused to do them on the basis that there was no evidence, after many years of clinical use, that 6-TG caused fibrosis.

Other Side Effects

Gastrointestinal complications occurred in 10 (12.2%) of the patients. Six experienced nausea, six had diarrhea, one developed a gastric ulcer, and one had exacerbation of a duodenal ulcer. Only two patients failed 6-TG because of gastrointestinal side effects; this was due to severe nausea in both.

A possible immunosuppressive effect of 6-TG is suggested by the occurrence of multiple skin cancers, both squamous and basal cell, in nonexposed as well as sun-exposed areas in four patients and herpes zoster and multiple warts in two patients each. Two patients developed a maculopapular eruption during the first 2 months of treatment requiring discontinuance of 6-TG. Other complications occurring in one patient each are listed in Table 1.

DISCUSSION

The median period of effective maintenance of 33 months in 76 patients indicates that 6-TG is an effective long-term treatment for plaque-type psoriasis. Additionally, most of our six patients with palmoplantar pustular psoriasis also benefited from 6-TG, although the median period of control of 10 months was considerably shorter than that obtained in plaque-type disease.

We emphasize that our cohort was comprised mostly of difficult-to-treat psoriasis. Almost half of our patients either had prior treatment with MTX or had been denied MTX because of liver or kidney disease. 6-TG is not considered to be a cause of liver fibrosis (4). Nevertheless, the occurrence of elevated liver enzymes in 25% of our patients indicates that close monitoring of transaminase levels is required.

Although MTX and cyclosporin are contraindicated in the presence of renal dysfunction, 6-TG may be used with caution in such patients because it is metabolized by the liver.

As expected, myelosuppression was the most frequent complication; however, this caused treatment failure in only one-fifth of the patients. Nevertheless, because of the hazard of severe myelosuppression we do not use 6-TG as a first-line treatment, and recommend its use only for patients who have failed other systemic therapies.

Snow and Gibson (5) and Anstey and Lennard (6) draw attention to the role of thiopurine methyltransferase (TPMT) in myelosuppression from thiopurine drugs such as azathioprine, 6-mercaptopurine, and 6-TG. Patients who have a relative TPMT deficiency are at increased risk for severe myelosuppression, and measurement of red blood cell TPMT activity is recommended to identify such patients.

A potentially fatal complication from 6-TG as well as from certain other antineoplastic agents is hepatic veno-occlusive disease (VOD) (4). As noted previously, one of our patients had a short-lived episode of acute hepatitis. However, he did not have the full-blown clinical features of VOD including jaundice, ascites, and right upper quadrant tenderness. Kao and Rosenblate (7) reported VOD in a patient with psoriasis while on 6-TG. However, this patient self-medicated when on vacation and took 320 mg daily, which is twice our maximum dose. He gradually recovered completely after discontinuing 6-TG.

REFERENCES

1. McCormack, J.J., and Johns, D.G. (1990). Purine and purine nucleoside antimetabolites. In *Cancer Chemotherapy: Principles and Practice.* B.A. Chabner and J.M. Collins (Eds.). J.B. Lippincott, Philadelphia, pp. 234–252.
2. Zackheim, H.S., Maibach, H.I., and Grekin, D.A. (1982). Thioguanine for psoriasis. In *Psoriasis. Proceedings of the 3rd International Symposium.* E.M. Farber and A.J. Cox (eds.). Grune & Stratton, New York, p. 405.
3. Zackheim, H.S., Glogau, R.G., Fisher, D.A., and Maibach, H.I. (1994). 6-Thioguanine treatment of psoriasis. *J. Am. Acad. Dermatol.* 30:452–458.
4. Perry, M.C. (1992). Chemotherapeutic agents and hepatotoxicity. *Semin. Oncol.* 19:551–565.
5. Snow, J.L., and Gibson, L.E. (1995). A pharmacogenetic basis for the safe and effective use of azathioprine and other thiopurine drugs in dermatologic patients. *J. Am. Acad. Dermatol.* 32:114–116.
6. Anstey, A., and Lennard, L. (1995). The role of genetic variation in thiopurine methyltransferase activity and efficacy and/or side effects of azathioprine therapy in dermatologic patients. *Arch. Dermatol.* 131:1087–1088.
7. Kao, N.L., and Rosenblate, H.J. (1993). 6-Thioguanine therapy for psoriasis causing toxic hepatic venoocclusive disease. *J. Am. Acad. Dermatol.* 28:1017–1018.

52

Cyclosporin for the Treatment of Psoriasis

John Y.M. Koo, Charles Gambla, and Jaeho Lee
University of California Medical Center, San Francisco, California

THE ORIGINAL FORMULATION OF CYCLOSPORIN

Cyclosporin is a neutral lipophilic undecapeptide first extracted from the fungus *Tolypocladium inflatum Gams* in 1970. In 1976, the profound immunosuppressive effect of cyclosporin was identified (1). It was first used in humans as an immunosuppressant in 1978. The official approval in the United States for use in kidney, heart, and liver transplantations was obtained in 1983. Its efficacy in the treatment of psoriasis was discovered fortuitously in 1979 (2). Since then, numerous clinical studies have demonstrated its efficacy in psoriasis (3,4). Cyclosporin has also been reported to be effective in the treatment of a variety of dermatological disorders, including pyoderma gangrenosum (5–8), atopic dermatitis (9,10), pemphigus and bullous pemphigoid (11–14), alopecia areata (15,16), pityriasis lichenoides chronica (17), Behcet's disease (18–21), photodermatoses (22), and dermatomyositis (23,24). In addition, successful cases of treatment with cyclosporin have been reported in androgenetic alopecia (25), epidermolysis bullosa acquisita (26–28), hidradenitis supparativa (17), ichthyosis (29), chronic urticaria (30), Darier's disease (17), bullous erythema multiforme (31), scleroderma (32), vitiligo (17), leprosy (33,34), and mycosis fungoides (35).

Cyclosporin holds two main advantages when treating psoriasis. First, cyclosporin compares favorably with some of the most efficacious treatments we have available, such as methotrexate and systemic PUVA therapy. Cyclosporin is thought to be significantly more efficacious than such treatment modalities as monotherapy etretinate, sulfasalazine, and hydroxyurea (Figs. 1–6). Second, cyclosporin has a very different side-effect profile from other treatment modalities, making it a viable alternative when other modalities are contraindicated.

Mechanisms of Action

The most established role of cyclosporin in psoriasis is its effects on T-lymphocytes. Cyclosporin inhibits interleukin-2 (IL-2) production of T-cells (36). This is thought to be accomplished by the inhibition of calcineurin, a calcium- and calmodulin-dependent phosphatase, by a complex formed between cyclosporin and cyclophilin, an intracellular receptor (37–39). Because IL-2 causes the proliferation of T helper cells and cytotoxic lymphocytes, impaired IL-2 production leads to a decline in the number of activated CD4 and CD8 cells in the epidermis (40). As cyclosporin inhibits T-cell secretion of lymphokines such as IFN-γ, which promotes release of proinflammatory cytokines by keratinocytes, infiltration and inflammation may also be reduced (36,41). Also, several in vitro studies have demonstrated that cyclosporin inhibits the growth of keratinocytes at high concentrations (42–45) although in actual usage the concentration of cyclosporin attained in vivo appears to be too low to exert a direct antiproliferative effect on keratinocytes

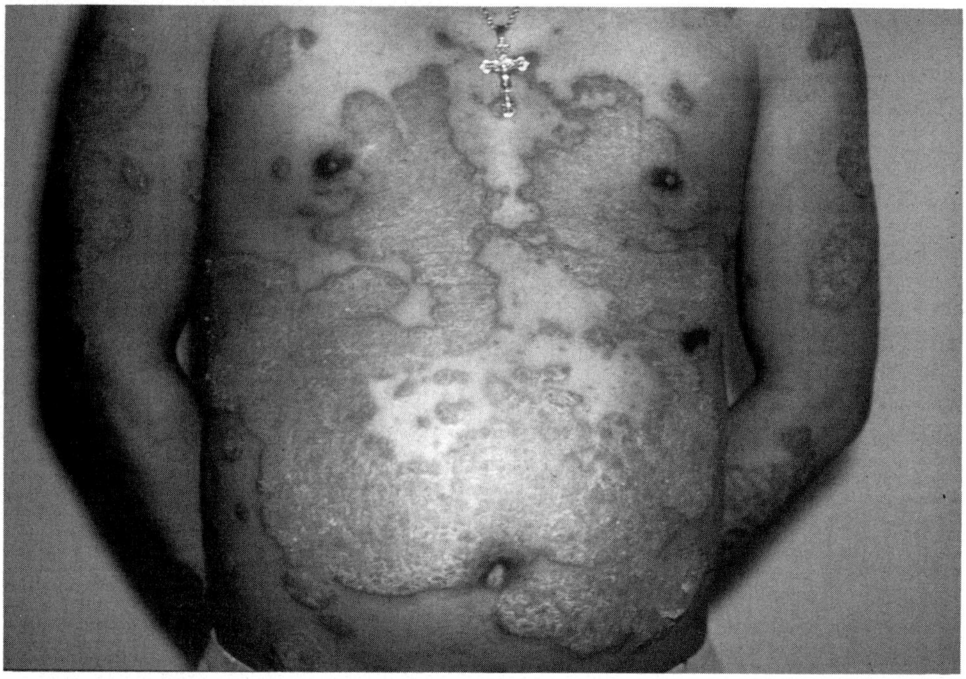

Figure 1 Pretreatment, anterior trunk.

(46). Cyclosporin also reduces the chemotactic ability of polymorphonuclear neutrophils through the modulation of cytokines (47). Cyclosporin's direct effect may extend to other cells, including antigen-presenting cells and mast cells (48–52).

Certain lymphokines such as IFN-γ are known to increase the expression of intercellular adhesion molecule 1(ICAM-1) (53,40). These molecules are expressed on the surface of various cells such as keratinocytes and dermal capillary endothelium and play a role in the immune process. Conceivably, they could enable the endothelium to attract circulating leukocytes more effectively and, once in the epidermis, inflammatory cells may stay near keratinocytes longer. Cyclosporin inhibits the production of IFN-γ (36,51,54) and, in turn, down-regulates ICAM-1.

Pharmacokinetics

Cyclosporin is available as a liquid with a concentration of 100 mg/mL or as a tablet in the dosages of 25, 50, and 100 mg. Approximately 40% of the oral dose is absorbed, with bioavailability of approximately 30%, owing to a 25% first-pass effect in the liver (55). Cyclosporin is metabolized by the hepatic enzyme cytochrome P450 3A isoform. The peak plasma level is generally reached in 2–4 h. The half-life of cyclosporin in serum is 19 h (range 8–24 h) (56). Cyclosporin is primarily excreted in bile. Because only approximately 6% of cyclosporin is excreted in urine, renal dysfunction does not significantly alter its pharmacokinetics (57,58).

Because cyclosporin is metabolized by the hepatic enzyme cytochrome P450 system, concomitant use of medications that compete for the P450 system (e.g., ketoconazole, erythromycin, norfloxacin, certain oral contraceptives, androgenetic steroids, high-dose corticosteroids, cimetidine, and danazol) may increase the serum concentration of cyclosporin (Table 1). In addition, certain calcium channel blockers such as diltiazem, nicardipine, and verapamil are also known to possibly increase the serum concentration of cyclosporin. On the other hand, there are medications that may decrease the serum concentration of cyclosporin by inducing cytochrome P450 activity. Many of the medications that fall into this category are antiepileptic medications such as phenytoin, phenobarbital, and carbamazepine. Certain antibiotics such as rifampin and sulfadimidine-trimethoprim are also known to induce hepatic cytochrome P450 activity, thereby possibly decreasing the serum concentration of cyclosporin.

Cyclosporin blood levels are generally determined 12–24 h after administration by either high-performance liquid chromatography or radioimmunoassay. The determination of cyclosporin blood levels may be useful to detect drug–drug interactions, noncompliance on the part of the patient, or patients with unusual pharmacokinetics owing to factors such as clinically silent disturbances of renal or hepatic functions. Cyclosporin, however, is known to share significant interpatient variation in blood levels for a given dosage, and there is no correlation between serum levels and efficacy in the treatment of psoriasis (59). Because of these considerations, routine monitoring of cyclosporin blood levels is not required in either the European or Canadian guidelines regarding its use (60).

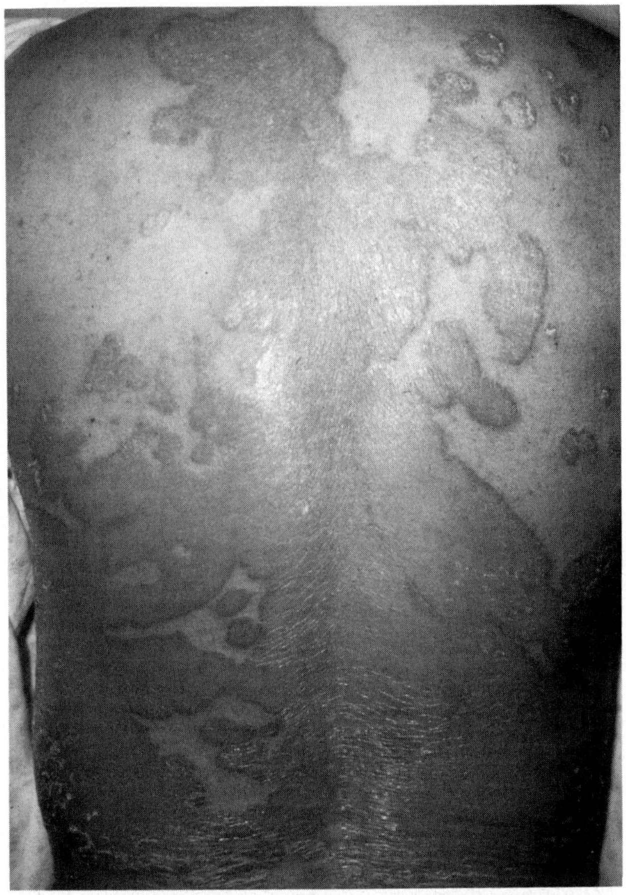

Figure 2 Pretreatment, posterior trunk.

Dosage

There are two schools of thought regarding the proper approach to dosing cyclosporin, that advocating the initial use of a high-dose regimen, with gradual transition to a lower dosage, and that advocating the initial use of a low dose, with upward adjustment as indicated. Even though dosages as high as 8 to 16 mg/kg/day are commonly used among nephrologists in the treatment of transplant patients, the highest dosage that is generally used for dermatologic purposes is 5 mg/kg/day, usually administered in two divided dosages. At least in treating psoriasis, it has been well demonstrated that 5 mg/kg/day dosing on the average is much more efficacious, in terms of both rapidity of the onset of therapeutic effect and the probability of clearing, compared with lower dosages such as 2.5 or 1.25 mg/kg/day (Figs. 7 and 8) (61). The Canadian consensus report generally recommends starting with a lower dosage such as 3 mg/kg/day, whereas the European consensus report takes the middle ground and recommends 3 to 4 mg/kg/day as a starting dose (62). In the multicenter research protocol conducted in the United States, the initial dosage of 5 mg/kg/day was used with the adjustment to a lower dose for the maintenance phase of the study.

Needless to say, much of the decision regarding the initial dosage depends on the clinical state of the patient. When one is faced with patients in acute distress such as those who are erythrodermic or who present with widespread, highly inflammatory flares of psoriasis, starting with the higher dosage, such as 5 mg/kg/day, is recommended in order to promptly control the intensity of the inflammation. On the other hand, in a patient who has widespread but relatively stable plaque-type psoriasis, it is reasonable to start with a lower dose and increase it as needed to determine the lowest possible effective dosage.

The ideal body weight, rather than the actual body weight, should be used to calculate the daily dosage of cyclosporin. This is especially critical for obese patients, because they may be overdosed if their actual body weight is used.

Once the patient achieves great improvement in clinical status, the dosage of cyclosporin should be decreased by decrements of 0.5 to 1 mg/kg/day until the lowest effective dose is reached for maintenance therapy, or cyclosporin is discontinued altogether, as other treatment modalities such as phototherapy are introduced and used for maintenance therapy.

Side Effects

The most troublesome side effects of cyclosporin involve nephrotoxicity and hypertension. These side ef-

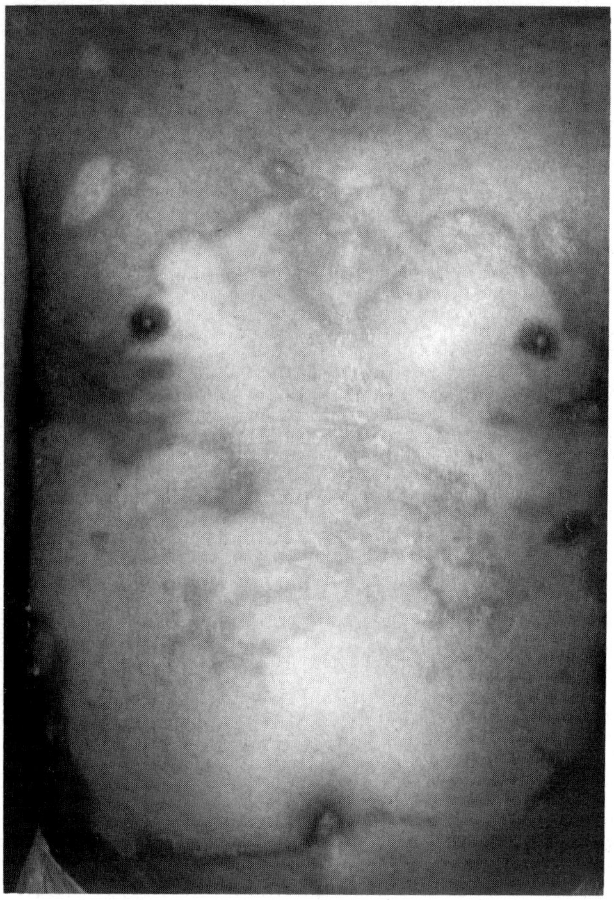

Figure 3 Anterior trunk after 2 weeks of cyclosporin at 4 mg/kg/day.

fects are dose-dependent; they usually develop gradually over time, in contrast to some rare side effects of methotrexate that can occur suddenly and catastrophically. The other possible metabolic side effects include imbalances in electrolytes, such as hyperkalemia and hypomagnesemia. Because cyclosporin may reduce the renal clearance of uric acid, there is a tendency toward hyperuricemia in susceptible patients. There are also neurological side effects associated with the use of cyclosporin, such as paresthesias, tremors, dysesthesisas, hyperesthesias, and headaches. In usage lasting 2 months or less, neurological side effects are most common because nephrotoxicity and hypertension are rarely encountered in short-term use. The use of cyclosporin is also associated with gingival hyperplasia, which is usually reversible on discontinuation of this medication. Some patients may experience elevated cholesterol and triglyceride levels, but much less so than with retinoids (62). Hypertrichosis may also occur. Other miscellaneous side effects include nausea, diarrhea, and anorexia, as well as fatigue, joint pains, and muscle aches. In contrast to the use of cyclosporin in high doses for transplant patients, the dermatological use of cyclosporin in low doses has not been reported to be associated with an increase in the incidence of internal malignancies, infection, or seizures. In a worldwide study involving more than 1000 research subjects who were exposed to cyclosporin for up to 1 year, the prevalence of internal malignancies, including lymphoma, was not significantly increased in comparison with the general public (data on file with Sandoz Clinical Research Division, East Hanover, NJ) or those on other modalities such as PUVA phototherapy. Consequently, the increased risk of developing malignancy and the risk of developing serious infections were thought to be both

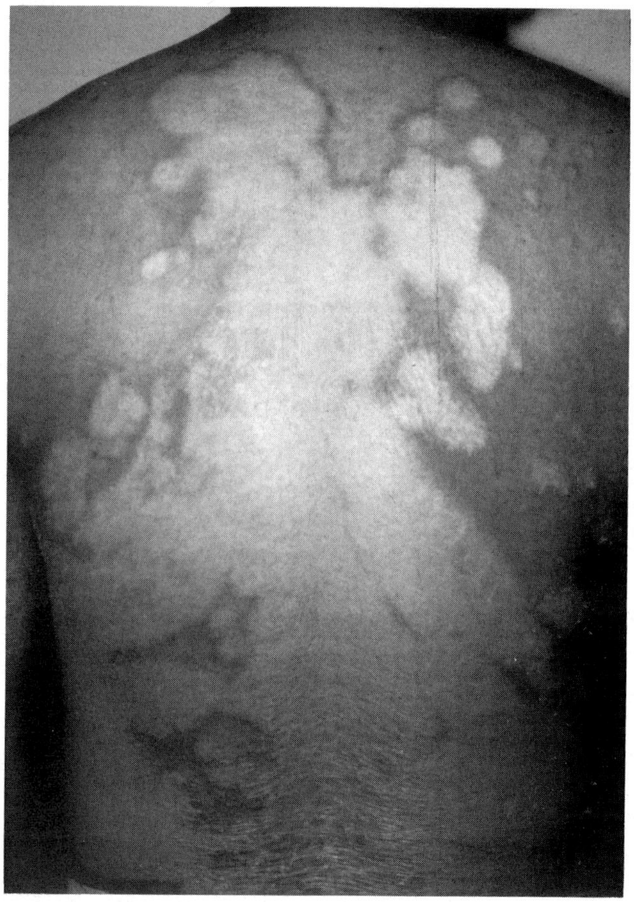

Figure 4 Posterior trunk after 2 weeks of cyclosporin at 5 mg/kg/day.

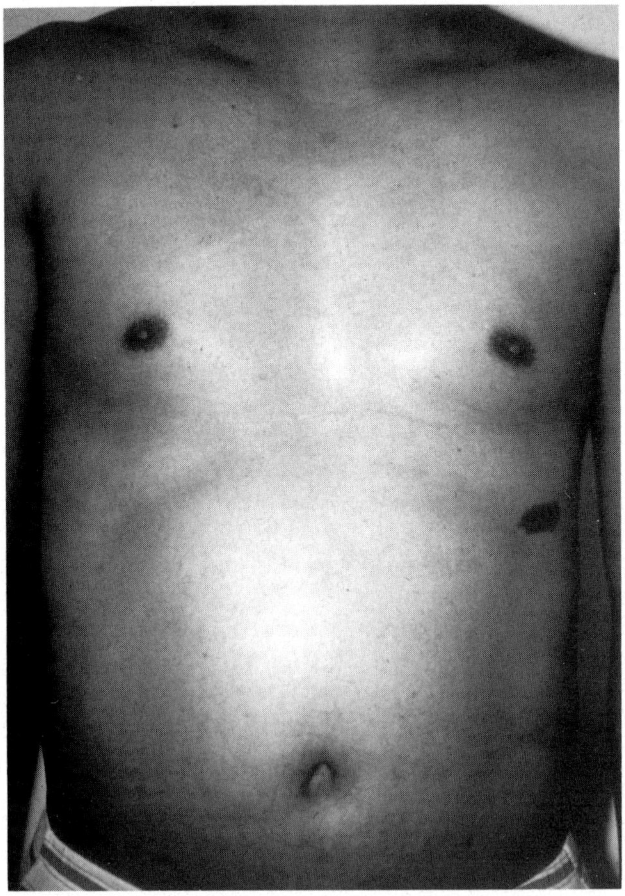

Figure 5 Anterior trunk after 1 month of cyclosporin at 5 mg/kg/day.

dose-dependent and contingent upon the depth of immunosuppression induced. Long-term data on the risks of malignancy associated with low-dose cyclosporin for psoriasis are not yet available.

In many cases, the development of hypertension during the use of cyclosporin was thought to be due to the direct vasoconstrictive effect of cyclosporin on the vascular smooth muscles of the kidneys (64). The development of hypertension, however, could also be secondary to renal dysfunction. If detected early, the development of hypertension is generally reversible by adjusting the dose of cyclosporin. The development of hypertension by itself does not constitute a contraindication to continuing therapy with cyclosporin, as long as the hypertension can be brought under control with appropriate antihypertensive agents. Currently, the antihypertensive agents of choice include nifedipine and isradipine because these two agents are known not to alter serum cyclosporin levels (65). Isradipine has one advantage over nifedipine in that it has not been associated with gingival hyperplasia, whereas nifedipine, by itself, has. Diltiazem and verapamil are not recommended, because these agents may alter cyclosporin blood levels (62). Also, the use of diuretics is controversial owing to the possibility of added nephrotoxicity (66,67).

The first 14 kidney biopsies of psoriatic patients treated with cyclosporin at 5 mg/kg/day for a mean duration of 15 months showed no cyclosporin-related structure abnormalities, compared with controls (68). A more recent report profiled eight patients who received an induction dosage of 5 mg/kg/day of cyclosporin and a mean maintenance dosage of 3.2 mg/kg/day for an average duration of 12 months. They exhibited persistent reduction in glomerular filtration rate (GFR) of 9.8% (range 5.5–21.5%) even 4 months after discontinuing cyclosporin (52). Nephrologists

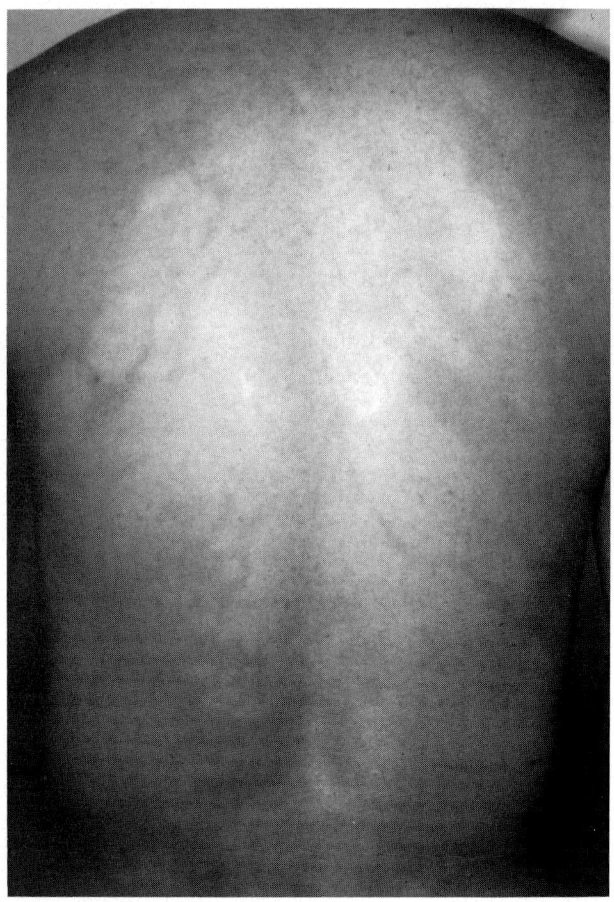

Figure 6 Posterior trunk after 1 month on cyclosporin at 5 mg/kg/day.

Table 1 Drugs That Interact with Cyclosporine

Drugs that may raise cyclosporine levels
Ketoconazole
Fluconazole
Itraconazole
Amphotericin B
Erythromycin
Norfloxacin
Cephalosporins
Doxycycline
Acyclovir
Oral contraceptives
Corticosteroids
Danazol
Cimetidine
Thiazide diuretics
Furosemide
Warfarin
Diltiazem
Nicardipine
Verapamil
Bromocriptine
Metoclopramide
Drugs that may reduce cyclosporine levels
Valproate
Phenytoin
Phenobarbital
Carbamazepine
Rifampin
Drugs that may increase nephrotoxicity
Gentamicin
Tobramycin
Vancomycin
Trimethoprim with sulfamethoxazole
Azapropazone
Cimetidine
Ranitidine
Diclofenac
Amphotericin B
Ketoconazole
Melphalan
Other interactions
Reduced clearance of lovastatin, digoxin, and prednisone

Source: Ref. 55.

accept that the use of cyclosporin may lead to a measurable decrease in GFR, which may persist, but generally they are of the opinion that this reduction in GFR is not seen every time cyclosporin is introduced; it may be seen initially and then the renal function usually appears to stabilize and show no further significant reduction in GFR as the treatment is reinitiated or maintained.

Last, there is a recent report regarding renal biopsy results in eight patients who were treated with the average dosage of 3.3 mg/kg/day of cyclosporin for an average duration of 5 years (69). This study reported that there were "biopsy features consistent with cyclosporin nephrotoxicity" in six of the eight patients. All six patients with abnormal biopsies had renal tubular atrophy and arteriolar hyalinosis, four had an increase in interstitium, and two showed an increased incidence of glomerular obsolescence. Because the duration of treatment in this study (i.e., an average of 5 years) is much longer than previously mentioned studies, these findings may be attributable to the prolonged continuous use of cyclosporin. This study unfortunately had no control population (i.e., renal biopsy results from psoriasis patients who were not on cyclosporin) and, therefore, the results are more difficult to interpret, whereas the first study of renal biopsies did have an appropriate control population of patients who were not exposed to cyclosporin-A treatment (68).

Certain precautions should be taken to minimize the risk of inducing irreversible renal damage form the use of cyclosporin. First, any patient who has preexisting renal disease should ordinarily not be given the drug. One needs to be careful in treating the elderly or those with preexisting hypertension. It is important to avoid concurrent use of nephrotoxic drugs such as nonsteroidal anti-inflammatory agents, aminoglycosides, and amphotericin B. Generally, the lowest effective dose of cyclosporin should be used for maintenance. Serum creatinine levels should be closely monitored. Pretreatment serum creatinine levels should be determined on two occasions within 2

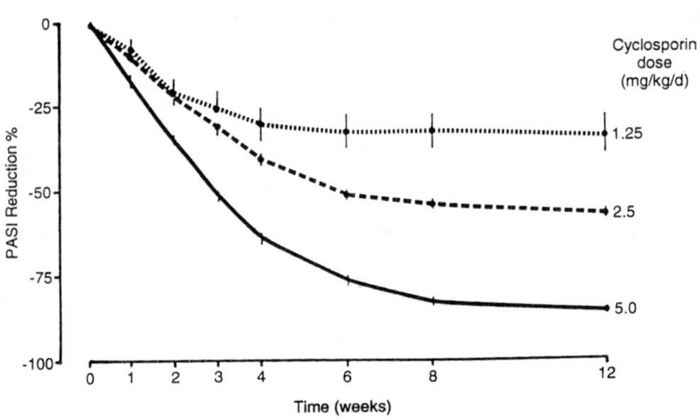

Figure 7 Percentage of psoriasis area and severity index (PASI) score reduction.

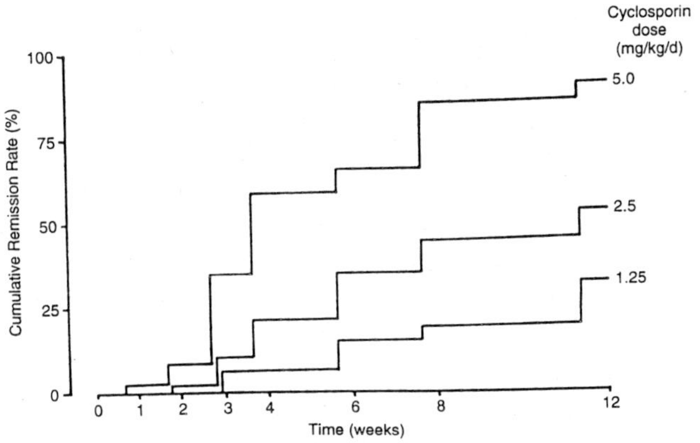

Figure 8 Cumulative success rate in the first 3 months of treatment.

weeks of starting cyclosporin. The cyclosporin dose should be decreased or the treatment discontinued if the serum creatinine level increases to greater than 30% of the baseline (Fig. 9). The comparison for serum creatinine is made against the patient's pretreatment serum creatinine level rather than against the upper limit of the normal range, because some patients with small body mass may in fact increase their baseline serum creatinine levels by 30% or more, yet the absolute value for creatinine may remain within normal limits. It is well recognized that serum creatinine may fluctuate depending on many factors, such as the type of food the patient consumed shortly before the blood test, the time of day when the sample was drawn, and the relative position of the patient (e.g., the patient's serum creatinine level taken right after the patient wakes up in the morning may be significantly different than the serum creatinine level taken in the late afternoon when the patient has been on his or her feet for a long period of time). Therefore, ideally, one should try to check the patient's serum creatinine under similar circumstances in terms of the time of day, activity levels, and diet. A rotational approach to the treatment of psoriasis should be employed whenever possible to avoid prolonged exposure to the nephrotoxic effect of cyclosporin. Last, whenever unusual difficulties arise, input from a nephrologist experienced in the use of cyclosporin should be obtained.

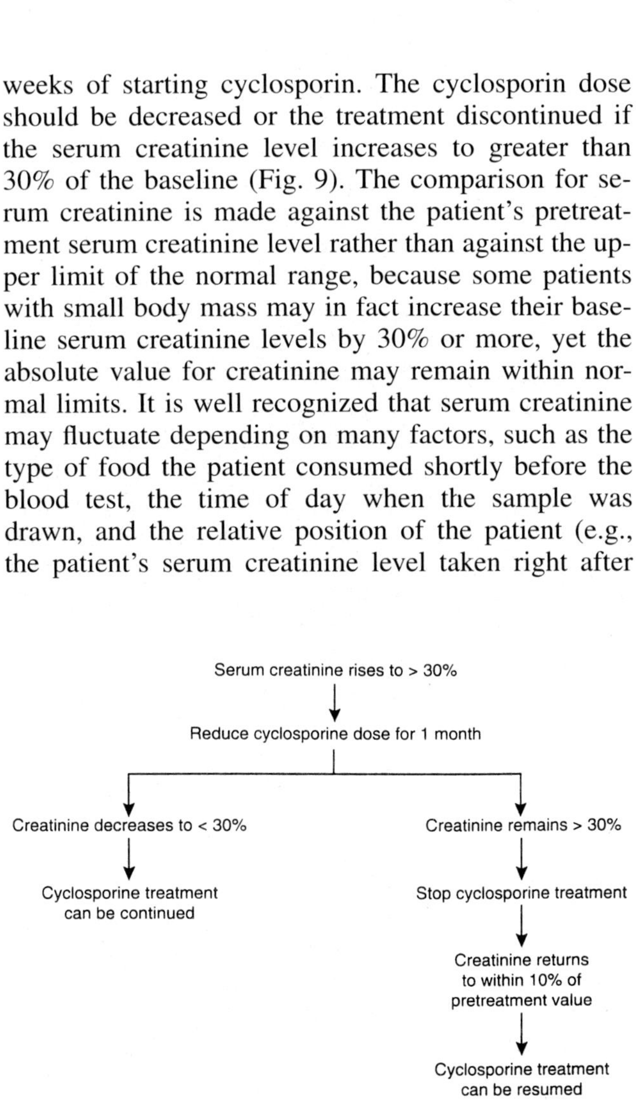

Figure 9 An algorithm for adjusting cyclosporin dosage.

Usage of Cyclosporin

The major indication for the use of cyclosporin is widespread or disabling psoriasis in patients who have failed other treatments such as topical steroids, outpatient Goeckerman therapy, or systemic PUVA therapy. The exceptions to this include those who present with widespread, intensely inflammatory, or frankly erythrodermic psoriasis who are not clinically ill (i.e., sepsis is not a concern), for whom cyclosporin may be the first-line treatment. It is well known that patients who present with widespread inflammation are liable to experience paradoxic reactions to phototherapy in which ultraviolet B or PUVA therapy exacerbates the inflammation rather than improves the clinical condition. In the recent past, when inpatient treatments for dermatologic diseases were commonly practiced, these patients were admitted into the dermatologic inpatient service to "cool down" with the use of intense topical treatments such as Aveeno bath, Hubbard tank, and triamcinolone acetonide 0.1% ointment every 2 h, in an occlusive garment. At times, even moist, cool towels were applied all over the body to reduce the intensity of erythema before patients could be started on phototherapy. Because of the current difficulties in obtaining insurance reimbursement for inpatient treatment of dermatologic patients, however, there is now a great need to find an alternative method of controlling the intense inflammation in these patients. Methotrexate can be used to control the inflammation among these erythrodermic or near-erythrodermic patients; however, if these patients have never been exposed to methotrexate before, definitive treatment with methotrexate may have to be postponed for at least 1 week to administer a test dose to make sure that the patient does not have unusual sensitivity to the drug. Moreover, methotrexate may take a few weeks to exert its maximal effects. Etretinate can also be used to calm an intense inflammatory reaction, but it is frequently less effective than cyclosporin or methotrexate. Moreover, in some patients, the erythema may in fact worsen on etretinate before it starts to improve. The other systemic agents available, such as hydroxyurea or sulfasalazine, have questionable efficacy. In view of these drawbacks, cyclosporin may be the most convenient and efficacious agent because of its profound anti-inflammatory effects and because it has no requirement for a test dose owing to the lack of sudden, serious, catastrophic side effects associated with its usage.

It should be noted that some patients who present with erythrodermic or near-erythrodermic psoriasis may in fact present with borderline elevated serum creatinine levels. If the patient has no previous history of renal disorder, this slight elevation in creatinine in clinically erythrodermic or near-erythrodermic patients may not represent a contraindication to the use of cyclosporin, because this may represent a temporary prerenal state found in patients with widespread inflammation in which a significant volume of blood flow is shunted to the skin. In fact, when cyclosporin therapy is initiated and the inflammation is brought under control, the prerenal state resolves and the serum creatinine level generally decreases.

Once the widespread inflammation is brought under control, the patient can be cautiously started on phototherapy, either ultraviolet B or PUVA. During the time necessary to optimize the ultraviolet exposure, cyclosporin can be maintained at the clearing dose. Once it is apparent that the phototherapy is well tolerated and its regimen has been optimized, the dose of cyclosporin can be tapered and eventually discontinued altogether. Even though it is generally not recommended to administer phototherapy and cyclosporin simultaneously for fear of increasing the risk of cutaneous malignancies, in actual practice, some period of overlap, which is usually no more than 2 to 3 weeks, may be necessary to provide a smooth transition from acute therapy with cyclosporine to long-term therapy with phototherapy.

The exclusion criteria include significant immunosuppression, preexisting renal or hepatic dysfunction (including postmethotrexate patients with significant hepatic damage), patients on cytotoxic or nephrotoxic medications or other medications that alter the bioavailability or metabolism of cyclosporin, a history of internal malignancies or, possibly, multiple cutaneous malignancies, uncontrolled hypertension, and active or latent infections, including tuberculosis. Patients who are unreliable, noncompliant, or cannot comprehend the complexity involved in the proper use of this medication should also be excluded.

The pretreatment cyclosporin workup (Table 2) generally includes a physical examination, with an emphasis on ruling out lymphadenopathy, active or latent infection, tumors, or evidence of immunosuppression such as the presence of HIV-related skin conditions. It is desirable to obtain several baseline serum creatinine levels, although this is not always possible owing to logistics and the urgency of starting treatment. It is also desirable to obtain at least two baseline blood pressure measurements. Laboratory evaluation should include serum creatinine and BUN, urinalysis with microscopic evaluation, serum electrolytes with serum magnesium and uric acid levels, cholesterol and triglyceride levels, liver function tests with bilirubin, and HIV testing, if there is such clinical suspicion and if the patient consents to having this performed. The need for creatinine clearance or GFR measurement is somewhat controversial in that neither European nor Canadian guidelines require these procedures as necessary prerequisites for starting or maintaining a patient on cyclosporin. The weight of their data suggests that close monitoring of serum creatinine level with strict guidelines for dosage adjustment or the discontinuation of cyclosporin as outlined previously (see Fig. 9) appears to be adequate in monitoring patients' renal function; however, the author still believes there is some utility in determining creatinine clearance for patients who are being considered for long-term treatment with cyclosporin, because occasionally patients have normal serum creatinine levels and unexpectedly compromised creatinine clearance. As a general screening method, CBC and chest radiography may be obtained.

For follow-up during the first 3 months, serum creatinine, BUN, urinalysis with microscopic evaluation, liver function tests with bilirubin, electrolytes, and CBC should be checked on a biweekly or at least a monthly basis. The patient should be evaluated with close attention to physical examination and blood pressure monitoring. After the first 3 months, monthly evaluations should be made, with comparisons of previous laboratory values, a physical examination, and blood pressure measurement, along with the occasional determination of serum uric acid, serum magnesium, cholesterol, and triglyceride levels. In a selected patient, creatinine clearance may be checked every 3 months.

Table 2 Suggested Minimum Monitoring of Patients Taking Cyclosporine

Parameter	Action
Pretherapy	
Serum creatinine	Obtain at least 2 measurements to determine baseline; range of values should be within 20% or additional determinations needed
At baseline, after 2 and 4 wk, and then at least monthly	
Blood pressure	Treat hypertension or, if possible, reduce cyclosporine dose
Serum	
Creatinine*	Reduce cyclosporine dose if value exceeds baseline by 30%
Urea nitrogen	Treat to correct if significantly abnormal
Lipids	Treat to correct if significantly abnormal
Bilirubin, liver function tests	Bilirubin usually increases with cyclosporine, but dose reduction usually not needed
Uric acid	Treat to correct if significantly abnormal
Magnesium	If low, give replacement therapy
Electrolytes	Treat to correct if significantly abnormal
A review of any new medications	Determine if new medication affects cyclosporine metabolism

*Outpatient creatinine clearance tests tend to be unreliable; creatinine clearance can be calculated from formulas based on the serum creatinine but this often adds little additional information. There is no consensus that routine glomerular filtration rates (GFRs) are necessary when cyclosporine is used in the manner discussed in this chapter.

CONCLUSION

Cyclosporin is known to be highly efficacious for the treatment of psoriasis as well as several other dermatologic conditions. Because of its profound anti-inflammatory properties and a side-effect profile that differs from other agents, such as methotrexate, the availability of cyclosporin confers certain advantages in meeting the challenges of treating recalcitrant psoriasis. In short-term use, cyclosporin can induce dramatic improvements in psoriasis, especially in those patients who present with intense inflammation. Because of nephrotoxicity and the possible development of hypertension, however, its long-term usage, especially if continued beyond 1 year, is still to be defined. With contemporary attempts to use combination and rotational therapies to maximize therapeutic efficacy and minimize risk of long-term side effects, cyclosporin is definitely a welcome addition to our current armamentarium in the treatment of psoriasis.

NEORAL: A NEW FORMULATION OF CYCLOSPORIN

Rationale for the Development of Sandimmune Neoral (SIM-Neoral)

The profound immunosuppressive effect of cyclosporin was first identified in 1976 (1). Official approval for use in kidney, heart, and liver transplants was obtained in the United States in 1983. Its benefit in the treatment of psoriasis was discovered in 1979 (2). Since then, clinical studies have demonstrated its efficacy in treating psoriasis (3,4,70), as well as a variety of other dermatologic diseases (71).

The pharmacokinetics, side-effect profile, and basis for rational use of cyclosporin for practicing dermatologists has also been reviewed (72,73). Guidelines for maximum dosing of cyclosporin in psoriasis have been established (62), and reasonable, effective maintenance doses have been recommended based on clinical trials (74).

However, since the introduction of cyclosporin to clinical medicine almost 15 years ago, wide variations have been noted in the absorption of the Sandimmune Soft Gelatin Capsules (SIM-SGC), both within and between patients. This variability of drug bioavailability has posed a dilemma to both patients and physicians. The average oral bioavailability is approximately 30%, with a range of variability from 5–90% (58,75,76). A certain subgroup of patients are poor absorbers of cyclosporin in its currently available formulation. These patients will be prevented by established safety guidelines (the ceiling of 5 mg/kg/day) from reaching drug levels needed for clinical efficacy in treating psoriasis.

With the current SIM-SGC formulation, drug exposure of the individual patient over time will vary and be unstable, even if the dosage remains unchanged (77). In addition, the pharmacokinetics of SIM-SGC varies widely with the fed versus the fasted state (see Table 4). This variation in drug absorption carries the risk of reduced efficacy, on the one hand, and increased side effects on the other. For patients with a non-life-threatening chronic disease for whom long-term treatment may be needed, such a risk needs to be minimized.

Pharmacokinetic Parameters of Interest

In comparing the standard formulation of cyclosporin (SIM-SGC) with the new formulation of cyclosporin (SIM-Neoral), several pharmacokinetic parameters will be compared and contrasted (78). The AUC (area under the curve) is defined as the area under the whole blood concentration versus time curve. The C_{av} is the average steady-state concentration of drug in whole blood. The C_{max} is the maximum measured concentration of drug at steady state. The C_{min} is the whole blood concentration at the end of a dosing interval (the steady-state trough concentration). The T_{max} is the time to reach C_{max}. The T ½ is the drug half-life and the %PTF equals the percentage of peak trough fluctuation.

Factors Affecting the Absorption of Cyclosporin (79,80)

There are several factors that affect the absorption of cyclosporin. These include the presence of bile in the gut, the administration of drug with or without food, and the presence or absence of gastrointestinal disease. Drug absorption of cyclosporin, otherwise known as the absorption window, seems to occur primarily in the duodenum, jejunum, and ileum, in contrast to the significantly decreased absorption in the colon (Fig. 10). Since the proposed mechanism of cyclosporin absorption is lipophilic, passive diffusion through biological membranes, a similar absorption pattern would be expected in the colon as well as the blood–brain barrier. However, penetration of cyclosporin through these latter areas is minimal. This suggests the possibility of interactions of cyclosporin with specific transmembranal carrier proteins in the duodenum, jejunum, and ileum, which enhances absorption in these regions. However, these transmembranal carrier proteins have not yet been identified.

SIM-SGC Pharmacokinetics

Cyclosporin is available as a liquid with a concentration of 100 mg/mL or as a tablet in the dosages of 25, 50, and 100 mg. Approximately 40% of the oral dose is absorbed, with bioavailability of about 30%, owing to a 25% first-pass effect in the liver (55). Cyclosporin is metabolized by the hepatic enzyme cytochrome P450 3A isoform. The peak plasma level is generally reached in 2–4 h. The half-life of cyclosporin in serum is 19 h (range, 8–24 h) (77). Cyclosporin is primarily excreted in bile. Because only approximately 6% of cyclosporin is excreted in urine, renal dysfunction does not significantly alter its pharmacokinetics (57,58). The elimination half-life (T ½) of the parent drug from the blood is 15.4 ± 6.8 h in rheumatoid arthritis patients and 12.1 ± 4.1 h in healthy volunteers (77).

Approximately 67% of SIM-SGC detectable in whole blood is bound to corpuscular elements (approximately 58% to erythrocytes, 9% to nucleated cells); only 33% are bound in the plasma (81). Within

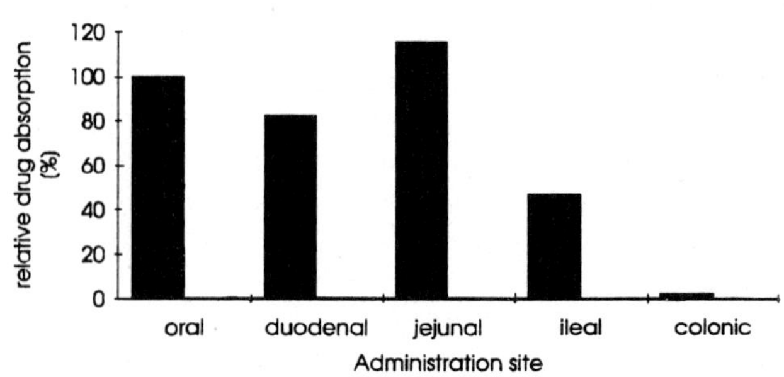

Figure 10 Rationale for the development of Sandimmune Neoral.

plasma, the major fraction of SIM-SGC is bound to lipoproteins (high-density lipoproteins 57%, low-density lipoproteins 25%, very low-density lipoproteins 2%), and albumin (10%). The distribution of SIM-SGC in the blood is dependent on lipoprotein concentrations, hematocrit, and temperature. For this reason, it is mandatory to use whole blood samples for drug concentration estimation rather than serum or plasma (82).

The currently available formulation of SIM-SGC must be physiologically "packaged" into a micelle form before absorption in the gut can occur. Although cyclosporin is an oligopeptide, it *does not* undergo prehepatic metabolism (83). In contrast to peptides, cyclosporin is not digested by peptidases in the epithelial cells lining the small intestinal villi. Cyclosporin is absorbed by the small intestine in a lipid/micelle "package" (79). Absorption by intestinal villi (lacteals) is concentration-dependent, primarily by passive lipid diffusion, although as mentioned earlier, facilitated diffusion may play a role that has not yet been clearly defined (80).

Role of Bile Salts

Bile salts accelerate lipid digestion and absorption by forming micelles (84). Micelles are spherical globules composed of bile salts, fatty acids, mono-, di-, and triglycerides, in addition to any drug that may be dissolved in the micelle. Micelles have a nonpolar, lipid-soluble center and a polar, water-soluble exterior. The negatively charged polar exterior of the micelles allows those substances suspended in the micelle (i.e., fatty acids, monoglycerides, or cyclosporin) to become dissolved in the water of the digestive fluids and to remain in stable solution (not precipitate) with lipid digestion.

The following steps in lipid digestion occur in the second portion of the duodenum. Ingested fat in the presence of bile plus agitation from intestinal peristalsis will yield emulsified fat. Emulsified fat in the presence of pancreatic lipase will yield breakdown products of fat, to include fatty acids and 2-monoglycerides. When this fat is broken down and processed into spherical micelles, the surface area of the fatty elements is increased tens of thousands of times and this increased surface area translated into increased absorption of particles by the brush border of the intestine.

Bile salt micelles act as a transport medium to carry monoglycerides, free fatty acids, and cyclosporin to the brush borders of the intestinal epithelial cells. These substances are then absorbed by the lacteals that comprise the brush border. Bile salts are then released back into the chyme to be used again.

SIM-SGC Absorption

When SIM-SGC is ingested, it then forms an oil and water emulsion in intestinal aqueous fluids. This cyclosporin is mainly distributed in oily droplets that have to be digested in order to release the drug for its absorption (80). The oily droplets have to be emulsified by bile salts to allow their digestion by pancreatic enzymes. During that digestive process, three drug phases are formed. The first drug phase that is formed is a small amount of calcium-cyclosporin precipitant, which is then taken out of the absorptive solution. A second drug phase that is formed is a mixed suspension phase containing cyclosporin solubilized by monoglycerides and bile salts. Only a low concentration of cyclosporin is dissolved in this phase. An oily phase from undigested lipids (tri- and diglycerides) with a high concentration of dissolved cyclosporin is the third phase that forms during in vivo intestinal digestion. This oily phase suspension of cyclosporin, which shows the greatest absorption in the small intestine, can be pharmacologically reproduced in vitro by combining standard cyclosporin with the cosolvents found in SIM-Neoral. These cosolvents are described later in this chapter.

Why SIM-SGC Is Poorly Absorbed

The *potential* "absorptive window" for cyclosporin consists of the entire duodenum, jejunum, and ileum. That is, intestinal villi or lacteals in these structures are fully capable of absorbing cyclosporin. However, *actual* cyclosporin digestion with SIM-SGC begins where the bile duct and the pancreatic duct enter the second portion of the duodenum at the ampulla of Vater (see Fig. 11). There cyclosporin is processed into lipid micelles at the second portion of the duodenum *below* the ampulla of Vater, where bile and pancreatic enzymes are released into the duodenum. Therefore, absorption of cyclosporin is not only delayed due to processing requirements, which include biochemical digestion of cyclosporin into the three phases mentioned previously, but the absorptive surface areas of the duodenal villi located *above* the ampulla of Vater are underutilized (85). Part of this underutilization is because intestinal peristalsis primarily

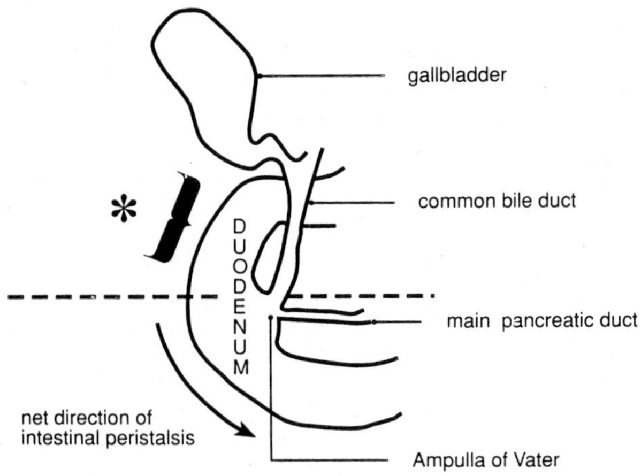

Figure 11 Schematic drawing of the gallbladder, common bile duct, etc. (Modified from Grant's Atlas of Anatomy.)

moves the intestinal chyme and micelles forward down the duodenum, jejunum, and ileum, thus further decreasing the probability of any cyclosporin being absorbed above the ampulla of Vater during in vivo intestinal digestion.

In addition, food affects SIM-SGC pharmacokinetics. This results in a decreased C_{max}, a decreased AUC, and an increased T_{max}. Thus, SIM-SGC is dependent on the physiological state of the GI tract, biodependency, and food effects. SIM-Neoral pharmacokinetics, on the other hand, are much less affected by the fed versus fasting state (Table 3) (86–88).

Why SIM-Neoral Has Better Absorption

SIM-Neoral is given as a soft gel capsule in 100- and 25-mg sizes. These capsules are filled with a preconcentrate of a microemulsion consisting of the active ingredient, cyclosporin, a surfactant, a lipophilic solvent (mono-, di-, and triglycerides), a hydrophilic solvent (propylene glycol), and ethanol as a hydrophilic cosolvent. Pharmaceutical research has shown that when medium-chain (C6-C12) fatty acids, mono-, di-, and triglycerides are incorporated in a microemulsion, significant enhancement of intraduodenal absorption can occur, especially when peptide drugs like cyclosporin are incorporated into these emulsions (85,89). The surfactant components and lipophilic solvents allow for increased absorption through the lipid layers of the intestinal brush border, as well as increased surface contact. This microemulsion simulates the micelle phase obtained after digestion of the cyclosporin lipid droplets.

Therefore, once ingested, Neoral releases cyclosporin rapidly for its absorption so that the entire length of the "absorption window" can be used. This includes the absorptive surface area (brush border) of the duodenal villi that lies above the ampulla of Vater (see Fig. 11). This microemulsion remains *in solution* during the entire absorption window so that no precipitation of cyclosporin occurs with bile salts, as is the case with digestion of classical cyclosporin (SIM-SGC). This Neoral microemulsion is thus ready for immediate absorption and its is not influenced by lipid digestion processes, bile flow, or pancreatic enzyme release. In addition, negligible food effect is observed on bioavailability of cyclosporin. With the increased consistency of the absorption from SIM-Neoral, the systemic exposure was shown to be almost completely dose-proportional. This dose proportionality is less evident with conventional SIM-SGC (see Fig. 12).

Table 3 Relative Bioavailability of Cyclosporine from Soft Gelatin Capsules of the Test Formulation (SIM-Neoral) Compared to the Reference Formulation (SIM-SGC) as Assessed in Healthy Volunteers at Four Dose Levels

Dose level (mg)	AUC_0 ratio (test/reference)[a]	95% confidence interval
200	1.74	1.58–2.07
400	2.20	1.95–2.87
600	2.20	1.96–2.71
800	2.39	2.12–2.95

[a]Geometric mean of intraindividual test/reference AUC_0, ratios.
Source: Ref. 87.

Study Populations

Most of the clinical pharmacology on Sandimmune Neoral to date derives from safety and tolerability studies from healthy subjects, renal, liver, and cardiac transplantation patients, and a limited number of patients with psoriasis and rheumatoid arthritis (77). Most of the data concerning safety and tolerability involve one-to-one switches from patients using the standard Sandimmune Soft Gel Capsules to Sandimmune Neoral.

Initial safety and efficacy studies performed by Sandoz involved 686 patients. Of these, 551 received a new formulation of SIM-Neoral; 46 patients were included in the experimental pharmacokinetic trials and their data are not included in this summary because of differences in recommended dosages. Pa-

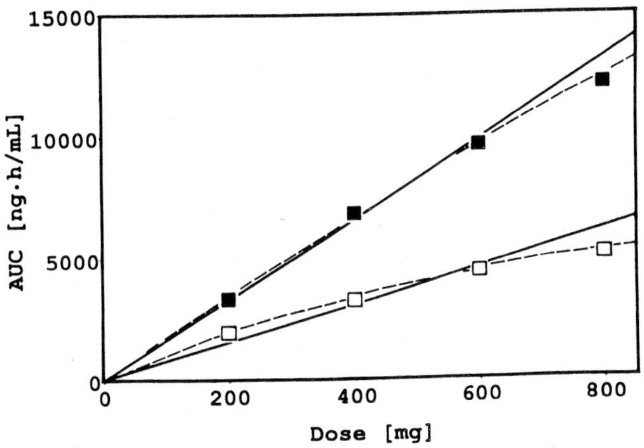

Figure 12 Relationship between dose and cyclosporin AUC. ■ SIM-Neoral; □ SIM-SGC.

tients were in the age range of 18–72 years, with a mean age of 45 years. No children were included in any of these initial preliminary studies. Thirty-three percent of the patients were female. Nearly all patients were Caucasians. Eighty-six patients received SIM-Neoral in 4-week studies and 418 patients were treated in 12-week studies. Stable renal transplant patients received mean doses of 3.5 mg/kg/day. Patients with rheumatoid arthritis and psoriasis received mean doses of 3 mg/kg/day. Newly transplanted patients received an average of 6 mg/kg/day, which had been reduced to 3.7 mg/kg/day at week 12. The pharmacokinetic data generated from these initial safety studies have been repeatedly confirmed through multiple clinical trails conducted primarily in the renal transplantation literature, but also in the cardiac and liver transplantation literature as well. The large multicenter Sandoz study comparing SIM-SGC with SIM-Neoral in the treatment of psoriasis has just been completed and the data from this multicenter study is discussed at the end of this page. However, several initial studies had been conducted prior to this large study which did look at the pharmacokinetics of SIM-SGC and SIM-Neoral in patients with both rheumatoid arthritis and psoriasis.

Results of Pharmacokinetic Studies

The following general conclusions can be drawn from previously completed pharmacokinetic studies (90–100) to date involving SIM-Neoral. SIM-Neoral is generally well-tolerated. The observed adverse events comprise the expected sensorial disturbances (heat sensation, hyperesthesia, dysesthesia, dry mouth, sore throat, tongue discomfort), GI complaints (stomach ache, nausea, pressure in the upper gastric area, loose stools), and central nervous system complaints (headaches, lightheadedness, dizziness, tiredness, weakness). The incidence of these adverse events increased in a dose-dependent manner for both formulations. The incidence at a given dose level was higher for SIM-Neoral than for SIM-SGC marketed form, which was probably the result of the higher exposure to cyclosporin after administration of SIM-Neoral. However, in subjects with a similar exposure to cyclosporin in terms of AUC, no difference in the incidence of adverse events was evident after the administration of SIM-SGC compared to SIM-Neoral.

In renal studies, sequential creatinine clearances (in stable renal transplant patients) were recorded over a steady-state dosing interval parallel to a 12-h pharmacokinetic assessment during treatment with SIM-SGC and after one-to-one switch to SIM-Neoral. Changes in creatinine clearance were similar with both treatments. Vital signs were frequently assessed during the studies and there was no difference between treatments. No difference in the effect of the formulations on blood pressure, serum concentrations of urea, uric acid, potassium, cholesterol, or triglycerides was apparent. The increases in C_{max} and AUC were not associated with decreased tolerability or changes in vital signs or clinical laboratory parameters.

After a one-to-one switch from SIM-SGC to SIM-Neoral, the bioavailability is increased on average by about 30%. C_{max} is increased on average by approximately 60%, while T_{max} is reduced by about 1 h. The intrapatient variability of all parameters is significantly reduced, and Neoral kinetics are much less affected by food administration (Table 4). The pharmacokinetic findings in the two small pharmacokinetic studies in rheumatoid arthritis and psoriasis patients are similar to those obtained in transplant patients. There are no statistically significant differences in adverse events in the two formulations. There were no statistically significant differences in laboratory safety parameters between the two formulations. The metabolism, elimination, and drug-drug interactions of SIM-SGC and SIM-Neoral are essentially the same.

Table 4 Mean (CV%) Pharmacokinetic Parameters Following Twice-Daily Dosing with SIM or Neoral by 11 Stable Renal Transplant Patients

Parameter	SIM Fasting	SIM Nonfasting	Neoral Fasting	Neoral Nonfasting
T_{max} (h)	2.1 (33.3)	2.6 (76.9)	1.5 (33.3)	1.2 (33.3)
C_{max} (μg/L)	663 (34.5)	528 (40.5)	997 (20.0)	892 (35.8)
C_{min} (μg/L)	78 (30.8)	92 (29.3)	94 (22.3)	100 (23.0)
AUC (μg h/L)	2645 (25.7)	2432 (24.3)	3454 (17.6)	3028 (19.7)
PIF%	261 (23.4)	212 (36.8)	317 (18.0)	309 (31.1)

All concentrations measured in whole blood at steady state AUC was measured over a dosing interval. jPIF% − percentage peak through fluctuation.
Source: Ref. 87.

Safety, Tolerability, and Efficacy of Two Formulations of Cyclosporin A in Patients with Severe Psoriasis: A Randomized, Double-Blind Study Comparing Neoral and Sandimmune

The safety, tolerability, efficacy and effective dosage of cyclosporin A (CyA [Sandimmune®, SIM]) and a new oral microemulsion formulation of CyA, Sandimmune Neoral® (Neoral), were compared in patients with severe, chronic, plaque-form psoriasis. This study was conducted in many centers in the United States and Europe (101).

Patients were randomized on a 1:1 basis to 24 weeks of treatment with Neoral (n = 152) or SIM (n = 157). The starting dose of each formulation was 2.5 mg/kg per day. Dose increases for lack of efficacy were allowed after 4 weeks; dose decreases for safety were allowed at any time. In patients who achieved remission [75% reduction in the Psoriasis Area and Severity Index (PASI) compared with baseline], the dose was down-titrated at 4-week intervals from week 16. The maximum permitted dose for each formulation was 5.0 mg/kg/day.

Both treatment groups showed improvement in efficacy parameters (change in PASI from baseline to week 16, time from baseline to remission and percentage of relapse-free patients), but Neoral appeared to produce a more rapid response; remission rates were higher for Neoral than SIM during the first 8 weeks of treatment when the same dosage was used (Fig. 13). The number of dose reductions for safety was similar in both treatment groups. Dose increases for lack of efficacy were more frequent in the SIM group (198) than the Neoral group (146), resulting in a higher mean dose for SIM (3.29 mg/kg/day) than for Neoral (3.04 mg/kg/day) at week 16. More dose reductions for stable remission were possible with Neoral (83) than SIM (73) after week 16. Hence the mean Neoral dose remained lower than the mean SIM dose from week 6 onward. As dose adjustments were permitted, relatively few patients (Neoral, n = 14; SIM, n = 8) discontinued treatment prematurely because of laboratory abnormalities or adverse events. The frequency and nature of adverse events were similar for both treatment groups.

In summary, due to its better bioavailability in many patients, Neoral has a more rapid onset of action and is just as well tolerated as SIM in the treatment of psoriasis.

Therapeutic Implications

Dosing with SIM-Neoral results in improved oral bioavailability. Consequently, there is less variability in trough cyclosporin blood concentrations. These concentrations are thus more closely related to the total drug exposure during a dosing interval (AUC) than is the case with SIM-SGC (Fig. 12). Evidence suggests that clinical efficacy of cyclosporin may be related to trough blood concentrations (C_{min}). Thus, if a patient shows poor absorption reflected by lower than expected trough concentrations, even at the maximum dose of 5 mg/kg/day of cyclosporin, this may reflect clinical inefficiency related to poor drug absorption. These "nonresponders" will probably do well once switched from the SIM-SGC to the SIM-Neoral preparation. Even the responders are likely to benefit from the more reliable dosing possible with SIM-Neoral. Since the use of SIM-Neoral instead of SIM-SGC makes a significant difference mainly to those patients who absorb SIM-SGC poorly, whereas for those who absorb SIM-SGC well switching to SIM-Neoral makes little or no difference, the maximum recom-

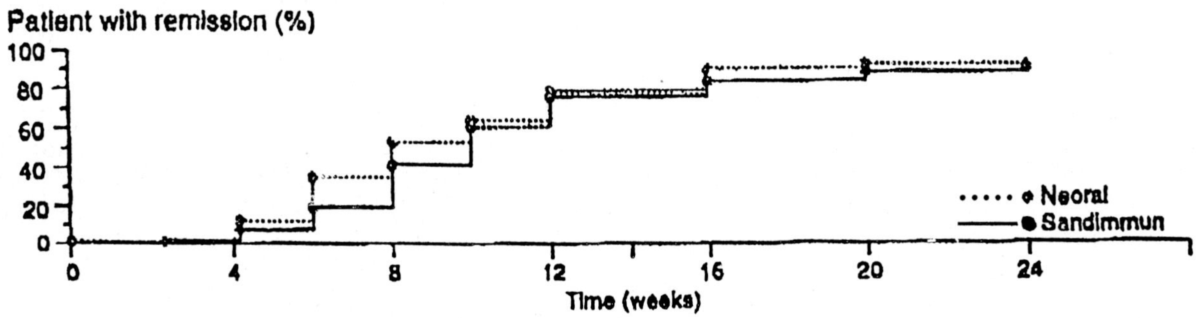

Figure 13 Remission rate, Neoral vs. Sandimmune.

mended dose for SIM-Neoral is still felt to be similar (i.e., approximately 5 mg/kg/day) to the maximum recommended dose for SIM-SGC. Some clinicians feel that we may get away with a slightly lower dosage of SIM-Neoral than of SIM-SGC. In the United States, where SIM-Neoral was approved by the Food and Drug Administration in June, 1997, the FDA, with their usual cautiousness, recommended 4 mg/kg/day as the maximum dermatological dosage to be used. The important point to realize is that patients can be switched from SIM-SGC to SIM-Neoral with the same dosage without having to worry about "overdosing the patient." Again, this is because such a switch will help those patients with a poor capacity for absorbing SIM-SGC but is not likely to overdose any patient with good absorption efficiency to SIM-SGC. In this sense, since SIM-Neoral is now available, it appears that there is no reason to use the old formulation (SIM-SGC), since it has no particular advantage in terms of safety and its efficacy is less reliable because of its less reliable bioavailability.

REFERENCES

1. Borel J.F., Feurer, C., Gubler, H.U. Biological effects of cyclosporin A: A new antilymphocyte agent. *Agents Actions* 1976; 6:468–475.
2. Mueller, W., Hermann, B. Cyclosporin A for psoriasis. *N. Engl. J. Med.* 1979; 301:555.
3. Ellis, C.N., Gorsulowsky, D.C., Hamilton, T.A., et al. Cyclosporin improves psoriasis in a double-blind study. *JAMA* 1986; 256:3110–3116.
4. van Joost, T.H., Bod, J.D., Heule, F., et al. Low-dose cyclosporin A in severe psoriasis. A double-blind study. *Br. J. Dermatol.* 1988; 118:193–190.
5. Curley, R.K., Macfarlane, A.W., Vickers, C.F.H. Pyoderma gangrenosum treated with cyclosporin A. *Br. J. Dermatol.* 1985; 113:601–604.
6. Magid, M.L., Gold, M.H. Treatment of recalcitrant pyoderma gangrenosum with cyclosporin. *J. Am. Acad. Dermatol.* 1989; 20:293–294.
7. Penmetacha, M., Navaratnam, A.E. Pyoderma gangrenosum. *Int. J. Dermatol.* 1988; 27:253.
8. Shelley, E.D., Shelley, W.B. Cyclosporin therapy for pyoderma grangrenosum associated with sclerosing cholangiitis and ulcerative colitis. *J. Am. Acad. Dermatol.* 1988; 18:1084–1088.
9. Taylor, R.S., Cooper, K.D., Headington, J.T., et al. Cyclosporin in atopic dermatitis. *J. Am. Acad. Dermatol.* (in press).
10. van Joost, T.H., Stolz, E., Heule, F. Efficacy of low-dose cyclosporin in severe atopic skin disease. *Arch. Dermatol.* 1987; 123:166–167.
11. Barthelemy, H., Frappaz, A., Cambazard, F., et al. Treatment of nine cases of pemphigus vulgaris with cyclosporin. *J. Am. Acad. Dermatol.* 1988; 18: 1262–1266.
12. Barthelemy, H., Biron, F., Claudy, A., et al. Cyclosporin: new immunosuppressive agent in bullous pemphigoid and pemphigus. *Transplant Proc.* 1986; 18: 913–914.
13. Cunliffe, W.F. Bullous pemphigoid and response to cyclosporin. *Br. J. Dermatol.* 1987; 117:113–114.
14. Cunliffe, W.J. Pemphigus foliaceus and response to cyclosporin. *Br. J. Dermatol.* 1987; 117:114–116.
15. Gebhart, W., Schmidt, J.B., Schemper, M., et al. Cyclosporin A-induced hair growth in human renal allograft recipients and alopecia areata. *Arch. Dermatol. Res.* 1986; 278:238–240.
16. Gupta, A.K., Ellis, C.N., Cooper, K.D., et al. Oral cyclosporin for the treatment of alopecia areata: a clinical and immunohistochemical analysis. *J. Am. Acad. Dermatol.* (in press).
17. Gupta, A.K., Ellis, C.N., Nickoloff, B.J., et al. Oral cyclosporin in the treatment of inflammatory and noninflammatory dermatoses. *Arch. Dermatol.* 1990; 126: 339–350.
18. French-Constant, C., Wolman, R., Geraint-James, D. Cyclosporin in Behcet's disease. *Lancet* 1983; 2:454.

19. Nussenblatt, R.B., Palestine, A.G., Chan C-C., et al. Effectiveness of cyclosporin therapy for Behcets disease. *Arthritis. Rheum.* 1985; 28:671–679.
20. Nussenblatt, R.B., Palestine, A.G., Rook, A.H., et al. Treatment of intraocular inflammatory disease with cyclosporin A. *Lancet* 1983; 2:235–238.
21. Sanders, M.D., Geraint-James, D., Graham, E., et al. Cyclosporin in Behcets disease. *Lancet* 1983; 2: 454–455.
22. Duschet, P., Schwarz, T., Oppolzer, G., et al. Persistent light reaction. *Acta. Dermatol. Venereol (Stockh.)* 1988; 68:176–178.
23. Ejstrup, L., Severe dermatomyositis treated with cyclosporin A. *Ann. Rheum. Dis.* 1986; 45:612–613.
24. Zabel, P., Leimenstoll, G., Gross, W.L. Cyclosporin for acute dermatomyositis. *Lancet* 1984; 1:343.
25. Picascia, D.D., Roenigk, H.H. Jr. Cyclosporin and male-pattern alopecia. *Arch. Dermatol.* 1987; 123: 1432.
26. Connolly, S.M., Sander, H.M. Treatment of epidermolysis bullosa acquisita with cyclosporin [Letter]. *J. Am. Acad. Dermatol.* 1987; 16:890.
27. Crow, L.L., Finkle, J.P., Gamman, W.R., et al. Clearing of epidermolysis bullosa acquisita with cyclosporin. *J. Am. Acad. Dermatol.* 1988; 19:937–942.
28. Zachariae, H. Cyclosporin A in epidemermolysis bullosa acquisita. *J. Am. Acad. Dermatol.* 1987; 17: 1058–1059.
29. Velthuis, R.J., Jesserun, R.F.M. Improvement of ichthyosis by cyclosporin. *Lancet* 1985; 1:335.
30. Frandin, M.S., Ellis, C.N., Goldfarb, M.T., et al. Cyclosporin for chronic urticaria. Submitted for publication.
31. Wilkel, C.S., McDonald, C.J. Cyclosporin therapy for bullous erythema multiforme. *Arch. Dermatol.* 1990; 126:397–398.
32. Vayssairat, M., Baudot, N., Biotard, C., et al. Cyclosporin therapy for severe systemic sclerosis associated with the anti-Scl-70 antibody. *J. Am. Acad. Dermatol.* 1990; 22:695–696.
33. Miller, R.A., Shen, J-Y, Rea, T.H., et al. Treatment of chronic erythema nodosum leprosum with cyclosporin A produces clinical and immunohistological remission. *Int. J. Lepr. Other Mycobact. Dis.* 1987; 55: 441–449.
34. Uyemura, K., Dixon, J.F.P., Wong, L., et al. Effect of cyclosporin A in erythema nodosum leprosum. *J. Immunol.* 1986; 137:3620–3623.
35. Tigalonowa, M., Bjerke, J.R., Gallari, H., et al. Immunological changes following treatment of psoriasis with cyclosporin. *Acta. Derm. Venereol. (Stockh.)* 1989; 146:142–146.
36. Granelli-Piperno, A. The effect of immunosuppressive agents on the induction of nuclear factors that bend to sites on the interleukin-2 promoter. *J. Exp. Med.* 1990; 171:533–544.
37. Flanagan, W.M., Corthesy, B., Bram, R.J., Crabtree, G.R. Nuclear association of a T-cell transcription factor blocked by FK-506 and cyclosporin. *Nature* 1991; 352:803–807.
38. Liu, J., Farmer, Jr. J.D., Lane, W.S., et al. Calcineurin is a common target of cyclophilin-cyclosporin and FKPP-FK5-6 complexes. *Cell* 1991; 66:807–815.
39. Schreiber, S.L., Crabtree, G.R. The mechanism of action of Cyclosporin and FK506. *Immunol. Today* 1992; 13:136–142.
40. Baker, B.S., Griffiths, C.E.M., Lambert, S., et al. The effects of cyclosporin A on T lymphocyte and dendritic cell sub-populations in psoriasis. *Br. J. Dermatol.* 1987;116(4):503–510.
41. Kalman, V.K., Klimpel, G.R. Cyclosporin A inhibits the production of gamma interferon (IFNγ), but does not inhibit production of virus-induced IFN$\alpha\gamma$. *Cell Immunol.* 1983; 78:122–129.
42. Fisher, G.J., Duell, E.A., Nickoloff, B.J., et al. Levels of cyclosporin in epidermis of treated psoriasis patients differentially inhibit growth of keratinocytes cultured in serum free versus serum containing media. *J. Invest. Dermatol.* 1988; 91:142–146.
43. Nickoloff, B.J., Fisher, G.J., Mitra, R.S., Voorhees, J.J. Additive and synergistic antiproliferative effects of cyclosporin A and gamma interferon on cultured human keratinocytes. *Am. J. Pathol.* 1988; 131: 12–18.
44. Sharpe, G.R., Fisher, C. Time-dependent inhibition of growth of human keratinocytes and fibroblasts by cyclosporin A: effect on keratinocytes at therapeutic blood levels. *Br. J. Dermatol.* 1990; 123:207–213.
45. Won, Y., Sauder, O.N., McKenzie, R.C. Cyclosporin A inhibits keratinocyte cytokine gene expression. *Br. J. Dermatol.* 1994; 130:312–319.
46. Wong, R.L., Winslow, C.M., Cooper, K.D. The mechanisms of action of cyclosporin A in the treatment of psoriasis. *Immunol. Today* 1993; 14:69–74.
47. Mozzanica, N., Pigatto, P.D., Finzi, A.F. Cyclosporin in psoriasis: pathophysiology and experimental data. *Dermatology* 1993; 187(Suppl. 1):3–7.
48. Demidem, A., Taylor, J.R., Grammer, S.F., Streilein, J.W. T-lymphocyte-activating properties of epidermal antigen-presenting cells from normal and psoriatic skin: evidence that psoriatic epidermal antigen-presenting cells resemble cultured normal Langerhans cells. *J. Invest. Dermatol.* 1991; 97:454–460.
49. Dupuy, P., Bagot, M., Michel, L., Descourt, B., Dubertret, L. Cyclosporin A inhibits the antigen-presenting functions of freshly isolated human Langerhans cells in vitro. *J. Invest Dermatol.* 1991; 96: 408–413.
50. Furue, M., Katz, S.I. The effect of cyclosporin on epidermal cells: cyclosporin inhibits accessory cell functions of epidermal Langerhans cells in vitro. *J. Immunol.* 1988; 140:4139–4143.

51. Hultsch, T., Rodriguez, J.L., Kaliner, M.A., Hohman, R.J. Cyclosporin A inhibits degranulation of rat basophilic leukemia cells and human basophils: Inhibition of mediator release without affecting PI hydrolysis or Ca^{2+} fluxes. *J. Immunol.* 1990; 144: 2659–2664.
52. Triggiani, M., Cirillo, R., Lichtenstein, L.M., Marone, G. Inhibition of histamine and prostaglandin D_2 release from human lung mast cells by cyclosporin A. *Interna. Arch. Allergy Appl. Immunol.* 1989; 88: 253–255.
53. Baadsgaard, O., Tong, P., Elder, J.T., et al. UM4D4+ (CDW60) T cells are compartmentalized into psoriatic skin and release lymphokines that induce a keratinocyte phenotype expressed in psoriatic lesions. *J. Invest. Dermatol.* 1990; 95:275–282.
54. Korstanje, M.J., Bilo, H.J.G., Stoof, T.J. Sustained renal function loss in psoriasis patients after withdrawal of low-dose cyclosporin therapy. *Br. J. Dermatol.* 1992; 127:501–504.
55. Wood, A.J., Maurer, G., Niederberger, W., et al. Cyclosporin: pharmacokinetics, metabolism and drug interactions. *Transplant Proc.* 1983; 15:2409–2412.
56. Gilman, A.G., Goodman, L.S., Rall, R.W., et al., eds. The pharmacologic basis for therapeutics, 7th ed. New York: Macmillan, 1985: 1682.
57. Follath, F., Wenk, M., Vozeh, S., et al. Intravenous cyclosporin kinetics in renal failure. *Clin. Pharmacol. Ther.* 1983; 34:638–643.
58. Ptachcinski, R.J., Venkataramanan, R., Burckart, G.J. Clinical pharmacokinetics of cyclosporin. *Clin. Pharmacokinet.* 1986; 11:107–132.
59. Feutren, G., Friend, D., Timonen, P. Barnes, A., et al. Predictive value of cyclosporin A level for efficacy or renal dysfunction in psoriasis. *Br. J. Dermatol.* 1990; 122(suppl. 36):85–93.
60. Mihatsch M.J., Wolff K: Report of a meeting: Consensus conference on cyclosporin A for psoriasis, February 1992. *Br. J. Dermatol.* 1992; 126:623.
61. Timonen P., Friend D., Abeywickrama K., Laburte C., et al. Efficacy of low-dose cyclosporin A in psoriasis; results of dose-finding studies. *Br. J. Dermatol.* 1990; 122 (suppl 36):33–39.
62. Mihatsch MJ, Wolff K. Report of a meeting: Consensus conference on cyclosporin A for psoriasis. *Br. J. Dermatol.* 1992; 126:621.
63. Rebora A. Cyclosporin A in psoriasis. *Clin. Dermatol.* 1992; 9:515–522.
64. Luke RG. Mechanism of cyclosporine-induced hypertension. *Am. J. Hypertension* 1991; 4:468–471.
65. Mihatsch MJ., Wolff K. Report of a meeting: Consensus conference on cyclosporin A for psoriasis, February 1992. *Br. J. Dermatol.* 1992; 126:622.
66. Deray G., Baumelou B., Letoang P., et al. Enhancement of cyclosporin nephrotoxicity by diuretic therapy. *Clin. Nephrol.* 1989; 32:47.
67. Whiting PH., Cunningham C., Thomson AW., et al. Enhancement of high dose cyclosporin A toxicity by frusemide. *Biochem. Pharmacol.* 1984; 33: 1075–1079.
68. Mihatsch M.J., Belghiti D., Bohman S.O., et al. Kidney biopsies in control or cyclosporin A-treated psoriatic patients. *Br. J. Dermatol.* 1990; 122 (suppl 36): 96–100.
69. Powles A.V., Cook T., Hulme B., et al. Renal function and biopsy findings after 5 years' treatment with low-dose cyclosporin for psoriasis. *Br. J. Dermatol.* 1993; 128:159–165.
70. Ellis C.N., Fradin M.S., Messana J.M., et al. Cyclosporin for plaque-type psoriasis: Results of a multidose, double-blind trial. *N. Engl. J. Med.* 1991; 324: 277–284.
71. Ellis C.N. (guest editor). Cyclosporin in dermatology. *J. Am. Acad. Dermatol.* 1990; 23:1241–1334.
72. Koo J., Lee J., Cyclosporin: What clinicians need to know. *Dermatol. Clin.* 1995; 13(4):897–907.
73. Koo J. Cyclosporin in dermatology: fears and opportunities. *Arch. Dermatol.* 1995; 131:842–845.
74. Ellis C.N., Fradin M.S., Voorhees J.J., Hamilton T.A. Duration of remission during maintenance cyclosporin therapy for psoriasis: Relationship to maintenance dose and degree of improvement during initial therapy. *Arch. Dermatol.* 1995; 131:791–795.
75. Linholm A. Factors influencing the pharmacokinetics of cyclosporin in man. *Ther. Drug Monit.* 1991; 13: 465–477.
76. Linholm A., Kahan B.D. Influence of cyclosporin pharmacokinetics, trough concentrations, and AUC monitoring on outcome after kidney transplantation. *Clin. Pharmacol. Ther.* 1993; 54:205–208.
77. Holt D.W., Mueller E.A., Kovarik J.M., van Bree J.B., Kutz K. The pharmacokinetics of Sandimmum Neoral: a new formulation of cyclosporin. *Transplant Proc.* 1994; 26(5):2935–2939.
78. Goodman L., Gilman A. The Pharmacological Basis of Therapeutics, 8th ed. Elmsford, New York. Pergamon Press, 1990:1–32.
79. Drewe D., Beglinger C., Thoma A. The absorption site of cyclosporin in the human gastrointestinal tract. *Clin. Pharm.* 1992; 33:29–43.
80. Vanderscher J., Meinzer A. Rationale for the development of Sandimmun Neoral. *Transplant. Proc.* 1994; 26(5):2925–2937.
81. Lemaire M., Tillement J.P. Role of lipoproteins and erythrocytes in vitro binding and distribution of cyclosporin in the blood. *J. Pharm. Pharmacol.* 1982; 34:715–718.
82. Niederberger W., Lemaire M., Maurer G., Nussbaumer K., Wagner O. Distribution and binding of cyclosporin in blood and tissues. *Transplant. Proc.* 1983; 15:2519.

83. Kovarik J.M., Vernillet L., Mueller E.A., Freiburghaus R., et al. Cyclosporin disposition and metabolite profiles in renal transplant patients receiving a microemulsion formulation. *Ther. Drug Monit.* 1995; 16(5):519–525.
84. Guyton A.C. *Textbook of Medical Physiology*, 8th ed. Philadelphia, P.A: W.B. Saunders, 1991:728–729, 734.
85. Drewe J., Meier R., Vonderscher J., Kiss D., Posanski U., et al. Enhancement of the oral absorption of cyclosporin in man. *Br. J. Clin. Pharm.* 1992; 34(1): 60–64.
86. Browne B.J., Jordan S., Welse M.S., Van Buren C., Kahan B.O. Diet and cyclosporin A—pharmacokinetic comparison between Neoral and Sandimmun gelatin capsules. *Transplant Proc.* 1994; 26(5): 2959–2960.
87. Mueller E.A., Kovarik J.M., van Bree J.B., Grevel J., et al. Influence of a fat-rich meal on the pharmacokinetics of a new oral formulation of cyclosporin in a crossover comparison with the market formulation. *Pharm. Res.* 1994; 11(1):151–155.
88. Tan KKC, Trull J.A., Ultridge S., Metcalfe C.S., et al. Effect of dietary fat on the pharmacokinetics and pharmacodynamics of cyclosporin in renal transplant recipients. *Transplant Proc.* 1994; 26(5):2855–2856.
89. Contantinides P.P., Scalart J.P., Lancaster C., Marcello J., et al. Formulation and intestinal absorption enhancement evaluation of water-in-oil microemulsions incorporating medium-chain glycerides. *Pharm. Res.* 1994; 11(10):1385–90.
90. Belli L.S., Slim O.R., De Carlis L., Rondinara G.F., et al. Neoral in liver transplant patients: pharmacokinetic study and clinical implications. *Transplant Proc.* 1994; 26(5):2981–2982.
91. Belli L.S., De Carlis L., Rondinara G.F., Riberti A., et al. Sandimmun-Neoral in liver transplantation: a remarkable improvement in long-term immunosuppression. *Transplant Proc.* 1994; 26(5):2983–2984.
92. Farber L., Maibucher A., Geissler F., Butzler F., et al. Favourable clinical results of Sandimmun-Neoral in malabsorbing liver and heart transplant recipients. *Transplant Proc.* 1994; 26(5):2988–2993.
93. Freeman D., Grant D., Levy G., Rochon J., et al. Pharmacokinetics of a new oral formulation of cyclosporin in liver transplant recipients. *Ther Drug Monit.* 1995; 17(3):213–216.
94. Kovarik J.M., Mueller E.A., van Bree J.B., Arns W., et al. Within-day consistency in cyclosporin pharmacokinetics from a microemulsion formulation in renal transplant patients. *Ther Drug Monit.* 1994; 16(3):232–237.
95. Kovarik J.M., Mueller E.A., van Bree J.B., Fluckiger S.S., et al. Cyclosporin pharmacokinetics and variability from a microemulsion formulation—a multicenter investigatoin in kidney transplant patients. *Transplantation* 1994; 58(6):658–663.
96. Kovarik J.M., Mueller E.A., van Bree J.B., Tetzloff W., et al. Reduced inter- and intraindividual variability in cyclosporin pharmacokinetics from a microemulsion formulation. *J. Pharm. Sci.* 1994; 83(3): 444–446.
97. Mikhail G., Eadon H., Leaver N., Yacoub M. Use of Neoral in heart transplant recipients. *Transplant Proc.* 1994; 26(5):2985–2987.
98. Mueller EA, Kovarik J.M., van Bree J.B., Lison A.E., Kutz K. Pharmacokinetics and tolerability of a microemulsion formulation of cyclosporin in renal allograft recipeints—a concentration-controlled comparison with the commercial formulation. *Transplantation* 1994; 57(8):1178–1182.
99. Neumayer H.H., Farber L., Haller P., Kohnen R., Maibucher A., et al. Clinical experience transferring kidney transplant patients from Sandimmun to Sandimmun Neoral—results after 3 months. *Clin. Nephrol.* 1995; 43(suppl 1): 527–532.
100. Taesch S., Niese D., Mueller E.A. Sandimmun neoral, a new formulation of cylcosporin A with improved pharmacokinetic characteristics: safety and tolerability in renal transplant patients. *Transplant Proc.* 1994; 26(6):3147–3149.
101. Poster presented at the 19th World Congress of Dermatology, Sydney, Australia.

53

Long-Term Use of Cyclosporin in Dermatology

Hugh Zachariae
Aarhus University Hospital, Aarhus, Denmark

The long-term safety of cyclosporin in the treatment of psoriasis has been discussed by Grossman et al. (1). However, cyclosporin is today used by dermatologists not only in psoriasis but increasingly in atopic dermatitis (2) as well as in a number of other conditions such as bullous disorders, pyoderma gangrenosum, lichen planus, dermatomyositis, systemic lupus erythematosus, and various forms of vasculitis. Cyclosporin has also received recognition as an effective disease-moderating agent in psoriatic arthritis. The time for evaluation of long-term safety seems appropriate, especially for psoriasis, since the drug has now been used for this condition for more than 10 years. The evaluation could then also, to a certain extent, give a basis for judgment regarding the use in other chronic dermatological diseases.

The basis for the use of cyclosporin in dermatology was first a series of encouraging observations, rather than a thorough understanding of its mechanism of action, which in general is both immunosuppressive and anti-inflammatory. Today the use in the two major diseases psoriasis and atopic dermatitis is clearly the result of well-planned, controlled studies together with a number of multicenter, dose-finding studies. In psoriasis these studies became the basis for clinical guidelines (3), which should help minimize the risk for side effects. These guidelines are referred to in the article by Grossman et al. (1) and they are now widely used in the management of dermatological conditions with cyclosporin.

RISKS AND SIDE EFFECTS

The important long-term risks in cyclosporin therapy are renal toxicity, hypertension, and an increased risk of malignancy. Infections can usually be encountered and the remaining other side effects may be bothersome but can be considered a fairly minor problem. The clinical material on which Grossman et al. (1) report has a special value for analysis, as it is based solely on patients who initially belonged to a prospective study population with strict inclusion criteria and strict rules for surveillance. Among these patients they found that 53 of 122 had an increase in serum creatinine greater than 30% above baseline. According to the guidelines, a dose reduction was enacted, but in one-fourth of the patients serum creatinine remained greater than the 30% after 1 month, which led to discontinuation of the drug. These data are important, as they indicate what should be expected in a great number of psoriatics, when a reasonable clearing of the disease is wanted.

The relatively high incidence of hypertension (29 of 122 patients) is also noteworthy. In this material 10 patients were treated with ACE inhibitors alone and five with β-blockers alone, while there is no mention of the use of calcium channel blockers, although nifedipine has been recommended as a first-line drug. Nifedipine has, together with felodipine, been suggested also to have a nephroprotective effect. In our hands this was established for felodipine in a double-blind crossover trial (4).

The two patients who developed cancer during the study period and the three malignancies reported after the study are probably within the limits of what can be expected in a group of 122 psoriatics, where many have had multiple other therapies over the years, which could all contribute to cancer. The patient who developed mycosis fungoides after 6 weeks of cyclosporin could have had concomitant parapsoriasis en plaque and thereby add to the evidence that cyclosporin should be contraindicated in cutaneous T-cell lymphoma (5). This is in contrast to the recommendations of Street et al. (6). At present we are waiting for the results of a long-term, multicenter, follow-up study introduced by Sandoz on what could be 1,000 psoriatics, to further elucidate this matter. So far, no studies on malignancy have given findings that should give rise to any alterations in the proposed risk/benefit ratio for cyclosporin in psoriasis.

The most important side effect is without doubt nephrotoxicity. Patients with psoriasis have been thought to be an ideal group to study as there is no known disease relation with renal pathology (7). However, psoriatics as a group have increased values of plasma endothelin, and the highest values are found in cyclosporin-treated individuals (8). Both cyclosporin and endothelins induce vasoconstriction, and endothelin antagonists have been shown in animal studies to produce a protective effect against cyclosporin nephrotoxicity (9). Whether the high plasma endothelin could explain a higher incidence of nephrotoxicity in psoriatics is at present unknown.

The effects of cyclosporin on the kidney may be functional and, in general, reversible or structural and partly reversible, partly irreversible. Of the structural changes, tubulopathy is mostly reversible while vasculopathy and interstitial fibrosis should be irreversible. Chronic cyclosporin nephrotoxicity is characterized by interstitial fibrosis and an obliterative vasculopathy (10). The basis for the guidelines was to a certain extent that if these were followed, only functional and reversible changes would be found. However, this no longer holds true. Although Grossman et al. (1) do comment on histological changes, they did not perform kidney biopsies. We, in early studies on cyclosporin-treated psoriatics, investigated pretreatment and posttreatment renal biopsy specimens from 12 patients treated for 6–18 months (11) and found that although 10 patients had normal pretreatment histology, only one of the patients had a normal posttreatment biopsy. Therapy was associated with a significant increase of interstitial connective tissue and focal fibrosis together with a nonsignificant increase in arteriolar hyalinosis. Morphological changes at the time did not reflect duration of therapy. Today our material consists of renal biopsies from 30 psoriatics studies from 6 months to 8 years (12) including pretreatment biopsies from 25 patients. No patient treated for 2 years or more had a normal kidney biopsy. There was a significant increase over the years of arteriolar hyalinosis, interstitial fibrosis, and, after 4 years, of glomerular sclerosis. The histology was evaluated blind in both studies. Of the 11 patients who were evaluated after 4 years, all but one had arteriolar hyalinosis and interstitial fibrosis was pronounced in five and moderate in the remaining six. One patient had 14% sclerotic glomeruli. There was also a negative correlation between glomerular filtration rate (GFR) and the degree of fibrosis. The long-term nephrotoxicity would probably have been even more pronounced if patients had not gradually been withdrawn from the study due to the toxicity. Our findings are, in general, in accordance with the data from a summary on the clinical aspects of cyclosporin and nephrotoxicity by Leaker and Cairns (13). The only difference is the relatively low doses of cyclosporin with which our psoriatic patients were treated (from 2.5 to 6 mg/kg/day, with one patient on 7 mg/kg/day for 2 weeks). Leaker and Cairns conclude that cyclosporin invariably produces a minimum of 25% reduction in GFR with chronic usage, which may only be partially reversible (30–50% in cardiac transplant patients), and that nephrotoxicity is dose related and that peak concentrations of drug may be responsible. The evidence of irreversible histological damage in a substantial proportion of our biopsied patients must raise doubt on the safety of long-term cyclosporin in nontransplant patients. We propose that all patients to be treated for more than 2 years deserve a kidney biopsy and that the good cooperation with the nephrologist should be encouraged when dermatological conditions are to be treated on a long-term basis.

Until a revision of the guidelines has taken place, these should be followed strictly. It is important that the physician in charge of the patient is aware of drug interactions. Patients with sustained hypertension should be treated with calcium antagonists such as nifedipine or felodipine, which partially protect against nephrotoxicity, but not with diltiazem or verapamil because of their interference with cyclosporin blood levels. Patients with psoriatic arthritis may need to continue to be on nonsteroidal anti-inflammatory drugs (NSAID). However, NSAID therapy should be discontinued when possible, because these drugs have a synergistic nephrotoxic effect with cyclosporin (14). Routine measurements of cyclosporin blood levels are not essential, but may be useful in detecting drug interactions, noncompliance, and unusual drug availability. The new oral formulation of cyclosporin Sandimmun Neoral, which incorporates the drug in a microemulsion preconcentrate (15), exhibits an improvement in dose linearity and a faster, more consistent rate of absorption with less pharmacokinetic variability. However, the formulation contains the identical active ingredient; therefore, pronounced changes in long-term toxicity should not be expected.

USE AS MAINTENANCE THERAPY

The use of cyclosporine as maintenance therapy in dermatology has previously been discussed (16,17). Nephrotoxicity is clearly the limiting factor for cyclosporin. The Newcastle group from the United Kingdom (18) have advocated the use of cyclosporin for short clearance of ordinary psoriasis. I do not agree that cyclosporin should be used for minor psoriasis. Minor psoriasis may turn out later to be severe psoriasis and any part of the cumulative cyclosporin dose should not have been "misused" in this way in patients who very well could be treated with less toxic agents. I agree that cyclosporin has its place in life-threatening dermatological conditions as part of combination therapy in pemphigus or in severe vasculitis. The capacity of cyclosporin as a steroid-sparing agent in these diseases has been impressive. In chronic diseases such as psoriasis and atopic dermatitis, I would not hesitate to use cyclosporin as a maintenance agent as part of a rational therapy for up to 2 years, provided the guidelines are followed. I would, however, in general not start out with cyclosporin as the first drug of choice. A subgroup of psoriatics have only minor changes in their kidney biopsies and GFR and seem to tolerate the drug much longer than others (12), but one would need a renal biopsy to establish if the patient belongs to this subgroup. The use of cyclosporin as crisis therapy in severe inflammatory psoriasis is another good indication. This should be used to prepare the patient for a switchover to other treatments. This can be done without expecting a rebound phenomenon.

It is true that until now, long-term follow-up studies have not demonstrated significant loss of renal function in nontransplant patients, but the experience from cardiac recipients (19) treated with cyclosporin over a 10-year period showing that 10% deteriorated to end-stage renal failure should not be wasted. Most of these patients progressed to this stage after at least 5 years of therapy. A second study (20) using "low-dose" cyclosporin (5 mg/kg/day) for cardiac transplant patients showed decreased renal function and typical histopathological changes of cyclosporin toxicity similar to what has been found in psoriasis (11,12,21,22) at approximately the same time after start of the drug.

I agree with Koo (17), who stated that it is necessary for the dermatologist to provide the best treatment available, especially for the worst cases. This is where the value of our specialty care is judged, and in this context cyclosporin is certainly a welcome addition to our armamentarium. However, we should also be fully aware of the long-term risks and constantly be willing to evaluate risk/benefit ratio.

REFERENCES

1. Grossman, R., Chevret, S., Abi-Rached, J., et al. (1996). Long-term safety of cyclosporine in the treatment of psoriasis. *Arch. Dermatol.* (in press).
2. Sowden, J., Berth-Jones, J., Ross, J., et al. (1991). Double-blind, controlled, crossover study of cyclosporin in adults with severe refractory atopic dermatitis. *Lancet* 338:137–140.
3. Mihatsch, M., and Wolff, K. (1992). Consensus conference of cyclosporin A for psoriasis, February 1992. *Br. J. Dermatol.* 126:621–623.
4. Pedersen, E., Madsen, J., Sørensen, S. and Zachariae, H. (1995). Improvement in renal function by felodipine during cyclosporine treatment in acute and short-term studies. *Proc. XIII International Congress of Nephrology, Madrid.*
5. Thomsen, K., and Wantzin, G. (1987). Extracutaneous spreading with fatal outcome of mycosis fungoides in a patient treated with cyclosporine A. A word of caution. *Dermatologica* 174:236–238.
6. Street, M., Muller, S., and Pittelkow, N. (1990). Cyclosporine in the treatment of cutaneous T-cell lymphoma. *J. Am. Acad. Dermatol.* 23:1084–1089.
7. Zachariae, H., Hansen, H., Søgaard, H., et al. (1990). Kidney biopsies in methotrexate-treated psoriatics. *Dermatologica* 181:273–276.
8. Zachariae, H., Bjerring, P., and Heickendorff, L. (1996). Plasma endothelins in psoriasis. *Acta Derm. Venereol. (Stockh.)* (in press).
9. Kon, V., Sugiura, M., Ingagami, T., et al. (1990). Role of endothelin in cyclosporine-induced glomerular dysfunction. *Kidney Int.* 37:1487–1491.
10. Mihatsch, M., Thiel G., and Ryffel, B. (1988). Histopathology of cyclosporin nephrotoxicity. *Transplant. Proc.* 20(Suppl. 3):759–771.

11. Zachariae, H., Hansen, H., Kragballe, K., and Olsen, S. (1992). Morphologic, renal changes during cyclosporine treatment of psoriasis. *J. Am. Acad. Dermatol.* 26:415–419.
12. Zachariae, H., Hansen, H., and Olsen, S. (1996). Long-term use of cyclosporine for psoriasis. Presented at the psoriasis symposium at American Academy of Dermatology, Washington, February.
13. Leaker, B., and Cairns, H. (1994). Clinical aspects of cyclosporin nephrotoxicity. *Br. J. Hosp. Med.* 52: 529–534.
14. Ludwin, D., and Alexopoulou, I. (1993). Cyclosporin A nephropathy in patients with rheumatoid arthritis. *Br. J. Rheumatol.* 32(Suppl. 1):60–64.
15. Kovarik, J., Mueller, E., van Bree, J., et al. (1994). Reduced inter- and-intraindividual variability in cyclosporine pharmacokinetics from a microemulsion formulation. *J. Pharm. Sci.* 83:444.
16. Ellis, C., Fradin, U., Hamilton, T., and Voorhees, J. (1995). Duration of remission during maintenance cyclosporine therapy for psoriasis: relationship to maintenance dose and degree of improvement during initial therapy. *Arch. Dermatol.* 131:791–795.
17. Koo, J. (1995). Cyclosporine in dermatology—fears and opportunities. *Arch. Dermatol.* 131:842–845.
18. Levell, N., Shuster, S., Monro, C., and Friedmann, P. (1992). Remission of ordinary psoriasis following a short clearance course of cyclosporin. Presented at British Association of Dermatology, Bournemouth, UK, July.
19. Myers, B., Sibley, R., Newton, L., et al. (1988). The long-term course of cyclosporine-associated chronic nephropathy. *Kidney Int.* 33:590–600.
20. Myers, B., and Newton, L. (1991). Cyclosporin induced chronic nephropathy: an obliteratory microvascular renal injury. *J. Soc. Nephrol.* 2(Suppl. 1): 545–552.
21. Powles, A., Cook, T., Hulme, B., et al. (1993). Renal function and biopsy findings after five years treatment with low-dose cyclosporin for psoriasis. *Br. J. Dermatol.* 128:159–165.
22. International Kidney Biopsy Registry of Cyclosporin (Sandimmun®) in Autoimmune Diseases. (1990). Kidney biopsies in control of cyclosporin A–treated psoriatic patients. *Br. J. Dermatol.* 122(Suppl. 336): 95–100.

54

Clinical Use of Etretinate and Acitretin

Michael T. Goldfarb and Charles N. Ellis
University of Michigan, Ann Arbor, Michigan

Vitamin A and chemically similar structures are collectively known as retinoids; those that occur in nature are also referred to as first-generation retinoids. Many molecules that are structurally related to vitamin A have been synthesized, including a series containing aromatic rings. The aromatic retinoids are also called second-generation retinoids. Two of the second-generation retinoids, etretinate and its principal metabolite, acitretin, have proved effective in the treatment of psoriasis (Fig. 1).

Etretinate is an aromatic retinoid that has been available in the United States since 1986 for the therapy of psoriasis. The drug was initially code-named Ro 10-9359; the brand name for etretinate in the United States is Tegison and it is sold as Tigason elsewhere. The acid metabolite of etretinate is acitretin, which is useful for the same indications. Acitretin was first identified as Ro 10-1670 and had the former generic term etretin; it is sold as Soriatane.

ETRETINATE

Pharmacological Considerations

The absorption of etretinate after oral administration is greater and is less variable when the drug is taken with whole milk or a meal with a high fat content. After a 6-month course of therapy with doses ranging from 25 mg once daily to 25 mg four times daily, peak serum concentrations of etretinate (102–389 ng/ml) occurred 2–6 hr after administration. With multiple dosing, etretinate accumulates in adipose tissues (Brazzell and Colburn, 1982; Massarella et al., 1985). The storage of etretinate in adipose tissue accounts for its prolonged elimination half-life of about 120 days after 6 months of daily administration. In some patients, etretinate has been detected in blood at concentrations of 0.5–12.0 ng/ml up to 3 years after completion of a course of etretinate therapy.

The persistence of etretinate in adipose tissue and blood after cessation of therapy has serious implications for women of childbearing potential; major congenital abnormalities were reported in some fetuses whose mothers had received etretinate therapy.

Efficacy

Etretinate has been rigorously tested as monotherapy for severe psoriasis in studies of different design, involving about 400 patients (Cunningham, 1985a, 1987; Ehmann and Voorhees, 1982). In double-blind studies designed to last up to 24 weeks, patients were randomly assigned to receive the drug or placebo for 8 weeks. After this initial phase, all patients could receive etretinate for the remaining time (thus, patients could be on active drug for a total of 16 or 24 weeks).

In these trials, the starting dose was 0.75–1.0 mg/kg/day and was adjusted up or down depending on the patient's response and ability to tolerate side effects.

Efficacy was evaluated in two ways: (1) The physician rated three disease parameters (scale, erythema,

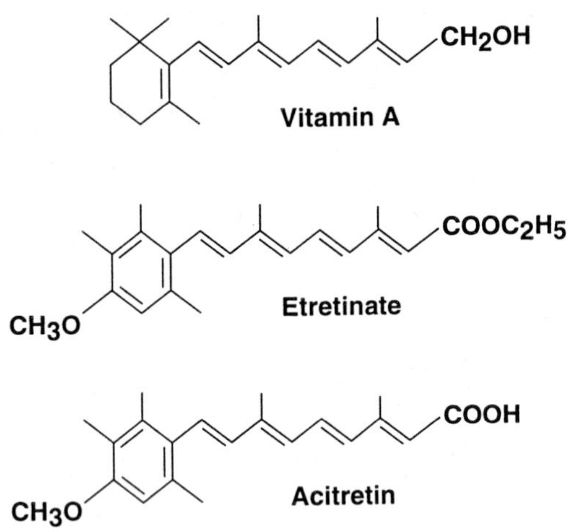

Figure 1 Structural formulas of vitamin A (retinol), etretinate, and acitretin. Etretinate and acitretin are aromatic derivatives of vitamin A, characterized by benzene in the cyclic portion of the molecule. Etretinate and acitretin vary only in the polar end group; etretinate is an ester whereas acitretin is an acid.

and induration or thickness) on a five-point scale, and (2) the physician and patient rated improvement generally (global evaluation) on a seven-point scale.

The first double-blind, placebo-controlled, multicenter protocol involved 129 psoriasis patients, of whom 15 had erythrodermic and seven had pustular psoriasis. At the end of 8 weeks, 97% of the etretinate-treated patients showed improvement compared with only 25% of the placebo-treated patients.

The second double-blind trial involved 30 psoriasis patients, including three with erythrodermic and one with pustular psoriasis. The results were similar. After 24 weeks, global evaluations showed that 96% had improved; 12 of the 27 patients evaluated were almost clear and two were totally clear. The disease parameters of scale, erythema, and induration decreased from baseline in both protocols by differences that were statistically significant. After drug treatment was discontinued, the psoriasis gradually returned.

Further efficacy studies with etretinate were conducted in an open-label fashion at five centers. Of the 280 patients with psoriasis who received 24 weeks of etretinate therapy, 94% showed some improvement; of these, 48% were either totally or almost clear and 13% were totally clear. In the subset of erythrodermic patients, 99% showed some improvement, 39% were almost to totally clear, and 6% were totally clear after therapy. In patients with pustular psoriasis, 100% showed some improvement and 34% were totally clear after etretinate therapy.

In a study of 20 patients with severe recalcitrant psoriasis vulgaris designed to evaluate the potential effect of etretinate on hepatic structure and function, most of the patients experienced an improvement in their psoriasis (Glazer et al., 1982). In another study of 20 patients with recalcitrant psoriasis, the authors found that 10 patients with erythrodermic psoriasis had a 62% improvement in their disease (percent surface involved), seven with plaque-type psoriasis had a 44% improvement, and two with inverse psoriasis had a 25–50% improvement (Kaplan et al., 1983). After etretinate therapy was stopped, maintenance therapy was required in most patients, since relapse of their psoriasis occurred on an average in about 8 weeks.

In 29 patients with chronic plaque psoriasis, etretinate was found to be superior to isotretinoin (Moy et al., 1985). After 8 weeks of treatment, 18 of the 19 patients treated with etretinate had either a complete or a moderate response, whereas only 4 of 10 patients treated with isotretinoin were moderate or complete responders. However, isotretinoin therapy appeared comparable to etretinate in a selected group of patients with pustular psoriasis.

In one report, two children 19 months of age were treated with etretinate under a compassionate plea protocol for recalcitrant, debilitating pustular psoriasis (Shelnitz et al., 1987). Both children showed remarkable improvement over a 3.5-year period of intermittent treatment with a maximum dosage of 1.5 mg/kg/day without experiencing any apparent drug effect on growth or development.

Etretinate had a beneficial effect in the therapy of acrodermatitis continua of Hallopeau in one patient, which is considered by many to be a variant of pustular psoriasis because of similar histological features (Pearson et al., 1984).

INSTRUCTIONS FOR USE

Dosing

Pustular Psoriasis

Etretinate may be the drug of first choice for pustular psoriasis. The initial dose is approximately 0.75–1 mg/kg/day with rapid resolution of the pustules in the first week of therapy (Ellis and Voorhees, 1987). After the pustules have cleared, patients may be controlled at a lower dose (0.25–0.5 mg/kg/day).

Erythrodermic Psoriasis

Erythrodermic psoriasis also responds favorably to etretinate and is frequently the first therapy considered. A lower initial dose of 0.25 mg/kg/day is recommended to avoid an early retinoid dermatitis that can flare the disease (Ellis and Voorhees, 1987). The dose can be increased by 0.25 mg/kg/day every few weeks until the disease is under control.

Plaque Psoriasis

Etretinate is effective for plaque psoriasis as both a monotherapy and in combination with other therapies (UVB, PUVA and topical corticosteroids, anthralin, and calcipotriene) (Ellis and Voorhees, 1987). The usual starting dose is 0.5–0.75 mg/kg/day. Initially the plaques may clear in the center, while they expand at the periphery, leading to an increase in the total body surface area involved. Improvement begins after approximately 1 month of therapy with initially a decrease in erythema and scaling followed by a decrease in thickness of the plaques. Maximum clearing often takes 4–6 months of therapy. Once the patient has cleared and achieved sufficient improvement, the dose may be tapered to 0.25–0.5 mg/kg/day. It may be advisable to give a "drug holiday" after 9 months of therapy for approximately 3 months. Patients often will stay in remission for 2 months and will be able to tolerate this time period off therapy. Occasionally after a course of etretinate, patients may be adequately controlled for months or even years with the use of topical corticosteroids, anthralin, calcipotriene, or ultraviolet therapy.

Etretinate, although effective as a monotherapy, is most frequently used with other therapies. Combining UVB or PUVA with etretinate often leads to lower doses of both ultraviolet and etretinate with greater clinical improvement. Even the addition of topical corticosteroids and anthralin can lower the dose of etretinate needed.

Evaluation of Patients

Etretinate is a potent medication and should be used only after careful evaluation of the patient, other treatments have been considered, and the patient has been given education and instruction on the intricacies of retinoid therapy. Etretinate should be reserved for patients who have moderate to severe psoriasis. It is not a therapy to be used for patients with mild disease that could be treated with less toxic topical therapy. The package insert in the United States recommends etretinate should not be used unless numerous other therapies including methotrexate and systemic steroids have been tried (*Physicians' Desk Reference*, 1995). We do not agree with this limitation as we do not use systemic steroids for psoriasis; furthermore, there are patients for whom etretinate is a better choice than methotrexate.

History

Before initiation of etretinate in a psoriasis patient, certain baseline information should be obtained. A family or personal history of atherosclerotic disease, diabetes mellitus, or hyperlipidemia suggests that the patient may be susceptible to the hyperlipidemic effects of etretinate. A family or personal history of psoriatic arthritis may be helpful in assessing the origin of musculoskeletal complaints during etretinate therapy. It is important to document any alcohol or tobacco use as well as the dietary habits of patients. Ingestion of alcohol can raise the liver function tests and serum triglycerides making it difficult to determine if etretinate is having a deleterious effect. Therefore, patients should abstain from heavy alcohol use during therapy and avoid any alcohol use for at least 3 days prior to laboratory testing. Also, we ask patients to limit their use of tobacco to decrease the risk of atherosclerosis and for their general health. Finally, we advise a low-fat diet as well as weight reduction in the obese.

Etretinate is a potent teratogen and absolutely contraindicated in pregnant women (Geiger et al., 1994). Because of its long half-life, there has been no safe time period established after stopping therapy after which a patient may become pregnant without risk. It should therefore be used in a woman of childbearing potential only in unusual circumstances. Use in lactating women is also undesirable.

Etretinate has not been shown to have any deleterious effects on semen. Even so, we do not recommend that men impregnate their partners while on therapy, so there is no concern that the etretinate was a factor if a spontaneous birth defect occurs. It has been suggested that men taking etretinate use a condom when having sexual intercourse with a pregnant woman to avoid any passage of etretinate in the semen. While there is no scientific justification for such recommendations, there is no harm in physicians protecting themselves from becoming involved in the random effects of gestation.

We have patients avoid additional vitamin A therapy while on etretinate. Because both etretinate and methotrexate may cause liver toxicity and etretinate may raise the serum level of methotrexate, we avoid the long-term combination of these two drugs (Larsen et al., 1990). Also, we avoid the concomitant use of drugs such as tetracycline, which, like etretinate, are associated with an increased risk of pseudotumor cerebri.

Side Effects

Both the patient and the physician should be familiar with the side effects of etretinate therapy (Cunningham, 1985b, 1987; Silverman et al., 1987). Numerous mucocutaneous side effects (Cunningham, 1987) are to be expected including cheilitis, dry mouth, dry nasal mucosa, epistaxis, diffuse xerosis, pruritus, peeling palms and soles, skin fragility, sticky-feeling skin, retinoid dermatitis, hair loss, change in hair texture, curling of hair, paronychial inflammation, nail thinning, and granulation tissue at the nail folds (Campbell et al., 1983; Peck et al., 1981). Patients should be instructed to keep their skin and mucous membranes well lubricated. We have patients apply petrolatum to the lips and nasal mucosa frequently as well as artificial tears to their eyes.

The retinoid dermatitis, which usually appears as an eczematous eruption on the back of the arms, can be treated by the application of topical corticosteroids or by reducing the dose of etretinate. It is important not to mistake this as a psoriasis flare and raise the etretinate dose, which may further worsen the retinoid dermatitis. Indeed, if the patient appears to worsen when the daily etretinate dose is increased, one should consider whether the effect is related to retinoid toxicity. Substantially reducing or stopping etretinate may have a surprising salutary effect.

Myalgias and arthralgias are common side effects of etretinate therapy. Even diffuse stiffness and hypertonia may occur (Ellis et al., 1986; Albin et al., 1988). These symptoms usually resolve rapidly with the discontinuation of therapy.

Long-term use of etretinate may lead to ligament and skeletal calcifications (Gerber et al., 1984; DiGiovanna et al., 1986). These changes are not usually demonstrated with short-term use (6–8 months) of etretinate (Gilbert et al., 1986). We recommend annual monitoring of skeletal x-rays of the spine, hips, knees, and ankle with chronic etretinate use. These areas have been shown to be more susceptible to calcifications. Also, radiographs should be obtained of symptomatic joints. Fortunately, the changes induced by retinoids are usually asymptomatic. However, patients should be kept informed of any calcifications on radiographs and they must assume the risk of any long-term disability that may develop if etretinate therapy is continued.

Etretinate caused an increase in serum cholesterol and triglyceride levels in some patients (Ellis, 1985; Ellis et al., 1982; Gerber and Erdman, 1982). Additionally, an undesirable decrease in high-density lipoprotein (HDL) levels occurred in some individuals. In most patients, lipid levels returned to normal promptly after etretinate therapy was stopped. In some patients, however, the lipid levels remained elevated, at least temporarily, after etretinate therapy was discontinued. Preliminary findings suggest that dietary fish oil supplements may ameliorate the lipid changes secondary to retinoids in some patients (Ashley et al., 1988). Studies of liver function tests during etretinate therapy indicate some abnormalities in about one-third of patients (Cunningham, 1987; Roenigk, 1985). These usually return to normal during continued therapy or once therapy is stopped. However, approximately 1.5% of patients have been reported to develop hepatitis that may be related to etretinate therapy (Cunningham, 1987). These cases resolved with the discontinuation of therapy, but rare cases of chronic hepatitis and hepatic-related deaths have been reported (Weiss et al., 1984, 1985).

To monitor for hyperlipidemia, liver abnormalities, and other systemic problems, blood and urine tests are recommended. A baseline complete blood count, fasting lipid profiles, liver function tests, electrolytes, blood urea nitrogen, creatinine, and urinalysis should be performed and repeated every 3 months during therapy. Also, liver function tests and fasting lipid profiles should be followed every 2–4 weeks until they are stable. Routine liver biopsies are not indicated (Glazer et al., 1982, 1984; Roenigk et al., 1985; Camuto et al., 1987).

Besides dry eyes, patients may experience a decrease in night vision. This may be best assessed by inquiring whether the patient has reduced vision after watching a movie; a patient with reduced night vision cannot quickly accommodate and has difficulty leaving the theater. Also, patients have experienced corneal erosion, superficial corneal opacities, lid infections, and conjunctivitis (Lichter, 1987). Fortunately, these problems resolve with the discontinuation of therapy.

Patients will frequently complain of fatigue during therapy. Also, headache occurs in over 25% of patients. A rare and dangerous side effect, pseudotumor cerebri, may present as headaches, nausea and vomiting, and visual disturbances. Patients with headaches should be evaluated for papilledema, and if it is present, referred immediately for neurological evaluation and treatment. Finally, patients may complain of depression and anxiety.

Owing to the toxicity of etretinoids, many physicians are rotating this treatment with other systemic treatments (PUVA, methotrexate, cyclosporin) for controlling severe psoriasis. Such a regimen may limit the toxicity of any of the therapies by reducing the length of time a patient continuously takes any one treatment. However, patients have been on long-term etretinate therapy for up to 4 years without substantially increased risk of major adverse effects (Stern et al., 1995).

ACITRETIN

Acitretin is the acid metabolite of etretinate. In this section, we include information extracted from the formal clinical trials to discuss the efficacy and side effects of acitretin.

Pharmacological Considerations

Acitretin does not accumulate in tissue, thus allowing rapid elimination from the body. It has about a twofold increase in, and more consistent, absorption when given with a meal. Peak plasma levels of 100–800 ng/ml occur within 4 hr after an oral dose of 50 mg. At steady state, the plasma concentration of the 13-*cis*-acitretin isomer is higher than that of acitretin. Both acitretin and the 13-*cis*-acitretin isomer have short half-lives of 50 and 75 hr, respectively, compared to the 4-month half-life of etretinate (Brindley, 1989). Therefore, neither form of acitretin is found in plasma at a level greater than 5 ng/ml after 3 weeks off therapy.

Unfortunately, high-performance liquid chromatography investigations have detected etretinate in the plasma of acitretin-treated patients. This esterification of acitretin to etretinate is enhanced by, but not completely dependent on, ethanol ingestion (Lambert et al., 1992, 1994; Larsen et al., 1993). Because acitretin is a metabolite of etretinate in humans that is rapidly eliminated from the body, it was hoped that acitretin would be acceptible for use in fertile (but not *pregnant*) women. The finding that acitretin can be converted to etretinate in the body dealt a blow to this expectation. Nevertheless, the relatively low levels of etretinate formed during acitretin therapy make acitretin a better choice for women of childbearing potential.

Efficacy

Clinical trials evaluating acitretin in the treatment of severe psoriasis parallel the investigation of etretinate (Goldfarb et al., 1988; Kingston et al., 1987; Madhok et al., 1987; Pilkington and Brogden, 1992). Acitretin was evaluated in two separate double-blind, placebo-controlled, multicenter trials. A total of 333 patients (240 men and 93 women), ranging in age from 20 to 80 years, with various types of psoriasis, including plaque (73%), guttate (13%), erythrodermic (6%), palmoplantar (6%), and pustular (2%), participated in these trials. The patients were randomly assigned to receive either placebo or a specific dose of acitretin for the first 8 weeks in a double-blind fashion. Between the two trials, the efficacy of acitretin in dosages of 10, 25, 50, or 75 mg/day was compared with placebo. After the initial 8 weeks of double-blind treatment, all patients, including those who had been treated with placebo, could receive acitretin for up to 24 weeks at a dose that best balanced efficacy and side effects for that individual. If needed, patients could continue to receive additional courses of acitretin therapy for up to 24 weeks.

The criteria used to evaluate the efficacy of acitretin in the treatment of psoriasis in these trials were (1) estimated extent of psoriasis (as a percentage of body surface area), (2) clinical appearance of lesions (scaling, thickness, and erythema), and (3) the physician's overall evaluation of the patient's psoriasis.

The effect of therapy on psoriasis in each dosage group was assessed by comparing each efficacy criterion before and after 8 weeks of treatment. In the placebo and 10 mg/day groups of patients, no statistically significant changes from baseline could be demonstrated in any of the efficacy variables after 8 weeks of treatment. In the 25 mg/day group, a statistically significant improvement over baseline was seen in the clinical appearance of lesions (scaling, thickness, and erythema) and in the physician's global evaluation of psoriasis, but not in the extent of body surface involved with psoriasis. However, in the 50 and 75 mg/day groups, all three efficacy parameters showed a statistically significant improvement over baseline.

The effect of therapy was also assessed by comparing the efficacy results in each dosage group with that of the placebo control group at the end of the 8-week double-blind period. The 10 mg/day acitretin group showed no difference from the placebo group for any of the efficacy criteria. In contrast, the 25, 50, and 75 mg/day groups showed a statistically significant improvement in all the efficacy parameters compared with the placebo group.

Other studies (Torok et al., 1989; Murray et al., 1991) concur that acitretin 25–50 mg/day provides the best therapeutic results for psoriasis with tolerable side effects. When comparing acitretin with etretinate, double-blind studies (Ledo et al., 1988; Bjerke and Geiger, 1989; Meffert and Sonnichsen, 1989) established these two drugs have essentially identical efficacy and side effects at comparable dosing for the treatment of psoriasis. Also, similar to etretinate, acitretin works better in conjunction with other psoriasis therapies, especially UVB and PUVA (Ruzicka et al., 1990; Lowe et al., 1991; Tanew et al., 1991). The degree of clearing of psoriasis is increased and the amount of ultraviolet is decreased when acitretin is added to either UVB or PUVA therapy.

INSTRUCTIONS FOR USE

Dosing

The use of acitretin mirrors the use of etretinate, although some suggest that acitretin has a higher response rate (Geiger and Saurat, 1993; Ho et al., 1995). Compared to etretinate, a slightly lower starting dose of acitretin of 0.5 mg/kg/day for plaque psoriasis is recommended. The dosage of acitretin for pustular psoriasis is slightly higher and for erythrodermic psoriasis, slightly lower. Psoriatic patients on acitretin will clear in a manner similar to those on etretinate therapy. Once adequate improvement is achieved, the dose of acitretin should be tapered to as low as possible and may eventually be discontinued. A relapse of the psoriasis is usually inevitable off therapy and requires the restart of treatment. When changing a patient from etretinate to acitretin, on a mg/kg basis two-thirds of the etretinate dose should be used initially.

Side Effects

Acitretin has an identical side effect profile to etretinate (Gupta et al., 1989; Kilcoyne, 1988). Therefore, when patients are being treated with acitretin, the same concerns regarding teratogenicity, hyperlipidemia, hepatotoxicity, and mucocutaneous, musculoskeletal, neurological, and ophthalmological side effects are pertinent. There is some evidence that the incidence of alopecia and mucocutaneous reactions with acitretin is higher than with etretinate at equivalent doses (Geiger and Saurat, 1993; Ho et al., 1995). This may be due to an increased potency of acitretin compared to etretinate. We recommend the same pretherapy evaluation and clinical laboratory and skeletal x-ray monitoring on acitretin as with etretinate.

Because acitretin is a potent teratogen and undergoes esterification to the lipophilic etretinate, an exact time period after which it is safe for a woman to become pregnant after therapy has not been established. In Europe, a time period of 2 years after discontinuing therapy before conception should be attempted is recommended for both etretinate and acitretin. After 2 years, patients on etretinate usually have blood levels at the lower limits of detection, 2 ng/ml, and patients on acitretin have etretinate levels that are far lower (Geiger et al., 1994). Also, when following the guideline of 2 years, it does not appear that there are more congenital malformations after retinoid therapy than occurs in the general population. In the United States labeling, women are instructed not to become pregnant "for at least 3 years" after stopping acitretin therapy.

It is our view that even though acitretin undergoes conversion into etretinate, the overall plasma levels and stores of etretinate are substantially lower and it will be useful for treating fertile women. However, until there are exact answers to the questions of what is a safe lower level of etretinate in the blood that is not a clinically significant teratogen and exactly how long after stopping acitretin it is safe to become pregnant, we will reserve the use of acitretin in the fertile woman for cases of psoriasis that are grave and where no other therapy would be appropriate. Also, we ask the patient to avoid ethanol intake to prevent as much etretinate formation as possible.

CONCLUSIONS

Both etretinate and acitretin have significant efficacy for the treatment of psoriasis. Owing to the side effects associated with these two drugs, their use is usually reserved for the more severe and recalcitrant cases of psoriasis. However, when both patient and physician are well informed on retinoid therapy, excellent results can be achieved without significant morbidity.

REFERENCES

Albin, R.L., Silverman, A.K., Ellis, C.N., Voorhees, J.J., and Albers, J.W. (1988). A new syndrome of axial muscle rigidity associated with etretinate therapy. *Movement Disord.* 3:70–76.

Ashley, J.M., Lowe, N.J., Borok, M.E., and Alfin-Slater, R.B. (1988). Fish oil supplementation results in decreased hypertriglyceridemia in patients with psoriasis undergoing etretinate or acitretin therapy. *J. Am. Acad. Dermatol.* 19:76–82.

Bjerke, J.R., and Geiger, J.-M. (1989). Acitretin versus etretinate in severe psoriasis. A double-blind randomized Nordic multicenter study in 168 patients. *Acta Derm. Venereol. (Stockh.)* Suppl. 146:206–207.

Brazzell, R.K., and Colburn, W.A. (1982). Pharmacokinetics of the retinoids isotretinoin and etretinate. *J. Am. Acad. Dermatol.* 6:643–651.

Brindley, C.J. (1989). Overview of recent clinical pharmacokinetic studies with acitretin (Ro 10-1670, etretin). *Dermatologica* 178:79–87.

Campbell, J.P., Grekin, R.C., Ellis, C.N., Matsuda-John, S.S., Swanson, N.A., and Voorhees, J.J. (1983). Retinoid therapy is associated with excess granulation tissue responses. *J. Am. Acad. Dermatol.* 9:708–713.

Camuto, P., Shupak, J., Ohrbuch, P., Tobias, H. Sidhu, G. and Feiner, H. (1987). Long-term effects of etretinate on the liver in psoriasis. *Am. J. Surg. Pathol.* 11:30–37.

Cunningham, W.J. (1985a). Clinical efficacy of retinoids. United States experience. In *Psoriasis*. H.H. Roenigk, Jr., and H.I. Maibach (Eds.). Marcel Dekker, New York, pp. 590–595.

Cunningham, W.J. (1985b). Side effects profile of etretinate. In *Psoriasis*. H.H. Roenigk, Jr., and H.I. Maibach (Eds.). Marcel Dekker, New York, pp. 631–633.

Cunningham, W.J. (1987). Clinical trials of etretinate. In proceedings of a symposium, "Retinoids and Therapy for Psoriasis," Jan. 20, 1987, Dallas, Texas. *Video J. Dermatol.* II (Suppl.).

DiGiovanna, J.J., Helfgott, R.K., Gerber, L.H., and Peck, G.L. (1986). Extraspinal tendon and ligament calcification associated with long-term therapy with etretinate. *N. Engl. J. Med.* 315:1177–1182.

Ehmann, C.W., and Voorhees, J.J. (1982). International studies of the efficacy of etretinate in the treatment of psoriasis. *J. Am. Acad. Dermatol.* 6:692–696.

Ellis, C.N. (1985). Retinoid toxicity: lipids. In *Psoriasis*. H.H. Roenigk, Jr., and H.I. Maibach (Eds.). Marcel Dekker, New York, pp. 593–595.

Ellis, C.N., and Voorhees, J.J. (1987). Etretinate therapy. *J. Am. Acad. Dermatol.* 16:267–291.

Ellis, C.N., Swanson, N.A., Grekin, R.C., Goldstein, N.G., Bassett, D.R., Anderson, T.F., and Voorhees, J.J. (1982). Etretinate therapy causes increases in lipid levels in patients with psoriasis. *Arch. Dermatol.* 118:559–562.

Ellis, C.N., Gilbert, M., Cohen, K.A., Albers, J.W., Ball, R.D., Albin, R.L., Silverman, A., and Voorhees, J.J. (1986). Increased muscle tone during etretinate therapy. *J. Am. Acad. Dermatol.* 14:907–909.

Geiger, J.-M., and Saurat, J.-H. (1993). Acitretin and etretinate. How and when they should be used. *Dermatol. Ther.* 11:117–129.

Geiger, J.-M., Baudin, M., and Saurat, J.-H. (1994). Teratogenic risk with etretinate and acitretin treatment. *Dermatology* 189:109–116.

Gerber, L.E., and Erdman, J.W., Jr. (1982). Changes in lipid metabolism during retinoid administration. *J. Am. Acad. Dermatol.* 6:664–672.

Gerber, L.H., Helfgott, R.K., Gross, E.G., Hicks, J.E., Ellenberg, S.S., Ellenberg, S.S., and Peck, G.L. (1984). Vertebral abnormalities associated with synthetic retinoid use. *J. Am. Acad. Dermatol.* 10:817–823.

Gilbert, M., Ellis, C.N., and Voorhees, J.J. (1986). Lack of skeletal radiographic changes during short-term etretinate therapy for psoriasis. *Dermatologica* 172:160–163.

Glazer, S.D., Roenigk, H.H., Yokoo, H., and Sparberg, M. (1982). A study of potential hepatotoxicity of etretinate used in the treatment of psoriasis. *J. Am. Acad. Dermatol.* 6:683–687.

Glazer, S.D., Roenigk, H.H., Yokoo, H., Sparberg, M., and Paravicini, U. (1984). Ultrastructural survey and tissue analysis of human livers after a 6-month course of etretinate. *J. Am. Acad. Dermatol.* 10:632–638.

Goldfarb, M.T., Ellis, C.N., Gupta, A.K., Tincoff, T., Hamilton, T.A., and Voorhees, J.J. (1988). Acitretin improves psoriasis in a dose-dependent fashion. *J. Am. Acad. Dermatol.* 18:655–662.

Gupta, A.K., Goldfarb, M.T., Ellis, C.N., and Voorhees, J.J. (1989). Side effect profile of acitretin therapy in psoriasis. *J. Am. Acad. Dermatol.* 20:1088–1093.

Ho, V.C., Cloutier, R.M.A., Griffiths, W.A.D., Gulliver, W.P., Lauzon, G.J., Marcoux, D., Miller, R.A.W., Murray, E.H., and Schacter, G.D. (1995). Acitretin for the treatment of psoriasis and disorders of keratinization. *Can. J. Dermatol.* 7:757–765.

Kaplan, R.P., Russell, D.H., and Lowe, N.J. (1983). Etretinate therapy for psoriasis: clinical responses, remission times, epidermal DNA and polyamine responses. *J. Am. Acad. Dermatol.* 8:95–102.

Kilcoyne, R.F. (1988). Effects of retinoids in bone. *J. Am. Acad. Dermatol.* 19:212–216.

Kingston, R.P., Matt, L.H., and Lowe, N.J. (1987). Etretin therapy for severe psoriasis. *Arch. Dermatol.* 123:55–58.

Lambert, W.E., Meyer, E., De Leenheer, A.P., De Bersaques, J., and Kint, A.H. (1992). Pharmacokinetics and drug interactions of etretinate and acitretin. *J. Am. Acad. Dermatol.* 27:S19–S22.

Lambert, W.E., Meyer, E., De Leenheer, A.P., and Kint, A.H. (1994). Pharmacokinetics of acitretin. *Acta. Derm. Venereol. (Stockh.)* Suppl. 86:122–123.

Larsen, F.G., Nielsen-Kudsk, F., Jakobsen, P., Schroder, H., and Kragballe, K. (1990). Interaction of etretinate with methotrexate pharmacokinetics in psoriatic patients. *J. Clin. Pharmacol.* 30:802–807.

Larsen, F.G., Jakobsen, P., Knudsen, J., Weismann, K., Kragballe, K., and Nielsen-Kudsk, F. (1993). Conversion of acitretin to etretinate in psoriatic patients is influenced by ethanol. *J. Invest. Dermatol.* 100:623–627.

Ledo, A., Martin, M., Geiger, J.M., and Marron, J.M. (1988). Acitretin (Ro 10-1670) in the treatment of severe psoriasis. *Int. J. Dermatol.* 27:656–660.

Lichter, P. (1987). Clinical trials of etretinate. In proceedings of a symposium, "Retinoids and Therapy for Psoriasis," Jan. 20, 1987, Dallas, Texas. *Video J. Dermatol.* II (Suppl.).

Lowe, N.J., Prystowsky, J.H., Bourget, B.S., Edelstein, P.A., Nychay, S., and Armstrong, R. (1991). Acitretin plus UVB therapy for psoriasis. *Am. Acad. Dermatol.* 24: 591–594.

Madhok, R., Muller, S.A., and Dicken, C.H. (1987). Treatment of psoriasis with etretin: a preliminary report. *Mayo Clin. Proc.* 62:1084–1089.

Massarella, J., Vane, F., Buffe, C., Rodriguez, L., Cunningham, W.J., Franz, T., and Colburn, W. (1985). Etretinate kinetics during chronic dosing in severe psoriasis. *Clin. Pharmacol. Ther.* 37:439–446.

Meffert, H. and Sonnichsen (1989). Acitretin in the treatment of severe psoriasis: a randomized double-blind study comparing acitretin and etretinate. *Acta Derm. Venereol. (Stockh.)* Suppl. 146:176–177.

Moy, R.L., Klingston, R.P., and Lowe, N.J. (1985). Isotretinoin vs. etretinate therapy in generalized pustular and chronic psoriasis. *Arch. Dermatol.* 121:1297–1301.

Murray, H.E., Anhalt, A.W., Lessard, R., Schacter, R.K., Ross, J.B., Stewart, W.D., and Geiger, J.-M. (1991). A 12-month treatment of severe psoriasis with acitretin: results of a Canadian open multicenter study. *J. Am. Acad. Dermatol.* 24:598–602.

Pearson, L.H., Allen, B.S., and Smith, J.G., Jr. (1984). Acrodermatitis continua of Hallopeau: treatment with etretinate and review of relapsing pustular eruptions of the hands and feet. *J. Am. Acad. Dermatol.* 11:755–762.

Peck, G.L., Gross, E.G., and Butkus, D. (1981). Comparative analysis of two retinoids in the treatment of disorders of keratinization. In *Retinoids.* C.E. Orfanos, O. Braun-Falco, E.M. Farber, et al. (Eds.). Springer-Verlag, Berlin, pp. 279–286.

Physicians' Desk Reference (1995), 49th ed. Medical Economics Co., Oradell, NJ, pp. 2061–2064.

Pilkington, T., and Brogden, R.N. (1992). Acitretin. A review of its pharmacology and therapeutic use. *Drugs* 43: 597–627.

Roenigk, H.H., Jr. (1985). Effects of retinoids on the liver. In *Psoriasis.* H.H. Roenigk, Jr., and H.I. Maibach (Eds.). Marcel Dekker, New York, pp. 593–595.

Roenigk, H.H., Jr., Gibstine, C., Glazer, S., Sparberg, M., and Yokoo, H. (1985). Serial liver biopsies in psoriatic patients receiving long-term etretinate. *Br. J. Dermatol.* 112:77–81.

Ruzicka, T., Sommerburg, C. Braun-Falco, O., Koster, W., Lengen, W., Lensing, W., Letzel, H., Meigel, W.N., Paul, E., Przybilla, B., Steinert, M., Winzer, M., and Wiskemann, A. (1990). Efficiency of acitretin in combination with UV-B in the treatment of severe psoriasis. *Arch. Dermatol.* 126:482–486.

Shelnitz, L.S., Esteriy, N.B., and Honig, J. (1987). Etretinate therapy for generalized pustular psoriasis in children. *Arch. Dermatol.* 123:230–233.

Silverman, A.K., Ellis, C.N., and Voorhees, J.J. (1987). Hypervitaminosis A syndrome: a paradigm of retinoid side effects. *J. Am. Acad. Dermatol.* 16:1027–1039.

Stern, R.S., Fitzgerald, E., Ellis, C.N., Lowe, N., Goldfarb, M.T., and Baughman, R.D. (1995). The safety of etretinate as long-term therapy for psoriasis: Results of the Etretinate Follow-Up Study. *J. Am. Acad. Dermatol.* 33: 44–52.

Tanew, A., Guggenbichler, A., Honigsmann, H., Geiger, J.-M., and Fritsch, P. (1991). Photochemotherapy for severe psoriasis without or in combination with acitretin: a randomized, double-blind comparison study. *J. Am. Acad. Dermatol.* 25:682–684.

Torok, L., Kadar, L., and Geiger, J.-M. (1989). Acitretin treatment of severe psoriasis. *Acta Dermatol. Venereol. (Stockh.)* Suppl. 146:104–106.

Weiss, V.C., West, D.P., Ackerman, R., and Robinson, L.A. (1984). Hepatotoxic reactions in a patient treated with etretinate. *Arch. Dermatol.* 120:104–106.

Weiss, V.C., Leyden, T., Spinowitx, A., Buys, C.M., Nemchausky, B.A., West, D.P., and Emmons, K.M. (1985). Chronic active hepatitis associated with etretinate therapy. *Br. J. Dermatol.* 112:591–597.

55

Acitretin and Etretinate: Strategy for Use and Long-Term Side Effects

Carle Paul and Louis Dubertret
Hôpital Saint Louis, Paris, France

The synthetic vitamin A derivative etretinate and its free aromatic acid acitretin are effective agents in the treatment of psoriasis. However, they have a relatively narrow therapeutic index and are teratogenic. Etretinate was first approved for the treatment of psoriasis but its use has been hampered by an extremely long elimination half-life of up to 120 days after repetitive dosing due to its lipophilic properties and storage in adipose tissue (1,2). Etretinate has been detected in the adipose tissue for as long as 2 years after drug discontinuation (3). Acitretin is less likely to be sequestered in adipose tissue and exhibits a considerably shorter terminal half-life (<3 days) than etretinate (3). Therefore, acitretin has recently replaced etretinate both in European countries and in the United States. However, recent studies have demonstrated the presence of etretinate in the plasma and the adipose tissue of patients treated with acitretin (4). Reesterification of acitretin to etretinate occurs in some patients, resulting in the loss of the metabolic advantages of acitretin. Concomitant alcohol intake appears to be an important contributing factor for the conversion of acitretin to etretinate (5). In this chapter we will focus on the clinical efficacy of etretinate and acitretin and on the best strategy for using retinoids in the treatment of severe psoriasis.

ETRETINATE AND ACITRETIN: STRATEGY FOR USE

Both etretinate and acitretin have proven to be effective in severe plaque psoriasis, erythrodermic psoriasis, pustular psoriasis, and arthropathic psoriasis (6–10). Several double-blind comparative clinical studies have shown that there is no difference between acitretin and etretinate with regard to efficacy (11–14 and Table 1). Acitretin and etretinate were found to produce similar reductions in severity scores with comparable improvement in the intensity of erythema, infiltration, and scaling (11–14). In general, systemic treatment with retinoids is indicated in patients with severe types of psoriasis with extensive involvement (PASI score >10–15) or major influence on quality of life.

Monotherapy

Plaque-Type Psoriasis

Place in Therapeutic Strategy

Retinoids produce complete remission in fewer patients with plaque-type psoriasis than other systemic treatments such as methotrexate, PUVA, or cyclosporin. Monotherapy with retinoids produces a

Table 1 Comparison of Efficacy of Acitretin and Etretinate in Plaque-Type Psoriasis

Study	Treatment duration (weeks)	% reduction in severity score		Mean dose (mg/day)		% of relapse		Number of patients in each group	
		A	E	A	E	A	E	A	E
Ledo, 1988 (12)	12	38	51	30	30	NA		10	10
Gollnick, 1988 (11)	8	54	61	50	50	NA		43	43
Kragballe, 1989 (13)	12	76	71	40	50	NA		127	41
Gollnick, 1993 (14)	12	60	60	48	48	42	48	71	74

A, acitretin; E, etretinate.

40–60% reduction in severity scores after 3 months of therapy and complete clearing is only obtained in approximately one-third of the patients (6,7). The clinical response is usually slow and maximum improvement can take as long as 3–4 months (15). Patients should be aware that initial worsening of psoriasis with an increase in plaque size can be observed during the first month of therapy (9,11). Studies comparing cyclosporin and etretinate in severe plaque psoriasis showed that the number and the speed of remissions were higher in the patients treated with cyclosporin than in the patients treated with etretinate (16,17). However, a higher relapse rate was observed after withdrawal of cyclosporin than after etretinate (17). Combination therapy with PUVA or UVB seems to be the best strategy in the initial treatment of plaque-type psoriasis, allowing a reduction both in retinoid dosage and in the amount of UV necessary for complete clearing.

Optimal Initial Dose

Great interindividual variability exists with regard to efficacy and tolerability. The mean effective daily dose varies greatly (range 20–50 mg). The experience from clinical studies with acitretin or etretinate indicates that approximately 10–20% of patients withdraw prematurely because of intolerable adverse effects or initial worsening of their psoriasis (9–15). Both clinical efficacy and side effects are dose dependent (18). In early studies with etretinate, high-dosage regimens of 1 mg/kg/day were used (19). We believe increased frequency and severity of side effects at high doses reduces patient acceptance and can impair quality of life (20). In one study comparing efficacy and safety of low initial dosage with high initial dosage of acitretin, efficacy was similar but the number and the intensity of adverse effects were significantly lower in patients treated with low initial dosage (18). The therapeutic goal in psoriasis is to improve the quality of life and to obtain the best balance between improvement of skin lesions and occurrence of side effects. We therefore recommend beginning treatment at a low dose. Acceptability of retinoids is better when treatment is started at a dose of 10–20 mg/day and then progressively increased with 10 mg/week increments over a 2–3-month period according to clinical improvement and the intensity of cheilitis (18,20,21). According to this strategy, the daily dosage of retinoid is progressively adjusted by the patient himself according to his own evaluation of efficacy and side effects. An alternative approach is to begin treatment with high doses (0.6–1 mg/kg/day) until complete clearing is achieved (6,22). This strategy yields a quicker response but it increases the frequency of severe adverse reactions and it discourages many patients from continuing therapy because of intolerable side effects.

Maintenance Therapy

Once psoriasis has been cleared by etretinate or acitretin, the need for maintenance therapy with retinoids remains a matter of debate. It has been shown that after clearing of chronic plaque-type psoriasis with etretinate, 60% of patients were maintained in remission for at least 4 months after stopping treatment (23). Gollnick et al. conducted a 24-week follow-up study comparing relapse rates in patients achieving good clinical response after treatment with acitretin or etretinate (14). The relapse rates after acitretin were not different compared to those of etretinate. By the end of the study approximately 50% of patients showed no relapse with no need for specific treatment. On the other hand, a 75% relapse rate was observed 1 year after clearing of psoriasis with etretinate in one study (24). Relatively few studies have questioned the efficacy of retinoids as a long-term treatment of plaque-type psoriasis. In a double-blind, placebo-controlled study, etretinate at 0.5 mg/kg/day was found to prevent relapse of psoriasis in 60% of patients after 1 year (24). These results can be compared to those of an unpublished multicenter, double-blind study evaluating the efficacy of acitretin or etretinate in the maintenance treatment of psoriasis (25). After skin clearing with etretinate or acitretin (combined with PUVA in refractory cases) 60 patients were included in the maintenance phase with etretinate or acitretin for 48 weeks. The mean daily dose during this maintenance phase was 38 mg with acitretin and 32 mg with etretinate. Remission was maintained in 55% of patients treated with acitretin and 48% of patients treated with etretinate. No significant difference in efficacy could be found between the two groups (25). In a 12-month open study of treatment of severe psoriasis, Murray et al. found acitretin to be effective in 70% of patients (15). Both acitretin and etretinate are useful in the long-term maintenance treatment of plaque-type psoriasis. We believe that long-term maintenance therapy with retinoids should only be initiated in patients undergoing rapid relapse after psoriasis clearing. The maintenance daily dose of retinoid should be determined individually by tapering the retinoid dose after the patient has been cleared for 2–3 months. The mean daily maintenance dose may vary from 30 to 50 mg. No rebound occurs when the drug is discontinued (14,15).

Erythrodermic Psoriasis

Place in Therapeutic Strategy

Retinoids are highly effective in the treatment of psoriatic erythroderma (26). Marked improvement can be observed in more than 80% of patients with erythroderma after 2–4 weeks of therapy. We believe retinoids are the treatment of choice in erythrodermic psoriasis. Retinoids are as effective as methotrexate and display less toxicity (27).

Optimal Initial Dose

Few clinical studies have been performed for this particular indication and the adequate initial dosage is still debated. We believe high initial dosage should be avoided as initial worsening of erythema and severe exudation may occur, resulting in life-threatening situations, especially in elderly patients. The recommended initial retinoid daily dose is 10 mg. Dosage can be progressively increased according to clinical response and tolerance.

Palmoplantar Pustular Psoriasis

Place in Therapeutic Strategy

Palmoplantar pustular psoriasis is responsive to retinoids treatment in a dose-dependent fashion (28–31). Retinoids represent a first-line treatment for palmoplantar pustular psoriasis although other modalities such as PUVA and low-dose cyclosporin are preferable in women of childbearing potential (29,32).

Optimal Initial Dosage

In early studies with etretinate it was suggested that higher initial dosages of about 1 mg/kg/day should be used (28,30). However Lassus and Geiger, in a double-blind trial comparing etretinate and acitretin, demonstrated that lower doses (30 mg/day) were highly effective, reducing the number of pustules by 90% at week 12 (31).

Maintenance Therapy

Maintenance treatment with low-dose retinoids is usually required to prevent relapses (29). The mean maintenance daily dose ranges from 20 to 30 mg. Discontinuation of smoking may be of interest in patients with palmoplantar pustulosis. Switching to low-dose cyclosporin or combination treatment with PUVA is helpful in recalcitrant cases (29,32).

Generalized Pustular Psoriasis

Place in Therapeutic Strategy

Retinoids have a dramatic effect on generalized pustular psoriasis and should be regarded as a first-choice therapy (26,33,34). Pustulation stops within 1–2 weeks and more than 90% of patients show marked improvement. Favorable results have also been reported in childhood pustular psoriasis (35,36). Complete clearing occurred within 3 weeks to 4 months of etretinate therapy in five patients (36).

Optimal Initial Dosage

Initial high dosages of 50–70 mg are recommended. Isotretinoin has proved to be effective in generalized pustular psoriasis but higher dosages (up to 2 mg/kg day) are required (37). In view of its short half-life, isotretinoin can represent a therapeutic alternative to acitretin or etretinate in women of childbearing age who want to avoid prolonged posttreatment contraception.

Maintenance Therapy

Maintenance therapy with the lowest possible dosage is necessary to prevent relapse in about 20% of patients (34). Relapses usually respond well to the reintroduction of retinoid therapy.

Arthropathic Psoriasis

Place in Therapeutic Strategy

Etretinate has been shown to improve arthropathic psoriasis in open studies (38,39). The clinical effects appear after 4–6 weeks of therapy and improvement in objective signs of arthritis is observed within 4–6 months of therapy. One controlled study comparing etretinate and ibuprofen, a nonsteroidal anti-inflammatory drug, was performed (40), but no conclusion could be drawn as many patients were withdrawn prematurely because of inefficacy or side effects. In one recent study comparing etretinate and cyclosporin, etretinate was shown to produce a 46% reduction in joint involvement score after 10 weeks of therapy as compared with 30% with cyclosporin (17). However, retinoids do not prevent joint deformation in severe cases of arthropathic psoriasis (41).

Optimal Dose

Many authors consider retinoids as a long-term adjuvant in psoriatic arthropathy (22,41,42). The recommended maintenance dose of retinoids is approximately 0.5 mg/kg/day (22). More aggressive therapy like methotrexate or azathioprine may be useful in severe arthropatic psoriasis (42).

Psoriasis and HIV

Psoriasis in HIV-infected patients is often severe and difficult to treat. Pustular psoriasis, erythroderma, palmoplantar keratoderma, and arthropathic psoriasis appear to be more frequent in HIV-infected patients than in the general population (43). Retinoids have proven to be useful in psoriasis associated with HIV (44). Therapeutic doses ranging from 30 to 50 mg/day are effective on skin lesions and arthritis but long-term maintenance treatment is usually required. Zidovudine has proved to be effective in HIV-associated psoriasis (45). Association of retinoids with zidovudine may produce better results without increasing toxicity.

Other Indications

Uncontrolled observations suggest that low-dose retinoids could be of value in nail psoriasis and Hallopeau acrodermatitis suppurativa (46,47). Good results with etretinate have been reported in the treatment of Reiter's disease associated with psoriatic skin lesions (48).

Combination Therapy

Combination therapy with PUVA or UVB appears to be a good strategy to clear psoriasis for patients with plaque-type psoriasis (49–53). Combination therapy with PUVA or UVB exhibits a synergistic effect allowing a reduction in both retinoid dosage and duration of therapy. After the psoriasis has been cleared with combination therapy, monotherapy with retinoid offers the advantage of a relatively safe and effective maintenance treatment (15,24,25,54). This strategy is particularly useful in patients undergoing rapid relapse after PUVA or UVB. Our previous study suggested that a good clinical response to PUVA treatment (i.e., clearing of psoriasis after less than 18 PUVA sessions) was a good predictor of the efficacy of maintenance therapy with etretinate (24). In this study, the percentage of relapse after 12 months of maintenance treatment with etretinate was 20% in patients cleared after less than 18 PUVA sessions and 45% in patients cleared after more than 18 PUVA sessions (24). The possibility that low doses of retinoids might be useful to prevent psoriasis relapse after clearing with other treatments remains to be determined. In one study, acitretin did not prevent psoriasis relapse after cyclosporin tapering (55).

SIDE-EFFECT PROFILE OF RETINOID THERAPY IN PSORIASIS

After more than 20 years of use, the side effect profile of retinoids is well established (52,54–57). In a 5-year prospective study of 956 patients treated with etretinate 34% of patients stopped etretinate before remission of psoriasis (54). The reason for discontinuation was because of side effects in 70% of the patients. Most side effects are not dangerous but are strongly uncomfortable and they may decrease quality of life. This situation opens a new concept: to evaluate not the efficacy of a drug but the efficacy of the maximal well-tolerated dose, stressing that the goal of the treatment is to improve quality of life and that the patient has to be able to adjust retinoid dosage by himself.

Nearly 100% of patients in clinical trials experienced adverse effects. Most side effects of etretinate are similar to those of acitretin (7). It is noteworthy that some differences in the safety profile of acitretin and etretinate have been found in comparative studies (12,13,25,31).

Mucocutaneous Side Effects

Type of Side Effects

Adverse effects affecting the mucocutaneous system account for approximately 90% of the total number of adverse effects in patients treated with etretinate or acitretin (6,7). Mucocutaneous side effects are dose related and reversible after stopping therapy. They appear to be the main reason for the premature cessation of retinoid treatment in clinical studies. Approximately 10% of patients are unable to complete treatment because of mucocutaneous adverse effects. The most frequently reported adverse event is cheilitis with an incidence of 90–100%. It can be considered a good clinical marker for observance and adequate drug absorption. It is also the most convenient marker for assessing the maximal well-tolerated dose (60). Dryness of other mucous membrane sites is reported in 70% of patients during long-term treatment (54): dry nose with epistaxis, dryness of the mouth with thirst and sore tongue, genital dryness with balanitis or vulvitis, eye irritation with blepharoconjunctivitis. Retinoid therapy can impair the ability to wear contact lenses. Thinning of the skin results in xerosis, pruritus, which can be severe, erythema, and increased skin fragility. Peeling of the palms and soles and thinning of fingertips may create a problem especially in manual laborers as mechanical traumatization with blister formation and erosions can easily occur. Patients sometimes complain of stickiness of the skin and an increase in apocrine sweat, which may cause otitis externa (61). Mucosal dryness induced by retinoids causes the nares to become colonized with *Staphylococcus aureus* and a propensity for staphylococcal and herpes virus infections can be seen. About 75% of patients experience diffuse hair loss, which increases gradually during the first 4 months of therapy (62). This is due in part to a decrease in the duration of anagen and is reversible on stopping the drug or reducing the dose (62). Retinoids may also induce nail changes such as nail thinning, paronychia-like changes, onychomadesis, and periungual exuberant granulation tissue (46). Pyogenic or sarcoid-like granuloma has rarely been reported during etretinate therapy (63). The spectrum of adverse effects with acitretin is somewhat different from the one observed with etretinate. In one short-term study involving 175 patients, physicians observed a good or very good acceptance in 91% of patients treated with etretinate 50 mg/day versus in 68% of patients treated with acitretin at the same dose (11). These findings were confirmed by Kragballe et al., who found that etretinate was better tolerated than acitretin in a comparative study in 168 patients (13). Scaling of palms and soles and hair loss were more frequent in patients treated with acitretin than in patients treated with etretinate in this study (13). In our double-blind study evaluating the efficacy of acitretin or etretinate in the maintenance treatment of psoriasis, side effects affecting mucous membranes were more common with etretinate than with acitretin (25). On the contrary, palmoplantar desquamation was more frequent in patients treated with acitretin (25) (Table 2). Thus acitretin appears to be more toxic for keratinized areas.

Practical Management

Patients should be carefully informed regarding the nature and the frequency of adverse effects affecting skin and mucous membranes. Cheilitis can be prevented by using a moisturizing lipstick (58). Pruritus and xerosis may be minimized by the concurrent use of an emollient cream or ointment. Artificial tears are helpful in patients wearing contact lenses, although most of them have to switch to regular glasses. If side

Table 2 Comparison of Side-Effect Profile of Acitretin and Etretinate in Maintenance Treatment of Plaque-Type Psoriasis

Type of side effect	Acitretin ($n = 30$)	Etretinate ($n = 29$)	p
Cheilitis	72%	84%	<0.01
Xerosis	28.5%	27.5%	NS
Dry mouth	14%	29%	<0.001
Dry nose	14%	30%	<0.001
Pruritus	22%	18%	NS
Palmoplantar desquamation	23%	13%	<0.01
Hair loss	16%	7%	NS
Blepharoconjunctivitis	15%	16%	NS

Source: From Ref. 25.

effects become unacceptable, patients should be advised to reduce drug dosage to find the maximal well-tolerated dose (18).

Teratogenicity

Type of Side Effects

Like vitamin A, acitretin and etretinate are potent teratogens and their administration to women of childbearing potential should be avoided. Abnormalities in children exposed in utero to etretinate include meningomyelocele, meningoencephalocele, cardiac malformations, facial dysmorphia, syndactyly, absence of terminal phalanges, malformations of hip and ankles, abnormalities of ears, and decreased cranial volume (64). Etretinate-associated malformations were detected in an infant born to a mother who stopped etretinate 51 weeks before conception (65). Therefore, a 2-year period of contraception after cessation of treatment is recommended in most countries (66). As detectable serum levels of etretinate can be found more than 2 years after cessation of therapy with etretinate due to storage in adipose tissue, the period during which pregnancy should be avoided after treatment with etretinate remains undetermined (3).

Practical Management

In rare cases retinoids may be indicated in women of childbearing age if other effective drugs are ineffective or contraindicated. Effective contraception is then essential during treatment and for at least 2 years thereafter. As the maximum risk of teratogenicity occurs within the first weeks of gestation it is of particular importance to begin contraception 1 month before the start of retinoid therapy. Treatment should be initiated after the first menstruation period and a serum pregnancy test should be performed before treatment initiation. Retinoids should be prescribed only after in-depth counseling and to patients able to comply with mandatory contraceptive measures. Reliable contraceptive measures include estroprogestative contraceptives and intrauterine devices. Condoms and spermicides appear not to be safe enough. Alcohol consumption must be avoided in women of childbearing age taking acitretin as it is a major promoting factor in reesterification of acitretin to etretinate (5). It has been suggested that monitoring etretinate and acitretin plasma concentrations could be of value in female patients at the end of and 2 years after treatment to confirm the complete elimination of the drug (67). However, it is noteworthy that acitretin and/or etretinate can be found in fat for up to 29 months after cessation of therapy even in the absence of detectable plasma concentration (68).

When pregnancy occurs during treatment or after exposure to acitretin or etretinate, clinical counseling is difficult. The problem is somewhat different with acitretin than with etretinate because acitretin is less lipophilic and exhibits a shorter elimination half-life. If pregnancy occurs during treatment or within 3 months after exposure to acitretin, the most reasonable action is to propose abortion because the fetal risk is high (69). If pregnancy occurs more than 3 months after treatment cessation, there is no definitive answer because the period of time during which pregnancy must be avoided and the risk of fetal outcome are not well determined (66). The decision to terminate the pregnancy or to carry it to term is highly individual and should be addressed with the parents on a case-by-case basis. Determination of retinoid serum levels could be of interest to better determine the teratogenic risk.

Ocular Side Effects

External eye problems (blepharoconjunctivitis, sticky eyes, keratitis) are common in both short-term and long-term treatment with retinoids. Impaired color and dark vision have rarely been reported to occur during long-term treatment with etretinate (56). It has been suggested that retinoids may induce retinal toxicity. However, a prospective study found no evidence of retinal toxicity during long-term treatment with etretinate (70). Similarly, a recent survey did not report a relationship between cataract development and long-term treatment with etretinate in contrast to previous anecdotal reports (54).

Musculoskeletal System

Type of Side Effects

Long-term treatment with retinoids has been associated with the development of spinal and extraspinal hyperostosis and calcifications of tendons and ligaments (58,59). Drug-induced calcifications may sometimes resolve spontaneously after withdrawal of retinoid therapy (71). The prevalence of retinoid-induced skeletal adverse effects is highly variable. Retrospective studies are difficult to interpret: as patients suffering from psoriasis have increased incidence of bone changes, some findings might be unrelated to treatment with retinoids. Kilcoyne found spine x-ray abnormalities in 86% of 236 patients treated with acitretin at the start of therapy (72). The percentage of patients developing bone abnormalities varies from 5 to 24% in prospective studies after 12–24 months of treatment with acitretin (71,73). In a recent retrospective study no relationship was found between spinal abnormalities and prolonged treatment with etretinate or acitretin (74). Moreover, the clinical significance of radiological bone abnormalities is not fully understood. In a prospective survey of 956 patients receiving long-term treatment with etretinate it appeared that continued use of etretinate was not a risk factor for the development of persistent symptomatic joint problems (54). Osteoporosis has been observed during hypervitaminosis A in humans. Some authors found a significant decrease in bone mineral density in patients who received long-term therapy with etretinate as compared with age-, sex-, and weight-matched controls (75,76). The clinical significance of this decrease in bone mineral density values is unknown and prospective studies are needed to assess the risk of developing symptomatic osteoporosis during long-term treatment with retinoids, particularly in patients who are at higher risk for osteoporosis (e.g., postmenopausal women or patients receiving systemic steroids).

In children, retinoids are usually well tolerated (36,77). A few cases of skeletal abnormalities including thickening of the periostum, bone resorption, and premature closure of the epiphyses have been reported (78,79). More recently, no premature closure of epiphyses was found in a study of 42 children undergoing long-term treatment with etretinate for ichthyosis (80). Musculoskeletal complications appear to be uncommon in children provided the initial dose is below 1 mg/kg/day and quickly reduced to the minimal effective dose, which is usually less than 0.5 mg/kg/day in our experience (77).

Practical Management

The usefulness of radiographic examination of bones remains controversial during long-term treatment with retinoids. Extensive radiographic or scintigraphic surveys are not recommended in adults. Patients over 50 and particularly psoriasis patients may develop skeletal abnormalities not related to treatment with retinoids and the results of x-ray examinations may be difficult to interpret. Moreover, we believe that hyperostosis or asymptomatic tendon calcifications are not absolute indications to discontinue treatment. On the other hand, the development of symptomatic joint problems in a patient under long-term retinoid therapy should prompt radiographs of the affected region.

When acitretin or etretinate is prescribed for a child, careful monitoring of the child's growth parameters is required (36,77). The frequency and the nature of radiological surveillance are not established in children.

Liver

Type of Side Effects

Both etretinate and acitretin therapy are associated with short-term elevation in liver enzymes (6,7). An increase in ASAT and ALAT above normal values is found in about 10% of patients either with acitretin or with etretinate (7). In other studies higher rates were found in 20–30% of all patients developing abnormal liver function tests but dosage regimens were higher (6,19). These changes are usually mild and reversible after cessation of treatment (18,57). They can resolve despite continued retinoid use. Occasionally acute hepatitis with fever and inconstant hypereosinophilia can occur early, after 1 month or less of acitretin or etretinate treatment (81). It is supposed to be an idiosyncratic hypersensitivity reaction and constitutes an absolute contraindication to continue treatment. Long-term treatment with retinoids is also associated with variations in liver enzymes (15,54,59). The incidence seems to be similar during acitretin and etretinate treatment. Low-grade hepatotoxicity is observed in about 1% of patients (54). In patients receiving long-term etretinate therapy for psoriasis, no consistent evidence of chronic toxicity was found in liver biopsy specimens (82). Cumulative data suggest that the hepatotoxicity with long-term treatment with etretinate or acitretin is less than with methotrexate. However, caution is necessary when the patient has other risk factors for the development of liver disease such as alcoholism, chronic viral hepatitis, or a history of previous treatment with methotrexate.

Practical Management

Monitoring serum for ASAT and ALAT at regular intervals is necessary. We recommend performing transaminases before and after 4 weeks of therapy. They should then be checked every 3 months thereafter. Patients at risk for hepatotoxicity may require more frequent evaluations. Excessive alcohol consumption should be avoided. In patients with continually elevated liver enzymes, treatment should be discontinued or a liver biopsy considered if treatment has to be continued. Any symptom suggesting a hypersensitivity reaction should prompt immediate withdrawal of the drug.

Serum Lipid Changes

Type of Side Effects

Hyperlipidemia is the most common biological side effect of etretinate and acitretin (6,7). Increases in serum triglycerides and cholesterol have been reported to occur in about 20% of patients during short-term treatment with either acitretin or etretinate. A decrease in high-density lipoprotein is observed in about one-third of the patients. Modifications of these parameters also occur during long-term treatment with retinoids. They may constitute an additional risk factor in cardiovascular diseases and atherosclerosis. This may be particularly true for high doses of retinoids as lipid elevations and cardiovascular events were found to be more frequent in patients receiving high doses of etretinate in one long-term prospective study (54). The hyperlipidemic potential of acitretin appears to be similar to that of etretinate (83).

Practical Management

Lipid abnormalities are important to consider in patients undergoing long-term treatment with retinoids. In an attempt to minimize the effects of retinoids on serum lipids, dietary recommendations are useful. Patients should avoid excessive alcohol intake and reduce dietary sugars (6,59). It has been suggested that fish oil supplementation may reduce hypertriglyceridemia and hypercholesterolemia due to etretinate (84). Patients with other risk factors such as smoking, alcoholism, familial hyperlipidemia, obesity, or diabetes mellitus have a greater incidence of lipid abnormalities during retinoid treatment (6). Dietary interventions and reduction in weight and in alcohol intake are particularly recommended in these patients. Cholesterol and triglycerides concentrations should be monitored before the start of therapy and 1 month thereafter. If lipid values are within normal limits, monitoring can be repeated every 3–4 months. Very high triglycerides values (above 800 mg/dl) may occur rarely in patients who have high pretreatment lipid levels. They should prompt the withdrawal of therapy as there is a risk of acute pancreatitis.

Rare Side Effects

Many rare side effects have been associated with treatment with etretinate or acitretin (11,12,56,85–96 and Table 3). Headache and dizziness are observed in less than 5% of patients (66). Benign intracranial hypertension has been rarely reported during treatment with etretinate (93,94). In children it can occur along with headache and abnormal irritability.

The imputability of retinoids in the development of some rare side effects is not always well established in individual case reports. For example, in the single case reported of toxic epidermal necrolysis associated with etretinate use, the patient also took indomethacin, a drug known to induce toxic epidermal necrolysis (89,97).

PRACTICAL GUIDELINES FOR MANAGEMENT OF PATIENTS ON RETINOIDS

Dosage Regimens

As discussed above, the problem of optimal initial dose is a controversial issue. One may bear in mind that the most frequent and severe side effects are observed in patients treated with high doses (0.6–1 mg/kg/day). We and others recommend that the lower dose range from 10–20 mg/day should be used to begin treatment in plaque-type psoriasis (18,20,21). This strategy is known to decrease the intensity of side effects and it may facilitate the patient's education and improve the quality of life. The suggested dosing reg-

Table 3 Rare Side Effects Reported During Therapy with Etretinate or Acitretin

Photosensitivity (85)
Edema of face and limbs (86)
Prurigo nodularis-like eruption (87)
Erythema multiformis (88)
Toxic epidermal necrolysis (89)
Muscle stiffness (56)
Gynecomastia (90)
Decreased libido (11,12)
Erectile dysfunction (91)
Peripheral neuropathy (92)
Intracranial hypertension (93,94)
Thrombocytopenia (95)
Acute renal impairment (96)

imens for the various types of psoriasis are listed in Table 4. In plaque-type psoriasis complete clearing is rarely obtained and combined therapy with PUVA or topical therapy (i.e., calcipotriol or topical steroids) may be useful to treat minimal flares of psoriasis during maintenance treatment with retinoids. Except for pustular psoriasis, clinical efficacy is slow to appear and maximal improvement is observed only after 2–4 months of therapy and even longer in some patients. For these reasons it seems advisable to inform patients that in most cases retinoids are not a short-term treatment in psoriasis. It is essential to instruct patients thoroughly about the adverse effects to be expected and the way to minimize them. Acitretin or etretinate should be taken with a meal to increase bioavailability (3).

Contraindications and Precautions

Contraindications

Etretinate and acitretin are completely contraindicated during pregnancy and lactation. Retinoids are not recommended in patients with severe hypertriglyceridemia or severe hepatic or renal dysfunction. Women of childbearing age represent a relative contraindication. As mentioned above, retinoids should only be prescribed to women with severe skin disease and after failure of other treatment modalities such as phototherapy, cyclosporin, or methotrexate.

Precautions

Women of childbearing potential should be able to maintain reliable contraceptive measures from 1 month before therapy to 2 years after its cessation. In children, etretinate and acitretin should be used cautiously and only in severe forms of psoriasis because relatively few studies have been published in childhood psoriasis and some concern remains about long-term side effects. Retinoids are usually well tolerated provided the maintenance dose is the lowest possible. We believe the maintenance dose of retinoids should be restricted to less than 0.5 mg/kg/day in children with severe psoriasis. Careful monitoring of the child's growth parameters is recommended. A baseline skeletal radiological examination can be performed in children if long-term treatment with retinoids is planned. Follow-up radiology should be restricted to children with pretreatment abnormalities and those developing musculoskeletal symptoms (80).

Clinical Monitoring and Laboratory Testing

A complete clinical examination including past medical history and determination of daily alcohol intake are necessary before treatment initiation. Serum levels of transaminases, triglycerides, and cholesterol should be evaluated before initiation of therapy and 1 month thereafter. If the values are within normal limits, we recommend monitoring of these parameters every 3–4 months. In the case of abnormal findings, more frequent determinations of these parameters are recommended. In fertile women a serum pregnancy test should be performed before the beginning of therapy.

Drug Interactions

Concomitant use of tetracyclines or vitamin A is contraindicated as there is a risk of intracranial hypertension and papilledema (94). Caution must be used concerning the combined used of retinoids and methotrexate because methotrexate plasma levels could rise (98). Moreover this association may increase methotrexate-induced hepatotoxicity. Combination of cyclosporin and etretinate or acitretin is not recommended because it can inhibit hepatic cyclosporin metabolism (99). An increase in cyclosporin concentration with renal toxicity has been reported in

Table 4 Place of Retinoids in the Treatment of Adult Psoriasis

Indication	Place of retinoids	Initial dose (mg/day)	Maintenance dose (mg/day)
Chronic plaque-type psoriasis	Second choice (after PUVA, UVB)	10–20	30–50
Palmoplantar pustular psoriasis	First choice	10–20	30
Generalized pustular psoriasis	First choice	50–70	30–50
Erythrodermic psoriasis	First choice	10	10–30

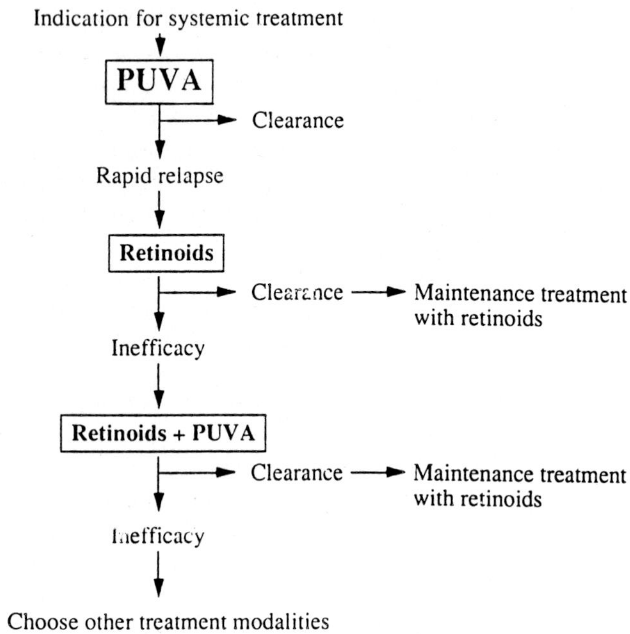

Figure 1 Algorithm showing the place of retinoids in the therapeutic strategy of plaque-type psoriasis.

a patient treated concomitantly with cyclosporin and etretinate (99). In fertile women using oral contraceptives, hepatic enzyme inducers such as rifampicine or anticonvulsants are contraindicated because these drugs can impair the effectiveness of estroprogestative contraceptives (66).

CONCLUDING REMARKS

Acitretin and etretinate are important antipsoriatic agents. They are particularly useful in pustular psoriasis and psoriatic erythroderma. Good results have also been obtained in plaque-type psoriasis in combination with PUVA and UVB and in psoriatic arthritis. Retinoids appear to be a good option for long-term maintenance treatment of plaque-type psoriasis after clearing with PUVA. Figure 1 is a proposed algorithm showing the place of retinoids in the therapeutic strategy of plaque-type psoriasis. Short-term side effects are dose related and must be explained to patients before initiation of therapy. Ideally, patients should be able to control mucocutaneous side effects by self-adapting retinoid dosage. Long-term side effects are acceptable and retinoids exhibit a good risk/benefit ratio provided guidelines are observed. Therapeutic dosage must be adapted individually and a compromise should be found between therapeutic benefit and side effects.

REFERENCES

1. Brindley, C.J. (1989). Overview of recent clinical pharmacokinetic studies with acitretin (Ro 10-1670, Etretin). *Dermatologica* 178:79–87.
2. Lambert, W.E., Meyer, E., De Leenheer, A.P., De Bersaques, J.D., and Kint, A.H. (1992). Pharmacokinetics and drug interactions of etretinate and acitretin. *J. Am. Acad. Dermatol.* 27:S19–S22.
3. Larsen, F.G. (1994). Pharmacokinetics of etretinate and acitretin with special reference to treatment of psoriasis. *Acta Derm. Venereol.* (*Stockh.*) Suppl. 190:5–33.
4. Meyer, E., De Bersaques, J., Lambert, W.E., De Leenheer, A.P., and Kint, A.H. (1994). Skin, adipose tissue and plasma levels of acitretin with rare occurrence of esterified acitretin during long-term treatment. *Acta Derm. Venereol.* (*Stockh.*) 73:113–115.
5. Larsen, F.G., Jakobsen, P., Knudsen, J., Weismann, K., Kragballe, K., and Nielsen-Kudsk, F. (1993). Conversion of acitretin to etretinate in psoriatic patients is influenced by ethanol. *J. Invest. Dermatol.* 100: 623–627.
6. Ellis, C.N., and Voorhees, J.J. (1987). Etretinate therapy. *J. Am. Acad. Dermatol.* 16:267–291.
7. Geiger, J.M., and Czarnetzki, B.M. (1988). Acitretin (Ro 10-1670, Etretin): overall evaluation of clinical studies. *Dermatologica* 176:182–190.
8. Geiger, J.M., and Saurat, J.H. (1993). Acitretin and etretinate. How and when they should be used. *Dermatol. Clin.* 11:117–129.
9. Goldfarb, M.T., Ellis, C.N., Gupta, A.K., Tincoff, T., Hamilton, T.A., and Voorhees, J.J. (1988). Acitretin improves psoriasis in a dose-dependent fashion. *J. Am. Acad. Dermatol.* 18:655–662.
10. Olsen, E.A., Wendel, W.W., Meyer, C.J., and Cobo, L.M. (1989). A double blind placebo-controlled trial of acitretin for the treatment of psoriasis. *J. Am. Acad. Dermatol.* 21;681–686.
11. Gollnick, H., Bauer, R., Brindley, C., Orfanos, C.E., Plewig, G., Wokalek, H., and Hoting, E. (1988). Acitretin versus etretinate in psoriasis. *J. Am. Acad. Dermatol.* 19:458–469.
12. Lebo, A., Martin, M., Geiger, J.M., and Marron, J.M. (1988). Acitretin (Ro 10-1670) in the treatment of severe psoriasis. A randomized double-blind parallel study comparing acitretin and etretinate. *Int. J. Dermatol.* 27:656–660.
13. Kragballe, K., Jansen, C.T., Geiger, J.M., Bjerke, J.R., Falk, E.S., Gip, L., Hjorth, N., Lauharanta, J., Mork, N.J., Reunala, T., Rosen, K., Schmidt, H., Thune, P.O., and Vahlquist, C. (1989). A double blind comparison

of acitretin and etretinate in the treatment of severe psoriasis. *Acta. Derm. Venereol. (Stockh.)* 69:35–40.
14. Gollnick, H.P.M., Zaun, H., Ruzicka, T., Sommerburg, C., Loew, S., Mahrle, G., Niedecken, H.W., Paul, E., Pfister-Wartha, A., and Reinel, D. (1993). Relapse rate of severe generalized psoriasis after treatment with acitretin or etretinate. Results of the first randomized double-blind multicenter half-year follow-up study. *Eur. J. Dermatol.* 3:442–446.
15. Murray, H.E., Anhalt, A.W., Lessard, R., Schacter, R.K., Baron Ross, J., Stewart, W.D., and Geiger, J.M. (1991). A 12-month treatment of severe psoriasis with acitretin: results of a Canadian open multicenter study. *J. Am. Acad. Dermatol.* 24:598–602.
16. Italian Multicenter Study Group on Cyclosporin in Psoriasis. (1993). Cyclosporin versus etretinate: Italian multicenter comparative trial in severe plaque-form psoriasis. *Dermatology* 187(Suppl. 1):8–18.
17. Mahrle, G., Schulze H-J., Färber, L., Weidinger, G., and Steigleder, G.K. (1995). Low-dose short-term cyclosporine versus etretinate in psoriasis: improvement of skin, nail, and joint involvement. *J. Am. Acad. Dermatol.* 32:78–88.
18. Berbis, P., Geiger, J.M., Vaisse, C., Rognin, C., and Privat, Y. (1989). Benefit of progressively increasing doses during the initial treatment with acitretin in psoriasis. *Dermatologica* 178:88–92.
19. Ehman, C.W., and Voorhees, J.J. (1982). International studies of the efficacy of etretinate in the treatment of psoriasis. *J. Am. Acad. Dermatol.* 6:692–696.
20. Dubertret L. (1985). Etretinate (Tigason, Europe; Tegison, USA) in psoriasis: advantages of low doses progressively increased. *J. Am. Acad. Dermatol.* 13:830.
21. Rosenbach, T., and Czarnetzki, B.M. (1994). Retinoids. In *Psoriasis*. L Dubertret (Ed.). ISED, Brescia, Italy, pp. 151–161.
22. Fritsch, P. (1992). Retinoids in psoriasis and disorders of keratinization. *J. Am. Acad. Dermatol.* 27:S8–S14.
23. Orfanos, C.E., and Goerz, G. (1978). Orale psoriasis therapie mit einem neuen aromatischen retinoid (Ro 10-9359). Eine multizentrische kontrollierte studie an 291 patienten in der Bundesrepublik. *Dtsche. Med. Wochenschr.* 103:195–199.
24. Dubertret, L., Chastang, C., Beylot, C., Bazex, J., Rognin, C., and Touraine, R. (1985). Maintenance treatment of psoriasis by Tigason: a double-blind randomized clinical trial. *Br. J. Dermatol.* 113:323–330.
25. Dubertret, L., Beylot, C., Baran, P., Souteyrand, P., Berbis, P., Meynadier, J., Ortonne, J.P., Daniel, F., Escande, J.P., Kalis, B., Chevrant-Breton, J., Grosshans, E., Bazex, J. A double-blind comparative study of acitretin and etretinate in the long-term treatment of psoriasis (in preparation).
26. Wolska, H., Jablonska, S., and Bounameaux, Y. (1983). Etretinate in severe psoriasis. *J. Am. Acad. Dermatol.* 9:883–889.
27. Lowe, N.J., Roenigk, H., and Voorhees, J.J. (1988). Etretinate. Appropriate use in severe psoriasis. *Arch. Dermatol.* 124:527–528.
28. White, S.I., Marks, J.M., and Shuster, S. (1985). Etretinate in pustular psoriasis of palms and soles. *Br. J. Dermatol.* 113:581–585.
29. Rosen, K., Mobacken, H., and Swanbeck, G. (1987). PUVA, etretinate, and PUVA-etretinate therapy for pustulosis palmoplantaris. A placebo-controlled comparative trial. *Arch. Dermatol.* 123:885–889.
30. Foged, E., Holm, P., Larsen, P.O., Lamberg, G., Reymann, F., Roesdahle, K., and Ullman, S. (1983). A randomized trial of etretinate (Tigason) in palmoplantar pustulosis. *Dermatologica* 166:220–223.
31. Lassus, A., and Geiger, J.M. (1988). Acitretin and etretinate in the treatment of palmoplantar pustulosis: a double-blind comparative trial. *Br. J. Dermatol.* 119: 775–759.
32. Reitamo, S., Erkko, P., Remitz, A., Lauerma, A.I., Montonen, O., and Harjula, K. (1993). Cyclosporine in the treatment of palmoplantar pustulosis. A randomized, double-blind, placebo-controlled study. *Arch. Dermatol.* 129:1273–1279.
33. Guilhou, J.J., Malbos, S., and Meynadier, J. (1978). Traitement oral des psoriasis graves par un nouveau rétinoide aromatique (Ro 10-9359). *Ann. Dermatol. Venereol.* 105:813–818.
34. Wolska, H., Jablonska, S., Langner, A., and Fraczykowska, M. (1985). Etretinate therapy in generalized pustular psoriasis (Zumbusch type). *Dermatologica* 171:297–304.
35. Zelickson, B.D., and Muller, S.A. (1991). Generalized pustular psoriasis in childhood. *J. Am. Acad. Dermatol.* 24:186–194.
36. Rosinska, D., Wolska, H., Jablonska, S., and Konca, I. (1988). Etretinate in severe psoriasis of children. *Pediatr. Dermatol.* 5:266–272.
37. Moy, R.L., Kingston, T.P., and Lowe, N.J. (1985). Isotretinoin versus etretinate therapy in generalized pustular and chronic psoriasis. *Arch. Dermatol.* 121: 1297–1301.
38. Kaplan, R.P., Russell, D.H., and Lowe, N.J. (1983). Etretinate therapy for psoriasis: clinical response, remission times, epidermal DNA and polyamines responses. *J. Am. Acad. Dermatol.* 8:95–102.
39. Chieregato, C.G., and Leoni, A. (1986). Treatment of psoriatic arthropathy with etretinate: a two-year follow-up. *Acta. Derm. Venereol. (Stockh.)* 66:321–324.
40. Hopkins, R., Bird, H.A., Jones, H., Hill, J., Surrall, K.E., Astbury, C., Miller, A., and Wright, V. (1985). A double blind controlled trial of etretinate (Tigason) and ibuprofen in psoriatic arthritis. *Ann. Rheum. Dis.* 44:189–193.
41. Braun-Falco, O., and Ruzicka, T. (1994). Psoriatic arthritis. *Int. J. Dermatol.* 33:320–322.

42. Goupille, P., and Valat, J.P. (1994). Le traitement du rhumatisme psoriasique. *Ann. Med. Int.* 145:205–214.
43. Duvic, M., Johnson, T.M., Rapini, R.P., Freese, T., Brewton, G., and Rios, A. (1987). Acquired immunodeficiency syndrome-associated psoriasis and Reiter's syndrome. *Arch. Dermatol.* 123:1622–1632.
44. Belz, J., Breneman, D.L., Nordlund, J.J., and Solinger, A. (1989). Successful treatment of a patient with Reiter's syndrome and acquired immunodeficiency syndrome using etretinate. *J. Am. Acad. Dermatol.* 20: 898–903.
45. Duvic, M., Crane, M.M., Conant, M., Mahoney, S.E., Reveille, J.D., and Nusinoff Lehrman, S. (1994). Zidovudine improves psoriasis in human immunodeficiency virus–positive males. *Arch. Dermatol.* 130: 447–451.
46. Baran, R. (1986). Etretinate and the nails (study of 130 cases) possible mechanisms of some side-effects. *Clin. Exp. Dermatol.* 11:148–152.
47. Rabinovitz, H.S., Scher, R.K., and Shupack, J.L. (1983). Response of psoriatic nails to the aromatic retinoid etretinate. *Arch. Dermatol.* 119:627–628.
48. Lassus, A., Eskelin, A., Sacha, K., Koenoenene, M., and Laurahanta, J. (1985). Treatment of Reiter's disease with etretinate. In *Retinoids: New Trends in Research and Therapy*. J.H. Saurat (Ed.). S. Karger, Munich, pp. 391–396.
49. Saurat, J.-H., Geiger, J.M., Amblard, P., Beani, J.-C., Boulanger, A., Claudy, A., Frenk, E., Guilhou, J.-J., Grosshans, E., Mérot, Y., Meynadier, J., and Tapernoux, B. (1988). Randomized double-blind multicenter study comparing acitretin-PUVA, etretinate-PUVA and placebo-PUVA in the treatment of severe psoriasis. *Dermatologica* 177:218–224.
50. Tanew, A., Guggenbichler, A., Hönigsmann, H., Geiger, J.M., and Fritsch, P. (1991). Photochemotherapy for severe psoriasis without or in combination with acitretin: a randomized, double-blind comparison study. *J. Am. Acad. Dermatol.* 25:682–684.
51. Lowe, N.J., Prystowsky, J.H., Bourget, T., Edelstein, J., Nychay, S., and Armstrong, R. (1991). Acitretin plus UVB therapy for psoriasis. *J. Am. Acad. Dermatol.* 24:591–594.
52. Green, C., Lakshmipathi, T., Johnson, B.E., and Ferguson, J. (1992). A comparison of the efficacy and relapse rates of narrowband UVB (TL-01) monotherapy vs. etretinate (re-TL-01) vs. etretinate-PUVA (re-PUVA) in the treatment of psoriasis patients. *Br. J. Dermatol.* 127:5–9.
53. Sommerburg, C., Kietzmann, H., Eichelberg, D., Goos, M., Heese, A. Hölzle, E., Koßmann, E., Wokalek, H., Przybilla, B., and Ruzicka, T. (1993). Acitretin in combination with PUVA: a randomized double-blind placebo-controlled study in severe psoriasis. *J. Eur. Acad. Dermatol.* 2:308–317.
54. Stern, R.S., Fitzgerald, E., Ellis, C.N., Lowe, N., Goldfarb, M.T., and Baughman, R.D. (1995). The safety of etretinate as long-term therapy for psoriasis: results of the etretinate follow-up study. *J. Am. Acad. Dermatol.* 33:44–52.
55. Salomon, D., Mesheit, J., Masgrau-Peya, E., Feldmann, R., and Saurat, J.-H. (1994). Acitretin does not prevent psoriasis relapse related to cyclosporine A tapering. *Br. J. Dermatol.* 130:257–258.
56. Halioua, B., and Saurat, J.H. (1990). Risk:benefit ratio in the treatment of psoriasis with systemic retinoids. *Br. J. Dermatol.* 122(Suppl. 36):135–150.
57. Gupta, A.K., Goldfarb, M.T., Ellis, C.N., and Voorhees, J.J. (1989). Side-effect profile of acitretin therapy in psoriasis. *J. Am. Acad. Dermatol.* 20:1088–93.
58. Saurat, J.H. (1992). Side effects of systemic retinoids and their clinical management. *J. Am. Acad. Dermatol.* 27:S23–S28.
59. Vahlquist, A. (1992). Long term safety of retinoid therapy. *J. Am. Acad. Dermatol.* 27:S29–S33.
60. Dubertret L. (1994). Therapeutic strategy. In *Psoriasis*. L. Dubertret (Ed.). ISED, Brescia, Italy, pp. 192–194.
61. Penney, N.S., Taylor, R., and Hernandez, D. (1992). Etretinate increases carcinoembryonic antigen in palmar scrapings. *J. Am. Acad. Dermatol.* 26:940–942.
62. Berth-Jones, J., and Hutchinson, P.E. (1995). Novel cycle changes in scalp hair are caused by etretinate therapy. *Br. J. Dermatol.* 132:367–375.
63. Fernandez-Redondo, V., Vazquez, J., Sanchez-Aguilar, D., and Toribio, J. (1994). Sarcoid-like granuloma following prolonged etretinate treatment. *Dermatology* 188:226–227.
64. Rosa, F.W. (1993). Retinoid embryopathy in humans. In *Retinoids in Clinical Practice. The Risk-Benefit Ratio*. G. Koren (Ed.). Marcel Dekker, New York, pp. 77–109.
65. Lammer, E.J. (1988). Embryopathy in an infant conceived one year after termination of maternal etretinate. *Lancet* 2:1080–1081.
66. Geiger, J.M., and Saurat, J.H. (1993). Acitretin and etretinate, how and when they should be used. *Dermatol. Clin.* 11:117–129.
67. Rink, G., Gollnick, H., and Orfanos, C.E. (1989). Duration of contraception after etretinate. *Lancet* 1: 845–846.
68. Sturkenboom, M.C., De Jong-Van Den Berg, L.T., Van Voorst-Vader, P.C., Cornel, M.C., Stricker, B.H., and Wesseling, H. (1994). Inability to detect plasma etretinate and acitretin is a poor predictor of the absence of these teratogens in tissue after stopping acitretin treatment. *Br. J. Clin. Pharmacol.* 38:229–235.
69. Kaiser, D.L. (1993). Retinoid embryopathy: epidemiological perspectives. In *Retinoids in Clinical Practice. The Risk-Benefit Ratio*. G. Koren (Ed.). Marcel Dekker, New York, pp. 209–223.

70. Pitts, J.F., Mackie, R.M., Dutton, G.N., McClure, E.A., and Allan, D. (1991). Etretinate and visual function: a 1-year follow-up study. *Br. J. Dermatol.* 125:53–55.
71. Mork, N.J., Kolbenstvedt, A., and Austad, J. (1992). Efficacy and skeletal side effects of two years acitretin treatment. *Acta Derm. Venereol. (Stockh.)* 72:445–448.
72. Kilcoyne, R.F. (1990). Acitretin effects on the spine. *Dermatologica* 181:359–360.
73. Kilcoyne, R.F. (1988). Effects of retinoids in bone. *J. Am. Acad. Dermatol.* 19:212–216.
74. Van Dooren-Greebe, R.J., Lemmens, J.A.M., De Boo, T., Hangx, N.M.A., Kuijpers, A.L.A., and Van De Kerkhof, P.C.M. (1996). Prolonged treatment with oral retinoids in adults: no influence on the frequency and severity of spinal abnormalities. *Br. J. Dermatol.* 134: 71–76.
75. Okada, N., Nomura, M., Morimoto, S., Ogihara, T., and Yoshikawa, K. (1994). Bone mineral density of the lumbar spine in psoriatic patients with long term etretinate therapy. *J. Dermatol.* 21:308–311.
76. DiGiovanna, J.J., Sollito, R.B., Abangan, D.L., Steinberg, S.M., and Reynolds, J.C. (1995). Osteoporosis is a toxic effect of long-term etretinate therapy. *Arch. Dermatol.* 131:1263–1267.
77. Bodemer, C., and De Prost, Y. (1994). Acitretin in children. *Acta Derm. Venereol. (Stockh.)* Suppl 186:124.
78. Prendiville, J., Bingham, E.A., and Burrows, D. (1986). Premature epiphysal closure—a complication of etretinate therapy in children. *J. Am. Acad. Dermatol.* 17:1259–1269.
79. Halkier-Sorensen, L., Laurberg, G., and Andresen, J. (1987). Bone changes in children on long-term treatment with etretinate. *J. Am. Acad. Dermatol.* 16: 999–1006.
80. Paige, D.G., Judge, M.R., Shaw, D.G., Atherton, D.J., and Harper, J.I. (1992). Bone changes and their significance in children with ichthyosis on long-term etretinate therapy. *Br. J. Dermatol.* 127:387–391.
81. Coschieri, M. Philippon, A., Quinsat, D., Dor, J.F., and Chichmanian, R.M. (1993). Atteinte hépatique aigue au cours de la prise d'acitretine. *Gastroenterol. Clin. Biol.* 17:769–770.
82. Roenigk, H.H., Gibstine, C., Glazer, S., Sparberg, M., and Yokoo, H. (1985). Serial liver biopsies in psoriatic patients receiving long-term etretinate. *Br. J. Dermatol.* 112:77–81.
83. Pilkington, T., and Brogden, R.N. (1992). Acitretin. A review of its pharmacology and therapeutic use. *Drugs* 43:597–627.
84. Frati, C., Bevilacqua, L., and Apostolico, V. (1994). Association of etretinate and fish oil in psoriasis therapy. Inhibition of hypertriglyceridemia resulting from retinoid therapy after fish oil supplementation. *Acta. Derm. Venereol. (Stockh.)* Suppl. 186:151–153.
85. Ferguson, J., and Johnson, B.E. (1986). Photosensitivity due to retinoids: clinical and laboratory studies. *Br. J. Dermatol.* 115:275–283.
86. Allan, S., and Christmas, T. (1988). Severe edema associated with etretinate. *J. Am. Acad. Dermatol.* 19: 140.
87. Boer, J., and Smeenk, G. (1987). Nodular prurigo-like eruptions induced by etretinate. *Br. J. Dermatol.* 116: 271–274.
88. David, M., Sandbank, M., and Lowe, N.J. (1989). Erythema multiforme-like eruptions associated with etretinate therapy. *Clin. Exp. Dermatol.* 14:230–232.
89. McIvor, A. (1992). Fatal toxic epidermal necrolysis associated with etretinate. *Br. Med. J.* 304:548.
90. Carmichael, A.J., and Paul, C.J. (1989). Reversible gynaeocomastia associated with etretinate. *Br. J. Dermatol.* 120:317.
91. Reynolds, O.D. (1991). Erectile dysfunction in etretinate treatment. *Arch. Dermatol.* 127:425–426.
92. Hammer, C.J., Carter, C., and Hanifin, J.M. (1993). Peripheral neuropathy during etretinate therapy for psoriasis. *J. Am. Acad. Dermatol.* 28:272–273.
93. Bonnetblanc, J.M., Hugon, J., and Dumas, M. (1983). Intracranial hypertension with etretinate. *Lancet* 2:974.
94. Viraben, R., Mathieu, C., and Fontan, B. (1985). Benign intracranial hypertension during etretinate therapy for mycosis fungoides. *J. Am. Acad. Dermatol.* 13: 515–517.
95. Naldi, L., Rozzoni, M., Finazzi, G., Pini, P., Marchesi, L., and Cainelli, T. (1991). Etretinate therapy and thrombocytopenia. *Br. J. Dermatol.* 124:395.
96. Cribier, B., Welsch, M., and Heid, E. (1992). Renal impairment probably induced by etretinate. *Dermatology* 185:266–268.
97. Roujeau, J.-C., Guillaume, J.-C., Fabre, J.-P., Penso, D., Fléchet, M.-L., and Girre, J.-P. (1990). Toxic epidermal necrolysis (Lyell syndrome). Incidence and drug etiology in France 1981–1985. *Arch. Dermatol.* 126:37–42.
98. Gollnick, H.P.M. (1995). Advances in retinoid therapy of psoriasis. *Retinoids Today Tomorrow* 39:3–12.
99. Ali Shah, I., Whiting, P.H., Omar, G., Ormerod, A.D., and Burke, M.D. (1993). The effects of retinoids and terbinafine on the human hepatic microsomal metabolism of cyclosporine. *Br. J. Dermatol.* 129:395–398.

56

Clinical Pharmacology of Acitretin

Ulf W. Wiegand and R. C. Chou
F. Hoffmann-La Roche, Ltd., Basel, Switzerland

Alice Bendix Gottlieb
University of Medicine and Dentistry of New Jersey—Robert Wood Johnson Medical School, New Brunswick, New Jersey

The efficacy of etretinate (Tegison, Tigason) in the treatment of psoriasis and disorders of keratinization has been well documented in therapeutic trials as well as in clinical practice (Gollnick et al. 1985; Ellis et al. 1987; Landow, 1988). A major disadvantage for the treatment of female patients, however, is the drug's teratogenicity. This effect is compounded by the high lipophilicity of etretinate resulting in its storage in adipose tissue. The slow release of etretinate from these tissues leads to a long elimination half-life with a mean value of approximately 120 days (Massarella et al. 1985). This pharmacokinetic characteristic necessitates a long period of posttherapy contraception. Outside the United States, this is set at 2 years, but the Food and Drug Administration has considered the contraception period as "undetermined" since the time of the drug's approval in 1986.

In vitro experiments have shown that etretinate (ethylester) is not the pharmacologically active molecule; the free acid acitretin (Soriatane, Neotigason) instead is responsible for the therapeutic effect (Bollag, 1985). The patient's body hydrolyzes etretinate to acitretin, which is then reversibly interconverted (Geiger and Brindley, 1988) to *cis*-acitretin, as shown in Figure 1. Acitretin was therefore developed to replace etretinate. Acitretin shows the same clinical efficacy as etretinate, but has more favorable pharmacokinetic properties, especially a much shorter half-life, and, as a consequence, it reduces the teratogenic risk for female patients of childbearing potential.

COMPARISON OF ACITRETIN AND ETRETINATE PHARMACOKINETICS

An understanding of the chemical properties of acitretin and etretinate will help to explain the data presented later in this chapter. At physiological pH etretinate is an uncharged, highly lipophilic molecule. This causes it to be retained in human adipose tissue, resulting in extensive accumulation during chronic administration. In contrast, acitretin carries a carboxylic acid group, which is negatively charged at normal blood pH. Consequently, acitretin is approximately 50 times more hydrophilic/water soluble than etretinate, so it does not accumulate in adipose tissue and is cleared much more rapidly from the body of a psoriatic patient.

It is important to understand that acitretin and its main metabolite, *cis*-acitretin, show different rates of elimination when acitretin is administered directly compared to the situation where they are formed as metabolites of etretinate. In the latter case the elimination does not depend on their own pharmacokinetic

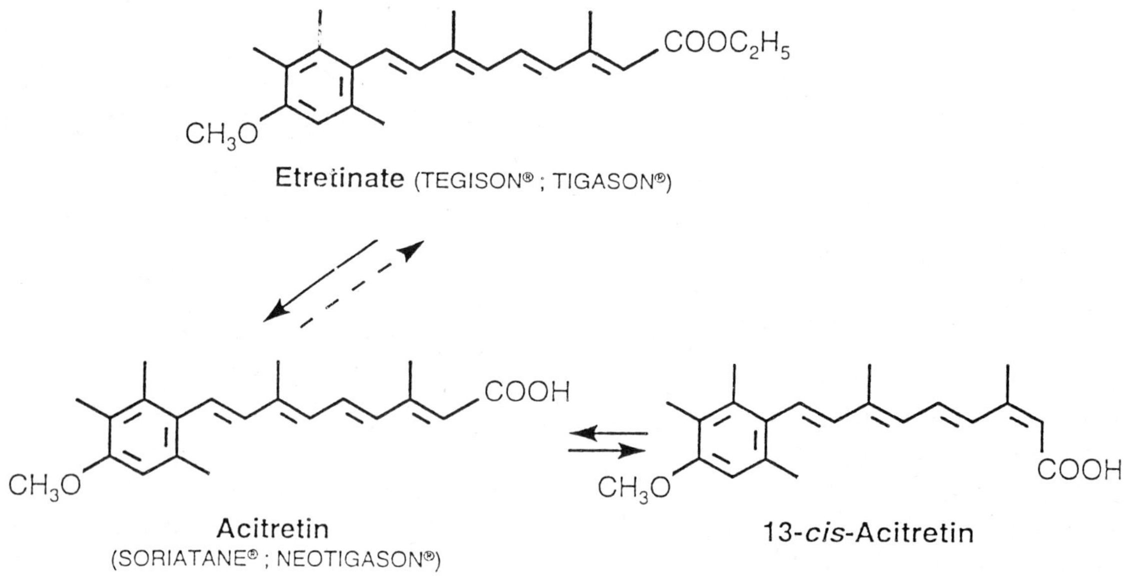

Figure 1 Chemical structure of acitretin and its metabolites.

properties but on the rate of their formation from etretinate. This characteristic is called "formation-rate limited elimination" and helps to explain differences in the kinetic behavior of acitretin. When acitretin and *cis*-acitretin are present in the body of a patient together with etretinate, their concentrations decline at the same rate as etretinate and they will continue to be detected in plasma for as long as etretinate is present in adipose tissue (although in this situation etretinate itself may not necessarily be detectable in plasma). Therefore, both compounds appear to show half-lives that are similar to those of etretinate. This phenomenon is often misunderstood when apparent long half-lives for acitretin and *cis*-acitretin are reported in psoriatic patients treated with acitretin.

It is generally accepted that the pharmacological effect is more closely related to the free drug concentrations in plasma than to the total concentrations. Therefore, studies to determine the extent of plasma protein binding of drugs and to estimate the free concentrations are important. Because of their high lipophilicity both acitretin and etretinate are very highly protein bound, with the values for both drugs exceeding 99%. Here again, there are differences between the binding proteins and the dispositions of acitretin and etretinate. Albumin is the major binding protein for acitretin and only 4–5% of the drug in plasma is associated with lipoproteins (Urien et al., 1992). In contrast, because of the difference in lipophilicity etretinate binds extensively to lipoproteins (Urien et al., 1992). The high protein binding of acitretin and *cis*-acitretin explains why neither compound is removed from the systemic circulation by hemodialysis (Stuck et al., 1989).

For quantification of acitretin and *cis*-acitretin in plasma samples the early methods involved an extraction with organic solvents followed by high-performance liquid chromatography using a normal phase column with UV detection at 360 nm and a quantification limit of 4 ng/ml (Paravicini and Busslinger, 1983). Later a very different chromatographic method was developed using a solid-phase extraction method and a reversed-phase column. This has a quantification limit of 0.3 ng/ml (Wyss and Bucheli, 1988, 1992; Wyss, 1990).

SINGLE-DOSE PHARMACOKINETIC STUDIES IN HUMAN VOLUNTEERS: CHARACTERIZATION OF ABSORPTION AND EFFECT OF FOOD

Figure 2 compares the mean plasma concentrations in healthy subjects after a single 50-mg oral dose of acitretin under fed and fasted conditions with a 19-mg intravenous infusion. After all three doses, the acitretin plasma concentrations decline rapidly and fall below the quantification limit of the chromatographic assay within 12–14 hr after drug administration. This prevents an accurate determination of the terminal

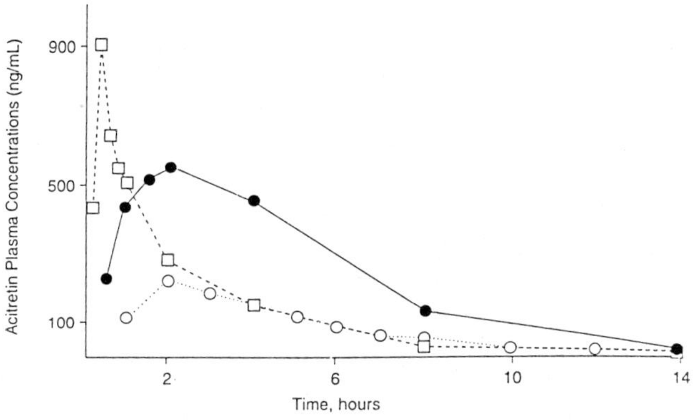

Figure 2 Mean acitretin plama concentrations in 12 healthy subjects after a 20-min intravenous infusion (19 mg; □) and single oral doses (50 mg) with (●) or without (○) food. (Adapted from Wiegand et al., 1993.)

elimination half-life for acitretin after single doses. For oral administration, the absorption of acitretin is variable and increases when it is given with food (McNamara et al., 1988). Although the mean maximum plasma concentrations (C_{max}) 400–500 ng/ml are reached with 4 hr of a single 50-mg oral dose when the drug is given with food, the intersubject variability is high, with the individual peak concentrations ranging from 87 to 1358 ng/ml. Under fed conditions the absolute bioavailability of acitretin is approximately 60%, with a range of 36–95% (Brindley et al., 1989).

In oral dose-ranging studies with 25–100 mg of acitretin (McNamara et al., 1988), the extent of absorption, assessed by C_{max} and area under the plasma concentration-time curve, increases in a dose-proportional manner when doses up to 100 mg are given with food. By contrast, the peak concentrations under fasted conditions are lower and less than dose-proportional for doses of more than 50 mg. For doses of 25 and 50 mg, coadministration with food produces an approximately twofold increase in oral absorption of acitretin, but at the higher doses of 75 and 100 mg, the oral absorption is three- to fourfold greater when the drug is given with food. It is therefore important that patients take acitretin together with food, since it improves oral bioavailability, reduces intersubject variability in absorption, and produces dose-proportional increases in plasma concentrations up to doses of 100 mg.

Several metabolites of acitretin are also present in plasma. *Cis*-acitretin (Fig. 1) is the main one. Three other minor metabolites (*cis*-acitretin with a hydroxy group and two compounds with shortened side chains and reduced double bonds) have also been detected. No unchanged acitretin is excreted in urine, but several metabolites have been observed. These are present in both the free and conjugated form of the products with the side chain shortened (Roche, data on file).

Following intravenous administration of radiolabeled acitretin, 53% of the dose was recovered in urine and 40% in feces with a total recovery of 93%. The high fecal recovery suggests biliary excretion. After oral administration only 83% of the radioactivity was recovered, 47% of which was excreted in the feces and 37% in urine (Brindley, 1989).

MULTIPLE-DOSE PHARMACOKINETIC STUDIES IN HUMAN VOLUNTEERS

Since patients whose psoriasis is being treated with acitretin need to take the drug for long periods, the multiple-dose pharmacokinetics of acitretin and *cis*-acitretin are very important. To characterize the pharmacokinetics under these conditions and to determine the elimination half-lives of acitretin and its main metabolite, 15 healthy volunteers were treated for 21 days with daily oral doses of 50 mg acitretin (Wiegand et al., 1993). Within 2–3 weeks of repeated oral dosing to these volunteers, steady-state conditions were reached for both acitretin and *cis*-acitretin, where plasma concentrations no longer increase with further dosing. As shown in Figure 3, the mean acitretin plasma concentrations at steady state are not much greater than those observed after the first dose. Mean concentrations of *cis*-acitretin are, however, considerably higher than those following single doses and reached levels of approximately 200–300 ng/mL. These higher steady-state concentrations are consistent with a longer half-life and lower clearance for *cis*-acitretin as compared to acitretin and should not be interpreted as an unusual accumulation of *cis*-acitretin. Since the pharmacological effect of *cis*-acitretin is much lower than that of acitretin, these higher systemic concentrations make only a limited contribution to the overall pharmacological effect. Since the metabolite *cis*-acitretin is interconverted back to form acitretin, during regular therapy acitretin tends to exhibit the longer half-life of its metabolite. However, this does not lead to significantly higher acitretin concentrations at steady state.

During daily oral administration of acitretin, the plasma concentrations of acitretin and *cis*-acitretin tend to be higher in elderly than young subjects, sug-

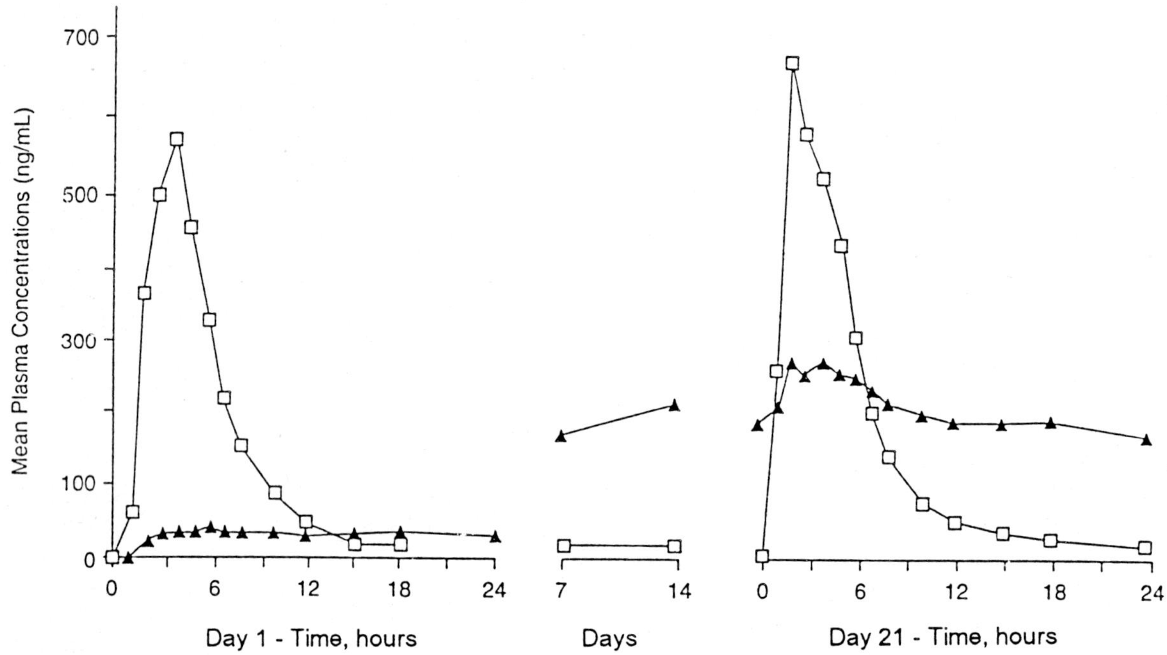

Figure 3 Mean plasma concentrations of acitretin (□) and cis-acitretin (▲) in 15 healthy subjects following daily oral doses of 50 mg for 21 days. Data on days 7 and 14 are mean trough concentrations. (Adapted from Wiegand et al., 1993.)

gesting a difference in clearance and/or volume of distribution in the elderly (Brindley, 1989). Contrary to these results, no significant correlation was found between acitretin steady-state plasma concentration and age (Gollnick et al., 1988). Since the therapeutic dose is based on efficacy and tolerability rather than plasma concentration of acitretin, no specific adjustment of the dose is suggested for elderly patients. In addition, no significant correlation was observed between acitretin plasma concentrations at steady state and body weight of patients during long-term therapy. A dose adjustment for body weight, which has been used for etretinate, is therefore not recommended for treatment with acitretin (Gollnick et al., 1988). The recommended treatment for each patient is to initiate therapy with a dose of 25–30 mg and then titrate up or down to the most effective dose with minimal adverse events.

MULTIPLE-DOSE PHARMACOKINETIC STUDIES IN PSORIATIC PATIENTS

The most extensive pharmacokinetic data on acitretin in patients were obtained from a multicenter trial conducted in several European hospitals during long-term treatment with acitretin (Wiegand and Jensen, 1991; Weigand et al., 1993, 1996b). This study reproduced the therapeutic situation in psoriatic patients by providing participants with a 2- to 12-month treatment period with individually optimized doses that ranged from 10 to 50 mg/day, which were optimized for clinical efficacy and adverse events. During that treatment, the trough plasma concentrations at steady state of acitretin and *cis*-acitretin varied considerably between individual patients. Typical plasma concentrations in the 65 patients evaluated so far were 10–30 ng/ml for acitretin and 50–70 ng/ml for *cis*-acitretin. The data for one individual patient are shown in Figure 4. Contrary to the experience with etretinate, no accumulation of acitretin was observed; thus the trough plasma concentrations during the first and last 4 weeks of treatment did not differ, despite a treatment period of more than 3 months. Identical information was obtained in all other patients of this trial even with treatment periods up to several months.

The higher steady-state concentrations of *cis*-acitretin are consistent with its longer half-life. Half-lives for acitretin and *cis*-acitretin in the patients evaluated so far were similar to those observed in other studies and ranged from 30 to 96 hr for acitretin and from 40 to 132 hr for *cis*-acitretin. These values were derived only from patients who did not show any etre-

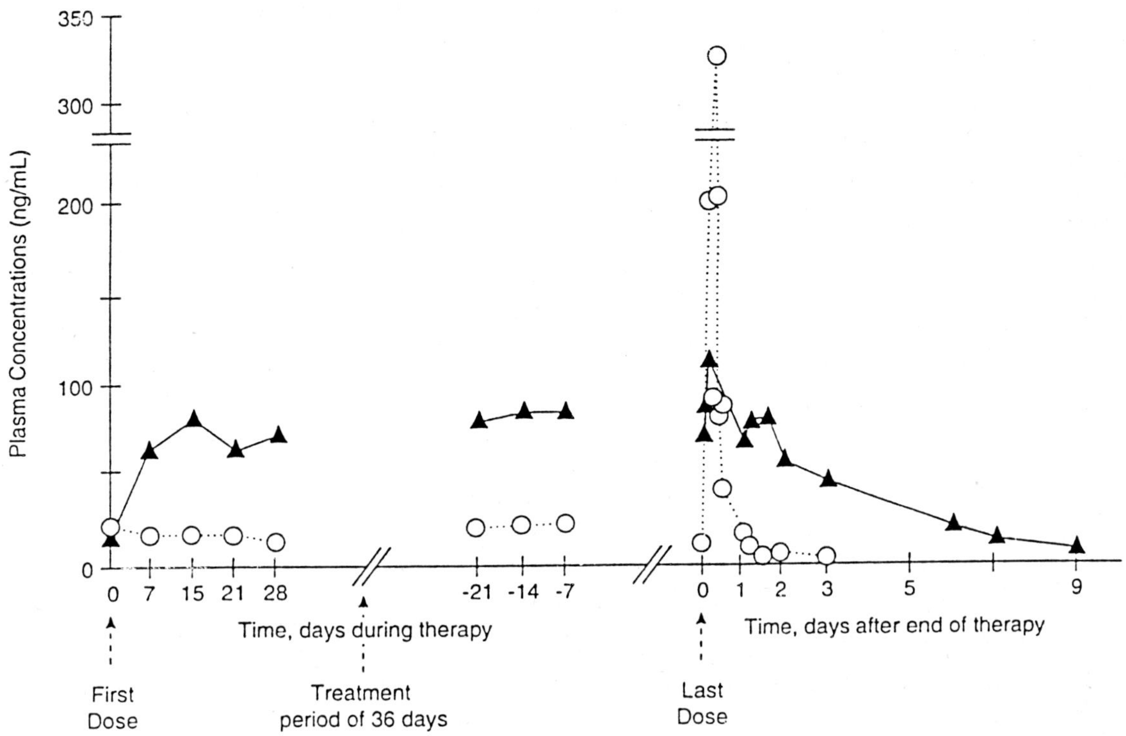

Figure 4 Plasma trough concentrations of acitretin (○) and *cis*-acitretin (▲) in an individual patient during daily 30-mg oral acitretin doses and plasma concentrations after the last dose. −21 represents 21 days before the last dose. (Adapted from Wiegand et al., 1993.)

tinate concentrations in their plasma. The half-lives in a few patients exceeded those observed in healthy volunteers, but these have to be considered with special caution, since it cannot be excluded that the longer half-lives of both compounds may be caused by etretinate residuals from a previous treatment in their adipose tissues. Although etretinate concentrations may not be detectable in their plasma, it would still influence the half-lives, due to formation-rate-limited generation of acitretin and *cis*-acitretin (cf. above).

Besides generating pharmacokinetic data for acitretin and *cis*-acitretin in a larger number of patients, this trial was important, since an interaction between acitretin and ethanol was documented for the first time. This will be discussed in more detail in the next section.

In another study retinoid plasma concentrations at steady state were compared in 43 patients treated with a daily dose of either 50 mg etretinate or acitretin (Gollnick et al., 1988). Etretinate concentrations during therapy with Tegison showed a mean value of about 100 ng/ml. Acitretin concentrations observed in these same patients were approximately 45 ng/ml. By contrast, the plasma concentrations of acitretin in patients treated with 50 mg/day of Soriatane were only approximately 20 ng/ml (Fig. 5). This is again consistent with the theory of formation-rate-limited elimination kinetics (cf. above). These differences in plasma concentrations continue to exist also after the end of treatment. Three weeks after the last Tegison dose, acitretin and etretinate showed mean plasma concentrations of 15 and 40 ng/ml, respectively, whereas after treatment with Soriatane, under identical conditions, acitretin and *cis*-acitretin were not detectable in plasma.

Additional pharmacokinetic data, which agree with the information reported above, were reported by Larsen in psoriatic patients (Larsen et al., 1991, 1993. The interested reader is referred to the original publications.

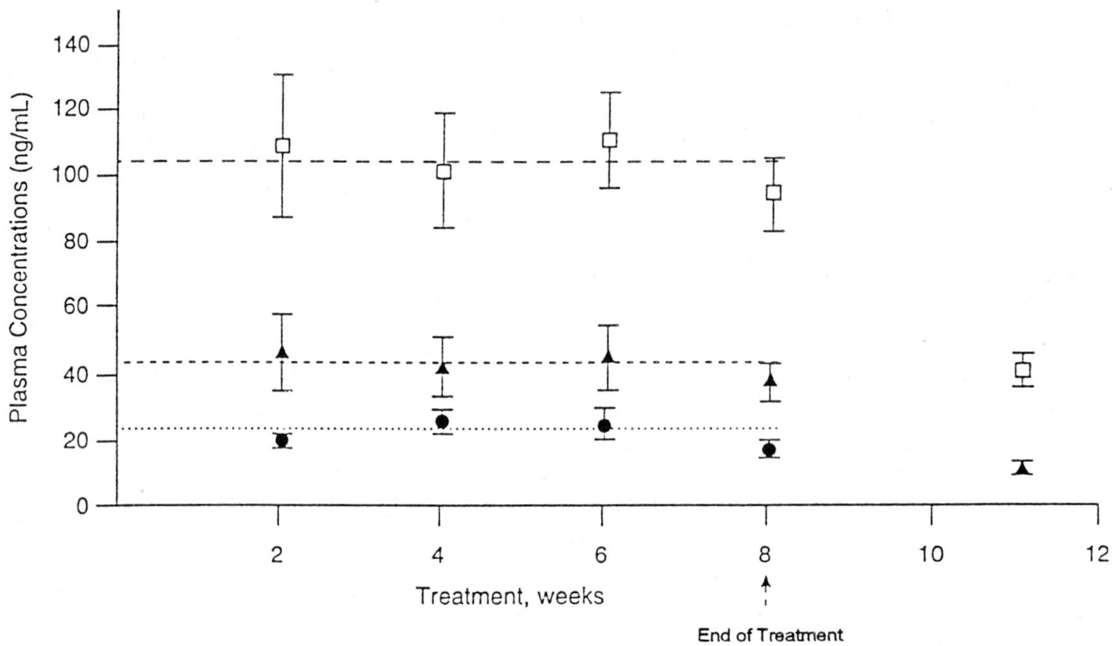

Figure 5 Trough retinoid plasma concentrations during treatment: (□) etretinate during treatment with Tegison; (▲) acitretin during treatment with Tegison; (●) acitretin during treatment with Soriatane.

FORMATION OF ETRETINATE BY AN INTERACTION BETWEEN ACITRETIN AND ETHANOL

A possible formation of etretinate from acitretin in patients treated with acitretin was considered from the beginning of the acitretin development, since from a theoretical perspective this reaction could not be totally excluded (see Fig. 1). However, the screening of many blood samples gave no indication that etretinate was present in plasma of volunteers or patients during acitretin treatment. Furthermore, based on thermodynamic principles, experts in the field of drug metabolism were convinced that etretinate would not easily be formed in acitretin-treated patients, and, if formed, would immediately be hydrolyzed back to acitretin.

Despite these predictions, an European Pharmacokinetic Multicenter Trial provided the first indications that etretinate might be formed as a metabolite of acitretin. This was conducted in 10 centers from seven European countries (Belgium, Denmark, Finland, France, Germany, United Kingdom, Sweden). The results from Finland and the United Kingdom provided the first hints of a potential formation of etretinate in some patients. The samples from this study were analyzed by the new analytical technology, which could measure lower concentrations of the retinoid in plasma (Wiegand and Jensen, 1991). In this study a considerable number of patients showed either traces or measurable etretinate plasma concentrations up to 48 ng/ml. The incidence of etretinate detection as well as the concentrations measured varied considerably not only between individual centers but also during the treatment period in the same patient. Etretinate plasma concentrations were again detected when patients were rechallenged with acitretin. (Wiegand et al., 1996b). An immediate and thorough follow-up excluded the possibility of artifact formation, but this did not prove that etretinate was formed in these patients.

In vitro experiments with isolated liver microsomes and studies in animals were needed to show without doubt that this unexpected metabolic reaction can indeed occur and that etretinate can be found from acitretin in the presence of ethanol (Chou et al., 1991, 1992).

A further study in human volunteers confirmed that this novel metabolic pathway can occur in humans (Jensen et al., 1992; Wiegand et al., 1996d). In this trial 10 healthy male subjects received a single oral dose of 100 mg acitretin with or without concomitant ethanol consumption (five drinks of vodka: approx. 100 ml ethanol = approx. 1.4 ethanol/kg bw) in a randomized crossover design. Etretinate plasma concentrations were observed in all subjects following intake of acitretin together with ethanol, whereas etretinate was not detectable when acitretin was administered alone. The mean peak etretinate concentration in plasma was 59 ng/ml (Fig. 6). Furthermore, the etretinate concentrations appeared to depend on the ethanol concentrations. Under the extreme conditions of this trial, the etretinate plasma concentrations observed would be equivalent to a 5-mg oral dose of etretinate as compared to a normal therapeutic dose of 50 mg.

The European Multicenter Trial cannot provide reliable conclusions regarding either the representative concentrations of etretinate in plasma or the number of patients who form etretinate when treated with acitretin. Although the inclusion of previous etretinate users was minimized, it cannot be totally excluded. Furthermore, patients were not advised to abstain from alcohol consumption and patients were not asked during the trial about their alcohol consumption. A common experience of many dermatologists who treat psoriatic patients is that quantification of their alcohol intake is very difficult. A retrospective evaluation of a patient's alcohol consumption is even less reliable and does not provide an appropriate basis to define the relationship between alcohol intake and etretinate formation.

Based on the data of the European Multicenter Trial, our laboratory ran a study with very strict inclusion criteria to ensure that there was no contamination by a previous etretinate treatment. A total of 36 acitretin-treated female patients (mean age: 31.9

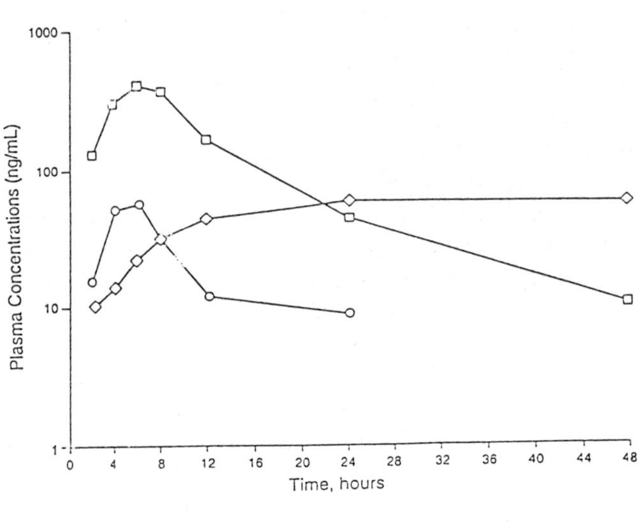

Figure 6 Plasma concentrations of acitretin (□), *cis*-acitretin (◇), and etretinate (○) in healthy volunteers following ingestion of acitretin with ethanol.

years) suffering from psoriasis or other disorders of keratinization were enrolled into an open study (Wiegand et al., 1995). Their intake of alcohol was variable. Thirteen patients were on therapy and 23 had discontinued acitretin treatment for 6 weeks to 60 months before entering the main study. Etretinate plasma concentrations were observed in three of 36 patients during acitretin treatment (0.30–4.7 ng/ml) and in two patients after the end of therapy (0.303 ng/ml and 5.28 ng/ml). By comparison etretinate plasma concentrations in patients treated with doses of 50 mg Tegison had values of approximately 100 ng/ml (Gollnick et al., 1988). In the second part of this study etretinate concentrations in plasma and subcutis of all etretinate-positive patients are being followed to determine the elimination of etretinate from the subcutis. This trial portion is still ongoing and final results are expected soon.

The main objective of this trial was to quantify etretinate concentrations in plasma and subcutis in the most important patient population: women of childbearing age. Etretinate was observed in plasma and subcutis (see next section) of all 36 patients. All have reported a consumption of alcohol, but one etretinate-positive patient claimed that she did not consume alcohol during the study. The concentrations showed some variation, which is not surprising considering the differences in duration of treatment, doses, and alcohol consumption. Most importantly, etretinate subcutis concentrations were substantially lower than those in etretinate-treated patients (898 ng/g vs. 16,000 ng/g), which is a relevant aspect in evaluation of safety concerns.

Also in this trial, a trend was observed linking higher alcohol consumption with higher etretinate concentrations. Even though these results are scientifically plausible, a real quantitative correlation would require a sophisticated psychology-based questionnaire.

Two centers (Larsen et al., 1993; Lambert et al., 1994) that participated in the European Multicenter Trial also published their results, which are in good agreement with the data presented here. As to their reports of a correlation between alcohol consumption and etretinate formation, the caveats mentioned above are still relevant.

Following the initial publication of etretinate formation in acitretin-treated patients (Wiegand and Jensen, 1991), several authors have reported similar results showing that etretinate can be formed when patients are being treated with acitretin, that etretinate also distributes into adipose tissue including subcutaneous fat, and that alcohol consumption influences the amounts of etretinate formed (Larsen et al., 1993; Laugier et al., 1994; Meyer et al., 1993; Sturkenboom et al., 1994).

The mechanism of the interaction between acitretin and ethanol is being elucidated at the moment by Dr. Knights from Flinders University in cooperation with our laboratories. The initial in vitro experiments provided evidence that enzymatic processes in the liver are responsible for etretinate formation (Chou et al., 1992; Schmitt-Hoffmann et al., 1995). In vitro, formation of the ethyl ester of acitretin was not solely dependent on ethanol, but several cofactors were required. The dependence on coenzyme A (CoA) and ATP suggested the participation of fatty-acid CoA ligases in the process. Formation of CoA conjugates by fatty-acid CoA ligases is not unusual for retinoids (Miller and DeLuca, 1985). Indeed, recent studies by Knights (personal communication) provide evidence that acitretin interacts with the microsomal long-chain fatty-acid ligase (palmitoyl-CoA ligase). Inhibition of palmitoyl-CoA formation was observed with human liver microsomal preparations at 500 ng/ml acitretin. Interestingly, in some human liver samples acitretin activated palmitoyl-CoA formation in the presence of low concentrations of palmitoic acid. This suggested that acitretin interacts not solely at the catalytic site of palmitoyl-CoA ligase, as expected for a substrate of the enzyme, but at the same time is capable of acting as a regulatory activator, which might explain the occasional elevation of blood lipids (see below).

The critical question from these findings is: what are the therapeutic consequences of the acitretin-ethanol interaction for female patients of childbearing potential? It is obvious that the initial short posttherapy contraceptive period of 2 months for acitretin has to be modified for safety reasons. Roche recommends a 2-year posttherapy contraceptive period for acitretin based on the pharmacokinetic parameters of acitretin and etretinate observed in clinical trials and on previous safety experience with etretinate. The pharmacokinetic advantages of acitretin as compared to etretinate still hold true for all female patients who strictly avoid alcohol consumption during treatment and for 2 months after the end of therapy. The treating dermatologist should stress the importance of strict alcohol abstinence, both during therapy and for 2 months after the end of treatment. We have no evidence at the moment that etretinate is formed if alcohol abstinence is strictly observed. For the dermatologist this information is particularly relevant for cases of unwanted pregnancies after the end of treatment.

RETINOID TISSUE CONCENTRATIONS

As outlined above, the main difference in the pharmacokinetics of acitretin and etretinate relates to the storage of etretinate in adipose tissue, due to its higher lipophilicity. Earlier studies by Vahlquist have documented that concentrations up to 16,000 ng/g were observed in subcutaneous fat and kidney patients treated with etretinate (Vahlquist et al., 1986). Following the documentation of an ethanol-acitretin interaction in psoriatic patients (see above), there is no doubt that etretinate would also be stored in adipose tissue when it is formed in a patient as a metabolite of acitretin. It is therefore important to have quantitative information on etretinate concentrations in plasma and subcutaneous fat of female patients treated with acitretin.

As mentioned in the preceding section, a study was conducted in 36 female patients treated with acitretin (Wiegand et al., 1995). As expected, etretinate was detected in several patients, in both their plasma and subcutaneous fat. Eleven of 36 patients showed measurable etretinate concentrations in subcutis and/or plasma whereas the other 25 patients showed traces of etretinate in subcutis. Measurable etretinate concentrations in the subcutis of these 11 patients ranged from 8.6 to 897.6 ng/g and they were, as expected from the high lipophilicity, higher than their plasma concentrations. For several of the patients, different etretinate concentrations were found in biopsies of involved and uninvolved skin. Based on previous experience, it is obvious that the relationship between etretinate concentrations in plasma and in subcutis is complex. To develop a model that will help predict etretinate concentrations in subcutis from those in plasma and vice versa, additional data in patients are now being generated. This information will be helpful in assessing the teratogenic risk for the outcome of an unforeseen pregnancy.

Some investigators suggest that the length of the contraceptive period should be based on the subcutis concentrations (Sturkenboom et al., 1994). Considering basic pharmacokinetic principles regarding the distribution of lipophilic compounds, as well as the anatomy of the subcutis and its blood circulation, a compound such as etretinate will accumulate rather extensively in subcutis. The diffusion of etretinate back into the systemic circulation is then very slow, as evidenced by the long elimination half-life. So far it has not been possible to influence this process, to generate a rapid release of etretinate back into the systemic circulation, by displacing etretinate from its binding sites in adipose tissue. Since etretinate stored in the subcutis or adipose tissue of a female patient can reach the embryo only via the systemic circulation and the placenta, measuring etretinate subcutis concentrations is of limited value in assessing the risk of a teratogenic outcome for a pregnancy in an individual patient. However, according to our experience with several cases from European countries during many years, retinoid plasma concentrations can help to estimate the risk for a potential birth defect in an unforeseen pregnancy. Since threshold plasma concentrations for the teratogenic effect of acitretin and etretinate are not known, however, a decision to continue or discontinue a pregnancy should not be based only on retinoid concentrations in plasma. Other considerations, such as the personal and medical situation of the individual patient, are an absolute requirement for assessing the potential risk.

Besides distribution into adipose tissues, concentrations of acitretin, *cis*-acitretin, and etretinate in placental tissue have been investigated using the isolated perfused human term placenta as a model (Dittrich et al., 1993, 1994). This information is very important to estimate the relationship between retinoid concentrations in plasma and the embryo. We were able to show that the factors that influence the concentration in placental tissue are: the lipophilicity of the retinoid, its protein binding, and the concentration of plasma proteins. Concentrations of *cis*-acitretin in placental tissue were lower than in perfusate. By contrast, at physiological albumin concentrations acitretin showed slightly higher concentrations in placental tissue than in perfusate. Furthermore, decreasing perfusate albumin concentrations increases the acitretin tissue concentrations. For therapeutic etretinate concentrations, however, the levels in placental tissue were approximately 160% higher than those of the perfusate. These results strongly suggest that the placenta may be able to bind the retinoids and thus protect the embryo. We are now developing a mathematical model for the transport of acitretin and etretinate from the mother to her embryo. This will also include information from appropriate animal species. It may enable us to predict retinoid concentrations in the embryo based on those in maternal plasma and will help to improve the assessment of the teratogenic risk in a female patient who unintentionally becomes pregnant.

A study from our laboratory evaluated the distribution of acitretin and *cis*-acitretin into the skin of psoriatic patients following not only systemic but also topical administration (Wiegand et al., 1996c). During 2 weeks of topical application in 32 patients, acitretin had no pronounced therapeutic effect, whereas oral treatment for the same time period markedly reduced the psoriatic lesions. During topical treatment, the concentrations of acitretin in skin (stratum corneum, epidermis, dermis, and subcutis) were very variable and ranged from 1405 ng/g to 131,025 ng/g. Plasma concentrations ranged from nondetectable to 8 ng/ml. *Cis*-acitretin concentrations were much lower in both skin and plasma while etretinate was not observed at all. During oral treatment, acitretin concentrations in skin were much lower than those during topical administration; they were highest in stratum corneum with a range of 121–1585 ng/g, while the plasma concentrations were similar to those observed in earlier studies with the same oral doses.

Larsen and colleagues also reported acitretin skin concentrations but only following systemic treatment with acitretin (Larsen et al., 1992). Steady-state concentrations of acitretin in epidermis were 17 ± 9 ng/g and were reached within 1 month of therapy. These authors found a correlation between the individual plasma trough value and the epidermal concentration of acitretin after 1 month of therapy. At the end of this treatment, the acitretin concentrations in subcutis varied from 15 to 1437 ng/g, but they had decreased to nondetectable concentrations in nine of 12 patients within 1 month.

Meyer et al. also evaluated the acitretin concentrations in skin during treatment with oral doses of 25 mg acitretin (Meyer et al., 1993). After 2 months of treatment they observed an increase from nondetectable concentrations to 28 ± 16 ng/g in 11 patients. Concentrations in subcutaneous fat exceeded those in skin with values of 98 ± 71 ng/g at 5 hr after dosing. In two patients, additional samples were taken 3 days after the end of therapy. Acitretin concentrations had decreased to nonquantifiable concentrations, confirming that acitretin is not stored in subcutaneous fat.

SAFETY ASPECTS OF ACITRETIN IN HEALTHY VOLUNTEERS AND PSORIATIC PATIENTS

Safety parameters such as vital signs [blood pressure, heart rate, and electrocardiogram (ECG)] and laboratory parameters (hematology, blood chemistry, creatinine clearance, and urinalysis) were assessed in all studies from our laboratories involving healthy volunteers.

There was no evidence in healthy volunteers of an effect of acitretin on blood pressure, heart rate, or

ECG or a change in creatinine clearance. Furthermore, no clinically relevant changes in hematological parameters were observed in any study with healthy volunteers. In vitro experiments with acitretin also did not induce aggregation of human blood platelets or show anticoagulating properties. Triglyceride and cholesterol levels in serum increased in several volunteers. These observations are in line with findings in patients during therapy with acitretin. Besides changes in lipid parameters there were no clinically significant changes in blood chemistry values that could be related to acitretin treatment. Urinalysis showed no pathological changes. Skin alterations, i.e., dry skin, cheilitis, desquamation, were common adverse events during multiple oral administration of acitretin. Several subjects also reported a headache even after the first dose of the drug.

During the course of therapy none of six male patients who were treated with acitretin for several months exhibited significant changes in andrological parameters (spermiogram, spermiocytogram) or sex hormones (FSH, LH, testosterone, DHEA). Despite the relative small number of patients, these results suggest that acitretin does not affect andrological parameters (Geiger and Czarnetzki, 1988).

Hypervitaminosis A–type signs and symptoms, specifically those affecting the mucocutaneous system, were observed in the majority of patients treated with acitretin (Geiger and Czarnetzki, 1988). These accounted for approximately 90% of the total number of adverse events in all patients. The most commonly reported adverse events were dry lips/cheilitis with an incidence of approximately 80%. Other adverse events affecting the mucocutaneous system with an incidence of greater than 15% were dryness of mouth, nose, or skin, conjunctivitis, scaling alopecia, and pruritus. Adverse events affecting other body systems were reported in less than 1% of the patients studied (Geiger and Czarnetzki, 1988). More detailed data on a large number of patients are reported in another chapter.

CONCLUSIONS

The clinical pharmacology of acitretin contributes important information for the therapeutic use of this drug in psoriatic patients. Four important features determine its pharmacokinetics: its comparatively low lipophilicity at physiological pH, the effect of food on its oral bioavailability, the reversible interconversion to *cis*-acitretin, and its interaction with ethanol. Owing to its negatively charged acid group, acitretin is not stored in adipose tissue even after multiple oral doses. It therefore has a much shorter terminal elimination half-life with a mean value of about 2 days in psoriatic patients as compared to 120 days reported for etretinate. Even at steady state, when it has assumed the half-life of its 13-*cis* metabolite, it is still only about 2 days. This property also considerably reduces the exposure of patients to this retinoid as seen for the low plasma concentrations of about 20 ng/ml. Acitretin absorption is improved by simultaneous ingestion with food. An interaction of acitretin with ethanol leads to formation of etretinate, which is stored in adipose tissue. Roche therefore recommends a 2-year contraceptive period for acitretin based on the pharmacokinetic parameters of acitretin and etretinate observed in clinical trials and on previous safety experience with etretinate. The pharmacokinetic advantage of acitretin as compared to etretinate still exists for all female patients who strictly avoid alcohol consumption during the course of treatment and for 2 months after the end of therapy. The treating dermatologist should thoroughly inform his female patients about the importance of strictly abstaining from alcohol.

REFERENCES

Bollag, W. (1985). New retinoids with potential use in humans. In *Retinoids*: *New Trends in Research and Therapy*. J.-H. Saurate (Ed.), Karger, Basel, 1985, pp. 274–288.

Brindley, C.J., (1989). Overview of recent clinical pharmacokinetic studies with acitretin (Ro 10-1670, Etretin). *Dermatologia* 178:79–87.

Brindley, C.J., Dubach, U.C., and Forgo, I. (1989). Absolute bioavailability of acitretin (Ro 10-1670). In *Pharmacology of Retinoids in the Skin*. U. Reichert and B. Shroot (Eds.), Karger, Basel, 1989, pp. 207–210.

Chou, R.C., Wyss, R., Huselton, C.A., and Wiegand, U.W. (1991). A newly discovered xenobiotic metabolic pathway: ethyl ester formation. *Life Sci*. 49:PL169–PL172.

Chou, R.C., Wyss, R., Huselton, C.A., and Wiegand, U.W. (1992). A potentially new metabolic pathway: ethyl esterification of acitretin. *Xenobiotica* 22:993–1002.

Dittrich, S., Malek, A., Schröder, S., Schneider, H., Nöschel, H., and Wiegand, U.W. (1993). Transport and tissue uptake of retinoids in the human placenta: acitretin. 5th Meeting of the European Placenta Group, September 8–11, Manchester, UK.

Dittrich, S., Schröder, S., Malek, A., Nöschel, H., Schneider, H., and Wiegand, U.-W. (1994). Transport and tissue uptake of retinoids in the human placenta: etretinate. 1st International Meeting of World Placenta Associations, October 24–28, Sydney, Australia.

Ellis, C.N., Voorhees, J.J., and Arbor, A. (1987). Continuing medical education (therapy). Etretinate therapy. *J. Am. Acad. Dermatol.* 16:267–291.

Geiger, J.M., and Brindley, C.J. (1988). *Cis-trans* Interconversion of acitretin in man. *Skin Pharmacol* 1:230–236.

Geiger, J.M., and Czarnetzki, B.M. (1988). Acitretin (Ro 10-1670, Etretin): overall evaluation of clinical studies. *Dermatologica* 176:182–190.

Gollnick, H., and Orfanos, C.E. (1985). Clinical efficacy of retinoids: European experience. In *Psoriasis*. H.H. Roenigk, Jr., and H.I. Maibach (Eds.), New York, Marcel Dekker, pp. 597–613.

Gollnick, H., Bauer, R., Brindley, C., Orfanos, C.E., Plewig, G., Wokalek, H., and Hoting, E. (1988). Acitretin versus etretinate in psoriasis. *J. Am. Acad. Dermatol.* 19: 458–469.

Jensen, B.K., Chaws, C.L., and Huselton, C.A. (1992). Clinical evidence that acitretin is esterified to etretinate when administered with ethanol. *FASEB J.* 6:A1570 (abstract no. 3669).

Lambert, W.E., Meyer, E., De Leenheer, A.P., De Bersaques, J., and Kint, A.H. (1994). Pharmacokinetics of acitretin. *Acta Derm. Venereol (Stockh.)* Suppl. (1994). 186: 122–123.

Landow, R.K. (1988). Etretinate. A clinician's view. *Dermatol. Clin.* 6:553–560.

Larsen, F.G., Jakobsen, P., Eriksen, H., Grønhøj, J., Kragballe, K., and Nielsen-Kudsk, F. (1991). The pharmacokinetics of acitretin and its 13-*cis*-metabolite in psoriatic patients. *J. Clin. Pharmacol.* 31:477–483.

Larsen, F.G., Vahlquist, C., Andersson, E., Torma, H., Kragballe, K., and Vahlquist, A. (1992). Oral acitretin in psoriasis: drug and vitamin A concentrations in skin and adipose tissue. *Acta Derm. Venereol. (Stockh.)* 72:84–88.

Larsen, F.G., Jakobsen, P., Knudsen, J., Weismann, K., Kragballe, K., and Nielsen-Kudsk, F. (1993). Conversion of acitretin to etretinate in psoriatic patients is influenced by ethanol. *J. Invest. Dermatol.* 100:623–627.

Laugier, J.P., de Sousa, G., Bun, H., Geiger, J.M., Surber, C., and Rahmani, R. (1994). Acitretin biotransformation into etretinate: role of ethanol on in vitro hepatic metabolism. *Dermatology* 188:122–125.

Massarella, J., Vane, F., Buggé, C., Rodriguez, L., Cunningham, W.J., Franz, T., and Colburn, W. (1985). Etretinate kinetics during chronic dosing in severe psoriasis. *Clin. Pharmacol. Ther.* 37:439–446.

McNamara, P.J., Jewell, R.C., Jensen, B.K., and Brindley, C.J. (1988). Food increases the bioavailability of acitretin. *J. Clin. Pharmacol.* 28:1051–1055.

Meyer, E., De Bersaques, J., Lambert, W.E., De Leenheer, A.P., and Kint, A.H. (1993). Skin, adipose tissue and plasma levels of acitretin with rare occurrence of esterified acitretin during long-term treatment. *Acta Derm. Venereol. (Stockh.)* 73:113–115.

Miller, D.A., and DeLuca, H.F. (1985). Activation of retinoic acid by coenzyme A for the formation of ethyl retinoate. *Proc. Natl. Acad. Sci. U.S.A.* 82:6419–6422.

Paravicini, U., and Busslinger, A. (1983). Determination of etretinate and its main metabolite in human plasma using normal-phase high-performance liquid chromatography. *J. Chrom. Biomed. Appl.* 276:359–366.

Schmitt-Hoffmann, A.H., Dittrich, S., Saulnier, E., Schenk, P., and Chou, R.C. (1995). Mechanistic studies on the ethyl-esterification of acitretin by human liver preparations in vitro. *Life Sci.* 57:407–412.

Stuck, A.E., Brindley, C.J., Bussinger, A., and Frey, F.J. (1989). Pharmacokinetics of acitretin and its 13-*cis* metabolite in patients of haemodialysis. *Br. J. Clin. Pharmacol.* 27:301–304.

Sturkenboom, M.C.J.M., De Jong-Van den Berg, L.T.W., Van Voorst-Vader, P.C., Cornel, M.C., Stricker, B.H.C.H., and Wesseling, H. (1994). Inability to detect plasma etretinate and acitretin is a poor predictor of the absence of these teratogens in tissue after stopping acitretin treatment. *Br. J. Clin. Pharmacol.* 38:229–235.

Urien, S., Claudepierre, P., Meyer, J., Brandt, R., and Tillement, J.P. (1992). Comparative binding of etretinate and acitretin to plasma proteins and erythrocytes. *Biochem. Pharmacol.* 44:1891–1893.

Vahlquist, A., Rollman, O., and Pihl-Lundin, I. (1986). Tissue distribution of aromatic retinoid (etretinate) in three autopsy cases: drug accumulation in adrenals and fat. *Acta Derm. Venerol (Stockh.)* 66:431–434.

Wiegand, U.W., and Jensen, B.K. (1991). Pharmacokinetics of acitretin in humans. In *Retinoids: 10 Years On*. J.-H. Saurat (Ed.), Karger, Basel, pp. 192–203.

Wiegand, U.W., Busslinger, A.A., Chou, R.C., and Jensen, B.J., (1993). The pharmacokinetics of acitretin in humans: an update. In *Retinoids. Progress in Research and Clinical Applications*. M.A. Livrea and L. Packer (Eds.), Dekker, New York, pp. 617–628.

Wiegand, U.W., De Bersaques, J., de la Brassinne, M., Hoenigsmann, H., Jansen, C., Marks, R., Salomon, D., and Wyss, R. (1995). Etretinate concentrations in plasma and subcutis of acitretin-treated female patients. *J. Eur. Acad. Dermatol. Venerol.* 5(Suppl. 1):S86.

Wiegand, U.W., Cunliffe, W., Wyss, R., and Crevoisier, C. (1996a). Treatment of female patients with isotretinoin: what is the safe post-therapy contraceptive period? Clinical Dermatology 2000 International Congress, May 28–31, Vancouver, Canada, p. 107 (abstract).

Wiegand, U.W., et al. (1996b). Pharmacokinetics of acitretin and its metabolites in psoriatic patients. (Manuscript submitted.)

Wiegand, U.W., et al. (1996c). Retinoid concentrations in plasma and skin during topical and systemic administration of acitretin. (Manuscript in preparation.)

Wiegand, U.W., et al. (1996d). Formation of etretinate in healthy subjects by an acitretin-ethanol interaction. (Manuscript in preparation.)

Wyss, R. (1990). Determination of retinoids in plasma by high-performance liquid chromatography and automated column switching. *Methods Enzymol.* 189:146–155.

Wyss, R., and Bucheli, F. (1988). Quantitative analysis of retinoids in biological fluids by high performance liquid chromatography using column switching. II. Simultaneous determination of etretinate, acitretin, and 13-*cis*-acitretin in plasma. *J. Chromatogr.* 431:297–307.

Wyss, R., and Bucheli, F. (1992). Use of direct injection precolumn techniques for the high-performance liquid chromatographic determination of the retinoids acitretin and 13-*cis* acitretin in plasma. *J. Chromatogr.* 593: 55–62.

57

Retinoid Combinations

Charles Grupper and Bruno Berretti
Polyclinique d'Aubervilliers, Aubervilliers, France

The introduction of synthetic retinoids has led to a veritable revolution in treatment for disorders of keratinization. Treatment of severe psoriasis constitutes their major clinical application. Two agents, etretinate and isotretinoin (1–10), have been the subject of studies worldwide, and their active antipsoriatic role is well-established. A third formulation, arotinoid (RO 13-6298) is currently undergoing preliminary studies the results of which, while limited, appear promising (11,12).

In the treatment of psoriasis, retinoids are administered by a systemic route; efficacy and side effects have been evaluated after use of these agents alone or in conjunction with other conventional antipsoriatic treatments.

The treatment of psoriasis with a *single-agent protocol* involving retinoids has shown that:

- These molecules have a clear and significant antipsoriatic activity.
- Etretinate shows better efficacy and safety than isotretinoin (3a).
- Required dosage and percentage clearing are a function of the clinical type of psoriasis treated.
- Side effects are numerous, of variable severity, sometimes troublesome, and dosage-related.

Studies on the treatment of psoriasis by retinoids with a single-agent protocol are discussed in another chapter.

Combinations of retinoids, essentially etretinate, with other conventional antipsoriatic treatments have opened up new treatment alternatives. Such a combination (in particular, etretinate plus PUVA: REPUVA) results in a more potent and rapid antipsoriatic efficacy. This combination allows a major reduction in both retinoid dosage and dosage of other conventional agents. Overall safety is thus better.

Since 1977, we have used etretinate (and occasionally isotretinoin) in our department, alone or in combination with other therapeutic modalities, for the treatment of more than 2000 psoriasis patients; our follow-up ranges from 6 months to 5 years. In light of this wide experience in a single center, as well as the principal published studies, we summarize therapeutic results with retinoid combinations in treatment of severe refractory psoriasis.

The retinoids (almost exclusively etretinate) have been used in conjunction with anthralin, local corticosteroids, ultraviolet B, and PUVA. These methods have been discussed in detail in other chapters; we will consider their combinations with retinoids. We will not discuss etretinate combined with antimitotic agents, since clinical experience is limited; however, in special cases, such as generalized von Zumbusch pustular psoriasis, this combination may be effective.

ANTHRALIN AND ETRETINATE

Anthralin and related agents have been part of the antipsoriatic arsenal for more than a century and concurrent administration of etretinate yields a more favorable response in patients resistant to anthralin alone (13). This combination has been suggested as a first line of treatment in severe psoriasis.

Our experience with use of anthralin alone for treatment of psoriasis has been disappointing. The classic preparations, undeniably efficacious, are poorly accepted by patients today. New low-strength regimens (14) were virtually inefficacious. Preparations with a high concentration (1–3%) in vehicles, which in theoretical and animal experimental study are highly efficacious when applied for short periods of time (short contact therapy) (15,16), have appeared to us to be of limited efficacy. Thus, we discontinued the use of anthralin-etretinate, preferring combinations of retinoids with other antipsoriatic treatments which, in our experience, are more effective and better tolerated.

ETRETINATE AND LOCAL CORTICOSTEROIDS

Several open and double-blind trials have shown the efficacy of these combinations (17–19). Addition of a fluorocorticosteroid (diflucortolone valerate, 0.1%, triamcinolone acetonide 0.1%, betamethasone valerate 0.1%) reduces the daily etretinate dosage required for clearing (0.50 mg/kg). A follow-up study over 3 years (20) showed that this combination allows 43% of patients to remain cleared, with a daily 0.3-mg/kg maintenance dose of etretinate, and a weekly local triamcinolone dose of 20 g.

In our study, we have combined active topical antipsoriatic agents (salicylic acid + tar + corticosteroids) (21,22) with the various systemic treatments (PUVA, etretinate). We maintain that this approach, which hypothetically increased the frequency of relapses at the end of systemic treatment, allows a reduction in clearing parameters for the principal treatment. Results are more rapid, and patient comfort is improved.

ETRETINATE AND UVB

This combination allows an improved *percentage of clearing* compared with results for the two methods used separately (23–30). It has allowed treatment of patients unresponsive to other regimens (UVB, PUVA, etretinate), with a reduction in parameters for clearing and good general tolerance. This method has the same efficacy as PUVA or REPUVA, but it eliminates the psoralen administration, and thus any possibility of chronic side effects theoretically attributable to prolonged and repeated PUVA.

We will not discuss possible long-term side effects of chronic UVB therapy, with or without etretinate. Frequency, clinical profile, and time to onset of such effects are currently as difficult to determine as those attributed to PUVA under the same conditions. We simply summarize our own clinical experience. We have treated more than 50 patients with severe or refractory psoriasis with UVB, alone or in combination with etretinate. Methods were entirely analogous with those described elsewhere (25–27); however, results have been disappointing by comparison with other studies, as well as by comparison with our usual results with PUVA and especially REPUVA. Only 40% of patients showed clearing; the time to clearing was always greater than that with REPUVA, and we were particularly impressed by the high frequency (50%) of phototoxic effects, which frequently required withdrawal of treatment. Thus, we currently reserve UVB for particularly REPUVA-resistant cases, in which addition of UVB frequently can be a deciding factor since it provides clearing without a major increase in total energy amount and psoralen or etretinate dosage.

ETRETINATE AND PUVA

Efficacy of PUVA for treatment of severe psoriasis has been fully demonstrated. Since 1978 (31), various protocols for combination etretinate-PUVA (REPUVA) treatment have been studied, the most efficacious being administration of etretinate alone at a mean dosage of 1 mg/kg per day for the first 2 weeks of treatment, followed by combination of PUVA, using the standard schedules. The daily etretinate dosage can then be reduced; however, administration is continued until complete clearing occurs. PUVA alone can then be continued as a maintenance treatment (22,31,45). This REPUVA combination shows major advantages compared with standard PUVA. Indeed, REPUVA allows salvage of failures of standard PUVA therapy, as well as clearing of clinical forms known to be highly refractory to treatment. Furthermore, there is a reduction in all parameters of PUVA required for clearing: decrease in the number of sessions and duration of treatment, and a reduction in the total accumulated UVA dosage. Finally, daily etretinate dosage can be rapidly diminished, thus decreasing the intensity and frequency of side effects associated with this drug. The most severe of the chronic side effects purportedly associated with PUVA is the possible development of

Table 1 Clearing Phase: Comparison of Four Protocols

	PUVA-5 MOP	PUVA-8 MOP	RE-PUVA-5 MOP	RE-PUVA-8 MOP
Number of patients	198	1259	75	80
(% of clearing) (>75%)	(82.3)	(84)	(92.1)	(82.4)
Number of treatments	20.6	21.1	13.6	16.5
Total dose (J/cm^2)	148	131	78.1	97.6
Duration (days)	44.6	42	25.9	38.9

Source: Ref. 53.

Table 2 Comparative Tolerance and Side Effects: PUVA-5-MOP vs. PUVA-8-MOP

	Number of patients (%)	No side effects	Nausea	Sunburn	Pruritus	Headache
PUVA-5-MOP	198 (100)	167 (84.34)	2 (1.01)	26 (13.18)	8 (4.04)	2 (1.01)
PUVA-8-MOP	1199 (100)	619 (51.62)	133 (11.09)	282 (23.51)	134 (11.17)	13 (1.08)

Source: Ref. 53.

chronic actinic cutaneous modifications, particularly skin cancers. While no convincing demonstration of this claim has yet been offered, if it does indeed occur, it would clearly be a function of total energy dosage received by the patient. Any modification in PUVA technique allowing reduction in such dosage would constitute a major improvement. Considering, moreover, that etretinate has been used with some degree of success for the prevention and treatment of precancerous states and cutaneous epitheliomas (46–48), REPUVA can be considered as a treatment of choice for severe, extensive, and resistant psoriasis with less risk of skin cancer.

Since 1976, we have used PUVA and REPUVA to treat more than 4000 patients with severe and extensive psoriasis, involving more than 40% of the total body surface (this minimum extension was imposed by the French Social Insurance Administration). In light of this wide monocentric experience, we would discuss the characteristics of this veritable therapeutic revolution in further detail (21,22,49–53). Our initial protocol for PUVA therapy was that proposed by the originators of the method. Subsequently, we have modified the technique in two important ways:

1. Replacement of the classic 8-methoxypsoralen (8-MOP) with 5-methoxypsoralen (5-MOP), which has the same efficacy but better safety (5-MOP-PUVA).
2. Combination of etretinate-PUVA (REPUVA). Initially, REPUVA was performed with 8-MOP (8-MOP-REPUVA), but this psoralen was replaced with 5-MOP (5-MOP-REPUVA).

In Tables 1 and 2, we summarize clinical results and safety at the end of the clearing phase. Table 3 summarizes results of our follow-up.

Replacement of 8-MOP with 5-MOP brought about an unarguable improvement in safety of standard PUVA, significantly reducing acute clinical side effects (nausea, pruritus, phototoxic accidents). Long-

Table 3 6-Month Follow-Up Study: Proportion of Patients Still Clear of Disease

Treatment	Number of patients clear	%
PUVA (8- and 5-MOP)	204/648	32
RE-PUVA (8- and 5-MOP)	53/67	61

Source: Ref. 53.

Figure 1 Infantile psoriasis of the face before and after REPUVA-5-MOP.

Figure 2 Infantile psoriasis of the palms before and after REPUVA-5-MOP.

Figure 3 Acral pustular psoriasis did not respond to 8-MOP-PUVA. Treatment with REPUVA-5-MOP was successful.

Figure 4 Pustular palmar psoriasis before and after REPUVA-5-MOP.

Figure 5 Pustular palmar psoriasis with arthritis before and after REPUVA-5-MOP.

Figure 6 Plantar hyperkeratotic psoriasis that did not respond to 8-MOP-PUVA was successfully treated with REPUVA-5-MOP.

term side effects still need to be evaluated. 8-MOP-REPUVA is superior to standard 8-MOP-PUVA. 8-MOP-REPUVA yielded a reduction in all clearing parameters, allowing salvage of patients whose disease was refractory to classic PUVA, as well as those with the most refractory clinical forms of psoriasis. Nevertheless, we are less optimistic about the performance of 8-MOP-REPUVA than certain authors who reported a reduction of more than 50% in all 8-MOP-PUVA parameters with this combination (32–38). Similarly, the purported action of 8-MOP-REPUVA on lesions of the scalp or psoriatic rheumatism (36–38) was virtually without basis in our patients. The only factor which we found to have some influence upon painful rheumatic symptomatology was the heat given off by whole-body PUVA units.

Substitution of 5-MOP for 8-MOP in the REPUVA combination yielded optimal results: a further reduction in the PUVA parameters, improvement in percentage clearing, and improvement in acute clinical tolerance. Our follow-up study, still somewhat limited, appears to show a supplementary advantage of REPUVA by comparison with PUVA; there is a reduction in frequency of recurrences 6 months after the end of all treatments. Thus, we consider that REPUVA, particularly 5-MOP-REPUVA, is the treatment of choice for severe and refractory psoriasis when constituting a major handicap to the patient. [Figures 1–12 (Color Plates 1–4)].

Some workers (54) have recommended an isotretinoin-PUVA combination, reporting results with this method in 30 psoriatic patients. They maintain that results were comparable with those obtained using etretinate-PUVA combination. By comparison with etretinate-PUVA, isotretinoin-PUVA would present the advantage of being more readily prescribed to women of child-bearing age. Both drugs are teratogenic, and require that patients use strict contraceptive protection. Isotretinoin is more rapidly eliminated than etretinate; duration of contraception would be shorter with the former. Other studies are needed to confirm initial observations.

Unlike the combination of etretinate with PUVA, isotretinoin PUVA has not yielded any improvement over standard PUVA in our preliminary studies. Isotretinoin has given rise to far more side effects than

Figure 7 Generalized pustular psoriasis before and after REPUVA-5-MOP.

Figure 8 Generalized pustular psoriasis before and after REPUVA-5-MOP.

Figure 9 Generalized plaque-type psoriasis before and after REPUVA-5-MOP.

Figure 10 Generalized plaque-type psoriasis before and after REPUVA-5-MOP.

Figure 11 Infantile erythrodermic psoriasis did not respond to 8-MOP-PUVA. Before and after successful treatment with REPUVA-5-MOP.

Figure 12 Psoriatic erythroderma was unresponsive to 8-MOP-PUVA and methotrexate treatment. Successful lasting treatment was effected with REPUVA-5-MOP.

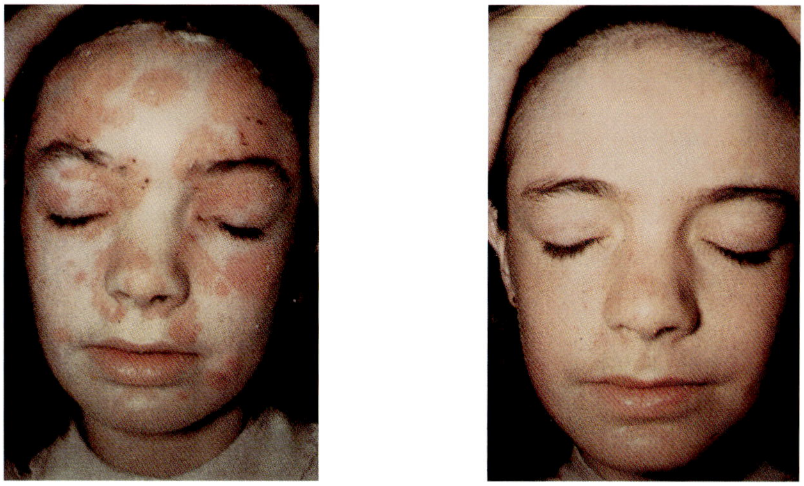

Figure 1

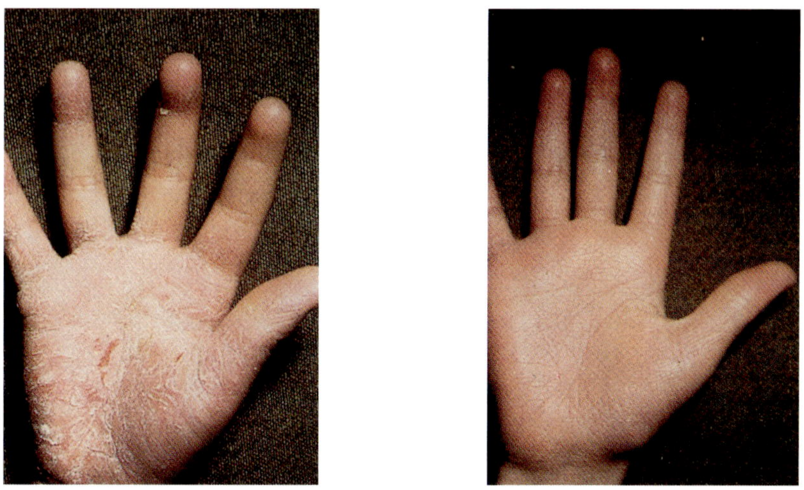

Figure 2

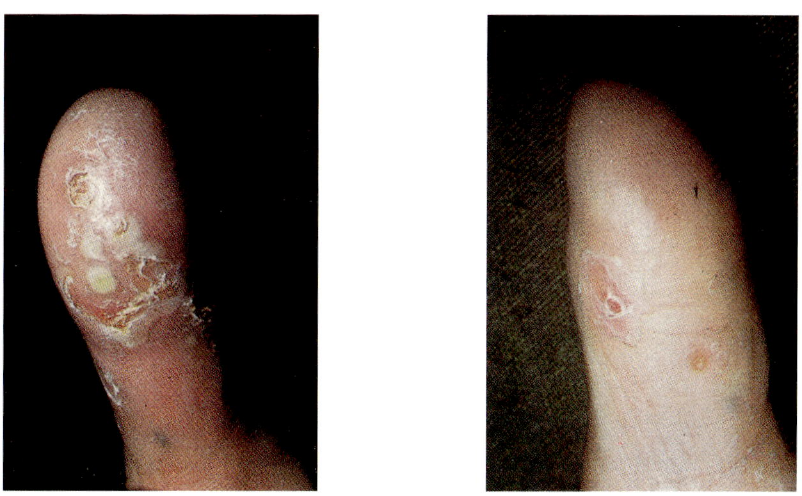

Figure 3

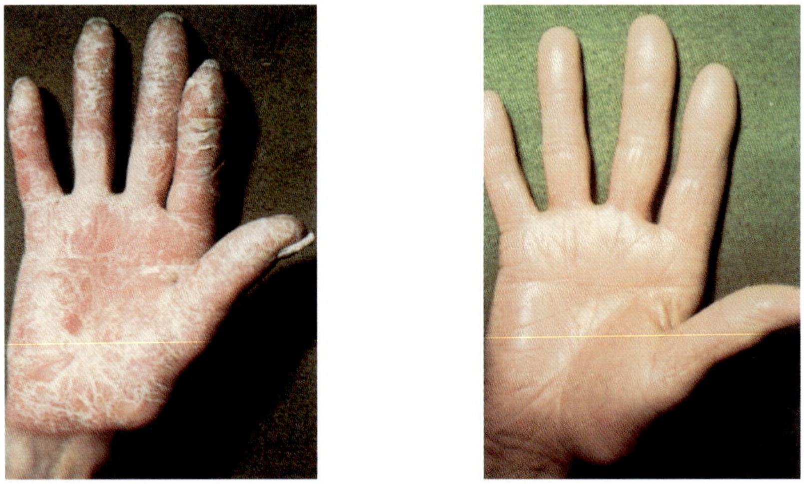

Figure 4

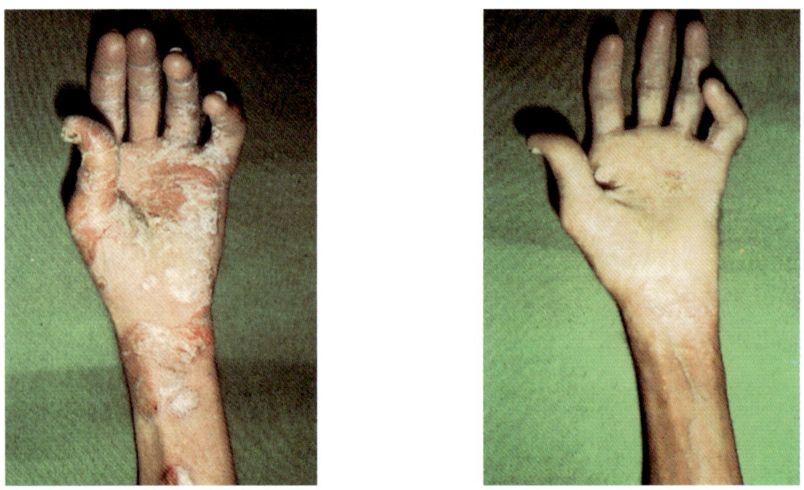

Figure 5

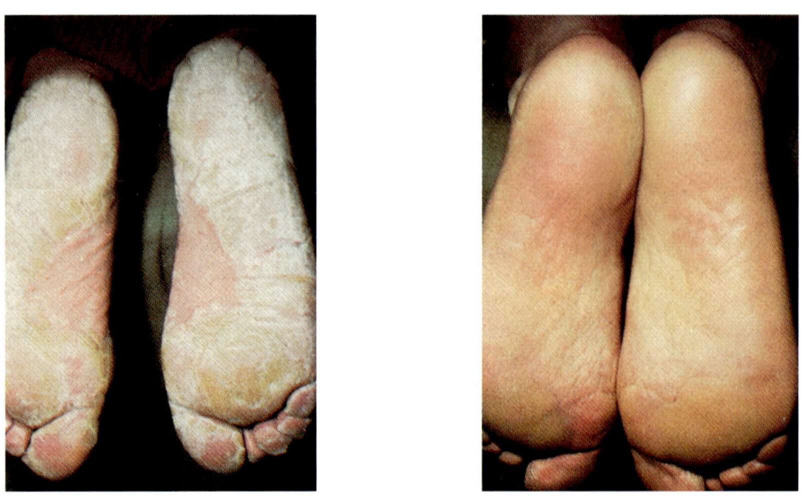

Figure 6

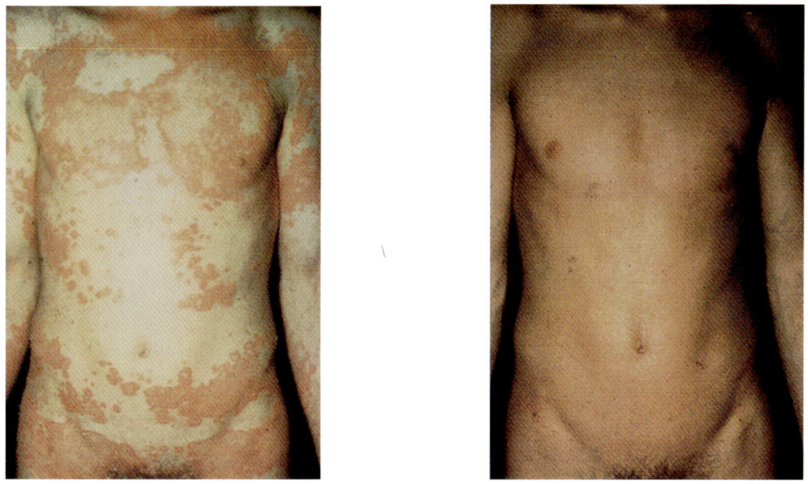

Figure 7

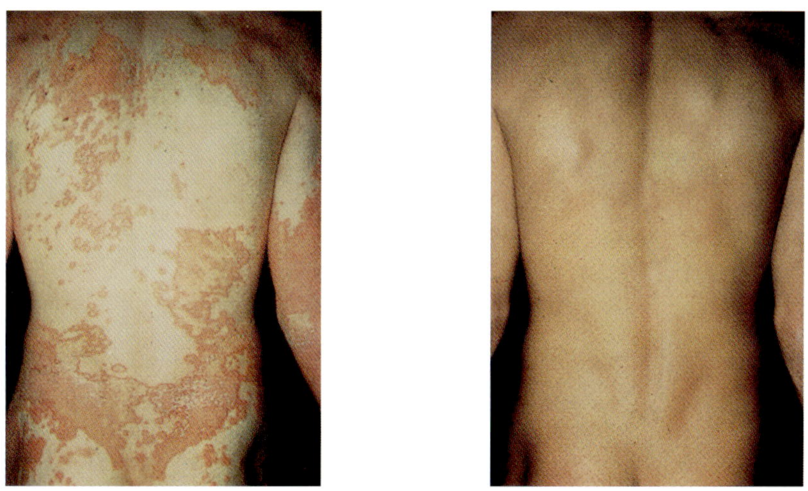

Figure 8

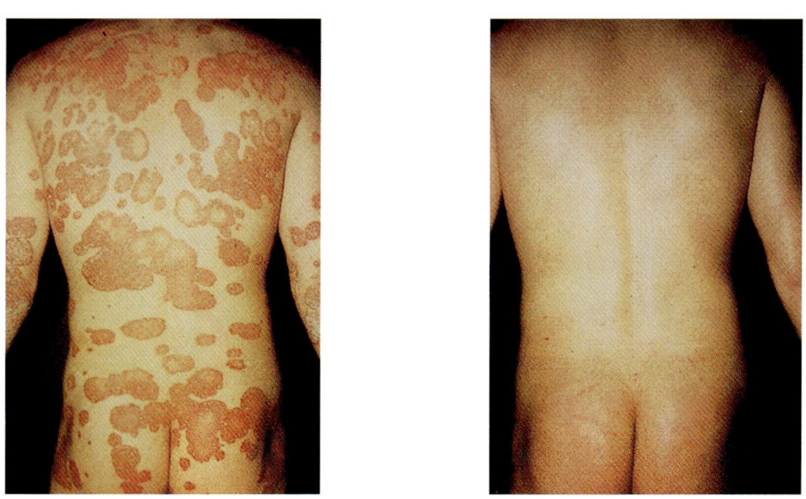

Figure 9

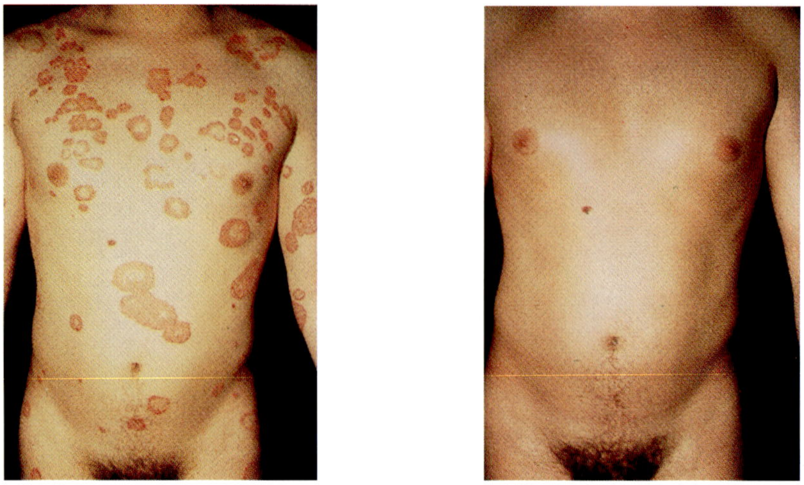

Figure 10

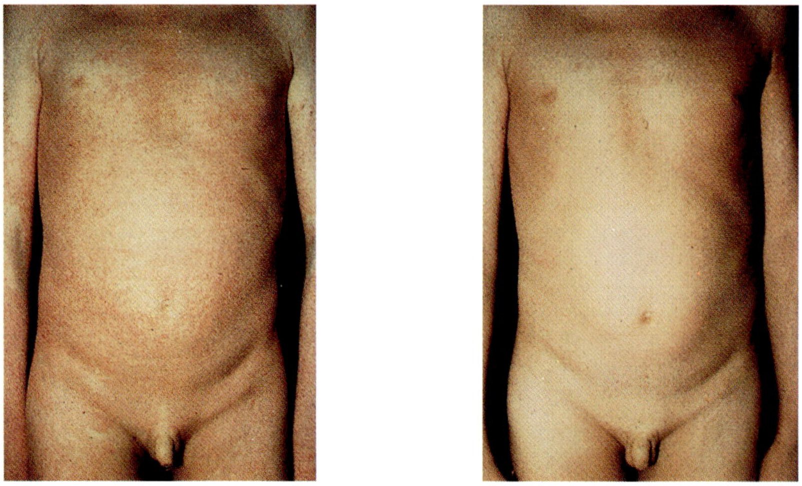

Figure 11

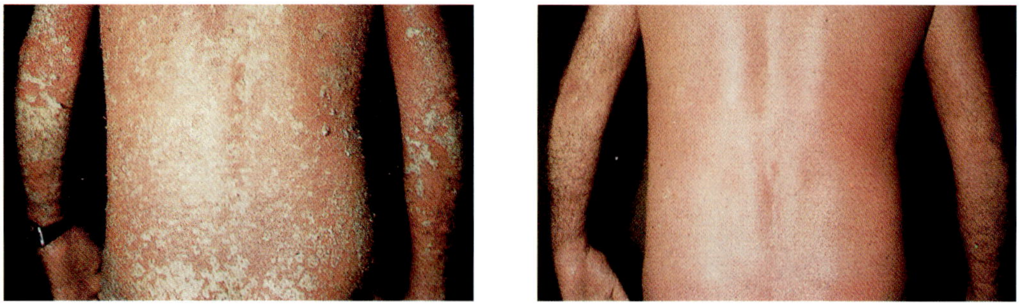

Figure 12

etretinate when conditions and dosage of the two agents were identical: severity of some side effects has required withdrawal of isotretinoin before clearing in several patients who were subsequently able to continue treatment with the classic etretinate-PUVA modality.

CONCLUSIONS

Combination of retinoids with certain conventional antipsoriatic techniques has allowed a further improvement of psoriasis while reducing the severity of side effects. Best results have been obtained with REPUVA. In our opinion, this combination therapy represents the fastest, most efficacious, best-tolerated, and most acceptable treatment. It is by far the safest approach to treating psoriasis that produces major disability. Development of new retinoids with better risk-to-benefit ratios, as well as more effective and better-tolerated photosensitizing agents, such as 5-MOP, will allow a further improvement in this method which already constitutes a revolution in psoriasis treatment.

REFERENCES

1. Orfanos, C.E. (1980). Oral retinoids—present status. *Br. J. Dermatol.* 103:473–481.
2. Editorial (1980). Retinoids in dermatology. *Arch. Dermatol.* 116:283–284.
3. Elias, P.M., and Williams, M.L. (1981). Retinoids, cancer, and the skin. *Arch. Dermatol.* 117:160–180.

3a. Orfanos, C.E., Braun-Falco, O., Farber, E.M., Grupper, C., Polano, M.K., and Schuppli, R. (Eds.). (1981). *Retinoids—Advances in Basic Research and Therapy.* Springer-Verlag, New York.

4. Peck, G.L. (1981). Retinoids in clinical dermatology. In *Progress in Diseases of the Skin.* R. Fleischmajer (Ed.). Grune & Stratton, New York, pp. 227–269.
5. Voorhees, J.J., and Orfanos, C.E. (1981). Oral retinoids. *Arch. Dermatol.* 117:418–421.
6. Pochi, P.E. (1982). Oral retinoids in dermatology. *Arch. Dermatol.* 118:57–61.
7. Orfanos, C.E. (1982). Oral retinoids in psoriasis: current clinical experiences and possible mechanisms of action. In *Psoriasis Proceedings of the 3rd International Symposium.* E.M. Farber and A.J. Cox (Eds.). Grune & Stratton, New York, pp. 197–209.
8. Ehmann, C.W., and Voorhees, J.J. (1982). International studies of the efficacy of etretinate in the treatment of psoriasis. *J. Am. Acad. Dermatol.* 6(part 2):692–696.
9. Dicken, C.H., and Connolly, S.M. (1982). Systemic retinoids in dermatology. *Mayo Clin. Proc.* 57:51–57.
10. Farber, E.M., Abel, E.A., and Charuworn, A. (1983). Recent advances in the treatment of psoriasis. *J. Am. Acad. Dermatol.* 8:311–321.
11. Tsambaos, D., and Orfanos, C.E. (1982). Arotinoid: a new potent oral retinoid: preliminary results. In *Psoriasis, Proceedings of the IIIrd International Symposium.* E.M. Farber and A.J. Cox (Eds.). Grune & Stratton, New York, pp. 519–524.
12. Fritsch, P.O. Rauschmeier, W., and Neuhofer, J. (1984). Response of psoriasis-arthropathy to arotinoid (Ro 139-6239). In *Retinoid Therapy.* W.J. Cunliffe and A. Miller (Eds.). MTP Press Limited, Lancaster, pp. 329–333.
13. Orfanos, C.E., and Runne, U. (1976). Systemic use of a new retinoid with and without local dithranol treatment in generalized psoriasis. *Br. J. Dermatol.* 95: 101–103.
14. Montes, L.F., Wilborn, W.H., and Brody, I. (1979). Low strength anthralin in psoriasis. *J. Cutan. Pathol.* 6:445–456.
15. Schaefer, H., Farber, E.M., Goldberg, L., and Schalla, W. (1980). Limited application period for anthralin in psoriasis and clinical efficacy. *Br. J. Dermatol.* 102: 571–573.
16. Runne, U., and Kunze, J. (1982). Short duration ("minute") therapy with dithranol for psoriasis—a new out patient regimen. *Br. J. Dermatol.* 106:135–139.
17. Van Der Rhee, H.J., Tijssen, J., Herrmann, W., Watermann, A., and Polano, M. (1980). Combined treatment of psoriasis with a new aromatic retinoid (Tigason) in low dosage orally and triamcinolone acetonide cream topically: a DB trial. *Br. J. Dermatol.* 102:203–211.
18. Binazzi, M., De Panfilis, G., and Landi, G. (1981). A controlled multicentric study of Ro 10-9359 in association with topical corticosteroid therapy in psoriasis. *Drugs. Exp. Clin. Res.* 7(1):57–64.
19. Christiansen, J.V., Holm, P., Moeller, R., Reymann, F., and Schmidt, H. (1982). Etretinate (Tigason) and Betamethasone valerate (Celeston valerate). *Dermatologica* 165(3):204–207.
20. Polano, M.K., and Van Der Rhée, H.J. (1982). A 3 year follow-up of psoriasis patients treated with low dosages of etretinate orally and corticosteroids topically. *Acta Dermatovenereol.* 62:361–364.
21. Berretti, B., and Grupper, C. (1979). La photochimiothérapie orale du psoriasis (Puva), résultats récents. *Gaz. Méd. Fr.* 83:3191–3197.
22. Grupper, C., Berretti B., and Forlot, P. (1980). Bilan de la puvathérapie à propos de 1400 cas personnels. Résultats et progrès récents en 1979. In *Ichtyoses, peau et lumière.* Proceedings of 16th Congrès de l'Association des Dermatologistes de Lángue Française. SAGEP, Tunis.
23. Beierdörfer, H., and Wiskemann, A. (1978). Combined therapy of psoriasis with aromatic retinoid (Ro 10-9359) an UVB-radiation. *Akt. Dermatol.* 4:183–187.

24. Streigleder, G.K., Orfanos, C.E., and Pullman, H. (1979). Retinoid—SUP—therapie der Psoriasis. *Z. Hautkr.* 54(1):19–23.
25. Orfanos, C.E., Pulmann, H., Steigleder, G.K., and Bloch, P.H. (1979). Oral retinoid and UVB radiation: a new alternative treatment for psoriasis on an outpatient basis. *Acta Dermatovener.* 59:241–244.
26. Lubach, D., Edmüller, M., and Rahm-Hoffmann, L.A. (1980). Kombinierte Retinoid—and UV—Phototherapie bei Pustulosis subcornealis (Sneddon-Wilkinson). *Hautarzt* 31(10):545–547.
27. Boer, J., and Suurmond, D. (1981). Combined UVB phototherapy and low dose oral retinoid Ro 10-9359 for psoriasis responding inadequately to UVB alone. In *Retinoids: Advances in Basic Research and Therapy.* C.E. Orfanos, O. Braun-Falco, E.M. Farber, C. Grupper, M.K. Polano, and R. Schuppli (Eds.). Springer-Verlag, New York, pp. 439–443.
28. Pullmann, H. (1981). Die Phototherapie in Verbindung mit aromatischen Retinoid. *Dtsche. Dermatol.* 29 Suppl. 1:36–38.
29. Schauder, S. (1981). Retinoid—und Phototherapie der Psoriasis. *Dermatologica* 162:236–242.
30. School, E. (1981). Ambulante Behandlund der Psoriasis mit UVB Bestrahlungen, aromatischen Retinoid und zehnprozntigen Solbädern. *Schweiz. Rundschau Med.* (*Praxis*) 70(41):1806–1816.
31. Fritsch, P., Honigsmann, H., Jaschke, E., and Wolff, K. (1978). Augmentation of oral methoxsalen—photochemotherapy with an oral retinoic acid derivative. *J. Invest. Dermatol.* 70:178–182.
32. Fritsch, P., Honigsmann, H., Jaschke, E., and Wolff, K. (1978). Photochemotherapie bei psoriasis: Steigerung der Wirksamkeit durch ein orales aromatisches Retinoid. *Dtsch. Med. Wochenschr.* 103:1731–1736.
33. Orfanos, C.E., Pullmann, H., Sterry, W., and Kunzig, M. (1978). Retinoid—Puva (Repuva): Systemische Kombinations—Behandlung bei Psoriasis. *Hautkr.* 53: 494–504.
34. Heidbreder G., and Christophers, E. (1979). Therapy of psoriasis with Retinoid + Puva: clinical and histological data. *Arch. Dermatol. Res.* 264:331–337.
35. Frenk, E. (1980). Traitement du psoriasis par l'association d'une rétinoide aromatique et de la photochimiothérapie orale 8-MOP. *Schweiz. Rundschau Med.* (*Praxis*) 9:221–224.
36. Thivolet, J., Robart, S., and Vignon, E. (1979). L'association rétinoide aromatique-PUVA dans de traitement des psoriasis arthropathiques. *Ann. Dermatol. Venéréol.* (*Paris*) 106:1037–1038.
37. Robart, S. (1980). La rétipuvathérapie dans le traitement du psoriasis et du rhumatisme psoriasique (à propos de 107 cas), *Thèse Université Claude Bernard,* Lyon I.
38. Thivolet, J., Robart, S., and Vignon, E. (1981). La rétinoide aromatique associée à la photochimiothérapie pour le traitement du psoriasis et du rhumatisme psoriasique. *Ann. Dermatol. Vénéréol.* 108:131–137.
39. Pullmann, H. (1981). Die Phototherapie in Verbindung mit aromatischem Retinoid. *Dtsche. Dermatol.* 29 Suppl. 1:36–38.
40. Lauharanta, J., Juvakonski, T., and Lassus, A. (1981). A clinical evaluation of the effects of an aromatic retinoid (Tigason), combination of retinoid and PUVA, and PUVA alone in severe psoriasis. *Br. J Dermatol.* 104:325–332.
41. Wolff, K., and Hönigsmann, H. (1981). Clinical aspects of photochemotherapy. *Pharmacol. Ther.* 12: 381–418.
42. Wolff, K., and Fritsch, P.O. (1982). Retinoid-PUVA chemophotochemotherapy. In *Psoriasis, Proceedings of the 3rd International Symposium,* E.M. Farber and A.J. Cox (Eds.). Grune & Stratton, New York, pp. 212–219.
43. Tsambaos, D., and Orfanos, C.E. (1982). Alterations of psoriatic epidermis under combined retinoid and PUVA treatment. In *Psoriasis, Proceedings of the 3rd International Symposium.* E.M. Farber and A.J. Cox (Eds.). Grune & Stratton, New York, pp. 509–514.
44. Lauharanta, J. (1982). Clinical, ultrastructural and biochemical effects of an aromatic retinoid (etretinate) on psoriasis and Darier's disease. *Acta Dermatol.* (*Stockh.*) Suppl. 101.
45. Michaelson, G., Noren, P., and Vahlquist, A. (1978). Combined therapy with oral retinoid and PUVA baths in severe psoriasis. *Br. J. Dermatol.* 99:221–222.
46. Schnitzler, L., and Verret, J.L. (1981). Retinoid and skin cancer prevention. In *Retinoids: Advances in Basic Research and Therapy.* C.E. Orfanos, O. Braun-Falco, E.M. Farber, C. Grupper, M.K. Polano, and R. Schuppli (Eds.). Springer-Verlag, New York, pp. 385–388.
47. Berretti, B., Grupper, C., Edelson, Y., and Bermejo, D. (1981). Aromatic retinoid in the treatment of multiple superficial basal cell carcinoma, arsenic keratosis and keratoacanthoma. In *Retinoids: Advances in Basic Research and Therapy.* C.E. Orfanos, O. Braun-Falco, E.M. Farber, C. Grupper, M.K. Polano, and R. Schuppli (Eds.). Springer-Verlag, New York, pp. 397–400.
48. Berretti, B., and Grupper, C. (1984). Cutaneous neoplasia and etretinate. In *Retinoid Therapy.* W.J. Cunliffe and A.J. Miller (Eds.). MTP Press, Lancaster, pp. 87–94.
49. Berretti, B., and Grupper, C. (1980). Qu'en est-il de la photochimiothérapie du psoriasis en 1980? *Rev. Méd.* 21(39):2091–2094.
50. Grupper, C., and Berretti, B. (1981). Treatment of psoriasis by oral PUVA therapy combined with aromatic retinoid. *Dermatologica* 162:404–413.
51. Grupper, C., and Berretti, B. (1981). Treatment of psoriasis by oral PUVA-therapy combination with aromatic retinoid (REPUVA). In *Retinoids: Advances in*

Basic Research and Therapy. C.E. Orfanos, O. Braun-Falco, E.M. Farber, C. Grupper, M.K. Polano, and R. Schuppli (Eds.). Springer-Verlag, New York, pp. 341–345.

52. Grupper, C., and Berretti, B. (1981). The Aubervilliers PUVA study. In *Psoralens in Cosmetics and Dermatology.* Scientific International Research (Ed.). Pergamon Press, Paris, pp. 223–231.

53. Grupper, C., and Berretti, B. (1981). 5-MOP in puva and REPUVA, 250 patients with a follow up of three years. In *Psoriasis, Proceedings of the 3rd International Symposium.* E.M. Farber and A.J. Cox (Eds.). Grune & Stratton, New York, pp. 503–508.

54. Honigsmann, H., and Wolff, K. (1983). Isotretinoin-PUVA for psoriasis. (Letter to Editor) *Lancet* 1:236.

Part VIII

NEW TREATMENTS AND INNOVATIONS

58

Bioengineering and Psoriasis

Enzo Berardesca and F. Distante
University of Pavia, Pavia, Italy
Howard I. Maibach
University of California School of Medicine, San Francisco, California

Bioengineering techniques are becoming popular among dermatologists by providing important information on different parameters of skin function and physiology. Psoriasis is one of the common dermatological diseases that has been investigated by noninvasive methods in recent years (1). This chapter reviews and updates the most recent advances in bioengineering techniques applied to diagnosis, treatment, and follow-up of psoriasis.

TRANSEPIDERMAL WATER LOSS (TEWL)

TEWL reflects the integrity of the water barrier function of the stratum corneum (2,3) and is used to study both normal and diseased skin (4,5).

In vivo, TEWL can be measured according to three different water-sampling techniques (6,7): the open-chamber method, providing continuous measurements in ambient air, with little alteration of the microclimate overlying the skin surface, is preferable and is currently used in commercially available devices. It has gained wide use in evaluation of the skin water barrier function and other related studies such as in vivo transcutaneous penetration (8,9).

A defective barrier function, expressed by alterations of TEWL, has been observed in certain inflammatory diseases with disturbance of proliferation and/or cheratinization (psoriasis, ichthyosis, erythrodermia, eczema). Ultrastructural studies in psoriatic skin have shown that the distribution, structure, and biochemistry of the intercellular lipid compartment of the stratum corneum, which are vital for the barrier function, are altered (10).

TEWL is increased in psoriasis, which indicates that the pathological horny layer has lost its water-retaining properties (11). TEWL values appear directly related to the clinical intensity of the lesion (11–13) and closely reflect the disappearance of the lesions. Frodin et al. reported the normalization of TEWL values parallel to progressive healing (13). TEWL and water content of the stratum corneum, when measured simultaneously, provide important information regarding skin function in physiological and pathological conditions (14). The psoriatic stratum corneum loses its water-holding properties and the skin becomes dry and scaly. This interpretation is supported by different investigators (11,15–17). An inverse relationship between the TEWL and the water content of the stratum corneum in psoriasis is reported (11,17), whereas these two parameters were considered directly proportional in normal skin (18). Serup and Blichmann (19) confirmed these results using the same method and suggested that the low hydration rate could be correlated to the abnormal cheratinization in psoriasis. A model allowing differentiation of dry senile skin from dry pathological skin has been suggested (2). Pathological dry skin, because of the impaired barrier function, is associated with increased TEWL and low stratum corneum water content. Senile skin, on the other hand, shows both decreased TEWL and stratum corneum water content. Uninvolved skin of psoriatic patients has normal TEWL levels (21).

TEWL measurements are also extremely useful to assess the progress of the psoriatic lesions during topical treatments and to compare the specific effects of different drugs and other topical or systemic treatments on involved skin. Hartop et al. (22) monitored TEWL on different psoriatic plaques treated topically with linoleic acid in comparison with clobetasol. TEWL in association with other noninvasive techniques has been used (23) to evaluate topical calcipotriol versus clobetasol: TEWL and laser Doppler velocimetry (LDV) were used to monitor restoration of water barrier and normalization of blood flow, respectively, in psoriatic plaques of the limbs of 24 male patients during 3 weeks of treatment. Data were compared to subjective evaluation using the PASI index of the same areas. Significant differences were recorded during treatment in both groups. The results correlated well with the PASI score. Clobetasol restored barrier function faster than calcipotriol. However, no significant differences were detected between the two groups. The authors confirmed the efficacy of vitamin D analogues in normalizing skin biophysical parameters and in avoiding the risks of side effects induced by potent topical corticoids in the treatment of psoriasis.

Contradictory findings have been reported on the usefulness of TEWL recordings in monitoring dithranol therapy: indeed, dithranol, a local irritant, may induce abnormally high TEWL values, not correlated with the clinical healing (24,25).

STRATUM CORNEUM HYDRATION

Electrical methods based on capacitance, conductance, or impedance are widely used to measure skin hydration (26,27). Several commercial instruments are available (28). Generally, pathological stratum corneum has a decreased water content as measured by these devices (19,27,29). This finding has been described as the paradox of skin hydration in psoriatic skin, since higher values of TEWL should indicate the presence of more water in such stratum corneum areas. Indeed, an inverse relationship between these parameters has been shown in psoriasis (11). Dynamic measurements of skin hydration can be used to provide a more complete understanding of water-binding properties of the horny layer (30,31); among these, the plastic occlusion stress test (POST) and the moisture accumulation test (MAT) have been used to study psoriasis (21,32,33).

The POST utilizes skin occlusion by the application of a plastic chamber for a lag of time (generally 24 hr). When the occlusion is removed, the excess water on the skin starts to evaporate and can be recorded using an evaporimeter. Analysis of the decay curve obtained with the POST technique gives information on stratum corneum (SC) hydration, integrity of the barrier function, and SC water-holding capacity (WHC). No particular differences between uninvolved psoriatic skin and normal skin are reported using the POST (21).

The MAT (32), is based on the increase of hydration consequent to occlusion induced by the probe of the device. Capacitance readings at regular intervals (1.5–3 sec) over a total of 45 sec describe a typical MAT curve, which shows a steep increase of capacitance within the first 20 sec that levels off afterward thus suggesting an exponential function. Elsner and Burg (33) evaluated both the MAT and the POST in uninvolved and lesional skin of the lateral upper arm in seven male psoriatic patients. In the MAT, capacitance values increased in both uninvolved and lesional skin. In the POST, SSWL decreased in uninvolved and lesional skin. The start and end points of MAT and the end points of POST were significantly different between uninvolved and lesional skin. Both accumulation of unbound water as expressed by the MAT and WHC as expressed by POST were increased in lesional psoriatic skin. Both the MAT and the POST can be useful dynamic parameters to assess therapeutic effects in psoriasis. Because no preocclusion is needed for the MAT and the measuring period is substantially lower for the MAT than the POST, the MAT may be more practical for use in larger populations. However, more studies are needed with this method to establish its scope and reproducibility.

MEASUREMENTS OF SKIN THICKNESS

Only few attempts to evaluate skin thickness have been reported in the literature before the development of ultrasound technique (34,35), which was made possible by the fundamental work of Alexander and Miller (36). Since then, ultrasound examination of skin has been successfully used to assess skin disorders (37) and represents a field of increasing interest as a noninvasive objective method to study skin pathophysiology for research and diagnosis. High-frequency A-mode scan, B-mode, C-mode, M-mode, three-dimensional (3D) scanning, or more advanced techniques (37–39) are available for investigating skin structure. The most widely used are A- and B-mode (20 MHz) scanning, the last considered more accurate as it provides a cross-sectional image of the object in two dimensions.

One of the most important features of high-frequency scanners is the opportunity to correlate sonograms with histological sections (40). Some important problems such as reliable differential diagnosis have not yet been solved, since scanning at that frequency does not provide resolution of histology (41). A common finding in any kind of inflammation is an echo-poor area underneath the entry echo, which increases under therapy and completely disappears with the resolution of a lesion (42,43). Echographic evaluation enables the identification of three characteristics of psoriatic lesions: an increase in skin thickness, the presence of a thick hyposonic subepidermal band, and an enhanced entrance echo. The hyposonic band can be caused by the presence of a homogeneous component such as an inflammatory infiltrate or edema. The enhancement of the entrance echo, on the other hand, corresponds to a thickening and a modification of psoriatic epidermis. The echogenicity increases parallel to the reduction of acanthosis and infiltrate (39,44–47). In pustular psoriasis the same type of abnormality is seen, with focal distribution (48).

Several studies (39,49–51) confirm the utility of ultrasound for objectively evaluating and characterizing the efficacy of various treatments. Scanners with high frequencies (50–150 MHz) and evaluation with image analysis provide additional information (52,53). In fact, while pathological processes in the dermis can be easily visualized, 20-MHz ultrasound scans have low resolution in the study of intraepidermal structures, making it impossible to correlate sonographic images with histological sections. El Gammal et al. (54) used 50-MHz B-scan ultrasound in the study of psoriatic plaques at different preamplification signals to visualize dermis and epidermis. Application of image-processing methods to the study of echographic images allows the characterization and quantification of echographic parameters, which vary during the course of the disease according to treatment (39,55). However, a major problem regarding image-processing methods is that information they provide, though quantitative in a relative sense, is highly instrument dependent, making data collected from different researchers with different equipment not comparable (53).

BLOOD FLOW

Psoriasis is characterized by changes in microvasculature of the upper dermis, with elongation and dilatation of skin capillaries. This is a prominent aspect of chronic psoriatic plaques, and correlates with disease activity (56,57). The microvascular alterations seem to regress during the healing process (58–61).

Several techniques that provide continuous quantitative or qualitative measurements of skin flux have been developed and are commercially available for clinical and research use. Among them are "in vivo" capillaroscopy, LDV, radioactive indicator washout technique (e.g., local ^{133}Xe washout), plethysmography, spectrophotometry, and thermography. Skin blood flow is greatly increased in psoriasis (62). Using a xenon washout technique, Klemp and Staberg (62) showed that mean blood flow in untreated lesional psoriatic skin is about 10 times higher than in normal skin and that mean perfusion in normal-appearing skin of psoriatic patients is significantly increased in comparison to that of normal subjects. The same authors (63) found no significant difference between nonlesional skin of patients with only mild psoriatic manifestations and skin of healthy individuals. They concluded that skin flux in psoriatic skin, both lesional and uninvolved, correlates well to the disease activity. Therefore, the severity of the disease can be monitored by cutaneous blood flow measurements in nonlesional skin.

Measurement of cutaneous blood flow by the ^{133}Xe washout method was elaborated by Sejrsen (64). However, the method has mostly been used to register relative changes in blood flow during various provocation tests (64). Real-time imaging of the skin microvasculature may be provided by means of an intravital capillaroscopy, based on a videomicroscopy system. The addition of fluorescein angiography improves contrast and detects aspects of blood vessel behavior, such as perfusion homogeneity and transcapillary solute diffusion, not detectable under native conditions. Bull et al. (65) evaluated whether the method can be applied to the investigation of capillary anatomy and dynamics in psoriatic skin, to define the role of blood vessels in the pathogenesis of the disease. Results are in agreement with other methods confirming higher perfusion in lesional skin compared to uninvolved skin and in uninvolved psoriatic skin compared to healthy control skin.

LDV is a widely used technique to monitor blood flow (66). The method consists of a He-Ne laser source of 632.5-nm wavelength applied to the skin via a small probe. The incident radiation enters the skin and is scattered and reflected by nonmoving tissue components and by mobile red blood cells encountered as the radiation penetrates to a depth of 1–1.5 mm. A portion of the scattered and reflected incident radiation exits the skin and is collected by a second optical fiber that carries the light back to a photodetector where it is converted into an electric signal. Stationary skin tissue reflects and backscatters light at the same frequency as the incident source, while moving erythrocytes reflect the frequency-shifted radiation. The shift increases with increasing velocity. The LDV extracts the frequency-shifted signal and derives an output proportional to the flux of erythrocytes in the blood flow.

Most antipsoriatic agents induce microvascular changes during and following therapy (67,68). The correlation of flux parameters measured instrumentally to the clinical course of the disease is useful to monitor the effectiveness of treatments and to understand the pathogenesis of the disease. Staberg and Klemp (69) compared blood flow during Goeckerman or beech tar therapy. Before therapy, skin blood flow was increased 9 times in psoriatic lesions as compared to uninvolved skin. During both treatments skin blood flow progressively reduced, approaching that of uninvolved skin in 3–4 weeks, and correlated strictly with visual assessment of the plaques ($P < 0.001$). Moreover, at the end of the treatment the values of involved skin were still 2–3 times higher than that of uninvolved skin. The same authors compared LDF to ^{133}Xe washout before and during treatment with tar (70). Their results confirmed the earlier finding of significantly higher perfusion levels in lesional versus uninvolved psoriatic skin, which declined during the course of therapy. Kahn et al. (71) confirmed that mean blood flow (as determined by LDV) is significantly higher in a psoriatic plaque ($P < 0.01$) than in uninvolved skin and in normal individuals. Blood flow of psoriatic plaques decreased to uninvolved skin levels after Goeckerman therapy. In contrast with the findings of Staberg and Klemp a nonsignificant linear correlation between LDV values and visual score was found. Blood flow decreased more rapidly than other morphological abnormalities. The decline in blood flow significantly preceded the clinical resolution 4–8 days after the beginning of treatment. The authors proposed that laser-Doppler flowmetry (LDF) measurements could predict disease improvement, which could be useful for the design and follow-up of new treatments. The comparison of visual estimation of irritation causes by dithranol with contact temperature and LDF of uninvolved skin of psoriatic patients (72) showed a dose-dependent correlation between all three methods.

Broby-Johansen and Kristensen (73,74), using LDF, proved that topical corticosteroid cream (clobetasol propionate), when combined with occlusion, is much more effective than the steroid cream alone. More recently, the same group (5) compared the effects on chronic psoriatic plaques of various topical corticosteroids applied for 1 week under a hydrocolloid dressing. Noninvasive measurements (ultrasound skin thickness, laser-Doppler flowmetry, colorimetry) were performed before and after treatment and compared to clinical score. The more potent the corticosteroid used, the closer to normality were the parameters measured and the clinical score. Berardesca et al. (23) showed the normalization of laser-Doppler values and other biophysical parameters after topically applied calcipotriol versus clobetasol.

Advanced methods for measuring skin flux have been proposed in the last few years. They offer further accuracy and precision in the assessment of skin flux, since they overcome some drawbacks of laser-Doppler technique. The utility of these new devices is complementary to preexisting techniques. Among them (75), the most important recent development is the scanning LDF (76,77), which quickly records the tissue perfusion in large areas of skin, without any contact with skin surface. It has been used in the assessment of vascular changes in psoriasis. Speight et al. (76,77) found mean blood flow flux within psoriatic plaques 4 times higher than in uninvolved skin. Auer et al. (78), using a two-dimensional laser-Doppler scanner, evaluated the effect of dithranol on blood flux during the course of therapy. They concluded that the increased perfusion of the psoriatic plaque is due to the combination of morphological (dilatation of vessels), dynamic (increased blood flow), and optical effects (reduced scattering and increased sampling depth of the laser beam in acanthotic tissue). A laser-Doppler perfusion imager was also used by some researchers to examine whether neurogenic mechanisms (axon reflexes) are important for blood flow regulation in the plaque (79).

COLORIMETRY

Reflectance spectrophotometry is an optical technique for the measurement of skin color. When a light is applied on the skin surface, a part of it is reflected and a part adsorbed. Diffuse reflectance (or remittance) is the fraction of incident radiation backscattered from the skin. Water, bilirubin, melanin, oxy- and reduced hemoglobin, carotenoids, and epidermal aromatic amino acids are the cromophores exerting the most important effects on diffuse reflectance spectra of human skin (80). Comparing the absorption at different wavelengths and the molecular characteristics of the cromophores, it is possible to calculate and quantify changes in skin color such as erythema and pigmentation. Ryatt et al. (81) thus calculated the hemoglobin content in 13 patients undergoing PUVA treatment. The final erythema index of the lesions 1 month after the last UVA dose was greater than that of normal sites, indicating that the vascular changes in psoriasis could remain despite the clearing of the plaques. The authors suggest that the marked change in the erythema response during treatment of psoriasis can be more efficiently detected by remittance spectroscopy rather than the naked eye and may be used as a basis to determine the length and the aggressiveness of treatment.

Chromametry is another method for determining skin color and/or erythema. The technique is based on the use of the tristimulus values of the Commission Internationale de l'Eclairage (CIE) (82). The CIE defined the L*a*b* color space (CIELAB) system, which easily measures reflected object color in an accurate and reproducible way. Several colorimeters based on this principle have been manufactured for medical and scientific use (83). The usefulness of this technique in combination with others has been reported (50,55).

COMMENT

Bioengineering techniques allow the noninvasive objective evaluation of psoriasis. They can give different biological information useful in comparing and monitoring the specific effects of different drugs or treatments. However, we are still unable to discriminate between diseases and make the exact diagnosis among different dermatoses. So far, the traditional techniques of investigation (visual assessment, palpation, biopsy, and histological examination) remain the most important tools for the dermatologist to recognize and classify skin disease.

REFERENCES

1. Berardesca, E., and Maibach, H. (1989). Noninvasive bioengineering assessment of psoriasis. *Int. J. Dermatol.* 28:157–160.
2. Grice, K., Sattar, H., Sharrat, M., and Baker, H. (1971). Skin temperature and transepidermal water loss. *J. Invest. Dermatol.* 57:108–110.
3. Dugard, P.H. (1977). Skin permeability theory in relation to measurements of percutaneous absorption in toxicology. In *Dermatotoxicology and Pharmacology.* F.N. Marzulli and H.I. Maibach (Eds.). Wiley, New York, pp. 525–550.
4. Hassing, J.H., Nater, J.P., and Bleumink, E. (1982). Irritance of low concentrations of soap and synthetic detergents as measured by skin vapour loss. *Dermatologica* 154:314–321.
5. Coenraads, P.J., and Pinnagoda, J. (1985). Dermatitis and water vapour loss in metal workers. *Contact Derm.* 13:347–348.
6. Maibach, H.I., Bronaugh, R., Guy, R., Turr, E., Wilson, D., Jacques, S., and Chaing, D. (1984). Noninvasive techniques for determining skin function. In *Cutaneous Toxicity.* V.A. Drill and P. Lazar (Eds.). Raven Press, New York, pp. 63–97.
7. Pinnagoda, J., Tupker, R., Agner, T., and Serup, J. (1990). Guidelines for transepidermal water loss (TEWL) measurement. *Contact Derm.* 22:164–168.
8. Rougier, A., Lotte, C., Corcuff, P., and Maibach H.I. (1988). Relationship between skin permeability and corneocyte size according to anatomical site, age and sex in man. *J. Soc. Cosmet. Chem.* 39:15–18.
9. Kompaore, F., Dupont, C., and Marty, J.P. (1991). "In vivo" evaluation in man by two noninvasive methods of the stratum corneum barrier function after physical and chemical modifications. *Int. J. Cosmet. Sci.* 13: 293–295.
10. Menon, G.K., and Elias, P.M. (1991). Ultrastructural localization of calcium in psoriatic and normal human epidermis. *Arch. Dermatol.* 127:57–63.
11. Tagami, H., and Yoshikuni, K. (1985). Interrelationship between water-barrier and reservoir functions of pathologic stratum corneum. *Arch. Dermatol.* 121: 642–645.
12. Marks, J., Rogers, S., Chadkirk, B., and Shuster, S. (1981). Clearance of chronic plaque psoriasis by anthralin-subjective and objective assessment and comparison with photochemotherapy. *Br. J. Dermatol.* 105(Suppl. 20):96–99.
13. Frodin, T., Helander, P., Molin, L., and Skogh, M. (1988). Hydration of human stratum corneum studied "in vivo" by optothermal infrared spectrometry, elec-

trical capacitance measurement, and evaporimetry. *Acta Derm. Venereol. (Stockh.)* 68:461–467.
14. Berardesca, E., and Maibach, H.I. (1990). Transepidermal water loss and skin surface hydration in the noninvasive assessment of stratum corneum function. *Derm. Beruf. Umwelt* 38:50–70.
15. Grice, K.A., and Bettley, F.R. (1967). Skin water loss and accidental hypothermia in psoriasis, ichthyosis and erythroderma. *Br. Med. J.* 4:195–198.
16. Grice, K.A. (1980). Measurement of transepidermal water loss in pathological skin. In *The Physiology and Pathophysiology of the Skin.* A. Jarret (Ed.). Academic Press, New York, p. 247.
17. Jacques, S. (1982). Water content and concentration profile in human stratum corneum. Thesis, University of California, Fullerton.
18. Leveque, J.L., Garson, J.C., and de Rigal, J. (1979). Transepidermal water loss from dry and normal skin. *J. Soc. Cosmet. Chem.* 50:333–343.
19. Serup, J., and Blichmann, C. (1987). Epidermal hydration of psoriasis plaques and the relation to scaling. *Acta Derm. Venereol.* 67:357–366.
20. Berardesca, E., and Maibach, H.I. (1990). Transepidermal water loss and skin surface hydration in the noninvasive assessment of stratum corneum function. *Derm. Beruf. Umwelt* Mar–Apr:50–53.
21. Berardesca, E., Fideli, D., Borroni, G., Rabbiosi, G., and Maibach, H.I. (1990). In vivo hydration and water-retention capacity of stratum corneum in clinically uninvolved skin in atopic and psoriatic patients. *Acta Derm. Venereol. (Stockh.)* 70:400–404.
22. Hartop, P.J., Allenby, C.F., and Prottey, C. (1978). Comparison of barrier function and lipids in psoriasis and essential fatty acid-deficient rats. *Clin. Exp. Dermatol.* 3:259–267.
23. Berardesca, E., Vignoli, G.P., Farinelli, N., Vignini, M., Distante, F., and Rabbiosi, G. (1994). Non-invasive evaluation of topical calcipotriol versus clobetasol in the treatment of psoriasis. *Acta Derm. Venereol.* 74(4): 302–304.
24. Rogers, S. (1993). Measurement of plaque thickness and evaporative water loss in psoriasis with PUVA and dithranol treatment. *Clin. Exp. Dermatol.* 18:21–24.
25. Snater, E., Janssen, E.A., van der Valk, P.G., and van de Kerkhof, P.C. (1995). Transepidermal water vapour loss is not increased during and following dithranol irritation. *Br. J. Dermatol.* 132(6):908–912.
26. Leveque, J.L., and de Rigal, J. (1983). Impedance methods for studying skin moisturization. *J. Soc. Cosmet. Chem.* 34:419–428.
27. Tagami, H. (1989). Impedance measurements for evaluation of the hydration state of the skin surface. In *Cutaneous Investigation in Health and Disease: Noninvasive Methods and Instrumentation.* J.L. Leveque (Ed.). Marcel Dekker, New York, pp. 79–111.
28. Blichmann, C.W., and Serup, J. (1988). Assessment of skin moisture. Measurement of electrical conductance, capacitance and transepidermal water loss. *Acta Dermatol. Venereol. (Stockh.)* 68:284–290.
29. Borroni, G., Berardesca, E., Gabba, P., and Rabbiosi, G. (1988). Skin impedance in psoriatic epidermis. *Bioeng. Skin* 4:15–22.
30. Tagami, H., Kanamaru, I., Inoue, K., Shehisa, S., Inoue, F., Iwatsuki, K., Yoshikuni, K., and Yamada, M. (1982). Water sorption-desorption test of the skin in vivo for functional assessment of the stratum corneum. *J. Invest. Dermatol.* 78:425–428.
31. Rietschel, R.L. (1978). A method to evaluate skin moisturizers in vivo. *J. Invest. Dermatol.* 70:152–155.
32. van Neste, H. (1990). In vivo evaluation of unbound water accumulation in stratum corneum. *Dermatology* 181:197–291.
33. Elsner, P., and Burg, G. (1991). Dynamic functional properties of psoriatic skin assessed by non-invasive bioengineering methods in vivo. Fifth Int. Psoriasis Symp., San Francisco, July.
34. Lee, M. (1957). Physical and structural age changes in human skin. *Anat. Rec.* 129:473.
35. Bliznack, J., and Staple, T.W. (1975). Roentgenographic measurement of skin thickness in normal individuals. *Radiology* 118:55–60.
36. Alexander, H., and Miller, D.L. (1979). Determining skin thickness with pulsed ultrasound. *J. Invest. Dermatol.* 72:17–19.
37. Sondergaard, J., Serup, J., and Tikjøb, G. (1985). Ultrasonic A- and B-scanning in clinical and experimental dermatology. *Acta Dermatovener.* 120:76–82.
38. Serup, J. (1992). Ten years' experience with high frequency ultrasound examination of the skin: development and refinement of technique and equipment. In *Ultrasound in Dermatology.* P. Altmeyer, S. el-Gammal, and K. Hoffmann (Eds.). Springer-Verlag, Berlin, pp. 41–54.
39. Di Nardo, A., Seidenari, S., and Giannetti, A. (1992). B-scanning evaluation with image analysis of psoriatic skin. *Exp. Dermatol.* 1:121–125.
40. Gassenmeier, G., Kiesewetter, F., Schell, H., and Zinner, M. (1990). Wertigkeit der hochaflosenden Sonographie fur dieBestimmnug des vertikalen Tumordurchmessers beim malignen Melanom der Haut. *Hautarzt* 41:360–364.
41. Hoffmann, K., el-Gammal, S., and Altmeyer, P. (1989) 20 MHz B-scan Sonographie an Handen und FuBen in Handsymposium: Dermatologische Erkrankungen der Hande und FuBe. P. Altmeyer et al. (Eds.). Edition Roche, pp. 285–300.
42. Hoffmann, K., el-Gammal, S., Schwarze, H., and Dirschka, T. (1992). Examination of psoriasis vulgaris using 20-Mhz B-scan ultrasound. In *Ultrasound in Dermatology.* P. Altmeyer, S. el-Gammal, and K. Hoffmann (Eds.). Springer, Berlin, pp. 207–220.

43. Kirsch, J.M., Hanson, M.E., and Gibson, J.R. (1984). The determination of skin thickness using conventional ultrasound equipment. *Clin. Exp. Dermatol.* 9:280–285.
44. Olsen, L.O., and Serup, J. (1993). High-frequency ultrasound scan for non-invasive cross-sectional imaging of psoriasis. *Acta Derm. Venereol.* 73(3):185–187.
45. Serup, J. (1984). Non-invasive quantification of psoriasis plaques-measurements of skin thickness with 15 mHz pulsed ultrasounds. *Clin. Exp. Dermatol.* 9: 502–508.
46. Hermann, R.C., Ellis, C.N., Fithing, D.W., Ho V.C., and Voorhees, J.J. (1989). Measurement of epidermal thickness in normal skin and psoriasis with high-frequency ultrasound. *Skin Pharmacol.* 1:128–136.
47. Rogers, S. (1992). Skin thickness in psoriasis. *Clin. Exp. Dermatol.* 17:324–327.
48. Krieg, P.H.G., Bacharach-Buhulers, M., el-Gammal, S., and Altmeyer, P. (1992). The pustule in palmoplantar psoriasis: transformed preside or mature microabscess? A three-dimensional study. *Dermatology* 185: 104–112.
49. Korting, H.C., Kerscher, M.J., and Shafer-Korting, M. (1992). Topical glucocorticoids with improved benefit /risk ratio: do they exist? *J. Am. Acad. Dermatol.* 27(1):87–92.
50. Broby-Johansen, U., Karlsmark, T., Petersen, L.J., and Serup, J. (1990). Ranking of the antipsoriatic effect of various topical corticosteroids applied under a hydrocolloid dressing—skin thickness, blood flow and colour measurements compared to clinical assessments. *Clin. Exp. Dermatol.* 15(5):343–348.
51. Kerscher, M.J., Hart, H., Korting, H.C., and Stalleicken, D. (1995). In vivo assessment of the atrophogenic potency of mometasone furoate, a newly developed chlorinated potent topical glucocorticoid as compared to other topical glucocorticoids old and new. *Int. J. Clin. Pharmacol. Ther.* 33(4):187–189.
52. Hoffmann, K., Dirting, K. Stucker, M., el Gammal, S., Wilmert, M., and Altmeyer, W.P. (1994). History of high frequency sonography. *Ultraschall Med.* 15(4): 192–197.
53. Seidenari, S. (1995). Ultrasound B-mode imaging and "in vivo" structure analysis. In *Handbook of Non-invasive Methods and the Skin.* J. Serup and G.B.E. Jemec (Eds.). CRC Press, Orlando, FL, pp. 257–268.
54. el Gammal, S., Auer, T., Popp, C., Hoffmann, K., Altmeyer, P., Passmann, C., and Ermert, H. (1994). Psoriasis vulgaris in 50 MHz B-scan ultrasound, characteristic features of stratum corneum, epidermis and dermis. *Acta Derm. Venereol. (Stockh.)* Suppl. 186: 173–176.
55. Hoffmann, K., Dirschka, T., Schwarze, H., el Gammal, S., Matthes, U., Hoffmann, A., and Altmeyer, P. (1995). 20 MHz sonography, colorimetry and image analysis in the evaluation of psoriasis vulgaris. *J. Dermatol. Sci.* 9(2):103–110.
56. Braverman, I.M., and Yen A. (1977). Ultrastucture of the capillary loops in the dermal papillae of psoriasis. *J. Invest. Dermatol.* 68:53–60.
57. Braverman, I.M., Keh, A., and Goldminz, D. (1990). Correlation of laser-Doppler wave patterns with underlying microvascular anatomy. *J. Invest. Dermatol.* 95(3):283–286.
58. Brody, I. (1984). Dermal and epidermal involvement in the evolution of acute eruptive guttate psoriasis vulgaris. *J. Invest. Dermatol.* 82:465–470.
59. Braverman, I.M., and Sibley, J. (1982). Role of the microcirculation in the treatment and pathogenesis of psoriasis. *J. Invest. Dermatol.* 78:12–17.
60. McKenzie, A.W. (1963). Histological changes in psoriasis treated with topical fluocinolone and occlusion. *Br. J. Dermatol.* 75:434–440.
61. Ross, J.B. (1964). The psoriatic capillary, its nature and value in the identification of the unaffected psoriatic. *Br. J. Dermatol.* 76:511–518.
62. Klemp, P., and Staberg, B. (1983). Cutaneous blood flow in psoriasis. *J. Invest. Dermatol.* 81:503–506.
63. Klemp, P., and Staberg, B. (1986). Cutaneous and subcutaneous blood flow in nonlesional skin of patients with minimal psoriatic skin manifestations. *J. Invest. Dermatol.* 86:582–584.
64. Kristensen, J.K., and Petersen, L.J. (1991). Measurement of cutaneous blood flow by the 133-Xenon washout method. Clinical applications in dermatology. *Acta Physiol. Scand.* Suppl. 603:67–73.
65. Bull, R.H., Bates, D.O., and Mortimer, P.S. (1992). Intravital video-capillaroscopy for the study of the microcirculation in psoriasis. *Br. J. Dermatol.* 126(5): 436–445.
66. Nilsson, G.E., Tenland, T., and Oberg, P.A. (1980). Evaluation of a laser Doppler flowmeter for measurement of tissue blood flow. *IEEE Trans. Biomed. Eng.* 27:597–604.
67. Gordon, M., Johnson, W.C., and Burgoon, C.F. (1967). Histopathology and histochemistry of psoriasis. II. Dynamics of lesions during treatment. *Arch. Pathol.* 84: 443–450.
68. Suurmond, D. (1966). Histochemical changes in treated and untreated psoriasis. *Dermatologica* 132: 237–247.
69. Staberg, B., and Klemp, P. (1984). Skin blood flow in psoriasis during Goeckermann or beech tar therapy. *Acta Derm. Venereol.* 64:331–363.
70. Klemp, P., and Staberg, B. (1985). The effects of antipsoriatic treatment on cutaneous blood flow in psoriasis measured by ^{133}Xe washout method and laser Doppler velocimetry. *J. Invest. Dermatol.* 85:259–263.
71. Khan, A., Schall, L.M., Tur, E., Maibach, H.I., and Guy, R.H. (1987). Blood flow in psoriatic skin lesions:

the effect of treatment. *Br. J. Dermatol.* 117(2): 193–201.
72. Mustakallio, K.K., and Kolari, P.J. (1983). Irritation and staining by dithranol (anthralin) and related compounds. *Acta Derm. Venereol.* 63:513–518.
73. Broby-Johansen, U., and Kristensen, J.K. (1989). Antipsoriatic effect of local corticosteroids—O_2-consumption and blood flow measurements compared to clinical parameters. *Clin. Exp. Dermatol.* 14: 137–140.
74. Broby-Johansen, U. and Kristensen, J.K. (1989). Antipsoriatic effect of semi-occlusive treatment—O_2-consumption, blood flow and temperature measurements compared to clinical parameters. *Clin. Exp. Dermatol.* 14:286–288.
75. Braverman, I.M., and Schechner, J.S. (1991). Contour mapping of the cutaneous microvasculature by computerized laser-Doppler velocimetry. *J. Invest. Dermatol.* 97:1013–1018.
76. Speight, E.L., Essex, T.J.H., and Farr, P.M. (1992). The measurement of plaques of psoriasis using a scanning laser-Doppler velocimeter. *Br. J. Dermatol.* 127 (Suppl.40):34 (abstract).
77. Speight, E.L., Essex, T.J.H., and Farr, P.M. (1993). The study of plaques of psoriasis using a scanning laser-Doppler velocimeter. *Br. J. Dermatol.* 128(5):519–524.
78. Auer, T., Bacharach-Buhles, M., el Gammal, S., Stucker, M., Panz, B., Popp, C., and Hoffmann, K. (1994). The hyperperfusion of the psoriatic plaque correlates histologically with dilatation of vessels. *Acta Derm. Venereol.* (*Stockh.*) Suppl. 186:30–32.
79. Krogstad, A.L., Swanbeck, G., and Wallin, B.G. (1995). Axon-reflex-mediated vasodilatation in the psoriatic plaque? *J. Invest. Dermatol.* 104(5):872–876.
80. Anderson, R.R., Hu, J., Parrish, J.A. (1981). Optical radiation transfer in the human skin and applications in "in vivo" remittance spectroscopy. In *Bioengineering and the Skin*. R. Marks and P. Payne (Eds.). MTP Press, Lancaster, pp. 253–265.
81. Ryatt, K.S, Feather, J.W., Dawson, J.B., and Cotterill, J.A. (1983). The usefulness of reflectance spectrophotometric measurements during psoralens and ultraviolet A therapy for psoriasis. *J. Am. Acad. Dermatol.* 9: 558–562.
82. Robertson, A.R. (1977). The CIE 1976 color difference formulas. *Color Res. Appl.* 2:7.
83. Weatherall, I.L., and Coombs, B.D. (1992). Skin color measurements in terms of CIELAB color space values. *J. Invest. Dermatol.* 99:468–473.

59

Pharmacological Models for Psoriasis Syndromes

Saqib J. Bashir and Howard I. Maibach
University of California School of Medicine, San Francisco, California

Determining the therapeutic efficacy of putative treatments of psoriasis requires reliable models of the disease upon which they can be tested as potentially toxic preparations cannot ethically be screened on humans. Here, the suitability of both established and potential in vivo and in vitro models is assessed in the context of their ability to predict potential treatments.

The value of an individual model is reflected in its ability to accurately mimic the disease studied. The further the features of a model are from human psoriasis, the less we can interpret the results in a human context. The more *psoriasiform* the resemblance, the more the model allows us to evaluate the drug. Psoriasis is a disease of many facets, and the interplay of immunological factors, cytokines, skin cells, and cellular markers must be replicated for a model to be truly comparative.

In the context of this discussion, the purpose of the model is to determine whether or not a drug is therapeutically active. Therefore, the broader issues of pharmacokinetics and pharmacodynamics will not be considered. Rather, the power of the model as a screen and as a predictor of human therapies is the focus.

HISTOLOGICAL CHANGES IN PSORIASIS

The degree by which a model resembles human psoriasis can be measured by comparing histological and biochemical features of the model to the human (Table 1). As molecular and immunological studies shed more light on the expression of cellular proteins and surface molecules, and the constituents of the extracellular matrix are identified, the precision of models can be elucidated.

Pharmacological models are used to determine the pharmacodynamic and pharmacokinetic properties of a drug as described above. In studies of antipsoriatic efficacy, many models simply test the antiproliferative and parakeratotic properties of the drug. It is thought that as these features are seen in human psoriasis, it may be possible to extrapolate experimental findings to humans. Without a good animal model, however, this can lead to hopeful estimations of a drug's efficacy: clearly a laboratory result cannot be equated to a human therapeutic response.

IN VIVO MODELS

Psoriasiform Models

The Mouse Tail Test

The normal structure of the tail of the adult mouse histologically resembles the histopathological structure of human psoriasis (1). Between the follicles, areas of epidermis are well defined, parakeratotic, and lack a granular layer. In between these *scale* areas are *hinge* regions, where hairs emerge underneath the scale. Here, the skin is orthokeratotic and possesses a granular layer, as does normal human skin. Putative antipsoriatic drug activity can be measured by the induction of a granular layer and orthokeratosis in the

Table 1 Histological Changes in Psoriasis

Elongation and dilatation of capillaries in papillary dermis
Perivascular dermal inflammatory infiltration of:
Histiocytes
Lymphocytes
Neutrophil
Leukocytes
Invasion of PML and mononuclear cells into epidermis
Epidermal hyperproliferation

scale region, the aim of human treatment. Clearly, the method utilizes a surrogate rather than a clinical endpoint.

Drugs can be administered orally, topically, and subcutaneously. Slides of the tail section are examined microscopically for the formation of a granular layer, the induction of orthokeratosis in parakeratotic regions, and measurement of epidermal thickness. This last assay is important in evaluating the atrophic action of corticosteroids. Although drugs have been administered for up to 1 month, for topical treatments 6–7 days appear sufficient for maximal changes in epidermal thickness and granular layer to formation (2).

The mouse tail test is a simple, reproducible, rapid, and convenient test that allows observation of a drug's effect on both parakeratotic and neighboring orthokeratotic regions of the tail. Both regions must be monitored as application to only the parakeratotic skin of a patient is impossible. Several drugs have been tested in this model (Table 2), and their effects are reviewed by Wrench (2).

However, drawbacks include the following: The "lesions" seen on the tail are normal mouse, while the lesions of psoriasis are pathological. Therefore, although drugs may be shown to be effective in this model, their cellular actions do not target the pathogenesis of the disease but interrupt the gross expression of signs. This fact also casts doubt on the value of biochemical assays in this model, although they have been performed (3). Finally, as this model is a qualitative assay, the effects of different drugs cannot be quantified for screening purposes, so we now consider a modified version.

The Modified Mouse Tail Test

Bosman et al. (4) modified the mouse tail test, allowing quantification of the orthokeratosis so that the efficacy of various treatments can be compared. Longitudinal sections of the tails skin were stained with hematoxylin and eosin and the length of the granular layer measured microscopically using a semiautomatic image evaluation unit. This length can be expressed as a percentage of the total length of the scale, 100% being extension of the granular layer of the whole scale length. The activity of the drug could be expressed as a percentage score to allow comparison of the efficacy of different drugs and also different doses.

This model, more powerful than its predecessor, provides dose-response data on individual compounds and aids the calculation of effective doses for antipsoriatic activity.

Bosman (5) compared the efficacy of various antipsoriatic drugs, finding that the mean orthokeratosis induced by 3% dithranol and 1% retinoic acid, respectively, was 85% and 86% orthokeratosis compared to 29% in controls. The lipoxygenase inhibitors 10% cathechol and 10% octyl gallate induced 96% and 72% orthokeratosis, respectively, while immunosuppressive drugs showed weaker effects. The drugs inducing orthokeratosis also induce epidermal thickening in this model (Table 2).

Qualitatively, results seen in this model appear to correlate with clinical findings, and its quantitative features mark it as a rational method for screening drugs. However, as with all animal models, experimental data cannot be directly extrapolated to humans. Also, this model provides no data on the anti-inflammatory and antiproliferative actions of drugs.

The Flaky Skin Mouse (*fsn*) Model

A new model is the flaky skin (*fsn*) mouse, which is a mutant mouse with naturally occurring psoriasiform disease. This mutation, which has been mapped to distal chromosome 17 (9), encodes for histopathological and biochemical features similar to those seen in psoriasis. The mouse, clinically normal at birth, develops a patchy, thick, white scale that becomes evident 4 weeks later (10). Microscopic features include prominent acanthosis, orthokeratosis with focal parakeratosis, subcorneal pustules, infiltration of mononuclear cells into the dermis, and dilation of dermal capillaries (11). Transmission and scanning electron microscopy reveals increased epidermal thickness, mitochondrial abnormalities, and other ultrastructural features consistent with psoriasis (12). The elicitation of the Koebner phenomenon in this model highlights its resemblance to human psoriasis.

Favoring this model are the following: it is a naturally occurring chronic disease model; the model is

Table 2 Effects of Drugs on the Mouse Tail Test and Modified Mouse Tail Test

Compound	Response	Comment	Author(s)
	Mouse Tail Test		
Retinoids	Induction of granular layer Induction of orthokeratosis Epidermal thickening	Epidermal thickening can be reduced if combined with Ledercort cream	
Corticosteroids	Epidermal thinning (i.e., mitosis inhibited)	Strongest: fluocinolone acetonide cream 0.025% Weakest: hydrocortisone cream 1%	Spearman and Jarrett (6)
	Epidermal thinning	Strongest: flucinonide 0.05% Weakest: hydrocortisone 1%	Wrench (7)
	Dermal atrophy: Dermovate and Metosyn Induction of granular layer: Locoid and Dermovate Ointments		
Coal tar fractions	Basic and neutral fractions: thickened epidermis Phenolic fractions: thickened epidermis + granular layer induction	Max. effect at fraction 330–340°C	Wrench and Britten (8)
	Modified Mouse Tail Test		
Drug	Mean orthokeratosis (%)		Bosman (5) Bosman et al. (4)
Dithranol 3%	85.0		
Retinoic acid 1%	86.4		
Fumaric acid 10%	32.8		
Catechol 10%	95.8		
Octyl gallate 10%	63.0		
Cyclosporin A	26.1		
Beech tar	42.9		
Control	29.1		
Vehicle control	29.5		

histologically similar to psoriasis and DNA synthesis is elevated (13); it is convenient and stable. However, this is a nonhuman model of which the pathogenesis and etiology are unknown, so care must be taken in the interpretation of its results.

The Chronic Proliferative Dermatitis (*cpdm*) Mouse Model

The *cpdm* mouse mutant suffers from progressive lesions, which appear 5 weeks after birth (14). Fine scaling, partial alopecia, and erythema reportedly characterize these lesions, which notably spare the ears, footpad, and tail. Light microscopy revealed hyperproliferation of keratinocytes, epidermal infiltration of neutrophils, and dermal capillary dilatation and proliferation. As these lesions are consistent with psoriasiform histology, this model may potentially be of use in the trial of novel therapies.

The Asebia Mouse

A mutant strain of the BALB/c mouse, the *asebia*, has been used as a model of psoriasiform disease as it exhibits chronic epidermal hyperplasia and dermal inflammation. However, this model has provided paradoxical results when tested with known antipsoriatic agents, and as the mouse is histologically different from the typical histology of psoriasis, it is a poor model (Table 3) (15–17).

Beta-Adrenoceptor Antagonist Models

Beta-adrenoceptor antagonists, rarely, can induce iatrogenic psoriasiform eruptions (18), encouraging attempts to induce psoriasis in an animal model with these drugs. Gaylarde et al. (19) experimented on the shaved backs of albino guinea pigs. Either propranolol or practolol was applied topically to one side and a vehicle control contralaterally. One week of daily application of propranolol led to scaling, hyperkeratosis, and parakeratosis. Practolol and the vehicle did not cause a psoriasiform eruption. This experiment was repeated by Tuzun et al. (20), who failed to demonstrate psoriasiform changes in response to topical propranolol. However, they did find psoriasiform changes after 30 days of oral propranolol, reporting microabscess formation and parakeratosis in four of seven guinea pigs, and acanthosis and dermal inflammatory infiltration in all seven. These findings are again contradicted by Wolf et al. (21), who failed to reproduce any characteristic signs of psoriasis after 30 days of oral propranolol, even when supplemented with intradermal propranolol injections (Table 4).

Such contradictory findings support the conclusion that this model may lack the reproducibility necessary for a consistent, reliable therapeutic assay.

Hyperproliferative Models

In hyperproliferative models, the animal is not histologically similar to psoriasis. Rather, the tissues have a high cellular turnover, which workers attempt to inhibit, in the hope that the drug will also inhibit the hyperproliferation seen in psoriasis and thus provide clinical relief. These models cannot, therefore, be employed in the study of remittive therapies, but only as possible suppressants of cell proliferation.

Essential fatty acid (EFA)-deficient mice (fed an EFA-free diet) have an increased rate of DNA synthesis and also demonstrate acanthosis. As reducing DNA synthesis may lead to reduction in epidermal cell proliferation and clinical improvement, this model has been used to study antipsoriatics (22). To evaluate this model and another model with increased DNA synthesis, the *ultraviolet irradiated mouse*, Lowe et al. (23) correlated the findings from clinically used topical antipsoriatics to reductions in DNA synthesis seen in the mice. Surprisingly, they found that normal hairless mice gave better predictive results of human data than either of the two models. EFA mice gave many false positive predictions of effective drugs, possibly because of increased drug absorption through their modified skin. The UV mice did not give consistent control values, so this model was abandoned. Therefore, the best predictor was the normal hairless mouse, which correctly predicted six clinically effective drugs and gave only three false positives out of 28 drugs (Table 5).

The *mouse vaginal mucosa model* has been used to investigate the effects of antimitotic agents as the vaginal epithelium is hyperproliferative during the estrus phase of its cycle. Although assays of mitotic activity can be performed by autoradiography and isotopic techniques (24), they have poor predictive value (25) and did not shed light on the drug's actions in a psoriasiform setting. The estrus phase lasts only 1 day, so the model cannot be used for chronic studies.

DNA Synthesis Suppression Model

Yoshino and Maibach (26) report that antipsoriatic DNA synthesis inhibitors have a different mechanism of action from DNA synthesis inhibitors that are not effective in psoriasis. Their study of ^{3}H-thymidine incorporation into normal hairless mice demonstrated different profiles of cellular activity on a linear time scale. All of the drugs initially suppressed synthesis within 3–12 hr of administration, but only drugs effective clinically induced a late increase in DNA synthesis above the original control values while nonantipsoriatic treatment DNA synthesis values returned to baseline (Table 6). As the rebound phenomenon resulting from clinically effective drugs was large, the authors postulate that effective antipsoriatic therapy may involve two components: suppression of DNA synthesis and its recovery in cycling cells, and the additional stimulation of a fraction of cells into the cell cycle for a limited period. Nonantipsoriatic treatments do not exhibit a rebound phenomenon, suggesting that there is no recruitment of additional cells into the cell cycle.

This difference between therapeutic and nontherapeutic drugs may be a basis for screening new therapies; potentially efficacious drugs may be identified by the rebound phenomenon, and others excluded. The repetition of these results with more drugs will demonstrate whether this model may be used as a standard bench test for novel antiproliferative drugs.

Table 3 Effects of Antipsoriatic Drugs on the Asebia Mouse Model

Drug	Effect (20 days, 21 days)	Comment	Author
Triamcinolone acetonide 0.25%	Decreased epidermal LI Increased epidermal thickness		Brown and Hardy (15)
Retinoic acid 0.25%/0.05%	Skin inflammation Increased epidermal thickness Increased epidermal LI	No inflammation at 0.05% Distant site involvement	
Anthralin 0.25%	Increased LI Increased epidermal thickness	Distant site involvement	
Anthralin 0.05%	As above at 10 days Control levels at 20 days	No distal involvement at 20 days	
UVB	No change in LI or epidermal thickness		Rogozinski et al. (18)
UVB + anthralin 0.25%	Increased LI Increased epidermal thickness		
Coal tar + UVB	Increased LI Increased epidermal thickness	Erythema	

LI = labeling index.

Xenographic Models

Transplanting human psoriatic tissue to animals for study aims to provide an ethical method of screening drugs on human tissue. Using an animal host potentially broadens the scope of study on human tissue without the complications of using people.

The Athymic (Nude) Mouse Model

Nude mice are congenitally athymic and thus unable to mount a cell-mediated immune response; they cannot reject transplanted skin grafts. Kruger et al. (27) transplanted punch biopsies of human psoriatic skin of variable thickness into nude mice. The skin survived for the life span of the mouse (approx. 11 weeks) and retained some psoriatic features. However, the value of this model is debatable. Although the skin does have some psoriasiform features, such as clubbing of the rete ridges, acanthosis, and parakeratosis, these features were not seen consistently. Kruger et al. (28) also demonstrated that although the rate of DNA synthesis in transplanted psoriatic skin was higher than in transplanted normal grafted skin, it had fallen markedly compared to its original level in the host. This demonstrates that maintenance of the xenograft is dependent on human host factors. Also, it has been shown that grafts are infiltrated by mouse lymphocytes. Thus, this model is of limited value in testing pharmacological preparations for human use: it requires a large volume of skin to be donated from human volunteers, and it remains uncertain whether the data would be relevant to human psoriasis as the tissue's behavior has changed. This model is of no value in long-term studies as athymic mice have a life expectancy of about 12 weeks.

The Severe Combined Immunodeficiency Mouse Model

Nickoloff et al. (29) report the maintenance of the psoriatic features of human skin transplants into severe combined immunodeficiency (SCID) mice. These mice are also incapable of mounting an immune response to xenografts, allowing in vivo study of human psoriatic skin. Both gross plaque characteristics and microscopic changes including hyperkeratosis, parakeratosis, acanthosis, elongation of rete ridges, dermal inflammatory infiltration, and dilatation of blood vessels were reported. However, the grafts were left in place for only 4–6 weeks, so the long-term gross and histological stability of the model remains to be proven. Although it is a potential tool for studying pathogenesis, this model is also beset by the drawbacks afflicting the nude mouse.

Transgenic Mouse Models

The expression of suprabasal integrins on the epidermis of transgenic mice results in abnormal histology. Psoriasiform changes including epidermal hyperplasia, acanthosis, and alternating regions of orthokera-

Table 4 Comparison of Guinea Pig Skin Changes After Beta Blockers

Drug, route and concentration	Effect
Gaylarde et al. (19)	
Topical propranolol 1%	Scaling; erythema; hyperkeratosis; parakeratosis
Topical propranolol 5%	Patchy, mixed cellular infiltrate around panniculus adiposus, scaling, erythema, hyperkeratosis, parakeratosis
Topical practolol 1%	No psoriasiform changes
Topical practolol 5%	No psoriasiform changes
Vehicle: emulsifying ointment	No psoriasiform changes
Tuzun et al. (20)	
Topical propranolol 5%	Acanthosis and papillomatosis (n = 6)
Oral propranolol 2 mg/day	Acanthosis and cellular infiltration at 30 days (n = 7) Parakeratosis and microabscesses (n = 4)
Oral saline control	Acanthosis and dermal cellular infiltration (n = 3) No change (n = 4)
Wolf et al. (21)	
Oral propranolol 2 mg/day	Normal epidermis and dermis at 30 days
Oral (2 mg/day) and intradermal propranolol injection (weekly)	Acanthosis, hypergranulosis, mild cellular infiltrate (no parakeratosis, no microabscesses or papillomatosis)
Control	Normal epidermis and dermis

tosis and parakeratosis have been reported in mice expressing the β_1 subunit, either alone or in combination with the α_2 or α_5 subunit (30). Further, neutrophil pustules similar to Munro microabscesses, a dermal inflammatory infiltrate, and capillary dilatation were also described. The resemblance is highlighted as ICAM-1 was induced and Ki-67 labeling was increased, as is the case in psoriasis (31). Carroll et al. (30) claim that this model most accurately resembles psoriasis; its predictive power for drug therapies remains to be demonstrated.

IN VITRO MODELS

Keratinocyte Culture Models

Cultures from Psoriasis Patients

Much work has been devoted to culturing keratinocytes from the involved and uninvolved cells of psoriasis patients in the hope that these cultures would form a large resource for experimental work. Rheinwald and Green (32) developed a successful culture technique by using mitomycin C–treated or irradiated mouse mesenchymal (3T3) cells as a feeder layer to enhance keratinocyte proliferation and suppress fibroblast growth. Improvements have been made, such as the addition of mitogens (epidermal growth factor, cAMP-elevating agents, and hydrocortisone) (33–35). Miyauchi et al. (36) have demonstrated that lesional psoriatic keratinocytes can be cultured, without fibroblasts, in high calcium concentrations by elevating the cells from the bottom of the culture dish with a collagen membrane. This technique allows the keratinocytes to be exposed to calcium concentrations similar to human extracellular fluid. Kragballe et al. (37) demonstrated that uninvolved psoriatic cells also maintained an increased DNA synthesis in vitro, suggesting that this defect was an inherent property of the keratinocytes. The workers also showed that terminal events of cellular differentiation did occur in their culture system as large-molecular-weight keratins could be found, unlike other culture systems in which these two properties could not be maintained.

Reconstitution of psoriasis biopsies in vitro without the use of epidermal separation or cell trypsinization has been employed to optimize maintenance of the psoriasiform phenotype in vitro. However, Mils et al. (38) demonstrate that normal and psoriatic reconstituted epidermis do not differ in their proliferation and differentiation markers, as they do in vivo. Indeed, they found that Ki-67 antigen expression was higher in normal cells than in psoriasis cells, indicating that the in vitro proliferation index of the normal epidermis was increased and that of psoriasis epidermis was decreased. It may be, therefore, that fibroblasts, inflammatory cells, or other nonskin factors are necessary for the maintenance of the psoriasiform phenotype in vitro. If this is the case, then doubt is cast over the

Table 5 Comparison of Drug Effects in Psoriasis Patients to Animal Models

Drug	Psoriasis patient response	Normal mouse model response	EFA-deficient mouse model
Betamethasone valerate	**	**	**
Cycloheximide	**	**	**
Emetine hydrochloride	**	**	—
Fluorouracil	**	**	*
Methyl GAG	**	—	—
Thiotepa	**	**	**
Azacytidine	*	—	—
Azaserine	*	—	—
Azathioprine	*	—	—
Cisplatin	*	—	*
Colchicine	*	—	—
Dactinomycin	*	—	—
Guanazole	*	—	—
Hydroxyurea	*	—	—
Vinblastine sulfate	*	*	**
Azaribine	—	—	*
Cyclocytidine	—	—	—
Cycloleucine	—	—	—
Dacarbarzine	—	**	—
Dichloromethotrexate	—	—	—
Etopside	—	—	—
Idoxuridine	—	—	—
Mercaptopurine	—	—	**
Scopolamine hydrobromide	—	—	—
Thioguanine	—	—	**
Vincristine sulfate	—	*	—

**Strong improvement; *weal improvement; —no improvement.
Source: Ref. 23.

Table 6 Comparison of the Effects of Antipsoriatic and Nonantipsoriatic Drugs on the Suppression of DNA Synthesis

Drug	Specific acitivty (% control) (DNA synthesis *suppression*)	Onset	Duration	Rebound specific activity (% control)	Duration
Antipsoriatics					
Anthralin 0.1%/1%	80–90% suppression	<6 hr	24 hr	300–500	6–8 days
Cyclohexamide 0.1%	80% suppression		6 hr	240	>8 days
1.0%	90% suppression		2 days	400	
Triamcinolone acetonide 0.1%	80% suppression		24 hr	150	6 days
1.0%	90% suppression		2 days	200	8 days
Nonantipsoriatics					
Ara-cytidine 1%/5%	75–80% suppression	<3 hr	24 hr	No effect	
Vincristine sulfate 0.03%/3%	50–60% suppression		2 days	No effect	

Source: Ref. 26.

role of current in vitro models in pharmacological evaluation. Skin organ culture has been extensively reviewed by Tammi et al. (39).

Organ Culture

Human organotypic cultures of outer root sheath (ORS) cells have been proposed as a model for evaluating antipsoriatics (40). These hair follicular cells express keratins 6, 16, and 17, which are associated with hyperproliferation and are absent in the nonpsoriatic epidermis. In culture, these cells form a psoriasiform stratified squamous epithelium, which is hyperplastic, has a poorly developed granular layer, and expresses hyperproliferative keratins. However, this model may be useful only in the study of antiproliferative agents and is not sufficiently psoriasiform to allow adequate study of drug effects on multiple disease characteristics.

Nonpsoriatic Cultures

Cultures of nonpsoriatic cells, used as an in vitro assay technique, measure the action of drugs on individual characteristics of the disease, such as hyperproliferation. For example, Sebök et al. (41) demonstrated that dimethylfumarate was the main antiproliferative agent in the fumaric acid therapy regime. However, it is unlikely that nonpsoriatic in vitro models can predict therapeutic efficacy, as their results cannot be interpreted in the context of psoriasis.

Summary

Despite these efforts to culture psoriatic keratinocytes, uncertainty remains when considering in vitro models for drug testing. Immunological dissimilarities to human skin have been demonstrated and the effects of removing the cells from their host are not clear. As the etiology of psoriasis is unknown, any potential therapeutic model must be as similar as possible to the human disease. It is not known which of the features of the disease are most relevant for pharmacological activity. Until this is known, we cannot target a particular mechanism but must employ macromodels for the blanket testing of drug efficacy.

HUMAN STUDIES

The use of humans is the ultimate evaluation of a drug's efficacy but raises ethical dilemmas. Any study done at the human level must be a double-blind, randomized, controlled clinical trial. A standard scale must be employed to assess the results objectively and patients must be matched for age, sex, life-style, and other social factors that may influence their motivation and compliance.

Tape Stripping

Tape stripping the epidermis of psoriatic patients has been shown to result in the formation of prepinpoint psoriatic papules (42). The effect of tape stripping is to induce the enzyme ornithine decarboxylase (ODC), which is the rate-limiting enzyme in the formation of polyamines, which are elevated in epidermal hyperplasia (43,44). Arnold et al. (45) used this model to study the effect of potential antipsoriatics on human skin. ODC activity was used to assay the activity of protein kinase C, as drugs that inhibit protein kinase C are thought to have an antipsoriatic action. Sphingosine did inhibit ODC, but showed no clinical improvement, and neither isoquinolone nor tannic acid inhibited ODC and neither showed clinical improvement. Indeed, sphingosine caused epidermal necrolysis. These results demonstrate the dangers and difficulties of extrapolating animal data into a clinical setting.

Gerritsen et al. (46) used repeated tape stripping to show that cyclosporin A did not directly modulate epidermal hyperproliferation and abnormal keratinization in vivo. Fisher and associates reported on the effect of physical modalities on stripped skin (47–50). These studies show that the tape-stripping model does have role in the evaluation of drug effects; however, it is seriously limited as a mass screening tool as patients cannot ethically be exposed to potential toxins.

Ultrasound

Vaillant et al. (51) reported the differences between normal and psoriatic skin on ultrasound: psoriatic skin had increased epidermal, dermal, and whole skin thickness, and a wide subepidermal nonechogenic band was seen. These changes were significantly different from controls, and were also significantly different from the disease state after treatment. As these changes can be quantified, it may be possible to use this model as an accurate, objective, noninvasive method of drug evaluation.

Vasoconstrictor Assay of Topical Corticosteroids

Studied by means of a randomized, double-blind, clinical trial, with both positive and negative controls, this model has been shown to correlate the efficacy of topical corticosteroids with degrees of vasoconstriction (52,53). A four-point visual measurement scale was used to assess blanching after 16 hr of occlusive application of topical corticosteroids: the degree of blanching correlated with the clinical efficacy for 20 of the 23 drugs tested. This model appears to be a simple and rapid method of evaluating a steroid's efficacy in an individual psoriasis patient. Additional details on corticosteroids are provided in another chapter.

CONCLUSION

Although many models have been presented, those that have been predictors of therapeutic ability are the mouse tail test, the modified mouse tail test, the normal hairless mouse model, the DNA synthesis suppression model, and the vasoconstrictor assay of topical corticosteroids. We suggest that a more systematic examination and refinement of these models might improve our ability to identify active compounds.

REFERENCES

1. Jarrett, A., and Spearman, R.I.C. (1970). Vitamin A and the skin. *Br. J. Dermatol.* 82:197–199.
2. Wrench, R. (1985). Assessing drugs for psoriasiform diseases and their anti-parakeratotic mechanisms using the mouse tail test. In *Models in Dermatology*, H.I. Maibach and N.J. Lowe (Eds.). Karger, Basel, pp. 76–91.
3. Bladon, P.T., Cooper, N.F., Wood, E.J., and Cunliffe, W.J. (1986). Biochemical markers in the mouse tail model of psoriasis. In *Skin Models. Models to Study Function and Disease of Skin*. R. Marks and G. Plewig. (Eds.). Springer-Verlag, Berlin, 1986.
4. Bosman, B., Matthiesen, T., Hess, V., and Frederichs, E. (1922). A quantitative method for measuring antipsoriatic activity of drugs by the mouse tail test. *Skin Pharmacol.* 5:41–48.
5. Bosman, B. (1994). Testing of lipoxygenase inhibitors, cyclooxygenase inhibitors drugs with immunomodulating properties and some reference antipsoriatic drugs in the modified mouse tail test, an animal model of psoriasis. *Skin Pharmacol.* 7:324–334.
6. Spearman, R.I.C., and Jarrett, A. (1975). Bio-assay of corticosteroids for topical application. *Br. J. Dermatol.* 92:581–584.
7. Wrench, R. (1980). Epidermal thinning: evaluation of commercial corticosteroids. *Arch. Dermatol. Res.* 267: 7–24.
8. Wrench, R., and Britten, A.Z. (1975). Evaluation of coal tar fractions for use in psoriasiform diseases using the mouse tail test. III. High boiling tar oil acids. *Br. J. Dermatol.* 93:67–74.
9. Pelsue, S.C., Schweitzer, P.A., Beamer, W.G., and Shultz, L.D. (1995). Mapping of the flaky skin (*fsn*) mutation on distal mouse chromosome 17. *Mammal. Genome* 6(10):758.
10. Sundberg, J.P., Boggess, D., Sundberg, B.A., Beamer, W.G., and Schultz, L.D. (1993). Epidermal dendritic cell populations in the flaky skin mutant mouse. *Immunol. Invest.* 22(5):389–401.
11. Sundberg, J.P., Beamer, W.G., Schultz, L.D., and Dunstan, R.W. (1990). Inherited mouse mutations as models of human adnexial, cornification and papulosquamous dermatoses. *J. Invest. Dermatol.* 95: 62S–63S.
12. Morita, K., Hogan, M.E., Nanney, L.B., King, L.E., Jr., Manabe, M., Sun, T.T., and Sundberg, J.P. (1995). Cutaneous ultrastructural features of the flakey skin (*fsn*) mouse mutation. *J. Dermatol.* 22(6):385–395.
13. Sundberg, J.P., Dunstan, R.W., Roop, D.R., and Beamer, W.G. (1994). Full thickness skin grafts from flaky skin mice to nude mice: maintenance of the psoriasiform phenotype. *J. Invest. Dermatol.* 102(5): 781–788.
14. Sundberg, J.P. (1996). Mouse models for scaly skin diseases. In *Dermatologic Research Techniques*. H.I. Maibach (Ed.). CRC Press, Orlando, FL.
15. Brown, W.R., and Hardy M.H. (1985). The asebia mouse: An animal model of psoriasiform disease. In *Models in Dermatology*, vol. 1. H.I. Maibach and N.J. Lowe. (Eds.). Karger, Basel, pp. 220–227.
16. Brown, W.R., and Hardy, M.H. (1984). Effects of topical triamcinolone acetonide, retinoic acid and anthralin on asebia mouse skin. *J. Invest. Dermatol.* 84: 412.
17. Arntzen, N., Kavli, G., and Volden, G. (1984). Psoriasis provoked by beta-blocking agents. *Acta Derm. Venereol. (Stockh.)* 64:346–348.
18. Rogozinski, T.T., Brown, W.R., and Ramsay, C.A. (1986). The effect of UVB, anthralin and tar on asebia mouse epidermis. *J. Invest. Dermatol.* 86:503.
19. Gaylarde, P.M., Brock, A.P., and Sarkany, I. (1987). Psoriatic changes in guinea pig skin from propranolol. *Clin. Exp. Dermatol.* 3:157.
20. Tuzun, B., Tuzun, Y., Gurel, N., Tuzuner, N., Altug, T., and Buyukdevrim, S. (1993). Psoriasis-like lesions in guinea pigs receiving propranolol. *Int. J. Dermatol.* 32(2):133–134.

21. Wolf, R., Shechter, H., and Brenner, S. (1994). Induction of psoriasiform changes in guinea pig skin by propranolol. *Int. J. Dermatol.* 33(11):811–814.
22. Lowe, N.J., and Stiughton, R.B. (1977). Essential fatty acid deficient hairless mouse: a model of chronic epidermal hyperproliferation. *Br. J. Dermatol.* 96:155.
23. Lowe, N.J., McCullough, J.L., and Weinstein, G.D. (1985). Topical antiproliferative and antipsoriatic drug assays. In *Models in Dermatology*, vol. 2. H.I. Maibach and N.J. Lowe (Eds.). Karger, Basel, pp. 43–52.
24. McCullough, J.L., and Weinstein, G.D. (1975). Mouse vaginal assay for topically effective chemotherapeutic agents. *J. Invest. Dermatol.* 65:394.
25. Hartman, M.E., McCullough, J.L., and Weinstein, G.D. (1981). Mechanisms of chemotherapeutic drug action in mouse vaginal epithelium. Predictive value for topical anti-psoriatic drugs. *Arch. Dermatol.* 117: 499–403.
26. Yoshino, K., and Maibach, H.I. (1991). Mechanism of topical chemotherapy. In *Psoriasis*, 2nd ed. H.I. Maibach and H.H. Roenigk, Jr. (Eds.). Marcel Dekker, New York, pp. 937–944.
27. Kruger, G., Manning, D.D., Malouf, J., and Ogden, B. (1975). Long term maintenance of psoriatic skin on congenitally athymic (nude) mice. *J. Invest. Dermatol.* 64:307–312.
28. Kruger, G., Chambers, D., and Shellby, J. (1981). Involved and uninvolved skin of psoriatic subjects: are they equally diseased? Assessed by skin transplanted into congenitally athymic (nude) mice. *J. Invest. Dermatol.* 68:1548–1557.
29. Nickoloff, B.J., Kunkel, S.L., Burdick, M., and Streiter, R.M. (1995). Severe combined immunodeficiency mouse and human psoriatic skin chimeras. Validation of a new animal model. *Am. J. Pathol.* 146(3): 580–588.
30. Carroll, J.M., Romero, M.R., and Watt, F.M. (1995). Suprabasal integrin expression in the epidermis of transgenic mice results in developmental defects and a phenotype resembling psoriasis. *Cell* 83(6):957–968.
31. Paukkonen, K., Naukkarinen, A., and Horsmanheimo, M. (1995). The development of manifest psoriatic lesions is linked with the appearance of ICAM-1 positivity on keratinocytes. *Arch. Dermatol. Res.* 287(2): 165–170.
32. Rheinwald, T.G., and Green, H. (1975). Serial cultivation of strains of human epidermal keratinocytes: the formation of keratinizing colonies from single cells. *Cell* 6:331–344.
33. Liu, S.C., and Karasek, M. (1978). Isolation and growth of adult human epidermal keratinocytes in cell culture. *J. Invest. Dermatol.* 71:157–162.
34. Rheinwald, J.G., and Green, H. (1977). Epidermal growth factor and the multiplication of cultured human keratinocytes. *Nature* 265:421–444.
35. Liu, S.C., and Parsons, S.C. (1983). Serial cultivation of epidermal keratinocytes from psoriatic plaques. *J. Invest. Dermatol.* 81:54–61.
36. Miyauchi, Y., Misuhashi, Y., Kikuchi, T., and Hashimoto, I. (1995). Feasibility of in vitro culturing of lesional psoriatic keratinocytes in medium containing high calcium concentrations. *Arch. Dermatol. Res.* 287:731–734.
37. Kragballe, K., Desjarkais, L., and Marcelo, C.L. (1985). Increased DNA synthesis of uninvolved psoriatic epidermis is maintained in vitro. *Br. J. Dermatol.* 112:263–270.
38. Mils, V., Basset-Séguin, N., Molès, J.-P., Tesnière, A., Leigh, I., and Guilhou, J.-J. (1994). Comparative analysis of normal and psoriatic skin both in vivo and in vitro. *Differentiation* 58:77–86.
39. Tammi, R., Saamanen, A.-M., Maibach, H.I., and Tammi, M. (1991). Degradation of newly synthesized high molecular mass hyaluronan in the epidermal and dermal compartments of human skin in organ culture. *J. Invest. Dermatol.* 97(1):126–130.
40. Limat, A., Hunziker, T., and Braathen, L.R. (1993). Effects of 1α,25-dihydroxy-vitamin D3 and calcipotriol on organotypic cultures of outer root sheath cells: a potential model to evaluate antipsoriatic drugs. *Arch. Dermatol. Res.* 285:402–409.
41. Sebök, B., Bonnekoh, B., Geisel, J., and Mahrle, G. (1994). Antiproliferative and cytotoxic profiles of antipsoriatic fumaric acid derivatives in keratinocyte cultures. *Eur. J. Pharmacol. Environ. Toxicol. Pharmacol.* 270:79–87.
42. Jablonska, S., Chowaniec, O., Beutner, E.H., Maciejowska, E., Jarzabek-Chorzelska, M., and Rzesa, G. (1982). Stripping of the stratum corneum in patients with psoriasis: production of prepinpoint papules and psoriatic lesions. *Arch. Dermatol.* 118:652–657.
43. Connor, M.J., and Lowe, N.J. (1982). The induction of ornithine decarboxylase activity and DNA synthesis in hairless mouse epidermis by retinoids. *J. Invest. Dermatol.* 79:189–193.
44. Lowe, N.J. (1988). Psoriasis. In vivo models for topical drug evaluation. *Drug Dev. Res.* 13:147–155.
45. Arnold, P.W., Glade, C.P., Mier, P.D., and van de Kerhof, P.C.M. (1993). Effects of sphingosine, isoquinolone and tannic acid on the human tape-stripping model and the psoriatic lesion. *Skin Pharmacol.* 6: 193–199.
46. Gerritsen, M.J.P., Rulo, H.F.C., Arnold, W.P., and van de Kerkhof, P.C.M. (1994). Response of the clinically uninvolved skin of psoriatic patients to repeated tape stripping during cyclosporin A treatment. *Br. J. Dermatol.* 130:180–188.
47. Fisher, L., and Maibach, H.I. (1972). Effect of occlusive and semipermeable dressings on the mitotic activity of normal and wounded human epidermis. *Br. J. Dermatol.* 86:593–599.

48. Fisher, L., and Maibach, H.I. (1973). Topical antipsoriatic agents and epidermal mitosis in man. *Arch. Dermatol.* 108:374–377.
49. Fisher, L., and Maibach, H.I. (1975). Effect of anthralin and its derivatives on epidermal cell kinetic. *J. Invest. Dermatol.* 64:338–341.
50. Fisher, L., Maibach, H.I., and Tracik, R. (1978). Effects of occlusive tape systems on the mitotic activity of epidermis. *Arch. Dermatol.* 114:384–386.
51. Vaillant, L., Berson, M., Machet. L., Callens, A., Pourcelot, L., and Lorette, G. (1994). Ultrasound imaging of psoriatic skin: a noninvasive technique to evaluate treatment of psoriasis. *Int. J. Dermatol.* 33(11): 786–790.
52. Cornell, R.C. (1992). Clinical trials of topical corticosteroids in psoriasis: correlations with the vasoconstrictor assay. *Int. J. Dermatol.* (Suppl. 1):38–40.
53. Cornell, R.C., and Stoughton, R.B. (1985). Correlation of the vasoconstriction assay and clinical activity in psoriasis. *Arch. Dermatol.* 121:63–67.

60

Psoriasis Small Plaque Assay for Assessment of Topical Drug Activity

Antti I. Lauerma
University of Helsinki, Helsinki, Finland

Howard I. Maibach
University of California School of Medicine, San Francisco, California

Psoriasis is a multifactorial disease of unknown etiology as well as a pathomechanism that has not been fully clarified (1). However, it is well established that inflammatory processes play a role in its manifestation. Psoriasis is unique to humans; no verified animal models are available. As in vitro systems have their limitations, it cannot be known whether a drug may be efficacious in psoriasis in vivo before documentation in humans.

Medications for psoriasis can be divided into two groups, systemic and topical. The psoriasis plaque assay screens for topical drug activity. Small areas of psoriatic lesions are exposed to different topical preparations under occlusion, which enhances drug delivery. Alternatively, open application may be used if considered more useful. The psoriasis microplaque assay permits the study of several different drug preparations at the same time, as well as having a low likelihood of systemic side effects from absorbed drugs.

The microplaque assay has been utilized in comparing the efficacy of corticosteroids (2) and topical immunosuppressants SDZ 281-240 (3) and tacrolimus (4). Additionally, it has been used in a multicenter study to prove its efficacy in detecting new potential antipsoriatic topical drugs (5). Its use as a standard may also enable development of better animal and in vitro psoriasis models.

PROTOCOL

Patient Selection

Patients with diagnosed plaque-type psoriasis are suitable for the assay. However, there is little experience with the assay in other types of psoriasis, such as pustular psoriasis, erythrodermic psoriasis, or inverse psoriasis. Psoriasis guttata patients are not suitable because the lesions are too small. Patients selected for study should have had a stable disease condition for at least several months.

Patients may be of either sex. Use of children is not recommended. The patients should have at least one plaque that is at least the size of the microplaque assay planned. The plaque should be homogeneous with respect to erythema and infiltration.

Female patients of childbearing age should use adequate birth control during the trial. The patients should understand the purpose of the trial, the protocol, and the possible risks involved. Pregnant patients, those who are breast feeding, or who have uncontrolled infections, a history of malignancy, HIV, or known hypersensitivity to study drug preparation components should not partake. A washout period of 4 weeks is recommended for systemic or UV radiation therapy and 1 week for topical treatment on plaques chosen for study. Other plaques may be treated topically during the washout period and trial.

Pretreatment

Selected target lesion(s) may be pretreated on the first visit overnight with 2% salicylic acid in white petrolatum to remove the scales. On the second visit (1 day later) the salicylic acid in petrolatum is removed.

Treatment Phase

The preparations are applied to target lesions with the microplaque assay for 5–14 days or longer. The patient is monitored for efficacy and safety of each preparation applied to the microplaques.

Posttreatment Phase

The patient is seen, if deemed useful, 7–28 days after discontinuation of the treatment for assessment of the microplaques and the general condition of the psoriasis.

Controls

A negative control (vehicle, placebo), positive control (such as a corticoid), and an untreated site (chamber control) provide useful benchmarks.

Microplaque Assay

The microplaque assay should be done in a controlled, double-blind manner. This is mandatory especially when only clinical assessment is done.

The microplaque assay method can be performed with 60-μl Finn Chambers (Epitest Ltd., Hyryla, Finland) with an outer diameter of 17 mm and inner diameter of 11 mm. Finn Chambers have been designed for patch testing; other patch test systems can also be used. Alternatively, other occlusive systems may be devised.

At the end of the second visit the chambers are filled with study medications, 60 μl for each Finn Chamber, according to a randomization code. Chambers are attached to paper tape and the tape with the chambers applied to the psoriasis plaque. The distance between chambers should be at least 15 mm, as such a distance would not allow horizontal spread of drugs to adjacent chamber sites to affect the result (6). Without changing the position of the tape and chambers on plaque, a plastic bandage (Tegaderm) may be applied on top of the plaque, tape, and chambers. The plastic bandage allows the patient to wash him/herself during study without wetting the tape or chambers.

At each exchange the bandages, tape, chambers, and medications are removed. Assessment (see below) can be done after removal of assay materials. After this, a new set of medications (according to code), chambers, tape, and plastic bandage are applied.

The application of the medications and assessment of efficacy should be done by separate personnel to avoid biased assessments.

Assessment of Efficacy

Assessment can be done on the plaques by clinical scoring (2–5), with laser-Doppler flow measurements of the superficial blood flow of the plaques (4), with ultrasound to measure the thickness of the skin (4), and/or by histological examination from punch biopsies (3,4) with possible in situ immunostainings (3) or hybridizations.

Clinical score may be done for both erythema and infiltration according to the following scale: 0 = no evidence; 1 = mild; 2 = moderate; 3 = severe; 4 = very severe. Scaling may also be graded.

Laser-Doppler measurement is done with standardized equipment after a rest of at least 10 min. The measurement should take place in controlled temperature (20–23°C) to avoid the influence of temperature on skin blood flow.

Ultrasound measurements should be done with specific skin ultrasound devices. A frequency of 30 MHz enables both adequate accuracy and depth of signal return.

Histopathological examinations may be done from 2–3-mm punch biopsies taken from microplaques at the last visit of the treatment phase. Routine staining methods are used but immunohistochemistry, as well as in situ hybridization, may provide further insights to the effects of drugs studied.

PSORIASIS MICROPLAQUE ASSAY WITH OPEN APPLICATION

As shown recently by Baadsgaard and colleagues (7), psoriasis plaques may be used in a similar manner as with the psoriasis microplaque assay when open application is studied. In their study, different concentrations of tacalcitol, a vitamin D derivative, were applied once a day. The application was performed as with the occluded microplaque assay, except that the study preparations were rubbed on the psoriasis plaque through a template hole of 2 cm in diameter, ensuring that the surrounding plaque area was not rubbed. The study enabled finding an optimal tacalcitol concentration for psoriasis treatment when open application once a day is used (7).

OTHER METHODS TO STUDY TOPICAL DRUG ACTIVITY FOR PSORIASIS

The details on in vitro and animal models for psoriasis drug study are provided in another chapter.

CONCLUSIONS

The psoriasis microplaque assay provides an accurate and relatively rapid method to assess the efficacy of topical drugs intended for psoriasis. The assay usually provides information in the occluded condition. Therefore, it cannot be known whether an efficacious drug in occluded microplaque assay would also be efficacious as an open application, until such application is performed, as an open application psoriasis plaque assay (7) or as such application on whole plaques.

In the absence of animal and in vitro models for psoriasis, microplaque assay should provide the safest way to predict the antipsoriatic potential of new compounds or the effect of delivery systems (e.g., vehicle). Further, it can serve as a standard method to develop alternative methods. It can also be used to study the effect of biological topical modulators to gain insight into psoriasis itself.

REFERENCES

1. Fry, L. (1988). Psoriasis. *Br. J. Dermatol.* 119: 445–461.
2. Dumas, K.J., and Scholtz, J.R. (1972). The psoriasis bio-assay for topical corticosteroid activity. *Acta Derm. Venereol. (Stockh.)* 52:43–48.
3. Rappersberg, K., Meingassner, J.G., Fialla, R., Fodinger, D., Sterniczky, B., Rauch, S., Putz, E., Stutz, A., and Wolff, K. (1996). Clearing of psoriasis by a novel immunosuppressive macrolide. *J. Invest. Dermatol.* 106:701–710.
4. Remitz, A., Reitamo, S., Erkko, P., Granlund, H., and Lauerma, A.I. (1996). A microplaque assay-based, double-blind trial to compare the efficacy of two tacrolimus ointment formulations with two active and two negative controls in patients with chronic plaque-type psoriasis vulgaris. Presented at Psoriasis: From Gene to Clinic, London, December 5–7.
5. Weinstein, G.D., McGullough, J.L., Eaglestein, W.H., Golub, A., Cornell, R.C., Stoughton, R.B., Clendenning, W., Zackheim, H., Maibach, H.I., Kulp, K.R., King, L., Baden, H.P., Taylor, J.S., and Deneau, D.D. (1981). A clinical screening program for topical chemotherapeutic drugs in psoriasis. *Arch. Dermatol.* 117: 388–393.
6. Bruze, M., Isaksson, M., and Dooms-Goossens, A. (1995). The influence of patch tests with clobetasol propionate on adjacent patch test reactions. *Contact Derm.* 32:167–170.
7. Baadsgaard, O., Traulsen, J., Roed-Petersen, J., and Jakobsen, H.B. (1995). Optimal concentration of tacalcitol in once-daily treatment of psoriasis. *J. Dermatol. Treat.* 6:145–150.

61

Topical Retinoids

Gerald D. Weinstein
University of California School of Medicine, Irvine, California

Roshantha A.S. Chandraratna
Allergan, Inc., Irvine, California

BRIEF HISTORY OF RETINOIDS IN DERMATOLOGY

Retinoids include retinol (vitamin A_1), the primary circulating form, and a variety of naturally occurring and synthetic derivatives of retinol (Marcus and Coulson, 1990). The structures of representative examples of the various "generations" of retinoids are shown in Figure 1, and their possible clinical applications are shown in Table 1.

Generations of Retinoids

Early attempts to use retinol or its ester, retinyl palmitate, to treat dermatoses such as psoriasis were largely unsuccessful because oral doses were too toxic and topical doses were ineffective (Kligman, 1987). Retinoic acid (vitamin A acid, tretinoin), the carboxylic acid derivative of retinol, is an endogenous metabolite and is believed to be responsible for many of the physiological functions of retinoids (Goss and McBurney, 1992). Both retinoic acid and its geometric isomer 13-*cis*-retinoic acid (iso-tretinoin) have been widely used clinically for the topical and oral treatment, respectively, of acne. Although an initial study of the use of topical retinoic acid in psoriasis was promising (Frost and Weinstein, 1969), subsequent investigations with both topical and oral forms have indicated that retinoic acid is of doubtful therapeutic value in psoriasis because of varying efficacy and unacceptable toxicity (Fredriksson, 1971; MacDonald et al., 1972; Günther, 1973; Orfanos et al., 1973).

Several different topical formulations of retinoic acid are currently being evaluated for acne and photoaging indications. An oral formulation (Vesanoid) has recently been approved for the treatment of acute promyelocytic leukemia. Also, another geometric isomer of retinoic acid, 9-*cis*-retinoic acid (ALRT 1057), has been tested in phase II clinical trials for the oral treatment of cancers and topical treatment of Kaposi's sarcoma (Boehm et al., 1995).

A second generation of retinoids, the aromatic retinoids, was developed by modifying the lipophilic end group of retinoic acid (Orfanos et al., 1985). Two derivatives of this class, etretinate and acitretin, have been used successfully for the oral treatment of psoriasis (Marcus and Coulson, 1990; Goss and McBurney, 1992). However, by the topical route, acitretin (1% cream) had no beneficial effects in psoriasis (Orfanos et al., 1987).

A third generation of highly potent retinoids, the arotinoids, was developed by structural modifications that incorporated the double bonds of the polyolefinic side chain of retinoic acid into aromatic rings (Loeliger et al., 1980). The arotinoid ethyl ester, Ro 13-6298, was an effective antipsoriatic agent at very low

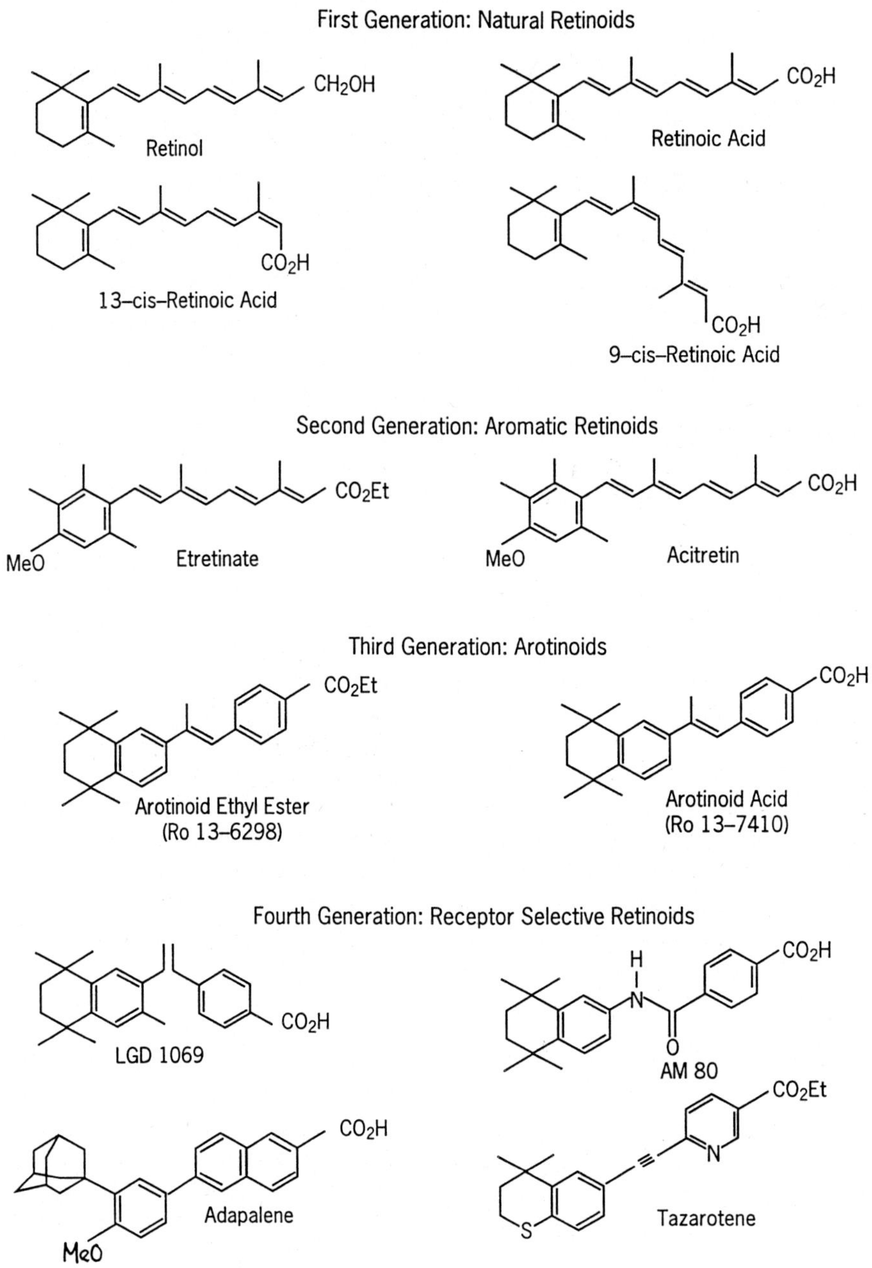

Figure 1 Generations of retinoids.

oral doses, but local application of ointment (up to 0.01%) was not effective in plaque psoriasis (Orfanos et al., 1985). The arotinoid acid, Ro 13-7410, was also effective in psoriasis by an oral route (Saurat et al., 1988). However, neither compound was developed further for dermatological indications because of a narrow margin between clinical efficacy and toxicity (Ott and Geiger, 1983).

Further modifications of the basic arotinoid structure have led to the development of a fourth generation of retinoids with varying degrees of selectivity for interaction with retinoid receptors. The advent of

Table 1 Generations of Retinoids and Their Potential Clinical Applications

Retinoid	Clinical application	Route of administration	Phase of development (U.S.)
First generation			
Tretinoin	Acne/photodamage	Topical	Launched
	Acute promyelocytic leukemia	Oral	Approved
Isotretinoin	Acne	Oral	Launched
Tretinoin/Topicare	Acne	Topical	Preregistration
ALRT-1057	Kaposi's sarcoma	Topical	Phase II
	Cutaneous T-cell lymphoma	Oral	Phase II
Second generation			
Etretinate	Psoriasis	Oral	Launched
Acitretin	Psoriasis	Oral	Preregistration
Third generation			
Ro 13-6298	Psoriasis	Oral	Not developed
Ro 13-7410	Psoriasis	Oral	Not developed
Fourth generation			
Tazarotene (AGN 190168)	Psoriasis/acne vulgaris	Topical	Preregistration
Adapalene (CD-271)	Acne vulgaris	Topical	Phase III
AM-80	Psoriasis	Topical	Unknown
LGD 1069	Cancer/Kaposi's sarcoma	PO/topical	Phase II

these receptor- and function-selective retinoids augurs well for the future of retinoid therapeutics in clinical medicine because such compounds are likely to have improved therapeutic indices in specific disease applications relative to the earlier generations of nonselective retinoids. Examples of these compounds are shown in Table 1. LGD 1069, a compound selective for the retinoid X receptor (RXR) family, is in phase II clinical trials for the topical treatment of Kaposi's sarcoma and the oral treatment of cancer. AM-80, a potent compound that is specific for the retinoic acid receptor (RAR) family and with some selectivity for the RAR_{α} subtype over the $RAR_{\beta\gamma}$ subtypes (Hashimoto and Shudo, 1991), has been shown to be effective in the topical treatment of psoriasis in phase II studies. Adapalene (CD 271), a compound selective for the $RAR_{\beta\gamma}$ subtypes (Boehm et al., 1995), is effective in the topical treatment of acne (Verschoore et al., 1991) and has recently been launched in Europe for this indication. Tazarotene (AGN 190168), a potent analog of the novel acetylenic class of retinoids, is completely specific for the RAR family and is selective for the $RAR_{\beta\gamma}$ subtypes in gene transactivation (Nagpal et al., 1995). Tazarotene is the first topical retinoid shown to be effective in the treatment of plaque psoriasis in well-controlled, phase III studies (Weinstein et al., 1995; Weinstein, 1996; Tazarotene Clinical Study Group, 1996). It is also effective in the topical treatment of acne vulgaris (Shalita et al., 1993) and a New Drug Application for both psoriasis and acne indications was approved by the FDA in 1997.

Retinoids: Clinical Experience

The physiological role of retinoids in growth, proliferation, differentiation, and cell death, in combination with the anti-inflammatory effect of these compounds, has been harnessed clinically in the treatment of dermatological diseases such as psoriasis, acne, photodamage, and various cancers. Three retinoids are currently approved in the United States for the treatment of dermatological diseases: tretinoin, isotretinoin, and etretinate.

Tretinoin is indicated for topical application in the treatment of acne vulgaris and photodamaged skin. Topical tretinoin was shown to exert some clinical benefit in the treatment of psoriasis, lamellar ichthyosis, and epidermolytic hyperkeratosis (Frost and Weinstein, 1969). However, further studies revealed that the therapeutic efficacy of tretinoin for the treatment of plaque psoriasis was limited, and local irritation severe enough to warrant discontinuation of therapy was common (Fredriksson, 1971; MacDonald et al., 1972; Orfanos et al., 1973; Günther, 1973).

Isotretinoin is indicated for oral administration in the treatment of severe recalcitrant cystic acne and, like etretinate, has also been valuable for acute pustular psoriasis. Topical isotretinoin is of limited use in the treatment of plaque psoriasis (Bischoff et al., 1992). Skin irritation (burning, stinging, redness, peeling) is the most common and frequently limiting adverse effect of topical tretinoin therapy, occurring in 80% of patients (Kamm et al., 1984).

TOPICALLY APPLIED "FOURTH-GENERATION" RETINOIDS: PHARMACOLOGICAL PROPERTIES RELATED TO PSORIASIS

Retinoids are very powerful biological mediators that elicit a variety of effects in many target tissues. This vast scope of retinoid action is the source of both therapeutic opportunity and many of the problems associated with the clinical use of currently available oral retinoids. The pleiotypic effects of retinoids facilitate their potential use in a wide variety of human diseases. However, drugs that indiscriminately elicit all of these retinoid actions are likely to be burdened with toxic side effects in many tissues that are not the targets of therapeutic action. An obvious partial solution to this problem is to deliver the drug to the diseased tissue. This approach is quite feasible in psoriasis, which is amenable to topical therapies. Unfortunately, the early attempts at using topical retinoids in psoriasis were complicated by variable efficacy and too much irritation. It was clear that newer approaches were required to achieve topical retinoids with sufficient potency to be effective in psoriasis, while exhibiting a manageable side effect profile. Recent advances in the molecular level understanding of the mechanism of action of retinoids have engendered such newer approaches involving receptor and function selectivity, and leading to "fourth-generation" retinoids.

Receptor Selectivity

Retinoids elicit their pleiotropic effects by regulating transcription of many genes through the intermediacy of specific nuclear receptors. The retinoid receptors belong to a superfamily of nuclear receptors that include the steroid, thyroid, and vitamin D receptors (Mangelsdorf et al., 1994). The six known retinoid receptors belong to two families, the RAR family (Petkovitch et al., 1987; Giguere et al., 1987) and the RXR family (Mangelsdorf et al., 1990), with three distinct isotypes (α, β, γ) in each. These receptors, upon activation by retinoid hormone binding, can regulate gene transcription in two ways: (1) up-regulation of transcription by binding directly to retinoid-responsive elements in the promoter regions of specific target genes, and (2) down-regulation of transcription of certain other genes by antagonizing the effects of nuclear transcription factors such as AP1, as schematically shown in Figure 2 (Nagpal and Chandraratna, 1996). The differentiation-inducing effects of retinoids are likely mediated primarily by the former, direct, gene-inducing effects. However, many of the antiproliferative and anti-inflammatory effects of retinoids are probably due to the antagonism of hyperproliferative and proinflammatory transcription factors.

In eliciting their transcriptional activation effects, the retinoid receptors always bind to their cognate response elements as dimers. RARs activate transcription of target genes as RAR-RXR heterodimers (Yu et al., 1991; Zhang et al., 1992a). Because there are three distinct subtypes in each retinoid receptor family, there are nine possible functional heterodimers. Binding of a ligand to the RAR portion of RAR-RXR heterodimers activates RAR hormonal pathways (Fig. 3). There is also recent evidence that binding of RXR ligands to the RXR portion of the heterodimer can modulate these RAR hormonal pathways (Roy et al., 1995).

RXRs can also function as homodimers (Zhang et al., 1992b), and RXR ligands can activate this putative RXR hormonal pathway. In addition, the vitamin D receptor (VDR), thyroid receptor (TR), and peroxisome proliferator-activated receptor (PPAR) hormonal pathways are all mediated by RXT heterodimers of the corresponding specific receptors. While each of these hormonal pathways is strongly activated by specific ligands for VDR, TR, and PPAR, respectively, all of these pathways can also potentially be affected by RXR ligands (Rosen et al., 1992).

Thus, it is apparent that the vast biology associated with retinoids is actually mediated by multiple discrete pathways. Retinoic acid, the hormone for the RARs, binds to RARs and specifically activates only RAR-RXR heterodimers. In contrast, 9-*cis*-retinoic acid, the putative hormone for the RXRs, binds to both RARs, and RXRs, activates both RAR-RXR heterodimers and RXR homodimers, and plausibly activates other heterodimeric pathways as well (Mangelsdorf et al., 1994). Additionally, these polyolefinic natural retinoids, as well as the second-generation aromatic retinoids, can readily be interconverted to the various geometrically isomeric forms. Thus, the phar-

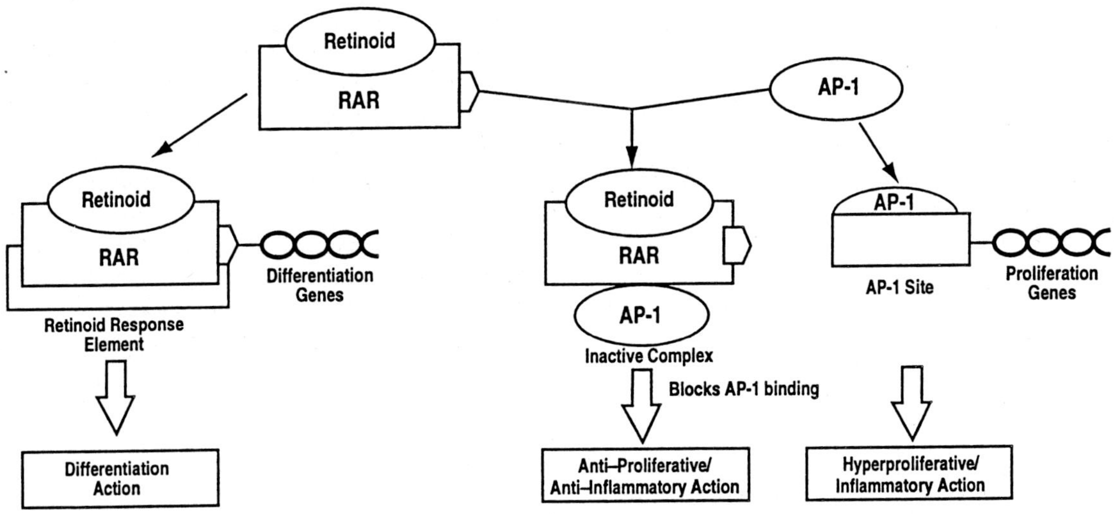

Figure 2 Molecular mechanism of action of retinoid receptors.

macological use of these first- and second-generation retinoids often results in the indiscriminate activation of all of these discrete retinoid pathways. As a consequence, these compounds, while being potentially useful in a wide spectrum of diseases, are likely to give rise to many toxic side effects.

Conceptually, an ideal retinoid drug would be one that would activate only those pathways that are required for efficacy in the target disease, such that the therapeutic use would be accompanied by few toxic effects. The differential distribution of retinoid receptor subtypes (Mangelsdorf et al., 1994) can facilitate this type of tissue/disease targeting. For example, the predominant RAR subtype in the skin is RAR_γ, and this subtype could well be the sole mediator of the antipsoriatic effects of retinoids. There is also emerging evidence that the individual RAR subtypes regulate distinct sets of genes, though with some overlap (Chambon, 1994). Thus, an RAR-subtype-specific retinoid will have biological effects only in tissues in which the particular subtype is expressed, and the type of effects obtained will be determined by the target genes that are regulated. Further targeting can be obtained by receptor functional selectivity, for example, by separation of receptor transactivation and AP1-antagonism functions (Nagpal et al., 1995). Thus, if most of the therapeutic benefit of a retinoid in a given disease stems from its ability to antagonize pathogenic nuclear transcription factors, then a compound that is selective for this type of effect will have a superior therapeutic index in that disease. In recent years, significant advances in the development of selective retinoids have been made possible by the availability of molecular level assays. These newer retinoids have included compounds that are specific for the RAR (Chandraratna et al., 1995) or RXR (Vuligonda et al., 1996) families, for an individual RAR subtype (Teng et al., 1996), as well as those that are specific for function (agonistic and antagonistic activity) (Nagpal et al., 1995; Johnson et al., 1995). Two of these fourth-generation, receptor-selective retinoids, AM-80 and tazarotene, have been evaluated for the topical treatment of psoriasis, and tazarotene has reached an advanced stage of clinical development with a pending new drug application.

Molecular Mechanisms of Topical Tazarotene Action

Tazarotene, a potent synthetic analog of the acetylenic class of retinoids, is rapidly converted to its free acid metabolite, tazarotenic acid, in vivo (Matsumoto et al., 1994). Tazarotene itself does not bind to any of the nuclear retinoid receptors and hence is a prodrug (Thacher et al., 1995). Tazarotenic acid, the active form of tazarotene, binds specifically to the RARs. In all culture assays, both tazarotene and tazarotenic acid activate gene transcription selectively through the RAR_β and RAR_γ subtypes, and have very little activity at RAR_α. Neither compound has any activity at any of the RXRs. Both tazarotene and tazarotenic acid are potent inhibitors of AP1-dependent gene expression in vitro and in vivo (Nagpal et al., 1995). Interestingly, these compounds are very active in AP1 inhibition

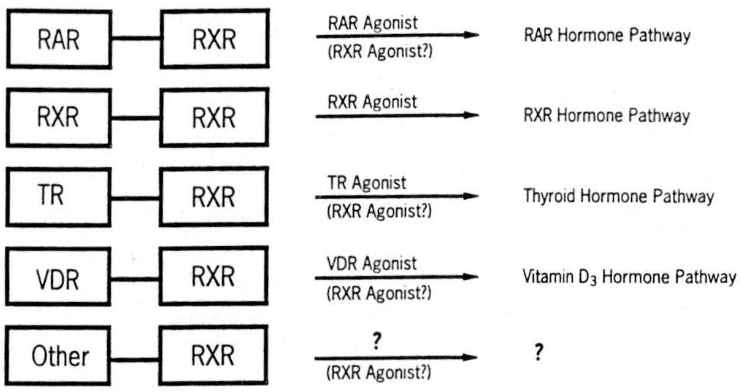

Figure 3 Multiplicity of retinoid pathways.

through RAR_{α}, but ineffective in corresponding transactivation assays indicating functional selectivity of RAR_{α}. Tazarotene is an effective and potent mediator of both the positive and negative gene regulatory effects of RAR_{γ}, the predominant RAR subtype in human keratinocytes.

Tazarotene has been shown to modulate three of the major pathogenic factors in psoriasis, namely, abnormal keratinocyte differentiation, keratinocyte hyperproliferation, and the influx of inflammatory cells into the skin (Chandraratna, 1996). The ability of tazarotene to beneficially affect all three of these factors may underlie the relatively long remissions observed after tazarotene treatment of psoriasis (Weinstein et al., 1995; Weinstein, 1996; Tazarotene Clinical Study Group, 1996). Several studies indicate that tazarotene has potent effects on human keratinocytes and it is probable that the psoriatic keratinocyte is the primary target for the therapeutic action of tazarotene in this disease, although an additional direct action on inflammatory immune cells cannot be ruled out. In this regard, the mechanism of action of tazarotene in psoriasis is likely to be quite distinct from that of topical glucocorticoids. However, if these drugs do impact psoriasis by distinct pathways, it would be interesting to speculate whether a combination of topical tazarotene and glucocorticoid would have a synergistic effect on the disease.

In Vitro/In Vivo Experiments with Tazarotene

The effects of tazarotene on keratinocyte differentiation have been demonstrated in both in vitro and in vivo models (Chandraratna, 1996). For example, tazarotene potently inhibits tumor promoter-induced cornified envelope formation in cultured human keratinocytes and reduces abnormal keratinization and utriculus size in rhino mice. The normal pattern of keratinocyte differentiation is altered in psoriasis and the disease is characterized by increased and/or precocious expression of involucrin, keratinocyte transglutaminase, and the hyperproliferative keratins, K6 and K16, and decreased expression of filaggrin. Tazarotene treatment of psoriatic lesions results in a normalization of the levels and patterns of expression of all of these differentiation markers (Esgleyes-Ribot et al., 1994; Nagpal and Chandraratna, unpublished data).

Migration inhibitory factor-related protein (MRP-8, or calgranulin A) is associated with chronic inflammatory diseases and also appears to be a marker of the abnormal, hyperproliferative differentiation of keratinocytes in psoriasis. MRP-8 is expressed at high levels in the suprabasal layers of psoriatic epidermis and is absent in normal skin, and hence it is a marker only of hyperproliferative psoriatic differentiation and not of normal differentiation of keratinocytes. The expression of MRP-8 is down-regulated by tazarotene in psoriatic lesions, and this is indicative of a reversal of the psoriatic differentiation state by the drug (Nagpal et al., submitted). Interestingly, interferon-γ, which is overexpressed in psoriasis and likely contributes to the disease process, up-regulates the expression of MRP-8 in cultured human keratinocytes, and tazarotene effectively antagonizes this induction. Thus, some of the therapeutic benefits of tazarotene may result from its ability to interdict the general pathogenic effects of interferon-γ in psoriasis.

Skin-derived antileukoproteinase (SKALP, or elafin) is an elastase inhibitor that also appears to be a marker of abnormal psoriatic differentiation, since it is expressed in the suprabasal layers of psoriatic epidermis but not in normal skin. SKALP is also a substrate for keratinocyte transglutaminase and is incorporated into epidermal crosslinked envelopes. The elevated expression of SKALP, together with that of other envelope precursors in psoriasis, may be a major cause for the excessive scale associated with the disease. Thus, the ability of tazarotene to down-regulate SKALP in psoriatic lesions is not only further indication of its differentiation normalizing functions but may directly contribute to its antiscaling effects in psoriasis.

Tazarotene has been shown to have antihyperproliferative effects in a variety of systems. Ornithine decarboxylase (ODC) is an essential enzyme in polyamine biosynthesis and is highly elevated in the hyperproliferative epidermis of psoriasis. Tazarotene is one of the most potent retinoids inhibiting tumor promoter-induced ODC activity in hairless mouse skin (Chandraratna, 1996). Tazarotene also has potent antiproliferative activity in a variety of transformed cell lines including those derived from squamous cell carcinomas, HPV-immortalized cervical cells, and Kaposi's sarcomas (Chandraratna, 1996). In psoriatic lesions, tazarotene down-regulates expression of the hyperproliferative keratins, K6 and K16, and of epidermal growth factor receptor (EGF-R). It is also likely that tazarotene has indirect effects on keratinocyte proliferation in psoriasis by its normalizing effects on differentiation.

The anti-inflammatory effects of tazarotene in psoriasis may stem largely from its ability to reduce the expression of inflammatory markers in keratinocytes. MRP-8, the hyperproliferative differentiation marker, appears to have proinflammatory properties since it is overexpressed in a variety of inflammatory conditions and has strong homology with a known murine chemokine, CP-10. Tazarotene effectively down-regulates MRP-8 in a variety of skin systems inducing psoriatic lesions. Interleukin-6 (IL-6), a potent proinflammatory cytokine that is overexpressed in psoriasis, is effectively down-regulated by tazarotene in cultured human keratinocytes and Kaposi's sarcoma cells, but effects in psoriasis have not yet been determined. In keratinocytes, tazarotene down-regulates the basal and induced levels of stromelysin, a member of the metalloprotease family that is associated with inflammatory conditions including arthritis and tumor metastases. However, a pathogenic role for metalloproteases in psoriasis has not been established. It has been proposed that the recruitment of T cells to the epidermis by the expression of adhesion molecules such as intercellular adhesion molecule 1 (ICAM-1) and HLA-DR contributes to the pathogenesis of psoriasis (Griffiths et al., 1989). Tazarotene treatment of psoriatic plaques results in decreased expression of these inflammatory markers, ICAM-1 and HLA-DR, in both the epidermis and dermis, and this type of effect could lead to a decreased trafficking of inflammatory T cells into the lesion (Esgleyes-Ribot et al., 1994).

A variety of molecular biology techniques, including subtractive hybridization and differential display polymerase chain reaction (PCR) assays, are being used in conjunction with ongoing clinical pharmacology studies to further elucidate the mechanisms of action of tazarotene in psoriasis. In addition to some of the results described above, these studies have led to the identification of three new genes, tazarotene-induced genes 1, 2, and 3 (TIG 1, TIG 2, TIG 3), which are up-regulated by tazarotene in psoriatic lesions. TIG 1 appears to be a transmembrane protein and has a hydropathic profile very similar to that of CD 38, an acutely up-regulated marker of retinoid action in immune cells (Nagpal et al., 1996a). CD 38 binds in vitro to hyaluronic acid, and a cell adhesion function has been suggested for it (Malavasi et al., 1994). Since TIG 1 also possesses a hyaluronic acid binding motif in its large extracellular domain, it might also function as a cell adhesion molecule and its induction by tazarotene might lead to normalization of differentiation and reduced proliferation in psoriasis. TIG 2, which is induced by tazarotene in psoriatic lesions and skin raft cultures, appears to be a secretory protein and has no significant homology to known proteins (Nagpal et al., 1996b). TIG 2 could be a ligand for a membrane receptor or itself be a soluble receptor but the establishment of these or other functions and its role in psoriasis need further study. TIG 3, which is induced by tazarotene in psoriatic lesions, skin grafts, and keratinocyte cultures, is an interesting molecule because it has significant homology to a known family of tumor suppressors (Nagpal and Chandraratna, unpublished data). If indeed TIG 3 is a tumor suppressor gene, then its induction by tazarotene may be crucial for the antiproliferative effects of the drug in psoriasis.

The potential molecular mechanisms of action of tazarotene in psoriasis are schematically summarized in Figure 4. Clearly, much work needs to be done to fully explain the therapeutic actions of this drug in psoriasis. A more complete understanding of its mechanisms of action would be of considerable value in the rational design and selection of newer, antipsoriatic topical retinoids.

Pharmacokinetics of Tazarotene

The majority of topically applied tazarotene remains on the skin surface. This produces significant drug concentrations in skin layers, but with limited systemic exposure. The small amounts of tazarotene and metabolites that are recovered in the plasma are eliminated rapidly.

Animal Studies

A study in minipigs indicated that topical application of ^{14}C-tazarotene to intact skin results in rapid penetration through the stratum corneum and into the viable epidermis, with only a minor degree of accumulation (Matsumoto et al., 1992).

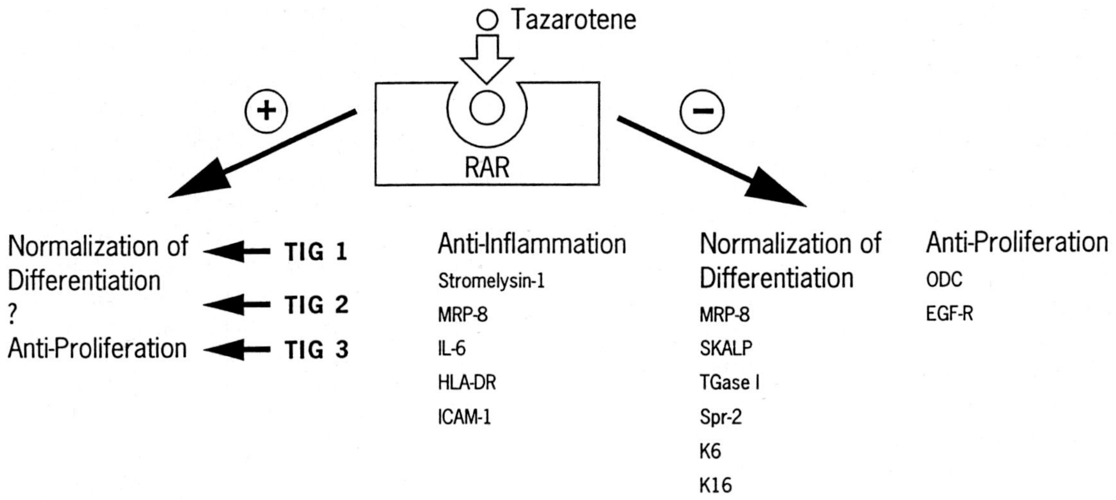

Figure 4 Molecular basis of tazarotene action: positive and negative gene regulatory activities.

Psoriatic Patients

Low potential for absorption was also reported among patients with psoriasis included in phase III controlled clinical efficacy studies. In one study, low plasma concentrations of tazarotene (up to 0.15 ng/ml) were detected in 2.7% (2/27) of patients treated with either tazarotene 0.1% or 0.05% once daily for 12 weeks (Weinstein, 1996). Tazarotenic acid was detected in the plasma samples of 47.2% (34/72) of the patients, in concentrations ranging from 0.05 to 6.1 ng/ml. Of the seven patients with plasma metabolite concentrations higher than 1 ng/ml, none experienced any systemic adverse events that were related to the study drug.

TOPICALLY APPLIED "FOURTH-GENERATION" RETINOIDS: CLINICAL TRIALS IN PLAQUE PSORIASIS

The clinical efficacy and safety of topically applied tazarotene gel in the treatment of mild to moderate plaque psoriasis has been confirmed by the results of phase III clinical studies, including a vehicle-controlled study and a comparison with fluocinonide cream.

Vehicle-Controlled Study

In a double-blind, randomized, parallel-group comparison, 318 patients (67% male, mean age 47 years) were treated once daily with either tazarotene 0.1% gel, tazarotene 0.05% gel, or vehicle gel for 12 weeks, followed by 12 weeks of posttreatment evaluation (Weinstein et al., 1995; Weinstein, 1996). In each patient, one target lesion from trunk or limbs and one target lesion from knees or elbows were evaluated for treatment success (good or excellent response or complete clearing; 50–100% improvement) and reduction in severity of psoriatic signs and symptoms, while nontarget lesions were evaluated for overall treatment success. Patients were allowed to use emollient on their nontarget lesions only.

Tazarotene gels were superior ($p < 0.05$) to vehicle, often as early as treatment week 1, in treatment success (for which a dose-response relationship was evident; Fig. 5). Maximum improvement was reached at 12 weeks for both trunk/limbs and elbows/knees lesions, for both tazarotene 0.1% (70%) and tazarotene 0.05% (59%). Improvement on the parameter of plaque elevation shows similar responses for trunk/limbs and elbows/knees, indicating drug activity on the clinically more-difficult-to-treat elbows/knees lesions (Fig. 6). A sustained therapeutic effect was observed for 12 weeks posttreatment. Tazarotene gel was cosmetically acceptable, and minimally absorbed systemically, limiting toxicity to local irritation.

Fluocinonide-Controlled Study

A total of 348 patients (57% male, mean age 46 years) participated in a multicenter, investigator-masked, randomized, parallel-group comparison of the efficacy,

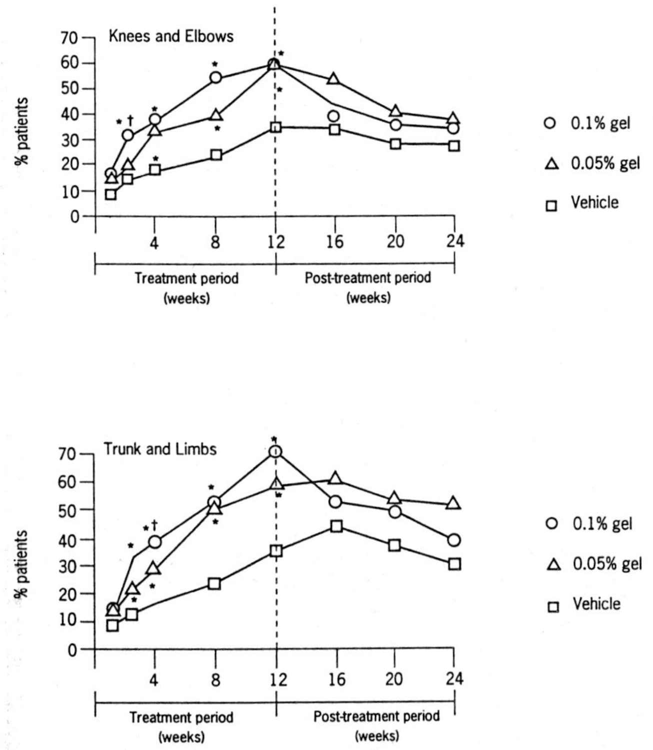

Figure 5 Tazarotene gel versus vehicle: treatment success, calculated from the numbers of patients achieving a good or excellent response, or complete clearing of psoriasis. $*p < 0.05$, tazarotene (either concentration) versus vehicle; $\dagger p < 0.05$, tazarotene 0.1% versus tazarotene 0.05%.

safety, and duration of therapeutic effect of 12 weeks' therapy with tazarotene 0.1% or 0.05% gel once daily, or fluocinonide 0.05% cream twice daily (Tazarotene Clinical Study Group, 1996).

Both concentrations of tazarotene gel were effective and safe for the treatment of plaque psoriasis. The therapeutic success obtained with tazarotene treatment was similar to that of fluocinonide 0.05% cream, especially for plaque elevation and scaling. However, relapse of psoriasis was more rapid with fluocinonide, particularly during the first 4 weeks posttreatment (Fig. 7). The probability of posttreatment relapse was greater for fluocinonide compared with tazarotene, with the difference between fluocinonide and tazarotene 0.1% gel being statistically significant ($p < 0.05$).

Signs and symptoms of local irritation due to tazarotene were consistent with the expected effects of a topical retinoid (predominantly mild to moderate pruritus, erythema, burning, or desquamation). As expected with a potent topical corticosteroid, minimal local irritation was associated with fluocinonide cream.

TOPICALLY APPLIED "FOURTH-GENERATION" RETINOIDS: SAFETY, TOLERABILITY, AND TERATOGENICITY

The most common adverse effect of tazarotene gel is mild-to-moderate local irritation. This is consistent with the known effects of other topical retinoids (Fredriksson, 1971; MacDonald et al., 1972; Günther, 1973; Orfanos et al., 1973). The cumulative irritation potential of tazarotene gel is concentration-dependent (Marks, 1996).

In phase III controlled clinical studies that included a total of more than 1000 psoriasis patients who were treated with tazarotene 0.1% or 0.05% gels, the most commonly encountered adverse reactions were signs

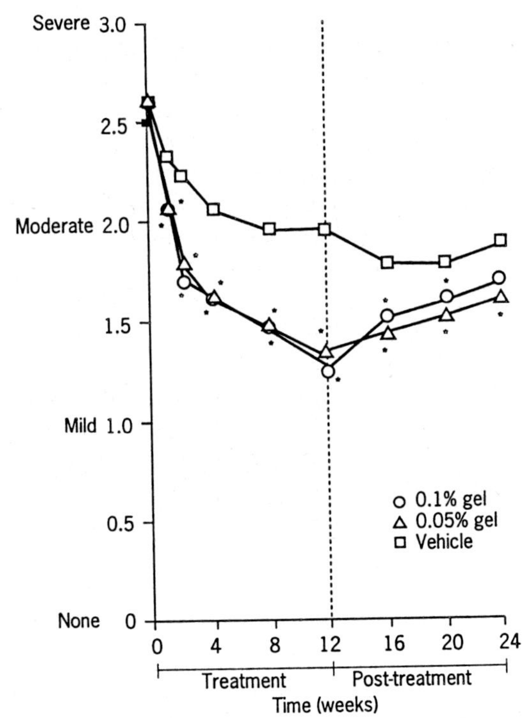

Figure 6 Tazarotene gel versus vehicle: severity of plaque elevation for elbows/knees target lesions. $*p < 0.05$, tazarotene (either concentration) versus vehicle. All mean severity scores were significantly decreased from baseline at all follow-up visits, including those during the posttreatment period ($p < 0.0001$).

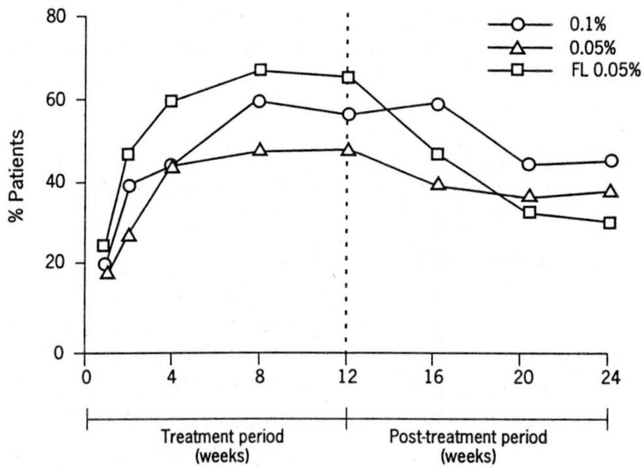

Figure 7 Tazarotene gel versus fluocinonide cream: treatment success for all lesions, calculated from the numbers of patients achieving a good or excellent response, or complete clearing of psoriasis. Significant differences ($p < 0.05$); fluocinonide versus tazarotene 0.1% at week 4; fluocinonide versus tazarotene 0.05% at weeks 2–8.

of local irritation, such as burning/stinging, pruritus, and erythema.

In standard laboratory and animal models, tazarotene applied topically was not found to be mutagenic, carcinogenic, or teratogenic, and the drug had no deleterious effects on male or female reproductive performance (Chandraratna, 1996).

DISCUSSION

In mild-to-moderate plaque psoriasis, the efficacy of systemic retinoid therapy is offset by the potential for serious systemic adverse effects and long-term toxicity. Topical retinoid therapy appears to offer a useful alternative by directing the retinoid therapy to the skin, but tretinoin has proven to be of limited therapeutic value.

Interaction with two families of nuclear receptors (RAR and RXR), each of which is encoded by three genes, results in the diverse biological effects of retinoids. Retinoids appear to act through nuclear RARs, primarily the γ subtype, to modulate pathogenic factors in psoriasis. The development of potent and receptor-selective fourth-generation retinoids, such as tazarotene, allows a more targeted clinical effect in the treatment of plaque psoriasis than did previous retinoids.

Tazarotene modulates three key pathogenic factors in psoriasis: abnormal keratinocyte differentiation, hyperproliferation, and inflammation. On the molecular level, tazarotene acts via a direct interaction with nuclear receptors and regulation of gene transcription. Tazarotene specifically activates the nuclear $RAR_{\beta,\gamma}$ subtypes and shows no affinity for RXR, which modulates other hormonal responses.

The down-regulated (MRP-8 and SKALP) and enhanced (TIG1) gene expression induced by tazarotene is associated with a positive clinical response in mild-to-moderate plaque psoriasis, suggesting that molecular markers may be developed to identify potential responders to tazarotene therapy.

Topical tazarotene used once daily is clinically effective on trunk/limb lesions, as well as the more difficult areas of elbows and knees. Beneficial therapeutic effects appear to continue in some patients for at least 3 months after discontinuation of therapy. Effectiveness is similar to that of a potent topical glucocorticoid, with a longer maintenance of the clinical response. Adverse effects include manageable, mainly mild-to-moderate local irritation.

In conclusion, increased understanding of the diverse receptor interactions of the retinoids has allowed the development of potent, receptor-selective fourth-generation retinoids such as tazarotene, which offers safe and effective treatment of mild-to-moderate plaque psoriasis.

REFERENCES

Bischoff, R., De Jong, E.M.G.J., Rulo, H.F.C., et al. (1992). Topical application of 13-*cis*-retinoic acid in the treatment of chronic plaque psoriasis. *Clin. Exp. Dermatol.* 17:9–12.

Boehm, M.F., Heyman, R.A., Patel, S., et al. (1995). Retinoids: biological function and use in the treatment of dermatological diseases. *Exp. Opin. Invest. Drugs* 4(7): 593–612.

Chambon, P. (1994). The retinoid signaling pathway: molecular and genetic analyses. *Semin. Cell Biol.* 5: 115–125.

Chandraratna, R.A.S. (1996). Tazarotene—first of a new generation of receptor-selective retinoids. *Br. J. Dermatol.* 135(Suppl. 49):19–26.

Chandraratna, R.A.S., Henry, E., Attard, J., Gillet, S.J., Song, T., et al. (1995). Development of RAR subtype selective retinoids for dermatological diseases. *Eur. J. Med. Chem.* 30(Suppl.):506–517.

Esgleyes-Ribot, T., Chandraratna, R.A., Lew-Kaya, D.A., et al. (1994). Response of psoriasis to a new topical retinoid, AGN 190168. *J. Am. Acad. Dermatol.* 30:581–590.

Fredriksson, T. (1971). Antipsoriatic activity of retinoic acid (vitamin A acid). *Dermatologica* 142:133–136.
Friant, S., Oda, R., Chandraratna, R.A.S., et al. (1995). Inflammatory cytokine release associated with retinoid cytotoxicity. Presented at 53rd Annual Meeting of the American Academy of Dermatology, February 4–9. Abstract.
Frost, P., and Weinstein, G.D. (1969). Topical administration of vitamin A acid for ichthyosiform dermatoses and psoriasis. *J.A.M.A.* 207:1863–1868.
Giguere, V., Ong, E.S., Segui, P., et al. (1987). Identification of a receptor for the morphogen retinoic acid. *Nature* 330:624–629.
Goss, G.D., and McBurney, M.W. (1992). Physiological and clinical aspects of vitamin-A and its metabolites. *Clin. Lab. Sci.* 29:185–215.
Griffiths, C.E.M., Voorhees, J.J., and Nicholoff, B.J. (1989). Characterization of intercellular adhesion molecule-1 and HLA-DR expression in normal and inflamed skin: modulation by recombinant gamma interferon and tumor necrosis factor. *J. Am. Acad. Dermatol.* 20:617–629.
Günther, S. (1973). The therapeutic value of retinoid acid in chronic discoid, acute guttate, and erythrodermic psoriasis: clinical observations on twenty-five patients. *Br. J. Dermatol.* 89:515–517.
Hashimoto, Y., and Shudo, K. (1991). Retinoids and their nuclear receptors. *Cell Biol. Rev.* 25(3):209–230.
Johnson, A.T., Klein, E.S., Gillett, S.J., Wang, L., Song, T.K., et al. (1995). Synthesis and characterization of a highly potent and effective antagonist of retinoic acid receptors. *J. Med. Chem.* 38:4764–4767.
Kamm, J.J., Ashenfelter, K.O., and Ehmann, C.W. (1984). Preclinical and clinical toxicology of selected retinoids. In *The Retinoids.* Academic Press, New York, pp. 287–326.
Kligman, A. (1987). Topical tretinoin: indications, safety, and effectiveness. *Cutis* 39(6):486–488.
Loeliger, P., Bollag, W., and Mayer, H. (1980). Arotinoids, a new class of highly effective retinoids. *Eur. J. Med. Chem.* 15:9–15.
MacDonald, A., McMinn, R.M.H., and Fry, L. (1972). Effect of retinoic acid in psoriasis. II. Long term study. *Br. J. Dermatol.* 87:256–260.
Malavasi, F., Funaro, A., Roggero, S., Horenstein, A., Calosso, L., et al. (1994). Human CD38: a glycoprotein in search of a function. *Immunol. Today* 15:95–97.
Mangelsdorf, D.J., Ong, E.S., Dyck, J.A., et al. (1990). Nuclear receptor that identifies a novel retinoic acid response pathway. *Nature* 345:224–229.
Mangelsdorf, D.J., Umeseno, K., and Evans, R.M. (1994). The retinoid receptors. In *The Retinoids: Biology, Chemistry, and Medicine.* H.B. Span, A.B. Roberts, and D.S. Goodman (Eds.). Raven Press, New York, pp. 319–349.
Marcus, R., and Coulson, A.M. (1990). Fat-soluble vitamins. In *The Pharmacological Basis of Therapeutics,* 8th ed. A.G. Gillman, T.W. Rail, A.S. Nies, and P. Taylor (Eds.). Pergamon Press, New York, pp. 1553–1571.
Marks, R. (1996). Early clinical development of tazarotene. *Br. J. Dermatol.* 135(Suppl. 49):27–32.
Matsumoto, R.M., Sun, H., Duff, S.B., et al. (1992). Skin distribution anbd metabolism of 14C-AGN 190168 in minipigs. *Pharm. Res.* 9(Suppl.):289 (abstract).
Matsumoto, R.M., Tang-Liu, D., Lew-Kaya, D., et al. (1994). Pharmacokinetics of AGN 190168, a novel retinoid, after topical dosing of a 0.1% or 0.05% gel in healthy male volunteers. *Pharm. Res.* 11(Suppl.):368 (abstract).
Nagpal, S., and Chandraratna, R.A.S. (1996). Retinoids as anti-cancer agents. *Curr. Pharmaceut. Design.* 2:295–316.
Nagpal, S., Athanikar, J., and Chandraratna, R.A.S. (1995). Separation of transactivation and AP1 antagonism functions of retinoic acid receptor α. *J. Biol. Chem.* 270: 923–927.
Nagpal, S., Patel, S., Asano, A.T., et al. (1996a). Tazarotene-induced gene 1 (TIG1), a novel retinoic acid receptor-responsive gene in skin. *J. Invest. Dermatol.* 106: 269–274.
Nagpal, S., Patel, S., Asano, A.T., Johnson, A., Duvic, M., et al. (1996b). TIG 1 and TIG 2 (tazarotene induced genes 1 and 2) are novel retinoic acid receptor-responsive genes in skin. *J. Invest. Dermatol.* 106:818.
Nagpal, S., Patel, S., Friant, S., Malhotra, M., Shafer, J., et al. (submitted). Negative regulation of two hyperproliferative keratinocyte differentiation markers by an RAR-selective retinoid: insight into the mechanism of retinoid action in psoriasis. *Cell Growth Different.*
Norris, D.A., Osborn, R., Robinson, W., and Tonnesen, G. (1987). Isotretinoin produces significant inhibition of monocyte and neutrophil chemotaxis in vivo in patients with cystic acne. *J. Invest. Dermatol.* 89:38–43.
Orfanos, C.E., Schmidt, H.W., Mahrle, G., et al. (1973). Retinoic acid in psoriasis: its value for topical therapy with and without corticosteroids. *Br. J. Dermatol.* 88:167–181.
Orfanos, C.E., Stadler, R., Gollnisk, H., and Tsambaos, D. (1985). Current developments of oral retinoid therapy with three generations of drugs. *Curr. Probl. Dermatol.* 13:33–49.
Orfanos, C.E., Ehlert, R., and Gollnick, H. (1987). The retinoids: a review of their clinical pharmacology and therapeutic use. *Drugs* 34:459–503.
Ott, F., and Geiger, J.M. (1983). Therapeutic effect of arotinoid Ro 13-6298 in psoriasis. *Arch. Dermatol. Res.* 275: 257–258.
Petkovitch, M., Brand, N.J., Krust, A., et al. (1987). A human retinoic acid receptor which belongs to the family of nuclear receptors. *Nature* 330:444–450.
Rosen, E.D., O'Donnell, A.L., and Koenig, R.J. (1992). Ligand-dependent synergy of thyroid hormone and retinoid X receptors. *J. Biol. Chem.* 267:22010–22013.

Roy, B., Taneja, R., and Chambon, P. (1995). Synergistic activation of retinoic acid (RA)-responsive genes and induction of embryonal carcinoma cell differentiation by an RA receptor α (RARα-), RARβ-, or RARγ-selective ligand in combination with a retinoid X receptor-specific ligand. *Mol. Cell Biol.* 15:6481–6487.

Saurat, J.-H., Merol, Y., Boskey, M., Abba, Z., and Hirschel-Scholz, S. (1988). Arotinoid acid (Ro 13-7410): a pilot study in dermatology. *Dermatologica* 176:191–199.

Shalita, A.R., Chalker, D.K., Griffith, R.F., et al. (1993). Double-blind study of AGN 190168, a new retinoid gel, in the topical treatment of acne vulgaris. *J. Invest. Dermatol.* 100:542 (abstract).

Tazarotene Clinical Study Group (1996). Tazarotene 0.1% and 0.05% gels compared with fluocinonide 0.05% cream in the treatment of plaque psoriasis: an investigator-masked study of safety, efficacy, and duration of effect. Presented at Clinical Dermatology 2000, Vancouver, BC, Canada, May 28–31.

Teng, M., Duong, T.R., Klein, E.S., Pino, M.E., and Chandraratna, R.A.S. (1996). Identification of a retinoic acid receptor α subtype specific agonist. *J. Med. Chem.* 39: 3035–3038.

Thacher, S.M., Klein, E., Arefieg, T., et al. (1995). The comparative pharmacology of the acetylenic retinoid tazarotene in skin and receptor-based assay. Presented at 53rd Annual Meeting of the American Academy of Dermatology, February 4–9. Abstract.

Verschoore, M., Langner, A., Wolska, H., Jablonska, S., Czermielewski, J., et al. (1991). Efficacy and safety of CD 271 alcoholic gels in the topical treatment of acne vulgaris. *Br. J. Dermatol.* 124:368–371.

Vuligonda, V., Lin, Y., and Chandraratna, R.A.S. (1996). Synthesis of highly potent RXR-specific retinoids: the use of a cyclopropyl group as a double bond isostere. *Bioorg. Med. Chem. Lett.* 6:213–218.

Weinstein, G., Jeffes, E., Duvic, M., Friedman, D., Jegasothy, B., et al. (1995). Tazarotene gel for the treatment of plaque psoriasis: a double-blind clinical study. *J. Invest. Dermatol.* 104:661.

Weinstein, G.D. (1996). Safety, efficacy and duration of therapeutic effect of tazarotene used in the treatment of plaque psoriasis. *Br. J. Dermatol.* 135(Suppl. 49):33–37.

Yu, V.C., Delsert, C., Andersen, B., et al. (1991). RXRβ: a coregulator that enhances binding of retinoic acid, thyroid hormone, and vitamin D receptors to their cognate response elements. *Cell* 67:1251–1266.

Zhang, X.-K., Hoffmann, B., Tran, P.B.-V., et al. (1992a). Retinoid X receptor is an auxiliary protein for thyroid hormone and retinoic acid receptors. *Nature* 355: 441–446.

Zhang, X.-K., Lehmann, J., Hoffmann, B., et al. (1992b). Homodimer formation of retinoid X receptor induced by 9-*cis*-retinoic acid. *Nature* 358:587–591.

62

Tacrolimus (FK506) in the Treatment of Psoriasis

Jan D. Bos
Academic Medical Center, University of Amsterdam, Amsterdam, The Netherlands

Tacrolimus (FK506) is a potent immunosuppressive agent that was isolated in 1984 from *Streptomyces tsukubaensis*, a microorganism found in a soil sample originating from the Tsukuba region of northern Japan. Tacrolimus is macrolide lactone and has a molecular weight of 822.05 daltons. In vitro, tacrolimus was shown to be 10–100 times more effective than cyclosporin in suppressing the human mixed lymphocyte reaction (1) while in vivo studies with mice demonstrated that the inhibitory effect of tacrolimus T-cell-dependent antibody production, the delayed hypersensitivity response, and induced graft-versus-host reactivity was 10-fold higher than that of cyclosporin (2). Tacrolimus has been used successfully in the field of transplantation to prevent and treat organ rejection (3–6) and is now licensed under the trade name Prograf in Japan, Canada, the United States, and several European countries. Furthermore, tacrolimus has proven to be an effective treatment for various autoimmune diseases (7).

MECHANISM OF ACTION

Although tacrolimus and cyclosporin have different chemical structures, they have a similar mechanism of action. Both immunosuppressive agents inhibit the activation and proliferation of T cells by interfering, at an early stage in the cell cycle, with the calcium-dependent transduction pathways that lead to gene expression.

Tacrolimus becomes biologically active when it forms a complex with the cytosolic FK-binding protein (FKBP), an immunophilin with peptidyl-prolyl *cis-trans* isomerase activity (cyclosporin, in contrast, binds to cyclophilin, a different cytosolic protein). The activated FKBP-tacrolimus complex subsequently binds to calcineurin, a calcium- and calmodulin-dependent protein phosphatase. Calcineurin is required for the calcium-dependent signal transduction pathway, which conveys the crucial information necessary for the initiation of interleukin-2 (IL-2) synthesis, from the cell membrane into the nucleus (8). Suppression of the phosphate activity of calcineurin by the FKBP-tacrolimus complex results in the inhibition of the T-cell-specific transcription factor (NF-AT), which regulates IL-2 transcription (9), so T-cell production is blocked.

Tacrolimus can also affect other cells involved in the immune response. B-cell activation is inhibited in the late phase of the cell cycle, not only because of the suppressive effect of tacrolimus upon lymphokine production by the T cells, but also by direct blockage of the induction of tumor necrosis factor-α (TNF-α) gene transcription by anti-Ig antibody (10). In addition, in vitro data from several studies have demonstrated that tacrolimus has strong anti-inflammatory activity and interferes with several IgE receptor-mediated processes, such as histamine and serotonin release in human skin mast cells and basophils, prostaglandin D_2 synthesis in human skin mast cells, and leukotriene C_4 secretion from human basophils and lung mast cells (11,12).

Tacrolimus has also been found to have a strong inhibitory effect upon the expression of IL-8, a cytokine believed to play an important role in the pathogenesis of psoriasis. IL-8 is expressed by several cell types as a consequence of IL-1 or TNF-α induction, but appears to be most prolific in hyperplastic keratinocytes (13). Elevated levels of mRNA for IL-8 have been detected in the lesions of patients with psoriasis, whereas IL-8 was absent in healthy skin (14). In Pittsburgh, the examination of skin biopsies from seven patients with severe recalcitrant psoriasis, who received oral treatment with tacrolimus (0.1–0.3 mg/kg/day), revealed that the circulating levels of IL-8 decreased in a time-dependent manner following tacrolimus treatment (15). The patients experienced a large reduction in Psoriasis Area Severity Index (PASI), but decreasing the dose of tacrolimus caused partial relapse in some of the patients, and an increase in the circulating levels of IL-8. Therefore, it seems that the therapeutic efficacy of tacrolimus in treating psoriasis is, among other mechanisms, correlated with the ability to interfere with the production of IL-8.

SYSTEMIC ADMINISTRATION OF TACROLIMUS

In animals, tacrolimus has only been administered orally or intravenously to obtain toxicology data (16) or as rejection prophylaxis following organ transplantation (17).

Clinical pharmacokinetics studies in healthy human subjects determined that a single oral dose of tacrolimus was rapidly absorbed throughout the gastrointestinal tract, and the mean time to peak concentration was approximately 1.5 hr (18). The mean oral bioavailability of tacrolimus was found to be about 16%. Tacrolimus is metabolized in the liver by the cytochrome P450 3A enzyme system and bile is the principal route of elimination.

The first clinical experience with tacrolimus as a treatment for psoriasis was in Pittsburgh (19) where tacrolimus was administered as rejection prophylaxis to one heart transplant and three liver transplant patients who had concurrent psoriasis (initial dose: 0.27–0.35 mg/kg/day; at 3 months: 0.20–0.40 mg/kg). Three nontransplanted patients with severe psoriasis (PASI range: 43–68) also received tacrolimus treatment (initial oral dose: 0.20–0.29 mg/kg/day; at 3 months: 0.10–0.32 mg/kg/day) for 5.5–14 months. All of the patients treated experienced a marked reduction in erythema and scaling by the end of the first week and had complete clinical remission within 4 weeks. In addition, psoriatic arthritis improved in the three patients whose primary diagnosis was psoriasis.

In common with systemic cyclosporin treatment (20), nephrotoxicity was the most serious side effect of tacrolimus therapy. Following a dose reduction in most of the patients, serum creatinine and serum urea nitrogen levels became stable, but remained higher than the pretreatment values. Another concern was that three patients developed arterial hypertension requiring treatment with antihypertensive medication. However, one patient had hypertension prior to tacrolimus treatment that was drug-controlled, and a second patient later become normotensive and required no further antihypertensive medication.

The oral dose of tacrolimus administered to the three nontransplant patients was relatively high, and in the range usually administered to liver transplant patients (3). Unfortunately, reducing the dose of tacrolimus resulted in swift reappearance of the psoriatic lesions in three patients.

More recently in a phase II, randomized, double-blind, placebo-controlled study, low oral doses of tacrolimus were investigated as a treatment for severe recalcitrant plaque-type psoriasis (21). The treatment phase lasted 9 weeks with a follow-up period of 3 weeks. Twenty-seven patients received an initial dose of 0.05 mg/kg/day tacrolimus, and the daily dosage could be adjusted upward after 3 and 6 weeks of treatment to 0.10 mg/kg/day and 0.15 mg/kg/day, respectively, if the therapeutic effect was insufficient and there were no adverse events. Continuous and progressive improvement in PASI and responder rates was observed in the patients receiving tacrolimus, and by the end of the treatment phase, these patients had significantly lower PASI compared with the patients receiving placebo treatment. The minimal effective dosage of tacrolimus was determined to be 0.10 mg/kg/day, and during the follow-up phase, when patients were no longer receiving tacrolimus, there was a high relapse rate, as would be expected.

In this study, the most frequently reported side effects that were considered to be related to tacrolimus treatment were diarrhea, paresthesia, and insomnia. All of these adverse events were assessed to be mild or moderately severe, and resolved without a decrease in the dose of tacrolimus. The problems normally associated with systemic immunosuppressive treatment, i.e., nephrotoxicity and hypertension, were not an important clinical concern for these patients, but of course, exposure to tacrolimus was limited in these patients. Two cases of renal dysfunction resolved without any dose reduction in tacrolimus being necessary, and one patient developed mild hypertension that also resolved without any change in the tacrolimus dosage.

It therefore appears that tacrolimus is an efficacious treatment for cases of severe, recalcitrant plaque-type psoriasis. In addition, several studies have demonstrated the success of systemically administered tacrolimus in treating other dermatological conditions such as epidermolysis bullosa (22), psoriatic arthritis (23), pyoderma gangrenosum (24), and Sézary syndrome (25).

TOPICAL APPLICATION OF TACROLIMUS

As mentioned previously, systemic immunosuppressive therapy can be associated with a number of important side effects, including both nephrotoxicity and hypertension. Topical formulations of immunosuppressive agents may be able to deliver therapeutic concentrations of the drug to the skin while minimizing systemic side effects. Unfortunately, topical applications of cyclosporin have not been effective in treating dermatological disorders in humans (26–28), and the lack of efficacy has been attributed to insufficient skin penetration by the large cyclosporin molecule (MW 1202 daltons; 26).

Topical applications of tacrolimus have been tested in several different animal models. In mice, tacrolimus ointment was found to reduce the extent of calcium-ionophore-induced skin inflammation (29), and studies in guinea pigs demonstrated that tacrolimus ointment was effective in decreasing sodium-lauryl-sulfate-induced skin irritation (30). Treatment was most effective when administered prior to the initiation of inflammation.

Pigs are a good experimental model for testing ointment formulations as their skin might be similar to that of human skin with respect to barrier properties (31). In domestic pigs, topical applications of 0.04–0.4% tacrolimus were found to inhibit inflammatory skin reactions caused by hypersensitivity to dinitroflurobenzene (32). The response to tacrolimus therapy was similar to that observed following treatment with superpotent topical glucocorticoid clobetasol proprionate, but skin atrophy, a dose-limiting side effect of superpotent topical corticosteroids, was not observed. These data indicated that, in animals, tacrolimus ointment was absorbed in sufficient amounts to be therapeutically efficacious.

Studies in healthy human subjects provided further evidence of the penetration of tacrolimus into the skin. Five male subjects, who were sensitized to 1-chloro-2,4-dinitrobenzene (DNCB), were treated with different concentrations of tacrolimus ointment. Tacrolimus treatment suppressed DNCB allergic reactions in a dose-dependent manner, and there was a marked decrease in inflammation, with no systemic side effects being observed (33). As tacrolimus has a smaller molecular size than cyclosporin, topical applications may be more efficacious because the smaller size of the tacrolimus molecule enables passage into deeper layers of skin (34). In addition, the greater immunosuppressive potency of tacrolimus compared with cyclosporin probably contributes to the larger therapeutic effect observed.

No published clinical data are currently available for the treatment of psoriasis with topical applications of tacrolimus, although studies are ongoing in Japan and Europe. However, tacrolimus ointment has been extremely efficacious in treating atopic dermatitis (35,36) and allergic contact dermatitis (37).

CONCLUSION

All systemic immunosuppressive agents have drawbacks as well as therapeutic benefits, and therefore the risk/benefit ratio has to be considered carefully by the physician prior to the prescription of these powerful drugs. Preliminary clinical data have indicated that systemic tacrolimus is a promising treatment for severe forms of psoriasis. There are some side effects associated with treatment, but these can be reduced or avoided by the administration of lower oral doses. Clinical studies of topical formulations of tacrolimus are ongoing and these may demonstrate equivalent therapeutic efficacy without the side effects associated with systemic treatment. For many patients whose quality of life is deleteriously affected by severe psoriasis resistant to other forms of therapy, tacrolimus may offer a ray of hope for the treatment of this debilitating disease.

ACKNOWLEDGMENT

The author gratefully acknowledges the assistance of Dr. Claire Foster, Fujisawa GmbH, in the preparation of this manuscript.

REFERENCES

1. Goto, T., Kino, T., Hatanaka, H., Nishiyama, M., Okuhara, M., Kohsaka, M., Aoki, H., and Imanaka, H. (1987). Discovery of FK506: a novel immunosuppressant isolated from *Streptomyces tsukubaensis*. *Transplant. Proc.* 23:2713–2717.
2. Kino, T., Hatanaka, H., Hashimoto, M., Nishiyama, M., Goto, T., Okuhara, M., Kohsaka, M., Aoki, H., and Imanaka, H. (1987). FK506, a novel immunosuppressant isolated from a *Streptomyces*. I. Fermentation, isolation and physico-chemical and biological characteristics. *J. Antibiot.* 40:1249–1255.
3. The US Multicenter FK506 Liver Study Group. (1994). A comparison of tacrolimus (FK506) and cyclosporine for immunosuppression in liver transplantation. *N. Engl. J. Med.* 331:1110–1115.
4. Fay, J.W., Nash, R.A., Wingard, J.R., Przepiorka, D., Collins, R.H., and Anasetti, C. (1995). FK506-based immunosuppression for prevention of graft-versus-host disease after unrelated donor bone marrow transplantation. *Transplant. Proc.* 27:1374.
5. Jain, A., Venkataramanan, R., Lever, J., Warty, V., Ebu-Elmagd, K., Furukawa, H., Reyes, J., Nour, B., Asrian, A., Tzakis, A., Todo, S., Fung, J., and Starzl, T.E. (1994). FK506 in small bowel transplant recipients: pharmacokinetics and dosing. *Transplant. Proc.* 26:1609–1610.
6. Ketel, B.L., Reed, K.M., and Barone, G.W. (1995). Initial results of tacrolimus maintenance therapy in combined kidney and pancreas transplantation. In: *7th Congress of the European Society for Organ Transplantation*, October 3-7, 1995. Book of Abstracts 215: Abstract 356.
7. Thomson, A.W., Carroll, P.B., McCauley, J., Woo, J., Abu-Elmagd, K., Starzl, T.E., and Van Thiel, D.H. (1993). FK506: a novel immunosuppressant for treatment of autoimmune disease. *Springer Semin. Immunopathol.* 14:323–344.
8. Bierer, B.E., Mattila, P.S., Standaert, R.F., Herzenberg, L.A., Burakoff, S.J., Crabtree, G., and Schreiber, S.L. (1990). Two distinct signal transmission pathways in T lymphocytes are inhibited by complexes formed between an immunophilin and either FK506 or rapamycin. *Proc. Natl. Acad. Sci. U.S.A.* 87:9231–9235.
9. Shaw, J-P., Utz, P.J., Durand, D.B., Toole, J.J., Emmel, E.A., and Crabtree, G.R. (1988). Identification of a putative regulator of early T-cell activation genes. *Science* 241:202–205.
10. Goldfeld, A.E., Flemington, E.K., Boussiotis, V.A., Theodos, C.M., Titus, R.G., Strominger, J.L., and Speck, S.H. (1992). Transcription of the tumor necrosis factor α gene is rapidly induced by anti-immunoglobulin and blocked by cyclosporin A and FK506 in human B-cells. *Proc. Natl. Acad. Sci. U.S.A.* 89:12198–12201.
11. De Paulis, A., Cirillo, R., Ciccarelli, A., de Crescenzo, G., Oriente, A., and Marone, G. (1991). Characterisation of the anti-inflammatory effect of FK506 on human mast cells. *J. Immunol.* 147:4278–4285.
12. De Paulis, A., Stellato, C., Cirillo, R., Ciccarelli, A., Oriente, A., and Marone, G. (1992). Anti-inflammatory effect of FK506 on human skin mast cells. *J. Invest. Dermatol.* 99:723–728.
13. Gillitzer, B., Berger, R., Mielke, V., Wolff, K., and Stingl, G. (1991). Upper keratinocytes of psoriatic lesions express high levels of NAP-1/IL-8 mRNA in situ. *J. Invest. Dermatol.* 97:73–79.
14. Lemester, B.H., Carroll, P.B., Rilo, H.R., Johnson, N., Nikaein, A., and Thomson, A.W. (1994). Effects of FK506 on IL-8 and IL-8R gene expression in lesional skin and on circulating IL-8 levels in psoriasis. *J. Immunol.* 6:3221.
15. Lemester, B.H., Carroll, P.B., Rilo, H.R., Johnson, N., Nikaein, A., and Thomson A.W. (1995). IL-8/IL-8 receptor expression in psoriasis and the response to systemic tacrolimus therapy. *Clin. Exp. Immunol.* 99: 148–152.
16. Ohara, K., Billington, R., James, R.W., Dean, G.A., Nishiyama, M., and Nouguch, I. (1990). Toxicologic evaluation of FK506. *Transplant. Proc.* 22: 83–86.
17. Todo, S., Ueda, Y., Demetris, J.A., Imventarza, O., Nalesnik, M., Venkataramanan R., Makowka, L., Starzl, T.E. (1988). Immunosuppression of canine, monkey, and baboon allografts by FK506: with special reference to synergism with other drugs and tolerance induction. *Surgery* 104:239–249.
18. Undre, N., Möller, A., Stadler, P. (1995). In *Clinical Pharmacokinetics of Tacrolimus*. W Zuckschwerdt Verlag, Munich pp. 13–19.
19. Jegasothy, B.V., Ackerman, C.D., Todo, S., Fung, J.J., Abu-Elmagd, K., and Starzl, T.E. (1992). Tacrolimus (FK506)—new therapeutic agent for severe recalcitrant psoriasis. *Arch. Dermatol.* 128:781–785.
20. Bos, J.D., Meinardi, M.M.H.M., Van Joost, Th., Heule, F., Powles, A.V., and Fry, L. (1989). Use of cyclosporin in psoriasis. *Lancet* 2:1500–1502.
21. European FK506 Multicenter Psoriasis Study Group. (1996). Systemic tacrolimus (FK506) is effective for the treatment of psoriasis in a double-blind, placebo-controlled study. *Arch. Dermatol.* 132:419–423.
22. Carroll, P.B., Rilo, H.L.R., Abu-Elmagd, K., Johnson, N., Carter, C., Wright, H., Jegasothy, B., Starzl, T.E., and Van Thiel, D.H. (1994). Effect of tacrolimus (FK506) in dystrophic epidermolysis bullosa: rationale and preliminary results. *Arch. Dermatol.* 130: 1457–1458.
23. Londino, A.V., Santora, D., Jegasothy, B.V., Abu-Elmagd, K., Fung, J.I., and Starzl, T.E. (1994). FK506 in the treatment of psoriasis and psoriatic arthritis. *Arthritis Rheum.* 37:207.

24. Abu-Elmagd, K., Jegasothy, B.V., Ackerman, C.D., Thomson, A.W., Rilo, H., Nikolaidis, N., Van Thiel, D., Fung, J.J., Todo, S., and Starzl, T.E. (1991). Efficacy of FK506 in the treatment of recalcitrant pyoderma gangrenosum. *Transplant. Proc.* 23:3328–3329.
25. Charley, M., Ackerman, C., Fung, J., Todo, S., Starzl, T.E., and Jegasothy, B. (1991). FK506—a new immunological agent to treat Sézary's syndrome. *J. Invest. Dermatol.* 4:571.
26. Hermann, R.C., Taylor, R.S., Ellis, C.N., Williams, N.A., Weiner, N.D., Flynn, G.L., Annesley, T.M., and Voorhees, J.J. (1988). Topical cyclosporin for psoriasis: in vitro skin penetration and clinical study. *Skin Pharmacol.* 1:246–249.
27. Bousema, M.T., Tank, B., Heule, F., Naafs, B., Stolz, E., and van Joost, T. (1990). Placebo-controlled study of psoriasis patients treated topically with a 10% cyclosporine gel. *J. Am. Acad. Dermatol.* 22:126–127.
28. De Rie, M.A., Meinardi, M.M.H.M., and Bos, J.D. (1991). Lack of efficacy of topical cyclosporin A in atopic dermatitis and allergic contact dermatitis. *Acta Derm. Venereol. (Stockh.)* 71:452–454.
29. Meingassner, J.G., and Stütz, A. (1992). Anti-inflammatory effects of macrophilin-interacting drugs in animal models of irritant and allergic contact dermatitis. *Int. Arch. Allergy Immunol.* 99:486–489.
30. Lauerma, A.I., Stein, B., Lee, H.L., Homey, B., Bloom, E., and Maibach, H.I. (1993). Topical tacrolimus (FK506): Percutaneous absorption and effect on allergic and irritant contact dermatitis. *J. Invest. Dermatol.* 110:491.
31. Bartek, M.J., LaBudde, J.A., and Maibach, H.I. (1972). Skin permeability in vivo: comparison in rat, rabbit, pig, and man. *J. Invest. Dermatol.* 58:114–123.
32. Meingassner, J.G., and Stütz, A. (1992). Immunosuppressive macrolides of the type FK506: a novel class of topical agents for treatment of skin diseases? *J. Invest. Dermatol.* 98:851–855.
33. Lauerma, A., Maibach, H.I., Granlund, H., Erkko, P., Kartamaa, M., and Stubb, S. (1992). Inhibition of contact allergy reactions by topical FK506. *Lancet* 340: 556.
34. Lauerma, A.I., and Maibach, H.I. (1994). Topical FK506—clinical potential or laboratory curiosity? *Dermatology* 188:173–176.
35. Aoyama, H., Tabata, N., Tanaka, M., Uesugi, Y., and Tagami, H. (1995). Successful treatment of resistant facial lesions of atopic dermatitis with 0.1% FK506 ointment. *Br. Assoc. Dermatol.* 133:494–495.
36. Nahagawa, H., Etoh, T., Ishibashi, Y., Higaki, Y., Kawashima, M., Torii, H., and Harada, S. (1994). Tacrolimus ointment for atopic dermatitis. *Lancet* 344: 833.
37. Funk, J.O., and Maibach, H.I. (1994). Horizons in pharmacologic intervention in allergic contact dermatitis. *J. Am. Acad. Dermatol.* 31:999–1014.

63

Clinical Use of Oral 1,25-Dihydroxyvitamin D_3 (Calcitriol) for the Treatment of Psoriasis and Psoriatic Arthritis

Michael F. Holick
Boston University Medical Center, Boston, Massachusetts

Vitamin D is a fat-soluble vitamin that is either made in the skin by the action of solar ultraviolet B radiation or ingested in the diet (1). Vitamin D is essential for regulating calcium and bone metabolism, and is important for the growth, development, and maintenance of a healthy skeleton. Vitamin D undergoes two obligate hydroxylations, first in the liver to 25-hydroxyvitamin D (25-OH-D) and then in the kidney where 25-OH-D is converted to 1,25-dihydroxyvitamin D (1,25$(OH)_2$D). The major physiological function of 1,25$(OH)_2$D is to increase the efficiency of intestinal calcium absorption and to mobilize calcium stores from bone to maintain the blood calcium level within the normal range (2).

1,25$(OH)_2$D carries out most, if not all, of its biological actions by interacting with a specific nuclear receptor, the vitamin D receptor (VDR), and forms a heterodimer with retinoic acid X receptor (RXR), which then interacts with specific vitamin D–responsive elements within the DNA to alter transcriptional activity.

During the past 16 years, it has been recognized that a variety of tissues and cells not associated with calcium metabolism, including the pancreas, gonads, stomach, breast, pituitary gland, thymus, mononuclear cells, and skin possess VDR and respond to 1,25$(OH)_2D_3$ (calcitriol) (3). The major noncalcemic activities of 1,25$(OH)_2D_3$ are inhibition of proliferation and enhancement of differentiation in cells that have VDR (4,5). Cultured human keratinocytes respond to 1,25$(OH)_2D_3$ in a similar fashion. 1,25$(OH)_2D_3$ decreases keratinocyte proliferation in a dose-dependent fashion and induces keratinocytes to terminally differentiate (6,7).

It was based on these observations and the serendipitous observation of a patient with osteoporosis who was treated with a 1,25$(OH)_2D_3$ analog, 1-hydroxyvitamin D_3, and also had her psoriasis improve that gave rise to the concept of using activated vitamin D compounds for the treatment of psoriasis (8,9). Topical 1,25$(OH)_2D_3$ and its analogs, calcipotriol and 1,24-dihydroxyvitamin D_3, have been shown to be very effective for treating psoriasis, especially psoriasis vulgaris (10–15).

EFFICACY AND SAFETY OF ORAL 1,25$(OH)_2D_3$ FOR THE TREATMENT OF PSORIASIS

Rationale

In the mid-1970s when it was realized that the kidney was the major organ responsible for producing the calciotropic hormone 1,25$(OH)_2D_3$, it was appreciated why patients with kidney failure suffered from severe disorders in calcium metabolism that often caused severe bone disease (renal osteodystrophy). It was demonstrated that orally administered 1,25$(OH)_2D_3$

(calcitriol) was very effective in reversing the calcium metabolic disorder of renal failure and prevented and treated renal osteodystrophy (2,16). Thus, $1,25(OH)_2D_3$ is available worldwide as an oral capsule for the treatment of renal osteodystrophy and other calcium and metabolic bone disorders (2).

We reasoned that for patients who have at least 10% of their body involved with psoriasis, it would be ideal if they could treat their psoriasis with orally administered $1,25(OH)_2D_3$. However, because $1,25(OH)_2D_3$'s major physiological action is to enhance the efficiency of intestinal calcium absorption and mobilize calcium stores from bone, there was great concern that oral $1,25(OH)_2D_3$ might be of limited value for treating psoriasis because of its potent calcemic effect, which could cause hypercalciuria, hypercalcemia, and soft tissue calcification.

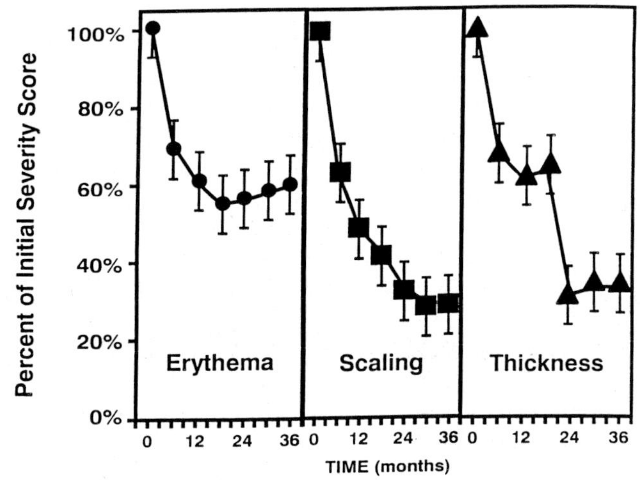

Figure 1 Changes in severity score using oral calcitriol before and during treatment. Vertical range bars indicate ± standard error of the mean (SEM). The severity scores during treatment with $1,25(OH)_2D_3$ were statistically significant ($p < 0.001$) in comparison with baseline values. (From Ref. 17.)

Therapeutic Efficacy

We enrolled 85 patients with no other significant illness (62 men and 23 women: mean age 46 years: range 19–76) with either stable plaque or erythrodermic psoriasis involving at least 15% of their body surface area. None of the patients had previously responded satisfactorily to at least one of the standard treatments for psoriasis. The patients were instructed to ingest no more than 800 mg of calcium from their diet in 24 hr. The patients were instructed to take 0.5 μg of $1,25(OH)_2D_3$ (calcitriol; Rocaltrol) at bedtime and at least 2 hr after the last meal. The patients had their $1,25(OH)_2D_3$ increased in increments of 0.5 μg every 2 weeks as long as the serum and 24-hr urinary calcium concentrations remained within the normal range. Most patients were maintained on 1.5–2.5 μg each night while a few patients needed up to 5 μg/night to control their psoriasis. Biyearly renal ultrasounds and bone mineral density measurements were conducted (17).

The baseline global severity score for the patients' lesions ranged from 5 to 9 with a mean value of 7.7 ± 1.2. The treatment period ranged from 6 months to 5 years. Twenty-five of the patients had been in the study for at least 3 years. At the last visit, the mean global severity score for all of the patients significantly decreased to 3.2 ± 1.9 ($p < 0.01$), which represented an almost 60% improvement. After 6 months on therapy, the patients showed significant decrease from baseline in the scaling, plaque thickness, and erythema. This improvement persisted as long as the patients remained on therapy (Fig. 1).

The mean baseline PASI score was 18.4 ± 1.0. At 6 and 36 months of treatment, the mean PASI score was reduced to 9.7 ± 0.8 and 7.0 ± 1.3, respectively (Fig. 2). The overall clinical assessment showed that 88% of all patients on oral calcitriol had some improvement in their disease (Fig. 3). Of these, approximately 27% had complete clearance, 37% had moderate improvement, and 25% had slight improvement in the activity of their disease. Twelve percent of the patients had no change in the activity of their disease and none of the patients had substantial worsening in their disease.

Patients with marked erythema as a component of their psoriasis often had the most dramatic improvement in their disease (Fig. 4). We have treated four patients with pustular psoriasis with oral $1,25(OH)_2D_3$ and found that one patient had dramatic improvement in the activity of her disease while on 1.0 μg of $1,25(OH)_2D_3$ each night.

Even for patients on oral $1,25(OH)_2D_3$ who experienced only moderate to slight improvement in their disease, they not only noted a decrease in scale production, but often found that the character of the scale changed and was more fine in nature. They also noted that the elasticity and comfortableness of the skin improved and there was often improvement in the nails of patients with nail involvement (Fig. 5).

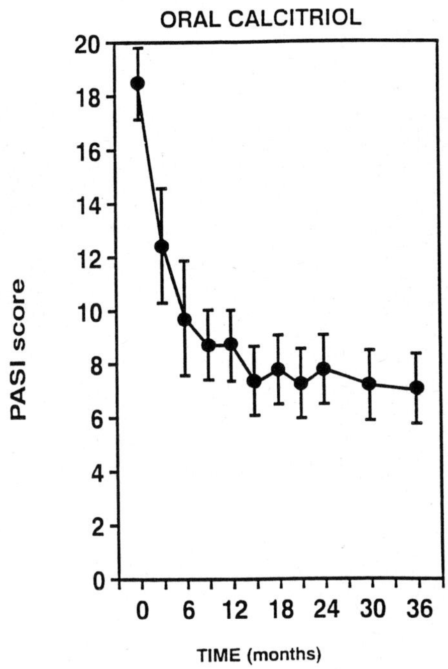

Figure 2 Mean values of the psoriasis area and severity index (PASI) scores using oral 1,25(OH)$_2$D$_3$ before and during treatment. Vertical range bars indicate mean ± SEM. PASI scores during treatment with 1,25(OH)$_2$D$_3$ were statistically significant ($p < 0.001$) in comparison with baseline values. (From Ref. 17.)

Safety Profile for Oral 1,25(OH)$_2$D$_3$

Patients were instructed to increase their 1,25(OH)$_2$D$_3$ intake in 0.5-μg increments at bedtime every 2 weeks until either they had significant improvement in the activity of their disease or their calcium/creatinine ratio in the urine reached 0.35 or their serum calcium was greater than 10.5 mg% (Fig. 6). The 24-hr urine collection for the determination of calcium/creatinine was the most useful marker for determining the calciuric activity of 1,25(OH)$_2$D$_3$ therapy. The patient's serum was also initially monitored for albumin and calcium every 2 weeks, and if the calcium went above the normal range, the therapy was either reduced or stopped. The therapeutic dose range was between 1.5 and 2.5 μg each night. However, some patients required higher doses and have tolerated up to 5.0 μg/night. Once the patient was on a therapeutic dose of 1,25(OH)$_2$D$_3$ and there were no significant changes in either the 24-hr urine calcium/creatinine or serum calcium, these evaluations decreased to once every 1–2 months. The serum concentrations of calcium increased 3.9 ± 7.1% and 0.7 ± 4.0% at 6 and 36 months, respectively. The mean baseline serum calcium value of 9.6 ± 0.4 mg/dl increased to 9.9 ± 0.5 mg/dl at 6 months during treatment. The mean serum calcium concentration at 36 months during treatment was similar to baseline value. The change in 24-hr urinary excretion of calcium from baseline averaged a 148% increase and the calcium/creatinine ratio increased from 0.11 ± 0.07 to 0.23 ± 0.1 ($p < 0.01$) and 0.20 ± 0.1 ($p < 0.1$) at 6 and 36 months, respectively (17).

The serum creatinine at 6 and 36 months during treatment increased by 11.8% and 25.7% from baseline, respectively. Intact parathyroid hormone (PTH) at 24 months during treatment decreased by 32.3 ± 8% from baseline. There were no significant changes in other blood chemistries and there was no effect on liver function.

All patients on oral 1,25(OH)$_2$D$_3$ therapy had renal ultrasounds performed semiannually to determine the presence of nephrocalcinosis and kidney stones. Of the 55 patients studied for a total period of 34,617 patient-days, two had positive renal ultrasounds for kidney stones. Both stones were radiopaqued while on treatment. One patient had a positive right kidney echogenic signal for a kidney stone on his first ultrasound study. As he did not have an ultrasound before treatment, we could not determine if the stone was new. This patient's calcium/creatinine ranged between 0.04 and 0.3, and his serum calcium was between 9.8 and 10.4 mg/dl. There were no observed changes in the size or number of kidney stones in his follow-up ultrasound studies while on oral 1,25(OH)$_2$D$_3$ (3 μg/night) for 6 years. The other patient with a normal baseline kidney ultrasound developed a kidney stone after 20 months. While on treatment, her calcium/creatinine ratio was between 0.1 and 0.4, and her serum calcium was between 9.7 and 10.8 mg/dl. When the patient developed hypercalcemia, the treatment was discontinued. The renal ultrasound studies have remained negative in the other 53 patients, who have been taking oral 1,25(OH)$_2$D$_3$ at a mean dose of 2.4 ± 0.6 μg for up to 6 years (17).

Effect of Oral 1,25(OH)$_2$D$_3$ on Renal Function and Bone Mineral Content

We were concerned that the creatinine clearance at 6 and 36 months decreased 13.4 and 13.3%, respectively, from baseline. The decrease in creatinine clear-

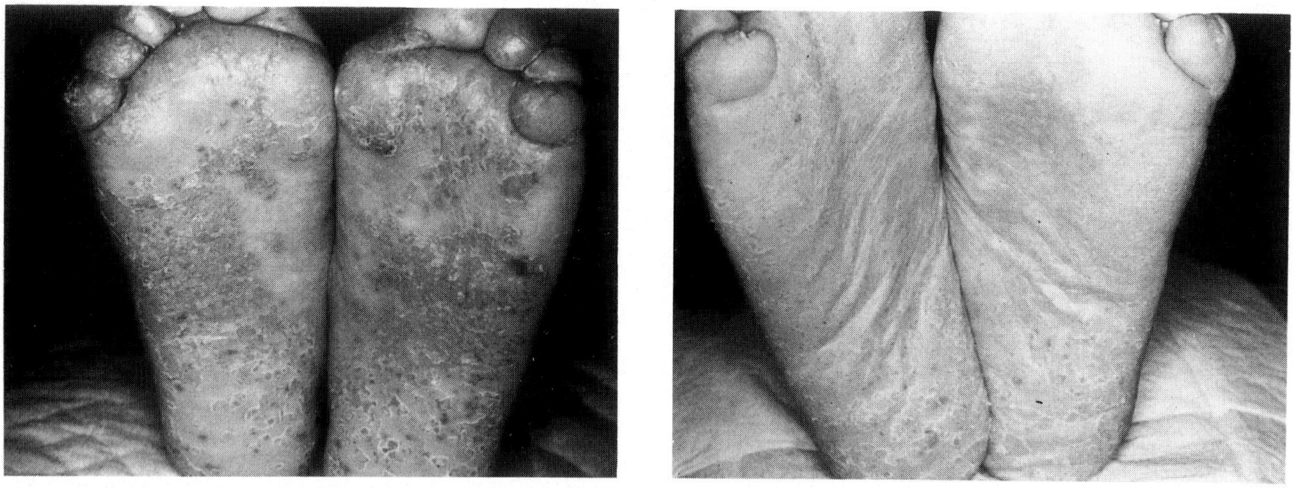

Figure 3 A 64-year-old man with plaque psoriasis for 18 years. Before (left) and 6 months after (right) oral $1,25(OH)_2D_3$ (1.5 μg).

ance was consistent with a similar percent increase in the serum creatinine values in these patients. To determine whether the oral $1,25(OH)_2D_3$ was causing renal dysfunction or altering creatinine metabolism or secretion in the kidney, we conducted creatinine and inulin clearances before and at 6 months of therapy in a group of eight patients with psoriasis. The age range for this group was 24–55 years. The creatinine clearance decreased by 23.3 $\pm$ 6% after 2 months of therapy while on oral $1,25(OH)_2D_3$ at 1.4 $\pm$ 0.3 μg/night. This decrease in creatinine clearance remained stable and unchanged during the next 4 months of treatment even while the patients were having their dose of $1,25(OH)_2D_3$ increased to 2.7 $\pm$ 0.3 μg/night. After 6 months, the creatinine clearance decreased by 24% (17).

We conducted an inulin (a nonreabsorbable sugar) clearance study and found that the inulin clearance in the same patients after 6 months of therapy was no different than baseline. To determine tubular function, we also conducted a para-aminohippuric acid (PAH) clearance. The maximum tubular secretion of PAH did not change between pretreatment and 6 months of $1,25(OH)_2D_3$ therapy.

Since $1,25(OH)_2D_3$ is a potent hormone that mobilizes calcium stores from bone, we were concerned that the large oral doses of $1,25(OH)_2D_3$ might cause bone loss and lead to osteoporosis. Patients who were begun on $1,25(OH)_2D_3$ therapy were followed semiannually to assess the bone mineral density of their lumbar spine and femoral neck. After 2 years of $1,25(OH)_2D_3$ therapy, all of the patients maintained their bone mineral density in their lumbar spine and hip (17).

TREATMENT OF PSORIATIC ARTHRITIS WITH ORAL $1,25(OH)_2D_3$

Some of the patients we treated with oral calcitriol also suffered with psoriatic arthritis. Since we anecdotally noted that some of the patients had some improvement in their psoriatic arthritis, we conducted a 6-month open trial and initially evaluated 10 patients with active psoriatic arthritis. The patients received oral $1,25(OH)_2D_3$ in a similar fashion as described above (17). Most of the patients were on at least 2.0 μg of oral $1,25(OH)_2D_3$ daily by the end of the study. There were statistically significant improvements in the tender joint count and physician's global impression (Fig. 7). Of the 10 patients, four had substantial ($\geq$50%) improvement and three had moderate

Figure 4 A 40-year-old man with psoriasis for 15 years. Before (a) and 6 months after (b) 2 μg each night of oral $1,25(OH)_2D_3$. (From Ref. 17.)

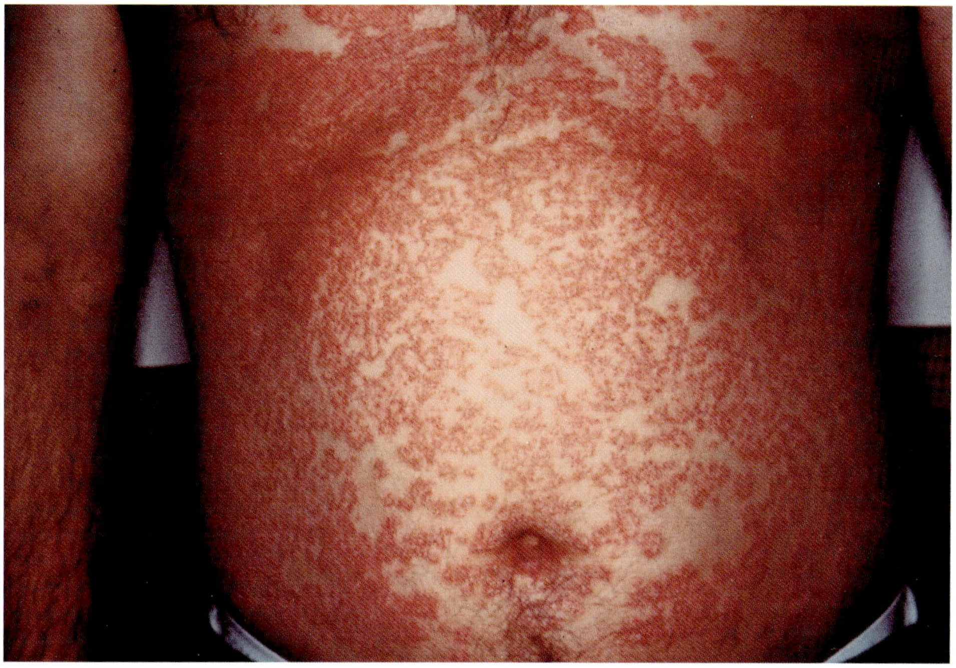

Figure 4a.

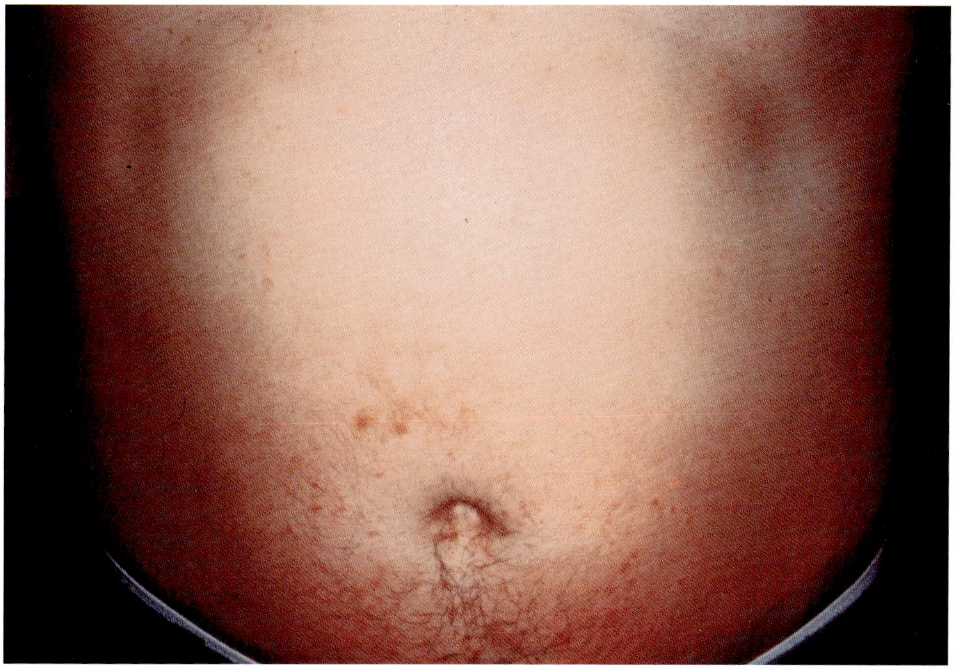

Figure 4b.

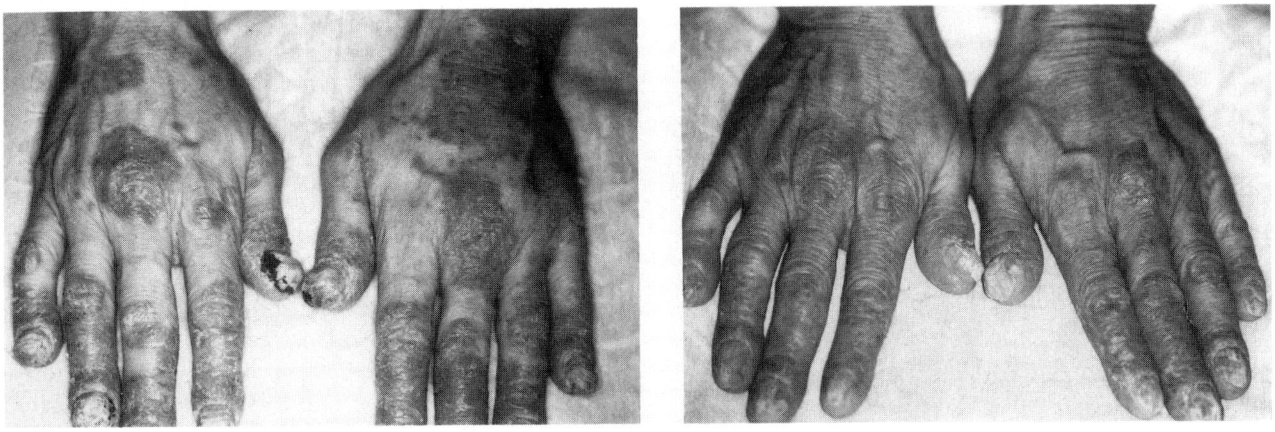

Figure 5 A 72-year-old man with plaque psoriasis for greater than 20 years with significant nail involvement. Before (left) and 4 months after (right) oral 1,25(OH)$_2$D$_3$ (2 μg).

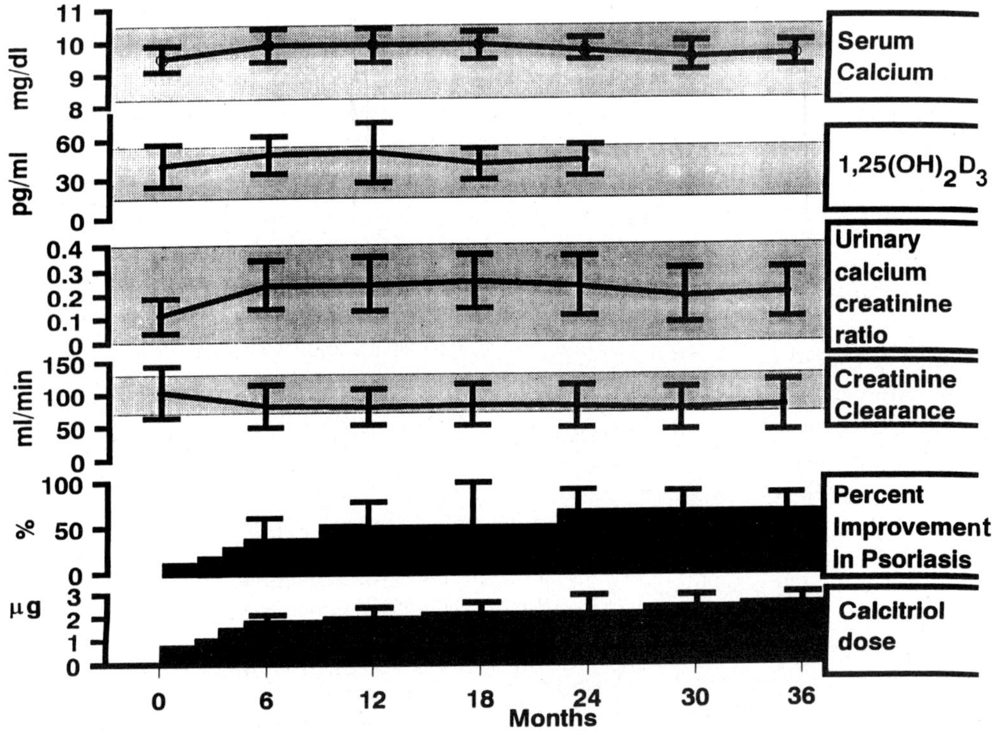

Figure 6 Sequence of clinical events over time. Changes in blood and urine calcium as well as serum 1,25(OH)$_2$D$_3$ (calcitriol) concentrations are shown at the same time as the clinical improvement occurred. (From Ref. 17.)

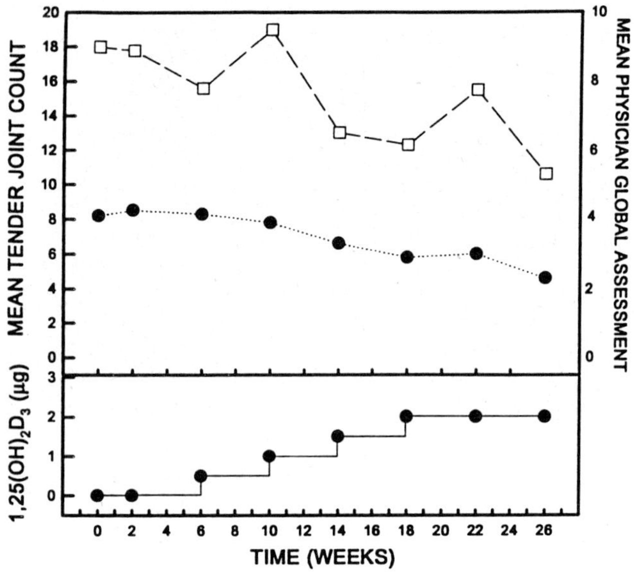

Figure 7 Changes in the mean tender joint count (□) and the mean physician global assessment (●) in six psoriatic arthritis patients who completed the 6-month oral trial of $1,25(OH)_2D_3$ (Rocaltrol: Hoffmann-La Roche, Nutley, NJ) (●), according to the mean daily dosage. (From Ref. 1.)

(≥25%) improvement in the tender joint count. Two patients were unable to receive therapeutic doses because of hypercalciuria (18).

CONCLUSION

For patients with less than 10% involvement of their skin with plaque psoriasis the choice of using an activated vitamin D ointment as the first line of therapy is becoming a widely accepted practice in dermatology. However, for patients with more extensive involvement, it becomes inconvenient for them to topically apply over a large surface area an ointment containing an activated vitamin D. For those patients, it is reasonable to consider treatment with a trial of oral $1,25(OH)_2D_3$. This medication and its analog, 1α-hydroxyvitamin D_3, are available worldwide for treating a variety of metabolic bone diseases including osteoporosis and renal osteodystrophy.

The major issues in considering oral $1,25(OH)_2D_3$ are: (1) the medication must be given in a stepwise manner, which means that the patient may not be on a therapeutic dosage for 1.5–3 months after initiating therapy, (2) the patient needs to limit his or her calcium intake to no more than 800 mg/day because of the calciotropic effect of $1,25(OH)_2D_3$ and (3) the patient requires frequent monitoring with a 24-hr urine calcium and creatinine and a serum calcium to make certain that the patient does not develop the major undesirable side effects of this medication, i.e., hypercalciuria or hypercalcemia.

In conclusion, oral administration of $1,25(OH)_2D_3$ or one of its active analogs should be considered for treating patients with widespread plaque psoriasis or erythrodermic psoriasis. It can be anticipated that most patients will have some improvement in the activity of their disease. The therapeutic dose begins at about 1.5 μg but may not be fully appreciated until the patient is on as much as 5 μg each night. It can be anticipated that most patients will continue to have a gradual decrease in scaling, erythema, and plaque thickness. This therapy will also cause significant improvement in how patients feel about their skin, i.e., being more flexible and less itching, as well as improvement in their nails. For patients who are considered for oral $1,25(OH)_2D_3$ therapy, frequent monitoring at least once or twice a month of blood and urine calcium levels should be practiced until a stable dose of $1,25(OH)_2D_3$ is attained. A renal ultrasound before initiation of therapy should be performed to rule out kidney stones and follow-up ultrasound at 6 months would be helpful to rule out the development of kidney stones. Yearly ultrasounds, thereafter, are all that are needed to ensure that the patients are not developing kidney stones as a result of therapy.

ACKNOWLEDGMENT

This work was supported in part by NIH grants RR00533 and AR36963.

REFERENCES

1. Holick, M.F. (1994). Vitamin D: new horizons for the 21st century. *Am. J. Clin. Nutr.* 60:619–630.
2. Holick, M.F. (1995). Vitamin D: photobiology, metabolism, and clinical applications. *Endocrinology*, 3rd ed. L. DeGroot et al. (Eds.). W.B. Saunders, Philadelphia, pp. 990–1013.
3. Stumpf, W.E., Sar, M., Reid, F.A., et al. (1979). Target cells for 1,25-dihydroxyvitamin D_3 in intestinal tract, stomach, kidney, skin, pituitary, and parathyroid. *Science* 206:1188–1190.
4. Abe, E., Miyaura, C., Sakagami, H., et al. (1981). Differentiation of rat *myc* leukemia cells induced by 1,25-

dihydroxyvitamin D_3. *Proc. Natl. Acad. Sci.* U.S.A. 78: 4990–4994.
5. Honma, Y., Hozumi, M., Abe, E., Konno, K., Fukushima, M., Hata, S., et al. (1982). 1α,25-Dihydroxyvitamin D_3 and 1α-hydroxyvitamin D_3 prolong survival time of mice inoculated with myeloid leukemia cells. *Proc. Natl. Acad. Sci.* 80:201–204.
6. Hosomi, J., Hosoi, J., Abe, E., Suda, T., and Kuroki, T. (1983). Regulation of terminal differentiation of cultured mouse epidermal cells by 1α,25-dihydroxyvitamin D_3. *Endocrinology* 113:1950–1957.
7. Smith, E.L., Walworth, N.D., and Holick, M.F. (1986). Effect of 1,25-dihydroxyvitamin D_3 on the morphologic and biochemical differentiation of cultured human epidermal keratinocytes grown in serum-free conditions. *J. Invest. Dermatol.* 86:709–714.
8. Morimoto, S., and Kumahara, Y. (1985). A patient with psoriasis cured by 1α-hydroxyvitamin D_3. *Med. J. Osaka Univ.* 35:51.
9. Smith, E.L., Pincus, S.H., Donovan, L., and Holick, M.F. (1988). A novel approach for the evaluation and treatment of psoriasis. *J. Am. Acad. Dermatol.* 19: 516–528.
10. Kragballe, K., Beck, H.I., and Sogaard, H. (1988). Improvement of psoriasis by a topical vitamin D_3 analogue (MC903) in a double-blind study. *Br. J. Dermatol.* 119:223–230.
11. Kato, T., Rokugo, M., Terui, T., and Tagami, H. (1986). Successful treatment of psoriasis with topical application of active vitamin D_3 analogue, 1α,24-dihydroxycholecalciferol. *Br. J. Dermatol.* 115:431–433.
12. el-Azhary, R.A., Peters, M.S., Pittelkow, M.R., Kao, P.C., and Muller, S.A. (1993). Efficacy of vitamin D_3 derivatives in treatment of psoriasis. *Mayo Clin. Proc.* 68:835–841.
13. Dubertret, L., Wallach, D., Souteyrand, P., Perussel, M., Kalis, B., Meynadier, J., et al. (1992). Efficacy and safety of calcipotriol (MC 903) ointment in psoriasis vulgaris: a randomized, double-blind, right/left comparative, vehicle-controlled study. *J. Am. Acad. Dermatol.* 27:983–988.
14. Henderson, C.A., Papworth-Smith, J., Cunliffe, W.J., et al. (1989). A double-blind placebo controlled trial of topical 1,25-dihydroxycholecalciferol in psoriasis. *Br. J. Dermatol.* 121:493–496.
15. Perez, A., Chen, T.C., Turner, A., Raab, R., Bhawan, J., Poche, P., and Holick, M.F. (1996). Efficacy and safety of topical calcitriol (1,25-dihydroxyvitamin D_3) for the treatment of psoriasis. *Br. J. Dermatol.* 134: 238–246.
16. Krane, S., and Holick, M.F. (1994). Metabolic bone disease. In *Harrison's Principles of Internal Medicine*, K.J. Isselbacher, E. Braunwald, J.D. Wilson, et al. (Eds.). McGraw-Hill, New York, pp. 2172–2183.
17. Perez, A., Raab, R., Chen, T.C., Turner, A., and Holick, M.F. (1996). Safety and efficacy of oral calcitriol (1,25-dihydroxyvitamin D_3) for the treatment of psoriasis. *Br. J. Dermatol.* 134:1070–1078.
18. Huckins, D., Felson, D.T., and Holick, M.F. (1990). Treatment of psoriatic arthritis with oral 1,25-dihydroxyvitamin D_3. A pilot study. *Arthritis Rheum.* 33:1723–1727.

64

Photodynamic Therapy of Psoriasis

Jerry L. McCullough and Gerald D. Weinstein
University of California School of Medicine, Irvine, California

Psoriasis is a skin disease with well-documented therapeutic responsiveness to various forms of light, both with and without chemical photosensitizers. Ultraviolet light (UVB) alone or in combination with coal tar is used to treat psoriasis, but both coal tar and ultraviolet light are potentially carcinogenic. Photo-"chemotherapy" using photosensitizing psoralen derivatives and long-wavelength (320–400 nm) UVA (PUVA) is one of the most effective and widely used therapies for the treatment of recalcitrant and severe psoriasis (1). As psoralen-mediated photosensitization involves direct interaction with DNA bases, PUVA is associated with an increased risk of squamous cell carcinoma (SCC), basal cell carcinoma (BCC), actinic keratoses, and cutaneous photodamage (2).

PORPHYRIN PHOTOSENSITIZERS

The porphyrins represent a different class of photosensitizers that are well known with respect to their cutaneous photosensitizing properties (human porphyria diseases, e.g., erythropoietic protoporphyria). Porphyrins are selectively taken up or retained in hyperproliferative tissue, where they are localized in different membrane structures (e.g., mitochondrial and plasma membranes). In contrast to the DNA target of cytotoxicity in psoralen photochemotherapy, photodynamic therapy (PDT)-induced cytotoxicity is mainly due to the singlet oxygen ($^1O_2$) pathway directed at these cellular membrane targets.

There have been several reports of the use of porphyrins as photosensitizers for the PDT of psoriasis. Oral doses of hematoporphyrin combined with ultraviolet light exposure was reported in 1937 to be beneficial in psoriasis (3). Systemically administered hematoporphyrin derivative (HPD) in combination with UVA was reported to improve psoriasis after 15 treatments with UVA (4). Systemic HPD in combination with visible red light (630 nm) administered by argon dye laser (20–40 J/cm^2) was shown to produce a selective tissue necrosis in psoriatic skin (5). More recent studies using Photofrin porfimer sodium, a purified form of HPD, and laser (630 nm, 15 J/cm^2) have resulted in long-term clearing of psoriatic lesions, without producing tissue necrosis (6). However, due to the extended length of time that Photofrin remains in the skin, patients are photosensitive for 2–3 months after treatment and must avoid sunlight and exposure to bright lights during this period. Recent phase I/II trials with a second-generation porphyrin photosensitizer, benzoporphyrin derivative mono acid (BPD-MA), have shown efficacy in the treatment of psoriasis (7). In contrast to Photofrin, BPD is rapidly cleared from the body and skin photosensitivity lasts only a few days. However, in its current use, BPD requires intravenous administration.

5-AMINOLEVULINIC ACID PDT

5-Aminolevulinic acid (ALA), the first committed intermediate in the heme biosynthesis pathway, results in the production of photosensitizing porphyrin precursors, particularly protoporphyrin IX (PpIX). When ALA is applied topically to target premalignant and malignant lesions, it produces a selective red fluorescence of the target tissue as compared to the surrounding normal skin. This may be due to selective penetration and/or selective enzymatic conversion to PpIX by the target tissue. Topical application of ALA to target skin lesions results in photosensitizing levels of PpIX, which, when followed by light exposure, produce a photodynamic effect. Topical ALA and visible red light have been used clinically in the PDT of a variety of cutaneous lesions, including superficial basal cell carcinoma, early invasive squamous cell carcinoma, precancerous actinic keratosis, and cutaneous T-cell lymphoma (8–10).

PpIX has a large absorption band in the 380–400-nm range, with less absorption in the visible spectrum. Red light is routinely used for PDT of malignant tumors with ALA owing to the greater tissue penetrance of this longer wavelength. In the treatment of psoriasis, where deep penetration is neither desirable nor necessary, the intense Soret band at 405 nm is useful for photoactivation of PpIX. Owing to this strong absorption band with a higher molar extinction coefficient, PpIX has a significant advantage in capturing any photons that penetrate into the tissue at 405 nm as opposed to 630 nm, resulting in much more efficient photosensitization. Long-wave UVA (380–420 nm) with photosensitizers, such as psoralens and hematoporphyrin derivative, has previously been shown to be effective in the PDT of psoriasis.

A pilot drug and light dose-ranging study was undertaken to evaluate the safety, tolerance, and clinical efficacy of UVA- and ALA-induced PpIX PDT of psoriasis. This was an open-label study that evaluated various concentrations of ALA (2%, 10%, 20%) in an optimized oil-in-water emulsion vehicle (M55A). A total of 14 patients with plaque psoriasis, with nine 2-cm psoriatic lesion sites per patient, were treated with topical ALA (2%, 10%, 20%) or vehicle emollient cream under occlusion. Three hours after drug application sites were treated with incremental dosages of UVA (2.5–30 J/cm^2 at an average power density of 15 mW/cm^2) with a HOUVA-LITE device (National Biological Corporation, Twinsburg, OH). Half of the treatment sites received only one PDT treatment, and the remaining sites were treated with ALA and UVA once weekly for 4 weeks.

Immediately prior to PDT, the treatment sites were examined by Wood's ultraviolet light. All concentrations of ALA produced an intense red fluorescence in the treated psoriatic lesions, reflecting the active conversion of ALA to PpIX in the lesional versus nonlesional skin. Fluorescence was markedly reduced (photobleached) during UVA treatment.

The results of this pilot study demonstrated approximately 50% improvement after four weekly treatments with 10% ALA (total UVA 80–120 J/cm^2) and 20% ALA (total 1–39 J/cm^2) (Fig. 1). Treatment with 2% ALA or vehicle was clinically ineffective with four weekly treatments at all UVA light dosages. Single treatment with ALA and UVA was also ineffective at all concentrations of ALA and UVA dosages. Clinical assessments of skin photosensitization and patient symptoms revealed that patients experienced a transient "burning" or "stinging" sensation of the treatment site during light irradiation. The discomfort was drug- and light-dose-dependent. Patients were able to tolerate treatment with 2% ALA and all light dosages (up to 30 J/cm^2). However, treatment with 10% and 20% ALA required reduction in the scheduled UVA dosing owing to the strong degree of discomfort. At the higher drug and light dosages there was localized erythema and edema at the treatment sites. Neither generalized (systemic) photosensitivity nor other adverse reactions were observed during the study.

CONCLUSION

This pilot study has established the potential for ALA PDT for the treatment of psoriasis. However, many variables are yet to be worked out, particularly relating to the reciprocity of drug and light dosimetry to minimize patient discomfort, and effective treatment/maintenance schedules. Other light sources may also be useful for PDT, as a recent study has reported the effectiveness of polychromatic light and topical 10% ALA for the treatment of plaque psoriasis (11). To optimize the multiplicity of treatment parameters for PDT, we must first have a better understanding of the basic mechanism(s) of PDT in psoriasis, which is distinctly different than in cutaneous malignancies where the goal is tissue eradication. Clearly, tissue destruction of psoriasis is not achieved in conjunction with the therapeutic responses observed in the present study. Jeffes et al. have recently reported the selective

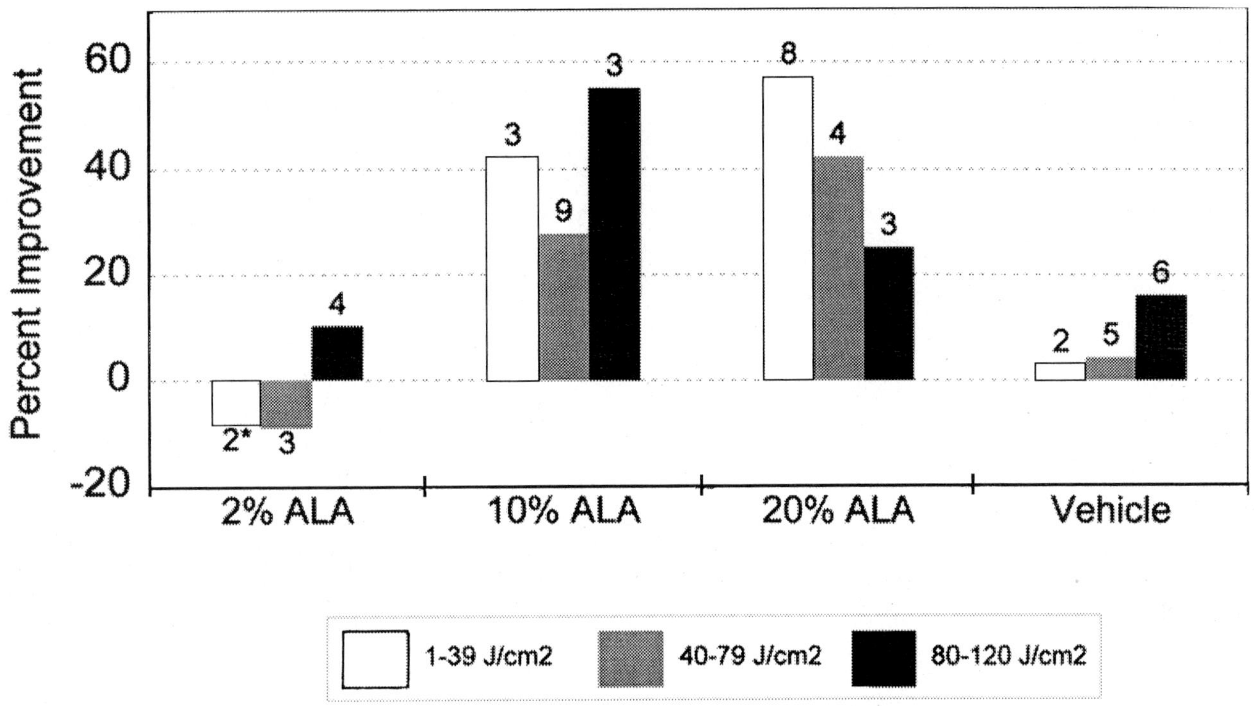

Figure 1 Clinical response of psoriasis to four weekly treatments with topical ALA photodynamic therapy. Mean percent improvement of lesion treated with ALA or vehicle and cumulative UVA (Joules/cm^2). *Number of treatment sites for each group.

killing effects of ALA PDT on lymphocytes versus keratinocytes (12). A selective killing of cutaneous immune cells may be a primary target of PDT, which modulates the cascade of events perpetuating psoriatic epidermal hyperproliferation and inflammation.

REFERENCES

1. Weinstein, G.D., Liem, W., and McCullough, J.L. (1995). Topical therapy for psoriasis: results of survey to U.S. dermatologists. *Cutis* 55:306–310.
2. Gupta, A.K., and Anderson, T.F. (1987). Psoralen photochemotherapy. *J. Am. Acad. Dermatol.* 17:703–734.
3. Silver, H. (1937). Psoriasis vulgaris treated with hematoporphyrin. *Arch. Dermatol. Syphilol.* 36: 1118–1119.
4. Diezel, W., Meffert, H., and Sonnichsen, N. (1980). Therapie der Psoriasis mit Hamatoporphyrin und Licht. *Dermatol. Monattschr.* 166:793–797.
5. Berns, M.W., Rettenmaier, M.A., McCullough, J.L., Coffey, J., Wile, A.G., Berman, M.L., DiSaia, P.J., and Weinstein, G.D. (1984). Response of psoriasis to red laser light (630 nm) following systemic injection of hematoporphyrin derivative. *Lasers Surg. Med.* 4: 73–77.
6. Weinstein, G.D., McCullough, J.L., Nelson, J.S., Berns, M.W., and McCormick, A. (1991). Low dose Photofrin II photodynamic therapy of psoriasis. *J. Invest. Dermatol.* 96:573.
7. Lui, H. (1994). Photodynamic therapy in dermatology with porfimer sodium and benzoporphyrin derivative: an update. *Semin. Oncol.* 21:11–14.
8. Kennedy, J.C., Pottier, R.H., and Pross, D.C. (1990). Photodynamic therapy with endogenous protoporphyrin IX: basic principles and present clinical experience. *J. Photochem. Photobiol. B Biol.* 6:143–148.
9. Wolf, P., Rieger E., and Kerl, H. (1993). Topical photodynamic therapy with endogenous porphyrins after application of 5-aminolevulinic acid: an alternative treatment modality for solar keratoses, superficial squamous cell carcinomas and basal cell carcinomas. *J. Am. Acad. Dermatol.* 28:17–21.
10. Svanberg, K., Andersson, T., Killander, D., et al. (1994). Photodynamic therapy of nonmelanoma malignant tumours of the skin using topical δ-amino levulinic acid sensitization and laser irradiation. *Br. J. Dermatol.* 130:743–751.

11. Boehncke, W.H., Sterry, W., and Kaufmann, R. (1994). Treatment of psoriasis by topical photodynamic therapy with polychromatic light. *Lancet* 343:801 (letter).
12. Jeffes, E., McCullough, J.L., Plowman, M., Herrod, R., Jadus, M.R., Horansky, E., and Weinstein, G.D. (1995). 5-Aminolevulinic acid (ALA) photosensitizes and kills lymphoid cells at concentrations easily achieved in the skin during photodynamic therapy (PDT). *Photochem. Photobiol.* 61:76S.

65

Antithyroid Thioureylenes in Psoriasis: A Novel Therapy

Alan Elias and Ronald Barr
University of California, Irvine, California

Psoriasis consumes approximately 2 billion dollars in health care costs annually in the United States (1). A significant portion of this expenditure is for drug costs. Current oral medications used to treat psoriasis consist of methotrexate, etretinate, and, more recently, cyclosporin. All these agents have significant side effects and some are effective only in specific forms of psoriasis. For instance, etretinate, a retinoid, is most effective in erythrodermic and pustular psoriasis but is less effective in chronic plaque psoriasis (2). Furthermore, its use is restricted to males and nonfertile female patients. Its long-term use has been associated with development of osteoporosis (3).

Severe psoriasis (>20% body surface area involved and resistant to topical therapy) affects less than 200,000 patients in the United States, and is often resistant to treatment with currently used medications because of the high risk-to-benefit ratio when these medications are used continuously. It is therefore imperative that newer, cheaper, and less toxic drugs be identified for the treatment of patients with psoriasis. Pilot studies suggest that the antithyroid thioureylenes, propylthiouracil (PTU) and methimazole (MMI), constitute such a new potential treatment for psoriasis (4–7). These drugs have well-documented immunemodulatory properties (8–11). In addition, PTU and MMI bind to the T_3 receptor (T3R) (12), a member of the superfamily of steroid receptors that includes retinoids and vitamin D (13). T3R, free of its natural ligand (triiodothyronine, T_3), may act as a gene repressor (14). It is likely that some of the beneficial clinical effects of antithyroid thioureylenes in psoriasis are based on interaction with the T3R.

PATHOGENESIS

The pathogenesis of psoriasis is unknown. Current hypotheses propose that T-cell recruitment of the endothelium of blood vessels in the skin following activation of autoreactive T cells is a potentiating event in the development of psoriasis (15–19). Release of interferon-gamma (IFN-γ) and tumor necrosis factor-α (TNF-α) by activated cells (T cells and macrophages) leads to enhanced expression of cellular adhesion molecules on the endothelium (intercellular adhesion molecule-1, ICAM-1) permitting retention of such activated T cells in the region of the dermal capillaries. Continued production of IFN-γ is believed to induce normal keratinocytes (KC) to express more receptors for ICAM-1 and produce enhanced amounts of transforming growth factor-α (TGF-α). Continued production of TGF-α by keratinocytes is associated with decreased negative feedback effects of IFN-γ on TGF-α production that appear to be linked to markedly decreased expression of type II histocompatibility antigen (HLA-DR) on the keratinocytes (17). This, in turn, is associated with less growth inhibition and development of the psoriatic plaque.

CHEMISTRY AND PHARMACOLOGY

Drugs that impair thyroid hormone synthesis fall into three major categories: thioureylenes, aniline derivatives such as sulfonamides, and polyhydric phenols such as resorcinol. All compounds in clinical use at the present time to treat hyperthyroidism belong to the class of thioureylenes. In the United States the most commonly used thioureylenes are propylthiouracil (PTU) and methimazole (MMI) (Fig. 1). Carbimazole, which is used in Europe, is converted to methimazole in the liver. Both PTU and MMI have prompt effects on thyroid hormone biosynthesis as measured by effects on radioiodine uptake. The effect of PTU is, however, much shorter than that of MMI: 6–8 hr versus 24 hr. The half-life of PTU in plasma is approximately 2 hr (20) while that of MMI is about 13 hr. Both drugs cross the placenta and trace amounts of PTU are found in breast milk.

IMMUNOLOGICAL EFFECTS OF PROPYLTHIOURACIL (PTU) AND METHIMAZOLE (MMI)

PTU and MMI are antithyroid drugs often used as the first form of therapy in patients with hyperthyroidism. In addition to their well-known effects on thyroid hormone biosynthesis, the drugs exhibit immunomodulatory activity (Table 1). This activity has been ascribed to their ability to act as free radical scavengers and to raise interleukin-2 (IL-2) levels in target tissue (21). IL-2 is the product of a T-cell subtype called the TH_2 (T-helper 2) cell, which is also the source of IFN-γ. The TH_2 cell inhibits proliferation of another class of T cells, the TH_1 cell, which is responsible for activation of B cells via TH_1-derived cytokines such as IL-4 and IL-5 (Fig. 2). Activated B cells in turn produce immune globulins, some of which have specific roles in autoimmune states. For instance, in Graves' hyperthyroidism, the hyperthyroid state is due to production of anti-TSH receptor antibodies, which have stimulatory and blocking properties. After binding to the TSH receptor, anti-TSH receptor stimulatory antibodies stimulate thyroid hormone synthesis and are therefore called thyroid-stimulating immunoglobulins (TSI). Antithyroid drugs impair TSI production, presumably by inhibiting TH_1 cell activation. In psoriasis, the antithyroid thioureylenes may act via a similar mechanism resulting in restoration of the cytokine signals in the skin to normal proportions, i.e., a balance between TH_2- and TH_1-derived cytokines.

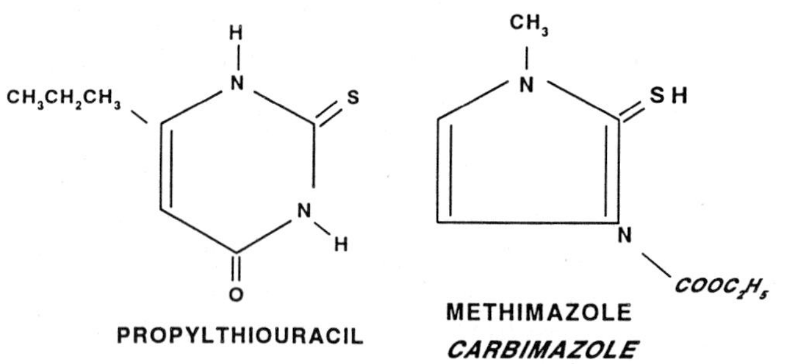

Figure 1 Antithyroid drugs of the thioureylene type. Chemical structures of propylthiouracil, methimazole, and carbimazole. Carbimazole is converted to methimazole after ingestion.

Table 1 Immunomodulatory Effects of PTU and MMI

PTU and MMI enhance the ratio of T-suppressor/cytotoxic cells to helper cells.
MMI enhances natural killer (NK) cell activity.
Thyroid antibodies and TSH-receptor antibody concentrations decline after treatment.
IL-2 production from peripheral blood lymphocytes (PBL) is increased in the presence of PTU and MMI.
PTU and MMI act as free radical scavengers.

THIOUREYLENES AS FREE RADICAL SCAVENGERS

Generation of free radicals in tissue results in tissue injury and causes an inflammatory response. In the skin such free radical generation may occur following environmental insult such as sun damage. Some patients with psoriatic flares can often relate exacerbation of their psoriasis to an episode of sunburn. The ability to protect from free radical injury may be an additional, albeit secondary, mechanism of action of the antithyroid thioureylenes.

The potential of antithyroid thioureylenes to act as free radical scavengers has been exploited in the treatment of patients with alcoholic liver disease (ALD). PTU given to patients with ALD for 2 years (22) has been shown to retard the development of hepatic fibrosis even when the patients continued to drink. The side effects of prolonged use of PTU in this already compromised population were minimal. Follow-up studies using PTU for as long as 4 years were also without significant side effects (23).

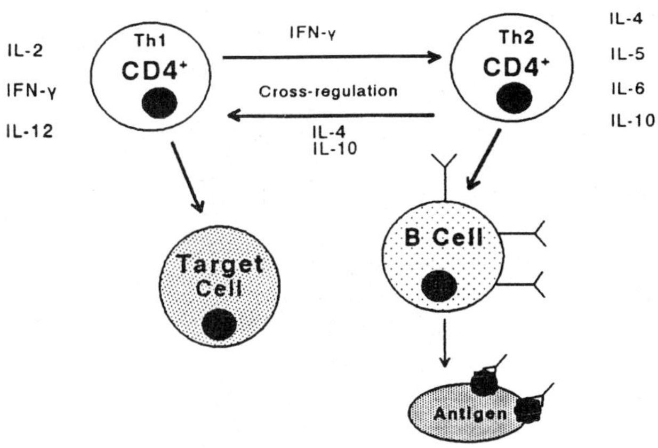

Figure 2 Interaction between TH_1 and TH_2 CD_4^+ (helper) T cells.

THIOUREYLENES AS ANTIPROLIFERATIVE AGENTS

In recent years the treatment of psoriasis, particularly topical therapy, has been accomplished using agents that belong to the superfamily of steroid receptor ligands. The most extensive experience has been with the use of topical glucocorticoids. This approach was followed by use of vitamin A derivatives (retinoids) and vitamin D_3 analogues such as calcipotriol (calcipotriene in the United States). T3R belongs to the same class of receptor as do the steroids, retinoids, and vitamin D (13). The T3R exists either as a homodimer or as a heterodimer with the non-T3R component being, most commonly, the retinoid-X receptor (RXR) whose natural ligand is 9-*cis*-retinoic acid (24). Binding of T_3 to its receptor results in activation of the promotor elements of genes that are concerned with cell differentiation and proliferation. Thyroid hormone is a classic morphogenic hormone being critically involved in the tadpole-to-frog metamorphosis. Vitamin A is also critical in activation of so-called homeobox genes that are involved in morphogenesis in many species (25,26). It is therefore not unreasonable to anticipate that some of the effects of vitamin A derivatives may be paralleled by T_3. Inactivation of T3R, either by a viral oncogene product such as the product of *v-erb*-A or by binding to an unnatural ligand, leads to loss of the promotional activity of genes dependent on T3R activation (13,14). PTU and MMI have been shown to effectively bind to T3R at concentrations of 10^{-4} to 10^{-5} M, which are achieved during systemic therapy of patients with hyperthyroidism on moderate doses of the drugs (13).

CLINICAL USE OF THIOUREYLENES IN PLAQUE PSORIASIS

PTU used in a dose of 100 mg every 8 hr and MMI used in a dose of 20 mg every 12 hr for 2 months produced significant improvement in the clinical (PASI) and histological scores of patients treated orally with these medications (4,5). These doses are comparable to moderate dose regimens employed in the treatment of patients with Graves' hyperthyroidism. Subsequent studies using much smaller doses (50–150 mg daily of PTU) for a longer period (3 months) produced similar improvement (6) (Fig. 3A and B). None of the patients treated with either the higher dose of PTU or MMI for 2 months of low-dose PTU for 3 months developed clinical hypothyroidism. Serum TSH concentration, which is considered the most sensitive marker of hypothyroidism, was not significantly elevated except in patients who were subsequently noted to have previously unsuspected subclinical hypothyroidism due to an underlying autoimmune thyroiditis. Thyroiditis was diagnosed on the basis of elevated antimicrosomal antibody (antithyroid peroxidase, anti-TPO) a relatively specific marker to thyroid autoimmune disease. In a patient with plaque psoriasis treated with 450 mg PTU daily for 3 months, serum TSH concentrations remained within the normal range (Fig. 4). Serum TSH concentration in this same patient after 6 months of treatment with 450 mg PTU daily also remained within the normal range.

Topical PTU (5% in propylene glycol and hydrophilic petrolatum) given to patients with plaque psoriasis in a double-blind manner produced significant improvement in the PTU-treated lesions (Fig. 5). None of the patients receiving topical PTU developed clinical hypothyroidism or showed any elevation of their serum TSH concentration (7).

Histological examination of skin biopsy specimens obtained from patients with plaque psoriasis prior to treatment with PTU or MMI shows abundant staining for proliferating cell nuclear antigen (PCNA), an auxiliary protein of DNA polymerase delta (27). Following treatment with PTU and MMI there is a marked reduction in PCNA staining in posttreatment skin biopsy specimens (28). PTU and MMI have no effect on p53 expression in skin biopsies (28). Native (nonmutant or wild-type) p53 is considered to have anti-

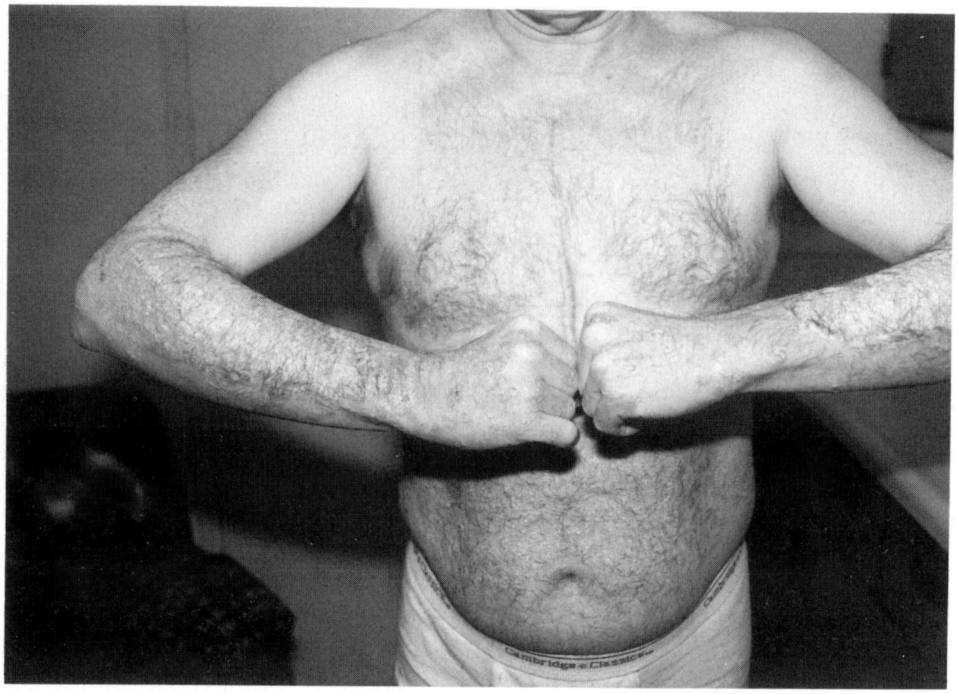

(A)

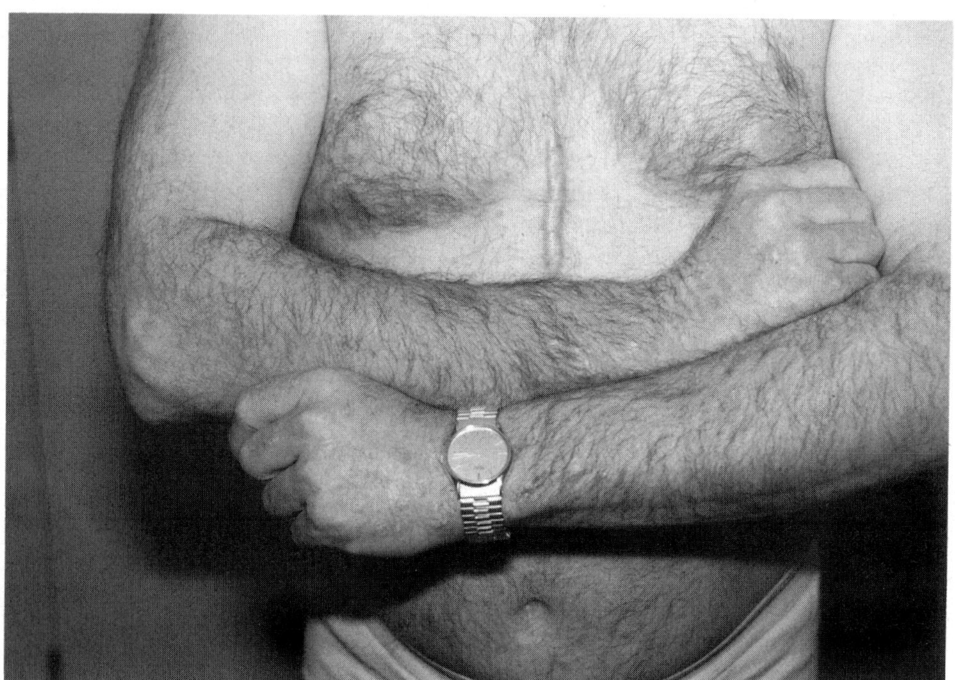

(B)

Figure 3 Appearance of patient before treatment (A) and after treatment (B) with propylthiouracil 100 mg every 8 h for 4 weeks followed by 50 mg every 8 h for an additional 8 weeks.

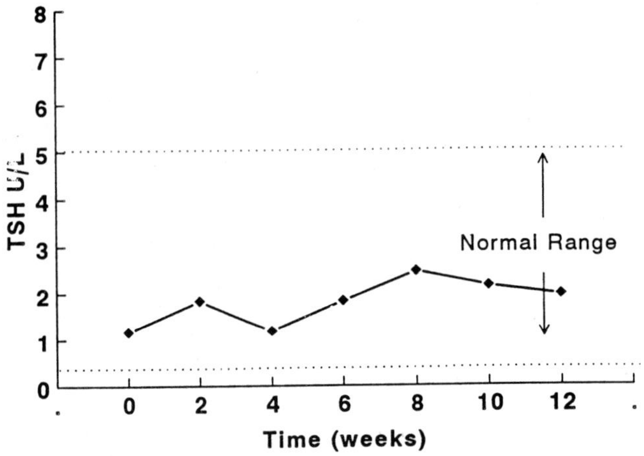

Figure 4 Serum TSH concentrations over a 3-month period in a euthyroid patient with stable plaque psoriasis receiving 150 mg of propylthiouracil every 8 h.

proliferative effects. Abnormalities in wild-type p53 have been associated with development of certain carcinomas such as colon cancer (29).

A number of locally produced cytokines inhibit keratinocyte proliferation. Such cytokines include TGF-β, interleukin-1 receptor antagonist peptide (IRAP), and parathyroid hormone–related peptide (PTHrP)(30–32). Using highly specific monoclonal antibodies, PTHrP is localized to the granular layer of the epidermis in skin biopsies taken from healthy subjects (30). In skin biopsy specimens from patients with untreated psoriasis stained with the same antibody no PTHrP is detected (30). Following treatment with glucocorticoids (betamethasone) or a vitamin D_3 analogue, PTHrP has been reported to reappear just above the granular layer in biopsy specimens taken from treated patients (30). Unlike the results reported after treatment with vitamin D_3 analogues or glucocorticoids, PTU and MMI do not enhance PTHrP expression in skin biopsies taken from patients treated with these drugs for 2 months, indicating that augmentation of PTHrP production is not a likely mechanism of action of these drugs when they are used in doses commonly employed in the treatment of patients with Graves' hyperthyroidism.

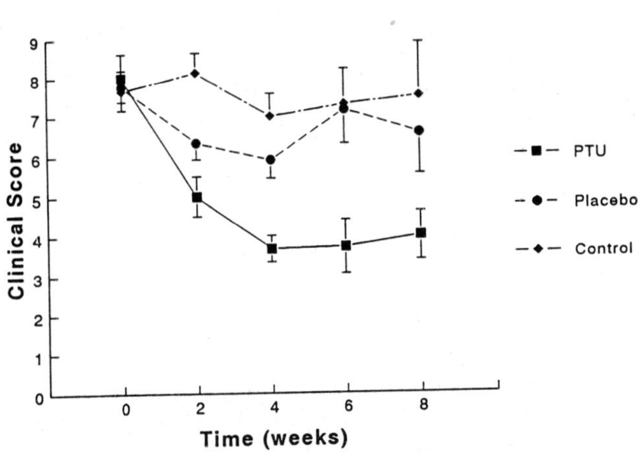

Figure 5 Clinical scores (means ± SE) in nine patients with plaque psoriasis treated for 4 to 8 weeks with 5% PTU, placebo, or nothing (control). Reproduced from *J. Am. Acad. Dermatol.* 1994; 31:455–458, with permission.

SIDE EFFECTS

PTU and MMI have been used for decades in the treatment of hyperthyroidism, so the toxicity and almost every conceivable side effect from the use of these medications are known. They constitute the primary treatment of hyperthyroidism in developing countries where they are often used for many years as the only form of treatment for this condition. In some instances, the drugs are used in large doses in combination with replacement doses of thyroid hormone to obviate the need for monitoring of thyroid function. Propylthiouracil has been used safely in pregnant patients who are maintained in a euthyroid or slightly hyperthyroid state on approximately 200 mg PTU daily in the third trimester (33).

The primary side effects of orally administered PTU and MMI consist of hypothyroidism and leukopenia. The latter occurs in 1:1000 to 1:500 patients and almost always abates when the medications are stopped. Hypothyroidism, if it does develop, can be readily reversed by the addition of supplemental thyroid hormone to patients while they are on PTU or MMI. Hypothyroidism also reverts to normal when the patient stops taking PTU or MMI since their primary effect on the thyroid is to inhibit thyroid hormone biosynthesis. The drugs therefore do not cause permanent damage to the thyroid gland. None of these side effects would be an issue if the preparations were used topically because such preparations can be formulated to limit systemic absorption from the skin.

Based on data in patients with psoriasis, it appears that nonhyperthyroid patients are more resistant to the inhibitory effects of PTU and MMI on thyroid hormone biosynthesis than are hyperthyroid patients such as those with Graves' disease. For instance, only

2/15 patients in oral studies showed biochemical evidence of mild hypothyroidism after 8 weeks of therapy with these drugs used in moderate dosage (300 mg daily for PTU and 40 mg daily for MMI) (4,5). Neither of the two patients became clinically hypothyroid. None of the patients treated with topical PTU developed either clinical or biochemical hypothyroidism. Furthermore, there were no reports of skin rash or increased itching with the topical preparation. In patients with alcoholic liver disease treated for 4 years with orally administered PTU, the incidence of either biochemical or clinical hypothyroidism was small (23).

CONCLUSIONS

The lack of cumulative toxicity of antithyroid thioureylenes in contrast to other oral treatments for psoriasis such as methotrexate and cyclosporin, and their effectiveness at low dose and after topical application where their potential side effects are negligible, should encourage use of these compounds in the treatment of patients with psoriasis, particularly in those patients who have failed other more conventional forms of treatment.

REFERENCES

1. Sander, H.M., Morris, L.F., Phillips, C.M., Harrison, P.E., and Menter, A. (1993). The annual cost of psoriasis. *J. Am. Acad. Dermatol.* 28:422–425.
2. Ellis, C.N., and Voorhees, J.J. (1987). Etretinate therapy. *J. Am. Acad. Dermatol.* 16:267–291.
3. DiGiovanna, J.J., Solitto, R.B., Abangan, D.L., Steinberg, S.M., and Reynolds, J.C. (1995). Osteoporosis is a toxic effect of long-term etretinate therapy. *Arch. Dermatol* 131:1263–1267.
4. Elias, A.N., Goodman, M.M., Leim, W., and Barr, R.J. (1993). Propylthiouracil in psoriasis—results of an open trial. *J. Am. Acad. Dermatol.* 29:78–81.
5. Elias, A.N., Goodman, M.M., Rohan, M.K., Alpern, K., and Barr, R.J. (1993). Methimazole (2-mercapto 1-methyl imidazole) in psoriasis—results of an open trial. *Dermatology* 187:26–29.
6. Elias, A.N., and Barr, R.J. (1995). Low-dose oral propylthiouracil in the treatment of psoriasis. *Int. J. Dermatol.* 34:519–520.
7. Elias, A.N., Goodman, M.M., and Rohan, M.K. (1993). Effect of propylthiouracil and methimazole on serum levels of interleukin-2 receptors in patients with psoriasis *Int. J. Dermatol.* 32:537–540.
8. Sharma, B.S., and Elias, A.N. (1987). Effects of methimazole on human lymphocyte proliferation and natural killer cell activity. *Gen. Pharmacol.* 18:449–453.
9. Signore, A., Pozzili, P., Di Mario, U., Sensi, M., Beales, P., and Andreani, D. (1985). Inhibition of the receptor for IL-2 induced by carbimazole: relevance for therapy of autoimmune thyroid disease. *Clin. Exp. Immunol.* 60:111–116.
10. Wall, J.R., Manwar, G.L., Greenwood, D.M., and Watters, B.A. (1983). The in vitro suppression of lectin induced [$_3$H]-thymidine incorporation into DNA of peripheral blood lymphocytes after the addition of propylthiouracil. *J. Clin. Endocrinol. Metab.* 56: 164–169.
11. Weetman, A.P. (1986). Effect of the antithyroid drug methimazole on interleukin-1 and interleukin-2 levels in vitro. *Clin. Endocrinol.* 25:133–142.
12. Takagi, S., Hummel, B.C.W., and Walfish P. (1990). Thionamides and arsenite inhibit T_3 binding to hepatic nuclear receptor. *Biochem. Cell Biol.* 68:616–621.
13. Evans, R.M. (1988). The steroid and thyroid hormone receptor superfamily. *Science* 240:889–895.
14. Baniahmad, A., Steiner, A., Kohne, A.C., and Renkawitz, R. (1990). Modular structure of a chicken lysosome silencer: involvement of an unusual thyroid hormone receptor binding site. *Cell* 61:505–514.
15. Barker, J.N.W.N., Allen, M.H., and MacDonald, D.M. (1989). The effect of in-vivo interferon-gamma on the distribution of LFA-1 and ICAM-1 in normal human skin. *J. Invest. Dermatol.* 93:439–442.
16. Barker, J.N. (1991). The pathophysiology of psoriasis. *Lancet* 338:227–230.
17. Baadsgaard, O., Fisher, G., Voorhees, J.J., and Cooper, K.D. (1990). The role of the immune system in the pathogenesis of psoriasis. *J. Invest. Dermatol.* 95: 32S–34S.
18. Barker, J.N.W.N., Allen, M.H., and MacDonald, D.M. (1989). The effect of in vivo interferon-gamma on the distribution of LFA-1 and ICAM-1 in normal human skin. *J. Invest. Dermatol.* 93:439–442.
19. Fry, L. (1988). Psoriasis. *Br. J. Dermatol.* 119: 445–461.
20. Kampmann, J., and Skovsted, L. (1974). The pharmacokinetics of propylthiouracil. *Acta Pharm. Toxicol.* 35:361–369.
21. Wilson, R., McKillop, J.H., Travers, M., Smith, J., Smith, E., and Thomson, J.A. (1990). The effects of antithyroid drugs on intercellular mediators. *Acta Endocrinol.* 122:605–609.
22. Orrego, H., Blake, J.E., Blendis, L.M., Compton, K.V., and Israel, Y. (1987). Long-term treatment of alcoholic liver disease with propylthiouracil. *N. Engl J. Med.* 317:1421–1427.
23. Orrego, H., Blake, J.E., Blendis, L.M., Compton, K.V., Volpe, R., and Israel, Y. (1994). Long-term treatment of alcoholic liver disease with propylthiouracil. Part 2.

Influence of drop-out rates and of continued alcohol consumption in a clinical trial. *J. Hepatol.* 20: 343–349.
24. Viera, A.V., Schneider, W.J., and Viera, P.M. (1995). Retinoids: transport, metabolism, and mechanisms of action. *J. Endocrinol.* 146:201–207.
25. Ogura, T., and Evans, R.M. (1995). A retinoic acid-triggered cascade of *HOX1* gene activation. *Proc. Natl. Acad. Sci. U.S.A.* 92:387–391.
26. Gudas, L.J. (1992). Retinoids, retinoid-responsive genes, cell differentiation, and cancer. *Cell Growth Different.* 3:655–662.
27. Atillosoy, E.J., Burtis, W.J., and Milstone, L.M. (1991). Immunohistochemical localization of parathyroid hormone-related protein (PTHRP) in normal human skin. *J. Invest. Dermatol.* 96:277–280.
28. Hayman, J.A., Danks, J.A., Ebeling, P.R., Moseley, J.M., Kemp, B.E., and Martin, T.J. (1989). Expression of parathyroid hormone related protein in normal skin and in tumours of skin and skin appendages. *J. Pathol.* 158:293–296.
29. Peller, S., Halevy, A., Slutzki, S., Kopilova, Y., Rotter, V. (1995). p53 mutations in matched primary and metastatic human tumors. *Mol. Carcinogen.* 13:166–172.
30. Juhlin, L., Hagforsen, E., and Juhlin, C. (1992). Parathyroid hormone related protein is localized in the granular layer of normal skin and in dermal infiltrates of mycosis fungoides but is absent in psoriatic lesions. *Acta Derm. Venerol. (Stockh.)* 72:81–83.
31. Kristensen, M., Deleuran, B., Eedy, D.J., Feldman, M., Breathnach, S.M., and Brennan, F.M. (1992). Distribution of interleukin 1 receptor antagonist protein (IRAP), interleukin 1 receptor, and interleukin 1α in normal and psoriatic skin. Decrease expression of IRAP in psoriatic lesional epidermis. *Br. J. Dermatol.* 127:305–311.
32. Sporn, M.B., Roberts, A.B., Wakefield, L.M., and Assoian, R.K. (1986). Transforming growth factor-β: biological function and chemical structure. *Science* 233: 523–534.
33. Sauder, D.N. (1990). The role of epidermal cytokines in inflammatory skin diseases. *J. Invest. Dermatol.* 95: 27S–28S.
34. Hamburger, J.I. (1992). Diagnosis and management of Graves' disease in pregnancy. *Thyroid* 2:219–224.

66

Ascomycins

Maximilian Grassberger, Josef G. Meingassner, and Anton Stütz
Novartis Research Institute, Vienna, Austria

Klemens Rappersberger and Klaus Wolff
Vienna General Hospital, Vienna, Austria

There is growing evidence that psoriasis is an immunogenic, autoreactive, inflammatory disorder based on a chronic ongoing Th-1 cell response (Baker and Fry, 1992; Uyemura et al., 1993; Schlaak et al., 1994). That psoriasis is mediated by immune mechanisms is suggested by its HLA association (B13, B17, Cw6, DR7) (for review see Christophers and Sterry, 1993; Elder et al., 1994), by an increased antigen-presenting cell activity and activated T cells within lesions that show a Th-1 cytokine pattern with lesional elevation of interferon-gamma and interferon-gamma-inducible adhesion molecules (Uyemura et al., 1993; Schlaak et al., 1994), by the acquisition or disappearance of psoriasis after bone marrow transplantation depending on whether donor or recipient has psoriasis (Eedy et al., 1990; Gardembas-Pain et al., 1990), by a clinical response of psoriasis to immunosuppressive drugs such as methotrexate (Weinstein and McCullough, 1976), cyclosporin A (Ellis et al., 1986), FK 506 (Jegasothy et al., 1992), and by the remission of psoriasis upon administration to the patients of anti-CD3 and anti-CD4 monoclonal antibodies (Weinshenker et al., 1989; Prinz et al., 1991) or lymphocyte-selective toxins (Gottlieb et al., 1995). The association of activated IL-2R-positive proliferating T cells in apposition to antigen-presenting cells suggests presentation of the T-cell receptor with a putative foreign or self antigen by these cells. It has been hypothesized that activated T cells release interferon-gamma, which together with TNF-alpha promotes ICAM-1 expression on keratinocytes to which T cells, which have been attracted to the epidermis by mediators and cytokines and arrested by activated endothelial cells, adhere through T-cell LFA-1/keratinocyte ICAM-1 interactions (Griffiths, 1994; Wakita and Takigawa, 1994). Since immunosuppressive agents such as cyclosporin A are capable of interrupting this process and thus induce a clinical remission of psoriasis and the long-term administration of these agents has led to concerns about potential side effects, there have been attempts to develop strategies of local immunosuppression by topically applied drugs. Despite the fact that intralesional cyclosporin A induces remissions of lesions (Baker et al., 1989), attempts to develop effective topical cyclosporin A treatment for psoriasis have been unsuccessful.

Ascomycins are a novel class of anti-inflammatory macrolactams acting on T cells. Based on current preclinical and clinical experience, they are as effective as potent and ultrapotent corticosteroids in the topical treatment of psoriasis and other inflammatory skin diseases in which T-cell activation is involved and have a low risk of local and systemic side effects. This chapter deals with this class of compounds and its effect on psoriatic lesions. We will show that these immunomodulatory macrolactams represent a novel class of topical agents for the treatment of this disease.

ASCOMYCINS

Ascomycin, the parent compound, is a 23-membered macrolactam. It was originally isolated from the fermentation broth of *Streptomyces hygroscopicus* var. *ascomyceticus* (Arai et al., 1962; Koyama et al., 1963). As with many other natural products that later developed into novel therapeutic principles for different indications, the discovery of ascomycin was based on its antifungal activity, which is mainly restricted to *Aspergillus* species (Arai et al., 1962). Ascomycin was reisolated later together with structurally related compounds from other *Streptomyces* strains (Hatanaka et al., 1988a; Monosghan et al., 1989). The structure and the effect of ascomycin on T-cell activation were revealed several years after its first isolation (Hatanaka et al., 1988b; Morisaki and Arai, 1992).

Ascomycin and structurally related compounds like FK 506 are inhibitors of T-cell activation. The compounds interfere with the signal transduction pathway leading from the T-cell receptor to the nucleus (Schreiber and Crabtree, 1992). More specifically, they prevent the Ca^{2+}-stimulated dephosphorylation of the constitutive cytoplasmic part of the transactivating factor NFAT by inhibiting the phosphatase calcineurin (Fruman et al., 1992; Liu et al., 1991). As a consequence, the translocation of cNFAT into the nucleus and thus the transcription of early cytokines such as IL-2 that are dependent on NFAT are blocked.

The effect of macrolactams on skin inflammation was first detected in animal models of allergic contact dermatitis (Grassberger et al., 1989; Meingassner and Stütz, 1992a,b). Potent topical anti-inflammatory activity was not only observed in mice (oxazolone-induced ear edema) but also in the more demanding model of DNFB-induced allergic skin reactions in pigs (Meingassner et al., 1992; Stütz, 1992). Cyclosporin A, for example, a drug that is established as an oral therapeutic in psoriasis, was found to be ineffective in the pig model after topical application. This correlated with the clinical experience that cyclosporin A, even in elaborated formulations, has failed to show efficacy after topical application in psoriasis or other skin disorders (Surber et al., 1992; Mrowietz, 1992; De Prost and Teillac, 1989; De Rie et al., 1991).

Based on these preclinical observations, ascomycin-type macrolactams were, therefore, expected to have a high therapeutic potential for the topical treatment of skin diseases that respond to corticosteroids or systemic cyclosporin A (Meingassner and Stütz, 1992a). This hypothesis was confirmed for the first time with SDZ 281-240, a novel ascomycin derivative, in a proof-of-concept study in psoriasis patients (Rappersberger et al., 1994, 1996). Topical activity in psoriasis was later also claimed for the related product FK 506 (Remitz et al., 1996), but there are no detailed published reports. A highly promising drug is the new ascomycin derivative SDZ ASM 981. It exhibits not only potent anti-inflammatory activity in animal models of skin inflammation (Meingassner et al., 1997) but also in proof-of-concept studies in psoriasis (Mrowietz et al., 1997), atopic dermatitis (Van Leent et al., 1997), and allergic contact dermatitis (Queille-Roussel et al., 1997) after topical application. In addition, SDZ ASM 981 has been shown to have a low potential for local and systemic side effects.

The anti-inflammatory activity of the ascomycin derivatives is probably primarily due to their effects on T cells. A screening of various ascomycin derivatives revealed, however, that binding to macrophilin and inhibition of T-cell activation do not always correlate with anti-inflammatory activity in vivo (Stütz et al., 1993). On the other hand, rapamycin, another macrocyclic compound that inhibits T-cell activation by a distinct mechanism, has turned out to be ineffective in models of allergic contact dermatitis (Meingassner et al., 1992; Stütz, 1992). There might be, therefore, additional but so far unknown effects that contribute to the overall anti-inflammatory activity of ascomycins.

PRECLINICAL ACTIVITIES OF SDZ 281-240 AND SDZ ASM 981

SDZ 281-240 and SDZ ASM 981 bind with high affinity to macrophilin-12, the cytosolic receptor of ascomycin-type macrolactams (Table 1) (Bevec et al., 1997). Binding to macrophilin-12 is a necessary but not sufficient prerequisite for the inhibition of T-cell activation (Schreiber and Crabtree, 1992). Both compounds inhibit the transcription of a reporter gene that is under the control of the IL-2 promoter in a stable transfected human T-cell line Jurkat at subnanomolar concentrations (Table 1) (Bevec et al., 1997). Inhibition of T-cell proliferation in a mouse two-way mixed-lymphocyte reaction is observed also at nanomolar concentrations, as determined by a block of ^{3}H-thymidine incorporation. The growth of other cells such as of the human keratinocyte cell line HaCaT,

Table 1 In Vitro Activities of SDZ 281-240 and SDZ ASM 981

	IC_{50} (nM) ± SD		
Assay	SDZ ASM 981	SDZ 281-240	Cyclosporin A
Macrophilin-12 binding	1.8 ± 0.3 (*n* = 3)	1.8 ± 0.2 (*n* = 4)	Not done
IL-2 reporter gene assay	0.4 ± 0.1 (*n* = 3)	0.5 ± 0.1 (*n* = 2)	9.0 ± 3.0 (*n* = 12)
Mixed-lymphocyte reaction	1.3 ± 0.7 (*n* = 6)	1.1 ± 0.2 (*n* = 2)	23.0 ± 13.2 (*n* = 10)
Mast cell degranulation	26.7 ± 3.3 (*n* = 9)	19.8 ± 7.1 (*n* = 4)	54.5 ± 24.5 (*n* = 92)
HaCaT proliferation	4800 ± 600 (*n* = 3)	10100 ± 280 (*n* = 2)	4700 ± 300 (*n* = 3)

n = number of experiments.

however, is not affected at up to micromolar concentration, demonstrating the specificity of the antiproliferative activity (Table 1). Both compounds inhibit, although at somewhat higher concentrations, also the antigen IgE-driven degranulation of the murine mast cell line CP2 (Table 1). This might contribute to their anti-inflammatory activity.

The two ascomycin derivatives potently inhibited allergic contact dermatitis in mice after topical application (Table 2) (Meingassner et al., 1997). Animals were sensitized by treating the abdomen with oxazolone and challenged 7 days later on the inner surface of the ear. Compounds were applied once 30 min after challenge and the effect was evaluated by determining the ear weight (reduction of ear swelling). Both, SDZ 281-240 and SDZ ASM 981 showed significant anti-inflammatory effects already at a concentration as low as 0.004%, similarly to dexamethasone. Cyclosporin A, in contrast, begins to be effective only at 10-fold higher concentrations (Table 2). Topical anti-inflammatory activity was also observed in TPA- and A 23187-induced irritant contact dermatitis in mice with a potency similar to that of hydrocortisone (Table 3 and 4).

In view of the very thin stratum corneum in the skin of mice or rats, however, results from topical treatment of skin inflammation in rodent models appear to have little predictive value for the clinical situation and might even be misleading. Indeed, cyclosporin A, which is clearly active in mice, has no effects at all on allergic contact dermatitis in humans when applied topically. Pig skin is much thicker than rodent skin and resembles human skin much closer. Therefore, allergic contact dermatitis in pigs was used for

Table 2 Topical Anti-inflammatory Activity of SDZ 281-240 and SDZ ASM 981 in a Murine Model of Allergic Contact Dermatitis in Comparison with Cyclosporin A and Dexamethasone

Concentration (%)	Inhibition of pinnal swelling (%)[a]			
	SDZ ASM 981	SDZ 281-240	Cyclosporin A	Dexamethasone
0.4	54%***[b]	67%***	49%***	73%***
	12.6 ± 5.5 (*n* = 8)[c]	9.0 ± 5.2 (*n* = 8)	13.8 ± 4.1 (*n* = 16)	7.4 ± 2.4 (*n* = 8)
0.13	61%***	52%***	46%***	65%***
	10.6 ± 4.5 (*n* = 8)	13.1 ± 5.4 (*n* = 8)	14.8 ± 5.7 (*n* = 32)	9.5 ± 3.9 (*n* = 16)
0.04	53%***	47%***	20%*	65%***
	12.9 ± 5.6 (*n* = 16)	14.3 ± 7.1 (*n* = 16)	21.7 ± 8.0 (*n* = 6)	9.4 ± 4.2 (*n* = 24)
0.01	35%***	53%***	5% n.s.	55%***
	17.7 ± 5.6 (*n* = 24)	12.8 ± 4.4 (*n* = 24)	25.9 ± 7.0 (*n* = 32)	12.2 ± 6.4 (*n* = 16)
0.004	37%***	32%***	−5% n.s.	37%***
	17.1 ± 5.6 (*n* = 8)	18.4 ± 7.0 (*n* = 16)	28.5 ± 5.7 (*n* = 16)	17.1 ± 5.7 (*n* = 16)
Controls	27.2 ± 5.5 (*n* = 48)			

[a]Data from one to six experiments.
[b]n.s. = not statistically significant; $*p < 0.05$; $***p < 0.001$ compared with controls.
[c]Mean (mg) of pinnal weight differences ± SD; *n* = number of animals.

Table 3 Topical Anti-Inflammatory Activity of SDZ 281-240 and SDZ ASM 981 in a Murine Model of TPA-Induced Irritant Contact Dermatitis in Comparison with Hydrocortisone

Concentration (mM)	Inhibition of pinnal swelling (%)[a]		
	SDZ ASM 981	SDZ 281-240	Hydrocortisone
100	84%***[b] 4.6 ± 3.02 (n = 8)[c]	92%*** 2.3 ± 2.49 (n = 8)	Not tested
30	55%*** 13.1 ± 3.76 (n = 8)	70%*** 8.8 ± 5.34 (n = 8)	61%*** 11.2 ± 4.49 (n = 24)
10	18% n.s. 23.5 ± 5.13 (n = 8)	49%*** 14.6 ± 6.52 (n = 8)	42%*** 16.6 + 6.10 (n = 32)
Vehicle controls		28.8 ± 5.42 (n = 48)	

[a]Data from one to six experiments.
[b]n.s. = not statistically significant; *** $p < 0.001$ compared with controls.
[c]Mean (mg) of pinnal weight differences ± SD; n = number of animals.

further evaluation of topical anti-inflammatory activity of ascomycin derivatives (Meingassner et al., 1997). Domestic pigs were sensitized with DNFB on both auricles and groins and challenge reactions elicited 12 days later at test sites arranged in four craniocaudal lines on the dorsolateral shaved back. Test sites were treated twice with solutions of the test compounds in ethanol/propylene glycol (3:7, v/v) or with galenical formulations of the compounds 30 min and 6 hr after challenge. The effect was assessed clinically by scoring the intensity and extent of erythema and infiltration 1 day after challenge (Meingassner and Stütz, 1992). Under these conditions, SDZ 281-240 and SDZ ASM 981 were found to be as potent and effective as clobetasol-17-propionate and fluticasone-propionate, when applied in solution (Table 5). Cyclosporin A, in contrast, even at 10%, was without any effect (data not shown).

Since the galenic formulation might have a significant influence on the overall performance of a topical drug, provisional 0.1% galenic formulations of the two ascomycins were prepared and compared to marketed glucocorticoid preparations in the pig model as well. Efficacy of SDZ 281-240 and SDZ ASM 981 proved to be in the same range as of a series of potent and ultrapotent glucocorticoid preparations including clobetasol-17-propionate and superior to that of clobetasone-17-butyrate and fluprednidene-21-acetate (Table 6).

Induction of skin atrophy is a common side effect of potent topical corticosteroids after repeated topical or oral application, affecting both dermis and epider-

Table 4 Topical Anti-Inflammatory Activity of SDZ 281-240 and SDZ ASM 981 in a Murine Model of A 23187–Induced Irritant Contact Dermatitis in Comparison with Hydrocortisone

Concentration (mM)	Inhibition of pinnal swelling (%)[a]		
	SDZ ASM 981	SDZ 281-240	Hydrocortisone
30	64%***[b] 10.1 ± 3.23 (n = 8)[c]	80%*** 5.6 ± 3.07 (n = 8)	Not tested
10	57%*** 11.9 ± 5.12 (n = 16)	57%*** 12.0 ± 5.07 (n = 8)	79%*** 5.9 ± 4.06 (n = 2)
1	45%*** 15.3 ± 6.26 (n = 16)	44%** 15.5 ± 6.91 (n = 8)	47%*** 14.8 ± 7.63 (n = 4)
Vehicle controls		27.7 ± 4.13 (n = 32)	

[a]Data from one to four experiments.
[b]** $p < 0.01$; *** $p < 0.001$ compared with controls.
[c]Mean (mg) of pinnal weight differences ± SD; n = number of animals.

Table 5 Topical Anti-Inflammatory Activity of Solutions of SDZ 281-240 and SDZ ASM 981 in Pig Model of Allergic Contact Dermatitis in Comparison with Clobetasol-17-Propionate and Fluticasone Propionate

Concentration (%)	Inhibition of gross changes (%)[a] SDZ ASM 981	SDZ 281-240	Clobetasol-17-propionate	Fluticasone propionate
0.4	61 ± 10.2%***[b] (1/16/4)[c]	50 ± 5.8%*** (1/8/2)	59 ± 1.0%*** (1/16/4)	Not tested
0.13	49 ± 6.8%*** (2/28/6)	44 ± 8.8%*** (2/32/8)	55 ± 6.4%*** (3/26/6)	56 ± 11.5%*** (2/24/6)
0.04	25 ± 12.4%*** (2/32/8)	16 ± 2.5%** (1/8/2)	35 ± 19.1%*** (2/20/5)	39 ± 9.8%*** (2/24/6)

[a]Mean values of percentage inhibition ± SD seen in animals by comparison of compound- and vehicle-treated test sites (four to six each per animal), assessed by clinical scoring.
[b]$**p < 0.01$; $***p < 0.001$ compared with controls.
[c]X/Y/Z: number of experiments/test sites/animals.

mis (Robertson and Maibach, 1992; Sillevis-Smitt and Winterberg, 1992; Marks, 1992). The atrophogenic potential of SDZ ASM 981 was assessed in comparison with clobetasol-17-propionate and diflucortolone-21-valerate in pigs. Small areas at the flank were treated daily for 6 hr (under occlusive conditions using Finn chambers) for 13 consecutive days with a formulation containing 0.3% SDZ ASM 981, placebo, or the reference drugs. Evaluation was performed by clinical observation, colorimetric measurement, and ultrasonographic measurement of skin thickness before treatment, during the application period, and after the last application. In addition, histomorphometry of test sites was performed 1 day after the last application by microscopy. Clobetasol-17-propionate and—less pronounced, diflucortolone-21-valerate—induced a blanching effect and changes in the skin texture (atrophy). By ultrasonography a significant inhibition of the normal increase of skin thickness was only observed with clobetasol-17-propionate (Fig. 1), which was confirmed by the histomorphometric analysis. SDZ ASM 981, in contrast, caused no visible or measurable effects (Meingassner et al., 1997).

Oral cyclosporin A shows excellent clinical efficacy in the treatment of psoriasis. Therefore, assess-

Table 6 Topical Efficacy of SDZ 281-240 and SDZ ASM 981 in Provisional Clinical Service Formulations in a Pig Model of Allergic Contact Dermatitis in Comparison with Marketed Preparations of Glucocorticoids

Active ingredient	Inhibition of gross changes (%)[a]	Number of experiments/ test sites/animals
SDZ ASM 981 (0.1%)	55 ± 9.2	2/24/5
Clobetasol-17-proprionate (0.05%)	63 ± 5.5	1/8/2
Betamethasone-17-valerate (0.10%)	36 ± 3.0	1/8/2
Diflucortolone-21-valerate (0.10%)	48 ± 12.0	2/20/4
Mometasone-17-(2-furoate) (0.10%)	41 ± 15.8	1/8/2
Clobetasone-17-butyrate (0.05%)	9 ± 26.0	1/8/2***[b]
Fluprednidene-21-acetate (0.10%)	7 ± 1.4	1/8/2***
Fluticasone propionate (0.05%)	46 ± 5.3	1/12/3

[a]Mean values ± SD of percentage inhibition in animals by comparison of compound-treated and untreated test sites.
[b]$***p < 0.001$ compared with SDZ ASM 981.

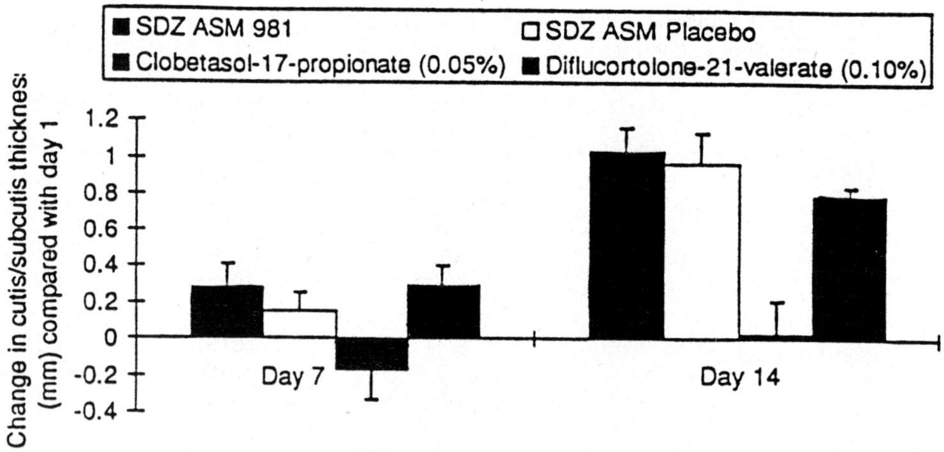

Figure 1 Effect of subchronic topical treatment of domestic pigs with SDZ ASM 981 ointment 0.3% on skin thickness, measured by ultrasonography, in comparison with clobetasol-17-propionate 0.05% and diflucortolone-21-valerate.

ment of the systemic anti-inflammatory potential SDZ ASM 981 in comparison with cyclosporin A was of particular interest. Rats, sensitized with DNFB, were challenged on both flanks 12 days after sensitization. Test compounds were applied orally 2 hr before and immediately after challenge. Inflammation was evaluated by measuring the thickness of the lifted skin fold at the test sites before challenge and 24 hr after challenge. SDZ ASM 981 proved to be four times as active as cyclosporin A, as judged by the lowest doses with statistically significant efficacy (Fig. 2).

The effects of oral SDZ ASM 981 and cyclosporin A on systemic immune reactions were then compared using a rat model of localized graft versus host reac-

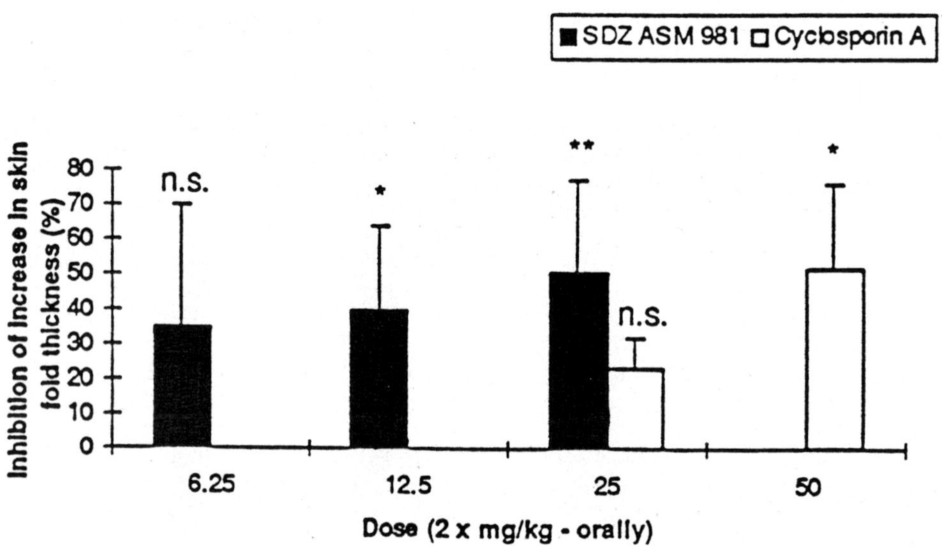

Figure 2 Oral anti-inflammatory activity of SDZ ASM 981 in a rat model of allergic contact dermatitis in comparison with cyclosporin A.

tion. Spleen cells from allogenic animals were injected into the footpad and the weight of the popliteal lymph nodes determined after 4 days. Test compounds were applied on the day of spleen cell injection and 1, 2, and 3 days later. Cyclosporin A inhibited lymph node weight increase with an ED_{50} of 5 mg/kg, whereas SDZ ASM 981 even at 30 mg/kg was without any effect.

These results indicate that SDZ ASM 981 has a larger therapeutic window in which skin inflammation may be treated with no adverse effects on the immune system compared with cyclosporin A.

CLINICAL STUDIES

SDZ 281-240

As reported elsewhere, clinical studies using SDZ 281-240 were performed in patients with plaque psoriasis employing the microplaque assay (Rappersberger et al., 1994, 1996). This assay is based on the application of the test drug to circumscribed test areas within one or more large psoriatic plaques using Finn chambers. Using a double-blind, placebo-controlled, within-patient protocol, the test substance SDZ 281-240 was employed at concentrations of 1% and 0.1% in an oil-water formulation and compared with placebo (vehicle) and 0.05% clobetasol-17-propionate (CP) cream as a positive control. Coded preparations of SDZ 281-240 in both concentrations and CP and placebo were randomly assigned to four test areas within the psoriatic plaques to be tested. Fifty milligrams of the test preparations were accommodated in each chamber, which corresponds to 0.5 mg and 0.05 mg of SDZ 281-240 in the respective formulations, and a semiocclusive dressing was applied to the entire plaque and left in place for 24 hr. Dressings were removed every 24 hr and coded study medications were reapplied to the respective test sites, the whole procedure being repeated daily for 10 days. All patients enrolled in this study showed a significant improvement of the test sites treated with the two concentrations of the ascomycin derivative and, as expected, with CP. There was a reduction of infiltration and erythema with both test preparations, which resulted in clearing of most test sites on day 11. A reduction of psoriatic erythema was observed within the first 4 days of treatment and was followed by a steady decline to almost complete blanching on day 11. Similarly infiltration improved in the initial phase of topical treatment and resolved by day 11. These results equal those obtained with the application of CP whereas placebo did not affect either parameter. The statistical analysis of the sum of scores confirmed the clinical observation whereby SDZ 281-240 and CP differed significantly ($p < 0.01$) from placebo-treated sites.

Histopathological examination of test and placebo-treated sites confirmed the clinical findings. SDZ 281-240 treatment induced an almost complete reversion of psoriatic epidermal hyperplasia to normal within 10 days at which time there was no more parakeratosis, hyperkeratosis, or papillomatosis, and this was true for both concentrations of SDZ 281-240 used. The inflammatory infiltrate was also markedly reduced and tortuous papillary capillaries were hardly observed. These changes were identical to those observed after corticosteroid application whereas placebo did not affect the histopathological parameters of psoriasis. Measurements of the thickness of hyperplastic psori-

---

Figure 3 Psoriatic plaque before (a) and on day 8 after (b) daily application of 1% SDZ 281-240 (test site 2), 0.1% SDZ 281-240 (test site 5), and placebo (test site 3). There is a pronounced (test sites 2 and 5) reversal of psoriasis to normal within 1 week of topical application of SDZ 281-240 in both concentrations. In contrast, placebo (test site 3) does not show any effect.

Figure 4 The clinical findings are paralleled by histopathological changes that show a preservation of the psoriatic phenotype with acanthosis, parakeratosis, papillomatosis, tortuous capillaries, and a dense inflammatory infiltrate in the placebo-treated test site (a), whereas macrolide-treated psoriasis shows almost normal skin (b). Epidermal hyperproliferation is characteristic of psoriasis and indicates the numerous Ki-67$^+$ keratinocytes are not influenced by a placebo (c), whereas in ascomycin-treated skin the number of Ki-67$^+$-proliferating keratinocytes is significantly reduced and positive cells are restricted to the basal cell layer (d). After 7 days of placebo treatment there is still a dense inflammatory infiltrate that is composed of CD4$^+$ leukocytes (e). SDZ 281-240 topically applied for 7 days leads to an almost complete depletion of CD4$^+$ leukocytes from the psoriatic plaque (f).

atic epidermis versus placebo-treated controls showed a significant reduction of epidermal thickness and also a significant reduction of proliferating, i.e., Ki-67$^+$, keratinocytes.

This reversion of the psoriatic phenotype as assessed histopathologically was also paralleled by epidermal differentiation markers as well as the composition of the inflammatory infiltrate. During treatment the staining patterns of involucrin and filaggrin reverted from that typical for psoriasis to that of normal epidermis, and keratinocyte activation, as expressed by focal staining for HLA-DR and ICAM-1, which were still present at the end of the study in placebo-treated psoriatic skin, was abolished by SDZ 281-240 treatment. Similar changes were apparent when verum- and placebo-treated sites were assessed for the extent and type of inflammatory cellular infiltrate: The inflammatory infiltrate in psoriasis predominantly consisting of CD3$^+$ activated HLA-DR$^+$ T lymphocytes, which was still evident in the placebo-treated sites at the termination of the study, was considerably changed by 10 days of SDZ 281-240 treatment. There was a significant reduction of CD3$^+$, CD4$^+$, and CD8$^+$ intraepidermal and dermal lymphocytes and there was a clear reduction of the number of CD25$^+$ leukocytes. By contrast, we observed a significant increase of CD1a$^+$ Langerhans cells, which suggested a repopulation of epidermis by these cells as the CD4$^+$ and CD8$^+$ lymphocytes decreased.

Involution of psoriasis in the SDZ 281-240-treated sites was also evident by staining for HLA-DR, ICAM-1, VCAM-1, ELAM-1, and PECAM molecules that are up-regulated in the superficial dermal microvasculature in psoriatic lesions but showed a pronounced reduction in SDZ 281-240-treated sites.

In summary, this study showed that the topical application of SDZ 281-240 under the conditions described abolishes the psoriatic phenotype, leading to clinically normal skin within 11 days, and that this is accompanied by reversion of the psoriatic histology to normal. In addition, the proliferative activity of keratinocytes is down-regulated and the expression and distribution pattern of epidermal maturation/differentiation markers are also reverted to normal. This is accompanied by normalization of the inflammatory infiltrate, the disappearance of activation markers from both epidermis and dermis.

SDZ ASM 981

Studies have been performed with SDZ ASM 981 using a similar study design (Mrowietz et al., 1997). In this study the therapeutic effect of 1% SDZ ASM 981 was comparable to that of 0.05% clobetasol-17-propionate (CP) ointment and was clearly dose-dependent. Total symptom scores decreased by 92% for CP, by 82% for 1% SDZ ASM 981, by 63% for 0.3% SDZ ASM 981, and by 18% for the ointment base. Whereas complete clearance of psoriasis (erythema and induration) was achieved in only two of 10 test sites treated with 0.3% SDZ ASM 981, it was achieved in six of 10 tests with 1% SDZ ASM 981, indicating a clear dose-effect relationship and was comparable to the clobetasol control, with complete clearing being obtained within 10–14 days (the median time to complete clearing was 12.5 days). All this shows that this macrolactam employed in an enhanced penetration formulation is also highly effective in chronic plaque psoriasis under the conditions employed (Mrowietz et al., 1997).

COMMENTS AND CONCLUSION

In the study described we show that a remission of plaque psoriasis can be induced by the topical application of novel semisynthetic derivatives of the immunomodulatory macrolactam ascomycin within 10–14 days as assessed by clinical, histopathological, and immunomorphological criteria (Rappersberger et al., 1996). These compounds are immunosuppressive but not antiproliferative in vitro (Rappersberger et al., 1996; Skehan et al., 1990). They interfere with early T-cell activation by blocking calcium-dependent intracellular signaling, ultimately leading to a suppression of the transcription of early lymphokines, such as IL-2, by binding to the common cytosolic receptor macrophilin (Schreiber and Crabtree, 1992). We thus show that an immunomodulatory agent that interferes with early T-cell activation can be designed to penetrate into psoriatic lesions when applied topically and can be functionally active within lesions suppressing the psoriatic process. We believe that the reduction of epidermal proliferation observed in our studies may not be a direct effect of the drug on keratinocytes but may result from a down-regulation of T-cell activation and consequent cytokine release. Thus a mode of action of these ascomycins could be envisaged in which the compounds down-regulate activated T-cells, and as the T-cell triggered and cytokine-mediated proliferation of keratinocytes subsides, the epidermis is allowed to revert to a normal state of proliferation and differentiation. This is in line with the observation that a systemically applied lymphocyte-selective toxin

(DAB_{398}-IL-2) induces remissions of psoriatic lesions indicating that psoriatic features are primarily linked to skin infiltrating IL-2 receptor-positive ($CD25^+$) leukocytes (Gottlieb et al., 1995). That the results observed in psoriasis, under the conditions employed, are mainly due to a down-regulation of activated T cells is further supported by the observation that both SDZ 281-240 and ASM 981 exhibit pronounced anti-inflammatory activities in animal models of allergic contact dermatitis (Meingassner et al., 1997) and that they are highly effective clinically in the suppression of atopic dermatitis (Van Leent et al., 1997) and allergic contact dermatitis (Queille-Roussel et al., 1997) in humans.

At this time we do not know how long the beneficial effect observed with both SDZ 281-240 and SDZ ASM 981 in psoriasis lasts and whether prolonged treatment will induce tachyphylaxis. Ongoing studies will show whether the agents are as effective in psoriasis when applied openly and to large areas as they are under the semiocclusive conditions employed in the microplaque assay. Also, there are no experimental data on potential systemic immunosuppressive effects of transcutaneous SDZ 281-240 and SDZ ASM 981 delivery, and although these appear unlikely from a quantitative viewpoint, this issue is presently being addressed in clinical studies. Data available so far have not revealed irritative or contact sensitizing potentials of the compounds. We acknowledge that therefore only clinical trials employing large-area or whole-body treatment will eventually determine the role these compounds will play in the treatment of psoriasis, but on the basis of the results obtained so far we believe that the development of these agents will lead to a new era in the treatment of psoriasis.

REFERENCES

Arai, T., Koyama, Y., Suenaga, T., and Honda, H. (1962). Ascomycin, an antifungal antibiotic. *J. Antibiot. Ser. A* 15:231–232.

Baker, B.S., Powles, A.V., Savage, C.R., McFadden, J.P., Valdimarsson, H., and Fry, L. (1989). Intralesional cyclosporin in psoriasis: effects on T lymphocytes and dendritic cell subpopulations. *Br. J. Dermatol.* 120:207–213.

Baker, B., and Fry, L. (1992). The immunology of psoriasis. *Br. J. Dermatol.* 126:1–9.

Bevec, D., Schuler, W., Schulz, M., Werner, F., Winiski, A., Wolff, B., Zenke, G., and Grassberger, M. (1997). SDZ ASM 981—a novel anti-inflammatory macrolactam: pharmacological activities in vitro. *Australasian J. Dermatol.* 38 (Suppl 2):285

Christophers, E., and Sterry, W. (1993). Psoriasis. In *Dermatology in General Medicine.* Fitzpatrick, Eisen, Wolff, Freedberg, Austen (Eds.). McGraw-Hill, New York, pp. 490–514.

De Prost, B.C., and Teillac, D. (1989). Randomized double blind placebo-controlled trial of local cyclosporine in atopic dermatitis. *Acta Derm. Venerol. (Stockh.)* 144: 136–138.

De Rie, M.A., Meinardi, M.M., and Bos, J.D. (1991). Lack of efficacy of topical cyclosporine A in atopic dermatitis and allergic contact dermatitis. *Acta Derm. Venerol. (Stockh.)* 71:452–454.

Eedy, D.F., Burrows, D., Bridges, J.M., and Jones, F.G.C. (1990). Clearance of severe psoriasis after allogeneic bone marrow transplantation. *Br. Med. J.* 300:908.

Elder, J.T., Naiv, R.P., and Voorhees, J.J. (1994). Epidemiology and the genetics of psoriasis. *J. Invest. Dermatol.* 102:24s–27s.

Ellis, C.N., Gorsulowsky, D.C., and Hamilton, T.A. (1986). Cyclosporin improves psoriasis in a double-blind study. *JAMA* 256:3110–3116.

Fruman, D.A., Klee, C.B., Bierer, B.E., and Burakoff, J. (1992). Calcineurin phosphatase activity in T lymphocytes is inhibited by FK-506 and cyclosporin A. *Proc. Natl. Acad. Sci. USA* 89:3686–3690.

Gardembas-Pain, M., Ifrah, N., Foussard, C., Boasson, M., Saint Andre, J.P., and Verret, J.L. (1990). Psoriasis after allogeneic bone marrow transplantation. *Arch. Dermatol.* 126:1523.

Gottlieb, S.L., Gilleandean, D., Johnson, R., Ester, L., Woodworth, T.G., Gottlieb, A.B., and Krueger, J.G. (1995). Response of psoriasis to lymphocyte-selective toxin (DAB_{389} IL-2) suggest a primary immune but not keratinocyte pathogenic basis. *Nature Med.* 1:442–447.

Grassberger, M., Meingassner, J.G., Stuetz, A., and Stuetz, P. (1989). Use of 11,28-dioxa-4-azatricyclo-[22.3.1.$0^{4,9}$]octacos-8-ene derivatives for the treatment of skin diseases, and pharmaceutical preparations containing them. Ger Offen DE 3:838-035 (Sandoz).

Griffiths, C.E.M. (1994). Cutaneous leucocyte trafficking and psoriasis. *Arch. Dermatol.* 130:494–499.

Hatanaka, H., Iwami, M., Kino, T., Goto, T., and Okuhara, M. (1988a). FR-900520 and FR-900523, novel immunosuppressants isolated from a streptomyces I. Taxonomy of the producing strain. *J. Antibiot.* 41:1586–1591.

Hatanaka, H., Kino, T., Miyata, S., Inamura, N., Kuroda, A., Goto, T., Tanaka, H., and Okuhara, M. (1988b). FR-900520 and FR-900523, novel immunosuppressants isolated from a streptomyces II. Fermentation, isolation and physico-chemical and biological characteristics. *J. Antibiot.* 41:1592–1601.

Jegasothy, B.V., Ackerman, C.D., Todo, S., Fung, J.J., Abu-Elmagd, K., and Starzl, T.E. (1992). Tacrolismus

(FK506): a new therapeutic agent for severe recalcitrant psoriasis. *Arch. Dermatol.* 128:781–785.

Koyama, Y., Hayashi, T., and Honda, H. (1963). Studies on ascomycin. *Annu. Rep. Inst. Food. Microbiol. Chiba Univ.* 15:79–83.

Krueger, G.G., and Duvic, M. (1994). Epidemiology of psoriasis: clinical issues. *J. Invest. Dermatol.* 102:14s–18s.

Liu, J., Farmer, J.D., Friedman, J., Weissman, I., and Schreiber, S.L. (1991). Calcineurin is a common target of cyclophilin-cyclosporin A and FKBP-FK-506 complexes. *Cell* 66:807–815.

Marks, R. (1992). Adverse side effects from the use of topical corticosteroids. In *Topical Corticosteroids.* H.I. Maibach and C. Surber (Eds.). Karger, Basel, pp. 170–183.

Meingassner, J.G., and Stütz, A. (1992a). Immunosuppressive macrolides of the type FK 506: a novel class of topical agents for treatment of skin diseases? *J. Invest. Dermatol.* 98:851–855.

Meingassner, J., and Stütz, A. (1992b). Anti-inflammatory effects of macrophilin-interacting drugs in animal models of irritant and allergic contact dermatitis. 19th Collegium Internationale Allergologicum, Capri, Italy, May, 3–7, Abstr. S 144.

Meingassner, J.G., Baumann, K., Grassberger, M., and Stuetz, A. (1994). Topical activity of the immunosuppressive macrolide SDZ 281-240 in animal models of allergic contact dermatitis. *J. Invest. Dermatol.* 102:599 (abstract).

Meingassner, J.G., Grassberger, M., Fahrngruber, H., Moore, H.D., Schuurman, H., and Stütz, A. (1997). A novel anti-inflammatory drug, SDZ ASM 981, for the topical and oral treatment of skin diseases: in vivo pharmacology. *Br. J. Dermatol.* 137:568–576.

Meingassner, J.G., Fahrngruber, H., Bavandi, A., and Grassberger, M. (1997). SDZ ASM 981—a novel anti-inflammatory macrolactam has high topical and systemic activity in animal models of skin inflammation. *Australasian J. Dermatol.* 38 (Suppl 2):287 (abstract).

Meingassner, J.G., Helm, A., Vit, P., and Grassberger, M. (1997). SDZ ASM 981—a novel anti-inflammatory macrolactam—does not induce skin atrophy. *Australasian J. Dermatol.* 38 (Suppl 2):285 (abstract).

Monasghan, R.L., Sigal, N.H., Kaplan, L., Byrne, R., Borris, F.T., Dumont, F.T., Garrity, G.M., and Zink, D.L. (1989). Novel immunosuppressant agent. Eur Pat 0 323 865A1 (Merck).

Morisaki, M., and Arai, T. (1992). Identity of immunosuppressant FR-900520 with ascomycin. *J. Antibiot.* 45: 126–128.

Mrowietz, U. (1992). The enigma of cyclosporine A treatment for psoriasis. Systemic efficacy versus topical nonresponsiveness. A review. *Acta Derm. Venerol.* [*Stockh.*] 72:321–326.

Mrowietz, U., Bräutigam, M., Gräber, M., Thurston, M., Wagenaar, A., Weidinger, G., and Christophers, E. (1997). Topical treatment with the anti-inflammatory macrolactam SDZ ASM 981 suppresses plaque-type psoriasis. *Australasian J. Dermatol.* 38 (Suppl 2):44 (abstract).

Queille-Roussel, C., Gräber, M., Wagenaar, A., Thurston, M., Lachapelle, J.M., Decroix, J., De Cuyper, Ch., and Ortonne, J.P. (1997). Topical treatment with the anti-inflammatory macrolactam SDZ ASM 981 inhibits established nickel contact dermatitis. *Australasian J. Dermatol.* 38 (Suppl 2):55 (abstract)

Prinz, J., Braun-Falco, O., and Meurer, M. (1991). Chimeric CD4 monoclonal antibody in treatment of generalized pustular psoriasis. *Lancet* 338:320–321.

Rappersberger, K., Meingassner, J.G., Födinger, D., Rehberger, A., Fiebiger, M., Putz, E., Tong, D., Stütz, A., and Wolff, K. (1994). Clearing of psoriasis by a novel macrolide. *J. Invest. Dermatol.* 102:532 (abstract 49).

Rappersberger, K., Meingassner, J.G., Fialla, R., Födinger, D., Sterniczky, B., Rauch, S., Putz, E., Stütz, A., and Wolff, K. (1996). Clearing of psoriasis by a novel immunosuppressive macrolide. *J. Invest. Dermatol.* 106: 701–710.

Remitz, A., Reitamo, S., Erkko, P., Granlund, H., Lauerma, A. (1996). A microplaque assay-based, double blind trial to compare the efficacy of two tacrolimus ointment formulations with two active and two negative controls in patients with chronic plaque-type psoriasis vulgaris. *Br. J. Dermatol.* 135:833 (abstract).

Robertson, D.B., and Maibach, H.I. (1992). Adverse systemic effects of topical corticoids. In *Topical Corticosteroids.* H.I. Maibach and C. Surber (Eds.). Karger, Basel, pp. 163–169.

Schlaak, J.F., Buslau, M., Jochum, W., Hermann, E., Girndt, M., Gallati, H., Meyer zu Büschenfelde, K.-H., and Fleischer, B. (1994). T cells involved in psoriasis vulgaris belong to the Th1 subset. *J. Invest. Dermatol.* 102: 145–149.

Schreiber, L., and Crabtree, G.R. (1992). The mechanism of action of cyclosporin A and FK 506. *Immunol. Today* 13: 136–142.

Sillevis Smitt, J.H., and Winterberg, D.H. (1992). Topical corticosteroids in children: local and systemic effects. In: *Topical Corticosteroids.* H.I. Maibach and C. Surber (Eds.). Karger, Basel, pp. 196–209.

Skehan, P., Storeng, R., and Scudiero, D. (1990). New colometric assay for anticancer-drug screening. *J. Natl. Cancer Int.* 82:1107–1112.

Stütz, A. (1992). Immunosuppressive macrolides. *Transplant. Proc.* 24 (Suppl 2):22–25.

Stütz, A., Grassberger, M., Baumann, K., Edmunds, A., Hiestand, B., Meingassner, J., Nussbaumer, P., Schuler, W., and Zenke, G. (1993). Immunophilin as drug targets. In *Perspectives in Medicinal Chemistry.* B. Testa and E. Kyburz (Eds.). Basel, Verlag Helvetica Chimica Acta, pp. 427–443.

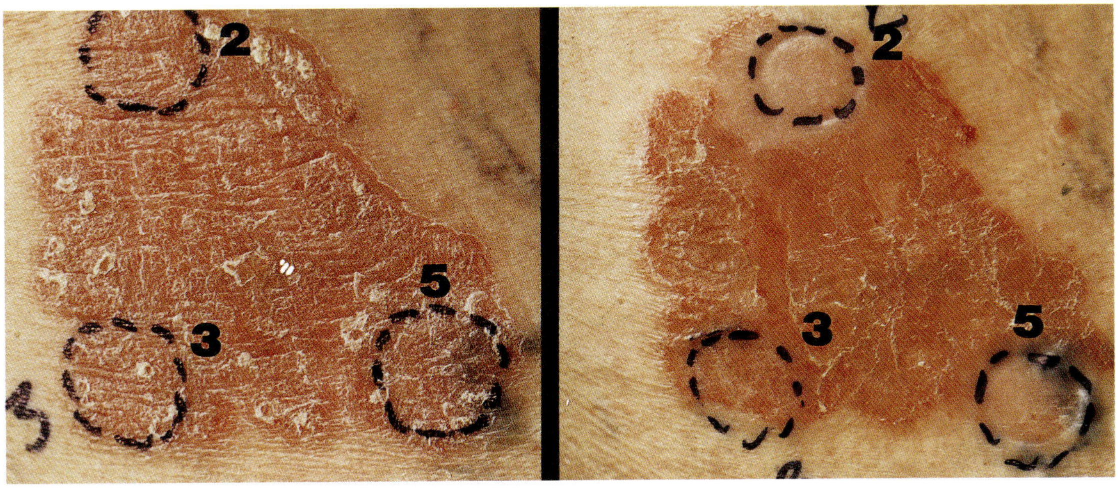

Figure 3.

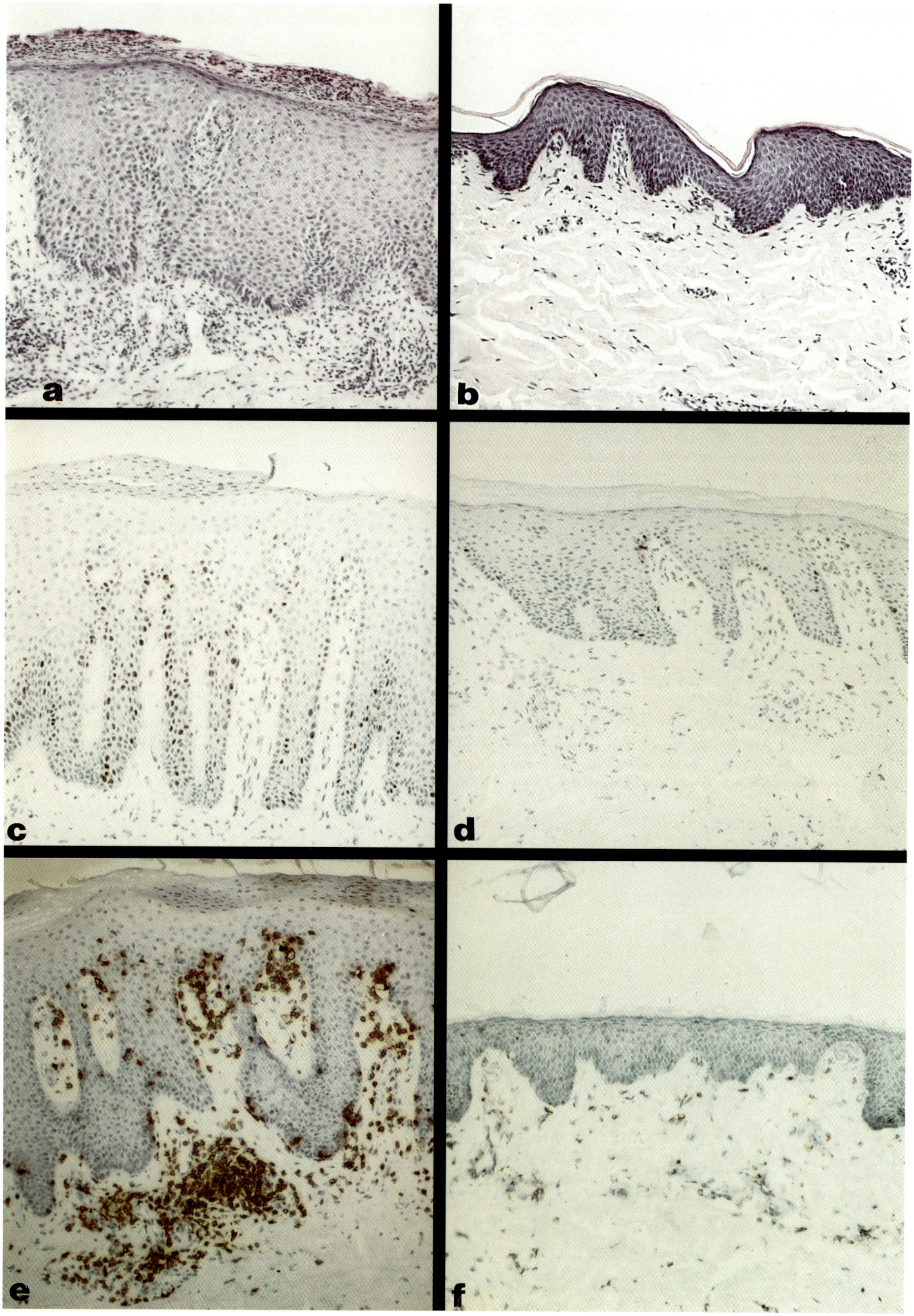

Figure 4.

Surber, C., Itin, P., and Büchner, S. (1992). Clinical controversy on the effect of topical cyclosporin: what is the target site? *Dermatology* 185:242–245.

Uyemura, K., Yamamura, M., Fivenson, D.F., Modlin, R.L., and Nickoloff, B.J. (1993). The cytokine network in lesional and lesion-free psoriatic skin is characterized by a T-helper type 1 cell-mediated response. *J. Invest. Dermatol.* 101:701–705.

Van Leent, E.J.M., Gräber, M., Thurston, M., Wagenaar, A., Spuls, Ph.I., and Bos, J.D. (1997). Topical treatment with the macrolactam SDZ ASM 981 is effective in atopic dermatitis. *Australasian J. Dermatol.* 38 (Suppl 2):234 (abstract).

Wakita, H., and Takigawa, M. (1994). E-selectin and vascular cell adhesion molecule-1 are critical for initial trafficking of helper-inducer/memory T cells in psoriatic plaques. *Arch. Dermatol.* 130:457–463.

Weinshenker, B.G., Bass, B.H., Ebers, G.C., and Rice, G.P.A. (1989). Remission of psoriatic lesions with muromonab CD3 (Orthoclone OKT3) treatment. *J. Am. Acad. Dermatol.* 20:1132–1133.

Weinstein, G.D., and McCullough, J.L. (1976). Cytokinetics and chemotherapy of psoriasis. *J. Invest. Dermatol.* 67: 26–30.

67

Purine Nucleoside Phosphorylase Inhibition: A Novel Therapy for Psoriasis

Gerald M. Walsh, George A. Omura, John A. Montgomery, Thomas J. Franz, Tacey X. Viegas, William J. Cook, Narra Reddy, and Alfred A. Bartolucci
BioCryst Pharmaceuticals, Inc., Birmingham, Alabama

Shanta Bantia and W. Mitchell Sams, Jr.
University of Alabama, Birmingham, Alabama

Howard I. Maibach
University of California School of Medicine, San Francisco, California

An early event in the development of psoriasis is infiltration of target tissue by activated T cells, which may play a crucial role in the maintenance of epidermal hyperplasia as suggested by the beneficial effects of selective T-cell suppressive agents such as anti-CD3 and anti-CD4 (1). Recently, a fusion protein DAB389IL-2, which selectively blocks the growth of activated T cells but not keratinocytes, produced moderate to striking improvement in psoriasis patients, suggesting a primary immunological basis in psoriasis (2). There appears to be a self-sustaining cycle of T-cell recruitment, intralesional activation, release of factors that preferentially stimulate psoriatic epidermal stem cells to proliferate, and further epidermal potentiation of T-cell-mediated lesions (1). Consequently, there has been increasing interest in developing inhibitors of T-cell function for the treatment of psoriasis.

To produce a relatively selective suppression of T-cell proliferation to treat psoriasis and other autoimmune disorders, a new class of drugs has emerged, purine nucleoside phosphorylase inhibitors (PNP, EC 2.4.2.1) (3). Inherited deficiency of PNP in humans produces a relatively selective depletion of T cells, suggesting that active PNP is required for human T-cell proliferation (4). PNP catalyzes the reversible phosphorolysis of purine ribo- or 2′-deoxyribonucleosides to the purine and ribose- or 2-deoxyribose-α-1-phosphate (5,6). The enzymology of PNP has been reviewed by Stoekler (7). PNP activity has been commonly determined enzymatically by a radiochemical assay in which radiolabeled inosine is converted to radiolabeled hypoxanthine (7). The selective inhibition of human T-cell proliferation produced by PNP inhibition is secondary to an accumulation of deoxyguanosine triphosphate (dGTP) in T cells, which apparently suppresses ribonucleotide reductase activity and, hence, DNA synthesis (4,8).

In 1981, in vitro studies with a relatively weak prototype PNP inhibitor, 8-aminoguanosine, showed that pharmacological PNP inhibition also selectively suppresses T-cell proliferation with respect to B-cell proliferation (9). A new class of PNP inhibitors, 9-deazaguanines, has recently been discovered (10,11). BCX-34 (Fig. 1) is a potent 9-deazaguanine PNP inhibitor currently in clinical trials for the dermal treat-

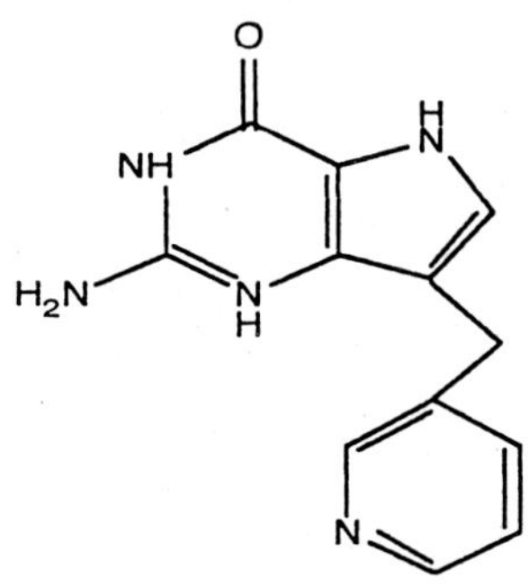

Figure 1 Structure of BCX-34 [peldesine; 2-amino-1,5-dihydro-7-(3-pyridinylmethyl)-4H-pyrrolo(3,2-d)pyrimidin-4-one].

ment of cutaneous T-cell lymphoma and psoriasis (12) as well as in oral dose-escalation studies.

PRECLINICAL STUDIES WITH BCX-34

The in vitro and in vivo pharmacology of BCX-34 has recently been described (13). BCX-34 inhibited human, rat, and mouse red blood cell (RBC) PNP in vitro with IC_{50}s of 36 ± 2.9, 5 ± 1.0, and 32 ± 2.9 nM, respectively. The K_i for BCX-34 against human RBC PNP was 23 ± 4 nM and analysis of the enzyme kinetics indicated that the compound was a competitive, reversible inhibitor of PNP with inosine as the substrate. BCX-34 inhibited in vitro proliferation of CCRF-CEM human T cells in the presence but not in the absence of deoxyguanosine (10 μM), associated with an intracellular accumulation of dGTP. The IC_{50} for this cell line was 0.57 ± 0.12 μM. The proliferation of rat and mouse T cells was not inhibited by BCX-34 up to 30 μM nor did these cells accumulate dGTP. Oral bioavailability of BCX-34 in rats was 76%. BCX-34 was orally active in elevating plasma inosine in rats (twofold at 30 mg/kg), in suppressing ex vivo RBC PNP activity in rats (98% at 3 hr, 100 mg/kg), and in suppressing ex vivo skin PNP activity in mice (39% at 3 hr, 100 mg/kg).

BCX-34 has been formulated in a triethanolamine-stearate-based oil/water dermal cream, containing glycerin as an emollient, for the topical treatment of psoriasis, cutaneous T-cell lymphoma, and atopic dermatitis. Dermal toxicity studies with 10% BCX-34 dermal cream showed no evidence of acute dermal irritation (rat) or delayed contact sensitization (guinea pig). Longer-term studies (14 and 91 days) in the rabbit also demonstrated no dermal irritation or systemic toxicity of the 10% BCX-34 dermal cream.

A dermal radiotracer ([^{14}C]-BCX-34) absorption study was performed in rats with 10% BCX-34 dermal cream. BCX-34 migrated from the vehicle and penetrated the skin. Approximately 3.6% of applied BCX-34 was absorbed into the skin. Most of the absorbed BCX-34 remained in the skin. A small amount (<10%) was slowly released from the skin into the systemic circulation where it was rapidly cleared and excreted. Resulting average blood levels were low, approximately 10 ng/ml.

In vitro dermal radiotracer ([^{14}C]-BCX-34) absorption studies were performed. In one in vitro study, human skin was selected from autopsy or surgical procedures, dermatomed to 500 μm thickness, and attached to a flow-through diffusion cell apparatus, providing a skin surface area of 1 cm^2. Dermal cream containing [^{14}C]-BCX-34 at 0.1%, 0.3%, 1%, 3%, and 5% was applied to the skin surface for 4 or 24 hr and then the skin was washed. Radioactivity in the reservoir fluid under the skin, in the skin, and remaining on the surface was measured. Small but detectable amounts of BCX-34 penetrated the skin into the reservoir over the 24-hr period (<0.1%). At both time points, theoretical concentrations in the skin reached 20–30 μM at 0.1% and 0.3% and approximately 150 μM at 1%, 3%, and 5%. Cellophane tape stripping of the skin after 24 hr indicated that BCX-34 was present to a large extent in the stratum corneum with about 15% in the epidermis and dermis. The results showed that BCX-34 in the dermal cream can penetrate through human skin and can achieve skin concentrations theoretically sufficient to inhibit PNP and T-cell proliferation. The data further suggested that the optimal concentration of BCX-34 in the dermal cream was 1% since higher concentrations in the selected cream base did not appear to produce greater skin concentrations of BCX-34.

A second in vitro study in human skin was performed to more clearly demonstrate whether BCX-34 penetrated into the dermis. Dermatomed, cryopreserved split-thickness human skin (250 μm) was obtained from a skin bank and attached to a diffusion cell apparatus, providing a skin surface area of 1 cm^2. BCX-34 dermal cream at a concentration of 1% was applied to the skin for 12 or 24 hr using a finite dosing technique. The skin was then removed and washed, the epidermis was separated from the dermis, and each portion was analyzed for the presence of BCX-34. The results are shown in Figure 2. At 12 hr 0.052 ±

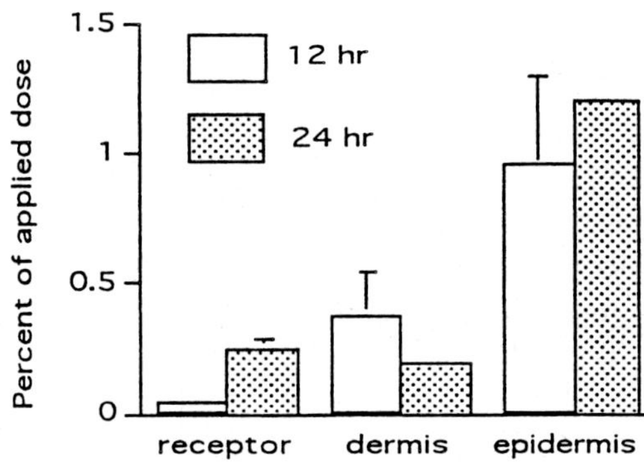

Figure 2 Diffusion [^{14}C]-labeled BCX-34 through cryopreserved split-thickness human skin (250 μm) following topical application of 1% BCX-34 dermal cream; values are means ± SE, n = 5–6.

0.009% of applied BCX-34 was in the receptor fluid, 0.378 ± 0.164% was in the dermis, and 0.958 ± 0.340% was in the epidermis. Corresponding values at 24 hr were 0.248 ± 0.038%, 0.105 ± 0.031%, and 1.089 ± 0.114%. The theoretical concentrations of BCX-34 in the epidermis and dermis at 24 hr were 250 and 28 μM, respectively. These results further suggested that BCX-34 in the dermal cream can penetrate through human skin and may achieve dermal and epidermal concentrations sufficient to inhibit PNP and T-cell proliferation. The data also demonstrated that BCX-34 persists to a greater degree in the epidermis than in the dermis.

Previous studies in the mouse demonstrated that oral BCX-34 at 50 mg/kg/day for 5 days could significantly reduce the dermal irritation produced by the application of dinitrofluorobenzene (DNFB) to the skin of the shaved abdomen (11). The mechanism of action of this effect is unknown but it is unlikely due to inhibition of T-cell proliferation. Rodent T cells are resistant to PNP inhibition and do not accumulate dGTP because of low kinase and high nucleotidase activity (13). The irritation induced by DNFB resulted mostly from the animals scratching themselves and the action of BCX-34 appeared to suppress this response. Studies were performed in mice to determine whether dermal application of BCX-34 would inhibit skin PNP and would also protect against DNFB dermal irritation.

The ex vivo inhibition of skin PNP activity was measured at several time points after dermal dosing with BCX-34 in adult male Balb/c mice. Separate groups of mice were used at each time point and at each dose. Mice were anesthetized with ketamine (100 mg/kg) and xylazine (1.8 mg/kg) ip. The abdomen was shaved and the remaining hair removed with a depilatory. A 1-cm^2 piece of pretreatment skin was removed from the abdomen and the blood vessels (panniculus) on the dermal layer were removed by scraping with a scalpel. The skin sample was kept on ice or frozen until analyzed ex vivo for PNP activity. After the pretreatment skin sample was obtained, dermal creams of varying BCX-34 concentrations were applied to the abdominal skin and left on the skin for varying durations, one concentration per group of mice. At various times after dermal application, the mice were anesthetized and the treated piece of abdominal skin was washed with soap and water. A 1-cm^2 piece of the skin was removed as before. The pretreatment and posttreatment skin samples were analyzed for PNP activity as described previously (13).

The results of dermal administration of BCX-34 on mouse skin PNP activity are shown in Figure 3. The 0.1% concentration was not effective up to 6 hr. The 0.3% concentration produced significant inhibition of PNP activity at 3 hr after application and this effect was maintained up to 18 hr (43 ± 2.7% inhibition). There was no inhibition at 24 hr (−7.9 ± 14.8%). The time of peak effect for the 0.3% concentration was 6 hr after application. The 1% and 5% concentrations inhibited PNP activity as early as 30 min after application and this effect was maintained up to 6 hr.

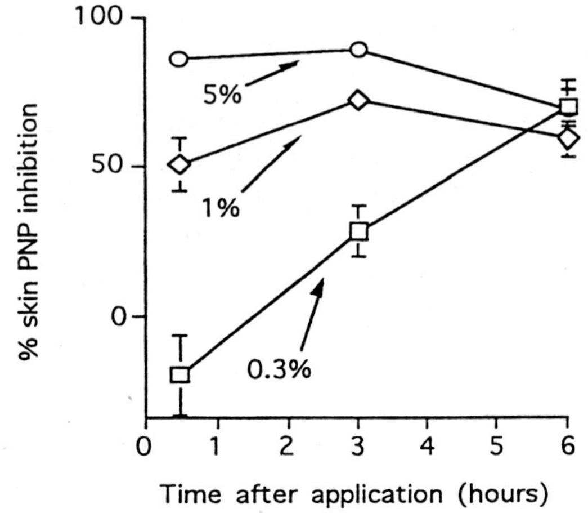

Figure 3 Time course of ex vivo skin PNP inhibition with topical BCX-34 dermal cream in mice at 0.3%, 1%, or 5% concentrations; values are means ± SE, n = 5/group.

There was little difference in the magnitude of PNP inhibition among the 0.3, 1, or 5% concentrations at 6 hr after application. However, clear dose-response relationships were seen at 30 min and 3 hr. The minimally effective concentration for dermal PNP inhibitory activity was 0.3%. At time of peak effect 0.3% also appeared to be a maximally effective concentration. The rate of onset of PNP inhibition may be a function of the concentration of BCX-34 in the dermal cream. BCX-34 has a relatively long duration of action in mouse skin after in vivo dermal application.

Male adult Balb/c mice were also used to evaluate the effects of BCX-34 dermal cream on contact dermatitis. The abdomens were shaved and remaining hair was removed with a depilatory. DNFB was applied topically to the abdomen, 20 μl 0.5% DNFB in acetone/olive oil (4:1). Three hours later BCX-34 dermal cream at 0.1%, 0.3%, 1%, or 5% or vehicle cream was applied to the DNFB-treated area. One group of mice received no treatment. There were five mice per treatment group. Treatments were applied once daily for 5 days. On the sixth day the abdomens were scored for redness, thickening, and excoriations with 0 = no effect, 1 = mild, 2 = moderate, and 3 = severe, with each variable given equal weight.

The results of this study are shown in Figure 4. The average irritation score in untreated mice was 2.5. The average score for mice treated with vehicle cream was 1.8, not statistically significantly different from the value in untreated mice. All BCX-34 treatment values were significantly reduced compared to the value in untreated mice; 1% and 5% BCX-34 treatment values were also significantly reduced compared to vehicle treatment values. There was no apparent difference in efficacy between the 1% and 5% BCX-34 treatments.

The data demonstrate a dose-related effect of BCX-34 dermal cream in reducing dermatitis produced by the dermal application of DNFB in mice. Concentrations of BCX-34 as low as 0.1% may be effective and maximum efficacy appears to be achieved at 1%. Higher concentrations may not produce a further significant benefit.

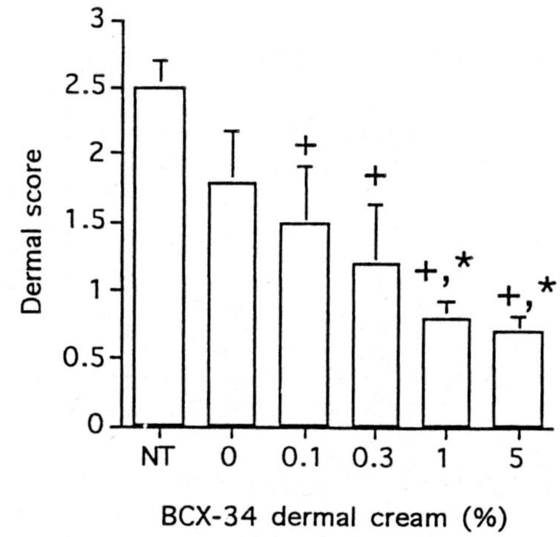

Figure 4 Effects of BCX-34 dermal cream on contact dermatitis in the mouse. BCX-34 dermal cream or vehicle was applied once per day for 5 days to skin previously exposed to DNFB. NT = no treatment. †$p < 0.05$ versus NT; *$p < 0.05$ versus vehicle (0 BCX-34).

An in vivo study to evaluate the absorption of BCX-34 into the stratum corneum was performed in human volunteers. BCX-34 dermal cream at 0.1%, 1%, 3%, or 5%, each containing [^{14}C]-BCX-34, was applied to a 1-cm^2 area of skin for 6 or 24 hr. At the end of the exposure periods the dosing area was washed and then stripped with tape to obtain stratum corneum samples. The amount of BCX-34 in the stratum corneum was calculated from radioactivity obtained in the skin stripings. The results are shown in Figure 5.

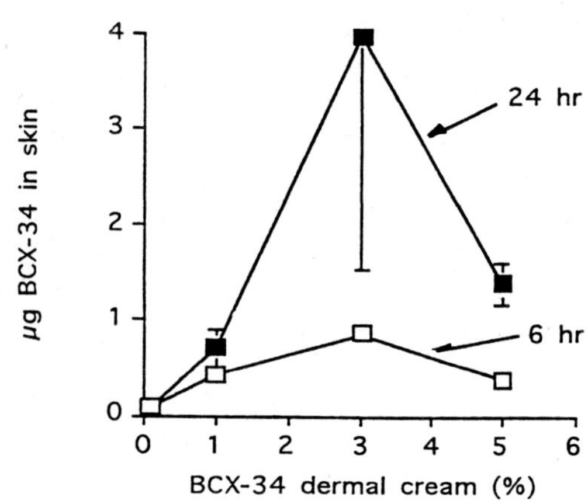

Figure 5 BCX-34 content in skin (1 cm^2) treated for 6 or 24 hr with BCX-34 dermal cream; values are means ± SE, n = 4/mean.

CLINICAL STUDIES WITH BCX-34

Dermal toxicity studies with 5% BCX-34 dermal cream were performed in human volunteers: In double-blind, placebo-controlled trials there was no evidence of cumulative (21 day) irritation, contact sensitization, phototoxicity, or photosensitization.

It was found that BCX-34 in the dermal cream penetrates the stratum corneum and application of a single dose provides a source of BCX-34 in the stratum corneum up to 24 hr. At 6 hr all concentrations of BCX-34 produced significant levels of BCX-34 in the stratum corneum in a concentration-dependent manner up to 3%. The 5% concentration delivered the same as the 1% concentration. At 24 hr, 0.1%, 1%, and 5% concentrations of BCX-34 produced significant levels of BCX-34 in the stratum corneum in a concentration-dependent manner. Results with the 3% dermal cream were highly variable at 24 hr. In view of this result with the 3% cream and the relative difficulty in formulating the 5% cream, BCX-34 1% dermal cream was considered suitable for clinical application.

The efficacy of BCX-34 dermal cream was evaluated in patients with psoriasis. Forty outpatients, 18 years of age or older, with stable plaque-stage psoriasis were studied. One of two matched lesions on each patient was randomly assigned treatments with BCX-34 dermal cream 0.1%, 0.3%, 1%, or 5% and the other lesion received treatment with vehicle (base cream without BCX-34). Ten patients were assigned to each dose of BCX-34 or vehicle. Treatments were applied twice daily for 6 consecutive weeks. Patients were evaluated clinically by two blinded investigators before (pretreatment), during, and at the end of 6 weeks. The evaluation comprised scoring the lesions for erythema, scaling, and thickness. These scores were added to give a total plaque score. A patient evaluation score was also obtained and was added to the total plaque score to give a global score. Pre- and posttreatment skin biopsies were obtained for evaluation by two blinded dermatopathologists for epidermal thickness, parakeratosis, and dermal lymphocytic infiltration.

The concentration-response relationship of BCX-34 dermal cream on the global score obtained at the end of 6 weeks is shown in Figure 6. The 5% dermal cream results are not included because this formulation was ineffective. In addition, it appeared to have less of an emollient effect than the vehicle alone. The scaling score for the vehicle was 1.67 ± 0.28 versus 1.28 ± 0.34 for BCX-34 5% dermal cream, $p = 0.02$. The large-scale production of the 5% dermal cream for the clinical trial produced a formulation that was relatively pasty and thick, and this formulation, as a consequence, may have produced little delivery of BCX-34 into the skin.

The concentration-response relationships were all positive for drug-treated lesions and the correlation coefficients were all high (>0.9) with the exception

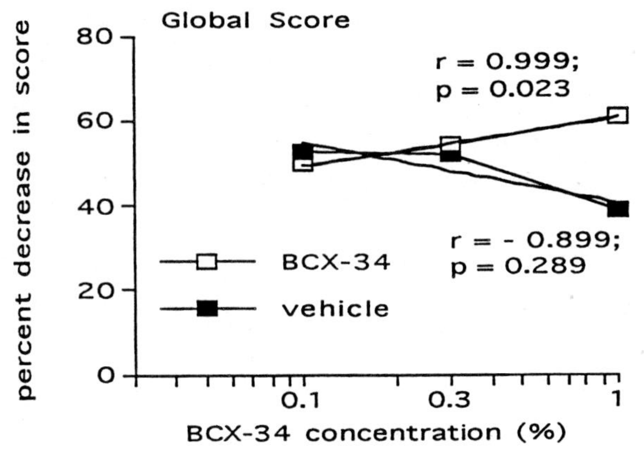

Figure 6 Concentration-response relationship of BCX-34 dermal cream in the treatment of psoriatic lesions.

of the patient evaluation score. The correlation was statistically significant with the global score, indicating a clear concentration-response relationship for BCX-34 dermal cream in reducing disease severity. On the other hand, the corresponding analysis of paired vehicle scores showed that all the scores, with the exception of the erythema score, were negatively related to the BCX-34 concentration. None of the correlations with vehicle were statistically significant. These data demonstrate a concentration-response relationship with BCX-34 that did not occur with the placebo. The 1% concentration was maximally effective in these studies.

The effects of treatment of psoriatic lesions with 1% BCX-34 dermal cream are shown in Tables 1 and 2. The 0.1%, 0.3%, and 5% formulations did not produce appreciable responses greater than the vehicle cream. The responses are expressed as absolute scores and as percent changes from baseline scores. The drug-induced responses ($n = 10$) are compared to corresponding vehicle responses ($n = 10$) as well as to all vehicle responses combined ($n = 40$). Paired and unpaired analyses were performed, taking into account unequal variance. When compared to paired vehicle responses, 1% BCX-34 produced a significantly greater reduction in total score, and greater reductions in thickness and global scores with borderline statistical significance. When compared to all vehicle responses combined, 1% BCX-34 produced significantly greater reductions in erythema, scaling, total score, and global score.

When compared to paired vehicle responses, BCX-34 produced a significantly greater reduction in lymphocytic infiltrate, and when compared to all vehicle

Table 1 Comparison of Clinical Dermal Scores Between Vehicle-Treated and 1% BCX-34 Dermal Cream-Treated Lesions in Psoriasis Patients

Score	BCX-34	Vehicle	*p*	All vehicles	*p*
Erythema					
Baseline	2.6 ± 0.16	2.6 ± 0.16	—	2.4 ± 0.09	0.33
6 weeks	1.2 ± 0.18	1.7 ± 0.32	0.11	1.6 ± 0.15	0.24
% change	56 ± 5.4	38 ± 10.3	0.15	24 ± 7.2*	0.006
Thickness					
Baseline	2.0 ± 0.26	2.0 ± 0.26	—	1.9 ± 0.09	0.66
6 weeks	0.79 ± 0.15	1.4 ± 0.34	0.08	1.3 ± 0.14	0.16
% change	55 ± 10.6	33 ± 10.5	0.18	35 ± 6.0	0.18
Scaling					
Baseline	2.0 ± 0.26	2.0 ± 0.26	—	2.3 ± 0.12	0.32
6 weeks	0.79 ± 0.10	1.3 ± 0.32	0.13	1.2 ± 0.16*	0.02
% change	56 ± 3.9	29 ± 15.9	0.14	43 ± 7.4	0.14
Total score					
Baseline	6.6 ± 0.58	6.6 ± 0.58	—	6.6 ± 0.25	0.96
6 weeks	2.8 ± 0.36	4.4 ± 0.87	0.08	4.1 ± 2.4*	0.02
% change	57 ± 4.4	35 ± 8.8*	0.05	37 ± 5.6*	0.01
Patient score					
Baseline	0.80 ± 0.36	0.80 ± 0.36	—	1.1 ± 0.18	0.48
6 weeks	0.14 ± 0.14	0.5 ± 0.33	0.25	0.16 ± 0.08	0.92
% change	92 ± 48.3	63 ± 26	0.29	85 ± 7.5	0.70
Global score					
Baseline	7.4 ± 0.69	7.4 ± 0.69	—	7.7 ± 0.31	0.71
6 weeks	2.9 ± 0.33	4.9 ± 0.94	0.07	4.3 ± 0.41*	0.017
% change	61 ± 4.2	39 ± 9.5	0.06	42 ± 5.7*	0.02

Values are means ± SE. Unaudited data.
*Significantly different from corresponding BCX-34 value.

Table 2 Comparison of Histopathological Dermal Scores Between Placebo-Treated and 1% BCX-34 Dermal Cream–Treated Lesions in Psoriasis Patients

Score	BCX-34	Vehicle	*p*	All vehicles	*p*
Epidermal thickness					
Baseline	28.2 ± 5.4	27.4 ± 4.4	0.91	30.2 ± 5.4	0.69
6 weeks	24.8 ± 7.3	29.3 ± 6.7	0.15	25.2 ± 2.2	0.95
% change	25 ± 13.2	27 ± 11.3	0.95	15 ± 8.0	0.57
Parakeratosis					
Baseline	2.4 ± 0.20	2.3 ± 0.29	0.69	2.3 ± 0.14	0.65
6 weeks	1.1 ± 0.26	1.7 ± 0.42	0.10	1.5 ± 0.19	0.37
% change	55 ± 8.7**	29 ± 18.8	0.23	19.6 ± 14.3*	0.04
Infiltrate					
Baseline	1.5 ± 0.33	1.6 ± 0.23	0.86	.13 ± 0.12	0.61
6 weeks	0.79 ± 0.18	1.3 ± 0.29*	0.02	0.97 ± 0.11	0.46
% change	43 ± 11.1**	18 ± 17.2	0.28	17 ± 9.81	0.28

Values are means ± SE. Unaudited data.
*Significantly different from corresponding BCX-34 value. **Significantly different from zero, $p < 0.05$.

responses combined, BCX-34 produced a significantly greater reduction in parakeratosis. The reductions in lymphocytic infiltrate and parakeratosis from baseline were statistically significant with BCX-34 treatment but not with vehicle treatment. There were no appreciable side effects related to BCX-34.

The results of these studies in patients with psoriasis suggest that topical application of 1% BCX-34 dermal cream for 6 weeks produces a moderate improvement in the clinical manifestations of the disease. This therapeutic effect of BCX-34 may be related to a decreased lymphocytic infiltration into the psoriatic lesion.

SUMMARY

BCX-34 is a new chemical entity with a novel mechanism of action for the suppression of T-cell proliferation. The dermal formulation of BCX-34 provides a reservoir of drug in the stratum corneum and facilitates penetration of the drug into the epidermis and, to some extent, the dermis. The formulation, however, produces little systemic absorption of the drug. Topical BCX-34 suppresses skin PNP and can reduce chemical-induced inflammation in the skin. In addition, the BCX-34 dermal cream formulation has an excellent dermal safety profile. The 1% concentration appears to be optimal for the present formulation and may produce a moderate therapeutic improvement in psoriatic lesions with little or no side effects.

REFERENCES

1. Bata-Csorgo, Z., Hammerberg, C., Voorhees, J.J., and Cooper, K.D. (1995). Intralesional T-lymphocyte activation as a mediator of psoriatic epidermal hyperplasia. *J. Invest. Dermatol.* 105(Suppl. 1):895–945.
2. Gottlieb, S.L., Gilleaudeau, P., Johnson, R., Estes, L., Woodworth, T.G., Gottlieb, A.B., and Krueger, J.G. (1995). Response of psoriasis to a lymphocyte-selective toxin (DAB389IL-2) suggests a primary immune, but not keratinocyte, pathogenic basis. *Nat. Med.* 1:442–447.
3. Stoeckler, J.D., Ealick, S.E., Bugg, C.E., and Parks, R.E., Jr. (1986). Design of purine nucleoside phosphorylase inhibitors. *Fed. Proc.* 45:2773–2778.
4. Markert, M.L. (1991). Purine nucleoside phosphorylase deficiency. *Immunodef. Rev.* 3:45–81.
5. Ealick, S.E., Babu, Y.S., Bugg, C.E., Erion, M.D., Guida, W.C., Montgomery, J.A., and Secrist, J.A. (1991). Application of crystallographic and modeling methods in the design of purine nucleoside phosphorylase inhibitors. *Proc. Natl. Acad. Sci. (U.S.A.)* 88: 11540–11544.
6. Montgomery, J.A. (1993). Purine nucleoside phosphorylase: a target for drug design. *Med. Res. Rev.* 13: 209–225.
7. Stoekler, J.D. (1994). Purine nucleoside phosphorylase: a target for chemotherapy. In *Developments in Cancer Chemotherapy.* R.I. Glazer (Ed.). CRC Press, Boca Raton, FL, pp. 35–60.
8. Eriksson, S., Thelander, L., and Kaerman, M. (1979). Allosteric regulation of calf thymus ribonucleoside diphosphate reductase. *Biochemistry* 18:2948–2952.
9. Kazmers, I.S., Mitchell, B.S., DaDonna, P.E., Wotring, I.I., Townsend, L.B., and Kelley, W.N. (1981). Inhibition of purine nucleoside phosphorylase by 8-aminoguanosine: selective toxicity for T-lymphocytes. *Science* 214:1137–1139.
10. Montgomery, J.A., Niwas, S., Rose, J.D., Secrist, J.A. III, Babu, Y.S., Bugg, C.E., Erion, M.D., Guida, W.C., and Ealick, S.E. (1993). Structure-based design of inhibitors of purine nucleoside phosphorylase: 9-(arylmethyl) derivatives of 9-deazaguanine. *J. Med. Chem.* 36:55–69.
11. Walsh, G.M., Reddy, N.S., Bantia, S., Babu, Y.S., and Montgomery, J.A. (1994). Development of inhibitors of purine nucleoside phosphorylase. *Hematol. Rev.* 8: 87–97.
12. Montgomery, J.A., Snyder, H.W., Walsh, D.A., and Walsh, G.M. (1993). BCX-34, purine nucleoside phosphorylase (PNP) inhibitor. *Drugs Future* 18:887–890.
13. Bantia, S., Montgomery, J.A., Johnson, H.G., and Walsh, G.M. (1996). In vivo and in vitro pharmacologic activity of the purine nucleoside phosphorylase inhibitor BCX-34: the role of GTP and dGTP. *Immunopharmacology* 1996; 35:53–63.

68

Potential Clinical Uses for Parathyroid Hormone–Related Peptide Analogues for Treating Psoriasis and Other Skin Disorders

Michael F. Holick
Boston University Medical Center, Boston, Massachusetts

Parathyroid hormone (PTH)-related peptide (PTHrP) has been identified as one of the major factors responsible for humoral hypercalcemia of malignancy, which occurs mostly in squamous cell tumors of the lung and kidney (1–3). The full-length cDNA clones of PTHrP have been shown to encode a 141-amino-acid protein that shares 70% homology with PTH in its first 13 amino acids but diverges completely in its primary structure thereafter (Fig. 1) (3). Studies using synthetic PTHrP amino-terminal fragments have demonstrated that these peptide fragments bind to the PTH receptor and cause biological effects on calcium and phosphorus metabolism similar to PTH in cultured bone and kidney cells. Thus, it has been postulated that a single receptor species mediates many of the physiological functions of PTH and PTHrP (4). A PTH/PTHrP receptor cDNA has been cloned (4). Using the cDNA probe for this PTH/PTHrP receptor, it was demonstrated that the PTH/PThrP mRNAs were widely expressed in many tissues besides classic PTH target organs (5). In addition to being a product of tumors that are associated with humoral hypercalcemia of malignancy, PTHrP is also expressed by a variety of normal and neoplastic tissues including the skin and hair follicles (6,7).

FRAGMENTS OF PTHrP AND THEIR BIOLOGICAL ACTIVITIES

Little is known about the actual secretory or circulating forms of PTHrP. It has been suggested that the full-length PTHrP is probably a precursor protein that is to be processed into several smaller peptides with different biological functions (2,3). A variety of PTHrP forms have been identified in cultured keratinocyte medium, in the circulation, in milk, and in tumor extracts (8). When cultured keratinocytes were protected from proteolysis, it was shown that the N-terminal species of PTHrP was secreted by human keratinocytes as a glycopeptide (9). A midregion PTHrP species has been purified from the medium and extracts from several cell types including human keratinocytes and a renal cell carcinoma cell line as well as two PTHrP (1–141)-transfected cell lines (rat insulinoma and Chinese hamster ovary cell lines) (10,11). These observations suggest that both midregion PTHrP species and N-terminal PTHrP fragments were present in conditioned media as well as in cell extracts and were possibly secretory forms of the peptide. A carboxy-terminal fragment of PTHrP containing PTHrP (109–138) immunoreactivity has also been

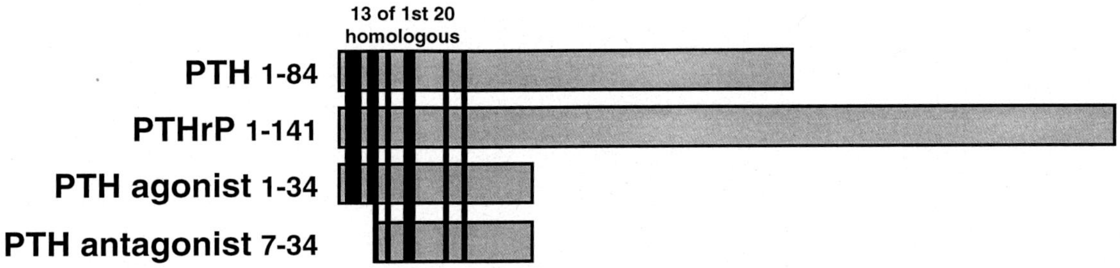

Figure 1 Structures and homology between PTHrP, PTH, PTH (1–34), and PTH (7–34).

found in four cell types that produced midregion fragments. Thus, it is likely that epidermal keratinocytes and dermal fibroblasts are exposed to and under the influence of not only a full-length PTHrP (1–141) but also different N-terminal, midregion, and C-terminal PTHrP fragments that may have separate biological actions in the skin (3).

It is well recognized that N-terminal fragments of PTHrP are capable of interacting with the PTH/PTHrP receptor and causing biological effects on calcium and phosphorus metabolism similar to PTH in cultured bone and kidney cells (12–17). It is also recognized, however, that a variety of tissues not related to calcium metabolism also produce PTHrP including human keratinocytes, stomach, islet cells, parathyroid glands, lactating mammary glands, brain, hypothalamus, thyroid, adrenal, and fetal liver. These observations along with the complex structure of the gene and the abundance of posttranslational processing sites have led to the hypothesis that PTHrP and its metabolites may have multiple physiological roles as autocrine and/or paracrine factors to regulate the growth and development of a variety of cells and tissues including the cells of the skin (3).

PTH/PTHrP RECEPTOR

The PTH/PTHrP receptor was cloned from rat osteosarcoma cells and opposum kidney cells (4). The PTH/PTHrP receptor is a seven-transmembrane-domain G-protein-linked receptor (Fig. 2). The PTH/PTHrP receptor has significant homology to the G-protein-linked secretin and calcitonin receptors and lacks homology to other G-protein-linked receptors. A variety of tissues, other than the traditional PTH-responsive tissues including bone and kidney, express the PTH/PTHrP receptor. In situ hybridization analysis for the expression of PTHrP and PTH/PTHrP receptor mRNAs in rodent fetuses revealed that in extraskeletal tissues such as the lungs and heart the PTHrP mRNA was expressed mainly in surface-lining cells whereas its receptor mRNA was expressed principally in adjacent mesenchymal cells (18).

An evaluation of the PTH/PTH receptor in keratinocytes and fibroblasts revealed that there was strong expression of the PTH/PTHrP receptor mRNA in cultured fibroblasts as well as in osteosarcoma cells and mouse kidney cells but there was no mRNA signal for the PTH/PTHrP receptor in cultured human keratinocytes (19). These observations are consistent with the observation that cultured dermal fibroblasts, when exposed to N-terminal fragments of PTH and PTHrP, had an increased adenylate cyclase activity (3,20) whereas there was no stimulation in cyclic AMP formation in cultured human keratinocytes (19). These data suggest that keratinocytes in the epidermis produce PTHrP, which acts in a paracrine fashion to interact with dermal fibroblasts to alter their biological activity (21). The fibroblasts, in turn, could regulate epidermal cell growth and differentiation.

BIOLOGICAL ACTIONS OF PTHrP IN THE EPIDERMIS

The presence of PTHrP bioactivity in nonmalignant cells was first demonstrated in conditioned medium harvested from confluent human cultured keratinocytes (22). Until recently, little was known about the physiological role of PTHrP in normal skin. The biological function of PTHrP in human skin was first suggested by studies that demonstrated that cultured human keratinocytes exposed to PTHrP agonists, PTHrP (1–34), and human PTH (1–34) (Fig. 1) caused a concentration-dependent decrease in the number of keratinocyte basal cells similar to 1,25-dihydroxyvitamine D_3 [$1,25(OH)_2D_3$] (21,23). To determine whether we could block the antiproliferative action of PTH (1–34) and $1,25(OH)_2D_3$ on cultured

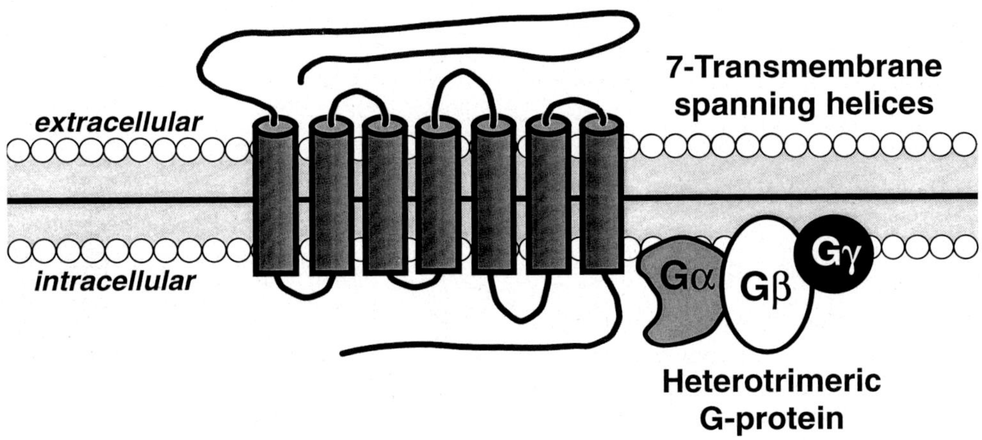

Figure 2 Schematic of the seven-transmembrane structure of the PTH/PTHrP receptor.

human keratinocytes, cultured keratinocytes exposed to PTH (1–34) or $1{,}25(OH)_2D_3$ were coincubated with the PTH/PTHrP receptor antagonist [$Nle^{8,18}Tyr^{34}$] bovine PTH (7–34)-amide [PTH(7–34)]. When keratinocytes were exposed to 10 nmol PTH (7–34), there was no significant effect on keratinocyte proliferation. However, when PTH (7–34) was coincubated with PTH (1–34) or $1{,}25(OH)_2D_3$, it reversed the antiproliferative and prodifferentiating activities of these hormones (Fig. 3) (21).

Milstone et al. (24) demonstrated that PTHrP (1–36) stimulated cornified envelope formation by 400% over control in cultured human keratinocytes. In contrast, using immortalized human keratinocyte cell line RHEK-1 grown in DMEM-supplemented medium with 5% fetal bovine serum albumin, Henderson et al. (25) showed a small (20%) increase in ^3H-thymidine incorporation into DNA in the presence of PTHrP (1–34). This observation was not supported by a study that demonstrated when the endogenous synthesis of PTHrP was blocked in a human keratinocyte cell line (HPK-1) by transfecting an antisense mRNA from PTHrP, there was an increase in ^3H-thymidine incorporation and an acceleration in growth (26). These data suggested that PTHrP was an endogenous inhibitor of cell growth. Furthermore, when Wysolmerski et al. (27) overexpressed the PTHrP protein in the skin of transgenic mice, they found a profound disturbance in hair follicle development especially in

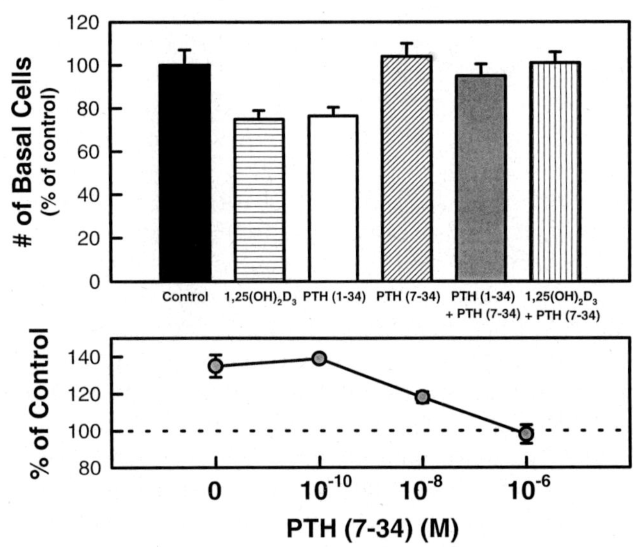

Figure 3 Effect of $1{,}25(OH)_2D_3$, a parathyroid hormone (PTH) agonist, and PTH antagonist on keratinocyte proliferation. (Top) Inhibition of cultured human keratinocyte proliferation in the presence of $1{,}25(OH)_2D_3$, PTH/PTHrP agonist PTH (1–34), or PTH/PTHrP antagonist PTH (7–34). Separate cultures of human keratinocytes were coincubated with $1{,}25(OH)_2D_3$ and PTH (7–34) or PTH (1–34) and PTH (7–34). (Bottom) Cornified envelopes as percentage of control from keratinocytes exposed to 10^{-8} M $1{,}25(OH)_2D_3$ with varying amounts of PTH (7–34), as described previously (28). Each of the data points and bars represents the mean ± SEM. (From Ref. 21, reproduced with permission.)

the ventral area of the skin where a complete lack of hair follicle formation was observed and there was decrease in the thickness of the skin in the same region.

EFFECT OF A PTH/PTHrP AGONIST AND ANTAGONIST ON EPIDERMAL PROLIFERATION AND HAIR GROWTH

The in vitro observations that PTHrP agonists inhibited keratinocyte proliferation and induced terminal differentiation (21,23,24) and the antagonist [PTH (7–34)] partially prevented the antiproliferative activity of a PTHrP agonist (21,23) suggested that PTHrP may have a fundamentally important role in the regulation of epidermal proliferation and differentiation (21). To determine whether these peptides had any biological effect on the skin in vivo, we used the SKH-1 hairless mouse for a model. SKH-1 hairless mice (5–6 weeks old) received either PTH (1–34), PTH (7–34), 1,25(OH)$_2$D$_3$, or control vehicle intraperitoneally for 3 days (28). On the third day, they received ^{3}H-thymidine intraperitoneally. An analysis of the skin samples revealed that the group of mice that received 0.5 μg of PTH (1–34) daily for 3 days showed a 59% decline in the incorporation of ^{3}H-thymidine into epidermal DNA compared to the control (Fig. 4). A similar degree of inhibition was observed with 1,25(OH)$_2$D$_3$ (0.1 μg). The PTH antagonist PTH (7–34) caused a dose-dependent increase in the incorporation of ^{3}H-thymidine into epidermal DNA. At a dose of 10 μg/day for 3 days, PTH (7–34) caused a 144% increase in ^{3}H-thymidine incorporation into epidermal DNA when compared to the control group. A separate group of mice that received 10 μg of PTH (7–34) intraperitoneally daily for 7 days had noticeably more hair on their bodies. There was a 188% increase in the number of hair shafts and 140% increase in the hair shaft length in the treated animals compared to the control group. The mice that received PTH (1–34) for 7 days showed no significant effect on hair shaft number or hair shaft length (28).

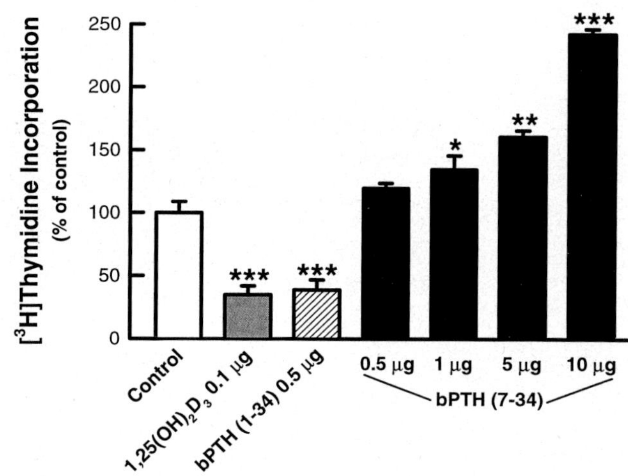

Figure 4 In vivo effects of 1,25(OH)$_2$D$_3$, hPTH (1–34), and bPTH (7–34) on incorporation of ^{3}H-thymidine into epidermal DNA. Data presented are mean ± SEM of three to seven animals. No statistically significant difference ($p > 0.1$) was observed between the control and the group given 0.5 μg of bPTH (7–34) daily. $^*p < 0.1$; $^{**}p < 0.01$; $^{***}p < 0.005$ compared with control. (From Ref. 28, reproduced with permission.)

POTENTIAL DEVELOPMENT OF PTH/PTHrP AGONISTS AND ANTAGONISTS FOR TREATING PSORIASIS AND OTHER SKIN DISORDERS

Based on all of the in vitro and in vivo data, it appears that PTHrP that is produced by the epidermis may have profound effects on skin and hair growth. It is now well recognized that activated vitamin D compounds, which inhibit the proliferation of cultured human keratinocytes, are effective as new therapeutics for treating psoriasis (21). Since PTH/PTHrP agonists have the same antiproliferative activity as 1,25(OH)$_2$D$_3$, it may be possible to develop highly potent PTH/PTHrP agonists that have marked antiproliferative activity and prodifferentiating activity and could be used for treating hyperproliferative skin disorders such as psoriasis, actinic keratoses, and some skin cancers. In addition, they could be developed for decreasing hair growth in unwanted areas and for hirsutism.

If PTHrP is an endogenous antiproliferative factor for the skin, then the ability to block its action in the skin provides an opportunity to regulate skin and hair growth. Therefore, PTH/PTHrP receptor antagonists such as PTH (7–34) could be developed to inhibit the endogenous antiproliferative activity of PTHrP thereby stimulating epidermal proliferation. Thus, PTH/PTHrP antagonists could be developed to help rejuvenate the epidermis damaged by topical steroid use, excessive exposure to sunlight, and aging. They could also be used to help preserve and maintain hair growth.

ACKNOWLEDGMENT

This work was supported in part by National Institutes of Health Grant STTR #CA 71119-01.

REFERENCES

1. Broadus, A.E., Mangin, M., Ikeda, K., Insogna, K.L., Weir, E.C., Burtis, W.J., and Stewart, A.F. (1988). Humoral hypercalcemia of cancer: identification of a novel parathyroid hormone-like peptide. *N. Engl. J. Med.* 319:556–563.
2. Thiede, M., Strewler, G.J., and Nissenson, R.A. (1988). Human renal carcinoma expresses two messages encoding a parathyroid hormone-like peptide: evidence for alternative splicing of a single copy gene. *Proc. Natl. Acad. Sci. U.S.A.* 85:4605–4609.
3. Orloff, J.J., Reddy, D., de Papp, A.E., Yang, K.H., Soifer, N.E., and Stewart, A.F. (1994). Parathyroid hormone–related protein as a prohormone: postranslational processing and receptor interactions. *Endocr. Rev.* 15:40–60.
4. Juppner, H., Abou-Samra, A.-B., Freeman, M., Kong, X.F., and Schipani, E. (1991). A G-protein-linked receptor for PTH and PTHrP. *Science* 254:1024–1026.
5. Urena, P., Kong, X.F., Abou-Samra, A.-B., and Juppner, H. (1993). Parathyroid hormone (PTH)/PTH-related peptide receptor messenger ribonucleic acids are widely distributed in rat tissues. *Endocrinology* 133:617–623.
6. Hayman, J.A., Danks, J.A., Ebeling, P.R., Moseley, J.M., Kemp, B.E., and Martin, T.J. (1989). Expression of parathyroid hormone-related protein in normal skin and in tumours of skin and skin appendages. *J. Pathol.* 158:293–296.
7. Atillasoy, E.J., Burtis, W.J., and Milstone, L.M. (1991). Immunohistochemical localization of parathyroid hormone-related protein (PTHrP) in normal human skin. *J. Invest. Dermatol.* 96:277–280.
8. Burtis, W.J. (1992). Parathyroid hormone-related protein: structure, function, and measurement. *Clin. Chem.* 38:2171–2183.
9. Wu, T.L., Soifer, N.E., Burtis, W.J., Milstone, L.M., and Stewart, A.F. (1991). Glycosylation of parathyroid-related peptide secreted by human epidermal keratinocytes. *J. Clin. Endocrinol. Metab.* 73:1002–1007.
10. Soifer, N.E., Dee, K.E., Insogna, K.L., Burtis, W.J., Matovcik, L.M., Wu, T.L., Milstone, L.M., Broadus, A.E., Philbrick, W.M., and Stewart, A.F. (1992). Parathyroid hormone–related peptide: evidence for secretion of a novel mid-region fragment by three different cell lines in culture. *J. Biol. Chem.* 267:18236–18243.
11. dePapp, A.E., Yang, K.H., Soifer, N., Bellantoni, M., Insogna, K., Burtis, W., Insogna, K., Broadus, A., Philbrick, W., and Stewart, A.F. (1993). Identification of a novel C-terminal secretory form of parathyroid hormone-related protein. Program of the 75th Annual Meeting of The Endocrine Society, Las Vegas, NV, p. 1978.
12. Kemp, B.E., Moseley, J.M., and Rodda, C.P. (1987). Parathyroid hormone–related protein of malignancy: active synthetic fragments. *Science* 238:1568–1570.
13. Horiuchi, N., Caulfield, M.P., and Fisher, J.E. (1987). Similarity of synthetic peptide from human tumor to PTH in vivo and in vitro. *Science* 238:1566–1568.
14. Stewart, A.F., Mangin, M., and Wu, T. (1988). Synthetic human parathyroid hormone–like protein stimulates bone resorption and causes hypercalcemia in rats. *J. Clin. Invest.* 81:596–600.
15. Yates, A.J.P., Gutierrez, G.E., and Smolens, P. (1988). Effects of a synthetic peptide of a parathyroid hormone–related protein on calcium homeostasis, renal tubular calcium reabsorption, and bone metabolism in vivo and in vitro in rodents. *J. Clin. Invest.* 81: 932–938.
16. Thorikay, M., Kramer, S., and Reynolds, F.H. (1989). Synthesis of a gene encoding parathyroid hormone–like protein-(1–141): purification and biological characterization of the expressed protein. *Endocrinology* 124:111–118.
17. Ikeda, K., Weir, E.C., Mangin, M., Dannies, P.S., Kinder, B., Deftos, L.J., Brown, E.M., and Broadus, A.E. (1988). Expression of messenger ribonucleic acids encoding a parathyroid hormone–like peptide in normal human and animal tissues with abnormal expression in human parathyroid adenomas. *Mol. Endocrinol.* 2:1230–1236.
18. Lee, K., Deeds, J.D., and Segre, G.V. (1995). Expression of parathyroid hormone related peptide and its receptor messenger ribronucleic acids during fetal development in rats. *Endocrinology* 136:453–463.
19. Hanafin, N.M., Chen, T.C., Heinrich, G., Segre, G.V., and Holick, M.F. (1995). Cultured human fibroblasts and not cultured human keratinocytes express a PTH/PTHrP receptor mRNA. *J. Invest. Dermatol.* 105: 133–137.
20. Goldring, S.R., Mahaffey, J.E., Rosenblatt, M., Dayer, J.M., Potts, J.T. Jr., and Krane, S. (1979). Parathyroid hormone inhibitors: comparison of biological activity in bone- and skin-derived tissue. *J. Clin. Endocrinol. Metab.* 48:655–659.
21. Holick, M.F., Chen, M.L., Kong, X.F., and Sanan, D.K. (1996). Clinical uses for calciotropic hormones 1,25-dihydroxyvitamin D_3 and parathyroid hormone-related peptide in dermatology: a new perspective. *J. Invest. Dermatol. Symp. Proc.* 1:1–9.
22. Merendino, J.J., Insogna, K.L., Milstone, L.M., Broadus, A.E., and Stewart, A.F. (1986). Cultured human keratinocytes produce a parathyroid hormone-like protein. *Science* 231:388–390.

23. Holick, M.F., Nussbaum, S., and Persons, K.S. (1988). PTH-like humoral hypercalcemia factor (HHF) of malignancy may be an epidermal differentiation factor: synthetic hHHF (1–34)NH_2 inhibits proliferation and induces terminal differentiation of cultured human keratinocytes. *J. Bone Mineral Res.* 3:S214.
24. Henderson, J.E., Kremer, R., Rhim, J.S., and Goltzman, D. (1992). Parathyroid hormone–like peptides increase intracellular calcium and differentiation of keratinocytes. *J. Cell Biol.* 107:73A.
25. Henderson, J.E., Kremer, R., Rhim, J.S., and Goltzman, D. (1992). Identification and functional characterization of adenylate cyclase–linked receptors for parathyroid hormone–like peptides on immortalized human keratinocytes. *Endocrinology* 130:449–457.
26. Kaiser, S.M., Laneuville, P., Bernier, S.M., Rhim, J.S., Kremer, R., and Goltzman, D. (1992). Enhanced growth of a human keratinocyte cell line induced by antisense RNA for parathyroid hormone-related peptide. *J. Biol. Chem.* 267:13623–13628.
27. Wysolmerski, J.J., Broadus, A.E., Zhou, J., Fuchs, E., Milstone, L.M., and Philbrick, W.M. (1994). Overexpression of parathyroid hormone–related protein in the skin of transgenic mice interferes with hair follicle development. *Proc. Natl. Acad. Sci. U.S.A.* 91: 1133–1137.
28. Holick, M.F., Ray, S., Chen, T.C., Tian, X., and Persons, K.S. (1994). A parathyroid hormone antagonist stimulates epidermal proliferation and hair growth in mice. *Proc. Natl. Acad. Sci. U.S.A.* 91:8014–8016.

69

DAB_{389} IL-2: A Lymphocyte-Targeted Fusion Toxin

James G. Krueger
The Rockefeller University, New York, New York

As discussed in another chapter, psoriatic lesional skin is infiltrated with activated, clonal, and proliferative T lymphocytes. Lymphocyte proliferation is regulated, in large part, by the binding of interleukin-2 (IL-2) to cell surface receptors via autocrine mechanisms. Antigen-initiated T-lymphocyte activation (1) stimulates synthesis and secretion of IL-2 in activated cells and (2) induces synthesis of the α subunit of the IL-2 receptor, a protein that increases affinity of this receptor for its ligand. Hence, unactivated T lymphocytes have cell-surface IL-2 receptors composed of β and γ subunits, while activated T lymphocytes have IL-2 receptors composed of α, β, and γ subunits (1). Synthesis of the α IL-2 receptor subunit increases overall receptor affinity for IL-2 by about 10-fold and produces a so-called "high-affinity" receptor complex (K_d for IL-2 approximately 10^{-11} M). The importance of this IL-2 receptor affinity shift is twofold. First, in a mixed population of unactivated and activated T lymphocytes, soluble IL-2 will bind preferentially to receptors on activated cells. Second, pathogenic lymphocyte clones in autoimmune and neoplastic diseases frequently have an activated cell phenotype and express the IL-2 receptor α subunit. Thus, at least theoretically, disease-mediating cells can be selectively targeted through increased receptor affinity for IL-2, which is contingent on expression of the α subunit of this receptor (1,2). Therapeutic strategies designed to exploit high-affinity IL-2 receptors include the use of monoclonal antibodies to the IL-2 receptor α subunit (the CD25 antigen) to block receptor activation or the use of radioactive conjugates with α-subunit antibodies to selectively kill activated cells (1). Another strategy, which is the focus of this chapter, uses an engineered protein or "fusion toxin," which combines IL-2 (as a targeting ligand) with toxic sequences of diphtheria toxin to selectively kill lymphocytes bearing high-affinity IL-2 receptors (2–4).

A number of fusion toxins have been constructed by genetic manipulation of diphtheria toxin (5,6). Figure 1 illustrates the structure of native diphtheria toxin and its modification into DAB_{389} IL-2, a fusion protein that combines IL-2 with a portion of the diphtheria

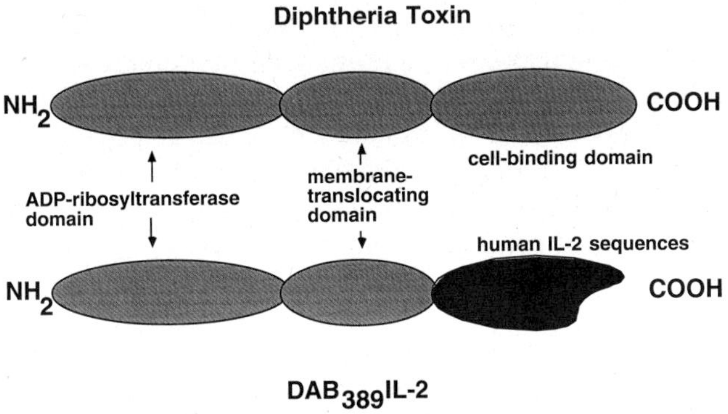

Figure 1 Diphtheria toxin.

toxin polypeptide. Native diphtheria toxin is composed of three functional regions or domains: an amino-terminal domain, which contains the enzymatic activity of this toxin (an ADP ribosyl transferase), a hydrophobic domain in the middle portion, which facilitates membrane translocation of the toxin, and a carboxyterminal cell-binding domain (7,8). DAB_{389} IL-2 is constructed from this native protein by fusion of gene sequences for the amino-terminal 389 amino acids (enzymatic and membrane-translocating domains) to gene sequences for the complete IL-2 protein (6,9) (see Fig. 1). This fusion toxin is thus composed of a single polypeptide chain, which is similar in overall size and structure to the native diphtheria toxin protein, except that it will bind only to cells that have IL-2 receptors on their cell surface (5,10). The DAB_{389} IL-2 fusion protein is a "second generation" construct that improves upon IL-2 receptor binding compared to DAB_{486} IL-2, an earlier fusion protein that contained unneeded amino acids from the native diphtheria toxin protein (2,11). Importantly, the DAB_{389} IL-2 fusion toxin (as well as the earlier DAB_{486} IL-2 version) binds only to certain leukocytes that have IL-2 receptors (T lymphocytes, NK cells, and some dendritic cells). Of these leukocytes, only T lymphocytes strongly up-regulate synthesis of the IL-2 receptor α chain in response to antigenic activation. Hence, activated T cells would then be the primary in vivo target of this fusion toxin.

DAB_{389} IL-2 interacts in a sequential fashion with activated T lymphocytes (Fig. 2). The first step in this interaction is the binding of soluble DAB_{389} IL-2 to high-affinity IL-2 receptors on the surface of activated lymphocytes (4). The second step is endocytosis of the DAB_{389} IL-2 (ligand)-receptor complex, as would normally occur for native IL-2 bound to high-affinity receptors. The third step is acidification of internalized endocytotic vesicles and proteolytic processing of the DAB_{389} IL-2 molecule so that a diphtheria toxin protein fragment is liberated from IL-2 sequences (12,13). The fourth step involves translocation of the diphtheria toxin enzymatic fragment across the membrane of the endocytotic vesicle to the cytoplasm of the T lymphocyte. This toxic fragment, which behaves as an enzyme, becomes active within the cytoplasm to inhibit protein synthesis through ADP ribosylation of EF-2, a ribosome subunit involved in polypeptide elongation (9). This sequence of events is fundamentally the same as native diphtheria toxin, except the entry of DAB_{389} IL-2 into cells is highly restricted by the selective expression of IL-2 receptors on a subset of leukocytes. The toxicity of DAB_{389} IL-2 for nonlymphoid cells is thus restricted through the use of IL-2 as a cellular targeting ligand and by the obligate intracellular activation of DAB_{389} IL-2 following receptor-mediated endocytosis (12). Accordingly, low-affinity cell surface interactions with other cell types would not activate the enzymatic actions of diphtheria toxin domains and thus cytotoxic effects would not occur (11,12). In cells that internalize the DAB_{389} IL-2 fusion toxin, rapid inhibition of protein synthesis is followed by inhibition of cellular proliferation and, eventually, by cell death occurring through apoptosis.

The first clinical application of fusion toxins (DAB_{486} IL-2 and DAB_{389} IL-2) was to lymphoid cancers in which malignant cells expressed the IL-2 receptor α chain (14). DAB_{389} IL-2 shows impressive ability to delay disease onset and to eradicate malignant T-cell clones in a xenogeneic transplantation model (15). In initial human studies conducted with relatively low-dose DAB_{389} IL-2 infusions, about 40% of patients with IL-2-receptor-positive neoplasms showed clear-cut clinical improvement or had remission of disease (9,14). At present, there are ongoing trials with DAB_{389} IL-2 in larger numbers of patients with lymphoid cancers and higher doses of the fusion toxin are being given in some patients. However, the initial studies are quite encouraging as numerous other effective chemotherapeutic agents, when given as single agents, produce disease improvements comparable to DAB_{389} IL-2 in initial malignancy trials.

Autoimmune diseases may be classified as related to humoral or cellular immunity, according to the hypothesized pathogenicity of autoantibodies versus self-reactive T-lymphocyte clones. Several otherwise unrelated human diseases—inflammatory bowel disease, thyroiditis, rheumatoid arthritis, type 1 diabetes, multiple sclerosis, and psoriasis, for example—are characterized by the accumulation of activated T lymphocytes in disease-associated target organs and/or by accumulations of clonal lymphocyte populations selectively in diseased tissues (16–19). It is generally postulated that aberrant T-cell proliferation in these conditions is triggered or sustained by inappropriate recognition of self-peptides, which are presented on MHC class I or class II molecules. Accordingly, the expansion of pathogenic T-lymphocyte clones would be mediated by normal signaling pathways, including up-regulation of IL-2 receptor α-chain protein and increased synthesis of IL-2. These activated lymphocyte clones would bind more DAB_{389} IL-2 (due to high-affinity conversion of the IL-2 receptor) compared to unactivated lymphocytes that are not disease-

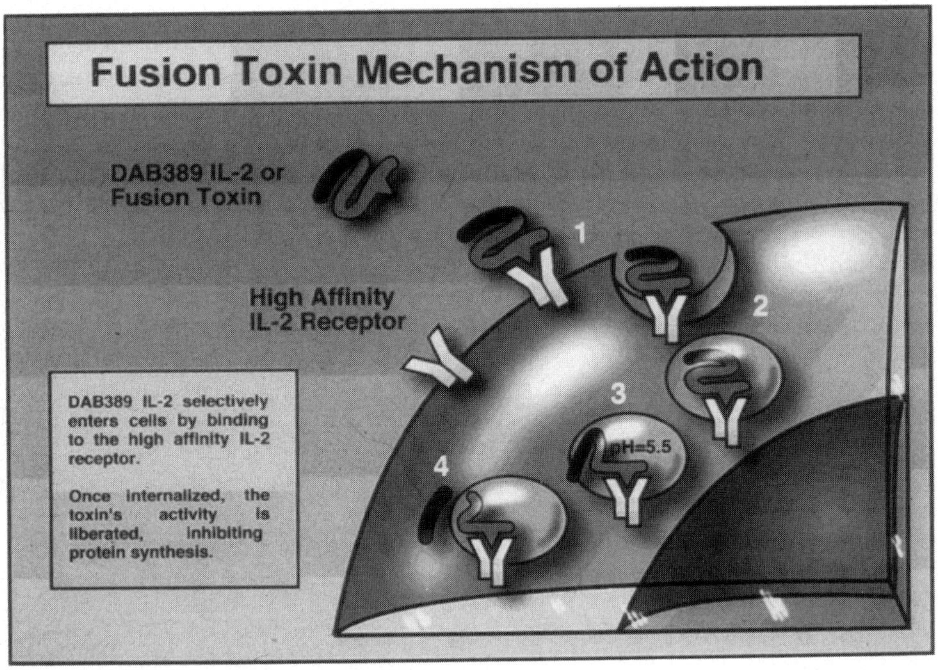

Figure 2 Fusion toxin mechanism of action.

associated. Based on this reasoning, clinical trials have been conducted in patients with rheumatoid arthritis (20) and psoriasis (21) using IL-2-based fusion toxins. The ability of DAB$_{389}$ IL-2 to improve psoriasis has been particularly striking and antipsoriatic actions are considered in more detail below.

A pilot study of the safety and potential efficacy of DAB$_{389}$ IL-2 in psoriasis was conducted in 10 patients with moderate-to-severe psoriasis by our research group (21). Patients received relatively low doses of DAB$_{389}$ IL-2 by intravenous infusion on a monthly schedule in which a 15-min infusion was given daily for 5 consecutive days and outcomes were monitored for a 23-day "rest" period. Each patient received at least two cycles of treatment on this protocol. Treatment outcomes were evaluated by clinical appearance (PASI scoring and photography) and by a series of qualitative and quantitative pathological disease markers. Eight patients showed disease improvements after DAB$_{389}$ IL-2 administration, and in four of these, clinical resolution of some or all psoriatic skin lesions occurred. Figure 3 illustrates the appearance of a psoriatic plaque in one patient before treatment and again after two cycles of treatment with DAB$_{389}$ IL-2. Clinical disease features (erythema, scaling, plaque elevation) disappeared completely following treatment with DAB$_{389}$ IL-2.

Treatment responses were also monitored by extensive histopathological analysis (21). Biopsies from psoriatic plaques before treatment were compared to biopsies obtained from plaque regions after two cycles of treatment (8 weeks after initiation of treatment). Psoriatic tissue was evaluated (1) for infiltrating T-lymphocyte subsets and for the presence of interferon-γ-induced inflammatory proteins in epidermal keratinocytes and (2) for increased epidermal thickness and for keratinocyte proliferation/differentiation abnormalities that distinguish psoriasis lesions from background skin (using markers to distinguish "regenerative" from "homeostatic" epidermal growth/differentiation).

Figure 4 shows photomicrographs of pre/posttreatment biopsies where tissue sections have been reacted with antibodies to identify (1) T lymphocytes infiltrating lesional tissue and (2) synthesis of keratin 16 by epidermal keratinocytes. Compared to dense T-lymphocyte infiltrates observed in lesional skin before treatment, posttreatment biopsies showed a marked depletion of lymphocytes from both the epidermal and dermal compartment. Depletion of intraepidermal T

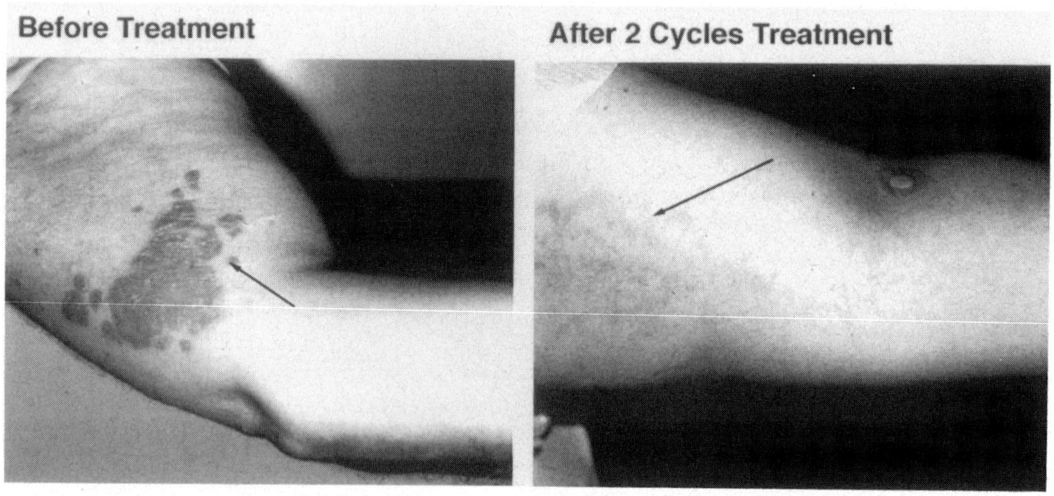

Figure 3 Psoriatic plaque.

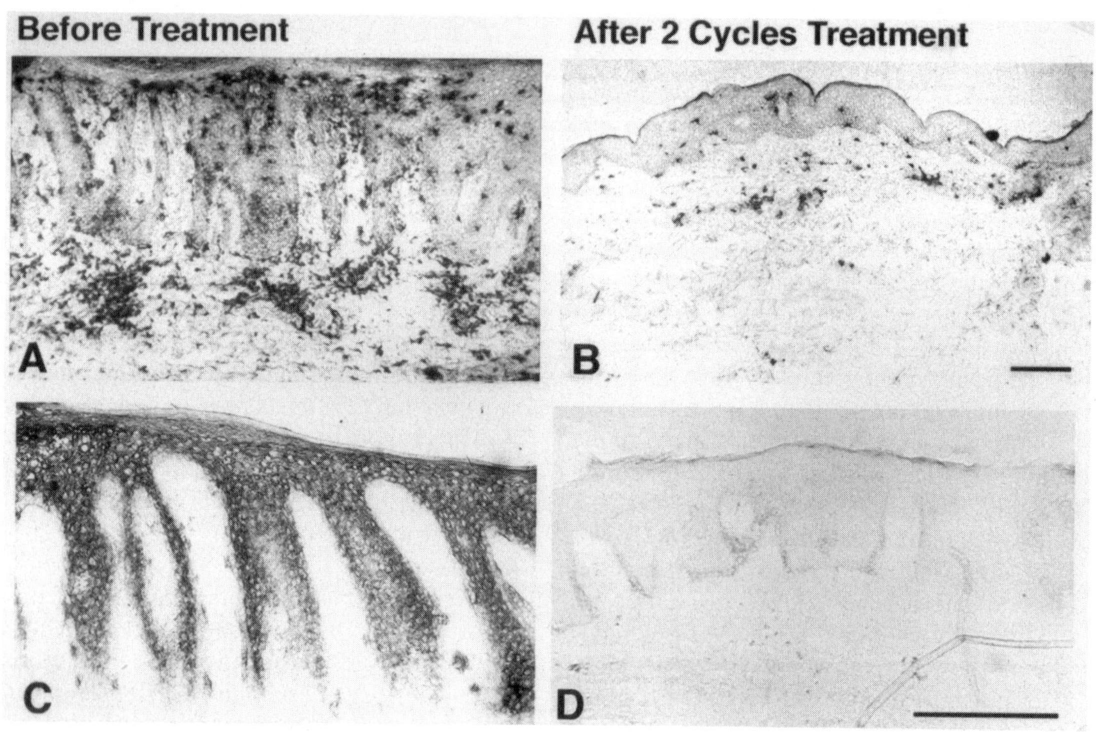

Figure 4 Pre- and posttreatment biopsies.

lymphocytes (which are predominantly CD8+) by DAB_{389} IL-2 was particularly striking and reductions in these cells correlated well with epidermal improvement and overall disease appearance (21). In cases where T lymphocytes were strongly depleted by treatment, a striking improvement in epidermal disease features also occurred. Improvements in the epidermis induced by DAB_{389} IL-2 included epidermal thinning (to nearly normal levels), reduction in psoriasiform patterning, restoration of a granular layer, elimination of parakeratosis, elimination of Munro microabscesses, a reduction in the number of hyperproliferative keratinocytes, and a restoration of the epidermal differentiation program back into the homeostatic mode (21). Figure 4 illustrates the expression of keratin 16 in psoriatic lesional epidermis before treatment and its lack of expression in psoriatic lesional tissue after DAB_{389} IL-2 treatment. The importance of this marker is that it distinguishes epidermal differentiation in the hyperproliferative or "regenerative" mode versus homeostatic growth, in which keratinocytes do not synthesize this keratin (22). With elimination of keratin 16 staining, and with other epidermal differentiation markers studied (21), one can classify the epidermal outcome following DAB_{389} IL-2 treatment as remittive, or eliminating all disease-defining histopathological markers. As DAB_{389} IL-2 showed no intrinsic antikeratinocyte actions in tissue culture systems, one can take these data as primary evidence that activated T lymphocytes induce and/or sustain an epidermal growth state in the alternate or "regenerative" pathway. This suggests that psoriasis is a disease state that is "autoimmune" or one in which the epidermal disease phenotype is dependent on the presence of activated T lymphocytes in lesional tissue.

The results obtained with DAB_{389} IL-2 in psoriasis have important implications for future therapy of psoriasis. First, DAB_{389} IL-2 could prove to be a useful and efficacious drug for the treatment of psoriasis. Of course, additional studies are required to examine its effectiveness in larger numbers of patients, to establish an optimal dosing schedule, and to determine its overall therapeutic index. Second, it appears that clinically effective psoriatic therapy can be achieved by selective targeting of activated T lymphocytes. At present, there are numerous pharmacological or biological approaches available to modulate T-lymphocyte actions and many of these may be applied as potential new therapies for the treatment of psoriasis.

ACKNOWLEDGMENTS

This research was supported in part by a General Clinical Research Center Grant (M01-RR00102) from the National Center for Research Resources at the National Institutes of Health (NIH); by an NIH FIRST Award (CA54215); by NIH Grant GM42461; by an NIH/NIAMS Training Grant (T32 AR07525); by an NIH Small Instrumentation Grant (ISI5-GM45521-01) to The Rockefeller University, by the Carl J. Herzog Foundation, the American Skin Association, and the Carson Family Charitable Trust; and by gifts from Dr. James Murphy and Ms. Sue Weil.

REFERENCES

1. Waldman, T.A. (1993). The IL-2/IL-2 receptor system: a target for rational immune intervention. *Immunol. Today* 14:264–270.
2. Strom, T.B., Kelley, V.R., Woodworth, T.G., and Murphy, J.R. (1992). Interleukin-2 receptor-directed immunosuppressive therapies: antibody- or cytokine-based targeting molecules. *Immun. Rev.* 129:131–163.
3. Derynck, R. (1986). Transforming growth factor-alpha: structure and biological activities. *J. Cell. Biochem.* 32: 293–304.
4. Waters, C.A., Schimke, P.A., Snider, C.E., Itoh, K., Smith, K.A., Nichols, J.C., Strom, T.B., and Murphy, J.R. (1990). Interleukin 2 receptor-targeted cytotoxicity. Receptor binding requirements for entry of a diphtheria toxin-related interleukin 2 fusion protein into cells. *Eur. J. Immunol.* 20:785–791.
5. Williams, D.P., Parker, K., Bacha, P., Bishai, W., Borowski, M., Genbauffe, F., Strom, T.B., and Murphy, J.R. (1987). Diphtheria toxin receptor binding domain substitution with interleukin-2: genetic construction and properties of a diphtheria toxin-related interleukin-2 fusion protein. *Protein Eng.* 1:493–498.
6. Shaw, J.P., Akiyoshi, D.E., Arrigo, D.A., Rhoad, A.E., Sullivan, B., Thomas, J., Genbauffe, F.S., Bacha, P., and Nichols, J.C. (1991). Cytotoxic properties of DAB486EGF and DAB389EGF, epidermal growth factor (EGF) receptor-targeted fusion toxins. *J. Biol. Chem.* 266:21118–21124.
7. Murphy, J.R. (1985). The diphtheria toxin structural gene. *Curr. Topics Microbiol. Immunol.* 118:235–251.
8. Choe, S., Bennett, M.J., Fujii, G., Curmi, P.M.G., Kantardjieff, K.A., Collier, R.J., and Eisenberg, D. (1992). The crystal structure of diphtheria toxin. *Nature* 357: 216–221.

9. vanderSpek, J., Cosenza, L., Woodworth, T., Nichols, J.C., and Murphy, J.R. (1994). Diphtheria toxin-related cytokine fusion proteins: elongation factor 2 as a target for the treatment of neoplastic disease. *Mol. Cell. Biochem.* 138:151–156.
10. Williams, D.P., Snider, C.E., Strom, T.B., and Murphy, J.R. (1994). Structure/function analysis of interleukin-2-toxin (DAB_{486}IL-2). *J. Biol. Chem.* 265:1185–1189.
11. vanderSpek, J.C., Mindell, J.A., Finkelstein, A., and Murphy, J.R. (1993). Structure/function analysis of the transmembrane domain of DAB_{389}-interleukin-2, an interleukin-2 receptor-targeted fusion toxin. *J. Biol. Chem.* 268:12077–12082.
12. Bacha, P., Williams, D.P., Waters, C., Williams, J.M., Murphy, J.R., and Strom, T.B. (1988). Interleukin 2 receptor-targeted cytotoxicity. Interleukin 2 receptor-mediated action of a diphtheria toxin-related interleukin 2 fusion protein. *J. Exp. Med.* 167:612–622.
13. vanderSpek, J., Hemard, A., Dautry-Varsat, A., Boquet, P., and Murphy, J.R. (1994). Epitope tagging of DAB_{389}IL-2: new insights into C-domain delivery to the cytosol of target cells. *Leukemia* 8:S144–S148.
14. LeMaistre, C.F., Meneghetti, C., Rosenblum, M., Reuben, J., Parker, K., Shaw, J., Deisseroth, A., Woodworth, T., and Parkinson, D.R. (1992). Phase I trial of an interleukin-2 (IL-2) fusion toxin (DAB_{486}IL-2) in hematologic malignancies expressing the IL-2 receptor. *Blood* 79:2547–2554.
15. Bacha, P.L., Forte, S.E., McCarthy, D.M., Estis, L., Yamada, G., and Nichols, J.C. (1991). Impact of interleukin-2-receptor-targeted cytotoxins on a unique model of murine interleukin-2-receptor-expressing malignancy. *Int. J. Cancer* 49:96–101.
16. Chang, J.C.C., Smith, L.R., Froning, K.J., Schwabe, B.J., Laxer, J.A., Caralli, L.L., Kurland, H.H., Karasek, M.A., Wilkinson, D.I., Carlo, D.J., and Brostoff, S.W. (1994). CD8+ T cells in psoriatic lesions preferentially use T-cell receptor Vβ3 and/or Vβ13.1 genes. *Proc. Natl. Acad. Sci. U.S.A.* 91:9282–9286.
17. Zouali, M., Kalsi, J., and Isenberg, D. (1993). Autoimmune diseases—at the molecular level. *Immunol. Today* 14:473–476.
18. Carnaud, C., and Bach, J.-F. (1993). Cellular basis of T-cell autoreactivity in autoimmune diseases. *Immunol. Res.* 12:131–148.
19. Davis, M.M., and Buxbaum, J. (Eds.). (1995). *T-Cell Receptor Use in Human Autoimmune Diseases*. New York Academy of Sciences, New York.
20. Strom, T.B., Kelley, V.R., Murphy, J.R., Nichols, J., and Woodworth, T.G. (1993). Interleukin-2 receptor-directed therapies: antibody- or cytokine-based targeting molecules. *Annu. Rev. Med.* 44:343–353.
21. Gottlieb, S.L., Gilleaudeau, P., Johnson, R., Estes, L., Woodworth, T.G., Gottlieb, A.B., and Krueger, J.G. (1995). Response of psoriasis to a lymphocyte-selective toxin (DAB_{389}IL-2) suggests a primary immune, but not keratinocyte, pathogenic basis. *Nature Med.* 1:442–447.
22. Mansbridge, J.N., and Knapp, A.M. (1987). Changes in keratinocyte maturation during wound healing. *J. Invest. Dermatol.* 89:253–263.

70

Surgical Treatment of Psoriasis

Michael H. Gold* **and Henry H. Roenigk, Jr.**
Northwestern University Medical School, Chicago, Illinois

Clinicians are often challenged with recalcitrant plaques of psoriasis which will not respond to conventional antipsoriatic therapy. Applying the theories of the Koebner phenomenon and the reverse Koebner phenomenon, investigators have treated resistant disease with various surgical techniques.

KOEBNER PHENOMENON

The Koebner phenomenon has been reported in a number of cutaneous diseases and is frequent in psoriasis. It is defined as the development of isomorphic cutaneous lesions in uninvolved skin which have been subject to trauma in patients who have the cutaneous disease (1,2). Studies have indicated an incidence of 24–54% of patients with psoriasis have developed psoriatic lesions secondary to a Koebner phenomenon (1–3).

Several types of injury have been shown to produce the Koebner phenomenon. These include irritation, physical injury, surgical wounds, and sunburn. Evidence has accumulated that both epidermal and dermal injury are needed to produce the reaction (3). Stankler (4) used superficial tape-stripping, subepidermal dissection, and full-thickness incisions in areas where both epidermal and dermal injury occurred. The subepidermal dissection spared the basement membrane and did not need to be damaged to evoke a reaction. Only when the dermal injury was accompanied by an epidermal injury, i.e., full-thickness incisions, could the Koebner phenomenon result.

Some investigators consider psoriasis an epidermal disease with lesions produced in part by an increase in epidermal cell turnover. The etiology of the epidermal hyperplasia remains unsolved (1). Others support a dermal component to be crucial, whereas some believe a vascular defect plays a major role. Van Scott and Ebel (5) have postulated that the epidermal hyperplasia occurs via expansion of the germinal cells through upward proliferation of the dermal papillae. Telner and Felske (6) have studied the capillary responses which have been observed in psoriatic lesions, and Braverman and co-workers (7–9) have further studied the microcirculation in psoriasis. They postulate that the epidermal hyperplasia occurs with accompanying vascular proliferation, and that the microvasculature plays a modulatory role in psoriasis.

The reverse Koebner phenomenon has been described as the clearance of a cutaneous lesion which has sustained a significant injury. This has been reported to occur in psoriasis, and is the premise via which surgical techniques have been used to treat recalcitrant psoriatic lesions (2,10–19). Table 1 lists the various surgical modalities which have been used in psoriasis to produce the reverse Koebner phenomenon.

**Current affiliation*: Gold Skin Care Center, Nashville, Tennessee.

Table 1 Surgical Modalities Used to Treat Psoriasis

Sandpaper abrasion
Electrodesiccation
Serial dermatomal shavings
Cryotherapy
Argon laser
Carbon dioxide laser
Dermabrasion

SURGICAL TREATMENTS

In 1972, Olson reported the successful use of abrasion in the treatment of psoriasis. He used fine- and medium-grade sandpaper to abrade chronic psoriatic lesions in 17 patients. Several days of oozing was common, and two patients discontinued therapy because of it. The remaining patients did respond favorably and were pleased with their results. Grekin and Van Scott (11) reported that 9 years following electrodesiccating a patient's initials, "ED," into a large plaque of psoriasis on the left upper arm, the scarred areas remained free of disease. They speculated that by destruction of the dermal papillae via the electrodesiccation technique epidermal hyperplasia over this site was prevented. Van Scott (20) also showed that in patients who suffer from both psoriasis and lineae atrophicans, an elastic tissue disorder in which dermal atrophy results in stretch marks, psoriasis spares areas where the dermal atrophy is present. This also supports a dermal role in producing epidermal hyperplasia.

Dermatomal shavings have been reported a successful method for the surgical treatment of psoriasis. Dellon (12) reported a partial thickness excision of psoriatic skin from the scalp using serial dermatomal shavings to the level of the reticular dermis. The surgical site healed uneventfully and no recurrence was noted in the area at 6 months. Because of this successful result, the patient had the remainder of her scalp lesions treated in a similar fashion. A biopsy specimen at 1 year postsurgery showed a "psoriasis-free scarlike epithelium." At 4.5 years following the procedures the scalp remained free of disease except for three small plaques. Dellon postulated that these areas were not shaved deep enough in the reticular dermis and represented persistent, not recurrent disease. Eyre and Krueger (2) studied involved and uninvolved psoriatic skin and reported results in 18 patients who had either partial or entire plaques removed via superficial dermatomal shavings. The shavings were split-thickness grafts taken as a shave biopsy with a hand-held keratome. In 12 of the patients, the psoriasis was noted to be clear from the area at 1 year follow-up.

Kill and his colleagues (13) reported on 24 patients with plaque-type psoriatic lesions who were treated by serial dermatomal shavings of involved skin. The best results, as with the others who used dermatomal shavings, were found when the shavings were into the level of the reticular dermis. More superficial dermatomal shavings resulted in recurrence of disease activity. Elberg and Brandrup (14) performed dermatomal shavings in 20 patients with chronic, recalcitrant plaque disease. Their shavings were to the level just beneath the superficial dermal vascular plexus; i.e., into the upper reticular dermis. In their study, 6 patients had no recurrence at 1 year, 10 had guttate lesions in the surgically treated areas, and 4 patients had "significant" recurrence. It is felt that the recurrences are related to residual acanthotic epidermis; this was confirmed histologically.

MOHS SURGERY AND SCARS

Fortier and Mikahil (15) reported two patients with widespread psoriasis who presented for Mohs micrographic surgery for basal cell carcinomas superimposed on the psoriasis. Both basal cell carcinomas were successfully removed and the remaining defects were left to heal via secondary intention. The scars which resulted remained free of psoriasis for 8 and 14 years, respectively. In one of the patients reported, an 8-mm full-thickness punch graft of psoriatic skin was transplanted into the surgical scar. The transplanted skin has shown persistent psoriasis; the remainder of the scar has no disease. The authors postulated that the dermis must play an important role in the development of psoriasis because if the Mohs defects healed only via an epidermal source from adjacent skin with psoriasis, scarred areas also should have had psoriasis. By the destruction of the dermal support, a reverse Koebner phenomenon was created and the psoriatic lesions were cleared.

CRYOSURGERY AND LASERS

Harrison and associates (16) used cryotherapy successfully in 7 of 10 patients with psoriasis and 19 patients treated with the argon laser. The response was variable in the cryotherapy group, but none of the laser-treated patients showed signs of recurrence at 1 year follow-up. One year prior, Colver and his colleagues (17) used a Bio-las D helium-neon laser to irradiate psoriatic plaques. This study was an attempt to inhibit angiogenesis; the psoriatic lesions were unaffected. Bekassy and Astedt (18) reported the successful use of the carbon dioxide (CO_2) laser in treating recalcitrant plaque psoriasis in three patients. The laser was used in a defocused mode with a spot size of 2 mm and a power density of 160–200 W/cm^2; this caused vaporization at a depth of about 1 mm. Following the procedure, the skin healed and was reported "similar" to normal skin and has remained psoriasis-free for a 3.5-year follow-up period. They postulated that the CO_2 laser destroyed the microvessels in the lesions, and since a vascular response may be important in the pathogenesis of the epidermal hyperplasia seen in psoriasis, a reverse Koebner phenomenon was elicited.

DERMABRASION

Gold and Roenigk (19) reported a reverse Koebner phenomenon using dermabrasion of very resistant, hypertrophic psoriatic plaques on the lower legs of a 65-year-old patient. The areas treated were dermabraded using a wire brush and a nitrogen-driven dermabrasion machine. The dermabraded sites remained clear 8 weeks postdermabrasion, but then began to show signs of evidence of small plaques of psoriasis. It was speculated that areas which had shown recurrence did not reach the level of the reticular dermis. A residual acanthotic epidermis was found histologically, and this may have prevented a full reverse Koebner phenomenon to occur.

CONCLUSIONS

The successful use of surgical techniques reviewed produced the reverse Koebner phenomenon. As noted in several reports, disease either persisted or recurred if the surgery performed did not reach a precise level of the reticular dermis. Paslin has reported psoriatic lesions on old surgical scars (21) and over cutaneous malignant metastases (22). Histologically, revisions in the dermis were seen; epidermal hyperplasia was not prevented, and the reverse Koebner phenomenon did not occur.

Psoriasis is a chronic papulosquamous disorder with numerous therapies which can be employed in order to control the disease process. Unfortunately, situations do arise where certain plaques will remain recalcitrant to proven antipsoriatic therapy. By applying the principles of the Koebner phenomenon and extending the premise to understand the reverse Koebner phenomenon, surgical techniques can become an aid to the patients with recalcitrant disease. The reports support the notion that dermal support and/or the microvasculature are required to produce psoriasis and if destroyed a reverse Koebner phenomenon results, and the disease can be successfully treated surgically.

REFERENCES

1. Millder, R.A. (1982). The Koebner phenomenon. *Int. J. Dermatol.* 21:192–197.
2. Eyre, R.W., and Krueger, G.G. (1982). Response to injury of skin involved and uninvolved in psoriasis and its relation to disease activity: Koebner and "reverse" Koebner reactions. *Br. J. Dermatol.* 106:153–159.
3. Eyre, R.W., and Krueger, G.G. (1985). The Koebner response in psoriasis. In *Psoriasis*. H. Roenigk and H. Maibach (Eds.). New York, Marcel Dekker, Inc., New York, pp. 105–116.
4. Stankler, L. (1969). An experimental investigation on the site of skin damage including Koebner reaction in psoriasis. *Br. J. Dermatol* 81:534–535.
5. Van Scott, E.J., and Ekel, T.M. (1963). Kinetics of hyperplasia in psoriasis. *Arch. Dermatol.* 88:373–381.
6. Telner, P., and Felske, Z. (1961). The capillary responses in psoriatic skin. *J. Invest. Dermatol.* 36: 225–229.
7. Braverman, I.M., and Yen, A. (1974). Microcirculation in psoriatic skin. *J. Invest. Dermatol.* 62:492–504.
8. Braverman, I.M., and Sibley, J. (1982). Role of the microcirculation in the treatment and pathogenesis of psoriasis. *J. Invest. Dermatol.* 78:12–17.
9. Braverman, I.M. (1985). Microcirculation. In *Psoriasis*. H. Roenigk and H. Maibach (Eds.). Marcel Dekker, Inc., New York, pp. 287–298.
10. Olson, E.S. (1972). Abrasive treatment of psoriasis. *Arch. Dermatol.* 105:292–293.
11. Grekin, D.A., and Van Scott, E.J. (1973). Dermal role and controls in psoriasis. *Arch. Dermatol.* 108:425.
12. Dellon, A.L. (1982). Long-term remission of psoriasis after dermatome shaving. *Plast. Reconstruct. Surg.* 70: 220–229.
13. Kill, J., et al. (1985). Surgical treatment of psoriasis. *Lancet* 2:16–18.
14. Elberg, J.J., and Brandrup, F. (1987). Dermatome shaving of psoriasis. *Br. J. Dermatol.* 117:745–750.

15. Fortier, L.J., and Mikhail, G.R. (1986). Psoriasis: disease of epidermis on dermis? *J. Dermatol. Surg. Oncol.* 12:480–482.
16. Harrison, P.V., et al. (1985). Trauma for psoriasis. *Lancet* 2:1063–1064.
17. Colver, G.B., Cherry, G.W., and Ryan, T.J. (1984). Lasers, psoriasis and the public. *Br. J. Dermatol.* 111: 243–244.
18. Bekassy, Z., and Astedt, B. (1986). Carbon dioxide laser vaporization of plaque psoriasis. *Br. J. Dermatol.* 114:489–492.
19. Gold, M.H., and Roenigk, H.H. (1987). Surgical treatment of psoriasis: a review including a case report of dermabrasion of hypertrophic psoriatic plaques. *J. Dermatol. Surg. Oncol.* 13:1326–1331.
20. Van Scott, E.J. (1972). Tissue compartments of the skin lesions of psoriasis. *J. Invest. Dermatol.* 59: 4–6.
21. Paslin, D.A. (1973). Psoriasis on scars. *Arch. Dermatol.* 108:665–666.
22. Paslin, D.A., and Spraque, E.A. (1975). Psoriasis on tumor. *Arch. Dermatol.* 111:622–624.

Part IX

PATIENT INVOLVEMENT IN PSORIASIS

71

Nursing for Psoriasis

Joan L. Shelk
Leone Dermatology Center, Arlington Heights, Illinois

Caring for the psoriasis patient is a multifaceted role; however, the primary nursing responsibility for the psoriatic is quality patient education. The opportunities to implement this responsibility are as endless as the disease itself. The educational process begins by obtaining information that offers an understanding of the individual's background, both personal and medical. This background aids both medical and nursing staff to formulate an appropriate treatment plan. Without ample information, the end result may fall short of its potential. The responsibility continues with the dispensing of information that helps the patient understand and cope with the disease.

AREAS OF PATIENT EDUCATION

Areas of patient education include:

- Primary skin care
- Medications—use and abuse
- Phototherapy basics
- Treatment options
- Realistic expectations and limitations of outcomes
- Treatment policies

Too often lack of time or resources has left the psoriasis patient to fend for himself. An investment in trained and caring staff reaps benefits far beyond the initial or ongoing outlay.

Very little attention is given to the integumentary system in nursing programs. In the majority of instances, training regarding psoriasis is received in a hands-on format, often from another staff member who has not had any formal training. For this reason, some of nursing for the psoriatic is science but a significant part is the art that develops over a period of time from listening to mentors, seeking training experiences, observing patient reactions, and pure instinct.

Intake Interview

When a psoriatic is seen in a practice, the success or failure of the ensuing relationship often depends on the intake interview. As in many areas of life, the first impression is very meaningful. The interviewer must make the patient comfortable. Without an adequate level of comfort, important information may not be forthcoming. The information gathering is the all-important act of collecting clues that will enable both practitioner and staff to understand not only the physical aspects of the patient's disease, but also the overall effect of any previous treatment and any emotional impact upon the patient.

The staff is gathering information for immediate needs, but also for future reference. Too often an interview begins and ends with only patient demographics. A great depth of knowledge is needed to provide successful therapeutic outcomes. The obvious first area of concern is the reason for the visit. Whatever the patient states as the assumed diagnosis, one must keep an open mind until the physician has completed the examination, as psoriasis has often been previously misdiagnosed. Throughout the interview, the staff should be on the alert for information volunteered or observed that is not part of the routine process. The initial interview needs to be both a receiving and giving of information.

INFORMATION NEEDED FROM AN INTAKE INTERVIEW

Presenting Complaint

Patients should be questioned about the initial onset of the disease, any precipitating factors such as streptococcal infection, and the treatment history. This history should include the type of treatment, frequency of use, length of use, and success rate. One should be wary of statements of failure of a particular treatment. Many treatments are judged a failure when in fact there was a failure to administer the therapies properly. This is generally the result when unrealistically conservative caps are placed on the use of medications or phototherapy doses.

Medical History

An overview of the patient's medical background provides valuable information that can impact on the current disease. For instance, a previous history of persistent polymorphous light reactions will make consideration of phototherapy an undesirable treatment option.

Questions should also be asked concerning family medical history. Areas of discussion should include the patient's presenting disease as well as history of skin cancers and of photodermatoses. A family history of a photodermatosis such as lupus may negate the utilization of phototherapy in the treatment program. Photodermatoses include:

Systemic lupus erythematosus
Chronic herpes
Xeroderma pigmentosum
Polymorphous light eruption
Persistent light reaction
Solar urticaria
Actinic reticuloid

Discussion of the family unit should include how it impacts on the patient's disease. Are they a positive support system? Do they provide stress? Are they knowledgeable about the disease and how it affects the patient's physical and emotional well-being?

Allergies

Investigating allergies or sensitivities is germane to any medical history. Psoriasis therapies often now include the use of antibiotics, as well as many other medications; therefore, allergy history is of paramount importance. Many patients have sensitivities to tar products or various ingredients contained in the vehicles of topical preparations. Avoiding these ingredients will avoid adding insult to injury.

Current Medications

A complete list of medications used by the patient for all reasons is advisable. Obviously one needs to know current and past preparations that were part of previous psoriasis therapies and their overall effect on the disease. The implications of other medications are also important. Are any of the current medications aggravators of psoriasis, such as beta-blockers or lithium? Are any potential photosensitizers? Groups of drugs that may cause photosensitivity are acne medications, anticancer drugs, antidepressants, antihistamines, antimicrobials, antipsychotic drugs, diuretics, and hypoglycemics. The word *potential* must be emphasized as all of the aforementioned medications will cause a sensitivity in only a limited number of patients.

Phototherapy shuld be adjusted when these drugs are involved, rather than discontinued. A booklet entitled *Medications that Increase Sensitivity to Light* is available.*

Keeping track of potential photosensitizers can be made easier by the creation of a Rolodex system. Each medication, along with any additional pertinent information, can be placed on an individual card. As new drugs need to be added, it is easy to add new cards. This is a much more efficient system than having to continually update a list of medications.

Medications are not the only potential photosensitizers. Adverse reactions can be caused by ingredients in certain foods and cosmetics. There are several reports of lime juice and ultraviolet light combining to cause blisters on the hands. Liberal use of colognes and perfumed lotions on the body prior to phototherapy has also led to severe erythema.

*It can be obtained from the Department of Health and Human Services, Public Health Service, HFZ-114, Food and Drug Administration, Rockville, Maryland 20857.

Life-Style

Social and cultural factors should be a significant part of information gathering. A person's life-style and occupation may influence compliance with a particular treatment regimen. Traveling will limit access to phototherapy and utilization of topical medications. Employment out-of-doors may make phototherapy somewhat complex. Students will be influenced by classroom experiences, particularly in the locker room and physical education setting.

Language barriers are an ever-increasing concern for practitioners. If the patient cannot understand directions or report factors necessary for complete treatment assessment, treatment management may become complex. Many facilities now require an interpreter for patients unable to communicate on their own.

Ethnic background may be a strong influence in the success of any treatment program because certain tasks or treatments are not acceptable. The ability to perform a complete examination may be restricted owing to unwillingness of a person to be examined, particularly by someone of the opposite gender.

Life-style questions should include the impact that psoriasis has on the patient's daily living. Useful questions include: Do you experience discrimination? Do you feel restricted by your feelings toward yourself? How would you describe yourself? Are you able to maintain a positive self-image? A patient was overheard stating, "When you have psoriasis, you always feel ugly and you never feel clean."

Skin Type

Skin typing seems simple; however, it is not always understood that various areas of the body have different skin types. Most phototherapy dosing is based on the patient's skin type; therefore, it is essential that it be calculated accurately, based on examination of an *unexposed* body surface (Table 1).

Nursing Assessment

Any observations on the part of the interviewer can be very helpful to the physician. All objective observations should be reported. Difficulty with speech, gait, or comprehension as well as unusual mannerisms need to be documented. Conditions not related to the patient's psoriasis may have an influence on his or her ability to function and to manage the disease. Many nurses have noted that objective observations have been helpful not only in the ultimate treatment of psoriasis, but other significant medical conditions have been noted and treated as well.

EXAMINATION

The nurse should set up the patient to facilitate a complete skin examination. The most frequently heard patient complaint is "The physician never even looks at me." On the other hand, many patients are so embarrassed and ashamed of their skin condition that they do not want even a physician to see them undressed. Nursing staff can be instrumental in helping raise the patient's comfort level. All areas of the body need to be checked for psoriasis because it may be evident in areas of which the patient is unaware such as the scalp. There are other benefits from a complete examination. Skin cancers or other skin disorders can be identified and treated. Explaining that a periodic skin check is an investment in overall good health may reassure the patient.

POST EXAMINATION

Once the examination is complete, the diagnosis made or confirmed, and a treatment plan selected, the staff's responsibility for patient education begins.

General Skin Care

Too often patients expect the selected treatment to perform miracles. They need to know that treatment will be expedited if they are compliant with a soaking and debridement routine. Heavy psoriatic scale impedes the penetration of medications and ultraviolet light. Debridement should not be vigorous. A multistep approach is advisable. What is not done easily today is best left to tomorrow. Tabs of skin should not be pulled off, they should be clipped. The best time to apply emollients and/or medication is after bathing. Moist skin requires less medication, facilitates easier application, and is absorbed more readily. Beneficial moisture is also sealed in the skin. The use of bland emollients prior to phototherapy is also recommended. This allows better penetration of ultraviolet rays.

Medications Instructions

How, why, when, and where to apply medications should be part of any instruction regarding medications. A brief explanation of the steroid classes is needed before a patient will accept that all corticoster-

Table 1 Skin Typing

Skin type	Skin reactions	Examples
1	Always burns easily and severely (painful burn); tans little or not at all and peels	People with fair skin; blue or even brown eyes; freckles; unexposed skin is white
2	Usually burns easily and severely (painful burn); tans minimally or lightly, also peels	People with fair skin; red blond or brown hair; blue hazel or brown eyes; unexposed skin is white
3	Burns moderately; tans about average	Average Caucasian; unexposed skin is white
	Burns minimally; tans easily and above average with each exposure: exhibits IPD reaction	People with white or light brown skin; dark eyes; unexposed skin is white or light brown
5	Rarely burns, tans easily and substantially; always exhibits IPD reaction	Brown-skinned persons; unexposed skin is brown
6	Never burns and tans profusely; exhibits IPD reaction	Blacks; unexposed skin is black

IPD = immediate pigment darkening.

oids are not the same. Where not to use medications should be included in any discussion of where they should be applied. When an excellent result is achieved with a class I steroid on resistant psoriasis, patients need to know that this medication is not an appropriate choice for their face or intertrigonous areas just because it was successful elsewhere.

Patients should be advised to apply all topical preparations in a downward stroke to reduce the possibility of inducing folliculitis.

If patients are not taught the proper use of their medications, they will not have good therapeutic results and they will run the risk of skin-damaging side effects including atrophy, purpura, and striae. Poor results are caused by underuse of topical medications. Damaging steroid side effects are the result of misuse of strong steroids and overuse of topical corticosteroids in general.

Phototherapy Education

When phototherapy is recommended as part of the treatment plan, patients need to understand that it is a commitment to a program of many weeks or months of therapy and not an instant miracle.

UVB usually will be administered three to five times weekly and topical preparations are customarily a part of the treatment. Many patients are unaware of this and it has to be reinforced.

PUVA usually will be administered two to three times weekly and topical preparations are optional and often omitted. The avoidance of topicals is one of the reasons patients are enthusiastic about this regimen. Perhaps the most important facet of education for the patient regarding PUVA is that it is a marriage of two elements, a chemical photosensitizer (psoralen) and long-wave ultraviolet light. One without the other is not PUVA. Even though this has been emphasized, there are reported cases of patients taking the oral medication on nontreatment days or those who have continued to come for their light sessions but have discontinued the medication, usually because of nausea.

Staff members are customarily responsible for advising the patient about pretreatment requirements. Before the patient is started on PUVA, an ophthalmological examination is required as a baseline, as well as certain blood studies. The exact studies vary from practice to practice, with a chemistry, complete blood count, and antinuclear antibody being the most routinely requested.

If an informed consent is required as a facility policy, it should be explained and signed by the physician and then reviewed again by staff who will then witness the patient's signature. The consent form will inform the patient of the risks and benefits of the designated treatment. If a consent form is not recommended by the practice, the risks and benefits should be part of the physician/patient interaction and so documented. Two copies should be signed. One copy should be placed in the patient's permanent record and the other can be given to the patient for reference.

Methotrexate or retinoids are often introduced in difficult cases of psoriasis. These are administered either independently or in combination with UBV or PUVA. Regular laboratory studies are customarily required for the management of these medications. Overseeing patient compliance with the policies of these programs is a staff responsibility. This will enable a practice to maintain prudent management of these effective, sophisticated medications.

ADDITIONAL EDUCATION

Options

Explanation of all therapies should include a discussion of treatment options, limitations of treatment, and realistic expectations.

Patients may be aware of another person who has tried a particular therapy with good results and they will request that regimen be prescribed for themselves. They must be made aware that the level of treatment selected for them must be appropriate for the level of need demonstrated by the extent and severity of their disease. The fact that not every patient can have complete clearing or a long-term remission is hard for the patient to accept. Staff can help the patient focus on accepting something less than perfection as a goal. They can discuss the options available should the current plan not bring remarkable results. This may prevent discouragement.

Levels of treatment are outlined in Table 2.

Photographs are helpful in establishing a baseline of disease activity. They should also be taken periodically to document treatment response and ultimate progress. Patients who are discouraged with what they perceive as lack of progress with their treatment are often amazed to see how much improvement they have made when they review their photographs.

Aggravating Factors

Very few patients are aware that psoriasis is aggravated by several factors including:

- Streptococal infection
- Medications (i.e., beta-blockers, lithium, prednisone)
- Excessive intake of alcoholic beverages
- Abrasion
- Stress
- Overexposure to ultraviolet light

Once patients are taught to avoid the stress factors, the progress of their treatment program may be greatly enhanced.

Table 2 Levels of Treatment

Level	Extent of involvement	Treatment
I	Minimal	Topicals and/or emollients only
II	Moderate	Topicals and/or emollients only UVB phototherapy
III	Extensive	PUVA only PUVA augmented by topicals Day treatment
IV	Resistant	PUVA with extra UVA to resistant areas PUVA with UVB Retinoids (with or without UVL) Methotrexate (with or without UVL) Day treatment Sulfasalazine
V	Severe	Day treatment Hospitalization (with or without methotrexate or retinoids) Cyclosporin Experimental drug programs Climatotherapy

Financial Considerations

In many practices, particularly those without business offices, the task of discussing the financing of treatment falls to the nursing staff. When patients are appraised of the cost of treatment before it is initiated, they seem to process the impact more successfully. In addition, it often is necessary to intervene on behalf of the patient with insurance carriers. Great detail to proper procedure coding will smooth the path for reimbursement. Staff need to become coding experts.

PHOTOTHERAPY

Training

Phototherapy training is available via the Dermatology Nurses' Association and the National Psoriasis Foundation; however, the majority of persons administering phototherapy have been trained by a co-worker. Unfortunately, much misinformation is included with appropriate information. The American Academy of Dermatology and the Dermatology Nurses' Association have guidelines for phototherapy that need to be the basis for any phototherapy program.

Administration and Supervision

Phototherapy should be administered by staff who are under the supervision of a dermatologist familiar with photomedicine. Patients must never be in a position of administering their own treatments.

Policies should be established that are clear-cut and enforceable regarding shielding and appointment compliance for both phototherapy and physician examination.

Prior to each session, patients should be evaluated for suitability for therapy. They should be questioned about the addition, deletion, or change in any medications in order to evaluate any impact on phototherapy. New medications should be checked for potential photosensitization.

The pretreatment evaluation should include general wellness, erythema, response to therapy, appropriate skin type treatment protocol, and the elapsed time since the last treatment.

ERYTHEMA RESPONSE

Erythema response is graded as follows:

Grade 0 No erythema
Grade 1 Minimally perceptible erythema—slightly pink
Grade 2 Marked (red) erythema without edema
Grade 3 Fiery (red) erythema with edema
Grade 4 Fiery (red) erythema with edema and/or blistering

Response to therapy is outlined in Table 3.

Administrators of phototherapy must be knowledgeable about treatment protocols and the operation of the equipment. They must always utilize a backup timer and be present to ensure the safe entry into and exit from phototherapy equipment. Often patients are placed into units and then the staff is required to perform duties elsewhere within the building. This is not an advisable or acceptable practice.

After treatment has been completed and before the patient leaves the facility, staff must be prepared to address any issues raised during the treatment session. If the patient has complained of erythema, pruritus, or nausea, a management protocol should be available.

Table 3 Response to Therapy

Grade	Criteria	% improvement compared to original extent of disease
−1	Psoriasis worse	0
0	No change	0
1	Minimal improvement; slightly less scale and/or erythema	5–20
2	Definite improvement; partial flattening of all plaques; less scaling and less erythema	20–50
3	Considerable improvement; nearly complete flattening of all plaques but borders of plaques still palpable	50–95
4	Clearing; complete flattening of plaques including borders; plaques may be outlined by pigmentation	95

Staff Issues

Not all staff responsibilities involve direct patient contact. How a treatment area and its equipment are maintained make a bold statement as to how the staff feel about themselves, their profession, and their patients. A clean environment and efficient equipment is essential to a successful practice.

Because psoriasis is chronic, capricious, and complex, it takes a certain type of individual to staff a unit treating this disease. The staff need to be committed, caring, and empathetic because patients not only need medical intervention, they need emotional support.

CONCLUSION

Interviewing patients and pushing the buttons on phototherapy equipment is only the beginning of nursing for the psoriatic patient.

Areas of nursing responsibility should include:

Patient education
Patient assessment
Phototherapy administration and supervision
Patient resource and support system
Treatment implementation and management
Unit maintenance

In general, when working with psoriasis patients, nurses and technicians must be able to build a sense of trust and confidence. Without it, patients become discouraged and failure often is the result. The goal of all psoriasis care should be to provide safe and effective therapy—not one without the other.

72

Using Art Therapy in the Treatment of Psoriasis: A Pilot Study*

Ruth S. Lewis
School of the Art Institute of Chicago, Chicago, Illinois

Approximately six million people in the United States have psoriasis. It is a skin disease that produces stigmatizing, chronic, recurrent lesions that often become emotionally and physically debilitating to the patient. It is an expensive disease and frequently requires lifelong treatment (Roenigk, 1977). Psoriasis is a common and recurring condition in which the skin develops red patches of various sizes, covered with dry, silvery scales. Though psoriasis is one of the oldest skin conditions known to mankind and was even around in biblical times, its cause is still unknown.

There is knowledge about its development. The epidermis, or outer layer of skin, is constantly manufacturing new cells and shedding old ones. In psoriasis, it is thought that some defect of the enzymes of the skin alters this process. Normally, the development of new cells, which grow out from the lower basal layer toward the skin surface, takes about 28 days. In psoriasis, this process is speeded up to 4 or 5 days. Instead of shedding inconspicuously, the outer cells form scales that remain heaped up on the skin.

> My torture is skin deep: there is no pain, not even itching; we lepers [psoriatics] live a long time, and are ironically healthy in other respects. . . . The name of the disease . . . is Humiliation.
>
> —John Updike

The onset of psoriasis can be traumatic. It is not necessarily the visibility or extensiveness of psoriasis that determines how a person is affected. A small patch of psoriasis may be more disturbing to one individual than extensive lesions are to another. The visibility of the lesions may affect occupational choice and professional activities. Marriage may be deferred or avoided, sexual activities may be impaired, and choice of clothing may be restricted. Complications may include development of a negative self-image with possible social separation. Preoccupation with physical appearance, treatment regimes, the anticipated reactions of others, and the construction of defense mechanisms to cope with anxieties may consume an inordinate amount of energy.

"The heartbreak of psoriasis" is not an advertising agency's empty, glib statement to encourage consumers to purchase one more remedy for psoriasis. There is no cure, and the most one can expect is a temporary remission. This remission can last from weeks to years, but eventually, the person knows that the psoriasis will return. I have had psoriasis for most of my adult life, and unless there is an enormous breakthrough in the medical treatment of psoriasis, I know I have to live with this condition forever.

*A thesis submitted in partial fulfillment of the requirements for the degree of Master of Arts in Art Therapy.

Much emphasis has been placed on the medical aspects of treatment, with little or no attention paid to the emotional problems concomitant with psoriasis. Having a good self-image is difficult when faced with a disfiguring condition. Fellow sufferers try to hide their condition from the world, and have no help in coming to terms with psoriasis either alone or with a supportive community.

Art therapy has the possibility of accessing those hidden inner feelings. I propose to access those feelings with art therapy, seeing patients of the clinic on an individual basis. If this therapeutic tool can be used successfully, it could be the beginning of an adjunctive treatment modality, alongside the various medical treatments now available. From my search of the literature, this has never been done with psoriasis patients.

LITERATURE REVIEW

> I cannot pass a reflecting surface on the street without glancing in, in hopes that I have somehow changed. Nature and the self . . . are each cloven in two by an ambivalent, fascinated attention. One hates one's abnormal, erupting skin but is led into a brooding, solicitous attention toward it. One hates the Nature that has imposed this affliction, but only this same Nature can be appealed to for erasure, for cure. Only Nature can forgive psoriasis; the sufferer in his self-contempt does not grant to other people this power.
>
> —John Updike

Psychological Views of Psoriasis

Approximately six million people in the United States have psoriasis. Psoriasis vulgaris is a scaling skin disease that classically produces stigmatizing, chronic, recurrent lesions that often become emotionally and physically debilitating. In addition, psoriasis is an expensive disease and frequently requires lifelong treatment.

Although the course of psoriasis is variable, trauma, obesity, alcoholism, emotional stress, infections, and drugs (indomethacin, beta blockers) are known to cause exacerbations. The tendency of the unaffected skin of psoriatics to develop lesions after injury may account for the localization of lesions to sites of repeated trauma. For treatment of psoriasis, the psychological approach must be stressed. Many psoriatics, even those with disease of long duration, do not understand the natural course of psoriasis and the many factors that may precipitate it. By spending a little time in instructing these patients in the basic pathophysiology of psoriasis, the attending physician can obtain a high degree of cooperation. This is essential for successful management of psoriasis (Roenigk, 1977).

McEvoy and Roenigk (1991) said that in biblical times, people were ostracized because of skin disease: "The one who bears the sore of leprosy shall keep his garments rent and his head bare, and shall muffle his bears; he shall cry out 'Unclean, unclean!' " (Lev. 13: 45–46). Ignorance and fear of contracting a skin disease led to the isolation of people with various skin conditions in leper colonies. Although we no longer isolate people with psoriasis, fear and ignorance persist and have an impact on the daily life of these individuals. Many feel isolated by their disease and become self-conscious and withdrawn. These reactions may lead to depression and, rarely, suicide. Fortunately, most patients with psoriasis compensate well, learning to live with and control their disease.

Dermatological disease has a strong impact on a patient's psyche because of its visibility. People infrequently die from skin disease; more importantly, they must live with their disease. Of all illness, skin disease most affects the psyche—it is what the world sees. Skin disease can be a great handicap in work and social settings. Many studies on the psychological aspects of psoriasis are subjective and are difficult to interpret objectively.

Patients with psoriasis also suffer the same range of psychiatric disorders as the general population. The use of lithium may precipitate or exacerbate psoriasis. Lithium-induced psoriasis is often resistant to conventional antipsoriatic therapy and may necessitate stopping use of the drug.

Studies on the relationship between stress and psoriasis are often at variance. Stress, in the broad sense, includes both emotional and physical stress. By elimination of these precipitating factors, longer remissions may be induced.

Covert alcoholism may be a problem among hospitalized patients with psoriasis and may contribute to an exacerbation of psoriasis either directly or indirectly through neglect.

Education of patients, their families, and the community will help to reduce feelings of isolation and stigmatization (McEvoy and Roenigk, 1991).

Psychosocial factors are important in the onset and/or exacerbation of psoriasis in 40–80% of cases. Yet psoriasis has received little attention in the recent psychiatric literature. A subgroup of psoriatics appear to be "stress reactors" and these patients may have a better long-term prognosis. Identification of such patients early in the course of treatment and incorporation of specific psychosocial interventions in their overall treatment regimen may improve the course of illness. The disturbances in body image perception and the effect of psoriasis on interpersonal, social, and occupational functioning can further contribute to the overall morbidity, especially if psoriasis first occurs during a developmentally critical period like adolescence (Gupta-Madhulika et al., 1987).

Disfigurement occurring during adolescence has been reported to have a great impact on body image in later life. This may be especially important in psoriasis, where 58% of patients develop psoriasis before age 30 years, 35% before age 20 years, and 10% before age 10 years. Presence of lesions on exposed body parts and increased severity have both been reported to adversely affect the patient's body image.

Psoriasis has been reported to affect sexual functioning in 72% of cases. When psoriasis is present in the "emotionally charged" areas of the body, such as the genital area, sexual functioning is more affected. Trauma to the genitals following sexual activity can result in new psoriatic lesions or an exacerbation of previous lesions as a result of the Koebner phenomenon, the appearance of new psoriatic lesions at sites of trauma. The fear of passing on psoriasis to the offspring and myths about the possibility of contagion may also lead to significant sexual problems. Marriage may be deferred as a result of these concerns.

Psoriasis has been associated with contagion, filth, and leprosy for centuries. The presence of psoriasis in areas of high visibility such as the face and hands can impair social and occupational functioning to a significant degree. Patients may be discriminated against in public places such as beaches and hotels and in hairdressing salons. They frequently give up swimming, sunbathing, and activities that necessitate exposure of their skin to others. Light-colored clothing may be chosen to cover the affected regions of the skin and camouflage the scales that are shed. Patients may develop a pervasive preoccupation with the anticipated negative response of others and, while dealing with these day-to-day problems, may experience a sense of losing control when faced with an unexpected exacerbation of their illness. "[B]rief hospitalization aimed at removing the patient from a stressful environment may lead to significant improvement of psoriasis in some cases" (Gupta et al., 1987).

Ginsburg and Link (1989) found that many people with moderate to severe psoriasis do feel stigmatized in specific ways, but others do not. On exploratory factor analysis, the 33 items formed six clusters, which permitted the identification of these facets of the experience of stigma: anticipation of rejection, feelings of being flawed (which include items relating to weakness and uncleanness), sensitivity to the opinions of others, guilt and shame, positive attitudes, and secretiveness. "We had not anticipated that 'positive attitudes' would be one factor; however, this cluster was present in an instrument designed to elicit other kinds of feelings. Clearly, feeling stigmatized by psoriasis is not a universal or monolithic experience" (Ginsberg and Link, 1989).

Different predictors emerged for the different dimensions of the stigma experience despite relatively high correlations among the latter. Thus, being older was a mitigating force for some aspects of stigma but not for others. Perhaps it should not be too surprising that the impact of a chronic, disfiguring disease that intrudes not only into the sufferer's daily routines and relationships but also into the most profound reaches of the sense of self might well be extremely complex.

Being older at the onset of psoriasis protects people against anticipating rejection, feeling sensitive to the opinions of others, feelings of guilt and shame, and secretiveness. Perhaps older persons, tending to have a more settled life-style and more extensive life experience, have a firmer sense of their own individuality, which mitigates the impact of the disease. Longer duration of illness is associated with less guilt and shame and less secretiveness.

Clearly these findings attest to the extreme vulnerability of those who experience an early onset of psoriasis and who would feel more shame and guilt, anticipate rejection more profoundly, and be more exquisitely sensitive to the opinions of others. A child or adolescent growing up with psoriasis has to come to terms with the psoriasis with regard to self-image, self-esteem, and relationships with others, as well as aspirations for the future. Perhaps younger patients, and even older patients whose illness started when they were young, might benefit from such interventions as group therapy or short-term individual therapy that focuses on their experience with psoriasis.

Actual experience of rejection that persons with psoriasis often report is a strong predictor of sensitivity to the opinions of others, which comprises an intensely experienced vulnerability but does not act as a predictor for anticipation of rejection, which elicits feelings about more external social experiences. Also, being rejected tends to leave the person with psoriasis feeling less positive about himself.

Being employed, a variable one might think would expose people to more actual experiences of rejection, is in fact associated with less anticipation of rejection, less guilt and shame, and less sensitivity to others' opinions when rejection experiences are controlled. Perhaps as the person with psoriasis works with colleagues in a positive context on a daily basis, self-esteem is likely to be high, thus diminishing a feeling of vulnerability. An alternative view, however, might be that some of those who are unemployed might have been unable to work because their psoriasis was disabling on a physical or emotional basis.

Secretiveness is an important component of the daily experience of the person with psoriasis, who may tend to wear concealing clothing and avoid situations where the lesions will be disclosed. It entails controlling the experience of psoriasis by hiding it. The fact that hospitalized patients are less secretive may be related to their being in an environment where all the patients have skin ailments and the regimen is totally focused on psoriasis. Also, family, co-workers, and insurance companies are more specifically aware of the disease and the patient's attempt to control it. As already noted, older age of onset, as well as longer duration, is related to less secretiveness. It is noteworthy, however, that whereas patients with parents or siblings afflicted with psoriasis tend to be less secretive, those who have a child with psoriasis are more secretive. It may be that in the first instance psoriasis is viewed as a family matter and a shared concern that is associated with such matters as help with treatment and willingness to discuss psoriasis. Greater secretiveness by a parent with psoriasis who has a child with psoriasis may relate to problems with identification and feelings of having borne a flawed offspring. There is a possibility of parental rejection because the onset usually occurs after parental bonding is completed.

Although bleeding is not a notable aspect of psoriasis, bleeding is a dismaying symptom in any ailment, and in psoriasis it is part of the experience of the disease mainly through patients' behavior toward their disease. Bleeding in psoriasis is strongly related to feelings of being flawed, as well as predicting sensitivity and guilt and shame. It is also strongly related to the despair associated with psoriasis; it is here that the experience of stigmatization may have enormous impact on treatment and perhaps even affect the course of the disease (Epstein, 1984).

The skin has long been acknowledged as an organ of emotion expression. Dungey and Buselmeier (1982) said that psoriatics can recall instances of blushing, sweating, or goose bumps, and of hearing such expressions as "getting under my skin," "thick-skinned," "makes my hair stand on end," "rubs me the wrong way," or "wouldn't want to be in his skin." There is no doubt that the feelings and moods of an individual can be related to the appearance of his or her skin, although sometimes inaccurately. An individual responds to and develops attitudes toward others based on their appearance.

Helping professionals and family members tend to withdraw both emotionally and physically from those afflicted with psoriasis. Similarly, psoriatic patients experience feelings of disgust and anger at their own body. Because psoriatics are generally healthy, the cosmetic disfigurement and uncleanliness of excessive scales perhaps weigh most heavily on their physiological and social adjustment.

The age of onset of psoriasis can determine the severity of psychological and social implications. Infantile eczema has been used as a model for analyzing the effects of skin disease on psychosocial development.

Family members are directly affected by the psoriatic's disease, but they may be misinformed about the disease and its causes. Parents may blame themselves because of the hereditary tendency, and siblings may fear that they too might develop psoriasis. Because the psoriatic is a constant reminder of this tendency, parents may resent him or her and react toward the condition in various detrimental ways. Family members may consciously or unconsciously shame the psoriatic as they try to cope with the psoriatic flaking and the greasy or tarry medications, which are usually odiferous and stain clothing and furniture.

The disruption of psychological development may occur as a result of skin disease in the various developmental periods leading to adulthood. Because adolescence in itself is a developmental period of highly charged emotions, it can present an even greater crisis to the young person who has or contracts psoriasis during this period. During adolescence, which is characterized by the influence of peers on an adolescent's sole behavior and definition of self, the adolescent with psoriasis may experience disturbances in his or her emotional well-being, family life, self-esteem, and social life. Because of the somewhat controllable nature of psoriasis, the adolescent may manifest the paradoxical behavior of overzealous regimentation or the imposition of self-destructive treatments. The adolescent may also use the disease as an excuse for social withdrawal.

The onset of psoriasis in adulthood can also be traumatic. It is not necessarily the visibility or extensiveness of psoriasis that determines how the adult may be affected. A small patch of psoriasis may be more disturbing to one individual than extensive psoriatic lesions are to another. For some, the visibility of the disease affects occupational choice and professional activities. Marriage may be deferred or avoided, sexual activities may be impaired, and choice of clothing may be restricted. The cost of various treatments and the lost income from work-related absenteeism may impose financial difficulties. Furthermore, the development of a negative self-image with possible social separation by oneself and others may be an additional psychosocial complication of the disease.

Preoccupation with physical appearance, treatment regimens, the anticipated reactions of others, and the construction of defense mechanisms to cope with anxiety may consume an individual's energies, which might otherwise be used to develop more positive aspects of the personality.

For those also afflicted with psoriatic arthritis, mobility may be impaired. Also significant are the perceived loss of control as well as hope for a cure and the interruption of previously made plans as a result of flare-ups. Daily living is affected by some of the treatment regimens that may require regular applications of tar and appointments for ultraviolet therapy.

Because there is no "cure" for the disease, psoriatics know that remission is perhaps only temporary. Knowledge that stress or illness might induce recurrence can be a constant concern and threat to their self-image. Thus, even during remission, psoriatics may benefit from supportive social work intervention. Although the lesions may appear minor or may even be in complete remission, and although psoriatics are generally physically healthy and often physically capable of accomplishing the basic routines of daily living, social workers should not dismiss the concerns, complaints, and coping difficulties of psoriatics (Dungey and Buselmeier, 1982).

> I feel my heart beginning to cramp. It hurt me so, I cover it with my hand. I think I might as well be under the table, for all they care. I hate the way I look. Before I know it, tears meet under my chin.
>
> —Alice Walker, *The Color Purple*, 1982

Body Image

Larose (1988) said that the mental pictures we hold of ourselves tend to externalize and affect our relationships and life experiences. As humans we grow up accruing an image of ourselves based on feedback from relevant others. We live out our self-images often without questioning their present suitability to our lives and goals.

We tend to treat people of certain physical attributes and psychological temperaments in certain ways. Thus a person's self-image is sculpted by his interactions with others. Our desires, conflicts, compensations, and social attitudes are somatically entrenched and influence self-projection through drawing the human figure as well as through ways of relating to others and the environment.

The creative process can serve as a means for going beyond the blockages of a learned self-image. In tapping the source of creativity, one can simultaneously become in touch with the true self and at least briefly have an expanded idea of what is potential.

Larose continues to say that a process of selection involving identification through projection and introjection enters at some point. The individual must draw consciously upon his whole system of psychic values. The body is the most intimate point of reference in any activity. We have in the course of growth come to associate various sensations, perceptions, and emotions with certain body organs. This investment in body organs or the perception of the body image as it has developed out of personal experience must somehow guide the individual who is drawing in the specific structure and content that constitutes his offering of a "person." Consequently, the drawing of a person in involving a projection of the body image provides a natural vehicle for the expression of one's body needs and conflicts.

Body image can be defined as the mental picture of one's own body painted by both conscious and unconscious attitudes toward one's body. These thoughts and feelings are developed through social experience and kinesthetic feedback.

Body image is known to become better integrated when self-esteem is enhanced and enhanced self-esteem is known to improve body image.

The distortions seen in schizophrenic children's art are exaggerations of distortions that occur in the fantasies and dreams of normals. It appears that body image disturbances occur along the psychological continuum from normal through severely disturbed states.

Play therapy and projective art therapy have been shown to be helpful in body image remediation work with latency-age children. Every symbol refers simultaneously to the body and to the outside. Every creative art expression is, in part, a projection of current and remembered body images and ego states. The use of figure drawing is an index of body image integration (Lincoln, 1987).

In the development of both body image and self-representations, a person's relationships are of great importance. These representations are formed through the assimilation of and comparison to representations of others.

To examine the relationships between self, interpersonal relationships, and body image two repertory grids were used to compare dysmorphophobic, psoriatic, and control subjects.

The correlation between body image and ideal body image was significantly higher for the control group than for the other two groups. The dysmorphophobics and psoriatics, therefore, were less satisfied with their body image than were the controls.

The relationships between body image and self-concept differed between the groups. The psoriasis group had a significantly lower correlation between body image and self than the controls.

The psoriatics and controls were significantly different in rating their body image. The psoriatics scored their body image as tougher. There were no other significant differences between the groups except between the dysmorphophobics and controls when rating their relationships. The controls scored their relationships as more gentle.

The dysmorphophobics and psoriatics rated their body image as significantly more sexually unattractive than did the controls (Hardy, 1982).

Body image and self-image are interrelated. Thus, it is not surprising that low self-esteem and a sense of ineffectiveness are commonly encountered in these patients. Therefore, treatment that focuses on improving body image should also result in improved self-concept and higher self-esteem.

Body image is "the picture of our own body which we form in our mind, that is to say the way in which our body appears to ourselves." Body image is the mental image or composite of body images people have of the physical appearance of their bodies. To this definition has been added the notion of the body as a psychological experience of the attitudes and feelings of individuals toward their bodies. Body image includes "the correctness or error in cognitive awareness of the bodily self, the accuracy in recognizing stimuli coming from without or within, the sense of control over one's own bodily functions, the affective reaction to the reality of the bodily configuration, and one's rating of the desirability of one's body by others." One's body image is crucial in the development of one's self-concept, and, in addition, body images are the "mental blueprints for the organization of our social behavior" contributing to the formation of our object relations.

Definitions of body image have incorporated perceptual, cognitive, affective, and interpersonal dimensions. Whereas this points to the lack of agreement on a clear and precise definition of body image, it points as well to the need for a multimodal therapeutic approach to disorders for which body image disturbance is significant.

Body image is developed partially in response to our perception of the relationship to the body that significant others hold (Kaslow and Eicher, 1988).

Body image can be defined as the mental picture of one's own body painted by both conscious and unconscious attitudes toward one's body. These thoughts and feelings are developed through social experience and kinesthetic feedback.

Body image is known to become better integrated when self-esteem is enhanced and enhanced self-esteem is known to improve body image.

Normally, body schema are constantly changing as a person shifts positions or passes from one state of alertness to another. Our mental pictures of ourselves change when we sit up or go to sleep. In states of ego disorganization, a variety of specific body image distortions are seen such as feelings of bodily deterioration, including feelings of invasion by alien material. It appears that body image disturbances occur along the psychological continuum from normal through severely disturbed states.

Play therapy and projective art therapy have been shown to be helpful in body image remediation work with latency-age children. Every symbol refers simultaneously to the body and to the outside. Every creative art expression is, in part, a projection of current and remembered body images and ego states. The use of figure drawing is an index of body image integration (Lincoln, 1987).

We tend to treat people of certain physical attributes and psychological temperaments in certain ways. Thus, a person's self-image is sculpted by his interactions with others. Our desires, conflicts, compensations, and social attitudes are somatically entrenched and influence self-production through drawing the human figure as well as through ways of relating to others and the environment.

The creative process can serve as a means for going beyond the blockages of a learned self-image. In tapping the source of creativity one can simultaneously become in touch with the true self and at least briefly have an expanded idea of what is potential.

A process of selection involving identification through projection and introjection enters at some point. The individual must draw consciously upon his whole system of psychic values. The body is the most intimate point of reference in any activity. We have in the course of growth come to associate various sensations, perceptions, and emotions with certain body organs. This investment in body organs or the perception of the body image as it has developed out of personal experience must somehow guide the individual who is drawing in the specific structure and content that constitutes his offering of a "person." Consequently, the drawing of a person in involving a projection of the body image provides a natural vehicle for the expression of one's body needs and conflicts (Larose, 1988).

Perhaps most significant in dealing with psoriatic patients is helping them adjust to their changed self- and body image. Because of the disease's obvious nature, the psoriatic may have a heightened mental and emotional awareness of the self.

The emotional task of the patient who has experienced an assault to self-image is adjustment to a new body image in which the loss or substitution of a part or function of the body is integrated into his individuality and self-esteem. If this does not occur during the recovery process, the self is perceived as mutilated in a world of nonmutilated, whole-bodied people. While replacement or regrowth of the physical part is unachieveable, the self-perception of wholeness based on the physiological incorporation of the loss is possible, a process analogous to, but more complicated than, the grieving process associated with the loss of a beloved person (Dungey and Buselmeier, 1982).

SETTING AND POPULATION

This was a pilot study on the feasibility of using art therapy as an adjunctive therapy for persons suffering from psoriasis.

The setting was the dermatology outpatient clinic of an urban major medical center. The complex included a medical school, so in addition to the dermatologists, there were always available residents in dermatology and medical students. The staff also consisted of nurses and technicians, all familiar with and knowledgeable about psoriasis.

The population using this clinic were adults with a variety of dermatological problems, with psoriasis being the major problem. The clinic was visited by hundreds of patients weekly with varying degrees of severity of psoriasis. The clinic was comprised of a series of consulting and treatment rooms. One of these rooms was offered to me for my use at each session. The sessions were private and confidential. Treatment for psoriasis consisted primarily of the use of light (ultraviolet A or B, UVA or UVB). Sometimes this light treatment was supplemented with topical and oral medications.

All patients were informed of this study and volunteers were requested. Space in the clinic was made available to me so that there would be no hardship (in travel) for the patients to avail themselves of the pilot study.

I was one of those patients. I could therefore empathize with everyone I met at the clinic and could communicate a great deal of understanding to those persons willing to become a part of this study.

METHODOLOGY

The subjects were seated at a desk in an office given to me for use in this project. They were first given a consent form to sign, and then I briefly explained the process of art therapy. The patients were then given a questionnaire to fill out. We briefly discussed the responses so that I was sure I understood what had been written.

Art supplies were placed on the table: Cray-pas, pastels, markers, pencils, watercolor pencils, watercolors, and crayons. The patients were asked to choose one or more of these materials and were given two sheets of paper. Then the task was described to them. The first task was to draw a picture of an animal, vegetable, or mineral that had psoriasis, and what it would be like if the animal, vegetable, or mineral had psoriasis. If there were questions about this, I answered as briefly as possible. When the patients indicated completion, I asked them to describe what they had done, to get a clear indication of their imagery. Then the second task was described to them.

Using, if they wished, just colors or shapes, they were to draw how it feels to have psoriasis. When completion was indicated, we talked about the images in both drawings. I limited our discussion to the amount of material the patient seemed comfortable discussing. Because this is a pilot study, I did not want to probe too deeply.

The sessions lasted from 0.5 to 2 hr. The length of time depended on how much the patient was willing to share with me and the length of time used to draw the image.

All sessions were audiotaped with the permission of the patients.

I had originally thought that I would receive an enthusiastic response, and the first few weeks after startup seemed to bear that out. However, responses were not forthcoming, and some persons with whom I had made appointments cancelled or did not show up. I began to hear remarks such as "I can't draw, not even stick figures," or "I don't want you to analyze me," or "I'm not an artist, I wouldn't fit in," or "I'm too busy." I therefore decided that in addition to the brief meeting that I had, I would meet with one patient over a period of several weeks to elicit more information and more art work. I also decided to draw my own two pictures. I felt, as a psoriatic, I had to know how the people felt, as well as expressing myself for my own benefit as a member of this group of fellow sufferers.

> Psoriatics should be given the opportunity to ventilate their feelings of fear, despair, anger, and the like, and appropriate channels for their expression as well as constructive coping mechanisms should be explored. Encouraging expressions of grief over their changed physical appearance may promote faster and more complete resolution of a new self-image. And the maintenance of previous social relationships should be encouraged (Dungey and Buselmeier, 1982).

CASE STUDIES

> Each drawing, it seemed, had some story or character behind it, some playacting that was crucial to its making. The result, Layton began to realize, was something like exorcism. Drawing was cathartic. She had noticed that her depression seemed to be withering, her grief over her son abating. Contour drawing is a wonderful way to get rid of anger or whatever you want to get rid of, she told Lambert. It's even one way to escape depression.
>
> —Lambert, 1984

Case Study 1

"E," a married woman, has had psoriasis for 15 years. She has two married children. Initially, she said she has accepted her psoriasis because of the diligence of the treatment, was diagnosed early, and was told it was treatable. But as the interview continued, she said, "I never say the word 'psoriasis'; I just say I have a skin problem when people ask." She travels into the Loop area, 1 h travel time from the suburb in which she lives, because she does not want to see a doctor in her own area.

Friends wonder why she does this, but she will not tell them. She is always looking around to see if others have noticed her skin, the psoriasis being on her elbows and legs. She has a swimming pool in her backyard and wears slacks there if others are around. She never wears shorts.

Her first drawing (Fig. 1) was a drooping, tiny flower, surrounded by other strong flowers, and the words "Why me?" The drawing was a direct contradiction of her words of denial only moments before.

Her second drawing (Fig. 2) was, she said, just a glob of color. Then she added she was trying to see which colors looked good with one another. She thought that there was too much green, and wondered if it was significant that green is not a primary color. When finished, she thought it looked like a boat, and said she enjoyed boating and was made happy through recreation. The shapes she drew seemed to be a metaphor for the scales of psoriasis. "No," she said, "I'm a square person, and everything goes together."

Case Study 2

"M" is a 72-year-old married man. He has had psoriasis for at least 10 years, starting about the time of divorce from his first wife. He has been retired for about 17 years. He had worked in real estate, and then at a succession of jobs including computer programming. After his "retirement" he took on various jobs, such as a security guard, bartender, starter at a golf course, and short-order cook. He has four grown children whom he sees on an irregular basis. He has remarried and celebrated his first anniversary recently.

When asked to draw an animal, vegetable, or mineral, he drew a rock with spots (Fig. 3). Why? "Because rocks are easy to do." It seemed a facile answer to a facile drawing, yet it did describe this man. Tall, of solid build, and seemingly at ease with himself and the world, he seemed secure and rock-like.

He said that he will talk to anyone about his psoriasis—family, friends, co-workers, acquaintances. Initially he said he did not cover his psoriasis except for the obvious, meaning it is primarily on his hands and feet, and shoes and stockings cover his feet.

He said that he has had the condition long enough so that he is not embarrassed. His first outbreak caused him to be admitted to an intensive care unit because it had spread all over his body. It finally cleared except for his hands and feet. He worked as a short-order cook and his boss asked him to wear gloves. He finally quit because people did not want food prepared by a person with "terrible things" on his hands.

He seems to have handled the problem of psoriasis very well. Yet, the rock is very small, and the figure in the bed is even smaller (Fig. 4). The words "Why me?" tell a story different than his presentation as self-assured.

Case Study 3

"W," a 25-year-old single woman, had a severe outbreak of psoriasis 9 years ago, but has actually had psoriasis since she was a baby. Her parents went to Mexico, leaving her in the care of her grandmother. When her parents returned, they discovered she had psoriasis in her scalp and she has had it ever since with the usual remissions and outbreaks. She said it is now getting worse. It is primarily on the trunk of her body, so clothing covers most of it, but she is getting tired of explaining it. Making explanations is difficult, but she guesses she always will be explaining. She has a wonderful boyfriend now who does not mind her condition.

She is a 1987 graduate of Indiana University and has worked in an advertising agency with personnel seeking directing jobs in television. She is now in a career transition. She has a brother 2 years younger than she and a sister 5 years younger. Neither has psoriasis.

Figure 1

Figure 2

Figure 3

Figure 4

Figure 5

Figure 6

Figure 7

Figure 8

Figure 9

She drew a forlorn-looking cheetah with spots. "The cheetah is unhappy, with closed eyes so that she can't see the spots" (Fig. 5).

The second drawing was a trunk with spots, covered with other colors so that the spots could not be seen, and then covered with black (Fig. 6).

He drawings were light in color and seemingly tentative.

Despite her initial statement that she has great difficulty discussing her condition, she was quite forthcoming in the session, discussing her situation freely. She said she felt relieved and somewhat unburdened by the end of the session.

Case Study 4

"L" is a 72-year-old woman, married for 51 years. Her husband is a professional artist; she has two married sons and three grandchildren.

In answer to my questionnaire, she said she has had psoriasis for 30 years and can talk about it only to her family and her doctor. She covers her psoriasis with clothing, i.e., slacks, her lesions being primarily on her legs.

She used to visit friends at their condo, with a community swimming pool. People there asked rude questions such as "Do you wear slippers, I hope?" or "Do you cover your chair when you sit down?" Her friends, she said, were more embarrassed than she was, so after a while she did not go back to the pool.

She began her drawing, saying, "I've got to be a cat. Cats are well taken care of."

After drawing a while, she said:

> This looks more like a dog—a Schnauzer. Well, he's a very unhappy dog (Fig. 7). I have been very unhappy. Without psoriasis, I may have been a happier, calmer person. I have trouble sleeping. I get up and scratch and bleed. Then I have to change the sheets. I get very upset at myself; it makes me nervous, very nervous.
>
> When I'm watching television my husband says to me, stop scratching. It makes me nervous and I start scratching again. It's very hard on my family. My husband feels sorry for me.

Asked to draw the second picture, she said:

> I'd like to use blue and yellow, they're nice, bright colors, but I don't feel nice and bright. Right now I'd like purple and black because that's the way I feel. They are sad colors. I feel very sad. My psoriasis is worse than it has ever been. My personality has changed. I find very few things fun. After 27 years in one place, we moved recently and there have been so many complications that I'm extremely unhappy.

I went back to the drawings and asked about the second. She said it was just a scribble with confusion and sad colors (Fig. 8).

I asked her to look again at the dog, and she exclaimed, "Why, there is only one tit!" She looked at the picture and then said:

> I worry about my sister-in-law. She has a tumor in one breast. I'm angry with her because she's running to doctors. I've had nightmares about what she's doing to herself. I worry about myself and feel sad. I feel better when I visit my sons and their families. They live in the East and we take Elder Hostel trips near them to be able to visit them. The trips are restful, and I don't go near the swimming pools. I think this has all been hardest on my husband.

Case Study 5

"G," a 73-year-old woman, was accompanied by her daughter to translate, since "G's" English is limited, and by her 18-year-old granddaughter. Both grandmother and granddaughter have psoriasis. "G" came to this country with her husband in 1977 from Iran. She worked for the Board of Education in Iran, and her husband was a policeman in that country. They had to leave because his life was in danger. They have five children—three boys and two girls. They had hoped to return to Iran, but they have no choice but to stay here. Her psoriasis began shortly after her arrival in this country. There is a subject, she says, that when she remembers it, her psoriasis gets worse. She would not discuss it. She has had psoriasis in her scalp, legs, and body, and because clothing has covered those areas, she has had no need to cover up. At times, she has had severe itching and bleeding. A pill she takes for itching has reduced the discomfort somewhat.

Her first picture (Fig. 9) was a bird, drawn, she said, because she likes birds. It is a small bird, with superimposed red spots, just like her, she said.

Her second picture (Fig. 10) was a small series of colors, black at the top, because she was very upset at being diagnosed as having psoriasis.

The next level was gray. She was beginning to adjust to it.

The bottom layer, yellow, represents the fact she is getting much better. She thinks she has gotten rid of it.

She has great confidence that she will be clear forever. She said when we finished that she would have liked another session.

Case Study 6

"S," the granddaughter of "G," is an 18-year-old, finishing high school this year, and has a 16-year-old sister who does not have psoriasis. She has had psoriasis for 12 years. She and her parents left Iran and spent some time in France before coming to this country in 1983. They were reunited with the entire family at that time. At first her psoriasis was limited to just a few spots, but has been increasing in intensity.

She had to swim at school for 6 weeks and hated it. She said it "wasn't good" and strangers made remarks.

She could not bear to wear shorts at a day camp where she worked. The parents of other campers would come up to her and make remarks, not good remarks, she added.

She does not want to do much about her psoriasis. It comes and goes. She said it feels good when it goes away, but "very crummy" when it returns. She would feel better if she could keep it all covered. She has a few friends with whom she can share her condition, but it makes her feel bad.

Her first drawing (Fig. 11) was small and portrayed a carrot—"It's my favorite vegetable." The black surrounding it is the psoriasis.

The second picture (Fig. 12) was also small. The inner black shows the negative aspect when the psoriasis was bad. White denotes when she got better. The purple shows that it began getting worse again, and the black shows it is back again to when it started; in fact, even worse now. It must be difficult for her to know at 18 years that she will have it all her life—her grandmother is a living example of the course her life will take, but her grandmother has more hope for herself than the granddaughter. That hope seems small when the size of the drawings is noted. I interviewed them at the same time so that it would be interesting to see if I were ever to meet with them again, separately, if their drawings would be similar in size and use of color.

Figure 10

Figure 11

Figure 12

Figure 13

Figure 14

Figure 15

Figure 16

Figure 17

Figure 18

Case Study 7

First Session

"D," a 63-year-old woman, filled out the questionnaire quickly, talking as she worked. She wrote that she had had psoriasis since 1975. She said that stress does bring it on, primarily on her legs, arms, and face. She said it slowly improves with light treatment. She uses dark glasses and makeup to cover her face, and rarely goes out in the evening because "it is odd to see someone wearing dark glasses in the evening." She loved to dance and misses it very much. She has a rough time in the summer because she used to wear shorts all the time, but now does not. She says that now she can talk about her psoriasis to whoever will listen, but that has happened only recently, and only because the treatments have somewhat reduced the severity of the psoriasis, but she still "has to be careful" of the clothing and makeup she wears. She pulled up her slacks to show me the condition of her legs (and I showed her mine). She has cut down the treatments from 3 days to 2 days, because she is exhausted.

She lives in a retirement home and has discussed the psoriasis with the director of the home, who has been encouraging her to wear seasonally appropriate clothing, i.e., shorts in summer. "D" says she cannot wear them yet. "Maybe someday."

She then was given materials for her drawings. I explained the tasks to her and she began immediately choosing felt tip markers and pencils for the first drawing—a large skunk drawn with the felt tip marker, and other figures and the trees with pencils. The following is her discussion of the drawing.

"This is a skunk—with the back to us, so that it can't see the other animals trying to get away (Fig. 13). Even the snake doesn't want to be near the skunk. The trees are healthy but the skunk can't get to them."

After a long pause, and very wistfully, she said, "But the skunk is a beautiful animal."

The skunk is very large, in comparison to the other animals, almost as though there is a spotlight on it, making it the focus of attention, and although the animals are turned away from it, there is still an awareness of the skunk.

The tail, while drawn in skunk-like colors, also seems to indicate, by the black lines, a thick skin covering, which is indeed what psoriasis looks like—a reddened thickening of the skin.

Given the second task, she thought for a short time, and again using felt tip markers, she began by saying, "This is going to be a maze." She worked carefully, beginning at one end of the paper, and gradually working up to the top. She took a very long time with this drawing, meticulously filling in each section, before going on to the next section. When finished, she said, "This is not a maze. In a maze, there is a way out. There is no way out of this. Down at the bottom it's not good, but the white up here is hope" (Fig. 14).

She gazed at both her drawings for a few moments, and then said, "I feel so relaxed. If you asked me to stand on my head, I would." And then, "I wish we could do this again."

The bottom of the drawing is indeed thick and the sections are next to each other, with no white spaces, but as one moves upward there are more white spaces, and some of the sections are thinner and lighter and brighter. It does seem to be a metaphor of the skin with its decreasing areas of psoriasis with treatment. I am sure that her statement "There is no way out" refers to the fact that there is no cure for psoriasis, only possible clearing and/or remission, but future flare-ups are an eventuality.

All of the statements made by "D" were spontaneous, with no prompting from me. She seemed very comfortable with me, and worked diligently on her drawings. Her affect was sad, yet there was a toughness of spirit that seemed to say, "I have problems, but that is what life is about."

In the second drawing I asked her to describe the various sections, and their significance.

The session took 2 hr and could easily have gone on for another 2 hr. This is a woman who has faced many problems in life, has solved some, but many remain unresolved. The question of facing society has been difficult for her. She has a sense of shame that is deeply rooted. Her skin has cleared somewhat, but in her eyes, the condition is as severe as ever, and she knows it will always be there.

Subsequently, I asked her if she would be interested in continuing the sessions several more times. She agreed to this with enthusiasm.

Second Session

At the second session, she gave me more information about herself. She has been a widow for 22 years with three children, two boys and one girl. There are six grandchildren, "three to each."

She worked as a cashier, then did clerical work, maintaining a one-woman office. She taught crafts and designed decorations for holiday tables. She invented tools to work with some of the materials, and holds two patents. Shortly before her husband died, her patterns for decorations were to be included in a crafts

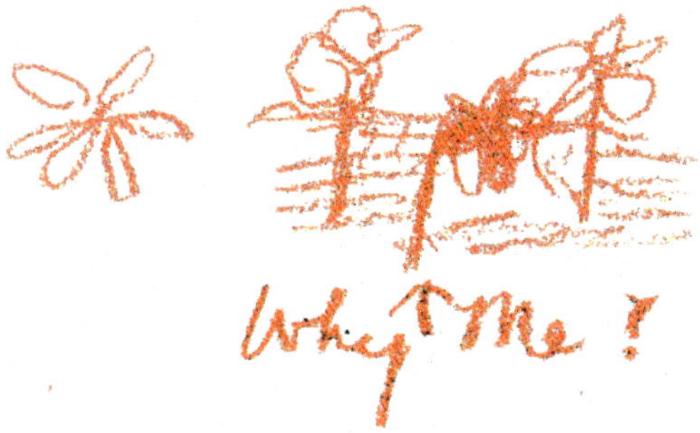

Figure 1.

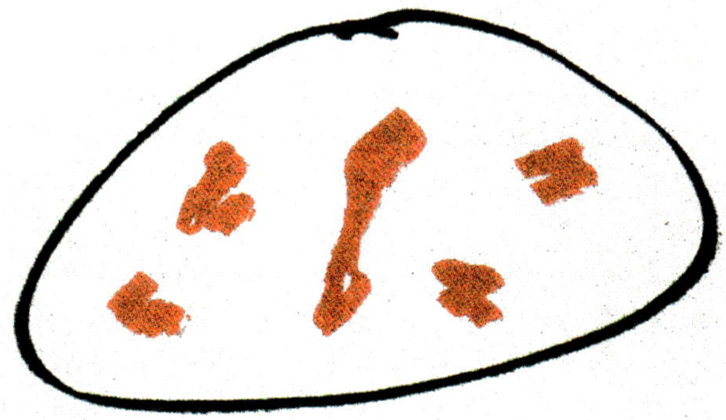

Figure 3.

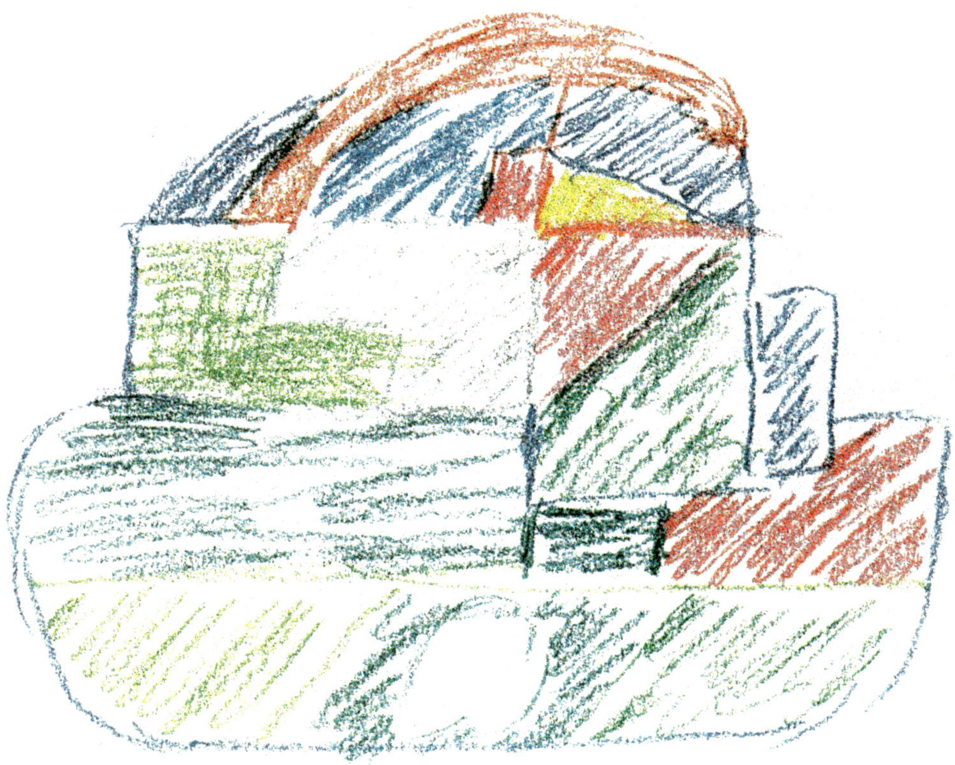

Figure 2.

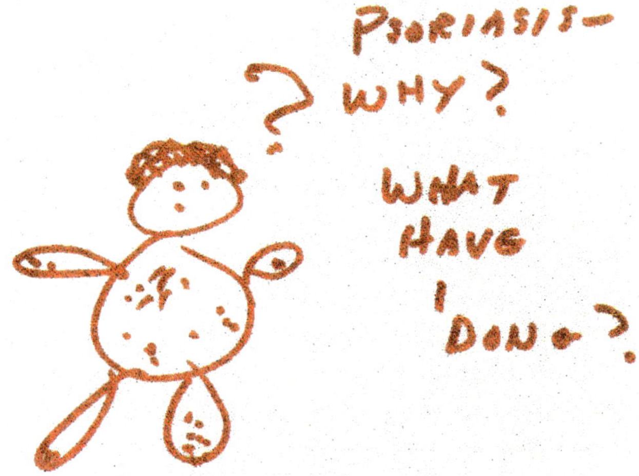

Figure 4.

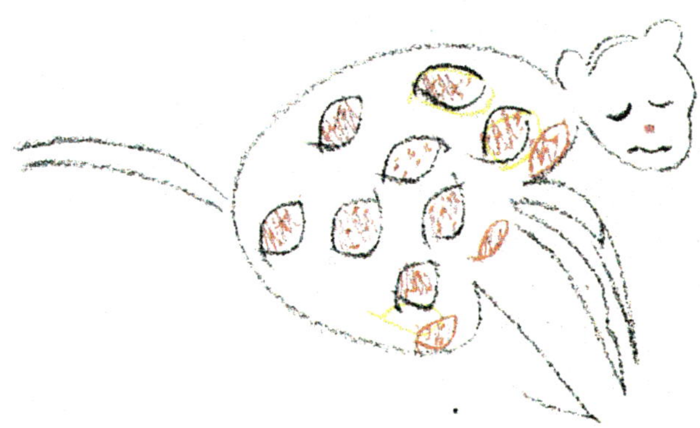

Figure 5.

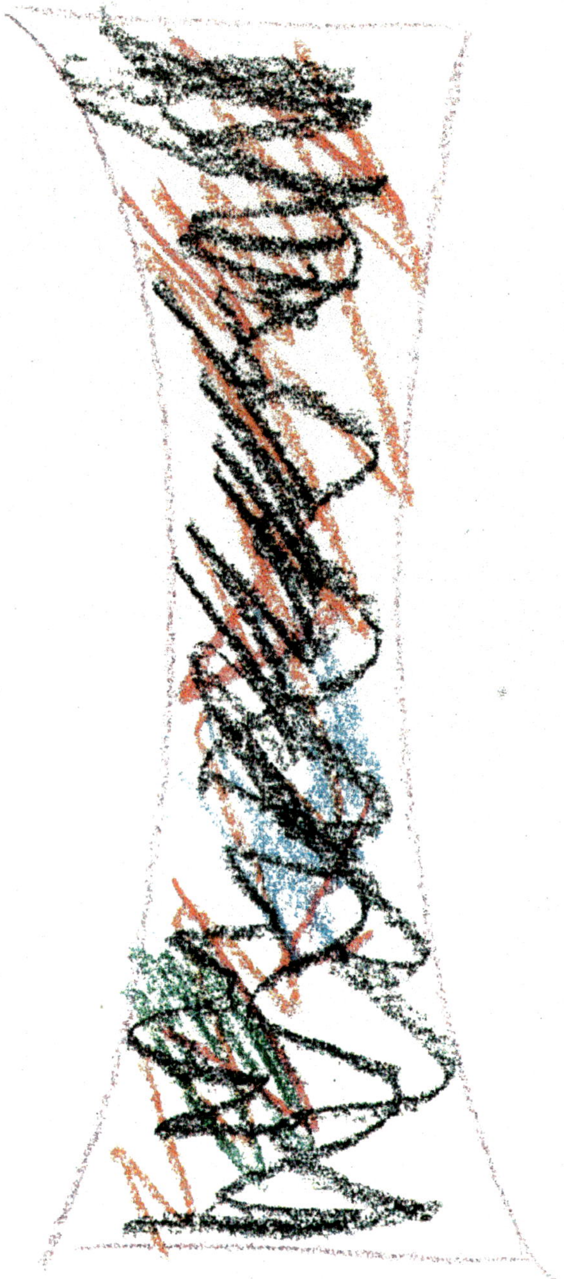

Figure 6.

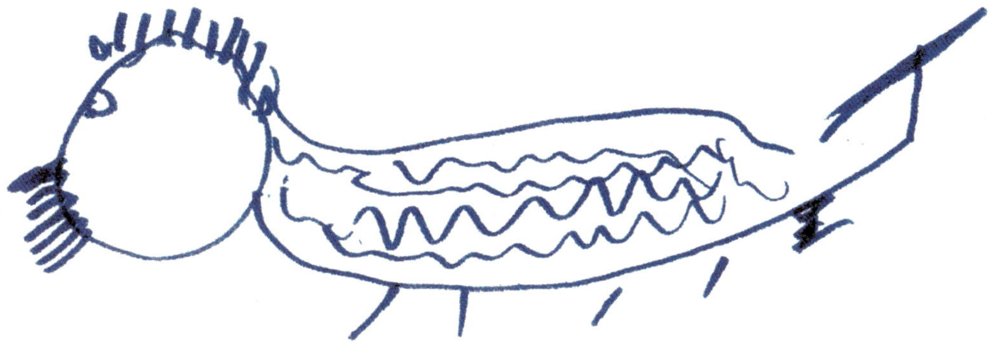

Figure 7.

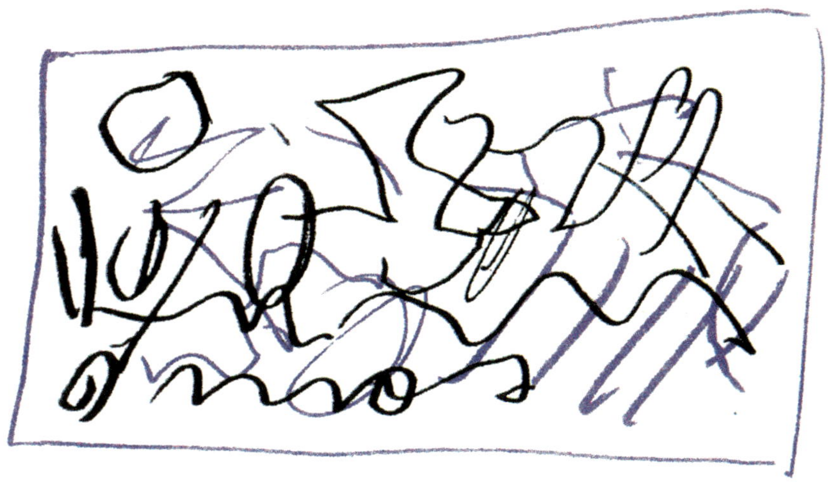

Figure 8.

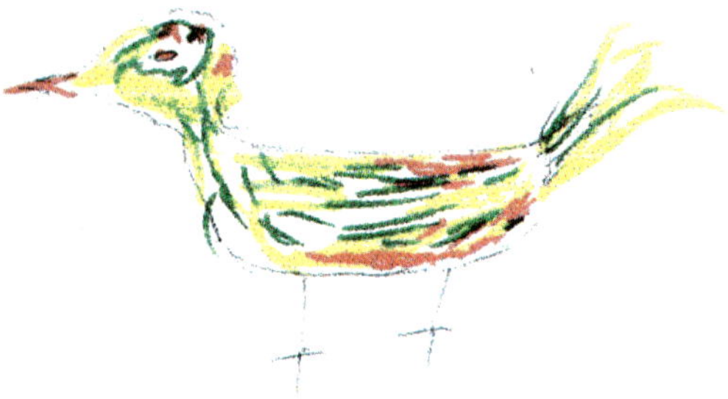

Figure 9.

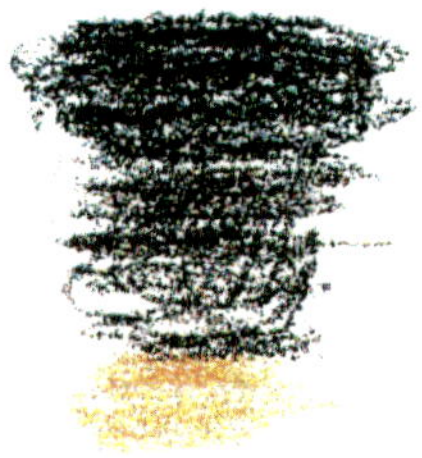

Figure 10.

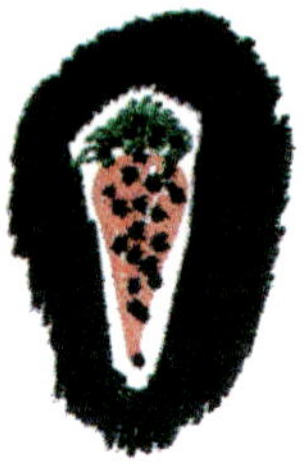

Figure 11.

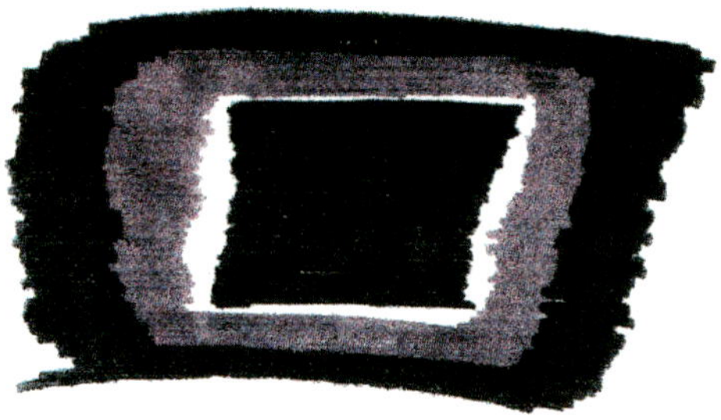

Figure 12.

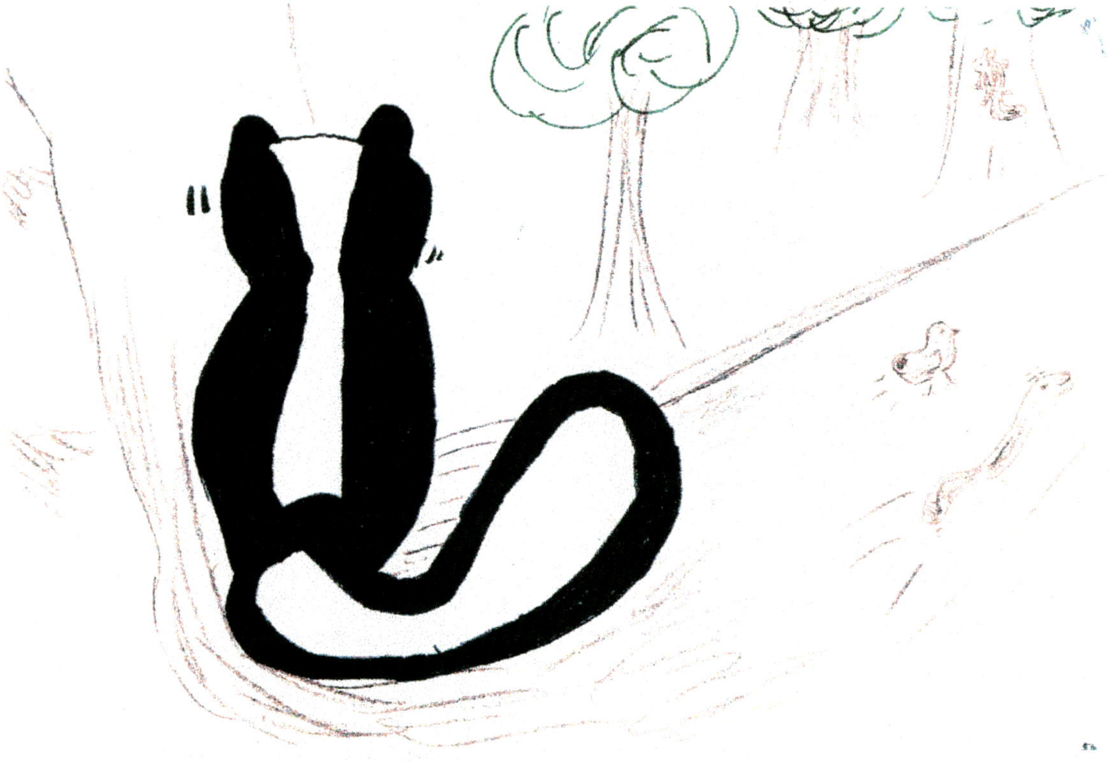

Figure 13.

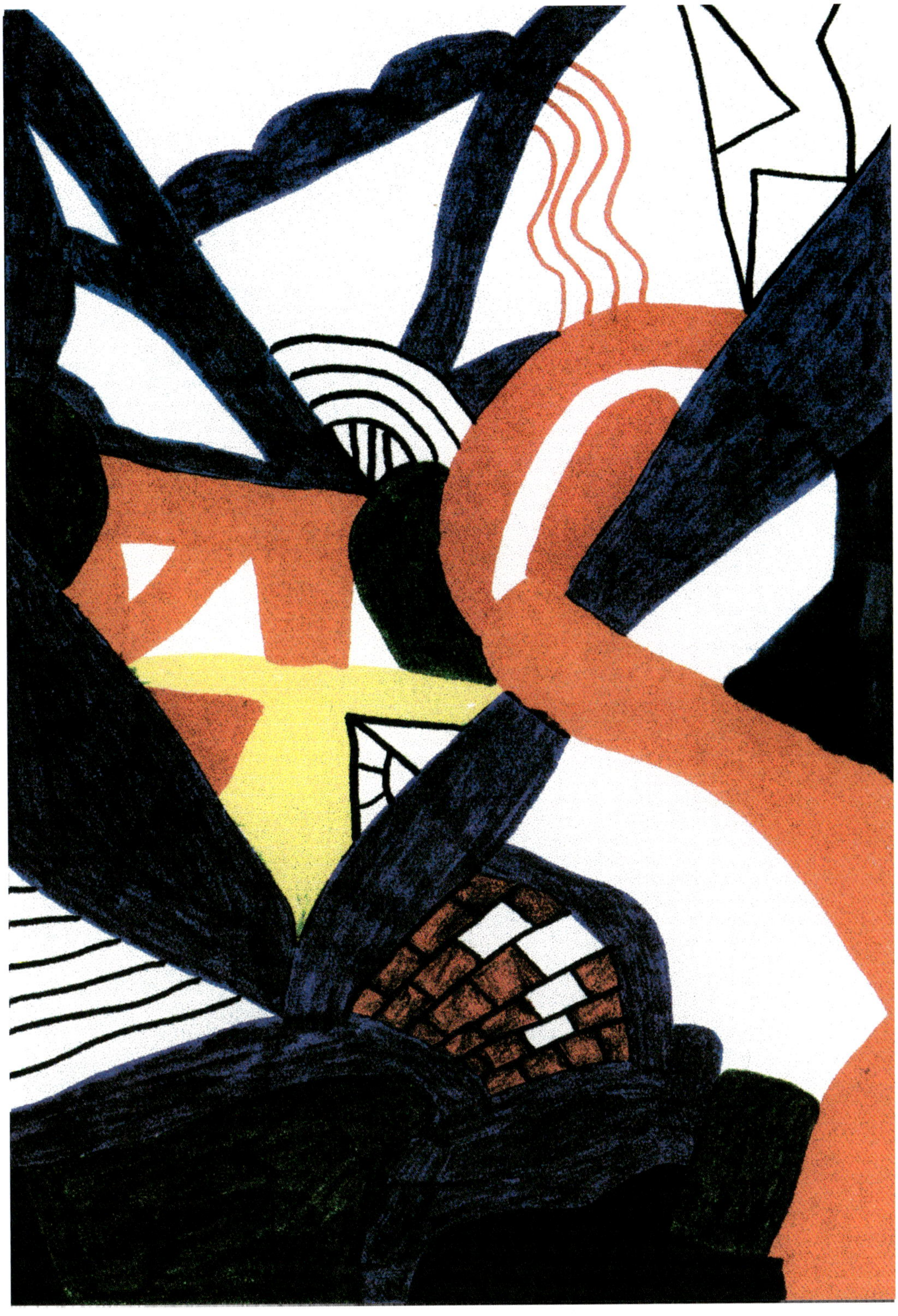

Figure 14.

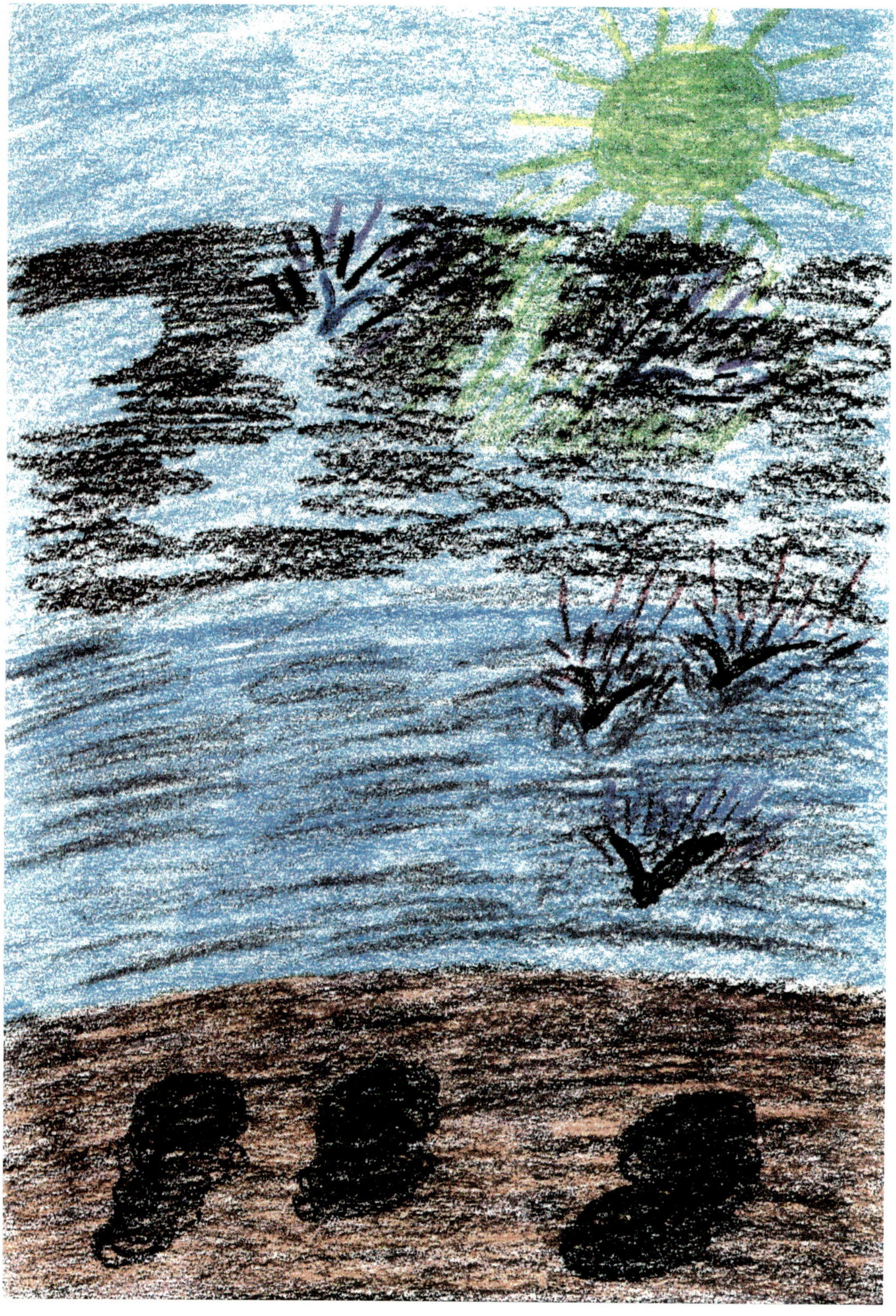

Figure 15.

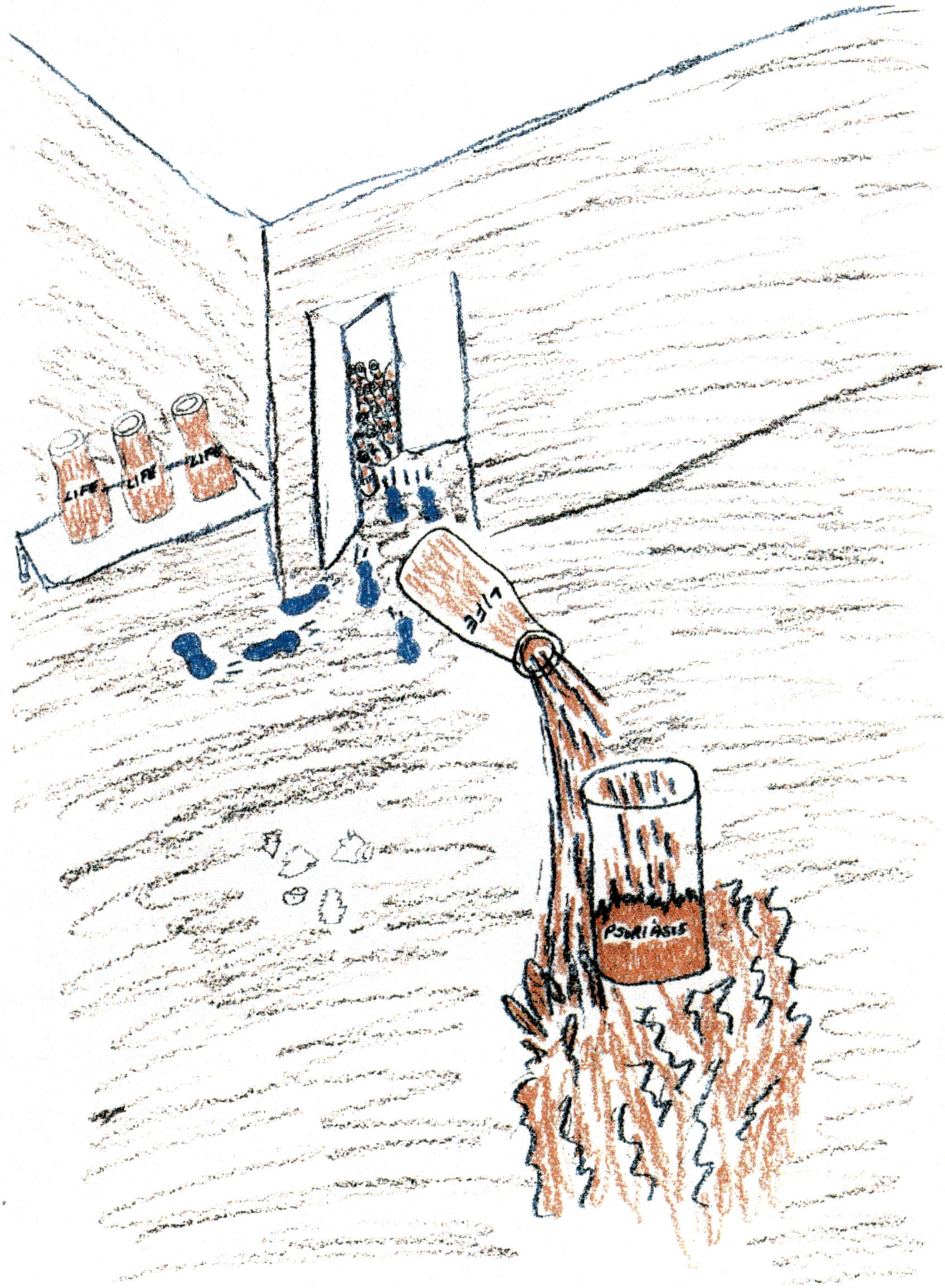

Figure 16.

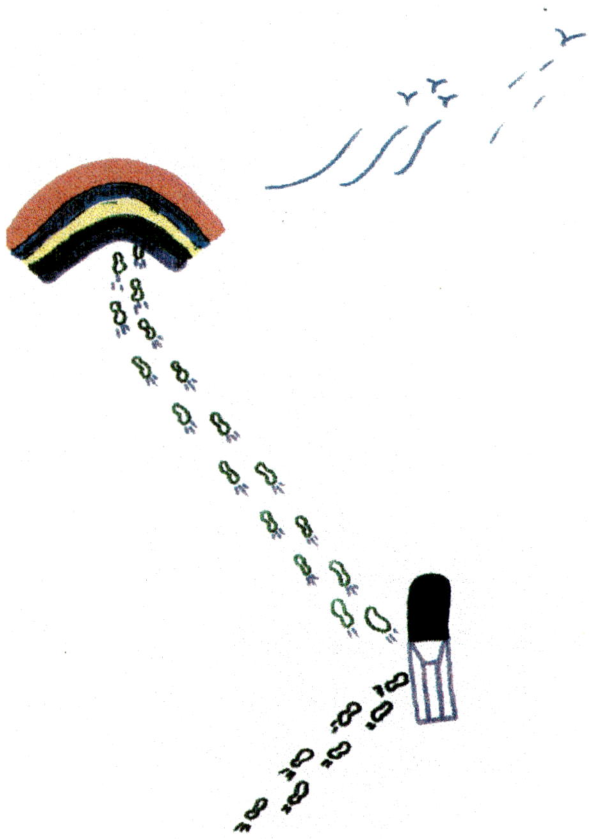

Figure 17.

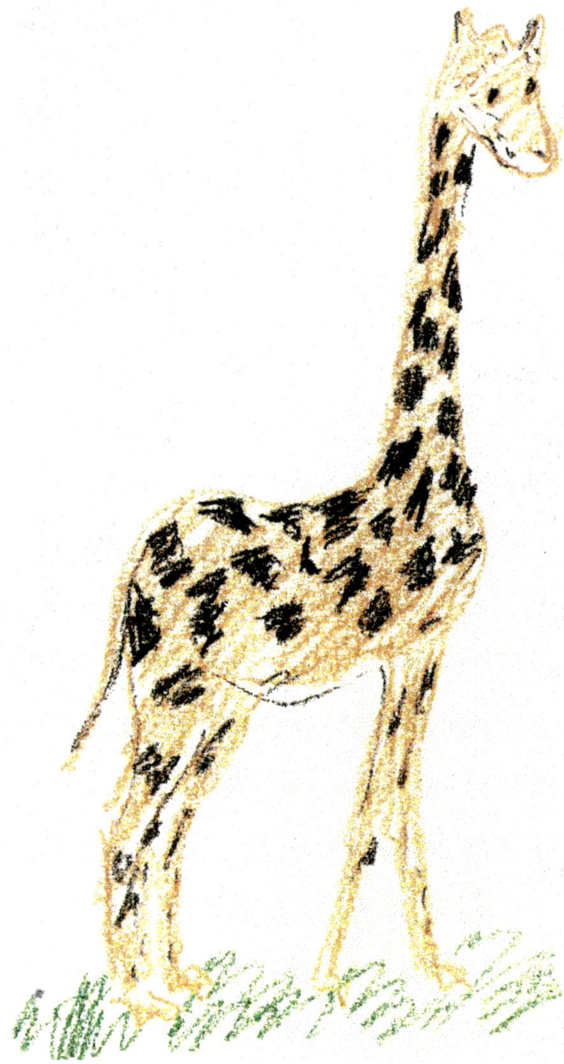

Figure 18.

catalogue, but problems with her partner and the death of her husband ended that phase of her life.

She began experiencing stress, with resulting physical problems, one after another. She describes her method of handling the crisis as "taking a breath until the crisis is over, and then coming apart."

Her mother died last July from complications of diabetes, and her father is dying of cancer. "I hate to say to him 'I love you,' but I do because I feel I should. My children have not been any help to me. I never realized until now, putting together my history, of the connection between stress and psoriasis."

At this point, and in subsequent sessions, I asked her to show me how she was feeling today. She drew a dark picture, finished it, and said:

> This did not turn out the way I wanted. I've put a lot of anger into it. I feel much better. I always do threes, pointing to the lower portion of the picture. I know they are my three children. It's supposed to be a nice beach, and water and sky, but it's not. The sky has heavy clouds, black, and 'icky' and fully of garbage. Birds are falling into dirty water and the garbage is killing the birds. The sun is trying to get through, but it got stuck in black clouds. There is a very small path for the sunshine, it's almost out. I understand a little better. I don't know all the answers but I'm getting there. The two top birds are my parents. The three middle birds are again my children (Fig. 15). This is how I feel—there is stress there. I think I've lost 5 lb of anger today.

Third Session

At this session when I offered her the usual array of media, she said, "I don't want to use those gloppy crayons" (Cray-pas). She then began drawing using pencils.

She described her drawing as follows:

> Outside the door are empty bottles. I'm pouring a bottle of life into the glass of psoriasis, which is not full. There are more bottles of life on the shelf, waiting to be used. Those are my footprints, rushing back to get more bottles, because I haven't given up. I feel better than I have in a long time. I'm rushing to get more bottles because I need more for the problem of psoriasis. I must have used a lot of bottles. There are so many outside the door. For many years, I didn't care, I wasn't trying. There is only one broken bottle (Fig. 16).

She then began talking again about her family, their estrangement, and the anger and stress that accompanied her. I told her the next session would be our last.

Fourth Session

I reminded her that this was our last session. She said she understood.

She has always talked throughout the sessions, while she was drawing, as well as after finishing her work. I again asked her to draw about her feelings today.

She first said that she had not been telling me the truth. The truth was that she was still angry, still stressed. In fact, for the first time, I felt that her affect was that of anger. She said she was finished, and I pointed out to her that she always began her drawings at the bottom. She said:

> This is where I thought I was headed—to an open grave—the grave is open because I'm not there yet, but the footprints show I'm right at the edge, but all of a sudden I'm heading away. Those footprints don't show how many there have been. I don't have enough paper to show how many footprints got me there. Then something turned me away. Those footprints represent a long time. That's my rainbow. I'm close, but I'm not coming out on the other side, because I'm not there yet. Well, here we are again—one, two, three—my children. They are free as the birds. That one at the top is my husband. He's almost out of the picture. I don't think about him too much any more. (Fig. 17.)

She then told me more about her earlier life. When her father told her to do something, she knew it was an order, and she would do it. This also meant that no matter how much pain or anger she was experiencing, she should not show it.

Her anger still has to do with her father and brother. Her brother, she says, is writing poetry, as therapy, but she feels art therapy is the best. "You can see more right here in the drawing. It opens a door."

DISCUSSION

I began to realize, as the cancellations, no-shows, and comments grew, that I was facing a barrier of fear and exposure. The literature was correct; there was so much shame and social stigmatization that the majority of the people seen at the clinic could not bear to talk to anyone besides the doctors and clinicians about their private horror and shame.

Those who did (seven people did come forward) were quite brave to have exposed themselves to me, and ultimately to others (with confidentiality assured).

Not only were they brave, they were very forthcoming in their art work, expressing themselves freely, but at the same time, expressing astonishment at what they had drawn, which was so expressive. They had no hesitation in engaging in the process I outlined. Their drawings were very quick and sure, which led me to believe they had been thinking of themselves in this way for some time. The shame expressed in the drawing of the skunk, and the sorrow in the drawing of the cheetah, tell us everything we have to know about psoriatics and their lives, without words. No comfort can be accepted until the skin is clear, and even then, there is apprehension that the psoriasis will reappear.

The person who drew the rock and the person who drew the wilted flower had some elements of denial in their discussion at first, but as the session for each progressed, there was a slight change of attitude that there is indeed a feeling of withholding the truth, perhaps from themselves, and particularly the world in which they move.

I drew a picture of a giraffe (Fig. 18). I did not know when I started that it would be that animal. As I looked at it, I realized the significance of what I had drawn. Not only did I have spots, but I was also sticking my neck out, by choosing this topic and then talking about it to others. But the more I talked about it and showed my own picture to others, the easier it became to discuss it until, at some point, I felt liberated. Part of that liberation came from what I sensed in my audiences, acceptance of me, with all my spots, real and potential. I hope that through art therapy, I can help convey that same feeling of liberation to others.

I had expected to see some evidence of the psoriatic condition in the drawings, but what emerged was startling and dramatic. There was no question that the drawings depicted not only the condition, but also the feelings associated with it. There was a pervasive feeling of sadness and in some cases depression.

There were primarily two images to be seen. The first, an animal, vegetable, or mineral, covered with spots, some object that is in fact spotty in nature—i.e., cheetah, giraffe—or covered with spots, i.e., the rock.

The other major symbol noted was the object surrounded by a thick black line, the thickness of that line and the solid blackness denoting the black despair that they discussed.

They all viewed their work with recognition and sadness. They had not, until then, faced the depth of their negative feelings about their bodies, which included feelings of shame and guilt. The guilt began to manifest itself in expressions of "Why did this happen to me? What did I do?"

A further reading of the images displays the body image of size and strength. The cheetah, which one normally associated with speed, strength, and dexterity, is drawn with light strokes and on legs that seemingly are immobile and will crumple at the first test of strength.

The rock, normally seen as hard and strong, looks tiny and ineffective. The flowers, which should be bright and with tensile strength, are wilting and dying; hence the words spoken in the session, "I am dying of shame."

The tiny carrot, the tiny sections of color, all bespeak the condition of living in a world of shame, guilt, poor self-image, of not feeling whole, and surrounded by people who seemingly are living their lives to the fullest, without problems.

All subjects recognized the stressors in their life, which could have led to the first outbreak of the lesions, as well as increases in the lesions from time to time in relation to the stressors they have faced. In addition to outside stressors is the daily knowledge and management of their bodies, which must be camouflaged from the hurtful responses of society.

Many of the subjects verbally expressed feelings of relief that they were able, for the first time, to discuss with someone how they really felt about their psoriasis. The drawing of the dog displays a third type of image—a scarred surface. The psoriatic skin is rarely smooth, feels rough to the touch.

It is also seen as flakes or plates of skin, peeling off. The drawing of the boat basically consists of plates, segments. This is also true of the maze drawing.

The one exception of size was the drawing of the skunk, which was so large that it seemed as though there was a spotlight, highlighting and enlarging the figure, as though everyone was looking at it, despite the other figures in the drawing turning away.

All of the drawings depict the skin of the psoriatic, the red spots, the white flakes. In addition, they all display the feelings engendered by the sufferers, which heretofore have been kept hidden.

"D"'s picture of the large skunk graphically portrays the feeling of the psoriatics that there is indeed a spotlight on all the spots and blemishes that the world can see. The effort to hide and/or camouflage is a burden that is lived with every day.

CONCLUSION

In one of the art therapy sessions, I was asked if the art therapy would aid the physical as well as the mental health of the individual. In all the sessions, opinions and feelings were expressed that the art therapy relaxed the subjects, enabling them to discuss their feelings about psoriasis, as opposed to their discussion in the clinic about their medical condition.

Insofar as art therapy is concerned, the relaxation and concomitant reduction in stress can be beneficial if stress is indeed one of the major factors in the psoriatic condition.

The subjects' relief at speaking of themselves was palpable. There has been a self-consciousness, a lack of self-esteem that permeates their lives. Some unburdened themselves with an affect of great relief; others were not so forthcoming, holding on to their denial despite the pain and sorrow that was showing up in the art work. The contradictory statements of acceptance and then denial seemed to be a construct of the psoriatics faced for the first time with a discussion of their feelings about their condition.

There is despair because of recognition that this is a lifelong condition that may go into remission, but sooner or later, treatment must begin again.

Body image suffers, no one feels a whole person. There is denial of this until faced with the drawings. Then there is sorrow and recognition.

As the foregoing presentation of the literature so amply demonstrates, there has been no attempt to address all the negative issues of the subjects' feelings that they must face every day. Every journal article discusses these premises of poor self-image, despair, anxiety, guilt, and so forth, but there has been no attempt to repair or to restore the whole person.

Medicine has made many advances in the treatment of psoriasis. There are many treatments to choose from determined by individual need.

Before I began this study, I had hoped the drawings would reflect some measure of the psoriatic condition. As the study progressed, I was constantly astonished by the power of art therapy to bring forth meaningful images heretofore hidden from the consciousness of the individual. The art work then can become the beginning of meaningful efforts to work with the individual in art therapy, concomitantly with medical procedures to relieve the suffering. Despite initial reluctance to become a part of this study, all those persons who did volunteer expressed themselves as being happy that they had done so, and all hoped that art therapy could be a continuous part of their lives.

As the study progressed, and I gathered more information and artwork, I was asked to make presentations of my work. As I did, I also began to talk about my reasons for doing this study. It is personal, it is based on my own lifelong struggle with psoriasis.

But the more I spoke of it—to friends, colleagues, audiences—it became more and more possible to speak out about myself. I found it easier and easier to say, "I have psoriasis." Indeed, at a recent session with my fellow thesis classmates, when they asked "What does psoriasis look like?" I was able to expose my skin to their view, and realized at that moment that it was the first time I had ever done so, and with no reluctance, or anxiety, or self-consciousness on my part. A year ago, before I began this study, I would not have thought it possible. By talking about it and showing my own artwork to accepting people, and talking about it, and talking about it, and showing my own artwork over and over—I became free.

ACKNOWLEDGMENTS

I wish to thank Patricia Allen, Ph.D., A.T.R., who encouraged me; Faith Townsend Attaguile, who made my words possible; and Barry, Barbara, Rachel, and Seth Lewis, whose love sustained me.

REFERENCES

Dungey, R.K., and Buselmeier, T.J. (1982). Medical and psychosocial aspects of psoriasis. *Health Soc. Work* 7(2): 140–147.

Epstein, E. (1984). Hand dermatitis: Practical management and current concepts. *J. Am. Acad. Dermatol.* 10(3): 395–424.

Ginsburg, I.H., and Link, B.G. (1989). Feelings of stigmatization in patients with psoriasis. *J. Am. Acad. Dermatol.* 20(1):53–63.

Gupta-Madhulika, A., Gupta, A.K., and Haberman, H.F. (1987). Psoriasis and psychiatry: An update. *Gen. Hosp. Psychiatry* 9(3):157–166.

Hardy, G.E. (1982). Body image disturbance in dysmorphophobia. *Br. J. Psychiatry* 141:181–185.

Kaslow, N.J., and Eicher, V.W. (1988). Body image therapy: A combined creative arts therapy and verbal psychotherapy approach. *Arts Psyhchother.* 15(3):177–188.

Larose, M.E. (1988). The use of art therapy with juvenile delinquents to enhance self-image. *Psychother. Patient* 4(2):161–167.

Lincoln, L. (1987). Body image remediation through creative arts therapy. *Pratt Inst. Creat. Arts Ther. Rev.* 8: 35–44.

McEvoy, M.T., and Roenigk, R.K. (1991). In *Psoriasis*, 2nd ed. H. Roenigk, Jr., and H. Maiback (Eds.). Marcel Dekker, New York, pp. 201–208.

Roenigk, H. (1977). Don't give up on the patient with psoriasis. *Mod. Med.* 45:59–76.

BIBLIOGRAPHY

Adler, R.F., and Fisher, P. (1984). Myself through music, movement and art. *Psychotherapy* 11(3):203–208.

Aissen-Crewett, M. (1987). Esthetic training of the elderly—With special reference to the therapeutic effects of pictorial creative activities. *Ztschr. Gerontol.* 20(5): 314–317.

Baer, B. (1985). The rehabilitative influence of creative experience. *J. Creat. Behav.* 19(3):202–214.

Barber, T.X. (1984). Changing unchangeable bodily processes by (hypnotic) suggestions: A new look at hypnosis, cognitions, imaging, and the mind-body problem. *Advances* 1(2):7–40.

Bolea, A.S. (1986). Treating loneliness in children. *Psychother. Patient* 2(3):15–27.

Breitenbach, N. (1984). Identity development during creative make-up sessions. *Arts Psychother.* 11(2):101–107.

Cameron, C.O., Juszczak, L., and Wallace, N. (1984). Using creative arts to help children cope with altered body image. *Child. Health Care* 12(3):108–112.

Cohen, Y. (1987). A creative group experience with blind and partially sighted children. *Pratt Inst. Creat. Arts Ther. Rev.* 8:14–26.

Corder, B.F., Haizlip, T., and DeBoer, P. (1990). A pilot study for a structured, time-limited therapy group for sexually abused pre-adolescent children. *Child Abuse Neglect* 14(2):243–251.

Darrell, E., and Wheeler, M. (1984). Using art therapy techniques to help underachieving seventh grade junior high school students. *Arts Psychother.* 11(4):289–292.

Davis, D.L., and Boster, L. (1988). Multifaceted therapeutic interventions with the violent psychiatric inpatient. *Hosp. Commun. Psychiatry* 39(8):867–869.

Davison, J. (1986). Dramatherapy for psychiatric patients. *Nurs. Times* 82(23):48–50.

Deb, S. (1988). Psychological body-choice anecdote of vitiligo. *Ind. J. Behav.* 1:1–25.

Dooley, C. J. (1986). Body stimulated imagery and syntegration. *Dissert. Abstr. Int.* 46(12-B, Pt. 1):4383–4383.

Dulical, D. (1984). The full rainbow: Symbol of individuation: Afterward. *Arts Psychother.* 11(1):42–43.

Elkin, E.M. (1984). Symbols and the development of language as transitional phenomena. *Pratt Inst. Creat. Arts Ther. Rev.* 5:49–62.

Elston, T., and Thomas, J.B. (1985). Anorexia nervosa. *Child Care Health Dev.* 11(6):355–373.

Famaey, J.P. (1988). Colchicine in therapy. State of the art and new perspectives for an old drug. *Clin. Exp. Rheumatol.* 6(3):305–317.

Farber, E.M. (1987). The natural course of psoriasis from infancy to adulthood. *Hautarzt* 38(1):53–56.

Farber, E.M. (1985). The office visit and the self-help concept in the treatment of psoriasis. *Cutis* 35(3):201–202.

Farber, E.M., and Nall, L. (1984). An appraisal of measures to prevent and control psoriasis. *J. Am. Acad. Dermatol.* 10(3):511–517.

Farber, E.M., and Nall, L. (1984). Psoriasis: A review of recent advances in treatment. *Drugs* 28(4):324–346.

Frampton, D.R. (1986). Restoring creativity to the dying patient. *Br. Med. J. Clin. Res. Ed.* 293(6562):1593–1595.

Fuller, J.R. (1988). Martial arts and psychological health. *Br. J. Med. Psychol.* 61(Pt. 4):327–328.

Geller, S.K., et al. (1986). Artbreak: Innovation in student life programming. *J. Coll. Stud. Person.* 27(3):229–233.

Green, B.L., Wehling, C., and Talsky, G.J. (1987). Group art therapy as an adjunct to treatment for chronic outpatients. *Hosp. Commun. Psychiatry* 38(9):988–991.

Haeseler, M.P. (1987). Censorship or intervention: "But you said we could draw whatever we wanted." *Am. J. Art Ther.* 26(1):11–20.

Hymer, S.M. (1983). The therapeutic nature of art in self reparation. *Psychoanal. Rev.* 70(1):57–68.

Jones, M.D., Pais, M.J., and Omiya, B. (1988). Bony overgrowths and abnormal calcifications about the spine. *Radiol. Clin. North Am.* 26(6):2213–2214.

Kelley, S.J. (1984). The use of art therapy with sexually abused children. *J. Psychosoc. Nurs. Men. Health Serv.* 22(12):12–18.

Leichtman, S.R., Burnell, J.W., and Robinsin, H.M. (1981). Body image concerns of psoriasis patients as reflected in human-figure drawings. *J. Personal. Assess.* 45(5): 478–484.

Lewis, P.P. (1988). The transformative process within the imaginal realm. Special issue: Creative arts therapists as contemporary shamans: Reality or romance? *Arts Psychother.* 15(4):309–316.

McIntyre, B.B. (1990). Art therapy with bereaved youth. *J. Palliat. Care* 6(1):16–25.

Morrison, J.K., and Holdridge, B. (1984). Emotive-reconstructive therapy and reduction of artists problem behaviors and negative self-constructs: A pilot study. *Psychol. Rep.* 54(2):505–506.

Panconesi, E., and Cossidente, A. (1986). Dermatological alternations, psychosomatic and sexual repercussions. *Psychol. Med.* 18(3):381–382.

Pilon, R.N. (1978). Laterality of body focus and digital skin temperature in patients with Raynaud's disease. *Psychophysiology* 15(4):320–323.

Porter, J.R., Beuf, A.H., Lerner, A., and Nordlund, J. (1986). Psychosocial effect of vitiligo: A comparison of vitiligo patients with "normal" control subjects, with psoriasis patients, and with patients with other pigmentary disorders. *J. Am. Acad. Dermatol.* 15(2 Pt. 1):220–224.

Purchard, P.R. (1967). Some psychiatric aspects of dermatology. *Psychiatr. Q.* 41(2):280–285.

Rabin, M. (1987). Phenomenal and nonphenomenal body image tasks in the treatment of eating disorders. *Dissert. Abstr. Int.* 48(5-B):1505.

Robbins, A. (1984). The struggle for self-cohesion: An analytically oriented art therapy case study. *Art Ther.* 1(3): 107–118.

Ryder, G.J. (1986). Expressive arts therapy with chemically dependent individuals. *Dissert. Abstr. Int.* 47(5-B):2144.

Schwartz, J.H., Bar, N.D., Almagor, B., and Iancu, T.C. (1984). Stimulation of self-image development in chronic familial hyperphosphatasemia. *Acta Paedopsychiatr.* 50(1):41–50.

Swan-Foster, N. (1989). Images of pregnant women: Art therapy as a tool for transformation. Special issue: Women and the creative arts therapies. *Arts Psychother.* 16(4):283–292.

Van-Moffaert, M. (1986). Training future dermatologists in psychodermatology. *Gen. Hosp. Psychiatry* 8(2): 115–118.

Virshup, D. (1985). Group art therapy in a methadone clinic lobby. *J. Subst. Abuse Treat.* 2(3):153–158.

Wadewon, H. (1987). Pursuit of the image: Paintings from poetry in a personal mid-life odyssey. *Arts Psychother.* 14(2):177–182.

Wadeson, H. (1985). A question of creativity: Paradigms—Facilitators or inhibitors? *Art Ther.* 2(1):39.

Wolff, K. (1986). Therapeutic photomedicine: History, state of the art, and perspectives. *Curr. Probl. Dermatol.* 15: 1–17.

Zimmerman, M.L., Wolbert, W.A., Burgess, A.W., and Hartman, C.R. (1987). Art and group work: Interventions for multiple victims of child molestation (Part II). *Arch. Psychiatr. Nurs.* 1(1):40–46.

APPENDIX: INDIVIDUAL RESPONSES TO PSORIASIS AS PROJECTED IN ARTWORK

Artwork

1. Self-portrait
2. How it feels to have psoriasis

Questionnaire

1. How long have you had psoriasis?
2. To whom can you talk about psoriasis?
   Doctor ____ Family ____ Friends ____
   Co-workers ____ Acquaintances ____
3. Do you cover your psoriasis with:
   Clothing ____ Makeup ____ Other ____

73

The National Psoriasis Organization: A Means to Educate and Advocate

Gail M. Zimmerman
National Psoriasis Foundation, Portland, Oregon

Until a cure is found for psoriasis, there will always be a need by the person with psoriasis for information. This need has led to the establishment of over 20 national lay organizations around the world to educate the public about psoriasis and provide patient support.

These organizations meet a critical need for people to understand their disease and the choices they have in treatment and in living with the disorder. All of these organizations were established by people whose lives were affected by psoriasis. Today, in almost every instance, they are the only comprehensive source of information of psoriasis in their respective countries. Each generally has a medical advisory board that reviews and approves the medical information distributed by the organization to the public and operates under the direction of a lay board of trustees or directors.

These organizations as resources of information provide a vital and unique service to psoriasis patients and their families. Studies have shown that knowledge increases the patient's ability to assist in the management of the disease, increases a patient's compliance with treatment regimens, and increases the patient's ability to cope in living with the disease. Dermatological treatment is only a part of psoriasis therapy. Psychological support and complete patient education regarding the disorder and its therapy are of critical importance. As one mother wrote to one of these organizations, "If my son and I have to battle this disease, we want to know the enemy."

The physician can play a major role in this educational process. For that reason, the lay organizations seek to work closely with the physician and nurse in offering information to the patient and family. The patient looks to the physician first for guidance in developing control over his skin disease. The lay organizations desire to work as an adjunct to the medical professional in supporting the educational process that is so necessary to patient care.

The organizations also seek to increase public awareness about psoriasis so as to eliminate fears or prejudice that can adversely impact the public and personal life of people with psoriasis. Public awareness is also important to ensure community support of insurance coverage of psoriasis therapies, funding of basic and clinical research into the disorder, and respect for the needs of people with psoriasis. All of the organizations have the goal of stimulating and supporting basic and clinical research in psoriasis and some provide research funding.

Of the national lay psoriasis organizations in existence today, the first to be established was the National Psoriasis Foundation (NPF) located in the United States. Since its founding in 1968, the NPF stimulated the first significant funding of psoriasis research by the National Institutes of Health; made psoriasis an eligible disease for social security disability income; funded the first psoriasis research fellowships; established the first comprehensive lay literature on psoriasis in the world; established the first international gene back in psoriasis; and has distributed over 2–3 million pieces of educational literature on psoriasis.

Today, over 20 similar organizations have been established and work with the NPF and one another through the International Federation of Psoriasis Associations (IFPA), an international organization whose goals are to advance efforts to lessen the suffering of people with psoriasis and to improve methods of treatments and research for finding the ultimate cause and cure of the disorder.

All of these organizations have patient educational materials and newsletters that are available by request and have an interest in working with the medical professional in serving the psoriasis patient. The reader may contact any or all of the organizations listed below for information on their services and programs.

MEMBER ORGANIZATIONS OF IFPA

Argentina
Contacto Psoriasis
Cucha Cucha 1075
(1405) Capital Federal
Buenos Aires, Argentina
Tel/Fax: 54-1-582-1029
Mensajes: 54-1-831-5400
Contact: Susana B. Iarmusch de Ficher

Australia
Psoriasis Association of NSW, Inc.
P.O. Box 1141
Penrith, N.S.W. 2751
Tel: 07-047-21-4166
Contact: Mrs. Sandra Freer, Secretary

Psoriasis Association of Victoria
P.O. Box 1151
Glen Waverley, Victoria 3150
Tel: (03) 9663-5983
Contact: Helen McNair, President

Belgium
Vlaamse Vereniging Psoriasis Patineten
Beervelde Darp 39
B9080 Lochristi
Tel: 32 2 452 67 16
Contact: Pol Labeeuw

Canada
Canadian Psoriasis Foundation
1306 Wellington St., Suite 500
Ottawa, Ontario K1Y 3B2
Tel: 613/728-4000
Fax: 613/728-8913
E-mail: CPFDONR@ISTAR.CA
Contact: Don Rutherford, Executive Director

Czech Republic
SPAE
Struharovská 2941, 141 00
Praha 4
Contact: Jana Brizová, President
Translator: Ms. Lenka Sajdlová
Pavrovského 5, 155 00
Prag 5
Czech Republic

Denmark
Danmarks Psoriasis Forening
Kloverprisvej 10 B
2650 Hvidovre
Contact: Mr. Karl Vilhelm Nielsen, Executive Director
Tel: 011-45-36-75-5400
Fax: 011-45-36-75-1403

England
Psoriatic Anthropathy Alliance
PO Box 111
St. Albans, Hertfordshire
England AL2 3JQ
Contact: Mr. & Mrs. David and Julie Chandler, Co-Directors

Estonia
Eesti Psoriaasi Liit
Box 674
EE0026, Tallinn
Contact: Vahur Joala
E-mail: vahur.joala@leica.fi

Finland
The Finish Psoriasis Association
Fredrikinkatu 27 A
FIN-00120 Helsinki
Tel: +358-0-641917
Fax: +358-0-608447
Contact: Pirkko Sotamaa

France
Association Pour La Lutte Contre Le Psoriasis
1 allee du Stade
95610 Eragny
Tel: +33-1-34-64-1768
Fax: +33-1-30-37-4581
Contact: Michele Allaire, Presidente

Iceland
Samtök Psoriasis
Spoex
Bolholt 6, 105 Reykjavik
Tel: 354-1-588-9666
Fax: 354-1-588-9622
Contact: Ms. Helga Ingölfsdöttir, Executive Director

Israel
Israel Psoriasis Association
P.O. Box 13275
Tel Aviv
Tel: +972-3-560-9711
Fax: +972-4-9855356
Contact: Chaya Apirion, Chairman

Italy
Associazione Salute Nature
Via Bergognone 43
20144 Milan
Fax: 39-6-32-40-281
Contact: Grazia Soldan, Presidente

Lithuania
Lithuanian Psoriasis Society
PO Box 2095
3000, Kaunas
Contact: Ms. V.J. Balciuniene, Secretary or Mr. S. Stasaitis, Chairman

Lietuvos Zyneline Liga
Serganciuju Draugija
Kairiukscio 2, AD 291 B
Vilnius

Netherlands
Nederlandse Bond van Psoriasis
Jansbuitensingel 32-1
68 MAE Arnhem
Tel: +085-514160
Fax: +085-420-552
Contact: Rosemary Boland

New Zealand
Psoriasis Association of NZ, Inc.
PO Box 44-007 VIC
Lower Hutt
Tel: 011-64-4-568-7139
64-9-278-6326
Fax: 64-9-309-4660
Contact: Carolyn McGonnell, Secretary

Norway
Norsk Psoriasisforbund
Hassellia 19
6523 Frei
Tel: 47-22-72-28-10
Fax: 47-71-52-82-36
Contact: Arne Jenssveen, Chairman

Singapore
Psoriasis Association of Singapore
National Skin Centre
c/o Phototherapy Unit
1 Mandalay Road Singapore 1130
Balestier Estate P.O. Box 0482
Singapore 9132
Tel: 65-3506-751

Slovak Republic
PhDr. Vlasta Husárová
Znievska 19
851 06 Bratislava

South Africa
South African Psoriasis Association
106 H Baker Street
Groenkloof
Pretoria 0181

Spain
ACCIÓ Psoriasi
Avgda. de Vallvidrera, 73
08017 Barcelona
Tel: 34-3-280-4622
Fax: 34-3-280-4280
Contact: Juana M. del Molino, President

Sweden
Svenska Psoriasisforbundet
Rokerigatan 19
S-121 62 JOHANNESHOV
Tel: +46-8-6003636
Fax: +46-8-6002284
Contact: Lars Ettarp, Chairman; Kristina Söderlind Penton, Executive Director

Switzerland
Schweizerisch Psoriasis & Vitiligo Gesellschaft
Postfach
CH 8048 Zurich
Tel/Fax: +41-30-2-4466
Contact: Peter Bischoff

United States
National Psoriasis Foundation
6600 S.W. 92nd, Suite 300
Portland, OR 97223
Tel: 503-244-7404
Fax: 503-245-0626
E-mail: corrine@npfusa.org
NPF World Wide Web Page: http://www.psoriasis.org
Contact: Gail Zimmerman, Executive Director

International Federation of Psoriasis Organizations
c/o National Psoriasis Foundation
6600 SW 92nd, Suite 300
Portland, OR 97223
Tel: 503-244-7404
Fax: 503-245-0626
E-mail: gail@npfusa.org
Contact: Gail M. Zimmerman, Chairman
Web Page: See NPF Web page for IFPA listings

Index

About the Editors

HENRY H. ROENIGK, Jr., is Professor of Dermatology, Northwestern University, Chicago, Illinois. He is past Chairman of Dermatology at Cleveland Clinic, Cleveland, Ohio, and Northwestern University Medical School. He has written extensively on numerous dermatology topics, including over 380 journal articles and book chapters, and is the coeditor, with Randall K. Roenigk, of *Dermatologic Surgery: Principles and Practice, Second Edition* (Marcel Dekker, Inc.) and three other textbooks. Dr. Roenigk serves on the editorial boards of *Cutis: Journal of Cutaneous Medicine*, the *Journal of Dermatological Surgery*, and *Skin and Allergy News*. Dr. Roenigk is a Fellow of the American College of Physicians and a member of the American Academy of Dermatology, the American Dermatological Association, the American Federation for Clinical Research, the American Society for Dermatologic Surgery, the Society for Investigative Dermatology, and many others. He is an honorary member of 10 foreign dermatologic societies. He received the M.D. degree (1960) from Northwestern University Medical School, Chicago, Illinois, and a dermatology fellowship from Cleveland Clinic, Cleveland, Ohio. Dr. Roenigk is currently in private practice in Phoenix, Arizona.

HOWARD I. MAIBACH is Professor of Dermatology, University of California School of Medicine, San Francisco. Dr. Maibach serves on the editorial boards of the *International Journal of Dermatology*, *Excerpta Medica*, and the *Journal of Toxicology: Clinical Toxicology* (Marcel Dekker, Inc.). His research includes work in dermatology, toxicology, pharmacology, and physiology, and he is the author of over 1400 papers in these and related fields, and coeditor of *Neonatal Skin* (with Edward K. Boisits), *Cutaneous Infestations and Insect Bites* (with Milton Orkin), *Percutaneous Absorption, Second Edition* (with Robert L. Bronaugh), and *Cutaneous Infection and Therapy* (with R. Aly and K.R. Beutner) [all titles, Marcel Dekker, Inc.]. Dr. Maibach is a Fellow of the American College of Physicians and a member of the American Academy of Dermatology, the Society for Investigative Dermatology, the American Federation for Clinical Research, the American Medical Association, and the American Dermatological Association. He received the M.D. degree (1955) from Tulane University, New Orleans, Louisiana.